Evidence-Based Imaging

L. Santiago Medina, MD, MPH

Co-Director, Division of Neuroradiology and Brain Imaging; Director of the Health Outcomes, Policy, and Economics (HOPE) Center, Department of Radiology, Miami Children's Hospital, Miami, Florida

C. Craig Blackmore, MD, MPH

Scientific Director, Center for Health Care Solutions, Department of Radiology, Virginia Mason Medical Center, Seattle, Washington

Kimberly E. Applegate, MD, MS, FACR

Vice Chair of Quality and Safety, Department of Radiology, Emory University School of Medicine, Atlanta, Georgia

Evidence-Based Imaging

Improving the Quality of Imaging in Patient Care

Revised Edition

With 264 Illustrations, 20 in Full Color

Foreword by Bruce J. Hillman, MD

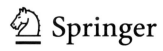 Springer

Editors

L. Santiago Medina, MD, MPH
Co-Director, Division of Neuroradiology
    and Brain Imaging
Director of the Health Outcomes, Policy,
    and Economics (HOPE) Center
Department of Radiology
Miami Children's Hospital
Miami, FL 33155, USA
santiago.medina@mch.com
Former Lecturer in Radiology
Harvard Medical School
Boston, MA 02114
smedina@post.harvard.edu

C. Craig Blackmore, MD, MPH
Scientific Director, Center for Health Care
    Solutions
Department of Radiology
Virginia Mason Medical Center
Seattle, WA 98111, USA
craig.blackmore@vmmc.org

Kimberly E. Applegate, MD, MS, FACR
Vice Chair of Quality and Safety
Department of Radiology
Emory University School of Medicine
Atlanta, Georgia 30322, USA
keapple@emory.edu

ISBN 978-1-4419-7776-2   e-ISBN 978-1-4419-7777-9
DOI 10.1007/978-1-4419-7777-9
Springer New York Dordrecht Heidelberg London

Library of Congress Control Number: 2011924338

Printed on acid-free paper

Springer is part of Springer Science+Business Media (www.springer.com)

To our patients, who are our best teachers,
and to the researchers, who made this book possible.
To our families, friends, and mentors.

Foreword

Despite our best intentions, most of what constitutes modern medical imaging practice is based on habit, anecdotes, and scientific writings that are too often fraught with biases. Best estimates suggest that only around 30% of what constitutes "imaging knowledge" is substantiated by reliable scientific inquiry. This poses problems for clinicians and radiologists, because inevitably, much of what we do for patients ends up being inefficient, inefficacious, or occasionally even harmful.

In recent years, recognition of how the unsubstantiated practice of medicine can result in poor-quality care and poorer health outcomes has led to a number of initiatives. Most significant in my mind is the evidence-based medicine movement that seeks to improve clinical research and research synthesis as a means of providing a more definitive knowledge basis for medical practice. Although the roots of evidence-based medicine are in fields other than radiology, in recent years, a number of radiologists have emerged to assume leadership roles. Many are represented among the authors and editors of this excellent book, the purpose of which is to enhance understanding of what constitutes the evidence basis for the practice of medical imaging and where that evidence basis is lacking.

It comes not a moment too soon, given how much is going on in the regulatory and payer worlds concerning health care quality. There is a general lack of awareness among radiologists about the insubstantiality of the foundations of our practices. Through years of teaching medical students, radiology residents and fellows, and practicing radiologists in various venues, it occurs to me that at the root of the problem is a lack of sophistication in reading the radiology literature. Many clinicians and radiologists are busy physicians, who, over time, have taken more to reading reviews and scanning abstracts than critically examining the source of practice pronouncements. Even in our most esteemed journals, literature reviews tend to be exhaustive regurgitations of everything that has been written, without providing much insight into which studies were performed more rigorously and hence are more believable. Radiology training programs spend inordinate time cramming the best and brightest young minds with acronyms, imaging "signs," and unsubstantiated factoids while mostly ignoring teaching future radiologists how to think rigorously about what they are reading and hearing.

As I see it, the aim of this book is nothing less than to begin to reverse these conditions. This book is not a traditional radiology text. Rather, the editors and authors have provided first a framework for how to think about many of the most important imaging issues of our day and then fleshed out each chapter with a critical review of the information available in the literature.

There are a number of very appealing things about the approach employed here. First, the chapter authors are a veritable "who's who" of the most thoughtful individuals in our field. Reading this book provides a window into how they think as they evaluate the literature and arrive at their conclusions, which we can use as models for our own improvement. Many of the chapters are coauthored by radiologists and practicing clinicians, allowing for more diverse perspectives. The editors have designed a uniform approach for each chapter and held the authors' feet to the fire to adhere to it. Chapters 5–40 provide, up front, a summary of the key points. The literature reviews that follow are selective and critical, rating the strength of the literature to provide insight for the critical reader into the degree of confidence he or she might have in reviewing the conclusions. At the end of each chapter, the authors present the imaging approaches that are best supported by the evidence and discuss the gaps that exist in the evidence that should cause us lingering uncertainty. Figures and tables help focus the reader on the most important information, while decision trees provide the potential for more active engagement. Case studies help actualize the main points brought home in each chapter. At the end of each chapter, bullets are used to highlight areas where there are important gaps in research.

The result is a highly approachable text that suits the needs of both the busy practitioner who wants a quick consultation on a patient with whom he or she is actively engaged or the radiologist who wishes a comprehensive, in-depth view of an important topic. Most importantly, from my perspective, the book goes counter to the current trend of "dumbing down" radiology that I abhor in many modern textbooks. To the contrary, this book is an intelligent effort that respects the reader's potential to think for himself or herself and gives substance to Plutarch's famous admonition, "The mind is not a vessel to be filled but a fire to be kindled."

Bruce J. Hillman, MD
Theodore E. Keats Professor of Radiology
University of Virginia

Preface

Medical imaging has grown exponentially in the last three decades with the development of many promising and often noninvasive diagnostic studies and therapeutic modalities. The corresponding medical literature has also exploded in volume and can be overwhelming to physicians. In addition, the literature varies in scientific rigor and clinical applicability. The purpose of this book is to employ stringent evidence-based medicine criteria to systematically review the evidence defining the appropriate use of medical imaging and to present to the reader a concise summary of the best medical imaging choices for patient care.

Since our prior version, we have added ten new chapters that cover radiation risk in medical imaging, economic and regulatory impact of evidence-based imaging in the new health care reform environment, and new topics on common disorders. The 40 chapters cover the most prevalent diseases in developed countries, including the four major causes of mortality and morbidity: injury, coronary artery disease, cancer, and cerebrovascular disease. Most of the chapters have been written by radiologists and imagers in close collaboration with clinical physicians and surgeons to provide a balanced and fair analysis of the different medical topics. In addition, we address in detail both the adult and pediatric sides of the issues. We cannot answer all questions – medical imaging is a delicate balance of science and art, often without data for guidance – but we can empower the reader with the current evidence behind medical imaging.

To make the book user-friendly and to enable fast access to pertinent information, we have organized all of the chapters in the same format. The chapters are framed around important and provocative clinical questions relevant to the daily physician's practice. A short listing of issues at the beginning of each chapter helps three different tiers of users: (1) the busy physician searching for quick guidance, (2) the meticulous physician seeking deeper understanding, and (3) the medical-imaging researcher requiring a comprehensive resource. Key points and summarized answers to the important clinical issues are at the beginning of the chapters, so the busy clinician can understand the most important evidence-based imaging data in seconds. Each important question and summary is followed by a detailed discussion of the supporting evidence so that the meticulous physician can have a clear understanding of the science behind the evidence.

In each chapter, the evidence discussed is presented in tables and figures that provide an easy review in the form of summary tables and flow charts. The imaging case series highlights the strengths and limitations of the different imaging studies with vivid examples. Toward the end of the chapters, the best imaging protocols are described to ensure that the imaging studies are well standardized and done with the highest available quality. The final section of the chapters is Future Research, in which provocative questions are raised for physicians and nonphysicians interested in advancing medical imaging.

Not all research and not all evidence are created equal. Accordingly, throughout the book, we use a four-level classification detailing the strength of the evidence and based on the Oxford-criteria: level I (strong evidence), level II (moderate evidence), level III (limited evidence), and level IV (insufficient evidence). The strength of the evidence is presented in parenthesis throughout the chapter so the reader gets immediate feedback on the weight of the evidence behind each topic.

Finally, we had the privilege of working with a group of outstanding contributors from major medical centers and universities in North America and Europe. We believe that the authors' expertise, breadth of knowledge, and thoroughness in writing the chapters provide a valuable source of information and can guide decision-making for physicians and patients. In addition to guiding practice, the evidence summarized in the chapters may have policy-making and public health implications. We hope that the book highlights key points and generates discussion, promoting new ideas for future research. Finally, regardless of the endless hours spent researching the multiple topics in-depth, evidence-based imaging remains a work in progress. We value your suggestions and comments on how to improve this book. Please email them to us, so we can bring you the best of the evidence over the years.

L. Santiago Medina, MD, MPH
C. Craig Blackmore, MD, MPH
Kimberly E. Applegate, MD, MS, FACR

Contents

Foreword.. vii
Preface.. ix
Contributors.. xv

Part I   Principles, Methodology, Economics, and Radiation Risk

1   Principles of Evidence-Based Imaging...................................   3
    L. Santiago Medina, C. Craig Blackmore, and Kimberly E. Applegate

2   Critically Assessing the Literature: Understanding Error and Bias........... 19
    C. Craig Blackmore, L. Santiago Medina, James G. Ravenel,
    Gerard A. Silvestri, and Kimberly E. Applegate

3   Radiation Risk from Medical Imaging: A Special Need to Focus on Children..... 27
    Donald P. Frush and Kimberly E. Applegate

4   The Economic and Regulatory Impact of Evidence-Based
    Medicine on Radiology... 43
    David B. Larson

Part II   Oncologic Imaging

5   Breast Imaging... 61
    Laurie L. Fajardo, Wendie A. Berg, and Robert A. Smith

6   Imaging of Lung Cancer... 89
    James G. Ravenel and Gerard A. Silvestri

7   Imaging-Based Screening for Colorectal Cancer........................... 109
    James M. A. Slattery, Lucy E. Modahl, and Michael E. Zalis

8   Imaging of Brain Cancer.. 127
    Soonmee Cha

9   Imaging in the Evaluation of Patients with Prostate Cancer.................. 147
    Jeffrey H. Newhouse

Part III   Neuroimaging

10   Neuroimaging in Alzheimer Disease   167
     Kejal Kantarci and Clifford R. Jack

11   Neuroimaging in Acute Ischemic Stroke   183
     Katie D. Vo, Weili Lin, and Jin-Moo Lee

12   Pediatric Sickle Cell Disease and Stroke   199
     Jaroslaw Krejza, Maciej Swiat, Maciej Tomaszewski, and Elias R. Melhem

13   Neuroimaging for Traumatic Brain Injury   217
     Karen A. Tong, Udochuckwu E. Oyoyo, Barbara A. Holshouser,
     Stephen Ashwal, and L. Santiago Medina

14   Neuroimaging of Seizures   245
     Byron Bernal and Nolan Altman

15   Adults and Children with Headaches: Evidence-Based Role
     of Neuroimaging   261
     L. Santiago Medina and Elza Vasconcellos

16   Imaging Evaluation of Sinusitis: Impact on Health Outcome   277
     Yoshimi Anzai

Part IV   Musculoskeletal Imaging

17   Imaging of Acute Hematogenous Osteomyelitis and Septic
     Arthritis in Children and Adults   297
     John Y. Kim and Diego Jaramillo

18   Imaging for Knee and Shoulder Problems   309
     William Hollingworth, Adrian K. Dixon, and John R. Jenner

19   Pediatric Fractures of the Ankle   327
     Martin H. Reed and G. Brian Black

20   Imaging of Adults with Low Back Pain in the Primary
     Care Setting   335
     Marla B. K. Sammer and Jeffrey G. Jarvik

21   Imaging of the Spine in Victims of Trauma   357
     C. Craig Blackmore and Gregory David Avey

22   Imaging of Spine Disorders in Children: Dysraphism
     and Scoliosis   369
     L. Santiago Medina, Diego Jaramillo, Esperanza Pacheco-Jacome,
     Martha C. Ballesteros, Tina Young Poussaint, and Brian E. Grottkau

Part V   Cardiovascular and Chest Imaging

23 Imaging of the Solitary Pulmonary Nodule   387
     Anil Kumar Attili and Ella A. Kazerooni

24 Cardiac Evaluation: The Current Status of Outcomes-Based
     Imaging   411
     Andrew J. Bierhals and Pamela K. Woodard

25 Imaging in the Evaluation of Pulmonary Embolism   425
     Krishna Juluru and John Eng

26 Aorta and Peripheral Vascular Disease   439
     Max P. Rosen

27 Imaging of the Cervical Carotid Artery for Atherosclerotic
     Stenosis   451
     Alex M. Barrocas and Colin P. Derdeyn

28 Blunt Injuries to the Thorax and Abdomen   465
     Frederick A. Mann

Part VI   Abdominal and Pelvic Imaging

29 Imaging of Appendicitis in Adult and Pediatric Patients   481
     C. Craig Blackmore, Erin A. Cooke, and Gregory David Avey

30 Imaging in Non-appendiceal Acute Abdominal Pain   491
     C. Craig Blackmore and Gregory David Avey

31 Intussusception in Children: Diagnostic Imaging and Treatment   501
     Kimberly E. Applegate

32 Imaging of Infantile Hypertrophic Pyloric Stenosis   515
     Marta Hernanz-Schulman, Barry R. Berch, and Wallace W. Neblett III

33 Imaging of Biliary Disorders: Cholecystitis, Bile Duct
     Obstruction, Stones, and Stricture   527
     Jose C. Varghese, Brian C. Lucey, and Jorge A. Soto

34 Hepatic Disorders: Colorectal Cancer Metastases, Cirrhosis,
     and Hepatocellular Carcinoma   553
     Brian C. Lucey, Jose C. Varghese, and Jorge A. Soto

35 Imaging of Inflammatory Bowel Disease in Children   571
     *Sudha A. Anupindi, Rama Ayyala, Judith Kelsen, Petar Mamula,
     and Kimberly E. Applegate*

36   Imaging of Nephrolithiasis and Its Complications in Adults
     and Children   593
     Lynn Ansley Fordham, Julia R. Fielding, Richard W. Sutherland,
     Debbie S. Gipson, and Kimberly E. Applegate

37   Urinary Tract Infection in Infants and Children   609
     Carol E. Barnewolt, Leonard P. Connolly, Carlos R. Estrada,
     and Kimberly E. Applegate

38   Current Issues in Gynecology: Screening for Ovarian Cancer
     in the Average Risk Population and Diagnostic Evaluation
     of Postmenopausal Bleeding   635
     Ruth C. Carlos

39   Imaging of Female Children and Adolescents with
     Abdominopelvic Pain Caused by Gynecological Pathologies   649
     Stefan Puig

40   Imaging of Boys with an Acute Scrotum: Differentiation
     of Testicular Torsion from Other Causes   659
     Stefan Puig

Index   669

Contributors

Nolan Altman, MD
Chief, Department of Radiology, Miami Children's Hospital, Miami, FL 33176, USA

Sudha A. Anupindi, MD
Assistant Professor, Department of Radiology, The Children's Hospital of Philadelphia, University of Pennsylvania School of Medicine, Philadelphia, PA 19104, USA

Yoshimi Anzai, MD, MPH
Professor of Radiology, Department of Radiology, University of Washington, Seattle, WA 98195, USA

Kimberly E. Applegate, MD, MS, FACR
Professor of Radiology, Vice Chair for Quality and Safety, Department of Radiology, Emory University School of Medicine, Atlanta, GA 30322, USA

Stephen Ashwal, MD
Chief, Division of Pediatric Neurology, Department of Pediatrics, Loma Linda University School of Medicine, Loma Linda, CA 92354, USA

Anil Kumar Attili, MD
Assistant Professor of Radiology, Cardiology, and Pediatrics, Department of Radiology, University of Kentucky, Lexington, KY 40536, USA

Gregory David Avey, MD
Department of Radiology, University of Wisconsin School of Medicine, Madison, WI 53711, USA

Rama Ayyala, BS, MD
Department of Radiology, Columbia University Medical Center, New York, NY 10032, USA

Martha C. Ballesteros, MD
Radiologist, Department of Radiology, Miami Children's Hospital, Miami, FL 33155, USA

Carol E. Barnewolt, MD
Assistant Professor of Radiology, Harvard Medical School; Staff Radiologist, Department of Radiology, Children's Hospital; Director, Division of Ultrasound, Children's Hospital Boston, Boston, MA 02115, USA

Alex M. Barrocas
Director of Interventional Neuroradiology and Endovascular Neurosurgery, Department
of Radiology, Mount Sinai Medical Center, Miami Beach, FL 33140, USA

Barry R. Berch, MD
Pediatric General Surgeon, Assistant Professor of Surgery, Department of Surgery, Blair E.
Batson Children's Hospital of Mississippi, University of Mississippi Medical Center, Jackson,
MS 39216, USA

Wendie A. Berg, MD, PhD, FACR
Breast Imaging Consultant and Study Chair, Johns Hopkins Greenspring, Lutherville,
MD 21093, USA

Byron Bernal, MD, CCTI
Clinical Neuroscientist, Department of Radiology, Miami Children's Hospital, Miami,
FL 33176, USA

Andrew J. Bierhals, MD, MPH
Assistant Professor of Radiology, Mallinckrodt Institute of Radiology, Washington University
School of Medicine, St. Louis, MO 63110, USA

G. Brian Black, BSc, MD, FRCS(C), FACS
Professor of Surgery and Pediatric Orthopedics, Department of Surgery, Winnipeg Children's
Hospital, University of Manitoba, Winnipeg, MB, Canada, R3A 1S1

C. Craig Blackmore, MD, MPH
Scientific Director, Department of Radiology, Center for Healthcare Solutions, Virginia Mason
Medical Center, Seattle, WA 98111, USA

Ruth C. Carlos, MD, MS
Associate Professor, Department of Radiology, University of Michigan Health System,
Ann Arbor, MI 48109, USA

Soonmee Cha, MD
Associate Professor, Department of Radiology and Biomedical Imaging, University of
California San Francisco Medical Center, San Francisco, CA 94117, USA

Leonard P. Connolly, MD
Associate Radiologist, Department of Nuclear Medicine and Radiology, Massachusetts
General Hospital, Boston, MA 02114, USA

Erin A. Cooke, MD
Assistant Staff, Department of Radiology, Ochsner Medical Center, New Orleans,
LA 70121, USA

Colin P. Derdeyn, MD
Professor of Radiology, Neurology, and Neurological Surgery, Director, Center for Stroke and
Cerebrovascular Disease, Mallinckrodt Institute of Radiology, Washington University School
of Medicine, St. Louis, MO 63110, USA

Adrian K. Dixon, MD, FRCR, FRCP, FRCS, FMedSci, FACR(Hon)
Professor Emeritus, Department of Radiology, University of Cambridge, Cambridge,
CB1 1RD, UK

John Eng, MD
Associate Professor of Radiology and Health Sciences Informatics, Department of Radiology and Radiological Science, Johns Hopkins University School of Medicine, Baltimore, MD 21287, USA

Carlos R. Estrada, MD
Assistant Professor of Surgery, Department of Urology, Harvard Medical School, Children's Hospital Boston, Boston, MA 02445, USA

Laurie L. Fajardo, MD, MBA
Professor and Chair, Department of Radiology, University of Iowa Hospitals and Clinics, University of Iowa Carver College of Medicine, Iowa City, IA 52240, USA

Julia R. Fielding, MD
Professor of Radiology, Department of Radiology, University of North Carolina, Chapel Hill, NC 27599, USA

Lynn Ansley Fordham, MD
Associate Professor, Chief of Pediatric Imaging, Department of Radiology, University of North Carolina, North Carolina Children's Hospital, Chapel Hill, NC 27599, USA

Donald P. Frush, MD
Professor of Radiology and Pediatrics, DUMC, Durham, NC, 27710, USA

Debbie S. Gipson, MD, MS
Associate Professor, Department of Pediatrics, University of Michigan, Ann Arbor, MI 48109, USA

Brian E. Grottkau, MD
Chief, Pediatric Orthopaedics, Department of Orthopaedic Surgery, Massachusetts General Hospital for Children, Harvard University, Boston, MA 02114, USA

Marta Hernanz-Schulman, MD, FAAP, FACR
Professor of Radiology and Radiological Sciences, Professor of Pediatrics, Radiology Vice-Chair for Pediatrics, Medical Director, Diagnostic Imaging, Department of Radiology, Monroe Carell Jr. Children's Hospital at Vanderbilt, Nashville, TN 37232, USA

William Hollingworth, PhD
Reader in Health Economics, School of Social and Community Medicine, University of Bristol, Bristol BS8 2PS, UK

Barbara A. Holshouser, PhD
Professor of Radiology, Department of Radiology, Loma Linda University Medical Center, Loma Linda, CA 92354, USA

Clifford R. Jack Jr., MD
Department of Radiology, Mayo Clinic, Rochester, MN 55905, USA

Diego Jaramillo, MD, MPH
Radiologist-in-Chief and Van Alen Chair of Radiology, The Children's Hospital of Philadelphia; Professor of Radiology, University of Pennsylvania School of Medicine, Philadelphia, PA 19104, USA

Jeffrey G. Jarvik, MD, MPH
Professor, Department of Radiology, University of Washington, Seattle, WA 98195, USA

John R. Jenner, MD, FRCP
Consultant in Rheumatology and Rehabilitation, Department of Rheumatology, Addenbrookes Hospital, Cambridge University Hospitals NHS Foundation Trust, Cambridge, CB2 0QQ, UK

Krishna Juluru, MD
Assistant Professor, Department of Radiology, Weill Cornell Medical College, New York, NY 10065, USA

Kejal Kantarci, MD, MSc
Associate Professor of Radiology, Division of Neuroradiology, Mayo Clinic, Rochester, MN 55902, USA

Ella A. Kazerooni, MD, MS
Professor, Associate Chair for Clinical Affairs, Director of Cardiothoracic Radiology Division, Department of Radiology, University of Michigan Health System, Ann Arbor, MI 48109, USA

Judith Kelsen, MD
Attending, Pediatric Gastroenterology, Hepatology, and Nutrition, Division of Gastroenterology, Department of Pediatrics, The Children's Hospital of Philadelphia, Philadelphia, PA 19146, USA

John Y. Kim, MD
Chairman, Department of Radiology, Texas Health Presbyterian Hospital of Plano, Plano, TX 75093, USA

Jaroslaw Krejza, MD, PhD
Professor, Department of Radiology, Hospital of the University of Pennsylvania, Philadelphia, PA 19104, USA

David B. Larson, MD, MBA
Staff Radiologist, Department of Radiology, Cincinnati Children's Hospital Medical Center, Cincinnati, OH 45229, USA

Jin-Moo Lee, MD, PhD
Associate Professor, Department of Neurology, Washington University School of Medicine, St. Louis, MO 63110, USA

Weili Lin, PhD
Professor, Department of Radiology, University of North Carolina at Chapel Hill, Chapel Hill, NC 27599, USA

Brian C. Lucey, MB, BCh, BAO, MRCPI, FFR(RCSI)
Clinical Director, Department of Radiology, The Galway Clinic, Doughiski, County Galway, Ireland

Petar Mamula, MD
Director of Kohl's Endoscopy Suite, Assistant Professor of Pediatrics, Department of Pediatrics, University of Pennsylvania School of Medicine, Children's Hospital of Philadelphia, Philadelphia, PA 19104, USA

Frederick A. Mann, MD
Assistant Chief of Radiology, Department of Radiology/Medical Imaging, APC, Swedish Medical Centers, 1229 Madison, Suite 900, Seattle, WA 98104, USA

L. Santiago Medina, MD, MPH
Co-Director, Division of Neuroradiology and Brain Imaging, Director of the Health Outcomes, Policy, and Economics (HOPE) Center, Department of Radiology, Miami Children's Hospital, Miami, FL 33155, USA; Former Lecturer in Radiology, Harvard Medical School, Boston, MA 02114, USA

Elias R. Melhem, MD, PhD
Vice-Chairman, Academic Affairs, Department of Radiology, University of Pennsylvania, Philadelphia, PA 19104, USA

Lucy E. Modahl
Radiologist, NightHawk Radiology Services, Sydney, 2000, NSW, Australia

Wallace W. Neblett III, MD
Professor, Chairman, Department of Pediatric Surgery, Vanderbilt University Medical Center, Nashville, TN 37232, USA

Jeffrey H. Newhouse, MD
Professor of Radiology and Urology, Department of Radiology, Columbia University College of Physicians and Surgeons, New York, NY 10032, USA

Udochuckwu E. Oyoyo, PhD(C), MPH
Research Associate, Department of Radiology, Loma Linda University Medical Center, Loma Linda, CA 92354, USA

Esperanza Pacheco-Jacome, MD
Co-Director of Neuroradiology, Department of Radiology, Miami Children's Hospital, Miami, FL 33155, USA

Tina Young Poussaint, MD
Attending Neuroradiologist, Associate Professor of Radiology, Department of Radiology, Harvard Medical School, Children's Hospital Boston, Boston, MA 02115, USA

Stefan Puig, MD, MSc
Associate Professor in Radiology, Research Program on Evidence-Based Medical Diagnostics, Paracelsus Medical University, Salzburg 5020, Austria

James G. Ravenel, MD
Professor of Radiology, Department of Radiology, Medical University of South Carolina, Charleston, SC 29425, USA

Martin H. Reed, MD, FRCP(C)
Head, Pediatric Radiology, Department of Diagnostic Imaging, Children's Hospital of Winnipeg, University of Manitoba, Winnipeg, Manitoba, Canada, R3A 1S1

Max P. Rosen, MD, MPH, FACR
Executive Vice Chairman, Department of Radiology, Beth Israel Deaconess Medical Center; Associative Professor of Radiology, Harvard Medical School, Boston, MA 02215, USA

Marla B. K. Sammer, MD
Radiologist, Department of Radiology, T. C. Thompson Children's Hospital, Chattanooga, TN 37403, USA

Gerard A. Silvestri, MD, MS
Professor of Medicine, Department of Radiology, Medical University of South Carolina, Charleston, SC 29425, USA

James M. A. Slattery
Midland Regional Hospital, Mullingar, County Westmeath, Ireland

Robert A. Smith, PhD
Director, Cancer Screening, Department of Cancer Control Science, American Cancer Society, Atlanta, GA 30303, USA

Jorge A. Soto, MD
Professor of Radiology, Department of Radiology, Boston University School of Medicine, Boston Medical Center, Boston, MA 02459, USA

Richard W. Sutherland, MD
Director, Pediatric Urology, Associate Professor, Department of Surgery/Urology, Pediatric Urology, University of North Carolina Children's Hospital, Chapel Hill, NC 27514, USA

Maciej Swiat, MD, PhD
Consultant Neurologist, Department of Neuroscience, University Hospitals Conventry and Warwickshire, Coventry, CV2 2DX, UK

Maciej Tomaszewski, MD, PhD
Division of Neuroradiology, Department of Radiology, University of Pennsylvania, Philadelphia, PA 19104, USA

Karen A. Tong, MD
Associate Professor, Department of Radiology, Loma Linda University Medical Center, Loma Linda, CA 92354, USA

Jose C. Varghese, MBChB
Associate Professor of Radiology, Department of Radiology, Boston University School of Medicine, Boston Medical Center and Quincy Medical Center, Boston, MA 02118, USA

Elza Vasconcellos, MD
Director, Headache Center, Department of Neurology, Miami Children's Hospital, Miami, FL 33155, USA

Katie D. Vo, MD
Associate Professor in Radiology, Director, Cerebrovascular Imaging, Director, Diagnostic Neuroradiology Fellowship, Mallinckrodt Institute of Radiology, Washington University School of Medicine, St. Louis, MO 63110, USA

Pamela K. Woodard, MD
Professor of Radiology and Biomedical Engineering, Head, Cardiac MR/CT, Department of Radiology, Washington University School of Medicine, St. Louis, MO 63110, USA

Michael E. Zalis, MD
Assistant Professor, Department of Radiology, Massachusetts General Hospital, Boston, MA 02114, USA

Part I

Principles, Methodology, Economics, and Radiation Risk

1

Principles of Evidence-Based Imaging

L. Santiago Medina, C. Craig Blackmore, and Kimberly E. Applegate

Medicine is a science of uncertainty and an art of probability.

Sir William Osler

I. What is evidence-based imaging?
II. The evidence-based imaging process
   A. Formulating the clinical question
   B. Identifying the medical literature
   C. Assessing the literature
      1. What are the types of clinical studies?
      2. What is the diagnostic performance of a test: sensitivity, specificity, and receiver operating characteristic curve?
      3. What are cost-effectiveness and cost-utility studies?
   D. Types of economic analyses in medicine
   E. Summarizing the data
   F. Applying the evidence
III. How to use this book
IV. Take home appendix 1: equations
V. Take home appendix 2: summary of Bayes' Theorem

Issues

I. What Is Evidence-Based Imaging?

The standard medical education in Western medicine has emphasized skills and knowledge learned from experts, particularly those encountered in the course of postgraduate medical education, and through national publications and meetings. This reliance on experts, referred to by Dr. Paul Gerber of Dartmouth Medical School as "eminence-based medicine" (1), is based on the construct that the individual practitioner, particularly a specialist devoting extensive time to a given discipline, can arrive at the best approach to a problem through his or her experience. The practitioner builds up an experience base over years and digests information from national experts who have a greater base of experience due to their focus in a particular area. The evidence-based imaging (EBI) paradigm, in contradistinction, is based

L.S. Medina (✉)

Department of Radiology, Miami Children's Hospital, 3100 SW 62 Ave, Miami, FL, 33155, USA

e-mail: smedina@post.harvard.edu

L.S. Medina et al. (eds.), *Evidence-Based Imaging: Improving the Quality of Imaging in Patient Care, Revised Edition*,
DOI 10.1007/978-1-4419-7777-9_1, © Springer Science+Business Media, LLC 2011

on the precept that a single practitioner cannot through experience alone arrive at an unbiased assessment of the best course of action. Assessment of appropriate medical care should instead be derived through evidence-based process. The role of the practitioner, then, is not simply to accept information from an expert, but rather to assimilate and critically assess the research evidence that exists in the literature to guide a clinical decision (2–4).

Fundamental to the adoption of the principles of EBI is the understanding that medical care is not optimal. The life expectancy at birth in the United States for males and females in 2005 was 75 and 80 years, respectively (Table 1.1). This is slightly lower than the life expectancies in other industrialized nations such as the United Kingdom and Australia (Table 1.1). In fact, the World Health Organization ranks the USA 50th in life expectancy and 72nd in overall health. The United States spent at least 15.2% of the gross domestic product (GDP) in order to achieve this life expectancy. This was significantly more than the United Kingdom and Australia, which spent about half that (Table 1.1). In addition, the US per capita health expenditure was $6,096, which was twice the expenditure in the United Kingdom or Australia. In conclusion, the United States spends significantly more money and resources than other industrialized countries to achieve a similar outcome in life expectancy. This implies that a significant amount of resources is wasted in the US health care system. In 2007, the United States spent $2.3 trillion in health care or 16% of its GDP. By 2016, the US health

percent of the GDP is expected to grow to 20% or $4.2 trillion (5). Recent estimates prepared by the Commonwealth Fund Commission (USA) on a High Performance Health System indicate that $1.5 trillion could be saved over a 10-year period if a combination of options, including evidence-based medicine and universal health insurance, was adopted (6).

Simultaneous with the increase in health care costs has been an explosion in available medical information. The National Library of Medicine PubMed search engine now lists over 18 million citations. Practitioners cannot maintain familiarity with even a minute subset of this literature without a method of filtering out publications that lack appropriate methodological quality. EBI is a promising method of identifying appropriate information to guide practice and to improve the efficiency and effectiveness of imaging.

Evidence-based imaging is defined as medical decision making based on clinical integration of the best medical imaging research evidence with the physician's expertise and with patient's expectations (2–4). The best medical imaging research evidence often comes from the basic sciences of medicine. In EBI, however, the basic science knowledge has been translated into patient-centered clinical research, which determines the accuracy and role of diagnostic and therapeutic imaging in patient care (3). New evidence may make current diagnostic tests obsolete and new ones more accurate, less invasive, safer, and less costly (3). The physician's expertise entails the ability to use the referring physician's clinical skills and

Table 1.1. Life expectancy and health care spending in three developed countries

	Life expectancy at birth (2005)		Percentage of GDP in health care (2007) (%)	Per capita health expenditure (2007)
	Male	Female		
United States	75.3	80.3	16.0	$6,096
United Kingdom	77.4	81.4	8.3	$2,560
Australia	79.5	84.5	9.1	$3,123

Sources: United Kingdom Office of National Statistics; Australian Bureau of Statistics; Per capita expenditures: *Human Development Report, 2007*, United Nations, hdr.undp.org; Life expectancy: Kaiser Family Foundation web site with stated source: WHO, World Health Statistics 2007, available at: http://www.who.int/whosis/en/.
Reprinted with kind permission of Springer Science+Business Media. Medina LS, Blackmore CC, Applegate KE. Principles of Evidence-Based Imaging. In Medina LS, Applegate KE, Blackmore CC (eds.): *Evidence-Based Imaging in Pediatrics: Optimizing Imaging in Pediatric Patient Care*. New York: Springer Science+Business Media, 2010.
GDP gross domestic product.

past experience to rapidly identify high-risk individuals who will benefit from the diagnostic information of an imaging test (4). Patient's expectations are important because each individual has values and preferences that should be integrated into the clinical decision making in order to serve our patients' best interests (3). When these three components of medicine come together, clinicians and imagers form a diagnostic team, which will optimize clinical outcomes and quality of life for our patients.

II. The Evidence-Based Imaging Process

The EBI process involves a series of steps: (A) formulation of the clinical question, (B) identification of the medical literature, (C) assessment of the literature, (D) summary of the evidence, and (E) application of the evidence to derive an appropriate clinical action. This book is designed to bring the EBI process to the clinician and imager in a user-friendly way. This introductory chapter details each of the steps in the EBI process. Chapter 2 discusses how to critically assess the literature. The rest of the book makes available to practitioners the EBI approach to numerous key medical imaging issues. Each chapter addresses common pediatric disorders ranging from congenital anomalies to asthma to appendicitis. Relevant clinical questions are delineated, and then each chapter discusses the results of the critical analysis of the identified literature. The results of this analysis are presented with meta-analyses where appropriate. Finally, we provide simple recommendations for the various clinical questions, including the strength of the evidence that supports these recommendations.

A. Formulating the Clinical Question

The first step in the EBI process is formulation of the clinical question. The entire process of EBI arises from a question that is asked in the context of clinical practice. However, often formulating a question for the EBI approach can be more challenging than one would believe intuitively. To be approachable by the EBI format, a question must be specific to a clinical situation,

a patient group, and an outcome or action. For example, it would not be appropriate to simply ask which imaging technique is better – computed tomography (CT) or radiography. The question must be refined to include the particular patient population and the action that the imaging will be used to direct. One can refine the question to include a particular population (which imaging technique is better in pediatric victims of high-energy blunt trauma) and to guide a particular action or decision (to exclude the presence of unstable cervical spine fracture). The full EBI question then becomes, in pediatric victims of high-energy blunt trauma, which imaging modality is preferred, CT or radiography, to exclude the presence of unstable cervical spine fracture? This book addresses questions that commonly arise when employing an EBI approach for the care of children and adolescents. These questions and issues are detailed at the start of each chapter.

B. Identifying the Medical Literature

The process of EBI requires timely access to the relevant medical literature to answer the question. Fortunately, massive on-line bibliographical references such as PubMed are available. In general, titles, indexing terms, abstracts, and often the complete text of much of the world's medical literature are available through these on-line sources. Also, medical librarians are a potential resource to aid identification of the relevant imaging literature. A limitation of today's literature data sources is that often too much information is available and too many potential resources are identified in a literature search. There are currently over 50 radiology journals, and imaging research is also frequently published in journals from other medical subspecialties. We are often confronted with more literature and information than we can process. The greater challenge is to sift through the literature that is identified to select that which is appropriate.

C. Assessing the Literature

To incorporate evidence into practice, the clinician must be able to understand the published literature and to critically evaluate the strength of the evidence. In this introductory chapter on the process of EBI, we focus on discussing types of research studies. Chapter 2 is a detailed discussion of the issues in determining the validity and reliability of the reported results.

1. What Are the Types of Clinical Studies?

An initial assessment of the literature begins with determination of the type of clinical study: descriptive, analytical, or experimental (7). *Descriptive* studies are the most rudimentary, as they only summarize disease processes as seen by imaging, or discuss how an imaging modality can be used to create images. Descriptive studies include case reports and case series. Although they may provide important information that leads to further investigation, descriptive studies are not usually the basis for EBI.

Analytic or *observational* studies include cohort, case–control, and cross-sectional studies (Table 1.2). Cohort studies are defined by risk factor status, and case–control studies consist of groups defined by disease status (8). Both case–control and cohort studies may be used to define the association between an intervention, such as an imaging test, and patient outcome (9). In a cross-sectional (prevalence) study, the researcher makes all of his measurements on a single occasion. The investigator draws a sample from the population (i.e., asthma in 5- to 15-year-olds) and determines distribution of variables within that sample (7). The structure of a cross-sectional study is similar to that of a cohort study except that all pertinent measurements (i.e., PFTs) are made at once, without a follow-up period. Cross-sectional studies can be used as a major source for health and habits of different populations and countries, providing estimates of such parameters as the prevalence of asthma, obesity, and congenital anomalies (7, 10).

In *experimental studies* or *clinical trials*, a specific intervention is performed and the effect of the intervention is measured by using a control group (Table 1.2). The control group may be tested with a different diagnostic test and treated with a placebo or an alternative mode of therapy (7, 11). Clinical trials are epidemiologic designs that can provide data of high quality that resemble the controlled experiments done by basic science investigators (8). For example, clinical trials may be used to assess new diagnostic tests (e.g., high-resolution CT for cystic fibrosis) or new interventional procedures (e.g., stenting for coronary artery anomalies).

Studies are also traditionally divided into retrospective and prospective (Table 1.2) (7, 11). These terms refer more to the way the data are gathered than to the specific type of study design. In *retrospective studies*, the events of interest have occurred before study onset. Retrospective studies are usually done to assess rare disorders, for pilot studies, and when prospective investigations are not possible. If the disease process is considered rare, retrospective studies facilitate the collection of enough subjects to have meaningful data. For a pilot project, retrospective studies facilitate the collection of preliminary data that can be used to improve the study design in future prospective studies. The major drawback of a retrospective study is incomplete data acquisition (10). Case–control studies are usually retrospective. For example, in a case–control study, subjects in the case group (patients with perforated appendicitis) are compared with subjects in a control group (nonperforated appendicitis) to determine factors associated with perforation (e.g., duration of symptoms, presence of appendicolith, size of appendix) (10).

Table 1.2. Study design

	Prospective follow-up	Randomization of subjects	Controls
Case report or series	No	No	No
Cross-sectional study	No	No	Yes
Case–control study	No	No	Yes
Cohort study	Yes/no	No	Yes
Randomized controlled trial	Yes	Yes	Yes

Reprinted with the kind permission of Springer Science+Business Media from by Medina and Blackmore (40).

In *prospective studies*, the event of interest transpires after study onset. Prospective studies, therefore, are the preferred mode of study design, as they facilitate better control of the design and the quality of the data acquired (7). Prospective studies, even large studies, can be performed efficiently and in a timely fashion if done on common diseases at major institutions, as multicenter trials with adequate study populations (12). The major drawback of a prospective study is the need to make sure that the institution and personnel comply with strict rules concerning consents, protocols, and data acquisition (11). Persistence, to the point of irritation, is crucial to completing a prospective study. Cohort studies and clinical trials are usually prospective. For example, a cohort study could be performed in children with splenic injury in which the risk factor of presence of arterial blush is correlated with the outcome of failure of nonmedical management, as the patients are followed prospectively over time (10).

The strongest study design is the prospective randomized, blinded clinical trial (Table 1.2) (7). The randomization process helps to distribute known and unknown confounding factors, and blinding helps to prevent observer bias from affecting the results (7, 8). However, there are often circumstances in which it is not ethical or practical to randomize and follow patients prospectively. This is particularly true in rare conditions, and in studies to determine causes or predictors of a particular condition (9). Finally, randomized clinical trials are expensive and may require many years of follow-up. Not surprisingly, randomized clinical trials are uncommon in radiology. The evidence that supports much of radiology practice is derived from cohort and other observational studies. More randomized clinical trials are necessary in radiology to provide sound data to use for EBI practice (3).

2. What Is the Diagnostic Performance of a Test: Sensitivity, Specificity, and Receiver Operating Characteristic Curve?

Defining the presence or absence of an outcome (i.e., disease and nondisease) is based on a standard of reference (Table 1.3). While a perfect standard of reference or so-called gold standard can never be obtained, careful attention should be paid to the selection of the standard that should be widely believed to offer the best approximation to the truth (13).

In evaluating diagnostic tests, we rely on the statistical calculations of sensitivity and specificity (see Appendix 1). Sensitivity and specificity of a diagnostic test are based on the two-way (2×2) table (Table 1.3). Sensitivity refers to the proportion of subjects with the disease who have a positive test and is referred to as the true positive rate (Fig. 1.1). Sensitivity, therefore, indicates how well a test identifies the subjects with disease (7, 14).

Table 1.3. Two-way table of diagnostic testing

| Test result | Disease (gold standard) | |
	Present	Absent
Positive	a (TP)	b (FP)
Negative	c (FN)	d (TN)

Reprinted with the kind permission of Springer Science+Business Media from by Medina and Blackmore (40). FN false negative; FP false positive; TN true negative; TP true positive.

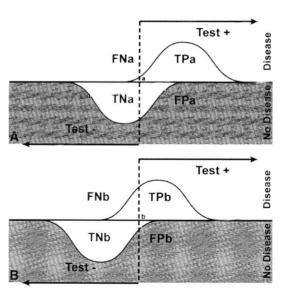

Figure 1.1. Test with a low (**A**) and high (**B**) threshold. The sensitivity and specificity of a test change according to the threshold selected; hence, these diagnostic performance parameters are threshold dependent. Sensitivity with low threshold (TPa/diseased patients) is greater than sensitivity with a higher threshold (TPb/diseased patients). Specificity with a low threshold (TNa/nondiseased patients) is less than specificity with a high threshold (TNb/nondiseased patients). FN false negative; FP false positive; TN true negative; TP true positive. (Reprinted with permission of the American Society of Neuroradiology from Medina (11).)

Specificity is defined as the proportion of subjects without the disease who have a negative index test (Fig. 1.1) and is referred to as the true negative rate. Specificity, therefore, indicates how well a test identifies the subjects with no disease (7, 11). It is important to note that the sensitivity and specificity are characteristics of the test being evaluated and are therefore usually independent of the prevalence (proportion of individuals in a population who have disease at a specific instant) because the sensitivity only deals with the diseased subjects, whereas the specificity only deals with the nondiseased subjects. However, sensitivity and specificity both depend on a threshold point for considering a test positive and hence may change according to which threshold is selected in the study (11, 14, 15) (Fig. 1.1A). Excellent diagnostic tests have high values (close to 1.0) for both sensitivity and specificity. Given exactly the same diagnostic test, and exactly the same subjects confirmed with the same reference test, the sensitivity with a low threshold is greater than the sensitivity with a high threshold. Conversely, the specificity with a low threshold is less than the specificity with a high threshold (Fig. 1.1B) (14, 15).

The effect of threshold on the ability of a test to discriminate between disease and nondisease can be measured by a receiver operating characteristic (ROC) curve (11, 15). The ROC curve is used to indicate the trade-offs between sensitivity and specificity for a particular diagnostic test and hence describes the discrimination capacity of that test. An ROC graph shows the relationship between sensitivity (*y* axis) and 1 – specificity (*x* axis) plotted for various cutoff points. If the threshold for sensitivity and specificity are varied, an ROC curve can be generated. The diagnostic performance of a test can be estimated by the area under the ROC curve. The steeper the ROC curve, the greater the area and the better the discrimination of the test (Fig. 1.2). A test with perfect discrimination has an area of 1.0, whereas a test with only random discrimination has an area of 0.5 (Fig. 1.2). The area under the ROC curve usually determines the overall diagnostic performance of the test independent of the threshold selected (11, 15). The ROC curve is threshold independent because it is generated by using varied thresholds of sensitivity and specificity. Therefore, when evaluating a new imaging test, in addition to the sensitivity and specificity, an ROC curve analysis should be

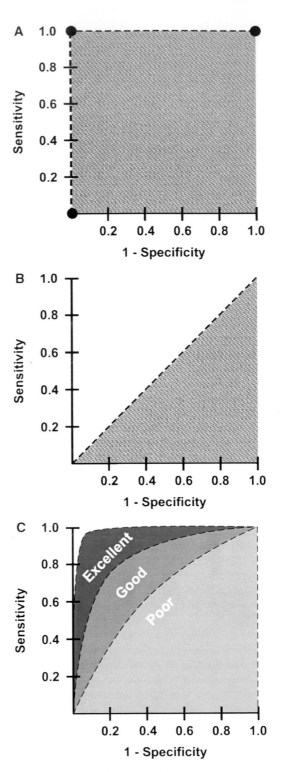

Figure 1.2. The perfect test (**A**) has an area under the curve (AUC) of 1. The useless test (**B**) has an AUC of 0.5. The typical test (**C**) has an AUC between 0.5 and 1. The greater the AUC (i.e., excellent > good > poor), the better the diagnostic performance. (Reprinted with permission of the American Society of Neuroradiology from Medina (11).)

done so that the threshold-dependent and threshold-independent diagnostic performance can be fully determined (10).

3. What Are Cost-Effectiveness and Cost-Utility Studies?

Cost-effectiveness analysis (CEA) is an objective scientific technique used to assess alternative health care strategies on both cost and effectiveness (16–18). It can be used to develop clinical and imaging practice guidelines and to set health policy (19). However, it is not designed to be the final answer to the decision-making process; rather, it provides a detailed analysis of the cost and outcome variables and how they are affected by competing medical and diagnostic choices.

Health dollars are limited regardless of the country's economic status. Hence, medical decision makers must weigh the benefits of a diagnostic test (or any intervention) in relation to its cost. Health care resources should be allocated so the maximum health care benefit for the entire population is achieved (10). Cost-effectiveness analysis is an important tool to address health cost-outcome issues in a cost-conscious society. Countries such as Australia usually require robust CEA before drugs are approved for national use (10).

Unfortunately, the term *cost-effectiveness* is often misused in the medical literature (20). To say that a diagnostic test is truly cost-effective, a comprehensive analysis of the entire short- and long-term outcomes and costs needs to be considered. Cost-effectiveness analysis is an objective technique used to determine which of the available tests or treatments are worth the additional costs (21).

There are established guidelines for conducting robust CEA. The US Public Health Service formed a panel of experts on cost-effectiveness in health and medicine to create detailed standards for cost-effectiveness analysis. The panel's recommendations were published as a book in 1996 (21).

D. Types of Economic Analyses in Medicine

There are four well-defined types of economic evaluations in medicine: cost-minimization studies, cost–benefit analyses, cost-effectiveness analyses, and cost-utility analyses. They are all commonly lumped under the term *cost-effectiveness analysis*. However, significant differences exist among these different studies.

Cost-minimization analysis is a comparison of the cost of different health care strategies that are assumed to have identical or similar effectiveness (16). In medical practice, few diagnostic tests or treatments have identical or similar effectiveness. Therefore, relatively few articles have been published in the literature with this type of study design (22). For example, a recent study demonstrated that functional magnetic resonance imaging (MRI) and the Wada test have similar effectiveness for language lateralization, but the later is 3.7 times more costly than the former (23).

Cost–benefit analysis (CBA) uses monetary units such as dollars or euros to compare the costs of a health intervention with its health benefits (16). It converts all benefits to a cost equivalent and is commonly used in the financial world where the cost and benefits of multiple industries can be changed to only monetary values. One method of converting health outcomes into dollars is through a contingent valuation or willingness-to-pay approach. Using this technique, subjects are asked how much money they would be willing to spend to obtain, or avoid, a health outcome. For example, a study by Appel et al. (24) found that individuals would be willing to pay $50 for low osmolar contrast agents to decrease the probability of side effects from intravenous contrast. However, in general, health outcomes and benefits are difficult to transform to monetary units; hence, CBA has had limited acceptance and use in medicine and diagnostic imaging (16, 25).

Cost-effectiveness analysis (CEA) refers to analyses that study both the effectiveness and cost of competing diagnostic or treatment strategies, where effectiveness is an objective measure (e.g., intermediate outcome: number of strokes detected; or long-term outcome: life-years saved). Radiology CEAs often use intermediate outcomes, such as lesion identified, length of stay, and number of avoidable surgeries (16, 18). However, ideally, long-term outcomes such as life-years saved (LYS) should be used (21). By using LYS, different health care fields or interventions can be compared.

Cost-utility analysis is similar to CEA except that the effectiveness also accounts for quality of life issues. Quality of life is measured as utilities that are based on patient preferences (16).

The most commonly used utility measurement is the quality-adjusted life year (QALY). The rationale behind this concept is that the QALY of excellent health is more desirable than the same 1 year with substantial morbidity. The QALY model uses preferences with weight for each health state on a scale from 0 to 1, where 0 is death and 1 is perfect health. The utility score for each health state is multiplied by the length of time the patient spends in that specific health state (16, 26). For example, let us assume that a patient with a congenital heart anomaly has a utility of 0.8 and he spends 1 year in this health state. The patient with the cardiac anomaly would have a 0.8 QALY in comparison with his neighbor who has a perfect health and hence a 1 QALY.

Cost-utility analysis incorporates the patient's subjective value of the risk, discomfort, and pain into the effectiveness measurements of the different diagnostic or therapeutic alternatives. In the end, all medical decisions should reflect the patient's values and priorities (26). That is the explanation of why cost-utility analysis is becoming the preferred method for evaluation of economic issues in health (19, 21). For example, in low-risk newborns with intergluteal dimple suspected of having occult spinal dysraphism, ultrasound was the most effective strategy with an incremented cost-effectiveness ratio of $55,100 per QALY. In intermediate-risk newborns with low anorectal malformation, however, MRI was more effective than ultrasound at an incremental cost-effectiveness of $1,000 per QALY (27).

Assessment of Outcomes: The major challenge to cost-utility analysis is the quantification of health or quality of life. One way to quantify health is descriptive analyses. By assessing what patients can and cannot do, how they feel, their mental state, their functional independence, their freedom from pain, and any number of other facets of health and well-being that are referred to as domains, one can summarize their overall health status. Instruments designed to measure these domains are called health status instruments. A large number of health status instruments exist, both general instruments, such as the SF-36 (28), and instruments that are specific to particular disease states, such as the Roland scale for back pain. These various scales enable the quantification of health benefit. For example, Jarvik et al. (29) found no significant difference in the Roland score between patients randomized to MRI versus radiography for low back pain, suggesting that MRI was not worth the additional cost. There are additional issues in applying such tools to children, as they may be too young to understand the questions being asked. Parents can sometimes be used as surrogates, but parents may have different values and may not understand the health condition from the perspective of the child.

Assessment of Cost: All forms of economic analysis require assessment of cost. However, assessment of cost in medical care can be confusing, as the term *cost* is used to refer to many different things. The use of charges for any sort of cost estimation, however, is inappropriate. Charges are arbitrary and have no meaningful use. Reimbursements, derived from Medicare and other fee schedules, are useful as an estimation of the amounts society pays for particular health care interventions. For an analysis taken from the societal perspective, such reimbursements may be most appropriate. For analyses from the institutional perspective or in situations where there are no meaningful Medicare reimbursements, assessment of actual direct and overhead costs may be appropriate (30).

Direct cost assessment centers on the determination of the resources that are consumed in the process of performing a given imaging study, including *fixed costs* such as equipment and *variable costs* such as labor and supplies. Cost analysis often utilizes activity-based costing and time motion studies to determine the resources consumed for a single intervention in the context of the complex health care delivery system. *Overhead*, or *indirect cost*, assessment includes the costs of buildings, overall administration, taxes, and maintenance that cannot be easily assigned to one particular imaging study. Institutional cost accounting systems may be used to determine both the direct costs of an imaging study and the amount of institutional overhead costs that should be apportioned to that particular test. For example, Medina et al. (31) in a vesicoureteral reflux imaging study in children with urinary tract infection found a significant difference ($p < 0.0001$) between the mean total direct cost of voiding cystourethrography ($112.7 \pm $10.33) and radionuclide cystography ($64.58 \pm $1.91).

E. Summarizing the Data

The results of the EBI process are a summary of the literature on the topic, both quantitative and qualitative. *Quantitative analysis* involves, at minimum, a descriptive summary of the data and may include formal *meta-analysis*, where there is sufficient reliably acquired data. *Qualitative analysis* requires an understanding of error, bias, and the subtleties of experimental design that can affect the reliability of study results. Qualitative assessment of the literature is covered in detail in Chap. 2; this section focuses on meta-analysis and the quantitative summary of data.

The goal of the EBI process is to produce a single summary of all of the data on a particular clinically relevant question. However, the underlying investigations on a particular topic may be too dissimilar in methods or study populations to allow for a simple summary. In such cases, the user of the EBI approach may have to rely on the single study that most closely resembles the clinical subjects upon whom the results are to be applied or may be able only to reliably estimate a range of possible values for the data.

Often, there is abundant information available to answer an EBI question. Multiple studies may be identified that provide methodologically sound data. Therefore, some method must be used to combine the results of these studies in a summary statement. *Meta-analysis* is the method of combining results of multiple studies in a statistically valid manner to determine a summary measure of accuracy or effectiveness (32, 33). For diagnostic studies, the summary estimate is generally a summary sensitivity and specificity, or a summary ROC curve.

The process of performing meta-analysis parallels that of performing primary research. However, instead of individual subjects, the meta-analysis is based on individual studies of a particular question. The process of selecting the studies for a meta-analysis is as important as unbiased selection of subjects for a primary investigation. Identification of studies for meta-analysis employs the same type of process as that for EBI described above, employing Medline and other literature search engines. Critical information from each of the selected studies is then abstracted usually by more than one investigator. For a meta-analysis of a diagnostic accuracy study, the numbers of true positives, false positives, true negatives, and false negatives would be determined for each of the eligible research publications. The results of a meta-analysis are derived not just by simply pooling the results of the individual studies, but instead by considering each individual study as a data point and determining a summary estimate for accuracy based on each of these individual investigations. There are sophisticated statistical methods of combining such results (34).

Like all research, the value of a meta-analysis is directly dependent on the validity of each of the data points. In other words, the quality of the meta-analysis can only be as good as the quality of the research studies that the meta-analysis summarizes. In general, meta-analysis cannot compensate for selection and other biases in primary data. If the studies included in a meta-analysis are different in some way, or are subject to some bias, then the results may be too heterogeneous to combine in a single summary measure. Exploration for such heterogeneity is an important component of meta-analysis.

The ideal for EBI is that all practice be based on the information from one or more well-performed meta-analyses. However, there is often too little data or too much heterogeneity to support formal meta-analysis.

F. Applying the Evidence

The final step in the EBI process is to apply the summary results of the medical literature to the EBI question. Sometimes the answer to an EBI question is a simple yes or no, as for this question: Does a normal clinical exam exclude unstable cervical spine fracture in patients with minor trauma? Commonly, the answers to EBI questions are expressed as some measure of accuracy. For example, how good is CT for detecting appendicitis? The answer is that CT has an approximate sensitivity of 94% and specificity of 95% (35). However, to guide practice, EBI must be able to answer questions that go beyond simple accuracy, for example, Should CT scan then be used for appendicitis? To answer this question it is useful to divide the types of literature studies into a *hierarchical framework* (36) (Table 1.4). At the foundation in this hierarchy is assessment of *technical efficacy*: studies that are designed to determine if a particular proposed imaging method or application has the underlying ability to produce an image that contains

Table 1.4. Imaging effectiveness hierarchy

Technical efficacy: production of an image or information
Measures: signal-to-noise ratio, resolution, absence of artifacts

Accuracy efficacy: ability of test to differentiate between disease and nondisease
Measures: sensitivity, specificity, receiver operator characteristic curves

Diagnostic-thinking efficacy: impact of test on likelihood of diagnosis in a patient
Measures: pre- and posttest probability, diagnostic certainty

Treatment efficacy: potential of test to change therapy for a patient
Measures: treatment plan, operative or medical treatment frequency

Outcome efficacy: effect of use of test on patient health
Measures: mortality, quality-adjusted life years, health status

Societal efficacy: appropriateness of test from perspective of society
Measures: cost-effectiveness analysis, cost-utility analysis

Adapted with permission from Fryback and Thornbury (36).

useful information. Information for technical efficacy would include signal-to-noise ratios, image resolution, and freedom from artifacts. The second step in this hierarchy is to determine if the image predicts the truth. This is the *accuracy* of an imaging study and is generally studied by comparing the test results to a reference standard and defining the sensitivity and the specificity of the imaging test. The third step is to incorporate the physician into the evaluation of the imaging intervention by evaluating the effect of the use of the particular imaging intervention on physician certainty of a given diagnosis (physician decision making) and on the actual management of the patient (*therapeutic efficacy*). Finally, to be of value to the patient, an imaging procedure must not only affect management but also improve outcome. *Patient outcome efficacy* is the determination of the effect of a given imaging intervention on the length and quality of life of a patient. A final efficacy level is that of society, which examines the question of not simply the health of a single patient, but that of the health of society as a whole, encompassing the effect of a given intervention on all patients and including the concepts of *cost* and *cost-effectiveness* (36).

Some additional research studies in imaging, such as clinical prediction rules, do not fit readily into this hierarchy. *Clinical prediction rules* are used to define a population in whom imaging is appropriate or can safely be avoided. Clinical prediction rules can also be used in combination with CEA as a way of deciding between competing imaging strategies (37).

Ideally, information would be available to address the effectiveness of a diagnostic test on all levels of the hierarchy. Commonly in imaging, however, the only reliable information that is available is that of diagnostic accuracy. It is incumbent upon the user of the imaging literature to determine if a test with a given sensitivity and specificity is appropriate for use in a given clinical situation. To address this issue, the concept of Bayes' theorem is critical. Bayes' theorem is based on the concept that the value of the diagnostic tests depends not only on the characteristics of the test (sensitivity and specificity), but also on the prevalence (pretest probability) of the disease in the test population. As the prevalence of a specific disease decreases, it becomes less likely that someone with a positive test will actually have the disease, and more likely that the positive test result is a false positive. The relationship between the sensitivity and specificity of the test and the prevalence (pretest probability) can be expressed through the use of Bayes' theorem (see Appendix 2) (11, 14) and the likelihood ratio. The positive likelihood ratio (PLR) estimates the likelihood that a positive test result will raise or lower the pretest probability, resulting in estimation of the posttest probability [where PLR=sensitivity/(1−specificity)]. The negative likelihood ratio (NLR) estimates the likelihood that a negative test result will raise or lower the pretest probability, resulting in estimation of the posttest probability [where NLR=(1−sensitivity)/specificity] (38). The likelihood ratio (LR) is not a probability but a ratio of probabilities and as such is not intuitively interpretable. The positive predictive value (PPV) refers to the probability that a person with a positive test result actually has the disease. The negative predictive value (NPV) is the probability that a person with a negative test result does not have the disease. Since the predictive value is determined once the test results are known (i.e., sensitivity and specificity), it actually represents a posttest probability; hence, the posttest probability is determined by both the prevalence (pretest probability) and the test information (i.e., sensitivity and specificity). Thus, the predictive values are affected by the prevalence of disease in the study population.

A practical understanding of this concept is shown in Examples 1 and 2 in Appendix 2. The example shows an increase in the PPV from 0.67 to 0.98 when the prevalence of carotid artery disease is increased from 0.16 to 0.82. Note that the sensitivity and specificity of 0.83 and 0.92, respectively, remain unchanged. If the test information is kept constant (same sensitivity and specificity), the pretest probability (prevalence) affects the posttest probability (predictive value) results.

The concept of diagnostic performance discussed above can be summarized by incorporating the data from Appendix 2 into a nomogram for interpreting diagnostic test results (Fig. 1.3). For example, two patients present to the emergency department complaining of left-sided weakness. The treating physician wants to determine if they have a stroke from carotid artery disease. The first patient is an 8-year-old boy complaining of chronic left-sided weakness. Because of the patient's young age and chronic history, he was determined clinically to be in a low-risk category for carotid artery disease-induced stroke and hence with a low pretest probability of 0.05 (5%). Conversely, the second patient is 65 years old and is complaining of acute onset of severe left-sided weakness. Because of the patient's older age and acute history, he was determined clinically to be in a high-risk category for carotid artery disease-induced stroke and hence with a high pretest probability of 0.70 (70%). The available diagnostic imaging test was unenhanced head and neck CT followed by CT angiography. According to the radiologist's available literature, the sensitivity and specificity of these tests for carotid artery disease and stroke were each 0.90. The positive likelihood ratio (sensitivity/1−specificity) calculation derived by the radiologist was 0.90/(1−0.90)=9. The posttest probability for the 8-year-old patient is therefore 30% based on a pretest probability of 0.05 and a likelihood

ratio of 9 (Fig. 1.3, dashed line A). Conversely, the posttest probability for the 65-year-old patient is greater than 0.95 based on a pretest

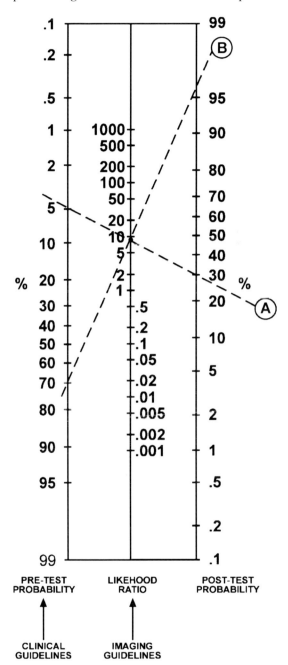

Figure 1.3. Bayes' theorem nomogram for determining posttest probability of disease using the pretest probability of disease and the likelihood ratio from the imaging test. Clinical and imaging guidelines are aimed at increasing the pretest probability and likelihood ratio, respectively. Worked example is explained in the text. (Reprinted with permission from Medina et al. (10).)

probability of 0.70 and a positive likelihood ratio of 9 (Fig. 1.3, dashed line B). Clinicians and radiologists can use this scale to understand the probability of disease in different risk groups and for imaging studies with different diagnostic performance. This example also highlights one of the difficulties in extrapolating adult data to the care of children as the results of a diagnostic test may have very different meaning in terms of posttest probability of disease in lower prevalence of many conditions in children.

Jaeschke et al. (38) have proposed a rule of thumb regarding the interpretation of the LR. For PLR, tests with values greater than 10 have a large difference between pretest and posttest probability with conclusive diagnostic impact; values of 5–10 have a moderate difference in test probabilities and moderate diagnostic impact; values of 2–5 have a small difference in test probabilities and sometimes an important diagnostic impact; and values less than 2 have a small difference in test probabilities and seldom have important diagnostic impact. For NLR, tests with values less than 0.1 have a large difference between pretest and posttest probability with conclusive diagnostic impact; values of 0.1 and less than 0.2 have a moderate difference in test probabilities and moderate diagnostic impact; values of 0.2 and less than 0.5 have a small difference in test probabilities and sometimes an important diagnostic impact; and values of 0.5–1 have small difference in test probabilities and seldom have important diagnostic impact.

The role of the clinical guidelines is to increase the pretest probability by adequately distinguishing low-risk from high-risk groups. The role of imaging guidelines is to increase the likelihood ratio by recommending the diagnostic test with the highest sensitivity and specificity. Comprehensive use of clinical and imaging guidelines will improve the posttest probability, hence increasing the diagnostic outcome (10).

III. How to Use This Book

As these examples illustrate, the EBI process can be lengthy (39). The literature is overwhelming in scope and somewhat frustrating in methodologic quality. The process of summarizing data can be challenging to the clinician not skilled in meta-analysis. The time demands on busy practitioners can limit their appropriate use of the EBI approach. This book can obviate these challenges in the use of EBI and make the EBI accessible to all imagers and users of medical imaging.

This book is organized by major diseases and injuries. In the table of contents within each chapter, you will find a series of EBI issues provided as clinically relevant questions. Readers can quickly find the relevant clinical question and receive guidance as to the appropriate recommendation based on the literature. Where appropriate, these questions are further broken down by age, gender, or other clinically important circumstances. Following the chapter's table of contents is a summary of the key points determined from the critical literature review that forms the basis of EBI. Sections on pathophysiology, epidemiology, and cost are next, followed by the goals of imaging and the search methodology. The chapter is then broken down into the clinical issues. Discussion of each issue begins with a brief summary of the literature, including a quantification of the strength of the evidence, and then continues with detailed examination of the supporting evidence. At the end of the chapter, the reader will find the take-home tables and imaging case studies, which highlight key imaging recommendations and their supporting evidence. Finally, questions are included where further research is necessary to understand the role of imaging for each of the topics discussed.

Acknowledgment: We appreciate the contribution of Ruth Carlos, MD, MS, to the discussion of likelihood ratios in this chapter.

IV. Take Home Appendix 1: Equations

Test result	Outcome	
	Present	Absent
Positive	a (TP)	b (FP)
Negative	c (FN)	d (TN)
a. Sensitivity	$a/(a+c)$	
b. Specificity	$d/(b+d)$	
c. Prevalence	$(a+c)/(a+b+c+d)$	
d. Accuracy	$(a+d)/(a+b+c+d)$	
e. Positive predictive value[a]	$a/(a+b)$	
f. Negative predictive value[a]	$d/(c+d)$	
g. 95% confidence interval (CI)	$p \pm 1.96\sqrt{\dfrac{p(1-n)}{n}}$ $p = \text{proportion}$ $n = \text{number of subjects}$	
h. Likelihood ratio	$\dfrac{\text{Sensitivity}}{1-\text{specificity}} = \dfrac{a(b+d)}{b(a+c)}$	

[a]Only correct if the prevalence of the outcome is estimated from a random sample or based on an a priori estimate of prevalence in the general population; otherwise, use of Bayes' theorem must be used to calculate PPV and NPV. TP true positive; FP false positive; FN false negative; TN true negative.

V. Take Home Appendix 2: Summary of Bayes' Theorem

A. Information before test × Information from test = Information after test

B. Pretest probability (prevalence) sensitivity / 1 – specificity = posttest probability (predictive value)

C. Information from the test also known as the likelihood ratio, described by the equation: sensitivity / 1 – specificity

D. Examples 1 and 2 predictive values: The predictive values (posttest probability) change according to the differences in prevalence (pretest probability), although the diagnostic performance of the test (i.e., sensitivity and specificity) is unchanged.

The following examples illustrate how the prevalence (pretest probability) can affect the predictive values (posttest probability) having the same information in two different study groups

Equations for calculating the results in the previous examples are listed in Appendix 1. As the prevalence of carotid artery disease increases from 0.16 (low) to 0.82 (high), the positive predictive value (PPV) of a positive contrast-enhanced CT increases from 0.67 to 0.98, respectively. The sensitivity and specificity remain unchanged at 0.83 and 0.92, respectively. These examples also illustrate that the diagnostic performance of the test (i.e., sensitivity and specificity) does not depend on the prevalence (pretest probability) of the disease. CTA, CT angiogram.

Example 1: Low prevalence of carotid artery disease

	Disease (carotid artery disease)	No disease (no carotid artery disease)	Total
Test positive (positive CTA)	20	10	30
Test negative (negative CTA)	4	120	124
Total	24	130	154

Example 2: High prevalence of carotid artery disease

	Disease (carotid artery disease)	No disease (no carotid artery disease)	Total
Test positive (positive CTA)	500	10	510
Test negative (negative CTA)	100	120	220
Total	600	130	730

Results: sensitivity = 500/600 = 0.83; specificity = 120/130 = 0.92; prevalence = 600/730 = 0.82; positive predictive value = 0.98; negative predictive value = 0.55.

References

1. Levin A. Ann Intern Med 1998;128:334–336.
2. Evidence-Based Medicine Working Group. JAMA 1992;268:2420–2425.
3. The Evidence-Based Radiology Working Group. Radiology 2001;220:566–575.
4. Wood BP. Radiology 1999;213:635–637.
5. Poisal JA et al. Health Aff 2007;26:w242–w253.
6. Davis K. N Engl J Med 2008;359:1751–1755.
7. Hulley SB, Cummings SR. Designing Clinical Research. Baltimore: Williams & Wilkins, 1998.
8. Kelsey J, Whittemore A, Evans A, Thompson W. Methods in Observational Epidemiology. New York: Oxford University Press, 1996.
9. Blackmore C, Cummings P. AJR Am J Roentgenol 2004;183(5):1203–1208.
10. Medina L, Aguirre E, Zurakowski D. Neuroimaging Clin N Am 2003;13:157–165.
11. Medina L. AJNR Am J Neuroradiol 1999;20: 1584–1596.
12. Sunshine JH, McNeil BJ. Radiology 1997;205: 549–557.
13. Black WC. AJR Am J Roentgenol 1990;154:17–22.
14. Sox HC, Blatt MA, Higgins MC, Marton KI. Medical Decision Making. Boston: Butterworth, 1988.
15. Metz CE. Semin Nucl Med 1978;8:283–298.
16. Singer M, Applegate K. Radiology 2001;219: 611–620.
17. Weinstein MC, Fineberg HV. Clinical Decision Analysis. Philadelphia: WB Saunders, 1980.
18. Carlos R. Acad Radiol 2004;11:141–148.
19. Detsky AS, Naglie IG. Ann Intern Med 1990; 113:147–154.
20. Doubilet P, Weinstein MC, McNeil BJ. N Engl J Med 1986;314:253–256.
21. Gold MR, Siegel JE, Russell LB, Weinstein MC. Cost-Effectiveness in Health and Medicine. New York: Oxford University Press, 1996.
22. Hillemann D, Lucas B, Mohiuddin S, Holmberg M. Ann Pharmacother 1997;31:974–979.
23. Medina L, Aguirre E, Bernal B, Altman N. Radiology 2004;230:49–54.
24. Appel LJ, Steinberg EP, Powe NR, Anderson GF, Dwyer SA, Faden RR. Med Care 1990;28:324–337.
25. Evens RG. Cancer 1991;67:1245–1252.
26. Yin D, Forman HP, Langlotz CP. AJR Am J Roentgenol 1995;165:1323–1328.
27. Medina L, Crone K, Kuntz K. Pediatrics 2001; 108:E101.
28. Ware JE, Sherbourne CD. Med Care 1992;30: 473–483.
29. Jarvik J, Hollingworth W, Martin B, et al. JAMA 2003;2810–2818.
30. Blackmore CC, Magid DJ. Radiology 1997;203: 87–91.

31. Medina L, Aguirre E, Altman N. Acad Radiol 2003;10:139–144.
32. Zou K, Fielding J, Ondategui-Parra S. Acad Radiol 2004;11:127–133.
33. Langlotz C, Sonnad S. Acad Radiol 1998;5 (suppl 2):S269–S273.
34. Littenberg B, Moses LE. Med Decis Making 1993;13:313–321.
35. Terasawa T, Blackmore C, Bent S, Kohlwes R. Ann Intern Med 2004;141(7):37–546.
36. Fryback DG, Thornbury JR. Med Decis Making 1991;11:88–94.
37. Blackmore C. Radiology 2005;235(2):371–374.
38. Jaeschke R, Guyatt GH, Sackett DL. JAMA 1994;271:703–707.
39. Malone D. Radiology 2007;242(1):12–14.
40. Medina LS, Blackmore DD. Evidence-Based Imaging: Optimizing Imaging in Patient. New York: Springer Science+Business Media, 2006.

2

Critically Assessing the Literature: Understanding Error and Bias

C. Craig Blackmore, L. Santiago Medina, James G. Ravenel, Gerard A. Silvestri, and Kimberly E. Applegate

Issues

I. What are error and bias?
II. What is random error?
   A. Type I error
   B. Confidence intervals
   C. Type II error
   D. Power analysis
III. What is bias?
IV. What are the inherent biases in screening?
V. Qualitative literature summary

The keystone of the evidence-based imaging (EBI) approach is to critically assess the research data that are provided and to determine if the information is appropriate for use in answering the EBI question. Unfortunately, the published studies are often limited by bias, small sample size, and methodological inadequacy. Further, the information provided in published reports may be insufficient to allow estimation of the quality of the research. Two recent initiatives, the CONSORT (1) and the STARD (2), aim to improve the reporting of clinical trials and studies of diagnostic accuracy, respectively. However, these guidelines are only now being implemented and are not well known to readers of the medical literature.

This chapter summarizes the common sources of error and bias in the imaging literature. Using the EBI approach requires an understanding of these issues.

I. What Are Error and Bias?

Errors in the medical literature can be divided into two main types. *Random error* occurs due to chance variation, causing a sample to be different from the underlying population. Random error is more likely to be problematic when the sample size is small. *Systematic error*, or *bias*, is an incorrect study result due to nonrandom

C.C. Blackmore (✉)
Department of Radiology, Center for Healthcare Solutions, Virginia Mason Medical Center,
1100 Ninth Avenue, Seattle, WA 98111, USA
e-mail: craig.blackmore@vmmc.org

L.S. Medina et al. (eds.), *Evidence-Based Imaging: Improving the Quality of Imaging in Patient Care, Revised Edition,*
DOI 10.1007/978-1-4419-7777-9_2, © Springer Science+Business Media, LLC 2011

distortion of the data. Systematic error is not affected by sample size, but is rather a function of flaws in the study design, data collection, and analysis. A second way to think about random and systematic error is in terms of precision and accuracy (3). Random error affects the precision of a result (Fig. 2.1). The larger the sample size, the more precision in the results and the more likely that two samples from truly different populations will be differentiated from each other. Using the bull's-eye analogy, the larger the sample size, the less the random error and the larger the chance of hitting the center of the target (Fig. 2.1). Systematic error, on the other hand, is a distortion in the accuracy of an estimate. Regardless of precision, the underlying estimate is flawed by some aspect of the research procedure. Using the bull's-eye analogy, in systematic error, regardless of the sample size, the bias would not allow the researcher to hit the center of the target (Fig. 2.1).

II. What Is Random Error?

Random error is divided into two main types: Type I, or alpha error, occurs when an investigator concludes that an effect or a difference is present when in fact there is no true difference. Type II, or beta error, occurs when an investigator concludes that there is no effect or no difference when in fact a true difference exists in the underlying population (3).

A. Type I Error

Quantification of the likelihood of alpha error is provided by the familiar p value. A p value less than 0.05 indicates that there is a less than 5% chance that the observed difference in a sample would be seen if there was in fact no true difference in the population. In effect, the difference observed in a sample is due to chance variation rather than a true underlying difference in the population.

There are limitations to the ubiquitous p values seen in imaging research reports (4). The p values are a function of both sample size and magnitude of effect. In other words, there could be a very large difference between two groups under study, but the p value might not be significant if the sample sizes are small.

Conversely, there could be a very small, clinically unimportant difference between two groups of subjects or between two imaging tests, but with a large enough sample size, even this clinically unimportant result would be statistically significant. Because of these limitations, many journals are underemphasizing the use of p values and encouraging research results to be reported by way of confidence intervals (CIs).

B. Confidence Intervals

Confidence Intervals are preferred because they provide much more information than p values. CIs provide information about the precision of an estimate (how wide are the CIs), the size of an estimate (magnitude of the CIs), and the statistical significance of an estimate (whether the intervals include the null) (5).

If you assume that your sample was randomly selected from some population (that follows a normal distribution), you can be 95% certain that the CI includes the population mean. More precisely, if you generate many 95% CIs from many data sets, you can expect that the CI will include the true population mean in 95% of the cases and not include the true mean value in the other 5% (4). Therefore, the 95% CI is related to statistical significance at the $p = 0.05$ level, which means that the interval itself can be used to determine if an estimated change is statistically significant at the 0.05 level (6). Whereas the p value is often interpreted as being either statistically significant or not, the CI, by providing a range of values, allows the reader to interpret the implications of the results at either end (6, 7). In addition, while p values have no units, CIs are presented in the units of the variable of interest, which helps readers to interpret the results. The CIs shift the interpretation from a qualitative judgment about the role of chance to a quantitative estimation of the biologic measure of effect (4, 6, 7).

CIs can be constructed for any desired level of confidence. There is nothing magical about the 95% that is traditionally used. If greater confidence is needed, then the intervals have to be wider. Consequently, 99% CIs are wider than 95, and 90% CIs are narrower than 95%. Wider CIs are associated with greater confidence but less precision. This is the trade-off (4).

As an example, two hypothetical transcranial circle of Willis vascular ultrasound studies in patients with sickle cell disease describe mean peak systolic velocities of 200 cm/s associated with 70% of vascular diameter stenosis and higher risk of stroke. Both articles reported the same standard deviation (SD) of 50 cm/s. However, one study had 50 subjects, while the other one had 500 subjects. At first glance, both studies appear to provide similar information. However, the narrower CIs for the larger study reflect greater precision and indicate the value of the larger sample size. For a smaller sample

$$95\%CI = 200 \pm 1.96\left(\frac{50}{\sqrt{50}}\right)$$

$$95\%CI - 200 \pm 14 = 186 - 214$$

For a larger sample

$$95\%CI = 200 \pm 1.96\left(\frac{50}{\sqrt{500}}\right)$$

$$95\%CI = 200 \pm 4 = 196 - 204$$

In the smaller series, the 95% CI was 186–214 cm/s, while in the larger series, the 95% CI was 196–204 cm/s. Therefore, the larger series has a narrower 95% CI (4).

C. Type II Error

The familiar p value alone does not provide information as to the probability of a type II or beta error. A p value greater than 0.05 does not necessarily mean that there is no difference in the underlying population. The size of the sample studied may be too small to detect an important difference even if such a difference does exist. The ability of a study to detect an important difference, if that difference does in fact exist in the underlying population, is called the power of a study. Power analysis can be performed in advance of a research investigation to avoid type II error. To conclude that no difference exists, the study must be powered sufficiently to detect a clinically important difference and have p value or CI indicating no significant effect.

D. Power Analysis

Power analysis plays an important role in determining what an adequate sample size is, so that meaningful results can be obtained (8).

Power analysis is the probability of observing an effect in a sample of patients if the specified effect size, or greater, is found in the population (3). Mathematically, power is defined as 1 minus beta $(1-\beta)$, where β is the probability of having a type II error. Type II errors are commonly referred to as false negatives in a study population. Type I errors, in contrast, are analogous false positives in a study population (7). For example, if β is set at 0.10, then the researchers acknowledge that they are willing to accept a 10% chance of missing a correlation between abnormal computed tomography (CT) angiographic findings in the diagnosis of carotid artery disease. This represents a power of 1 minus 0.10, or 0.90, which represents a 90% probability of finding a correlation of this magnitude.

Ideally, the power should be 100% by setting β at 0. In addition, ideally α should also be 0. By accomplishing this, false-negative and false-positive results are eliminated, respectively. In practice, however, powers near 100% is rarely achievable, so, at best, a study should reduce the false negatives (β) and false positives (α) to a minimum (3, 9). Achieving an acceptable reduction of false negatives and false positives requires a large subject sample size. Optimal power, α and β, settings are based on a balance between scientific rigorousness and the issues of feasibility and cost. For example, assuming an α error of 0.10, your sample size increases from 96 to 118 subjects per study arm (carotid and noncarotid artery disease arms) if you change your desired power from 85 to 90% (10). Studies with more complete reporting and better study design will often report the power of the study, for example, by stating that the study has 90% power to detect a difference in sensitivity of 10% between CT angiography and Doppler ultrasound in carotid artery disease.

III. What Is Bias?

The risk of an error from bias decreases as the rigorousness of the study design and analysis increases. Randomized controlled trials (RCTs) are considered the best design for minimizing the risk of bias because patients are randomly allocated. This random allocation allows for unbiased distribution of both known and unknown confounding variables between the study groups. In nonrandomized studies, appropriate study design and statistical analysis can control only for known or measurable bias.

Detection of and correction for bias, or systematic error, in research is a vexing challenge for both researchers and users of the medical literature alike. Maclure and Schneeweiss (11) have identified ten different levels at which biases can distort the relationship between published study results and truth. Unfortunately, bias is common in published reports (12), and reports with identifiable biases often overestimate the accuracy of diagnostic tests (13). Careful surveillance for each of these individual bias phenomena is critical, but may be a challenge. Different study designs are also susceptible to different types of bias, as will be discussed in this section as well. Well-reported studies often include a section on limitations of the work, spelling out the potential sources of bias that the investigator acknowledges from a study as well as the likely direction of the bias and steps that may have been taken to overcome it. However, the final determination of whether a research study is sufficiently distorted by bias to be unusable is left to the discretion of the user of the imaging literature. The imaging practitioner must determine if results of a particular study are true, are relevant to a given clinical question, and are sufficient as a basis to change practice.

A common bias encountered in imaging research is that of *selection bias* (14). Because a research study cannot include all individuals in the world who have a particular clinical situation, research is conducted on samples. Selection bias can arise if the sample is not a true representation of the relevant underlying clinical population (Fig. 2.2). Numerous subtypes of selection bias have been identified, and it is a challenge to the researcher to avoid all of these biases when performing a study. One particularly severe form of selection bias occurs if the diagnostic test is applied to subjects with a spectrum of disease that differs from the clinically relevant group. The extreme form of this spectrum bias occurs when the diagnostic test is evaluated on subjects with severe disease and on normal controls. In an evaluation of the effect of bias on study results, Lijmer et al. (13) found the greatest overestimation of test accuracy with this type of spectrum bias.

A second frequently encountered bias in imaging literature is that of *observer bias* (15, 16), also called test-review bias and diagnostic-review

bias (17). Imaging tests are largely subjective. The radiologist interpreting an imaging study forms an impression based on the appearance of the image, not based on an objective number or measurement. This subjective impression can be biased by numerous factors including the radiologist's experience; the context of the interpretation (clinical vs. research setting); the information about the patient's history that is known by the radiologist; incentives that the radiologist may have, both monetary and otherwise, to produce a particular report; and the memory of a recent experience. But because of all these factors, it is critical that the interpreting physician be blinded to the outcome or gold standard when a diagnostic test or an intervention is being assessed. Important distortions in research results have been found when observers are not blinded vs. blinded. For example, Schulz et al. (18) showed a 17% greater outcome improvement in studies with unblinded assessment of outcomes versus those with blinded assessment. To obtain objective scientific assessment of an imaging test, all readers should be blinded to other diagnostic tests and final diagnosis, and all patient-identifying marks on the test should be masked.

Bias can also be introduced by the *reference standard* used to confirm the final diagnosis. First, the interpretation of the reference standard must be made without knowledge of the test results. Reference standards, like the diagnostic tests themselves, may have a subjective component and therefore may be affected by knowledge of the results of the diagnostic test. In addition, it is critical that all subjects undergo the same reference standard. The use of different reference standards (called differential reference standard bias) for subjects with different diagnostic test results may falsely elevate both sensitivity and specificity (13, 16). Of course, sometimes it is not possible or ethical to perform the same reference standard procedure on all subjects. For example, in a recent meta-analysis of imaging for appendicitis, Terasawa et al. (19) found that all of the identified studies used a different reference standard for subjects with positive imaging (appendectomy and pathologic evaluation) than for those with negative imaging (clinical follow-up). It simply would not be ethical to perform appendectomy on all subjects. Likely the sensitivity and specificity of imaging for appendicitis was overestimated as a result.

IV. What Are the Inherent Biases in Screening?

Investigations of screening tests are susceptible to an additional set of biases. Screening case–control trials are vulnerable to *screening selection bias*. For example, lung cancer case–control studies have been performed in Japan, where long-running tuberculosis control programs have been in place. This allowed for the analysis of those who were screened to be matched with a database of matched unscreened controls to arrive at a relative risk of dying from lung cancer in screened and unscreened populations. Because screening is a choice in these studies, selection bias plays a prominent role. That is, people who present for elective screening tend to have better health habits (20). In assessing the exposure history of cases, the inclusion of the test on which the diagnosis is made, regardless of whether it is truly screen or symptom detected, can lead to an odds ratio greater than 1 even in the absence of benefit (21). Similarly, excluding the test on which the diagnosis is made may underestimate screening effectiveness. The magnitude of bias is further reflected in the disease preclinical phase; the longer the preclinical phase, the greater the magnitude of the bias.

Prospective nonrandomized screening trials perform an intervention on subjects, such as screening for lung cancer, and follow them for many years. These studies can give information on the stage distribution and survival of a screened population; however, these measures do not allow an accurate comparison to an unscreened group due to lead time, length time, and overdiagnosis bias (22) (Fig. 2.3). *Lead-time bias* results from the earlier detection of the disease, which leads to longer time from diagnosis and an apparent survival advantage, but does not truly impact the date of death. *Length-time bias* relates to the virulence of tumors. More indolent tumors are more likely to be detected by screening, whereas aggressive tumors are more likely to be detected by symptoms. This disproportionally assigns more indolent disease to the intervention group and results in the appearance of a benefit. *Overdiagnosis* is the most extreme form of length-time bias in which a disease is detected and "cured," but it is so indolent that it would have never caused symptoms during life. Thus, survival alone is not an appropriate measure of the effectiveness of screening (23).

For this reason, a RCT with disease-specific mortality as an end point is the preferred methodology. Randomization should even out the selection process in both arms, eliminating the bias of case–control studies and allowing direct comparison of groups that underwent the intervention and those that did not, to see if the intervention lowers deaths due to the target disease. The disadvantage of the RCT is that it takes many years and is expensive to perform. There are two biases that can occur in RCTs and are important to understand: *sticky diagnosis* and *slippery linkage* (24). Because the target disease is more likely to be detected in a screened population, it is more likely to be listed as a cause of death, even if not the true cause. As such, the diagnosis "sticks" and tends to underestimate the true value of the test. On the other hand, screening may set into motion a series of events in order to diagnose and treat the illness. If these procedures remotely lead to mortality, such as a myocardial infarction during surgery with death several months later, the linkage of the cause of death to the screening may no longer be obvious (slippery linkage). Because the death is not appropriately assigned to the target disease, the value of screening may be overestimated. For this reason, in addition to disease-specific mortality, all-cause mortality should also be evaluated in the context of screening trials (24). Ultimately, to show the effectiveness of screening, not only more early-stage cancers need to be found in the screened group, but also there must be fewer late-stage cancers (stage shift) (22).

V. Qualitative Literature Summary

The potential for error and bias makes the process of critically assessing a journal article complex and challenging, and no investigation is perfect. Producing an overall summation of the quality of a research report is difficult. However, there are grading schemes that provide a useful estimation of the value of a research report for guiding clinical practice. The method used in this book is derived from that of Kent et al. (25) and is shown in Table 2.1. Use of such a grading scheme is by nature an oversimplification. However, such simple guidelines can provide a useful quick overview of the quality of a research report.

Conclusion

Critical analysis of a research publication can be a challenging task. The reader must consider the potential for type I and type II random errors, as well as systematic error introduced by biases including selection bias, observer bias, and reference standard bias. Screening includes an additional set of challenges related to lead time, length bias, and overdiagnosis. These challenges may seem daunting, yet without an understanding of them, a medical practitioner can not learn efficiently from the literature and in so doing, help their patients with the best evidence we have to offer them.

Take Home Tables and Figures

Table 2.1 and Figs. 2.1–2.3 serve to highlight key recommendations and supporting evidence.

Table 2.1. Evidence classification for evaluation of a study

Level I: Strong evidence
Studies with broad generalizability to most patients suspected of having the disease of concern: a prospective, blinded comparison of a diagnostic test result with a well-defined final diagnosis in an unbiased sample when assessing diagnostic accuracy or blinded randomized control trials or when assessing therapeutic impact or patient outcomes. Well-designed meta-analysis based on level I or II studies

Level II: Moderate evidence
Prospective or retrospective studies with narrower spectrum of generalizability, with only a few flaws that are well described so that their impact can be assessed, but still requiring a blinded study of diagnostic accuracy on an unbiased sample. This includes well-designed cohort or case-control studies and randomized trials for therapeutic effects or patient outcomes

Level III: Limited evidence
Diagnostic accuracy studies with several flaws in research methods, small sample sizes, or incomplete reporting, or nonrandomized comparisons for therapeutic impact or patient outcomes

Level IV: Insufficient evidence
Studies with multiple flaws in research methods, case series, descriptive studies, or expert opinions without substantiating data

Reprinted with kind permission of Springer Science+Business Media from Blackmore CC, Medina LS, Ravenel JG, Silvestri GA. Critically Assessing the Literature: Understanding Error and Bias. In Medina LS, Blackmore DD (eds): *Evidence-Based Imaging: Optimizing Imaging in Patient Care.* New York: Springer Science+Business Media, 2006.

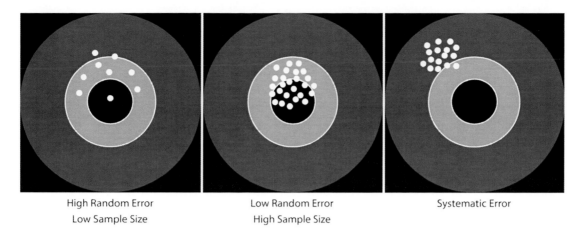

High Random Error   Low Random Error   Systematic Error
Low Sample Size   High Sample Size

Figure 2.1. Random and systematic errors. Using the bull's-eye analogy, the larger the sample size, the less the random error and the larger the chance of hitting the center of the target. In systematic error, regardless of the sample size, the bias would not allow the researcher to hit the center of the target. (Reprinted with kind permission of Springer Science+Business Media from Blackmore CC, Medina LS, Ravenel JG, Silvestri GA. Critically Assessing the Literature: Understanding Error and Bias. In Medina LS, Blackmore DD (eds): *Evidence-Based Imaging: Optimizing Imaging in Patient Care.* New York: Springer Science+Business Media, 2006.)

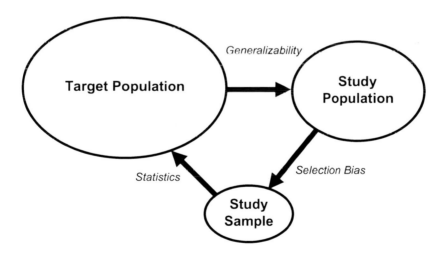

Figure 2.2. Population and sample. The target population represents the universe of subjects who are at risk for a particular disease or condition. In this example, all subjects with abdominal pain are at risk for appendicitis. The sample population is the group of eligible subjects available to the investigators. These may be at a single center or group of centers. The sample is the group of subjects who are actually studied. Selection bias occurs when the sample is not truly representative of the study population. How closely the study population reflects the target population determines the generalizability of the research. Finally, statistics are used to determine what inference about the target population can be drawn from the sample data. (Reprinted with kind permission of Springer Science+Business Media from Blackmore CC, Medina LS, Ravenel JG, Silvestri GA. Critically Assessing the Literature: Understanding Error and Bias. In Medina LS, Blackmore DD (eds): *Evidence-Based Imaging: Optimizing Imaging in Patient Care.* New York: Springer Science+Business Media, 2006.)

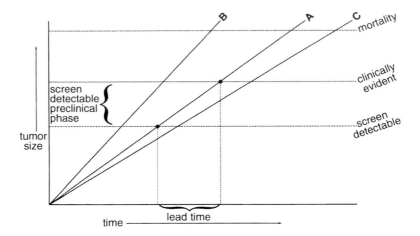

Figure 2.3. Screening biases. For this figure, cancers are assumed to grow at a continuous rate until they reach a size at which death of the subject occurs. At a small size, the cancers may be evident on screening, but not yet evident clinically. This is the preclinical screen-detectable phase. Screening is potentially helpful if it detects cancer in this phase. After further growth, the cancer will be clinically evident. Even if the growth and outcome of the cancer is unaffected by screening, merely detecting the cancer earlier will increase apparent survival. This is the screening lead time. In addition, slower growing cancers (such as C) will exist in the preclinical screen-detectable phase for longer than do faster growing cancers (such as B). Therefore, screening is more likely to detect more indolent cancers, a phenomenon known as length bias. (Reprinted with kind permission of Springer Science+Business Media from Blackmore CC, Medina LS, Ravenel JG, Silvestri GA. Critically Assessing the Literature: Understanding Error and Bias. In Medina LS, Blackmore DD (eds): *Evidence-Based Imaging: Optimizing Imaging in Patient Care.* New York: Springer Science+Business Media, 2006.)

References

1. Moher D, Schulz K, Altman D. JAMA 2001;285: 1987–1991.
2. Bossuyt PM, Reitsma J, Bruns D, et al. Acad Radiol 2003;10:664–669.
3. Hulley SB, Cummings SR. Designing Clinical Research. Baltimore: Williams and Wilkins, 1998.
4. Medina L, Zurakowski D. Radiology 2003;226: 297–301.
5. Gallagher E. Acad Emerg Med 1999;6: 1084–1087.
6. Lang T, Secic M. How to Report Statistics in Medicine. Philadelphia: American College of Physicians, 1997.
7. Gardener M, Altman D. Br Med J 1986;292: 746–750.
8. Medina L, Aguirre E, Zurakowski D. Neuroimag Clin North Am 2003;13:157–165.
9. Medina L. AJNR Am J Neuroradiol 1999;20: 1584–1596.
10. Donner A. Stat Med 1984;3:199–214.
11. Maclure M, Schneeweiss S. Epidemiology 2001;12:114–122.
12. Reid MC, Lachs MS, Feinstein AR. JAMA 1995;274:645–651.
13. Lijmer JG, Mol BW, Heisterkamp S, et al. JAMA 1999;282:1061–1066.
14. Blackmore C. Acad Radiol 2004;11:134–140.
15. Ransohoff DF, Feinstein AR. N Engl J Med 1978;299:926–930.
16. Black WC. AJR Am J Roentgenol 1990;154:17–22.
17. Begg CB, McNeil BJ. Radiology 1988;167: 565–569.
18. Schulz K, Chalmers I, Hayes R, Altman D. JAMA 1995;273:408–412.
19. Terasawa T, Blackmore C, Bent S, Kohlwes R. Ann Intern Med 2004;141:537–546.
20. Marcus P. Lung Cancer 2003;41:37–39.
21. Hosek R, Flanders W, Sasco A. Am J Epidemiol 1996;143:193–201.
22. Patz E, Goodman P, Bepler G. N Engl J Med 2000;343:1627–1633.
23. Black WC, Welch HG. AJR Am J Roentgenol 1997;168:3–11.
24. Black W, Haggstrom D, Welch H. J Natl Cancer Inst 2002;94:167–173.
25. Kent DL, Haynor DR, Longstreth WT Jr, Larson EB. Ann Intern Med 1994;120:856–871.

3

Radiation Risk from Medical Imaging: A Special Need to Focus on Children

Donald P. Frush and Kimberly E. Applegate

Issues

I. Is there a cancer risk from low-level radiation used in medical imaging? What are the uncertainties in the data?
    A. Cancer risk and radiation following diagnostic medical imaging
    B. CT scan and risk
    C. Assumption in estimating radiation risks
    D. Increased radiosensitivity in children
    E. Nonfatal cancers
    F. Additional confounders in risk estimation
    G. Radiation doses from medical imaging and uncertainty in cancer risks
II. What is the estimated risk from a single chest X-ray in a child?
III. What is the estimated risk from a single abdominal CT scan in a child?
    A. The changing landscaping of radiation dose for medical imaging
    B. Lowering CT dose in children
IV. Understanding benefit versus risk of imaging tests in well-indicated studies versus those that have very low probability of disease
    A. The example of CT in children with headache
V. How should I communicate radiation risk from imaging to parents and patients?
VI. Special situation: Increased cancer risk following therapeutic medical radiation

D.P. Frush (✉)
DUMC, Durham, NC, 27710, USA
e-mail: frush943@mc.duke.edu

L.S. Medina et al. (eds.), *Evidence-Based Imaging: Improving the Quality of Imaging in Patient Care, Revised Edition*,
DOI 10.1007/978-1-4419-7777-9_3, © Springer Science+Business Media, LLC 2011

■ **Key Points**Medical radiation currently accounts for an increasing percentage (approximately 50%) of the total radiation exposure for the US population (previously about 15%) (moderate evidence).

■ Children are 2–5 (some cite up to 10) times more sensitive to radiation than adults (moderate evidence).

■ There are no data that prove a direct link between low-level radiation from diagnostic imaging and cancer. The best data regarding long-term effects of low-level radiation (100–150 mSv) exposure come from the longitudinal survivor study (LSS) of atomic bomb survivors (moderate evidence).

■ Most major medical and scientific organizations accept the linear, no-threshold model as the preferred model for low-level radiation and cancer risk estimation.

■ The lifetime risk of fatal cancer from a single (relatively high dose) CT in a child has been estimated to be 1:1,000 (limited to moderate evidence).

Definition and Pathophysiology

Medical radiation is used for both diagnostic and therapeutic purposes. The X-ray is an invisible beam of ionizing radiation that passes through the body and is altered by different tissues to create images. Imaging tests that use ionizing radiation include the plain X-ray (or radiograph), fluoroscopy, and the CT scan. Diagnostic imaging uses low-level radiation that is defined, for the purposes of radiation risk, as <100–150 mSv.

Radiation Terminology

Measurements are presented in standard international units (SI = *Systeme Internationale*) (1) (Table 3.1). Incident X-ray radiation *intensity* can be characterized by exposure in coulombs/kg (ionizations in coulombs per mass) or the preferred air kerma in Gray (Gy) (kinetic energy transferred per unit mass). The *absorption* of this radiation intensity is then, simply, the *absorbed dose*, also measured in Gy (the energy transfer will depend on factors including physical properties of the material and depth in the body), including skin and other organ doses. The biological *impact* to tissue is represented by *equivalent dose* in Sieverts (Sv), the product of the absorbed dose and a weighting factor (value depends on the type of radiation that causes ionization in tissue, with the factor being 1.0 for medical imaging). Finally, the

effective dose equivalent (alternatively, effective dose) in Sv is the sum of products of dose equivalents multiplied by weighting factors depending on the radiosensitivity of organs exposed. Effective doses represent a whole body equivalent (as if the whole body were exposed) for exposures that may be regional. Because absorbed dose and effective dose represent energy deposition and ionization in tissues, these terms are typically used in discussions of radiation risk in humans.

Radiation Mechanisms of Effect

Ionizing radiation particles include X-rays (photons). These high-energy photons interact with tissue depositing energy at the nuclear level causing ionizations. Ionizations then damage DNA either directly or secondarily through generation of free radicals, especially hydroxyl free radicals. Single-stranded DNA damage is usually repaired but double-stranded DNA damage is more difficult to repair completely. Biological effects may be immediate, causing *cell death* (such as radiation necrosis), which may lead to organism death, or consist of *cell damage*, leading to other effects such as birth defects or cancer. Cell damage could not only be due to direct DNA damage but may also be due to other effects such as genomic instability (with additional DNA aberrations in cell progeny) and regulatory mechanisms. For diagnostic imaging levels of radiation dose, the most pertinent bioeffect is carcinogenesis. In short, the development of radiation-induced cancer is a multistep process. In addition to these generalized mechanisms of radiation bioeffects, there are other factors determining susceptibility; for example, there is a genetic basis of cancer in up to 10–15% of childhood cancer (Table 3.2) (2).

Types of Biological Effects

There are two types of biological effects: stochastic and deterministic. Deterministic effects have a threshold below which the effect is not seen (Table 3.3). These effects include cataracts, skin burns, and epilation (hair loss). These types of effects are almost all seen in imaging when interventional procedures are performed with doses well above the low-level radiation doses seen in diagnostic imaging. Recently, however, epilation was noted with a diagnostic perfusion and computed tomography angiography (CTA) examination (3). Stochastic effects do not have a threshold. The risk of a particular effect increases with increasing radiation dose; however, the severity of the effect is independent of dose. Radiation carcinogenesis and radiation-induced genetic damage are stochastic phenomena. For the purposes of this chapter, the stochastic effect of carcinogenesis will be discussed as most literature and attention have been focused on this effect. While other biological effects of low-level radiation have been assessed (4, 5), the overwhelming majority of investigation with low-level radiation deals with cancer risk.

Radiation Doses in Medical Imaging

Radiation doses for the imaging modalities of radiography, fluoroscopy/angiography, and computed tomography vary depending on the type of dose measurement, age of the patient, examination, and techniques used. A detailed discussion of dose ranges for these various modalities is beyond the intent of this chapter; however, readers are referred to the UNSCEAR report (6) for a comprehensive review of dose ranges for many of these modalities.

Fluoroscopy and angiography procedures are better described in terms of dose rates, since the dose from these procedures will depend on imaging time, as well as on the number of radiographs (CR, DR, or conventional screen film) (7). For the purposes of clinical practice, it can be helpful to describe these common fluoroscopic (and other diagnostic imaging) procedures in terms of dose equivalents compared with the number of chest radiographs (Table 3.4). Recently, Thierry-Chef et al. (8) estimated that lifetime risk for developing brain cancer following a variety of neurointerventional procedures in children ranged from 2 to 80% (relative risk of 1.02–1.8).

It is worth mentioning, since CT is a relatively large component contributing to total medical dose, that there are methods for estimating patient dose based on the CT dose index (CTDI) in mGy and the dose length product (DLP) in mGy cm (the product of CTDI and the length of the scan). It is important to realize that this dose represents only the determination from a phantom and has nothing to do with the individual patient on the scanner. However, conversion factors to change the DLP into an effective dose estimate are available and have been recently well reviewed by Thomas and Wang (9). In addition, Huda et al. have described a method for converting pediatric CT examination parameters into effective dose estimates for a variety of pediatric CT examinations (10).

Epidemiology and Medical Utilization of Ionizing Radiation

We all are exposed to small amounts of radiation from soil, rocks, building materials, air, water, and cosmic radiation. This naturally occurring background radiation dose is about 3.0 mSv annually. When medical radiation is added to this background, the average dose for the US population is about 6.2 mSv (11). The largest contributors to medical radiation dose are CT scanning (up to one-half of medical exposure) followed by nuclear medicine (about one-quarter of medical exposure). Medical imaging is predominantly used in developed rather than developing nations.

Medical imaging is an extremely important diagnostic tool; in a recent survey, leaders in internal medicine ranked CT and MR imaging as the most important medical innovations in the twentieth century (12). With increased technological advances and potential applications, the benefits to the patients and society will continue to become more diverse and increase. However, there are inherent risks in those modalities which depend on ionizing radiation for imaging formation, consisting primarily of radiography, fluoroscopy/angiography, and computed tomography in the pediatric population. One of these risks is the potential for cancer development. While there are clearly established relationships between cancer development and radiation from studies of Hiroshima atomic bomb survivors at medium- and high-level exposures (>100–150 mSv), the risks in the lower range are debated. In general, assignment of this risk follows a linear, no-threshold model. This model is accepted by most major medical imaging organizations. There are no data from medical exposures in this range of low-level exposure that directly link diagnostic imaging with cancer development; our understanding of this potential link comes from atomic bomb data, with some additional contribution from epidemiologic studies from higher dose of radiation used for both diagnostic and therapeutic purposes. With these data, there is growing evidence supporting the association between lower level radiation and a significant increased risk of cancer development as predicted by the linear, no-threshold model. This adds support for subscribing to the As Low As Reasonably Achievable (ALARA) principle. This principle of ALARA means that we should use as low a radiation dose as possible to answer the clinical question asked.

Increased Dose from Medical Imaging

While increased use is part of the reason for increasing radiation exposure to the population, technologic advances have also resulted in some of this increase in radiation exposure. Digital technology is now nearly standard for all diagnostic imaging modalities that use ionizing radiation, including radiography, fluoroscopy/angiography, and computed tomography. When properly performed, digital technology for radiography should provide for lower (or similar) radiation exposures as the traditional film-based systems. This is not always the case. Often, dose information from computed radiography (CR), digital radiography (DR), and computed tomography images is neither displayed nor apparent, and monitoring dose based on annotation on the image is difficult. In the past, with film, an overexposure resulted in a dark image serving as a quality control. This does not happen with digital technology; there is no visual manifestation or "penalty" for overexposures. Collimation can reduce the field of view for the final image and the exposure outside this field is no longer accounted for as with traditional film-based technology. Similarly, since there is no "film repository" for poor-quality studies, a digital radiograph which is unacceptable may essentially vanish into an unmonitored, electronic wastebasket despite the fact that the patient did receive the dose.

Increased Use of CT Scans

CT scans contribute the highest dose of radiation from medical imaging in developed nations. Worldwide, an estimated 272,000,000 CT studies are performed annually. USA accounts for an estimated 25% of all CT examinations worldwide, representing 68,000,000 CT examinations each year (6, 13). If we apply a year 2000 estimate that 11% of CT examinations being performed are in children, then there are at least 7.1 million children scanned each year in USA (14).

Assessing Risk Versus Benefit when Using Medical Imaging in Children

Medical imaging is often now the first line in the diagnosis of injury and illness in children as well as in adults. More simply stated, information obtained from imaging alone can be lifesaving. However, the decision to obtain imaging examinations needs to balance this potential benefit with both established and potential risks. Risks for several of these imaging modalities include bioeffects due to exposure to ionizing radiation. The bulk of pediatric diagnostic imaging that exposes children to ionizing radiation consists of radiography, fluoroscopy/angiography, and computed tomography; radionuclide scintigraphy contributes relatively little to medical dose in children since examinations are relatively infrequent and employ lower dose of radiation compared with that in adults (i.e., cardiac imaging). As will be discussed later, the radiation dose from imaging can vary and may be relatively high. This is particularly important since imaging use has grown. For example, medical imaging, especially computed tomography, currently accounts for up to or more than 50% of all of the radiation exposure in the US population (11). This increased use has not gone without continued scrutiny. Brenner and Hall outlined the growing use of CT with respect to potential cancer development late in 2007 (13).

While the topic of medical imaging, radiation exposure, and potential risk is important at all ages, this is especially topical for children. Children are more sensitive to radiation than adults. Accordingly, imaging applications and techniques may need to differ from those in adults to minimize the radiation exposure, in keeping with the ALARA principle (15). However, adult techniques, for example, in CT (16), have traditionally been the default. A lack of understanding of radiation risks in children coupled with a neglect of the unique considerations in applications and techniques may shift the balance away from patient benefit.

Therefore, this chapter will discuss radiation risks with medical imaging in children. This material will primarily address what is known about low-level radiation – 100–150 mSv (17) – resulting from diagnostic imaging rather than oncologic radiation treatment where radiation bioeffects are clearly present and risks are more definitively established due to doses which may be orders of magnitude greater. Some data on radiation therapy for non-oncologic conditions in children will be presented as these doses are lower and approach low-level radiation. While cumulative doses from diagnostic imaging may exceed the low-level threshold, most material will focus on low-level doses.

The topic of radiation and biological impact is extensive and discussion will be focused on diagnostic imaging in the pediatric population, and will not address fetal exposures. Information will be provided from a perspective of radiology rather than radiation biology, health or radiation physics, or epidemiology. More extensive information on radiation and the potential effects can be found in other comprehensive sources (18). Finally, discussion will not include

strategies for dose management, including radioprotectants (19).

Overall Cost to Society

The American health care system costs more than $2.3 trillion annually, more per capita than any other developed nation. The cost of medical imaging is estimated at $100 billion per year and is the fastest growing segment of the health care system, growing at approximately 10–15% annually. CT and medical imaging use is primarily in USA and developed nations. Compared to USA, other developed nations have much lower use and spending on health care in general and on imaging in particular, yet have similar life expectancy. The main issue is the number of either unindicated or borderline indicated studies in USA for ionizing (CT, radiography, and fluoroscopy) and non-ionizing (MRI, sonography) imaging studies. Furthermore, there is under-recognition of the harm from false-positive imaging tests.

Goals

The goal of imaging is to diagnose or exclude medical conditions that concern the patient, family, or clinician. Imaging, like any test, should ideally improve patient health outcomes and reduce the intensity and use of resources, especially cost, of care. Diagnostic imaging guides clinicians in the management of patients. Imaging tests have both risks and benefits that must be weighed for each patient.

Methodology

Information for this chapter was obtained primarily through a MEDLINE search using PubMed (National Library of Medicine, Bethesda, Maryland, http://www.ncbi.nlm.nih.gov/sites/entrez) from 1968 to January 2010. Keywords are *ALARA (As Low As Reasonably Achievable), pediatric, radiation, radiation risk, CT, diagnostic imaging*, and the resultant related fields from this original database.

I. Is There a Cancer Risk from Low-Level Radiation Used in Medical Imaging? What Are the Uncertainties in the Data?

Summary of Evidence: There is strong research evidence for cellular and organism damage from high levels of ionizing radiation (strong evidence). At lower levels of radiation (<100–150 mSv), the linear, no-threshold model suggests increased cancer risk. Although most major medical and scientific organizations accept the linear, no-threshold model as the preferred model for low-level radiation and cancer risk estimation, direct evidence linking medical use of low-level radiation is lacking (insufficient evidence).

In analyzing potential radiation biological effects, there are other considerations in addition to the modeling discussed above, including type of radiation, site (e.g., organ or organ system)-specific risks, regional versus whole body exposure, acute versus protracted exposure, and gender and age sensitivity.

Supporting Evidence: Dose from CT represents the largest contribution from medical radiation to developed nation populations. The risk of radiation-induced cancer from CT should be put into context against the statistical risk of developing cancer in the entire population. The average risk of fatal cancer developing over a person's lifetime is approximately 18–22%. So, for every 1,000 children, 180–220 will develop fatal cancer in their lifetime regardless of exposure to medical radiation. The estimated increased risk of cancer over a person's lifetime from a single CT scan is controversial but has been estimated to be a fraction of this risk (0.03–0.05%); this estimate is based on the model showing that 1 in 1,000 children who undergo abdominal CT may have later fatal cancer induction. It is important to remember that these estimates are population based rather than for the individual child.

A. Cancer Risk and Radiation Following Diagnostic Medical Imaging

Gonzulea and Darby estimated cancer risk from diagnostic imaging and concluded that the attributable risk in developed countries varied from 0.6, to as high as 3.2% (20), similar to projections reported by Brenner and Hall (11). These projections come under the same scrutiny as with any that base conclusions on LSS Hiroshima data and may not reflect contemporary imaging techniques, particularly in children. In addition, there is no provision for the benefit achieved by diagnostic imaging. Ron et al. discuss development of leukemia, thyroid, and breast cancer from diagnostic X-rays (21). For example, one investigation by Doody et al. reported on the association of breast cancer and scoliosis radiography follow-up in childhood, concluding that with a mean dose of 110 mGy, mean exposure age 10.6 years, that there were 70 observed breast cancers versus nearly 36 expected (22). These data are in agreement with those of atomic bomb survivors.

For fluoroscopic and angiographic evaluations, increases in breast cancer in girls undergoing fluoroscopic evaluation for tuberculosis have been summarized (14). However, three investigations of cardiac catheterizations in children have not shown an increased risk of cancer (23–25). Doses up to 500 mGy showed no effect (26).

Finally, diagnostic imaging exposes the medical community to radiation dose. Bearrington et al. reported cancer and other causes of mortality for British radiologists from 1897 to 1997 and found no significant increase in morality from all causes reviewed except for cancer in those radiologists in early years (5).

B. CT Scan and Risk

CT examinations, as noted above, provide a relatively high dose per examination compared with other forms of ionizing radiation used in diagnostic medical imaging. The potential risks of cancer development have been outlined by Brenner, Hall, and colleagues (13, 17, 27). In summary, depending on the age of exposure and the technique used, Brenner reports a risk of fatal cancer in up to 1 in 500 children from a single CT examination. Of note, the techniques assumed for this analysis were well beyond those currently advocated as standard (28, 29). Using lower dose (1.0 mSv) biennial screening CT predictions from 2 years of age until death in the cystic fibrosis population, de Jong et al. concluded that while the risk of cancer was small, projected excess relative risk could be 13% at 65 years of age. Again, assumptions are based on LSS data and they point out that there is no assumption of benefit from screening CT (30). Chodick et al. also estimated an excess risk of 0.29% in a population under 18 years of age in Israel (31). Although a large population (in the millions) would likely be needed to assess low-level radiation risk in children, there are an estimated 7,000,000 CT examinations performed in children per year in USA (32). While these large numbers provide an opportunity for study of low-level doses from diagnostic imaging, the cost of this type of investigation would be prohibitively high, given the decades of follow-up required. Alternatively, a retrospective evaluation of children who have had multiple examinations could be culled for those that have total estimated effective doses at more than 100–150 mSv to see if this subgroup demonstrates the same risk for cancer as that shown in the atomic bomb population.

C. Assumptions in Estimating Radiation Risks

In general, medium- and high-level radiation dose effects are linear, although recent reports suggest that there may be some nonlinearity at higher effects (33). The issue with radiation from diagnostic imaging is that these doses are low level, and because of potentially small effects, the data have been less conclusive. There are several possible extrapolation models for cancer risk with low-level radiation. The linear, no-threshold model is in general the most accepted model, being supported by scientific committees, major imaging organizations, and other scientific bodies including the Committee on the Health Risks from Exposure to Low Levels of Ionizing Radiation, Biological Effects of Ionizing Radiation of the National Academy of Sciences (BEIR VII), National Council on Radiation Protection and Measurement (NCRP), International Commission on Radiological Protection (ICRP), American Academy of Pediatrics (AAP), Radiological Society of North America (RSNA), and the Society for Pediatric Radiology (SPR).

D. Increased Radiosensitivity in Children

Children are more radiosensitive than adults. The range quoted is 2–10 times. Preston et al. note that children are 2–5 times more sensitive (33, 34), and Hall (35) indicates that children are up to 10 times more sensitive. Infants are more sensitive than older children, and girls are more radiosensitive than boys. Preston et al. (33) notes that the most recent LSS data not only indicate that the female to male ratio is 1.4 (90% confidence interval 1.1; 1.8) but also point out that this difference disappeared when non-gender-specific cancers were analyzed.

E. Nonfatal Cancers

In addition, it should be understood that non-fatal cancer incidence is higher than that of cancer resulting in fatality. This frequency is about two times (21). Part of this is due to the fact that some cancers, such as that of breast and thyroid, have relatively successful treatment regimes with improved survival.

F. Additional Confounders in Risk Estimation

Finally, these estimations represent an imperfect science due to other confounding variables. Prasad argues that health risks of doses <100 mGy (absorbed dose) in "…humans may not be accurately estimated by any current mathematical model because of numerous inherit environmental, dietary and biological variables that cannot be accounted for in epidemiologic studies. In addition, the expression of radiation-induced damage depends not only on dose, dose rate, LET, fractionation, and protraction but also on repair mechanisms, bystander effects, an exposure to chemical and biological mutagens, carcinogens, tumor promoters, and other toxins as well as radioprotective substances, such as antioxidants" (36).

G. Radiation Doses from Medical Imaging and Uncertainty in Cancer Risks

There is still debate as to whether the linear, no-threshold model is an acceptable model for low-level radiation (recall that this is generally the accepted model) and, what, if any, potential risks exist for the levels of radiation seen with diagnostic imaging. Currently, *there are no data from diagnostic medical imaging modalities that prove the connection between low-level radiation doses and risk of cancer development.* What is discussed, then, are data from other sources, predominantly the atomic bomb LSS data, for cancer risk in this low-level range. Brenner et al. goes on to summarize that "the epidemiologic study with the highest statistical power for evaluating low dose risk is the LSS cohort atomic bombs survivors" (17). As discussed previously, the radiation exposure in this population has potential variations from medical imaging exposure, in that the atomic bomb radiation consisted of other than just gamma (X-ray equivalent) radiation, acute versus protracted (such as with multiple CT examinations) exposures, and whole body versus regional exposures. That said, the following supports a significant risk of cancer development at low-level exposure.

"For x- or gamma-rays, good evidence of an increase and risk for cancer is shown at acute doses >50 mSv, and reasonable evidence for an increase and some cancer risks at doses above [approximately] 5 mSv. As expected from basic radiobiology … the doses above which statistically significant risks are seen are somewhat higher for protracted exposures than for acute exposures; specifically, good evidence of an increase in some cancer risks is shown for protracted doses >100 mSv, and reasonable evidence for an increase in cancer risks at acute doses above [approximately] 50 mSv" (17) (Table 3.5). From Preston et al. (33) "…furthermore, there is statistically significant dose response when analyses were limited to cohort members with doses of 0.15 Gy (150 mGy) or less."

One of the difficulties in determining if there is a significant risk of cancer development or mortality from low-level exposures is that this would take a very large population study over a long period of time. For example, solid tumors may take more than three decades to develop. To find an effect may take a long-term study of an exposed population of several million individuals for doses near the 10 mSv range (17). According to Kleinerman (26), "Large population size is usually required to evaluate the risk of cancer, because cancer is a rare outcome, especially in children. In addi-tion, the lower the radiation dose, the large the population size required to detect a radiation effect" (Tables 3.6 and 3.7).

II. What Is the Estimated Risk from a Single Chest X-Ray in a Child?

Summary of Evidence: The dose to a child from a single plain radiograph is very low. Unless these low-dose examinations are repeatedly performed in young children, the risk is considered negligible. There is little concern to terminally ill children or to older adults whose life expectancy is less than the latency time to develop cancer from the radiation exposure (several years for leukemia and several decades for solid cancers).

Supporting Evidence: The effective radiation dose from a single chest X-ray in a child is approximately 0.02 mSv (Table 3.4), a very small dose. It is the equivalent of 1 day of natural background radiation and less than the dose from a cross-country flight. Table 3.8 provides a comparison of radiation dose from a single chest radiograph to that from air travel across USA.

III. What Is the Estimated Risk from a Single Abdominal CT Scan in a Child?

Summary of Evidence: The dose to a child from a single abdominal CT is approximately 100 times higher than that from a plain X-ray but still low. When these CT examinations are repeatedly performed in children, the risk may be significant. There is little concern in terminally ill children or to older adults whose life expectancy is less than the latency time to develop cancer from the radiation exposure (several years for leukemia and several decades for solid cancers).

Supporting Evidence: As noted above, Table 3.8 shows the dose from a single abdominal CT compared to that from natural background, a chest radiograph, and a cross-country flight. When the CT parameters are adjusted for children, the dose is approximately 5 mSv. This represents up to 20 months of natural background dose. Another way of assessing the relative risk of having a CT scan is to compare the theoretical risk of one abdominal CT scan with other risks. The estimated risk of one abdominal CT has been compared to driving a car 7,500 miles (accident risk) or even less distance on a motorcycle. This information shows that the risk of developing cancer related to a single CT scan is very small and helps to put risk in the context of everyday life experiences.

A. The Changing Landscaping of Radiation Dose for Medical Imaging

The use of medical imaging is increasing in developed nations. This does depend somewhat on the modality as radiography and fluoroscopy rates have remained relatively stable. However, there has been a substantial increase in the use of CT in both children and adults. For example, Broder et al. examined CT use in the emergency department and found that, in children, the use of chest CT increased more than 435% during a 6-year period (2000–2006), while the frequency of emergency room visits increased by only 2% during the same period (Fig. 3.1) (37).

B. Lowering CT Dose in Children

There are a few simple strategies that can lower the radiation exposure to children undergoing CT. These concepts include the following: using pediatric protocols – adjusting the kVp and mA settings based on the child's weight; performing a single scan rather than multiple passes through the child's body – this is usually adequate to answer the clinical question, and scanning only the indicated area of the child's body.

IV. Understanding Benefit Versus Risk of Imaging Tests in Well-Indicated Studies Versus Those that Have Very Low Probability of Disease

Summary of Evidence: It is critical to weigh both the benefits and the risks when using any test, including medical imaging with ionizing radiation. The benefit to a patient should outweigh risks. Risk from an imaging test must include the potential for false-positive (and false-negative) results that lead to unnecessary intervention and anxiety, as well as lifetime cancer risk. Because children are more radiosensitive than adults and have longer expected life spans, these considerations may alter the diagnostic work-up and management plan for children undergoing imaging.

What is the benefit–risk of CT in high-versus very low-risk groups? High-risk children for disease, such as acute trauma, have relatively low risk from CT or its radiation compared to its potential benefit. In low-risk groups for a disease such as low-impact trauma, there is little benefit in using CT and the risk of short-term-increased false-positive results plus long-term radiation risk outweigh any benefit.

Supporting Evidence: Health benefit or lifesaving use of CT has been shown in certain populations including those with acute motor vehicle trauma, non-accidental trauma, acute infection, and acute abdominal pain. The appropriate use of imaging has not been well researched or well funded by research agencies.

A. The Example of CT in Children with Headache

Medina and colleagues investigated the clinical role and cost of head CT and MR in children with headache (38). They compared three diagnostic strategies: (a) magnetic resonance imaging (MRI), (b) computed tomography followed by MRI for positive results (CT-MRI), and (c) no neuroimaging with close clinical follow-up in the evaluation of children suspected of having a brain tumor.

They also grouped the children's risk into low, medium, and high for brain tumor prior to imaging. With a high pretest probability of brain tumor (4% risk), MRI of the head was the recommended and cost-effective imaging strategy. When there was an intermediate pretest probability of brain tumor (0.4%), imaging was very expensive (CT then MR, if CT was positive).

When children had chronic headache, the pretest probability of tumor was low (0.01%), and neither CT nor MR was recommended. Even with high sensitivity and specificity of CT (95%, 95%), the posttest probability of tumor was only 16%. In the short term, this means children are being submitted to a false-positive rate (low positive predictive value). MRI would have the same results but avoids ionizing radiation exposure to the child. On the contrary, there is a small risk from sedation or anesthesia in young children undergoing MR that would not be needed with CT. If, however, the study is well indicated, CT has more benefit than risk in the high-risk group of children with headache: CT would reduce short-term morbidity and mortality.

So we emphasize the importance of weighing benefit versus risk. For many other diseases in children, there are low-risk subgroups that get studies ordered that expose them to both high false-positive rates and radiation.

V. How Should I Communicate Radiation Risk from Imaging to Parents and Patients?

Summary of Evidence: There are growing numbers of web sites and published literature that provide both appropriate language and data to discuss the benefits and risk of medical imaging to consumers. There are survey data that suggest that parents and families both want to know and can understand these issues (39).

Supporting Evidence: The Internet has revolutionized access to scientific and medical information for consumers. There are growing numbers of both scientific and medical web sites that target consumers, including the Image Gently Campaign (http://www.imagegently. org) for children, the International Atomic Energy Agency (IAEA) radiation protection of patients (http://rpop.iaea.org/RPoP/RPoP/ Content/index.htm), the National Cancer Institute (http://www.cancer.gov/cancertopics/causes/radiation-risks-pediatric-CT), the Health Physics Society (http://hps.org), the American Academy of Pediatrics (http://www. aap.org), and the American College of Radiology (http://www.acr.org).

The "Image Gently Campaign" is an educational and awareness campaign created by the Alliance for Radiation Safety in Pediatric Imaging that was formed in July 2007. It is a coalition of health care organizations dedicated to providing safe, high-quality pediatric imaging nationwide. There are four founding members – the Society for Pediatric Radiology, the American Association of Physicists in Medicine, the American College of Radiology, and the American Society of Radiologic Technologists – as well as 58 national and international societies in this coalition, representing over 700,000 health care professionals in radiology, pediatrics, medical physics, and radiation safety. The site provides information for all stakeholders in medicine. As an example, Table 3.8 shows the relative radiation doses to children for common imaging examinations compared to that from background and airline flight.

Information about radiation and the role of all stakeholders to improve radiation safety in medicine is summarized in a Blue Ribbon Panel article (15). The American College of Radiology (ACR) guidelines now include dose estimates for imaging tests and reference levels for acceptable doses in all appropriateness criteria.

Larson and colleagues surveyed parents about their understanding of the benefits and risks from CT for their children. They found that two of three parents knew that CT used ionizing radiation. After they were given an informational brochure, 99% reported understanding that CT used ionizing radiation. After reading the brochure, 86% of parents reported that there was a risk of cancer induction from CT, yet they remained willing to have their child undergo CT when appropriate (39). They concluded that "A brief informational handout can improve parental understanding of the potential increased risk of cancer related to pediatric CT without causing parents to refuse studies recommended by the referring physician." Families and patients should be encouraged to ask questions about the risks and benefits of CT scans and other imaging tests (40).

The risk of radiation-induced cancer from CT should be put into context against the statistical risk of developing cancer in the entire population. The average risk of fatal cancer developing over a person's lifetime is approximately 18–22%. So, for every 1,000 children, 180–220 will develop cancer in their lifetime regardless of exposure to medical radiation. The estimated increased risk of cancer over a person's lifetime from a single CT scan is controversial but has been estimated to be a fraction of this risk (0.03–0.05%) or 1 in 1,000 children who undergo CT. It is important to remember that these estimates are population based rather than for the individual child.

VI. Special Situation: Increased Cancer Risk Following Therapeutic Medical Radiation

Summary of Evidence: There are known risks of secondary cancer development after medical radiation treatment for both neoplastic and non-neoplastic conditions in children (41) (strong evidence).

Supporting Evidence: There are a number of studies showing increased risk of cancers after radiotherapy including leukemia, lymphoma, and solid cancers (42). The risk is variable and is related to the primary cancer treatment and other factors. The Children's Oncology Cancer group provides medical recommendations for lifelong follow-up in these children (43).

According to Kleinerman (26) "many of the classic epidemiologic studies of cancer following medical radiation exposure are distinguished by a cohort design, large population size, long-term follow-up of the cohort, well-characterized dose estimates for individuals, and a wide range of doses in order to estimate a dose–response relationship; studies based on a cohort design are generally less likely to be biased than case control studies that depend on the retrospective collection of data." Ron and colleagues also discuss the advantages and disadvantages of assessing cancer risks in patients who have relatively high doses for medical therapy of both neoplastic and non-neoplastic conditions (Table 3.9) (44). The advantages of these types of data include that the records are relatively accurate, with data on other potentially confounding medical problems. Radiation is generally always an X-ray (gamma ray) exposure and the region radiated is known. However, disadvantages include confounding factors that include underlying diseases, chemotherapy treatment, genetics, nutrition, and other environmental factors. Long-term effects from radiation therapy for cancer in children have recently been reviewed (42).

There are illustrative reports for cancer risk from non-oncologic treatment that are worth reviewing. For example, in a review of six investigations dealing with thyroid cancer, all cohort studies, the author concludes "these studies demonstrate that the thyroid gland is very sensitive to the carcinogenic effects of radiation, characterized by a strong linear dose response." In three of these investigations, the risk was seen with doses as low as 100 mGy. In an additional investigation, a thyroid dose of 90 mGy was associated with a 400% increase in malignant tumors and a 200% increase in tumors that were benign. A linear dose response was demonstrated in children exposed under the age of 5 years, and these children were significantly more likely to develop tumors than older children (44). Brenner et al. discussed data from pooled studies, including that of Ron et al. (44), and noted that the thyroid cancer risk was significant at glandular doses as low as 50 mSv (17). Kleinerman also summarizes data demonstrating increased risk of breast cancer seen with therapeutic doses as low as 300 mGy (26).

Take Home Tables and Figures

Tables 3.1–3.9 and Fig. 3.1 serve to highlight key recommendations and supporting evidence.

Table 3.1. Radiation dose units

Absorbed dose – Gray (Gy) – rad (rad) is prior
Unit
1 Gy = 100 rad
1 cGy = 1 rad
1 mGy = 100 mrad
Equivalent dose – Sievert (Sv) – rem (rem) is prior
Unit
Sv = Gy × quality factor (=1)
1 Sv = 100 rem
10 mSv = 1 rem
1 mSv = 100 mrem

Reprinted with permission of Elsevier from Frush DP, Slovis TL. Biological effects of diagnostic radiation on children. In Slovis TL (ed.): Caffey's Pediatric Diagnostic Imaging. Philadelphia: Elsevier, 2007;29–41 (2).

Table 3.2. Inherited human syndromes associated with sensitivity to X-rays

Ataxia–telangiectasia
Basal cell nevoid syndrome
Cockayne's syndrome
Down syndrome
Fanconi's anemia
Gardner's syndrome
Nijmegan breakage syndrome
Usher's syndrome

Reprinted and adapted with permission of Elsevier from Frush DP, Slovis TL. Biological effects of diagnostic radiation on children. In Slovis TL (ed.): Caffey's Pediatric Diagnostic Imaging. Philadelphia: Elsevier, 2007;29–41 (2), and from Hall (45).

Table 3.3. Deterministic effects: relatively high-radiation doses needed compared to what is used in diagnostic imaging

Injury	Approximate	Threshold
Skin Transient erythema	2 Gy	(200 rad)
Eyes Cataracts (acute)	>2.0 Gy	(>200 rad)

Reprinted and adapted with permission of Elsevier from Frush DP, Slovis TL. Biological effects of diagnostic radiation on children. In Slovis TL (ed.): Caffey's Pediatric Diagnostic Imaging. Philadelphia: Elsevier, 2007, 29–41 (2), and from Hall (45).

Table 3.4. Estimated medical radiation doses for a 5-year-old child

Imaging area	Effective dose (mSv)	Equivalent number of CXRs
Three-view ankle	0.0015	1/14th
Two-view chest	0.02	1
Anteroposterior and lateral abdomen	0.05	2–1/2
Tc-99m radionuclide cystogram	0.18	9
Tc-99m radionuclide bone scan	6.2	310
FDG PET scan	15.3	765
Fluoroscopic cystogram	0.33	16
Head CT	4	200
Chest CT	3	150
Abdomen CT	5	250

CXR chest radiograph; *Tc-99m* technetium 99m; *FDG PET* fluorodeoxyglucose positron emission tomography. Data were provided by R. Reiman, MD (Duke Office of Radiation Safety (http://www.safety.duke.edu/RadSafety), written communication, 2006).
Reproduced with permission of the AAP from Brody et al. (40).

Table 3.5. Atomic bomb (longitudinal survivor study) data showing excess solid cancers linked to radiation exposure doses. These data combine children and adults. Atomic bomb (longitudinal survivor study) data 1950–1997

Dose (Sv)	People	1950–1997 Deaths	Expected background	Fitted excess	1991–1997 Deaths	Expected background	Fitted excess
<0.005	37,458	3,833	3,844	0	742	718	0
0.005–0.1	31,650	3,277	3,221	44	581	596	12
0.1–0.2	5,732	668	622	39	137	109	10
0.2–0.5	6,332	763	678	97	133	118	24
0.5–1	3,299	438	335	109	75	62	28
1–2	1,613	274	157	103	68	31	27
2+	488	82	38	48	20	8	13
Total	86,572	9,335	8,895	440	1,756	1,642	114

Reprinted with permission from Preston et al. (34).

Table 3.6. Hematopoietic cancer risks and adult diagnostic X-rays

Kaiser-Permanente, Oregon and California, 1956–1982
565 Leukemias (358 non-CLL)
318 Non-Hodgen's
208 Multiple myeloma
Various diagnostic procedures
Exposure data from medical records
RR[a]   Non-CLL = 1.4 (0.9–2.2)   NHL = 0.99 (0.6–1.6)   MM = 1.3 (0.6–3.0); *P*-trend 0.03

Reprinted with the kind permission of Springer Science + Business Media from Ron (21).
CLL chronic lymphatic leukemia; *NHL* non-Hodgkin's lymphoma; *MM* multiple myeloma; *RR* relative risk.
[a]Two-year lag.

Table 3.7. Childhood cancer risks and diagnostic X-ray examinations

Population-based study: Shanghai 1981–1991; 642 cancer cases (<15 years), 642 controls; postnatal diagnostic X-ray exposure risks:		
Cancer	**OR**	**95% CI**
Total cancer	1.3	1.0–1.7
Acute leukemia	1.6	1.0–2.6
Brain cancer	1.5	0.8–3.0
Lymphoma	1.3	0.6–22

Cases included prenatal and postnatal diagnostic radiation exposure in children. The odds ratios for total cancer and acute leukemia are significant. Given large confidence intervals for brain cancer and lymphoma, these are not significant. Reprinted with the kind permission of Springer Science + Business Media from Ron (21).
OR odds ratio; *CI* confidence interval.

Table 3.8. Relative radiation doses for children

Source	Estimated effective dose (mSv)
Natural background radiation	3 mSv per year
Airline passenger (cross-country)	0.04 mSv
Chest X-ray (single view)	0.01 mSv
Head CT	Up to 2 mSv
Chest CT	Up to 3 mSv
Abdominal CT	Up to 5 mSv

Based on US data and adapted from http://www.imagegently.org.
Reprinted with the kind permission of Springer Science + Business Media from Frush and Applegate (46).

Table 3.9. Cancer risks following childhood therapeutic irradiation for benign diseases

Cancer site	Benign condition, cohort	No. of irradiated subjects	Mean age (years)	Mean dose (Gy)	ERR/Gy (95% CI)
Thyroid	Tinea capitis, Israel	10,834	7.1	0.1	32 (14–57)
	Tinea capitis, New York	2,224	7.8	0.1	7.7 (<0–60)
	Hemangioma[a], Gotenburg	11,914	<1.5	0.1	7.5 (0.4–18)
	Hemangioma[a], Stockholm	14,435	<1.5	0.3	4.9 (1.3–10)
	Enlarged tonsils, Chicago	2,634	4	0.6	2.5 (0.6–26)
	Thymus, Rochester, NY	2,650	<1	1.4	9.1 (3.6–29)
Breast	Hemangioma (pooled)[a]	17,202	0.5	0.3	0.4 (0.2–0.6)
	Thymus, Rochester, NY	1,201	<1	0.7	2.5 (1.1–5.2)
Leukemia	Tinea capitis, Israel	10,834	7.1	0.3	Not available
	Hemangioma (pooled)[a]	28,008	0.5	0.1	1.6 (–0.6 to 5.5)
Brain	Tinea capitis, Israel	10,834	7.1	1.5	4.6 (2.4–9.1)[b]
				1.5	2.0 (0.7–4.7)[c]
	Hemangioma (pooled)[a]	28,008	0.5	0.1	2.7 (1.0–5.6)[d]
Skin	Tinea capitis, Israel	10,834	7.1	6.1	0.7 (0.3–1.4)
	Tinea capitis, New York	2,224	7.8	4.3	1.6 (1.3–2.1)

Reprinted with the kind permission of Springer Science + Business Media from Kleinerman (26).
Note that ERR is the excess relative risk (where relative risk = excess relative risk + 1).
[a]Radium-226 treatment.
[b]Benign tumor only.
[c]Malignant tumor only.
[d]Benign and malignant tumors combined.

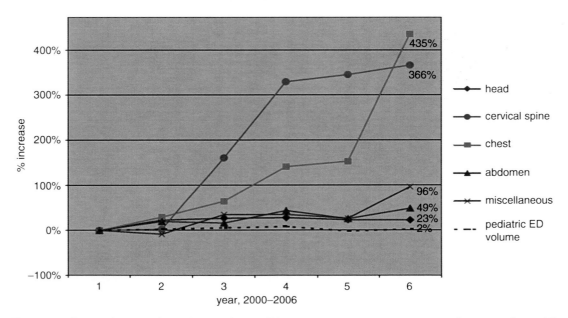

Figure 3.1. Percent increase in various pediatric CT examinations over a 6-year period compared to a 2% increase in visits over the same time period (years 2000–2006). (Reprinted with kind permission of Springer Science + Business Media from Broder and Fordham. (37))

References

1. Huda W. Medical Radiation Dosimetry. Categorical Course in Physics: Radiation Dose and Image Quality. Chicago, IL: Radiological Society of North America, 2006;167–182.
2. Frush DP, Slovis TL. In Slovis TL (ed.): Caffey's Pediatric Diagnostic Imaging. Philadelphia: Elsevier, 2007;29–41.
3. Imanishi Y et al. Eur Radiol 2005;15:41–46.
4. Hall HA et al. BMJ 2004;328:1–5.
5. Berrington A et al. Br J Radiol 2001;74:507–519.
6. UNSCEAR. Medical Radiation Exposures, Annex D. United Nations Scientific Committee on the Effects of Atomic Radiation Report to the General Assembly. New York: UNSCEAR, 2000.
7. Gaca AM. Pediatr Radiol 2008;38:285–291.
8. Thierry-Chef I, Simon SL, Miller DL. Pediatr Radiol 2006;36(14):159–162.
9. Thomas KE, Wang BB. Pediatr Radiol 2009;39:668–676.
10. Huda W, Vance A. AJR Am J Roentgenol 2007;188:540–546.
11. NCRP report no. 160. Ionizing Radiation Exposure of the Population of the United States. http://www.ncrponline.org/Publications/160press.html [last accessed June 1, 2010].
12. Fuchs VR, Sox HC. Health Aff 2001;20:30–42.
13. Brenner DJ, Hall EJ. N Engl J Med 2007;357:2277–2284.
14. Mettler FA, Wiest PW, Locken JA et al. J Radiol Prot 2000;20:353–359.
15. Amis ES Jr. et al. J Am Coll Radiol 2007;4:272–284.
16. Paterson A, Frush DP, Donnelly LF. AJR Am J Roentgenol 2001;176(2):297–301.
17. Brenner DJ et al. Proc Natl Acad Sci USA 2003;100(24):13761–13766.
18. BEIR VII. Health risks from exposure to low levels of ionizing radiation 2006. http://www.nap.edu/openbook.php?isbn=030909156X. Last accessed 1-1-08.
19. Prasad KN, Cole WC, Hasse GM. Exp Biol Med 2004;229:378–382.
20. Gonzalea AB, Darby S. Lancet 2004;363:345–351.
21. Ron E. Pediatr Radiol 2002;32:232–237.
22. Doody MM et al. Spine 2000;25:2052–2063.
23. Modan B et al. Int J Epidemiol 2000;29:424–428.
24. Spengler RF et al. Pediatrics 1983;71:235–239.
25. McLaughlin JR et al. Int J Epidemiol 1993;22:584–591.
26. Kleinerman RA. Pediatr Radiol 2006;36(2):121–125.
27. Brenner DJ et al. AJR Am J Roentgenol 2001;176:289–296.
28. Donnelly LF et al. AJR Am J Roentgenol 2001;176:303–306.
29. Frush DP. In Kalra M, Saini S, Rubin G (eds.): MDCT: Form Protocols to Practice. New York: Springer, 2008;333–354.
30. De Jong PA et al. Am J Respir Crit Care Med 2006;173:199–203.
31. Chodick G et al. Isr Med Assoc J 2007;9(8):584–587.
32. Frush DP, Applegate K. J Am Coll Radiol 2004;1:113–119.
33. Preston DL et al. Radiat Res 2007;168:1–64.
34. Preston DL et al. Radiat Res 2003;160:381–407.
35. Hall EJ. Pediatr Radiol 2002;32:700–706.
36. Prasad KN, Cole WC, Haase GM. Br J Radiol 2004;77:97–99.
37. Broder J, Fordham L, Warshaver D. Emerg Radiol 2007;14:227–232.
38. Medina LS, Kuntz KM, Pomperoy S. Pediatrics 2001;108:255–263.
39. Larson DB, Rader SB, Forman HP, Fenton LZ. AJR Am J Roentgenol 2007;189(2):271–275.
40. Brody AS, Frush DP, Huda W, Brent RL. Pediatrics 2007;120(3):677–682.
41. http://www.ncrponline.org/
42. Larrier N, Lawrence T, Halperin EC. In Slovis T (ed.): Caffey's Pediatric Diagnostic Imaging. Philadelphia: Elsevier, 2007;13–25.
43. http://www.childrensoncologygroup.org/.
44. Ron E et al. Radiat Res 1989;120:516–531.
45. Hall EJ. Radiobiology for the Radiologist, 5th ed. Philadelphia: Lippincott Williams & Wilkins, 2000.
46. Frush DP, Applegate KE. Radiation risk from medical imaging in children. In Medina LS, Applegate KE, Blackmore CC (eds.): Evidence-Based Imaging in Pediatrics: Optimizing Imaging in Pediatric Patient Care. New York: Springer Science Business Media, 2010.

4

The Economic and Regulatory Impact of Evidence-Based Medicine on Radiology

David B. Larson

Issues

I. What political and economic forces influence the United States' healthcare system?
II. What is the impetus driving US healthcare reform now?
III. How are rising costs of healthcare affecting governments and individuals?
IV. Do increased health expenditures lead to better care?
V. How does supplier-driven demand influence imaging utilization?
VI. What can be learned from "high-value" systems?
VII. Cost-control strategies: rationing versus reducing inappropriate care
   A. Reimbursement cuts
   B. Intermediaries (RBM organization)
   C. Accountable care organization
VIII. How is the recently passed US healthcare reform initiative expected to influence cost and quality?
   A. Learning what works
   B. Coming changes
IX. What are the challenges and opportunities for evidence-based imaging?

Key Points

- US healthcare expenditures have nearly continuously increased over the past 40 years, not only in real dollars, but also in almost every other measurable term.

D.B. Larson (✉)
Department of Radiology, Cincinnati Children's Hospital Medical Center,
3333 Burnet Avenue, ML 5031, Cincinnati, OH 45229, USA
e-mail: David.Larson@cchmc.org

Parts of this chapter used with permission of the ARRS from ARRS 2010 Categorical Course: The Financial and Regulatory Aspects of Evidence-Based Medicine, 2010.

- If current rates of increase were to continue, long-term growth in medical spending would eventually consume all growth in per capita income and in 30 years, more than one third of the US gross domestic product (GDP) would be devoted to healthcare costs.
- According to some analyses, much of the stagnation of standard of living of the working-class can be explained by the continued rise in medical costs, without which American working families would continue to enjoy a rising standard of living.
- Most other industrialized countries routinely use cost-effectiveness analysis (CEA) to improve the value of medical care, decreasing both inappropriate underutilization and overutilization.
- Example of overutilization: self-referral. From 2001 to 2006, the volume of CT imaging performed at in-office facilities owned by radiologists rose by 85%. The volume of imaging performed at in-office facilities in which nonradiologist referring clinicians had a financial stake rose by 263%.
- Some physician groups have had success both lowering costs and improving quality. Whatever their organizational structure, the so-called accountable care organizations tend to have certain elements in common: physicians and hospitals tend to have a close working relationship, most of them use electronic medical record systems to track and improve care, and they generally encourage a culture of restrained spending and collaboration with competitors for the benefit of patients.
- The two main thrusts of policy makers' efforts are (1) to pay for appropriate care that, based on the evidence, is most likely to improve health outcomes, and (2) to encourage providers to work more closely together to make sure that evidence-based care is provided consistently and efficiently. Ideas that are taking root include decreasing reimbursement, using third parties to help decrease inappropriate imaging, and changing the reimbursement incentive structure.
- The recently enacted US healthcare reform statute has two main priorities: to expand coverage and control costs. While the coverage provisions of the act have received the majority of the attention in the press, the second priority of the statute, that of cost control, probably has more potential to affect radiologists and other physicians.
- The challenge has been issued to the medical community, including radiology, to move evidence-based imaging (EBI) from a theory or a collection of anecdotes to one that can be effectively implemented on a broad scale.

I. What Political and Economic Forces Influence the United States' Healthcare System?

Summary of Evidence: The US healthcare system is widely perceived to be a "free-market" system. However, two major factors substantially limit the efficiency of the US healthcare market: employer-based health insurance and the sizeable role of government payers.

On one hand, many US voters strongly oppose government involvement in the regulation and administration of medical care. On the other hand, many of the same voters adamantly support current government-sponsored programs.

This has led to political division and, in the absence of consensus, has resulted in a system in which no single payer or set of cohesive market rules control healthcare expenditures (1).

Supporting Evidence: The US healthcare system is based on a disparate mix of private and government payers. The healthcare system is widely perceived to be a "free-market" system. However, two major factors substantially limit the efficiency of the US healthcare market. First, the majority of individuals with private health insurance (159 million Americans) obtain it through an employer (2). Thus, at least two intermediaries – the employer and the insurance company – are placed between the customer (the patient) and the supplier (the provider). This profoundly alters the normal interaction between supply and demand that is expected in a free market. Second, government sources contribute 48% of all health expenditure payments (Fig. 4.1) (3). While, ostensibly, the United States is the only major industrialized country without a government-sponsored healthcare system, only the governments of two other such countries, Norway and Denmark, pay more for their citizens' healthcare on a per capita basis (4).

The disconnection between the perception of a market-based US healthcare system versus the reality of a government- and insurance-financed system has created predictable problems. On one hand, many voters strongly oppose government involvement in the regulation and administration of medical care. On the other hand, many of the same voters adamantly support current government-sponsored programs. One constituent reportedly told President Barack Obama, "I don't want government-run health care, I don't want socialized medicine, and don't touch my Medicare" (5). Compounded by the disproportionate influence of special-interest groups, politicians find themselves facing incompatible demands to ensure widespread access to advanced medical care, while at the same time limiting government intervention and expenditures. This has led to political division and, in the absence of consensus, has resulted in a system in which no single payer or set of cohesive market rules control healthcare expenditures (1).

If current rates of increase were to continue, long-term growth in medical spending would eventually consume all growth in per capita income (6), and, in 30 years, more than one-third of the US gross domestic product (GDP) would be devoted to healthcare costs (7).

Supporting Evidence: Sustained market-style demand without the usual market-style constraints has led to continued increases in spending. US healthcare expenditures as a percentage of GDP are nearly double those of any other major developed country, and the per capita expenditures are more than double. At the same time, US health outcomes are not significantly better, and, in many cases are worse, than those of other major developed countries (8).

US healthcare expenditures have nearly continuously increased over the past 40 years, not only in real dollars, but also in almost every other measurable term. Figure 4.2 demonstrates US national health expenditures from 1965 to 2018 (2008–2018 projected). National health expenditures increased 57-fold from $42 billion in 1965 to $2.4 trillion in 2008, and are projected to reach $4.4 trillion in 2018. This represents an average yearly increase of 9.6% from 1965 to 2008, which is 4.9% greater than the rate of inflation (9). Adjusted for population growth, the annual increase is 3.9% (10). This indicates that the portion of economic output spent on healthcare for the average person in the USA is five times that of the amount spent for a person in 1965. Spending is expected to continue to escalate in the coming years. If current rates of increase were to continue, long-term growth in medical spending would eventually consume all growth in per capita income (6), and, in 30 years, more than one-third of the US GDP would be devoted to healthcare costs (7). Economists, business executives, and government officials are urgently reporting that this constitutes a major threat to the US economic well-being and ability to compete in a global marketplace (11).

II. What Is the Impetus Driving US Healthcare Reform Now?

Summary of Evidence: US healthcare expenditures have nearly continuously increased over the past 40 years, not only in real dollars, but also in almost every other measurable term.

III. How Are Rising Costs of Healthcare Affecting Governments and Individuals?

Summary of Evidence: According to some analyses, much of the stagnation of standard of living of the working-class can be explained by the continued rise in medical costs, without which American working families would continue to enjoy a rising standard of living (12).

In its summary of the 2009 annual reports, the Medicare trustees projected that, unless changes to the revenue or payment system or both are made, the HI trust fund, which has already begun to contract, will be exhausted by 2017 while spending commitments will continue to increase.

Supporting Evidence: Escalating costs are increasingly impacting individual American families. The total annual medical cost for the average family of four is approximately $16,771, of which the employee pays $6,824 and the employer pays $9,947 (13). For a family with a median income of approximately $52,233, health insurance premiums and out-of-pocket costs make up approximately 13% of household take-home salary. However, when benefits paid by the employer are taken into consideration, health costs for the median worker account for approximately 25% of total compensation ($17,000 of $66,570) (12).

Adjusting for inflation, after-medical-cost compensation of households in the median income level and below has essentially remained flat for the last 30 years, and is projected to decrease in coming years. According to some analyses, much of this stagnation of standard of living of the working-class can be explained by the continued rise in medical costs, without which American working families would continue to enjoy a rising standard of living (12).

Costs that are burdensome for healthy families with medical insurance can be financially devastating for those with a family member who becomes ill. Medical costs for hospitalized individuals quickly reach the hundreds of thousands of dollars and those without insurance can expect to be charged, on average, two to three times that of a person with insurance (14). Families of those without insurance or with insufficient insurance are commonly held liable for most, if not all, of this amount. In 2007, 62% of all bankruptcies were linked to medical expenses. Nearly 80% of persons involved in such bankruptcies had health insurance (15). Furthermore, each year approximately 1.5 million US families lose their homes to foreclosure due to medical crises (16).

In addition to the increasing financial burden on individual families, rising healthcare costs are also increasingly straining government budgets. Medicare, the US federal government's insurance program for the elderly, is financed from two trust funds: the Hospital Insurance (HI) fund, which pays for hospital services and related inpatient care, and the Supplemental Medical Insurance (SMI) fund, which pays for physician and outpatient services (part B) and prescription drugs (part D). In its summary of the 2009 annual reports, the Medicare trustees projected that, unless changes to the revenue or payment system or both are made, the HI trust fund, which has already begun to contract, will be exhausted by 2017 while spending commitments will continue to increase. The SMI fund is more difficult to project, since the projections incorporate two unlikely assumptions. First, current law calls for continued physician reimbursement rate cuts of more than 20%; Congress has overridden adjustments to the sustainable growth rate for the past 7 years and will likely do so again. Second, premium increases for most enrollees are disallowed under the current law, and the deficit is compensated by unusually large premium increases for the unprotected minority of enrollees; the resulting disparity would likely be very unpopular. Therefore, while the trustees do not directly project the SMI fund status, it is likely to follow a similar course as the HI fund, with depletion by around 2017 (17).

Increasing healthcare expenditures have been the main driving force behind the 2009 legislative efforts to overhaul healthcare. In a White House speech in March 2009, President Obama remarked, "the greatest threat to America's fiscal health is not Social Security, though that's a significant challenge; it's not the investments that we've made to rescue our economy during this crisis. By a wide margin, the biggest threat to our nation's balance sheet is the skyrocketing cost of health care. It's not even close" (18). In his address to a joint session of Congress in September 2009, he stated, "If we do nothing to slow these skyrocketing costs, we will eventually be spending more on Medicare and Medicaid than every other government program combined. Put simply, our health care problem is our deficit problem. Nothing else even comes close" (11). While rising healthcare costs have been a source of concern by policy makers for many years, the recently passed healthcare reform law indicates that we have finally reached the point that such concerns outweigh the considerable political resistance to changing the system.

IV. Do Increased Health Expenditures Lead to Better Care?

Summary of Evidence: Wide regional variation in US healthcare expenditures cannot be adequately explained by illness severity, cost of living, quality of care, or improved health outcomes.

Because of this apparent overutilization, many experts believe that the opportunity exists to simultaneously improve quality and decrease costs.

Most other industrialized countries routinely use CEA to improve the value of medical care, decreasing both inappropriate underutilization and overutilization.

Supporting Evidence: While rising healthcare costs are the major driver for the recent healthcare reform initiative, an additional major cause of concern for payers and policy makers is that much of the healthcare spending is not contributing to improved health outcomes. Awareness of this possibility was first raised by Dr. John Wennberg and his group at Dartmouth Medical Center. Beginning in the 1970s, Wennberg and his colleagues demonstrated that Medicare spending varied considerably by region (19). This finding naturally led to questions of appropriateness of care and medical spending, which has been summed up by Princeton health economist Uwe Reinhardt, who asks, "How can it be that 'the best medical care in the world' costs twice as much as the best medical care in the world?" (20). Further research has shown that this variation cannot be adequately explained by illness severity, cost of living, quality of care, or improved health outcomes. Fisher found that, at the regional level, increased spending on healthcare is actually associated with *worse* health outcomes (21). Because of this apparent overutilization, many experts believe that the opportunity exists to simultaneously improve quality and decrease costs. Peter Orszag, then the director of the Congressional Budget Office, stated in 2008 that "researchers have estimated that nearly 30% of Medicare's costs could be saved without negatively affecting health outcomes if spending in high- and medium-cost areas could be reduced to the level in low-cost areas – and those estimates could probably be extrapolated to the health care system as a whole" (22). In other words, the US healthcare system does not necessarily need to look to foreign countries for examples of how to decrease costs, but can look at regions within its own borders.

The causes for the wide variation in healthcare expenditures have been elusive. The factor which seems to best explain variation in healthcare utilization is capacity (21). The most reliable way to predict the per capita healthcare expenditures in a region is to measure the per capita availability of hospital beds, specialists, and capital equipment. The other predictor, which is more difficult to measure, is the local "culture." In other words, in terms of recommending more office visits, ordering more tests, and directing longer hospital admissions, physicians tend to behave similarly to other physicians in his or her region (23). These are likely highly correlated with one another and neither is especially surprising to many authors, given the current reimbursement environment that financially rewards increased utilization, punishes decreased utilization, and virtually ignores quality and appropriateness of care (21).

Not only does the system reward more care rather than better care, it is further flawed in that physicians and physician groups are rewarded for working alone and in competition rather than as members of cooperative teams. It is not surprising that the result is an expensive, fragmented health care system. In an article in *The New Yorker* magazine in June 2009, Atul Gawande (24) likens the provision of health care to the building of a house in which the electrician, plumber, and carpenter are paid for each outlet, faucet and cabinet they install, without a subcontractor to oversee the project. You would not be surprised, he contends, if the final product resulted in a home containing "a thousand outlets, faucets, and cabinets, at three times the cost you expected, and the whole thing fell apart a couple of years later." This lack of coordination remains a major problem, he argues, no matter how competent the providers are or who pays for their work.

From the perspective of the federal government and other US payers, misaligned provider incentives result in inappropriate overutilization of care much more often than inappropriate underutilization. However, some screening procedures and other public health initiatives are inappropriately underutilized, even though they have proven to be cost-effective. For example, mammographic screening has a very competitive cost-effectiveness ratio (CER) of $10,000–$25,000 per quality adjusted life-years; interventions with a CER of less than $100,000 are generally considered to be worthwhile. However, utilization rates of mammography are only 50–70% (1). Osteoporosis screening has similar CER, but even lower implementation of 35% (1).

Most other industrialized countries routinely use CEA to improve the value of medical care, decreasing both inappropriate underutilization and overutilization (1) (see Chap. 1). However the Center for Medicare and Medicaid Services (CMS) has deliberately avoided CEA, largely due to political considerations. Nevertheless, as we will discuss later in this chapter, this is likely to change with recently enacted healthcare reform legislation.

V. How Does Supplier-Driven Demand Influence Imaging Utilization?

Summary of Evidence: From 2001 to 2006, the volume of CT imaging performed at in-office facilities owned by radiologists rose by 85%. The volume of imaging performed at in-office facilities in which nonradiologist referring clinicians had a financial stake rose by 263% (25).

Supporting Evidence: One of the most obvious examples of so-called supplier-driven demand, where the sales of goods or services are highly influenced by the seller, occurs when physicians refer patients for imaging in which the same physician stands to gain financially from the imaging study. Radiologists refer to this as "self-referral." It has been a recognized conflict of interest for many years, and legislation has been enacted to prevent this from occurring (known as Stark laws). However, imaging performed in the physician's own office is exempted from the restriction. Imaging volume in these offices has increased substantially in the past few years. For example, from 2001 to 2006, while the volume of CT imaging performed at in-office facilities owned by radiologists rose by 85%, it rose by 263% in facilities owned by nonradiologists (25). Another study showed that physicians who referred patients to themselves or those of the same specialty were up to twice as likely to refer a patient for imaging as those who referred patients to radiologists (26). The June 2009 Medicare Payment Advisory Commission (MedPAC) report to Congress found that self-referring physicians ordered between 5 and 104% more imaging than nonself-referring physicians (27).

Not surprisingly, self-referral is a controversial issue. The issue of self-referral has been a focus of discussion by the ACR leaders on Capitol Hill for years, but no significant changes have occurred in regulations. Self-referral has typically been viewed by lawmakers as a turf-battle between radiologists and other imaging providers. The Patient Protection and Affordable Care Act only indirectly addresses self-referral, with a provision that requires physicians to inform patients that they may obtain imaging services from other providers and to supply patients with a list of such providers (28).

While it is unclear whether self-referral will be more regulated in the near future, judging from the number of times the subject has been highlighted in recent policy reports and major news articles, it at least has gained increasing attention by lawmakers. An entire report from the Government Accountability Office (GAO) in June 2008 was dedicated to the subject, which urged CMS to consider further expansion of imaging management practices or utilization of intermediary companies to restrict overutilization (29). Private insurers have already realized the role of self-referral in increased utilization and, through radiology benefit management (RBM) companies, are beginning to limit self-referral, which may obviate the need for further legislative action (30).

VI. What Can Be Learned from "High-Value" Systems?

Summary of Evidence: Whatever their organizational structure, so-called accountable care organizations (ACOs) tend to have certain elements in common: physicians and hospitals tend to have a close working relationship, most of them use electronic medical record systems to track and improve care, and they generally encourage a culture of restrained spending and collaboration with competitors for the benefit of patients.

Supporting Evidence: Historically, research on variation in care has highlighted examples of overuse of healthcare services, like self-referred imaging. However, by documenting variation, researchers at Dartmouth and elsewhere recently have begun to highlight regions that consistently demonstrate improved health outcomes at lower costs than the national average. Increasing attention has been paid to these regions to discover how they are able to achieve such remarkable results. The theme that commonly resurfaces is that they are dominated by groups of clinicians who work together in a cooperative way to study and systematically improve care from the perspective of the patient. Elliott Fisher has termed these types of organizations "ACOs" (31). They may be highly organized into an integrated delivery system, like the Mayo Clinic in Rochester, or they may be a community of unaffiliated care providers like that in Grand Junction, Colorado (32).

Whatever their organizational structure, these groups of providers tend to have certain elements in common: physicians and hospitals tend to have a close working relationship, most of them use electronic medical record systems to track and improve care, and they generally encourage a culture of restrained spending and collaboration with competitors for the benefit of patients. They also are dominated by non-profit health systems (33).

Under the fee-for-service system, organizations that achieve improved outcomes at lower costs often do so at their own financial peril. For example, large investments that improve coordination of care, like implementation of a multi hundred-million-dollar electronic medical record system, have been borne by the hospital or health system. When physicians choose to avoid unnecessary imaging and procedures, they forgo the potential income. And when hospitals work together to discharge patients sooner, arranging better postdischarge care, resulting in decreased readmission rates, all of the savings are retained by the payer, and lost to the care provider (24). Hence, the fee-for-service payment structure incentivizes behavior that is not necessarily optimal for the patient.

VII. Cost-Control Strategies: Rationing Versus Reducing Inappropriate Care

Summary of Evidence: The two main thrusts of policy makers' efforts are (1) to pay for appropriate care that, based on the evidence, is most likely to improve health outcomes, and (2) to encourage providers to work more closely together to make sure that evidence-based care is provided consistently and efficiently. Ideas that are taking root include decreasing reimbursement, using third parties to help decrease inappropriate imaging, and changing the reimbursement incentive structure.

Supporting Evidence: Spiraling healthcare costs in the face of budget constraints have finally pushed lawmakers to tackle this issue legislatively. While this is not the first attempt at healthcare cost control, it differs in significant ways from prior attempts. Policy makers have realized that simply limiting access to healthcare or attempting to pay providers less for the same service is not politically palatable, does nothing to address inefficiencies in the system, and is not sustainable. While across-the-board reimbursement cuts are likely to be used in some cases, policy makers are beginning to realize the perversity of the financial incentives inherent in the current reimbursement structure and are seeking payment systems that reward appropriate care and discourage inappropriate care (22).

In general, the two main thrusts of their efforts are (1) to pay for appropriate care that, based on the evidence, is most likely to improve health outcomes, and (2) to encourage providers to work more closely together to make sure that evidence-based care is provided consistently and efficiently. While there are many ideas circulating regarding how to accomplish these objectives as they relate to imaging, ideas that are taking root include decreasing reimbursement, using third parties to help decrease inappropriate imaging, and changing the reimbursement incentive structure.

A. Reimbursement Cuts

In its annual report to Congress in March 2009, MedPAC specifically examined reimbursement rates for diagnostic imaging. While recognizing the rapid technological progress in diagnostic imaging which enables physicians to more rapidly and precisely diagnose and treat illness, the Commission expressed concern that "the rapid volume growth of costly imaging services over the past several years may signal that they are mispriced" (29).

CMS reimburses providers separately for performing imaging studies (technical component) and interpreting the studies (professional component). The technical component is generally larger than the professional component, often much larger; for example, for MRI of the brain, the technical component accounts for 88% and the professional component accounts for 12% of the total reimbursement. Under a fee-for-service arrangement, a practice is reimbursed according to the volume of imaging performed. Therefore, once a practice has invested in a scanner, it has a strong incentive to perform as many scans as possible to recoup the investment and then to make a profit. MedPAC argues that the technical component for expensive services such as MRI and CT scans likely are too high, encouraging practices that would otherwise have insufficient volume to justify purchasing a scanner to make the investment and over-utilize it. The Commission believes that, if the reimbursement were lowered, fewer scanners would be purchased, decreasing the pressure for overutilization.

Part of CMS' decision regarding how much to reimburse practices and institutions for direct costs of the technical component was based on how much of the time the equipment was estimated to be utilized. CMS set rates based on the estimation that equipment is utilized 25 h/week. MedPAC states in its report that this estimate was not based on empirical data and is not accurate (29). In 2006, MedPAC sponsored a survey that found that CT scanners are in operation an average of 42 h/week (median 40 h) and MRI scanners 52 h/week (median 46 h). In order to discourage the purchase of excessive equipment, MedPAC recommended that the equipment-use factor be changed. This was incorporated into the Patient Protection and Affordable Care Act (28), which changed the utilization factor from one based on 25 h/week to one based on 37.5 h/week (28). This has the effect of decreasing the technical component by 33% as soon as the provision takes effect on January 1, 2011.

The act also decreases continuous body part reimbursement. Currently, when an imaging study is performed on two continuous body parts, the technical component of the examinations is discounted by 25%. Under the new law, this discount will be increased to 50% (28). This continues a trend of recent reimbursement cuts and limitations, including those imposed under the Deficit Reduction Act of 2005, recent imaging-based RVU adjustments, and Medicare conversion factor changes (34).

B. Intermediaries (RBM Organizations)

Responding to escalating costs, many payers have contracted with third-party RBM organizations that assist in decreasing inappropriate utilization on a case-by-case basis. The RBM model is derived from the pharmacy benefit management programs that emerged in the 1990s to control the growth of spending on prescription medications. RBM programs attempt to limit overutilization of imaging in a variety of ways. For more expensive imaging procedures, most RBMs utilize prior authorization to approve or deny payment on the basis of predetermined criteria. RBM organizations also may grant privileges to physicians and sites based on training and equipment, especially for in-office imaging. Many RBMs establish their own network of imaging providers, independently negotiating discounts with and processing medical claims from physicians and physician groups and then passing on those discounts and claims to the payer. RBM organizations also evaluate the practice patterns of ordering clinicians compared to a standard or benchmark and provide feedback and incentives to change ordering behavior (27).

RBM organizations have been effective in controlling imaging utilization and associated costs (35, 36), making the model an extremely attractive option for payers and regulators. To the extent that they are able to do this using evidence-based guidelines makes them even more attractive. The model gives payers an option to decrease spending by decreasing inappropriate utilization rather than cutting reimbursement rates (29).

The American College of Radiology (ACR) has responded to the growth of such organizations by issuing a set of best practices guidelines for the organizations (37). The report calls for judicious use of preauthorization (including an after-hours approval process), simplification of administrative processes, and transparency of decision-making and reporting procedures. The ACR does not, however, endorse the RBM model; rather, it believes that cost and quality goals can be reached through alternative processes, including order entry decision support and referring physician education, without the added administrative complexity of third-party RBM organizations.

Despite the position of the ACR, payers are increasingly embracing the RBM model. In 2007, at least five major firms provided RBM service in the USA, covering an estimated 88 million persons (36). In a 2008 report, the GAO recommended that CMS either adopt practices used by RBMs, including privileging and prior authorization, or simply contract with RBM companies directly (29). This was not included in the healthcare reform act, but, as we will see, this could very quickly become a reality without the approval of congress.

The RBM model is likely to have a mixed effect on individual radiologists. On one hand, RBM organizations constitute an extra layer of administration between the ordering physician and the radiologist. On the other hand, if using an RBM leads to more consistent use of evidence-based ordering practices, then this loss of individual control may be worth the potential to decrease costs in a way that is not detrimental to health outcomes. At the same time, RBM organizations provide an infrastructure for limiting inappropriate imaging by prospectively applying evidence in individual cases. RBM organizations also are able to objectively argue against costly self-referral practices – an argument that is often perceived as turf protection when delivered by radiologists (30).

RBM organizations are likely to increase in prevalence, at least in the short run. Radiologists have essentially three options for dealing with RBM growth: do nothing with the hope that market forces will naturally encourage RBM organizations to behave in patients' best interest (which is not inconceivable); attempt to replicate the functions of RBM organizations (preventing their penetration into local markets) through processes such as computerized physician order entry and physician feedback; and either form partnerships with RBM organizations that are more receptive to radiologists' input or become involved with the selection of an RBM organization before the decision is made for them. Active opposition to the RBM model without a viable alternative is not likely to be successful at this point, given the track record of decreasing costs and the level of market penetration already achieved by RBM organizations.

C. Accountable Care Organizations

The idea of the ACO was first proposed in 2006 (31) and was included in expanded form in MedPAC's annual report to Congress in 2009 (27). The overall objective is to find a way to provide financial incentives for greater cooperation between physician groups and hospitals by rewarding them for minimizing cost increases and maintaining quality. As proposed by MedPAC, each ACO would be centered around an individual hospital or local hospital network. Primary care physicians and specialists would be assigned to the same ACO as the hospital caring for most of their patients. The size of the organization might range from a single hospital with local physicians to a large hospital network and affiliated physician groups. The relationships could also vary, from unaffiliated physician groups and hospitals to staff-model integrated delivery systems. Regardless of the affiliation, the ACO would need to meet two criteria: have a minimum number of patients – in order to distinguish improvement from random variation, MedPAC recommends a minimum of 5,000 patients – and have a formal organizational structure that would allow it to make decisions regarding capacity. Once the ACO is recognized, each member would accept joint responsibility for the quality and cost of care received by the ACO's panel of patients.

The underlying philosophy of the ACO is that organizations should share in the savings when they make appropriate utilization decisions that save costs and preserve quality of care. MedPAC proposed that 80% of those savings be given to the organizations and 20% be retained by Medicare. A fixed dollar amount of spending growth targets would be established for all organizations. A bonus would be allotted to physicians and hospitals in those ACOs with lower than average spending increases (27). The MedPAC report provides an example of a low-use, average-use, and high-use ACO with baseline spending per capita of $7,000, $10,000, and $12,000, respectively. Each would be given an allowance for growth of $500. Therefore, in order to meet the spending targets, they would need to spend less than $7,500, $10,500, and $12,500 per beneficiary, respectively. This is a percent increase of 7.1, 5.0, and 4.2%, respectively. As shown in the example, while the opportunity to meet the spending-target is equal from the perspective of dollar growth, the low-use ACO enjoys an advantage from the perspective of percentage growth.

The ACO model attempts to balance the incentives of capitation and fee-for-service plans. A major criticism of the capitation plans common in the 1990s was that they created incentives for providers and hospitals to underutilize services since spending for care financially penalized the provider, regardless of necessity. On the other hand, the currently predominant fee-for-service model incentivizes overutilization, with reimbursement dependent on the volume of services provided. The ACO model combines elements of both capitation and fee-for-service, with additional rewards for provision of evidence-based care.

The MedPAC report entertains both voluntary and mandatory participation models for ACOs. Voluntary participation would be more politically palatable, but may be less incentivizing, as physician and hospital groups may enroll with little intention of changing behavior, hoping that they happen to meet the spending targets based on their current practice.

In addition to spending targets, ACOs would also need to meet quality targets. Initially, these would be based on process measures, with more limited outcomes measures. Eventually, outcomes measures would be incorporated, which might include mortality rates, avoidable hospital admissions, readmissions, patient satisfaction, etc. A weighted quality score would likely be established, and the ACO would need to meet the target to be eligible for the bonus. Quality measures would likely include assessments of how well their organizations adhere to evidence-based guidelines. Rather than micromanage utilization behavior, the objective of the ACO structure is to provide incentives for the practice of evidence-based medicine at the level at which clinicians make decisions – at the local, regional, or health system level – and let the clinicians and hospitals work together to determine how to make it happen. The desired result is that when clinicians and hospitals work together to provide the best care for the lowest cost, the care will naturally become more evidence-based.

The Patient Protection and Affordable Care Act provides for the establishment of ACO pilot projects by organizations that meet certain criteria. If they meet cost and quality criteria, they will share in the Medicare savings averaged over a 3-year period (28).

VIII. How Is the Recently Passed US Healthcare Reform Initiative Expected to Influence Cost and Quality?

Summary of Evidence: The US healthcare reform statute has two main priorities: to expand coverage and control costs. While the coverage provisions of the act have received the majority

of the attention in the press, the second priority of the statute, that of cost control, probably has more potential to affect radiologists and other physicians.

The Patient Protection and Affordable Care Act provides for the establishment of a large number of demonstration projects and initiatives that will be carried out over the next few years.

The question of whether the provisions contained in the Patient Protection and Affordable Care Act will go forward likely depend to a great extent on the current administration's ability to execute its provisions.

Supporting Evidence: Concepts of simultaneous cost control have played a prominent role in the Patient Protection and Affordable Care Act signed into law on March 30, 2010. It was passed by a narrow majority in the US Congress after more than a year of bitter partisan politics, having been nearly defeated on several occasions. It represents a considerable political risk on the part of the President and Democratic lawmakers; it is now in their interest to make it work.

The statute has two main priorities: to expand coverage and control costs. The Democrats felt that it was important to expand coverage first, since without that protection, cost-control mechanisms would likely exclude large elements of the population. The statute expands coverage through a variety of mechanisms, including health insurance exchanges, penalties for nonparticipants, assistance for low-income individuals, increases in insurance oversight, and expansion of Medicaid (28). While the coverage provisions of the act have received the majority of the attention in the press, the second priority of the statute, that of cost control, probably has more potential to affect radiologists and other physicians.

A. Learning What Works

The cost-control provisions reflect the desire to move beyond across-the-board reimbursement cuts and to change the incentive structure to one that rewards quality rather than quantity. However, there are few examples of practical ways to accomplish this. Therefore, the Act provides for the establishment of a large number of demonstration projects and initiatives that will be carried out over the next few years. Examples are listed in Table 4.1.

Most of these projects and initiatives will involve a limited number of healthcare networks, providers, and patients at first. However, evidence gathered from these projects will guide implementation of changes that will affect a broader cross-section of the US population. Therefore, while the effects of cost-control initiatives are not likely to be felt immediately, after a few years of study, we may witness waves of sweeping changes driven by research that is currently getting underway.

B. Coming Changes

A comprehensive discussion of the projects and initiatives included in the PPACA is beyond the scope of this chapter. Several of these provisions have already been discussed. One more deserves special attention: the Independent Payment Advisory Board (IPAB).

The IPAB provision was a relatively low-profile element of PPACA that has high potential impact on the future of the US healthcare system. In 1997, Congress established the MedPAC and tasked them with advising Congress on issues affecting Medicare, primarily dealing with access, cost, and quality (28). MedPAC has provided many recommendations to Congress since that time. However, once they are put before Congress, they are subjected to political processes that make it difficult to enact the unpopular changes that are often put forth. Having witnessed this for over a decade, authors of the healthcare reform act saw the need for a body that not only was independent of Congress, but whose recommendations could be insulated from the political process.

The IPAB will be made up of 15 members, nominated by the president and confirmed by Congress to 6-year terms. Beginning in 2014, any year in which the Medicare per capita financial growth rates exceed targeted rates (which is likely to occur most years), the Board will be required to recommend Medicare spending reductions. These recommendations will automatically become law unless Congress passes an alternative. Furthermore, the president can veto Congress' alternative. While the board has some limitations – it may not recommend provisions that ration care, raise taxes or beneficiary premiums, or change Medicare benefits, eligibility, or cost-sharing standards – it may have significant authority to quickly enact politically charged changes needed to control costs.

C. Political Outlook

The Patient Protection and Affordable Care Act is widely considered to be one of the most sweeping, but politically divisive, US legislative initiative in decades. Legal challenges to several provisions in the law have already begun to mount. However, most experts feel that such challenges are unlikely to prevent the statute from being implemented. Most of the beneficial provisions take effect relatively soon, while implementation of many of the controversial decisions has been intentionally delayed. The authors of the statute hope that this will help garner political support for the act before legal or legislative challenges can overturn it (38).

Given the current political makeup of Congress, it is unlikely that the bill will be overturned legislatively any time soon. Even if opponents of the bill, who are currently dominated by "Tea-Party" Republicans, were able to overturn the statute, they would essentially be taking upon themselves the task of controlling escalating healthcare costs that dominate the US budget deficit. After witnessing the political damage inflicted on the Democratic Party, it is unlikely serious cost-control efforts will be taken up by anyone in Congress any time soon. Therefore, the question of whether the provisions contained in the Act will go forward likely depend to a great extent on the current administration's ability to execute its provisions.

IX. What Are the Challenges and Opportunities for Evidence-Based Imaging?

Summary of Evidence: The common element of nearly all of the concepts discussed in this chapter is a desire to encourage and enable the use of evidence-based medical care and to discourage use of care that is not evidence-based. Policy makers have learned that it is not sustainable to enforce blunt cuts in reimbursement and services, and have placed their faith in what they have been told by quality and evidence-based practiced advocates – that we can both decrease costs and improve healthcare quality at the same time.

The challenge has been issued to the medical community, including radiology, to move EBI from a theory or a collection of anecdotes to one that can be effectively implemented on a broad scale.

Supporting Evidence: While it may not be obvious now, these developments provide a significant opportunity for the advancement of evidence-based medicine. The common element of nearly all of the concepts discussed in this chapter is a desire to encourage and enable the use of evidence-based medical care and to discourage use of care that is not evidence-based. Policy makers have learned that it is not sustainable to enforce blunt cuts in reimbursement and services, and have placed their faith in what they have been told by quality and evidence-based practiced advocates – that we can both decrease costs and improve healthcare quality at the same time. The next few years will provide an opportunity for organizations to demonstrate whether that can be achieved. The challenge has been issued to the medical community, including radiology, to move EBI from a theory or a collection of anecdotes to one that can be effectively implemented on a broad scale. This will require research to determine how to do this effectively. In other words, wide adoption of EBI will require evidence-based EBI implementation.

Relative to other specialties, radiology finds itself in a favorable position. The ACR has taken a role in terms of evidence-based image utilization with the ACR Appropriateness Criteria®. These are a set of guidelines that were developed to assist referring physicians and other providers in making the most appropriate imaging or treatment decision. While they have their shortcomings, they constitute a relatively objective and comprehensive set of criteria that can serve as the basis for local implementation of image utilization (39, 40). For example, Appropriateness Criteria® are established through committee consensus through the modified Delphi process – a valuable technique for group decision making (41). However, consensus methodology renders the distillation of evidence susceptible to political influences. Nevertheless, although the Appropriateness Criteria are not formed through accepted EBI methods, a critical review of the evidence forms the basis for many of the panel recommendations. The evidence tables and narrative literature reviews prepared by the panel leaders thus constitute a valuable starting point for EBI (42). Furthermore, what the Appropriateness Criteria lack in depth

they make up for in breadth, covering over 170 topics (42). The appropriateness criteria have been incorporated into at least some RBM algorithms (30) and into the computerized physician order entry system of at least one large academic medical center, with resultant decreased growth in utilization of imaging (43).

An alternative method for guideline generation is that used by the National Institute for Clinical Evidence, whereby EBM experts develop the guidelines, and stakeholders from different groups are permitted to provide input. The final guidelines reflect the stakeholder input only at the discretion of the guideline developers (41). With few exceptions, imaging strategies recommended by most radiology textbooks do not incorporate accepted EBI methodology. The purpose of this text is to provide systematic reviews of clinical issues in imaging, presenting concise summaries of the best imaging choices for patient care, along with evaluations of the strength of the evidence (42).

Government and private payers are likely to continue to encourage incorporation of such criteria, guidelines, and protocols into local healthcare information systems. Under such a financial incentive structure, those providing and interpreting imaging services are likely to be in a better financial position if they follow evidence-based guidelines. One could argue that radiologists are at an advantage in that, since they only rarely refer patients for imaging, radiologists themselves are rarely the direct cause of overutilization.

As these initiatives move forward, radiologists have an opportunity to take a strong position locally and nationally in promoting the use of EBI. On a national level, the simultaneous efforts of radiology researchers in investigating the effects of self-referral on image utilization with the development of evidence-based appropriateness criteria place radiologists in a favorable light as an interested but relatively objective party. By continuing to develop the evidence base and continually refining imaging criteria, radiology can continue to be a recognized national leader in this regard.

A similar opportunity exists at the local level. Financial incentive structures are likely to move increasingly toward rewarding radiologists who actively cooperate with other physicians to implement evidence-based guidelines and ordering systems in local health networks. Radiology groups who are active in promoting such guidelines and implementing such systems within their own hospitals are likely to be prepared for such an evolution. However, they may find it difficult spending the time and effort on such activities that do not provide direct reimbursement in the short run. Even simple efforts such as standardization of imaging protocols and increased coordination with ordering clinicians are likely to be well-received as financial incentives increasingly move toward rewarding a more teams- and evidence-based practice of medicine.

Take Home Tables and Figures

Table 4.1 and Figs. 4.1–4.2 serve to highlight key recommendations and supporting evidence.

Table 4.1. Examples of demonstration projects and initiatives included in the Patient Protection and Affordable Care Act

Establishment of an independent payment advisory board
Extension of the physician quality reporting initiative (PQRI) through 2014
Establishment of a national strategy to improve health care delivery, patient outcomes, and population health
Interagency working group on health care quality convened by the President
Establishment of a center for Medicare & medicaid innovation
Accountable care organizations (ACOs) demonstration projects
Bundled payments demonstration projects
Medical home demonstration projects
Medicare value-based purchasing program for hospitals
Preventable Medicare readmissions adjustment
Reimbursement adjustments for imaging services and power-driven wheelchairs
Medicare advantage (MA) quality bonus payments
Medicare hospital productivity adjustment
Establishment of a health delivery-system research center
Use of medication management services
Establishment of a patient-centered outcomes research institute
Uniform standards for financial and administrative health care transactions

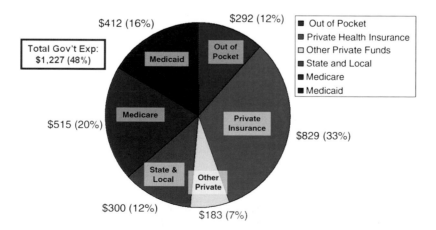

Figure 4.1. Source of payment of US health expenditures, 2010. Source: created from data at http://www.cms.gov/NationalHealthExpendData/downloads/proj2009.pdf

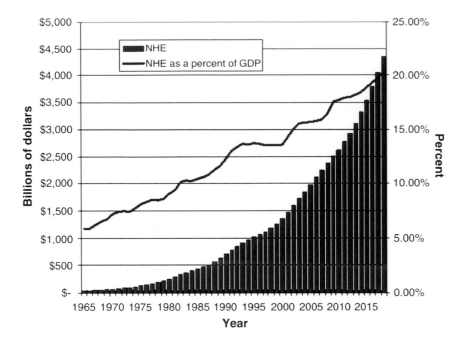

Figure 4.2. National Health Expenditures, in dollars and as a percent of GDP. Data for 2008 and greater are projections. Source: created from data from (44) and (45)

References

1. Neumann PJ, Rosen AB, Weinstein MC. N Engl J Med 2005;353(14):1516–1522.
2. Kaiser Family Foundation, Kaiser Commission on Medicaid and the Uninsured. The Uninsured: A Primer, October 2008.
3. http://www.cms.gov/NationalHealthExpend Data/downloads/proj2009.pdf.
4. World Health Organization. World Health Statistics, 2009.
5. http://www.whitehouse.gov/the_press_office/ Remarks-by-the-President-in-AARP-Tele-Town-Hall-on-Health-Care-Reform/.
6. Chernew ME, Hirth RA, Cutler DM. Health Aff (Millwood) 2009;28(5):1253–1255.
7. Executive Office of the President of the United States. The Economic Case for Health Care Reform, 2009, http://www.whitehouse.gov/ assets/documents/CEA_Health_Care_Report. pdf [accessed September 30, 2009].
8. Davis K et al. Slowing the Growth of U.S. Health Care Expenditures: What are the Options? The Commonwealth Fund, January 2007. http:// www.commonwealthfund.org/usr_doc/Davis_ slowinggrowthUShltcareexpenditureswhatare-options_989.pdf.
9. United States Department of Labor Website. Databases, Tables & Calculators by Subject. Bureau of Labor Statistics. http://www.bls.gov/ data/inflation_calculator.htm [accessed September 30, 2009].
10. Population Estimates Program. United States Census Bureau, 2000. http://www.census.gov/ popest/archives/1990s/popclockest.txt [accessed September 30, 2009].
11. Office of the Press Secretary, the White House. Remarks by the President to a Joint Session of Congress on Health Care, September 9, 2009. White House Website. http://www. whitehouse.
12. Polsky D, Grande D. N Engl J Med 2009;361(5): 437–439.
13. Milliman I. Milliman Medical Index 2009, 2009. http://www.milliman.com/expertise/healthcare/ products-tools/mmi/pdfs/milliman-medical-index-2009.pdf.
14. Anderson GF. Health Aff (Millwood) 2007;26(3): 780–789.
15. Himmelstein DU et al. Am J Med 2009;122(8): 741–746.
16. Robertson CT, Egelhof R, Hoke M. Health Matrix: J Law Med 2008;18(1):65–104.
17. Publications A. Status of the Social Security and Medicare Programs. Social Security Online, 2009. http://www.ssa.gov/OACT/TRSUM/index. html [accessed September 30, 2009].
18. Administration of Barack H. Obama. Remarks at the White House Forum on Health Reform. GPO Access Website. http://www.gpoaccess.gov/ presdocs/2009/DCPD200900130.pdf [accessed November 11, 2009].
19. The Dartmouth Institute for Health Policy and Clinical Practice. Q&A with Dr. Jack Wennberg.

http://www.dartmouthatlas.org/press/ Wennberg_interviews_DartMed.pdf [accessed September 30, 2009].

20. Kolata G. Sharp Regional Incongruity Found in Medical Costs and Treatments. The New York Times on the Web, January 30, 1996. http://www.nytimes.com/specials/women/warchive/960130_1576.html.

21. Fisher ES. J Am Coll Radiol 2007;4(12):879–885.

22. Orszag P. Opportunities to Increase Efficiency in Health Care. Congressional Budget Office, 2008. http://finance.senate.gov/healthsummit2008/Statements/Peter%20Orszag.pdf [accessed September 30, 2009].

23. Sirovich B et al. Health Aff (Millwood) 2008;27(3):813–823.

24. Gawande A. The Cost Conundrum. The New Yorker 2009:11.

25. Levin DC et al. J Am Coll Radiol 2008;5(12):1206–1209.

26. Gazelle GS et al. Radiology 2007;245(2):517–522.

27. Hackbarth G. Report to Congress: Improving Incentives in the Medicare Program. Medicare Payment Advisory Commission (MedPAC) Report to Congress, 2009. http://www.MedicarePayment Advisory Commission (MedPAC).gov/documents/Jun09_EntireReport.pdf.

28. H.R. 3590: Patient Protection and Affordable Care Act, 111th Congress, 2009–2010.

29. G U.S. Government Accountability Office. Medicare Part B Imaging Services: Rapid Spending Growth and Shift to Physician Offices Indicate Need for CMS to Consider Additional Management Practices. Washington, DC: U.S. Government Accountability Office, 2008. http://www.gao.gov/new.items/d08452.pdf [accessed November 11, 2009].

30. Farnsworth C. Personal Communication, September 29, 2009.

31. Fisher ES et al. Health Aff (Millwood) 2007;26(1):w44–w57.

32. Nichols L, Weinberg M, Barnes J. Grand Junction, Colorado: A Health Community That Works. New America Foundation, 2009. http://www.newamerica.net/files/GrandJunctionCOHealth CommunityWorks.pdf [accessed September 30, 2009].

33. Galewitz P. Local Hospitals and Doctors Join Forces to Improve Health Care, Restrain Costs. Kaiser Health News, 2009. http://www.kaiserhealthnews.org/Stories/2009/July/22/Hospital.aspx.

34. Hackbarth G. Report to the Congress: Medicare Payment Policy, 2009. http://www.MedicarePaymentAdvisoryCommission(MedPAC).gov/documents/Mar09_March%20report%20testimony_WM%20FINAL.pdf.

35. Senate Committee on Finance. America's Healthy Future Act of 2009 [Chairman's Mark], September 22, 2009. http://finance.senate.gov/sitepages/leg/LEG%202009/091609%20Americas_Healthy_ Future_Act.pdf [accessed September 30, 2009].

36. Mitchell JM, Lagalia RR. Med Care Res Rev 2009;66(3):339–351.

37. American College of Radiology and Radiology Business Management Association. Best practices Guidelines on Radiology Benefits Management Programs. Reston, VA: American College of Radiology, January 24, 2009. http://www.acr.

38. Farrington B. "White House, Experts: Health Care Suit Will Fail". The San Diego Union-Tribune. Associated Press, March 23, 2010. http://www.signonsandiego.com/news/2010/mar/23/white-house-experts-health-care-suit-will-fail/ [accessed April 7, 2010].

39. Blackmore CC, Medina LS. Evidence-Based Radiology and the ACR Appropriateness Criteria. J Am Coll Radiol 2006;3(7):505–509.

40. Bettmann MA. J Am Coll Radiol 2006;3(7):510–512.

41. Blackmore CC, Medina LS. J Am Coll Radiol 2006;3:505–509.

42. Medina LS, Blackmore CC. Radiology 2007;244(2):331–336.

43. Sistrom CL et al. Radiology 2009;251(1):147–155.

44. Centers for Medicare and Medicaid Services, U.S. Department of Health and Human Services. National Health Expenditure Projections: Forecast Summary 2008–2018. Baltimore, MD: Centers for Medicare and Medicaid Services, 2008. http://www.cms.hhs.gov/NationalHealthExpendData/downloads/proj2008.pdf. [accessed September 30, 2009].

45. Center for Medicare and Medicaid Services, National Health Expenditure Data. "NHE Historical and Projections, 1965–2018 (ZIP, 32 KB)". https://www.cms.gov/NationalHealthExpendData/03_NationalHealthAccounts Projected.asp [accessed September 30, 2009].

Part II

Oncologic Imaging

5

Breast Imaging

Laurie L. Fajardo, Wendie A. Berg, and Robert A. Smith

Mammography Screening

I. How effective is mammographic screening?
II. Who should undergo screening?
III. How frequently should women be screened?
IV. How cost-effective is mammographic screening?

Breast Ultrasound

V. How should ultrasound be applied to breast cancer screening?
VI. How accurate is ultrasound in evaluating palpable breast masses?
VII. How accurate is ultrasound in evaluating nipple discharge?
VIII. How accurate is ultrasound in determining local extent of disease?

Diagnosis of Nonpalpable Breast Cancer by Percutaneous Image-Guided Biopsy

IX. Which lesions (BIRADS 1–6) should undergo biopsy?
    A. Special case: radial sclerosing lesions (radial scars)
X. What is the performance of percutaneous image-guided breast biopsy compared with standard surgical excisional biopsy?
XI. What type of imaging guidance is best suited for breast lesions that manifest as masses or as microcalcifications?
    A. Special case: biopsy of breast lesions detected on breast MRI
XII. How cost-effective is image-guided biopsy?

Issues

L.L. Fajardo (✉)
Department of Radiology, University of Iowa Hospitals and Clinics, University of Iowa
Carver College of Medicine, 200 Hawkins Drive, 3966 JPP, Iowa City, IA, 52240, USA
e-mail: L-Fajardo@uiowa.edu

L.S. Medina et al. (eds.), *Evidence-Based Imaging: Improving the Quality of Imaging in Patient Care, Revised Edition*,
DOI 10.1007/978-1-4419-7777-9_5, © Springer Science+Business Media, LLC 2011

Mammography

- Prospective randomized controlled trials (RCT) have demonstrated reduced breast cancer mortality of approximately 30% associated with mammography screening (strong evidence).
- Evaluations of mammography screening in community settings have shown greater mortality reductions associated with participating in screening (moderate evidence).
- Women aged 40–54 years should be screened at intervals of 12–18 months in order to achieve similar mortality reductions compared with women who are 55 years of age and older due to faster tumor growth in younger women (moderate evidence).

Ultrasound

- Data from single center studies of screening ultrasound suggest that it has a detection benefit as a supplement to screening mammography in patients with dense (at least 50% of the breast is not fatty) breast parenchyma (moderate evidence).
- Reports from single-institution studies found that a high percentage (91%) of breast cancers identified on supplemental screening sonography are stage I invasive cancers. Detecting this subset of breast cancers is most likely to reduce breast cancer mortality (moderate evidence).
- In patients with dense breast parenchyma, mammography and sonography appear complementary, in that ductal carcinoma in situ (DCIS) is better depicted by mammography and small, <1 cm, invasive breast cancers are better detected sonographically (moderate evidence).
- Women with dense breast parenchyma on mammography, contemplating a supplemental sonographic screening examination, should consider the risk of a false-positive sonogram, possibly resulting in the recommendation for a breast biopsy (moderate evidence).
- Sonography is appropriate in the evaluation of palpable breast masses (moderate evidence).
- Sonography is appropriate in the evaluation of mammographically circumscribed, obscured, or indistinctly marginated masses and focal asymmetries (moderate evidence).
- The combination of mammography and sonography depicts 96–97% of palpable breast cancer and 92% of nonpalpable breast cancer (moderate evidence).
- Sonography can help identify the invasive component of mixed invasive and intraductal carcinoma and guide optimal percutaneous biopsy (limited evidence).
- Sonography is a useful supplement to mammography in depicting the extent of invasive carcinoma in dense breasts (moderate evidence).
- Sonography is useful in the evaluation of the patient with nipple discharge (limited evidence).

Biopsy

- Percutaneous image-guided breast biopsy is not indicated for nonpalpable lesions classified as BIRADS 3. For these lesions, short-term interval follow-up, generally at 6-month intervals, is recommended (strong evidence).

> - For BIRADS 4 and 5 lesions, image-guided percutaneous biopsy is cost-effective as the initial strategy for diagnosing nonpalpable breast lesions (strong evidence).

Pathophysiology and Epidemiology

Breast cancer takes a tremendous toll in the United States. For 2004, the American Cancer Society (ACS) predicted that 217,440 new cases of breast cancer would be diagnosed, and 40,580 individuals would die from the disease (1). Mammographic screening remains controversial, as reflected in greatly varying national policies. The specificity and positive predictive value of mammography are limited because of overlap in the appearance of benign and malignant breast lesions (2–4). However, until research uncovers a way to better cure or prevent breast cancer, early detection is viewed as the best hope for reducing the burden of this disease.

The risk of breast cancer increases with increasing age. A family history of breast cancer confers a variable degree of increased risk. The Gail (5–8), Claus (9), and other models have been developed to calculate a woman's risk of breast cancer primarily as a function of age and family history. The risk of developing breast cancer nearly doubles with a family history of breast cancer in a first-degree relative (10). Women with a personal history of breast cancer, and those with prior biopsies showing atypical ductal hyperplasia (ADH) or atypical lobular hyperplasia (ALH), are at a four- to fivefold increased risk of breast cancer (10). Women with prior lobular carcinoma in situ are also at high risk of breast cancer, with rates of eight- to tenfold than women without such risk (11). Such high-risk women are candidates for chemoprevention with agents such as tamoxifen. The National Surgical Adjuvant Breast and Bowel Project (NSABP) P-1 chemoprevention trial demonstrated that tamoxifen lowered the rate of invasive breast cancer by 49% in women at high risk (12).

Women with a history of prior axillary, chest, or mediastinal irradiation, usually for Hodgkin's disease, are another group at high risk of developing breast cancer. The relative risk of breast cancer is approximately 7-fold in women irradiated at 20–30 years of age and as high as 56-fold if exposure was after puberty and before age 20 (13–15).

The perception of cancer on mammography requires a difference in density compared to surrounding tissue, architectural distortion, or presence of microcalcifications. There are four grades of breast density: fatty (<25% dense), minimal scattered fibroglandular densities (25–50% dense), heterogeneously dense (51–75% dense), and extremely dense (>75% dense) (16). Identification of a mass against a background of equally dense tissue is problematic. In heterogeneously dense and extremely dense breasts, the sensitivity of mammography in several series is under 50% (17–19). Methods to supplement mammography, such as screening breast ultrasound, are being sought in women with dense breasts (>50% dense), and especially those women with higher rates of breast cancer (e.g., high-risk women) with dense breasts.

Ultrasound uses sound waves to penetrate tissue. Differences in the time to reflect the echo back to the transducer are used to create the image. With current high-frequency linear array transducers with a center frequency of 10–12 MHz, detailed images are produced at tissue depths of 0.2–4 cm, with lateral resolution (in effect, slice thickness) of 1 mm or less. The performance of ultrasound in dense breast tissue is equivalent (20) or superior to its performance in fatty breasts.

Biopsy remains the definitive method of confirming the diagnosis of breast cancer, and physicians perform millions of breast biopsies each year. Selecting the most appropriate method of biopsy for each patient has distinct health and economic benefits. Approximately 75% (range 65–86%) of breast abnormalities detected at mammography and referred for biopsy ultimately prove benign histopathologically (2, 21–26). The fact that most breast biopsies are benign necessitates that the method of diagnosis be minimally invasive, have the best possible cosmetic outcome, and have high accuracy.

Overall Cost to Society

The cost of breast cancer to society can never fully be estimated because there are so many dimensions for which measurement in economic and social terms is indefinable. Nonetheless, a common approach to measuring the economic dimension of disease burden is cost-of-illness (COI) methodology, which encompasses direct costs (costs associated with procedures, therapy, and care), morbidity costs (work-related costs associated with disability and absenteeism), and mortality costs (lost income, including the value of household work, due to premature death) (27). Based on previous estimates of the proportion of the direct costs of cancer attributable to breast cancer (27) and current estimates from the National Heart Lung and Blood Institute for the direct costs of all neoplasms (28), in 2004 direct costs of breast cancer were approximately $9.85 billion. This estimate does not include the costs of oral medications, such as tamoxifen, which in 1995 were estimated to be $400 million per year (27), or the annual cost of screening and diagnostic evaluations of women. Since there are no current indirect cost estimates by cancer site, if we assume that indirect costs as a percentage of COI in 2004 are the same for all cancers, then in 2004 the indirect cost of breast cancer was $26.94 billion, for a total COI of approximately $37 billion. The COI for all cancers in 2004 was estimated to be $198.8 billion (28).

Goals

The next section of this chapter is a summary of the evidence supporting the use of mammography to screen for breast cancer. The following section is a compilation of the evidence regarding the use of ultrasound in imaging the breast. Available evidence on the use of ultrasound in a variety of clinical scenarios, including screening, is analyzed and is used to present criteria that physicians can apply to individual patients. The final section is a compilation of the evidence regarding the selection of the method of breast biopsy for patients who have a suspicious nonpalpable breast lesion that should be biopsied. The evidence analyzed addresses nonpalpable lesions only and is used to present criteria that physicians can apply to

these individual patients. By incorporating the evidence into clinical decision making, practitioners can develop personal or organizational guidelines that will assist in choosing the biopsy method that is best for each patient.

Methodology

Medline searches were performed using PubMed (National Library of Medicine, Bethesda, Maryland) for original research publications discussing the diagnostic performance and effectiveness of mammography, breast ultrasound, and imaging-guided percutaneous biopsy of nonpalpable breast lesions. The searches covered the years 1980–2004 (1997–2004 for mammography, 1980–2004 for breast ultrasound, and 1980–2002 for breast biopsy) and were limited to human studies and the English-language literature. The search strategies employed different combinations of the following terms: (1) *breast biopsy*, (2) *stereotactic* OR *ultrasound* OR *imaging guided*, (3) *nonpalpable breast lesion*, (4) *mammography*, (5) *ultrasound* OR *sonography* AND *breast*, (6) *breast screening*, (7) *breast screening guidelines*, (8) *harms and anxiety*, and (9) *cost-effectiveness*. Additional articles were identified by reviewing the reference lists of relevant papers and by including recently published studies not yet indexed in Medline. The authors performed an initial review of the titles and abstracts of the identified articles followed by review of the full text in articles that were relevant.

I. How Effective Is Mammographic Screening?

Summary of Evidence: The fundamental goal of mammographic screening is to reduce the incidence rate of advanced breast cancer by detecting the disease early in its natural history (29). There is strong evidence for the benefit of mammography from a series of prospective RCT and meta-analyses (30–34) and moderate evidence of benefit from institutional-based case series studies (35) and recent evaluations of population-based service screening (36, 37). Results from individual trials showed significant mortality reductions ranging from 22 to

32% (38). A smaller level of benefit is observed in meta-analysis results that combine all trials, due to variability in end results (38, 39). Results from service screening with modern mammography have shown greater mortality reductions (40–50%) among women who participate in regular screening (37, 40).

Supporting evidence: There have been eight prospective RCTs of breast cancer screening. As can be seen in Table 5.1, the first of these studies, the Health Insurance Plan (HIP) of Greater New York Study, was initiated in the early 1960s, while the most recent RCTs were initiated in Canada in 1980 (31, 34, 41–50). Each RCT followed a somewhat different protocol, and the outcome in each has been influenced by a number of design and protocol factors that have important implications for the interpretation of study end results. These factors include the study methodology, the clinical protocol, adherence to the randomization assignment (compliance and contamination), and the number of screening rounds before an invitation was extended to the control group. Other factors that likely influenced end results include the quality of the screening process, thresholds for diagnosis, and follow-up mechanisms for women with an abnormality. Individual RCT results and meta-analysis results should be interpreted in the context of study methodology to demonstrate efficacy rather than a measure of the potential effectiveness of mammography, since the classic intention-to-treat analysis compares breast cancer mortality in a group invited to screening with breast cancer mortality in a group receiving usual care rather than a screened vs. unscreened group. Moreover, variability in RCT outcomes is consistent with the performance of each study's success at reducing the risk of being diagnosed with an advanced breast cancer compared with the control group. Specifically, those RCTs that significantly reduced the risk of being diagnosed with a node-positive breast cancer showed similar reductions in the risk of breast cancer death in the group invited to screening (38, 51).

Over the years, there have been numerous studies reporting the results from the individual RCTs and meta-analyses, although screening policy in the USA began to take shape based on initial findings from the HIP study. The trials now have a substantial amount of follow-up time ranging from 12 to 20 years. In a recent overview of the RCTs, a meta-analysis of the most current data showed an overall relative risk of breast cancer death associated with an invitation to screening of 0.80 [95% confidence interval (CI), 0.75–0.86], with corresponding relative risks of 0.85 (95% CI, 0.73–0.98) for women randomized to an invitation between ages 39 and 49, and 0.78 (95% CI, 0.70–0.85) for women aged 50 years and older at the time of randomization (38). These estimates are lower than some of the individual RCTs, due to RCT variability, and considerably lower than mortality reductions observed in service screening, in large part due to measuring the benefit of an invitation to screening rather than actually being screened.

The breast cancer RCT data have recently undergone several independent reevaluations for the purpose of updating screening guidelines (33, 39, 52), and several evidence-based reviews (42, 53–56). A recent review by the Cochrane Collaboration was sharply critical of the RCTs that had shown a benefit from mammographic screening, and concluded that there was insufficient evidence to recommend screening with mammography (53). Representatives from the RCTs and others responded to these criticisms and showed them to be either incorrect, inconsequential, or, if true, previously and satisfactorily addressed by the authors in original publications (34, 50, 55, 57–61). Although the RCTs of breast cancer screening had some shortcomings, there is widespread agreement that they have provided solid and valid evidence regarding the efficacy of early breast cancer detection with mammography (42).

As noted above, while the breast cancer screening RCTs demonstrated the efficacy of screening, they provide a less clear measure of the effectiveness of screening. There has been increasing interest in evaluating the impact of screening in the community setting, also referred to as *service screening*, and to measure the effectiveness of screening among women who participate in screening. The evaluation of screening outside of research studies poses a set of unique methodologic challenges, including identifying when screening is introduced, the duration of time required to invite the eligible population to screening, the rate of screening uptake in a population, and finally the importance of distinguishing between screened and unscreened cohorts in mortality analysis since deaths resulting from cases diagnosed before the introduction of screening may predominate for 10 years or longer (62). In three recent reports evaluating Swedish data, investigators were able to classify breast cancer cases before and after the introduction to screening on the basis of exposure to screening in order to measure the benefit of screening among those women who attended screening (37, 40, 62). In a recent report that expanded an earlier analysis of two Swedish counties to seven counties in the Uppsala region, Duffy and colleagues (62) compared breast cancer mortality in the prescreening and postscreening periods among women aged 40–69 in six counties, and 50–69 in one county. Overall, they observed a 44% mortality reduction in women who actually underwent screening, and a 39% reduction in overall breast cancer mortality after adjustment for selection bias, associated with the policy of offering screening to the population. Greater breast cancer mortality reductions were observed in those counties that had offered screening longer than 10 years (−32%) compared with counties that had offered screening less than 10 years (−18%). Finally, in a separate analysis, the investigators examined the effectiveness of mammography based on age at diagnosis, comparing mortality reductions in women diagnosed between ages 40 and 49 with women diagnosed after age 50 (37). They observed a 48% mortality reduction in women aged 40–49 years at diagnosis based on an 18-month screening interval, and a 44% mortality reduction in women aged 50–69 at diagnosis based on a 24-month screening interval. These data demonstrate that organized screening with high rates of attendance in a setting that achieves a high degree of programmatic quality assurance can achieve breast cancer mortality reductions equal to or greater than observed in the randomized trials.

II. Who Should Undergo Screening?

Summary of Evidence: It is generally accepted that women should begin regular screening mammography in their forties, and continue regular screening as long as they are in good health (39, 52).

Supporting evidence: There is widespread acceptance of the value of regular breast cancer screening with mammography as the single most important public health strategy to reduce mortality from breast cancer. For many years, breast cancer screening in women aged 40–49 was controversial based on the absence of a statistically significant mortality breast cancer reduction compared with women aged 50+ (63–66). Further, the benefit that was evident appeared much later in younger women, leading some to argue that the appearance of benefit was attributable to cases diagnosed after age 50 in the women who were randomized in their forties (67). This argument persisted despite contrary evidence (40), and the eventual observation of statistically significant mortality reductions for this age group in two individual trials (Malmo II and Gothenburg) (44, 47) and favorable meta-analysis results were also obtained (32). Further, Tabar and colleagues (68, 69) showed that the 24- to 33-month interval between screening exams in the Two County Study had been sufficient to reduce the incidence rate of advanced ductal grade 3 cancers in women aged 50+, but not in women aged 40–49 years. The appearance of a delayed benefit was due to the similar performance of mammography in younger and older women to reduce breast cancer deaths among women diagnosed with less aggressive tumors. These and other findings showing higher interval cancer rates in younger women (70) led the Swedish Board of Health and Welfare to set shorter screening intervals for younger women (18 months) compared with older women (24 months). As noted above, when the screening interval is tailored to women's age, similar benefits are evident. Recent analysis of service screening data also has shown similar mortality reductions in women aged 40–49 years at diagnosis compared with women aged 50 years and older (37).

Setting an age to begin and end screening is admittedly arbitrary, although the HIP investigators were led to include women in their forties because they observed that more than a third of all premature mortality associated with breast cancer deaths was attributable to women diagnosed between age 35 and 50 (30). This is less of an issue for guidelines today than the fact that the evidence base from RCTs is for average-risk women aged 39 and older. The ACS recommends that women at higher risk for diagnosis of breast cancer at a younger age due to family history could begin screening as early as age 25 depending on their risk profile, and also consider additional imaging modalities (52). An age at which screening could be stopped, for instance age 70, based on risk or potential benefit also has been proposed (71), although several observations argue against setting a specific age at which all women would no longer be invited to screening. First, risk of developing and dying of breast cancer is significant in older women. The age-specific incidence of breast cancer rises until age 70–74, and then declines somewhat, but not below the average risk of women aged 60–64 (72, 73). Approximately 45% of new breast cancer cases and deaths occur in women aged 65 and older (1, 46). Second, although tumor growth rate is slower (31), and breast cancers tend to be less aggressive in older women (31, 74), it is important to emphasize that breast cancer is a potentially lethal disease at any age, and these tumor characteristics combined with declining breast density with age mean screening is somewhat less of a challenge in older women compared with younger women. Third, although only one RCT included women over age 69, observational studies have concluded that the effectiveness and performance of mammography in women over age 70 is equivalent to, if not better than, the screening of women under age 70 (75, 76). Finally, although rates of significant comorbidity increase with increasing age (77) and longevity declines, the average 70-year-old woman is in good health with an *average* life expectancy to age 85 (78). Thus, a significant percentage of the population, of women age 70 and older, has the potential to still benefit from early breast cancer detection.

The ACS recommends that chronological age alone should not be the reason for the cessation of regular screening, but rather screening decisions in older women should be individualized by considering the potential benefits and risks of mammography in the context of current health status and estimated life expectancy (52). If a woman has severe functional limitations or comorbidities, with estimated life expectancy of less than 3–5 years, it may be appropriate to consider cessation of screening. However, if an older woman is in reasonably good health and would tolerate treatment, she should continue to be screened with mammography.

III. How Frequently Should Women Be Screened?

Summary of Evidence: Current guidelines for breast cancer screening recommend breast cancer screening intervals of either 1 year (52) or 1–2 years (39). Current evidence suggests that adherence to annual screening has greater importance in premenopausal women compared with postmenopausal women.

Supporting evidence: Current recommendations for the interval between screens are influenced by different approaches to evidence-based medicine. Insofar as there has not been a trial directly comparing annual vs. biannual screening in women of different age groups, some guideline groups recommend intervals of 1–2 years based on favorable results from trials that screened at intervals of 12 or 24 months. Other guideline groups have drawn inferential guidance from the RCTs, including the proportional incidence of interval cancers in the period after a normal screening, and estimates of the duration of the detectable preclinical phase, or *sojourn time*, to define screening intervals. Tabar and colleagues (31) used data from the Swedish Two County study and estimated the mean sojourn time for women by age as follows: 40–49, 2.4 years; 50–59, 3.7 years; 60–69, 4.2 years; and 70–79, 4 years. Since the average sojourn time properly should define the upper boundary of the screening interval, it becomes clear that annual screening is more important for younger women. Data from two trials (44, 47) and inferential evidence used to estimate sojourn time (29, 79) have provided persuasive evidence that younger women likely will benefit more from annual screening compared with screening at 2-year intervals. The evidence review accompanying the most current U.S. Preventive Services Task Force reached a similar conclusion (33). Recent data from the National Cancer Institute's (NCI) Breast Cancer Screening Consortium also concluded that women under age 50 derive greater benefit from annual screening compared with biannual screening, as measured by lower rates of detection of advanced disease (80). White and colleagues (80) concluded that annual screening offered no measurable advantage to women over age 77, but other studies support an advantage with shorter screening intervals for postmenopausal women. Estimating that tumor characteristics are associated with screening intervals of 24, 12, and 6 months, Michaelson et al. (81) showed that shorter screening intervals were associated with greater reductions in the proportion of cases diagnosed with distant metastases. Similar findings were reported by Hunt et al. (82) comparing tumor outcomes among women aged 40+ undergoing screening at intervals of 10–14 months vs. 22–26 months.

IV. How Cost-Effective Is Mammographic Screening?

Summary of Evidence: Mammography screening in women aged 40–79 years of age has been shown to meet conventional criteria for cost-effectiveness (55). The marginal cost per year of live saved (MCYLS) varies with age, with greater MCYLS in age groups between ages 40 and 79 with lower incidence or lower longevity.

Supporting evidence: Cost-effectiveness studies in screening are focused on the net cost of achieving a particular health-related outcome, typically years of life gained expressed as the MCYLS, or the cost of a death avoided. Costs may be expressed in monetary terms, or in terms of the number of women needed to screen once or over some number of years, or number of screening exams conducted, to save one life. Although most cost-effectiveness analyses have concluded that screening for breast cancer is cost-effective, results have been highly variable overall and within age-specific subgroups due to differences in the underlying methodology (83–87); different assumptions about costs, amount, and timing of benefits from screening; whether costs and benefits are discounted against future value; and whether or not benefits are quality adjusted. Even though there have been formal efforts to create some common guidelines for conducting cost-effectiveness analysis (88), the current literature estimating MCYLS shares little in common with respect to methodology, model inputs, and end results beyond the finding that screening is somewhat less cost-effective in women under age 50 and older than age 70 compared with women aged 50–69 years. There also has been variability in estimates of the number needed to screen to save one life, but here the explanation for wide differences in estimates has been due to the manner in which RCT data

have been applied to estimate the fraction. It has been common to confuse the number invited to screening with the number of women actually screened, and to confuse the period of time women underwent screening with the tumor follow-up period, which usually is considerably longer. For example, a recent evidence review concluded that with 14 years of observation, the number needed to screen to save one life was 1,224.5. However, when the number needed to screen is calculated on the basis of women actually attending screening, and the duration of the screening period, Tabar and colleagues (89) estimated that the number of women needed to screen for 7 years to save one life over 20 years is 465 (95% CI, 324–819). The number of mammographic examinations needed to save one life was 1,499 (95% CI, 1,046–2,642). Put another way, on average 465 women needed just over three rounds of screening to prevent one death from breast cancer. With annual screening over a longer duration, say 10 years, the number needed to screen to save one life would be even lower.

V. How Should Ultrasound Be Applied to Breast Cancer Screening?

Summary of Evidence: Moderate evidence exists to support sonographic screening for breast cancer, though its efficacy is incompletely demonstrated by existing single-center studies (18, 20, 90–93). The studies to date have been limited to women with mammographic or clinical abnormalities (90), negative mammography and clinical examination (92, 93), a combination of the two (20, 91), or women presenting for screening (18, 94). The results of mammography were known to the individual performing the sonogram in every case (not blinded). This creates potential bias in that areas of vague asymmetry may be unintentionally targeted sonographically, or there may be a tendency to dismiss otherwise subtle mammographic findings as negative.

Women with nonfatty breast parenchyma and average risk for breast cancer comprised the study populations with the exception of the Taiwan study of first-degree relatives of women with breast cancer invited to screening (94). Studies have focused on the application of ultrasound (US) as an adjunct or supplemental test to screening mammography. Supplemental screening with sonography (or magnetic resonance imaging (MRI)), after mammography, increases the rate of early detection of breast cancer in women with dense breast parenchyma. The degree to which this additional testing adversely affects women is being studied (95). Whether or not additional detection of breast cancer by supplemental sonographic screening alters the outcome of the disease has not been established directly. Advocates hypothesize that surrogate end points, such as tumor size and presence of metastases to local lymph nodes, will inform future discussions and guidelines. Such end points have been shown to closely parallel survival outcomes (96).

Supporting evidence: Across six series of average risk women, totaling 42,838 exams, 150 (0.35%) additional cancers have been identified only on sonography in 126 women (18, 20, 90–93) (Table 5.2). Of the 150 cancers seen only on sonography, 141 (94%) were invasive and nine (6%) DCIS (Table 5.3). Of the 141 invasive cancers, 99 (70%) were 1 cm or smaller. The detection benefit of supplemental sonography increased with increasing grades of breast density. Indeed, of the 126 women with sonographically detected cancers, 114 (90.5%) had either heterogeneously dense or extremely dense parenchyma. When results of mammography were also reported across 26,753 examinations (Table 5.3), another 56 cancers were seen only mammographically, of which 42 (75%) were DCIS and 14 (25%) invasive. Women at higher risk of breast cancer were two- to threefold more likely to have a cancer seen only sonographically. Overall sensitivity of US was slightly lower than mammography, at 66% compared to 77% where both exams were performed.

Biopsy of benign lesions seen only sonographically and the induced short term interval follow-up sonograms are the riskd of undergoing screening ultrasound. Across the five series where specifics are detailed (Table 5.2), after 38,602 screening sonograms, 1,137 (2.9%) resulted in biopsy and 134 (11.8%) biopsies showed malignancy. In the four series with details (18, 90, 92, 93), short interval follow-up was recommended in another 6.6% of women. It should be noted that in all but one series (18), only a single prevalence screen was performed; these rates of false positives are likely higher than would be seen on annual incidence screens.

A prospective multicenter trial funded by the Avon Foundation and the NCI, Screening Breast Ultrasound in High-Risk Women was opened April 19, 2004 through the American College of Radiology Imaging Network (ACRIN) (95). Importantly, sonography will be performed blinded to the results of mammography. Tumor size, grade, and nodal status will be determined.

Another point of controversy in sonographic screening is generalizability across investigators. For a sonogram to depict a cancer, the sonographer must perceive it as an abnormality while scanning. No amount of subsequent review of images will correct for lack of real-time detection. Optimal technique requires appropriate real-time adjustments of pressure, angle of insonation, focal zones, dynamic range, time-gain compensation, and depth. Methods to automate scanning may facilitate standardization of technique and documentation. Consistent interpretation is another area of concern as with any imaging technique (97). To assure high standards of performance in both detection and interpretation, investigator qualification tasks have been developed for ACRIN Protocol 6666, including a phantom lesion detection task, and interpretive skills tests for proven sonographic and mammographic lesions. Materials to complete these tasks are available to interested individuals through ACRIN (http://www.acrin.org).

In the screening series (Table 5.2) as above, mammography showed better overall performance than ultrasound, with invasive cancer overrepresented among cancers seen only sonographically and DCIS overrepresented among cancers seen only mammographically (Table 5.3). Among invasive cancers, 17 (28%) of the 61 seen only sonographically were invasive lobular type, which is often especially subtle mammographically. Where detailed, supplemental US is the greatest detection benefit in dense parenchyma (19, 98). DCIS is most often manifested mammographically as microcalcifications (99) and is therefore problematic for US. In the reported US series, 62% of DCIS was detected sonographically, compared to 78% for mammography.

VI. How Accurate Is Ultrasound in Evaluating Palpable Breast Masses?

Summary of Evidence: Moderate evidence supports the use of US in addition to mammography in the evaluation of women with palpable masses or thickening.

Supporting evidence: In addition to its potential use in screening, US can also be used to evaluate palpable breast masses. Ultrasound is the initial test of choice in evaluating a lump in a young woman (under 30 years old) (100). The most common cause of a palpable mass in a woman under age 30 is a fibroadenoma (101). A palpable, circumscribed, oval mass with no posterior features or minimal posterior enhancement is most likely a fibroadenoma. If the mass has clinically been known to the patient and stable for a period of months, then follow-up is a reasonable alternative to biopsy. Since 15% of fibroadenomas are multiple, bilateral whole breast US is reasonable as part of the initial evaluation. Many women prefer excision of a palpable lump, and direct excision of a probable fibroadenoma is reasonable in a young woman. The finding of a sonographically suspicious mass, or a clinically suspicious mass without a sonographic correlate, should prompt bilateral mammographic evaluation to better define the extent of malignancy if any. At age 30 and over, breast cancer is increasingly common, and mammography is the initial test of choice for symptomatic women.

Moderate evidence supports the use of US in addition to mammography in the evaluation of women with palpable masses or thickening. The combination of US and mammography is especially effective in evaluating women with palpable masses (Table 5.4). In the multiinstitutional study of Georgian-Smith et al. (102), 616 palpable lesions were evaluated sonographically and all 293 palpable cancers were depicted sonographically. Across several series, of 545 cancers in women with symptoms, 529 (97.1%) were depicted. A negative result after both mammography and US is highly predictive of benign outcome with 98.6% negative predictive value across these series (102–106). Nevertheless, final management of a clinically suspicious mass must be based on clinical grounds.

VII. How Accurate Is Ultrasound in Evaluating Nipple Discharge?

Summary of Evidence: Bloody nipple discharge and spontaneous unilateral clear nipple discharge merit imaging and clinical evaluation, with malignancy was found in 13% of patients on average (range 1–23%) across multiple series (reviewed in (107)).

Supporting evidence: Papilloma is the most common cause of nipple discharge, found in 44–45% of patients (107, 108), with fibrocystic changes accounting for the rest. Milky discharge is almost always physiologic or due to hyperprolactinemia (107) and does not warrant imaging workup. Injection of contrast into the discharging duct, followed by magnification craniocaudal and true lateral mammographic views (galactography), has been the standard for imaging evaluation of nipple discharge (109). Ultrasound has the advantage of being noninvasive. A few studies have compared US and galactography, with promising but limited evidence for the utility of US in this setting (110, 111). The visualization of intraductal masses on US is facilitated by distention of the duct. Whether or not the full extent of multiple intraductal lesions is well depicted on US has not been systematically studied (insufficient evidence).

VIII. How Accurate Is Ultrasound in Determining Local Extent of Disease?

Summary of Evidence: Sonography may aid in determining the local extent of breast cancer when used in conjunction with mammography and clinical exam (moderate evidence).

Supporting evidence: Moderate evidence from several unblinded prospective series supports a detection benefit of sonography after mammography and clinical examination in evaluating the preoperative extent of breast cancer (Table 5.5). When MRI was used in addition, the limitations of combined US, mammography, and clinical examination became evident. In particular, an extensive intraductal component was often underestimated without MRI in one series (19). On average, 48% of breasts with cancer will have additional tumor foci not depicted on mammography or clinical examination (112). If US is being used to guide biopsy, there is an advantage to at least scanning the quadrant containing the cancer as 89–93% of additional tumor foci are within the same quadrant as the index lesion (19, 112, 113), and over 90% of malignant foci will be detected by combined mammography and US in this setting.

Ultrasound is not particularly sensitive to lesions manifest solely as calcifications due to their small size and speckle artifact present in tissue (114). Nevertheless, US can help identify the invasive component of malignant calcifications. Soo et al. (115) evaluated 111 cases of suspicious calcifications and only 26 (23%) could be seen sonographically. Of those seen on US, 69% were malignant compared to only 21% of those not seen on US (115). Those cancers seen on US were more likely invasive (72% vs. 28%), and underestimation of disease was less common when biopsies were performed with US guidance than stereotactic guidance. Similarly, Moon et al. (116) showed that 45 (45%) of 100 suspicious microcalcifications were sonographically visible, including 31 (82%) of 38 malignant calcifications and 14 (23%) of 62 benign calcifications.

IX. Which Lesions (BIRADS 1–6) Should Undergo Biopsy?

Summary of Evidence: The widespread use of screening mammography has resulted in the detection of clinically occult and probably benign lesions in up to 11% of patients (117). One concern regarding the dissemination and utilization of image-guided percutaneous biopsy was that unnecessary sampling of probably benign lesions would result in an unacceptably low positive predictive value. There has also been concern that it might replace the short-interval, 6-month imaging follow-up that has been demonstrated as effective management of probably benign [Breast Imaging and Reporting and Data Systems (BIRADS) category 3] masses and microcalcifications. The positive biopsy rate of mammography is improved when the procedure is performed primarily on lesions categorized by BIRADS (16) as category 4 (suspicious) or 5 (highly suspicious) and when short-interval, 6-month follow-up mammography is judiciously used in place of biopsy for the majority or probably benign (BIRADS category 3) lesions (117–121).

Supporting evidence: Early studies reporting the low yield of breast cancer in BIRADS category 3, probably benign, nonpalpable lesions were

largely level II (moderate evidence) investigations, both prospective and retrospective from single institutions (122–124) that were limited by small patient populations, incomplete mammographic follow-up, and short durations of follow-up (6–20 months).

A single level I (strong evidence) report was published by Sickles (117) in 1991. This prospective trial included 3.5 years of mammographic follow-up in a population of 3,184 probably benign breast lesions, of which 17 (positive predictive value for cancer, 0.5%) were found to be malignant. These results established the validity of managing mammographically depicted, probably benign (BIRADS category 3) lesions with periodic mammographic surveillance (117).

A. Special Case: Radial Sclerosing Lesions (Radial Scars)

The reported incidence of radial scar is 0.1–2.0 per 1,000 screening mammograms and 1.7–14% of autopsy specimens (125) (Fig. 5.1). Their major significance pertains to an association with ADH and carcinoma that is seen in up to 50% of cases (Table 5.6) (126). However, multi-institutional studies of larger patient populations evaluating percutaneous biopsy find a much lower incidence of cancer associated with radial scar than previously reported (127–129). Although the largest published studies are retrospective level II (moderate evidence), excisional biopsy is recommended when percutaneous biopsy results show radial scar, especially when associated with atypical hyperplasia.

X. What Is the Performance of Percutaneous Image-Guided Breast Biopsy Compared with Standard Surgical Excisional Biopsy?

Summary of Evidence: Percutaneous, image-guided breast biopsy has been found to be an accurate, safe, well-accepted, reliable method for diagnosing nonpalpable breast abnormalities. When a carcinoma is initially diagnosed by percutaneous biopsy significantly fewer surgical procedures are required to achieve clear margins when breast conservation is the therapeutic goal (130).

Supporting evidence: There have been several studies evaluating percutaneous breast biopsy guided by both stereotactic (Fig. 5.2) or ultrasound (Fig. 5.3) imaging guidance (Table 5.7) (131–145). The majority were prospective, single-institution studies, but three were multiinstitutional (139, 143, 145). Several studies were limited by small study populations (defined as less than 200 subjects). All studies having a pathologic gold standard (i.e., all patients went to surgical biopsy after percutaneous image-guided biopsy) were less than 200 patients in size. In all studies over 200 patients in size, those with a benign percutaneous biopsy result were followed with either mammography or US. No study had complete imaging follow-up on this category of patients, and delayed cancers were diagnosed in the follow-up groups. For six studies evaluated as level II (moderate evidence) and two studies evaluated as level I (strong evidence), percutaneous imaging-guided biopsy diagnosed cancer in 72–98% of malignant lesions.

XI. What Type of Imaging Guidance Is Best Suited for Breast Lesions that Manifest as Masses or as Microcalcifications?

Summary of Evidence: Any lesion that is adequately visualized by US is best biopsied using this guidance method. US biopsy is less costly than stereotactic biopsy and more comfortable for the patient. However, most microcalcification clusters are not visualized with US and require stereotactic guidance for tissue acquisition. Radiography of the core biopsy specimens should be performed whenever microcalcifications are biopsied to document adequate retrieval of calcifications in the biopsy specimens (145).

Supporting evidence: The only major prospective randomized study that attempted to study which type of imaging guidance was best suited for percutaneous breast biopsy was the Radiology Diagnostic Oncology Group (RDOG) trial (145). In this study, 1,103 subjects were assigned to stereotactic core biopsy (SCB) and 578 were assigned to US core biopsy. However,

86 (8%) of subjects assigned to stereotactic biopsy were changed to US-guided biopsy by the physician performing the procedure, and 415 (72%) of subjects assigned to US biopsy were changed to stereotactic biopsy. All patients changed from stereotactic to US biopsy had a solid breast mass, and the most frequent reasons for change were lesion inaccessibility by the stereotactic system or a breast that was very thin on compression in the stereotactic biopsy device. Among patients where the breast lesion was calcifications, none were switched from stereotactic to US biopsy, while 99% (255 of 257) of subjects with calcifications assigned to US biopsy were switched to stereotactic biopsy because the calcifications were not well seen with US.

The RDOG5 trial reported summary measures for sensitivity, specificity, and predictive values for image-guided biopsy by the type of lesion biopsied (masses or calcifications) and imaging guidance used (US or stereotactic) (145). The overall sensitivity, specificity, and accuracy for all breast lesions by either imaging guidance method in this trial were 0.91, 1.00, and 0.98, respectively. The combined sensitivity, negative predictive value, and accuracy for US and stereotactic biopsy for diagnosing masses (0.96, 0.99, and 0.99, respectively) were significantly greater ($p < .001$, Chi-square) than for calcifications (0.84, 0.94, and 0.96, respectively) (145). The sensitivity (0.89) of stereotactic biopsy for diagnosing all lesions was significantly lower ($p = .029$, Fisher's exact) than that of US biopsy (0.97) because of the preponderance of calcifications biopsied by stereotactic vs. US guidance (718 vs. 2) (130). There was no difference between US and stereotactic guidance in sensitivity, specificity, or accuracy for the diagnosis of masses (0.97, 1.00, 0.99, respectively, for US core biopsy (USCB) and 0.96, 100, and 0.99, respectively, for SCB) (131). The calculated overall false-negative rate for percutaneous image-guided biopsy in this trial was 0.093 (145). Figure 5.4 is an algorithm of decision support regarding the use of imaging-guided biopsy for diagnosing nonpalpable breast lesions.

A. Special Case: Biopsy of Breast Lesions Detected on Breast MRI

With increasing use of magnetic resonance to image the breast, investigators are reporting that MRI finds lesions that are not detected by mammography or physical examination (50). Although MRI has a high sensitivity in detecting breast cancer, approaching 100% in some series, the reported specificity has ranged from 37 to 97% (146–150). Biopsying the lesions seen by MRI has gained attention in recent years. In some cases, a focused breast US examination, guided by the MRI findings, permits biopsy using US guidance. Some investigators report limited, single-institution experience with different approaches to performing percutaneous biopsy guided by MRI (146–150); however, there is insufficient evidence to substantiate its use. The cost-effectiveness of using MRI for the breast poses additional concerns. At present, there is insufficient evidence and there are currently are no level I, II, or III studies to guide which patient populations should undergo breast MRI.

XII. How Cost-Effective Is Image-Guided Biopsy?

Summary of Evidence: Percutaneous biopsy of a nonpalpable breast lesion using either stereotactic of US guidance is less expensive than surgical biopsy. The cost savings are greater if the biopsy is performed with US guidance (151); however, most calcification lesions are not visualized by US and are better evaluated with stereotactic biopsy guidance (145).

Supporting evidence: Previous studies of the cost-effectiveness of imaging-guided biopsy have involved analysis of both stereotactic and US biopsy (145, 151–156). Lindfors and Rosenquist (154) reported that the marginal cost per year of life saved with screening was reduced by 23% with the use of stereotactic rather than open surgical breast biopsy. Liberman et al. (151, 153) found that stereotactic biopsy decreased the cost of diagnosis by more than 50%; if these results were generalized to the national level, annual savings in the USA would approach $200 million. Liberman et al. (153) and Lee et al. (155) found that the savings were greater with breast masses than with calcifications, probably due to underestimation of pathology when ADH and DCIS are associated with microcalcifications. When a lesion is visible by US – and many microcalcification clusters are not – biopsy is least expensive using this imaging guided modality. This is in part due to the fact that US equipment is less costly than stereotactic systems and US can be used for imaging purposes other than guiding biopsy. When data by Liberman et al. (151) were used to estimate what the annual national cost savings would be if US rather than open surgical biopsy was used to diagnose breast masses, a figure of $59,523,000 was derived.

Take Home Tables and Figures

Tables 5.1–5.7 and Figs. 5.1–5.4 serve to highlight key recommendations and supporting evidence.

Table 5.1. The randomized controlled trials of breast cancer screening

Study (duration)	Screening protocol — Invited vs. control group	Frequency — No. rounds	Study population — Age	Subgroup	Invited	Control	Years of follow-up	RR (95% CI)
HIP study (1963–1969)	2VMM+CBE vs. usual care	Annually, Four rounds	40–64	40–49	14,432	14,701	18	0.77 (0.52–1.13)
				50–64	16,568	16,299		0.79 (0.58–1.08)
Edinburgh (1979–1988)	1 or 2VMM + initial CBE vs. usual care	24 months, Four rounds	45–64	45–49	11,755ᵃ	10,641ᵃ	13	0.75ᵃ (0.48–1.18)
				50–64	11,245	12,359		0.79 (0.60–1.02)
Two county (1977–1985)	1VMM vs. usual care	40–49: 24 months, 50–69: 33 months, Four rounds	40–74	40–49	9,650	5,009	20	0.93 (0.63–1.37)
				50–74	28,939	13,551		0.65 (0.55–0.77)
Malmo (1976–1990)	1 or 2VMM vs. usual care	18–24 months, Five rounds	45–69	45–49	13,528ᵇ	12,242ᵇ	16	0.70ᵇ (0.49–1.00)
				50–69	17,134	17,165		0.83 (0.66–1.04)
Stockholm (1981–1985)	1VMM vs. usual care	28 months, Two rounds	40–64	40–49	14,185	7,985	15	1.52 (0.8–2.88)
				50–64	25,815	12,015		0.70 (0.46–1.07)
Gothenburg (1982–1988)	1 or 2VMM vs. usual care	18 months, Five rounds	39–59	39–49	11,724	14,217	18	0.65 (0.40–1.05)
				50–59	16,394	9,276		0.91 (0.61–1.36)
CNBSS-1 (1980–1987)	2VMM+CBE+BSE vs. initial CBE	12 months, Four to five rounds	40–49	40–49	25,214	25,216	12	0.97 (0.78–1.33)
CNBSS-2 (1980–1987)	2VMM+CBE+BSE vs. CBE+BSE	12 months, Four to five rounds	50–59	50–59	19,711	19,694	12	1.02 (0.74–1.27)

Reprinted with kind permission of Springer Science+Business Media from Fajardo LL, Berg WA, Smith RA. Breast Imaging. In Medina LS, Blackmore DD (eds): *Evidence-Based Imaging: Optimizing Imaging in Patient Care*. New York: Springer Science+Business Media, 2006.

1MM one-view mammography of each breast, 2VMM two-view mammography of each breast, CBE clinical breast examination, BSE breast self-examination, CNBSS Canadian National Breast Screening Study.

ᵃThe Edinburgh trial included three separate groups of women aged 45–49 years at entry: the first had 5,949 women in the invited group and 5,818 in the control group (with 14 years' follow-up); the next had 2,545 in the invited group and 2,482 in the control group (12 years' follow-up); and the third had 3,261 in the invited group and 2,341 in the control group (10 years' follow-up) (6). Only the first group's results had been reported previously.

ᵇThe Malmo trial included two groups of women aged 45–49 at entry: one group (MMST-I) received first-round screening in 1977–1978 and had 3,954 women in the invited group, 4,030 women in the control group; the second group (MMST-II) received first-round screening from 1978 to 1990 and had 9,574 women in the invited group, 8,212 women in the control group (2). Only the first group's results had been reported previously.

Table 5.2. Breast cancers detected by sonography and mammography

Study	No. of examinations	No. of cancers	No. of cancers detected		Ultrasound-induced biopsy	
			Mammography	Ultrasound	Number of biopsies	Number of cancers (%)
Gordon and Goldenberg (90)	12,706	n/a	n/a	44	279	44 (16)
Buchberger et al. (91)	8,970	182	142	160	405	40 (10)
Kaplan (92)	1,862	n/a	n/a	6	57	6 (11)
Kolb et al. (18) (all women)	13,547	246[a]	191	110	358	37 (10)
Crystal et al. (93)	1,517	n/a	n/a	7	38	7 (18)
LeConte et al. (20)	4,236	50	34	44	n/a	n/a
Overall	42,838	478	367 (76.8%)	371, with 314/478 (65.7%) where mammography also reported	1,137	134 (12)

Reprinted with kind permission of Springer Science+Business Media from Fajardo LL, Berg WA, Smith RA. Breast Imaging. In Medina LS, Blackmore DD (eds.): *Evidence-Based Imaging: Optimizing Imaging in Patient Care*. New York: Springer Science+Business Media, 2006.

n/a not available, not reported (90), or not applicable as patients are selected because of negative mammogram (92, 93).

[a]Includes four invasive cancers detected only on clinical breast examination. In 5,826 examinations in women <50 years of age, 42 cancers were identified including 21 seen on mammography and 33 on ultrasound.

Table 5.3. Histopathology of breast cancer seen only on ultrasound[a]

	No. of cancers	Invasive			DCIS	Size (range), mm
		Total	Ductal	Lobular		
Gordon and Goldenberg (90)	44	44[b]	n/a[a]	n/a	0	Mean 11, median 10 (4–25)
Buchberger et al. (91)	40	35	26	9	5	Mean 9.1 (4–20)
Kaplan (92)	6	5	3	2	1	Mean 9 (6–14) – US size
Kolb et al. (18)	37	36[b]	n/a	n/a	1	Mean 9.9
Crystal et al. (93)	7	7	6	1	0	Median 10 (4–12)
LeConte et al. (20)	16	14	9	5	2	Mean 11, median 9 (2–30)
Overall	150	141 (94%)	44 (29%)	17 (11%)	9 (6%)	

Reprinted with kind permission of Springer Science+Business Media from Fajardo LL, Berg WA, Smith RA. Breast Imaging. In Medina LS, Blackmore DD (eds.): *Evidence-Based Imaging: Optimizing Imaging in Patient Care.* New York: Springer Science+Business Media, 2006.*n/a* not available.
[a]Women had both whole breast ultrasound and mammography.
[b]Cancers are listed only as invasive with no further details available; 26 of 37 cancers were 1 cm or smaller with range not available.

Table 5.4. Sensitivity and negative predictive value of combined mammography and US in symptomatic women

	No. of cancers	Sensitivity (%)	NPV (%)	Purpose of study/patient population	Detection of misses	Cancers missed
Georgian-Smith et al. (102)	293	293 (100)	n/a	Palpable, sensitivity of US to cancers	Biopsy	None
Dennis et al. (103)	0	n/a	600/600 (100)	Palpable, biopsy avoidance	Biopsy or 2-year follow-up	None
Moy et al. (104)	6	0	227/233 (97.4)	Palpable	Tumor registry, 2-year follow-up	2 DCIS, 1 ILC, 3 IDC
Kaiser et al. (105)	6	6 (100)	117/117 (100)	Thickening	Biopsy or 14-month follow-up	n/a
Houssami et al. (106)	240	230 (95.8)[a]	174/184 (94.6)	Symptoms[a]	Tumor registry, 2-year follow-up	n/a
Overall	545	529 (97.1)	1,118/1,134 (98.6)			

Reprinted with kind permission of Springer Science+Business Media from Fajardo LL, Berg WA, Smith RA. Breast Imaging. In Medina LS, Blackmore DD (eds.): *Evidence-Based Imaging: Optimizing Imaging in Patient Care.* New York: Springer Science+Business Media, 2006.*NPV* negative predictive value, *n/a* not applicable, *DCIS* ductal carcinoma in situ, *ILC* invasive lobular carcinoma, *IDC* invasive ductal carcinoma.
[a]In the series of Houssami et al. (106), 157 women with cancer had a lump and 114 without cancer had a lump.

Table 5.5. Use of combined mammography and US in evaluating local extent of breast cancer

	No. of cancers	Sensitivity (%)	Detection of misses	Cancers missed
Fischer et al. (157)	405	366[a] (90.4)	MRI	4 DCIS, 3 ILC, 32 IDC
Berg and Gilbreath (158)[b]	64	62 (97)	Some surgery, details not specified	2 ILC
Hlawatsch et al. (98)	105 breasts with cancer	94/105 (90%) accurate extent	MRI	7 invasive NOS, 1 DCIS
Moon et al. (116)	289	276 (95.5)[a]	Some surgery, details not specified	5 IDC, 1 ILC, 7 DCIS
Berg et al. (19)[b]	96 breasts with cancer	81 (84%)[a]	MRI, 2-year follow-up	7 DCIS, 6 IDC, 2 ILC
Berg et al. (19)	177	162 (91.5)	MRI, 2-year follow-up	8 DCIS, 4 IDC, 3 ILC

Reprinted with kind permission of Springer Science+Business Media from Fajardo LL, Berg WA, Smith RA. Breast Imaging. In Medina LS, Blackmore DD (eds.): *Evidence-Based Imaging: Optimizing Imaging in Patient Care.* New York: Springer Science+Business Media, 2006.
MRI magnetic resonance imaging, *DCIS* ductal carcinoma in situ, *ILC* invasive lobular carcinoma, *IDC* invasive ductal carcinoma.
[a]Includes clinical breast examination.
[b]References (152) and (19) are nonoverlapping series.

Table 5.6. Published reports and evidence classification of radial scar (RS): association with malignancy and diagnostic accuracy by percutaneous biopsy (PB)

Authors, year	No. of RS diagnosed by PB	No. of gold standard correlation	Incidence of cancer	Cancer missed by PB	Study characteristics	Evidence classification
Brenner et al. 2002 (127)	198	Surgical excision: 102 mammography: 55	8.2% cancer 28% ADH	3% overall 5% for spring loaded 0% for vacuum device	2, 3, 4, 6	Level II
Philpotts et al. 2000 (128)	9	8	0% cancer 50% ADH		2, 3, 5, 7	Level II
Alleva et al. 1999 (126)	N/A	Surgical excision: 22	41%	N/A	2, 5	Level II
Orel et al. 1992 (129)	4	Surgical excision: 4	0% cancer 0% ADH	N/A	2, 5, 7	Level II

Reprinted with kind permission of Springer Science+Business Media from Fajardo LL, Berg WA, Smith RA. Breast Imaging. In Medina LS, Blackmore DD (eds.): *Evidence-Based Imaging: Optimizing Imaging in Patient Care*. New York: Springer Science+Business Media, 2006.
Study characteristics: 1, prospective; 2, retrospective; 3, nonpalpable lesions only; 4, multiinstitutional; 5, single institution; 6, lack of follow-up in some cases; 7, small population; *ADH* atypical ductal hyperplasia.

Table 5.7. Published reports and evidence classification: image-guided breast biopsy compared to surgical biopsy

Authors, year	Method	Needle size (gauge)	No. of patients	No. of PB	Gold standard (GS)		% of cancers diagnosed on PB compared with GS	Other	Evidence classification
					F/U M or US	Surgical biopsy			
Parker et al. 1990 (131)	S	14, 16, 18	103	102	102	102	14/16 (88%)	1, 3, 5, 7	III
Parker et al. 1991 (132)	S	14	102	102	102	102	22/23 (96%)	1, 5, 7	III
Parker et al. 1993 (133)	US	14	164	181	112	49	48/49 (98%)	1, 5, 6, 7	III
Elvecrog et al. 1993 (134)	S	14	100	100	n/a	100	34/36 (94%)	1, 3, 5, 7	III
Brendlinger et al. 1994 (135)	S	14	75	75	65	15	13/15 (87%)	1, 3, 5, 7	III
Burbank et al. 1994 (136)	US/S	14	105	105	NG	24	13/13 (100%)	1, 5, 6, 7	III
Gisvold 1994 (137)	S	14	158	160	n/a	160	55/67 (82%)	1, 3, 7	III
Jackman et al. 1994 (138)	S	14	379	450	NG	116	99/116 (85%)	1, 3, 5	II
Parker et al. 1994 (139)	US/S	14	6152	6152	3765	1363	910/925 (98%)	1, 4, 6	II
Meyer et al. 1998 (140)	S	14	1032	1032	706	214	196/214 (96%)	1, 3, 5, 6	II
Jackman et al. 1999 (141)	S	14	483	483	259	221	55/76 (72%)	1, 3, 5, 6	II
Meyer et al. 1999 (142)	S	14, 14V, 11V	1643	1836	855	614	412/444 (93%)	1, 3, 5, 6	II
Brenner et al. 2001 (143)	S	14	1003	1003	596	307	242/254 (95%)	1, 3, 4	I
Margolin et al. 2001 (144)	S/US	16	1183	1333	963	175	135/147 (92%)	1, 3, 5, 6	II
Fajardo et al. 2004 (145)	US/S	14, 14V, 11V	2403	1174	1051	631	410/452 (91%)	1, 3, 4, 6, 8	I

Reprinted with kind permission of Springer Science+Business Media from Fajardo LL, Berg WA, Smith RA. Breast Imaging. In Medina LS, Blackmore DD (eds.): *Evidence-Based Imaging: Optimizing Imaging in Patient Care*. New York: Springer Science+Business Media, 2006.

S stereotactic, M mammography, US ultrasound, V vacuum-assisted, PS percutaneous biopsy, NA not applicable, NG not given. Other: 1, prospective; 2, retrospective; 3, nonpalpable lesions only or could separate data for nonpalpable lesions from palpable; 4, multiinstitutional; 5, single institution; 6, follow-up incomplete in some cases; 7, small population; 8, randomized.

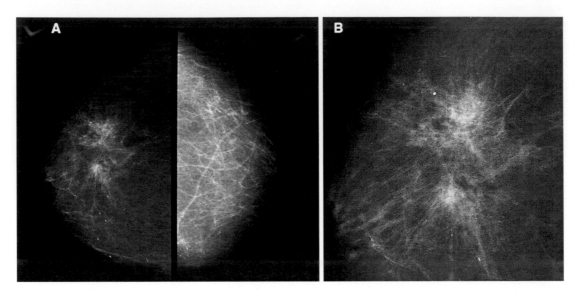

Figure 5.1. Radial scar. Right and left cranial-caudal (CC) (**A**) and coned right CC (**B**) mammography images demonstrate an ill-defined mass associated with architectural distortion in the left breast (*right*). Image-guided percutaneous biopsy demonstrated sclerosing radial lesion associated with sclerosing adenosis, ADH, and fibrosis histopathologically. Surgical excision demonstrated a 7-mm tubular carcinoma in addition to the aforementioned findings. (Reprinted with kind permission of Springer Science+Business Media from Fajardo LL, Berg WA, Smith RA. Breast Imaging. In Medina LS, Blackmore DD (eds.): *Evidence-Based Imaging: Optimizing Imaging in Patient Care*. New York: Springer Science+Business Media, 2006.)

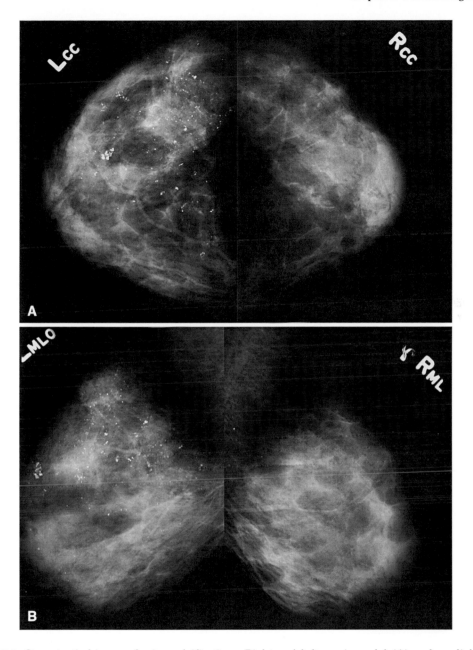

Figure 5.2. Stereotactic biopsy of microcalcifications. Right and left craniocaudal (**A**) and medial-lateral oblique (**B**) mammography images demonstrate suspicious microcalcifications in the upper outer and upper inner quadrants of the left breast. (**C**) Patient positioning for stereotactic biopsy. X-ray and biopsy equipment are located beneath the table. (**D**) Stereotactic images of calcifications (*arrows*) performed for targeting (*upper row of images*) of a microcalcification cluster are shown above and images performed after placement of the biopsy probe (*curved arrows in lower images*) are shown below (biopsy probe obscured the cluster of interest in lower right image). (**E**) Biopsy probe positioned within breast for retrieval of tissues samples from microcalcifications that were targeted with computer assistance from stereotactic images acquired digitally. (**F**) Radiographs of the biopsy specimens document presence of microcalcifications (*arrows*) within the tissue. DCIS was diagnosed histopathologically. (Reprinted with kind permission of Springer Science+Business Media from Fajardo LL, Berg WA, Smith RA. Breast Imaging. In Medina LS, Blackmore DD (eds.): *Evidence-Based Imaging: Optimizing Imaging in Patient Care.* New York: Springer Science+Business Media, 2006.)

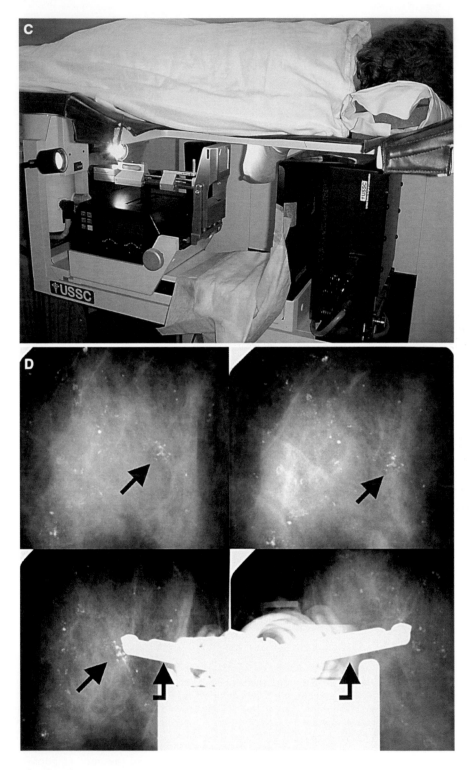

Figure 5.2. *Continued*

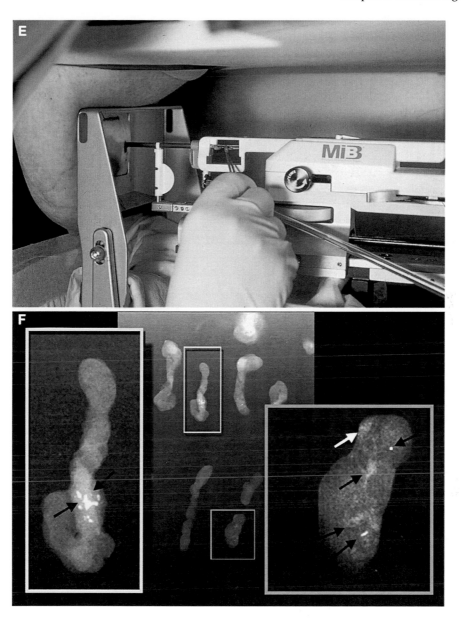

Figure 5.2. *Continued*

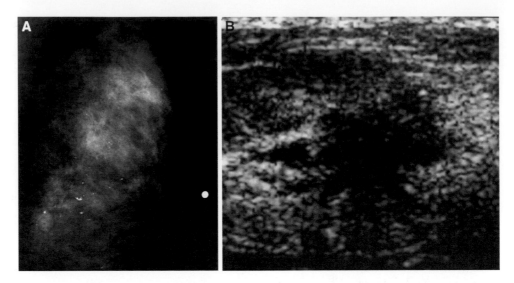

Figure 5.3. Ultrasound of mammographically occult malignancy. (**A**) Mediolateral oblique mammogram with dense parenchyma in a 53-year-old with a palpable mass (marked with radiopaque marker). No discrete mammographic correlate is seen. (**B**) Transverse sonogram over the palpable abnormality demonstrates a spiculated hypoechoic mass highly suggestive of malignancy. Sonographically guided core biopsy showed infiltrating and intraductal carcinoma. (Reprinted with kind permission of Springer Science+Business Media from Fajardo LL, Berg WA, Smith RA. Breast Imaging. In Medina LS, Blackmore DD (eds.): *Evidence-Based Imaging: Optimizing Imaging in Patient Care.* New York: Springer Science+Business Media, 2006.)

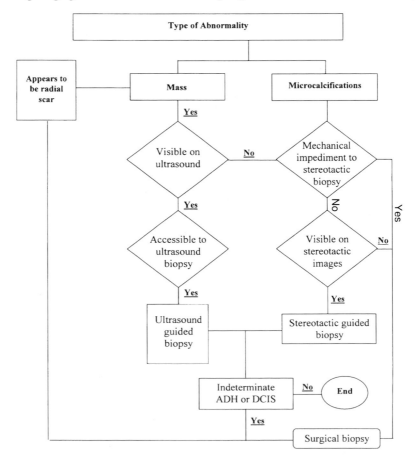

Figure 5.4. Decision support: determining the method of diagnostic breast biopsy for nonpalpable abnormalities. (Reprinted with kind permission of Springer Science+Business Media from Fajardo LL, Berg WA, Smith RA. Breast Imaging. In Medina LS, Blackmore DD (eds.): *Evidence-Based Imaging: Optimizing Imaging in Patient Care.* New York: Springer Science+Business Media, 2006.)

Future Research

- Data evaluating the performance of digital mammography relative to conventional screen film mammography for breast cancer screening are currently being analyzed from the recently completed ACRIN Digital Mammographic Imaging Screening Trial (DMIST). Information from this trial, which recruited approximately 49,520 women, should be reported in mid- to late 2005 (http://www.acrin.org/6652_protocol.html).
- The efficacy of whole breast US imaging as a screening tool or adjunct to screening mammography is currently undergoing evaluation in the ACRIN 6666 trial, Breast Cancer Screening in High-Risk Women (http://www.acrin.org/6666_protocol.html). Results may be reported in early 2006.
- Data evaluating the efficacy of breast MRI to screen women at high risk for breast cancer are also undergoing analysis and may be reported in mid- to late 2005 (ACRIN 6667 trial, Breast Cancer: Screening of Contralateral Breast with MRI, http://www.acrin.org/6667_protocol.html).

References

1. American Cancer Society Surveillance Program. Estimated New Cancer Cases by Sex and Age. Atlanta: American Cancer Society, 2003.
2. Elmore JG, Barton MB, Moceri VM, Polk S, Arena PJ, Fletcher SW. N Engl J Med 1998;16:1089–1096.
3. Kerlikowske K. J Natl Cancer Inst Monogr 1997;22:79–86.
4. Kerlikowske K, Grady D, Barclay J, Sickles EA, Eaton A, Ernster V. JAMA 1993;270:2444–2450.
5. Gail MH, Costantino JP. J Natl Cancer Inst 2001;93(5):334–355.
6. Gail MH, Brinton LA, Byar DP et al. J Natl Cancer Inst 1989;81(24):1879–1886.
7. Gail MH. Ann N Y Acad Sci 2001;949:286–291.
8. Gail MH, Benichou J. J Natl Cancer Inst 1994;86(8):573–575.
9. Claus EB, Risch N, Thompson WD. Breast Cancer Res Treat 1993;28(2):115–120.
10. Page DL, Dupont WD, Rogers LW, Rados MS. Cancer 1985;55(11):2698–2708.
11. Page DL, Kidd TE Jr, Dupont WD, Simpson JF, Rogers LW. Hum Pathol 1991;22(12):1232–1239.
12. Fisher B, Costantino JP, Wickerham DL et al. J Natl Cancer Inst 1998;90(18):1371–1388.
13. Hancock SL, Tucker MA, Hoppe RT. J Natl Cancer Inst 1993;85(1):25–31.
14. Aisenberg AC, Finkelstein DM, Doppke KP, Koerner FC, Boivin JF, Willett CG. Cancer 1997;79(6):1203–1210.
15. Clemons M, Loijens L, Goss P. Cancer Treat Rev 2000;26(4):291–302.
16. American College of Radiology. Illustrated Breast Imaging Reporting and Data System (BI-RADS): Mammography, 4th ed. Reston, VA: ACR, 2003.
17. Mandelson MT, Oestreicher N, Porter PL et al. J Natl Cancer Inst 2000;92(13):1081–1087.
18. Kolb TM, Lichy J, Newhouse JH. Radiology 2002;225(1):165–175.
19. Berg WA, Gutierrez L, NessAiver M et al. Radiology 2004;233(3):830–849.
20. LeConte I, Feger C, Galant C et al. Am J Roentgenol 2003;180(6):1675–1679.
21. Ciatto S, Cataliotti L, Distante V. Radiology 1987;165:99–102.
22. Hall FM, Storella JM, Silverstone DZ, Wyshak G. Radiology 1988;167:353–358.
23. Sickles EA, Ominsky SH, Sollitto RA, Galvin HB, Monticciolo DL. Radiology 1990;175:323–327.
24. Skinner MA, Swain M, Simmons R, McCarty KS Jr, Sullivan DC, Iglehart JD. Ann Surg 1988;208:203–208.
25. Spivey GH, Perry BW, Clark VA, Coulson AH, Coulson WF. Am Surg 1982;48:326–332.
26. Molloy M, Azarow K, Garcia VF, Daniel JR. J Surg Oncol 1989;40:152–154.
27. Brown ML, Lipscomb J, Snyder C. Annu Rev Public Health 2001;22:91–113.
28. National Heart Lung and Blood Institute. NHLBI Year 2003 Fact Book. Washington, DC: National Institutes of Health, 2003.
29. Tabar L, Duffy SW, Vitak B, Chen HH, Prevost TC. Cancer 1999;86(3):449–462.
30. Shapiro S, Venet W, Strax P, Venet L. Periodic Screening for Breast Cancer: The Health Insurance Plan Project and Its Sequelae. Baltimore: Johns Hopkins Press, 1988.
31. Tabar L, Vitak B, Chen HH et al. Radiol Clin North Am 2000;38(4):625–651.
32. Hendrick RE, Smith RA, Rutledge JH III, Smart CR. J Natl Cancer Inst Monogr 1997;22:87–92.
33. Humphrey LL, Helfand M, Chan BK, Woolf SH. Ann Intern Med 2002;137(5 pt 1):347–360.
34. Nystrom L, Andersson I, Bjurstam N, Frisell J, Nordenskjold B, Rutqvist LE. Lancet 2002; 359(9310):909–919.
35. Michaelson J, Satija S, Moore R et al. Cancer 2002;94(1):37–43.
36. Paci E, Duffy SW, Giorgi D et al. Br J Cancer 2002;87(1):65–69.

37. Tabar L, Yen MF, Vitak B, Chen HH, Smith RA, Duffy SW. Lancet 2003;361(9367):1405–1410.
38. Smith RA, Duffy SW, Gabe R, Tabar L, Yen AM, Chen TH. Radiol Clin North Am 2004;42(5): 793–806, v.
39. U.S. Preventive Services Task Force. Ann Intern Med 2002;137(5 pt 1):344–346.
40. Tabar L, Vitak B, Tony HH, Yen MF, Duffy SW, Smith RA. Cancer 2001;91(9):1724–1731.
41. Shapiro S. Health insurance plan. J Natl Cancer Inst Monogr 1997;22:27–30.
42. IARC Working Group on the Evaluation of Cancer-Preventive Strategies. Breast Cancer Screening, vol. 7. Lyon: IARC Press, 2002.
43. Alexander FE, Anderson TJ, Brown HK et al. Lancet 1999;353(9168):1903–1908.
44. Andersson I, Janzon L. J Natl Cancer Inst Monogr 1997;22:63–67.
45. Frisell J, Lidbrink E. J Natl Cancer Inst Monogr 1997;22:49–51.
46. Frisell J, Lidbrink E, Hellstrom L, Rutqvist LE. Breast Cancer Res Treat 1997;45(3):263–270.
47. Bjurstam N, Bjorneld L, Duffy SW et al. Cancer 1997;80(11):2091–2099.
48. Bjurstam N, Bjorneld L, Warwick J et al. Cancer 2003;97(10):2387–2396.
49. Miller AB, To T, Baines CJ, Wall C. J Natl Cancer Inst 2000;92(18):1490–1499.
50. Miller AB, To T, Baines CJ, Wall C. Ann Intern Med 2002;137(5 pt 1):305–312.
51. Organizing Committee and Collaborators. Int J Cancer 1996;68:693–699.
52. Smith RA, Saslow D, Sawyer KA et al. CA Cancer J Clin 2003;53(3):141–169.
53. Olsen O, Gotzsche P. Lancet 2001;358:1340.
54. Swedish Board of Health and Welfare. Vilka Effekter Har Mammografiscreening? Referat av ett expertmöte anordnat av Socialstyrelsen och Cancerfonden. Stockholm: 2002.
55. Health Council of the Netherlands. The Benefit of Population Screening for Breast Cancer with Mammography. Health Council of the Netherlands, 2002.
56. Veronese U, Forrest P, Wood W, Boyle P. Statement from the chair: Global Summit on Mammographic Screening, June 3–5, 2002. European Institute of Oncology, 2002.
57. Duffy SW, Tabar L, Vitak B et al. Ann Oncol 2003;14(8):1196–1198.
58. Tabar L, Smith RA, Duffy SW. Lancet 2002;360 (9329):337, discussion 39–40.
59. Duffy SW, Tabar L, Vitak B et al. Eur J Cancer 2003;39(12):1755–1760.
60. Smith RA, Cokkinides V, Eyre HJ. CA Cancer J Clin 2003;53(1):27–43.
61. Freedman DA, Petitti DB, Robins JM. Int J Epidemiol 2004;33(1):43–55.
62. Duffy S, Tabar L, Chen HH et al. Cancer 2002;95: 458–469.
63. U.S. Preventive Services Task Force. Ann Intern Med 2002;137(5 pt 1):I47.
64. Fletcher SW, Black W, Harris R, Rimer BK, Shapiro S. J Natl Cancer Inst 1993;85(20): 1644–1656.
65. U.S. Preventive Services Task Force. Guide to Clinical Preventive Services, 2nd ed. Baltimore: Williams & Wilkins, 1996.
66. National Institutes of Health Consensus Development Panel. J Natl Cancer Inst 1997; 89(14):1015–1026.
67. de Koning HJ, Boer R, Warmerdam PG, Beemsterboer PM, van der Maas PJ. J Natl Cancer Inst 1995;87(16):1217–1223.
68. Tabar L, Duffy SW, Chen HH. J Natl Cancer Inst 1996;88(1):52–55.
69. Tabar L, Chen HH, Fagerberg G, Duffy SW, Smith TC. J Natl Cancer Inst Monogr 1997;22:43–47.
70. Tabar L, Faberberg G, Day NE, Holmberg L. Br J Cancer 1987;55(5):547–551.
71. Kerlikowske K, Salzmann P, Phillips KA, Cauley JA, Cummings SR. JAMA 1999;282(22): 2156–2163.
72. Ries L, Eisner M, Kosary C et al. SEER Cancer Statistics Review, 1975–2001. National Cancer Institute, 2004.
73. National Cancer Institute. SEER*Stat 4/2, ed. 4.2. Bethesda: National Cancer Institute, 2002.
74. Nixon AJ, Neuberg D, Hayes DF et al. J Clin Oncol 1994;12(5):888–894.
75. McCarthy EP, Burns RB, Freund KM et al. J Am Geriatr Soc 2000;48(10):1226–1233.
76. McPherson CP, Swenson KK, Lee MW. J Am Geriatr Soc 2002;50(6):1061–1068.
77. Walter LC, Covinsky KE. JAMA 2001;285(21): 2750–2756.
78. Arias E. United States Life Tables, 2002. Center for Health Statistics, 2004.
79. Duffy SW, Day NE, Tabar L, Chen HH, Smith TC. J Natl Cancer Inst Monogr 1997;22:93–97.
80. White E, Miglioretti DL, Yankaskas BC et al. J Natl Cancer Inst 2004;96(24):1832–1839.
81. Michaelson JS, Halpern E, Kopans DB. Radiology 1999;212(2):551–560.
82. Hunt KA, Rosen EL, Sickles EA. Outcome analysis for women undergoing annual versus biennial screening mammography: a review of 24,211 examinations. Am J Roentgenol 1999;173(2): 285–289.
83. Rosenquist CJ, Lindfors KK. Cancer 1998;82(11): 2235–2240.
84. Rosenquist CJ, Lindfors KK. Radiology 1994;191(3):647–650.
85. Lindfors KK, Rosenquist CJ. JAMA 1995;274(11): 881–884.
86. Salzmann P, Kerlikowske K, Phillips K. Ann Intern Med 1997;127(11):955–965.
87. Mandelblatt J, Saha S, Teutsch S et al. Ann Intern Med 2003;139(10):835–842.

88. Gold M. JAMA 1996;276:1253–1258.

89. Tabar L, Tony Chen HH, Amy Yen MF et al. Cancer 2004;101(8):1745–1759.

90. Gordon PB, Goldenberg SL. Cancer 1995;76(4): 626–630.

91. Buchberger W, Niehoff A, Obrist P, DeKoekkoek-Doll P, Dunser M. Semin Ultrasound CT MR 2000;21(4):325–336.

92. Kaplan SS. Radiology 2001;221(3):641–649.

93. Crystal P, Strano SD, Shcharynski S, Koretz MJ. Am J Roentgenol 2003;181(1):177–182.

94. Hou MF, Chuang HY, Ou-Yang F et al. Ultrasound Med Biol 2002;28(4):415–420.

95. Berg WA. Am J Roentgenol 2003;180:1225–1228.

96. Michaelson JS, Silverstein M, Wyatt J et al. Cancer 2002;95(4):713–723.

97. Baker JA, Kornguth PJ, Soo MS, Walsh R, Mengoni P. Am J Roentgenol 1999;172(6): 1621–1625.

98. Hlawatsch A, Teifke A, Schmidt M, Thelen M. Am J Roentgenol 2002;179(6):1493–1501.

99. Dershaw DD, Abramson A, Kinne DW. Radiology 1989;170(2):411–415.

100. Bassett LW. Radiol Clin North Am 2000;38(4): 669–691.

101. Bartow SA, Pathak DR, Black WC, Key CR, Teaf SR. Cancer 1987;60(11):2751–2760.

102. Georgian-Smith D, Taylor KJ, Madjar H et al. J Clin Ultrasound 2000;28(5):211–216.

103. Dennis MA, Parker SH, Klaus AJ, Stavros AT, Kaske TI, Clark SB. Radiology 2001;219(1): 186–191.

104. Moy L, Slanetz PJ, Moore R et al. Radiology 2002;225(1):176–181.

105. Kaiser JS, Helvie MA, Blacklaw RL, Roubidoux MA. Radiology 2002;223(3):839–844.

106. Houssami N, Irwig L, Simpson JM, McKessar M, Blome S, Noakes J. Am J Roentgenol 2003; 180(4):935–940.

107. Paterok EM, Rosenthal H, Sabel M. Eur J Obstet Gynecol Reprod Biol 1993;50(3):227–234.

108. Leis HP Jr, Greene FL, Cammarata A, Hilfer SE. South Med J 1988;81(1):20–26.

109. Cardenosa G, Doudna C, Eklund GW. Am J Roentgenol 1994;162(5):1081–1087.

110. Yang WT, Tse GM. Am J Roentgenol 2004; 182(1):101–110.

111. Hild F, Duda VF, Albert U, Schulz KD. Eur J Cancer Prev 1998;7(suppl 1): S57–56.

112. Liberman L, Morris EA, Dershaw DD, Abramson AF, Tan LK. Am J Roentgenol 2003;180(4): 901–910.

113. Holland R, Veling SH, Mravunac M, Hendriks JH. Cancer 1985;56(5):979–990.

114. Anderson ME, Soo MS, Bentley RC, Trahey GE. J Acoust Soc Am 1997;101(1):29–39.

115. Soo MS, Baker JA, Rosen EL. Am J Roentgenol 2003;180(4):941–948.

116. Moon WK, Noh DY, Im JG. Radiology 2002; 224(2):569–576.

117. Sickles EA. Radiology 1991;179:463–468.

118. Varas X, Leborgne F, Leborgne JH. Radiology 1992;184:409–414.

119. Sickles EA. Radiology 1994;192:439–442.

120. Sickles EA. Radiology 1998;208:471–475.

121. Vizcaino I, Gadea L, Andreo L et al. Radiology 2001;219:475–483.

122. Hall FM. Arch Surg 1990;125:298–299.

123. Wolfe JN, Buck KA, Salane M, Parekh NJ. Radiology 1987;165:305–311.

124. Helvie MA, Pennes DR, Rebner M, Adler DD. Radiology 1991;178:155–158.

125. Rosen PP. Rosen's Breast Pathology. Philadelphia: Lippincott-Raven, 1997:76–82.

126. Alleva DQ, Smetherman DH, Farr GH Jr, Cederbom GJ. Radiographics 1999;19:S27–35.

127. Brenner RJ, Jackman RJ, Parker SH et al. Am J Roentgenol 2002;179(5):1179–1184.

128. Philpotts LE, Shaheen NA, Jain KS, Carter D, Lee CH. Radiology 2000;216:831–837.

129. Orel SG, Evers K, Yeh IT, Troupin RH. Radiology 1992;183:479–482.

130. Smith DN, Christian RL, Meyer JE. Arch Surg 1997;132:256–259.

131. Parker SH, Lovin JD, Jobe WE et al. Radiology 1990;76:741–747.

132. Parker SH, Lovin JD, Jobe WE, Burke BJ, Hopper KD, Yakes WF. Radiology 1991;180:403–407.

133. Parker SH, Jobe WE, Dennis MA et al. Radiology 1993;187:507–511.

134. Elvecrog EL, Lechner MC, Nelson MT. Radiology 1993;188:453–455.

135. Brendlinger DL, Robinson R, Sylvest V, Burton S. Va Med Q 1994;121(3):179–184.

136. Burbank F, Kaye K, Belville J, Blumenfeld M. Radiology 1994;191:165–171.

137. Gisvold JJ, Goellner JR, Grant CS et al. Am J Roentgenol 1994;162:815–820.

138. Jackman RJ, Nowels KS, Shepard NJ, Finkelstein SI, Marzoni FA. Radiology 1994;193:91–95.

139. Parker SH, Burbank F, Jackman RJ et al. Radiology 1994;193:359–364.

140. Meyer JE, Smith DN, Lester SC et al. Radiology 1998;206:717–720.

141. Jackman RJ, Nowels KW, Rodriquez-Soto J, Marzoni FA Jr, Finkelstein SI, Shepard MJ. Radiology 1999;210:799–805.

142. Meyer JE, Smith DN, Lester SC et al. JAMA 1999;281:1638–1641.

143. Brenner RJ, Bassett LW, Fajardo LL et al. Radiology 2001;218:866–872.

144. Margolin FR, Leung JWT, Jacobs RP, Denny SR. Am J Roentgenol 2001;177:559–564.

145. Fajardo LL, Pisano ED, Caudry DJ et al. Acad Radiol 2004;11:293–308.

146. Orel SG, Schnall MD, Newman RW, Powell CM, Torosian MH, Rosato EF. Radiology 1994;193: 97–102.

147. Orel SG, Schnall MD, Powell CM et al. Radiology 1995;196:115–122.

148. Doler W, Fisher U, Metzger I, Harder D, Grabbe E. Radiology 1996;200:863–864.
149. Daniel BL, Birdwell RL, Black JW, Ikeda DM, Glover GH, Herfkens RJ. Acad Radiol 1997;4: 508–512.
150. Kuhl CK, Elevelt A, Leutner CC, Gieseke J, Pakos E, Schild HH. Radiology 1997;204:667–675.
151. Liberman L, Feng TL, Dershaw DD, Morris EA, Abramson, AF. Radiology 1998;208:717–723.
152. Hillner BE, Bear HD, Fajardo LL. Acad Radiol 1996;3:351–360.
153. Liberman L, Fahs MC, Dershaw DD et al. Radiology 1995;195:633–637.
154. Lindfors KK, Rosenquist CJ. Radiology 1994;190: 217–222.
155. Lee CH, Egglin TK, Philpotts L, Mainiero MB, Tocino I. Radiology 1997;202:849–854.
156. Fajardo LL. Acad Radiol 1996;3:521–523.
157. Fischer U, Kopka L, Grabbe E. Radiology 1999;213(3):881–888.
158. Berg WA, Gilbreath PL. Radiology 2000;214(1): 59–66.

6

Imaging of Lung Cancer

James G. Ravenel and Gerard A. Silvestri

Issues

I. Is there a role for imaging in lung cancer screening?
   A. What is the role of chest X-ray?
   B. What is the role of computed tomography?
II. How should lung cancer be staged?
   A. How is the primary tumor evaluated?
   B. How is the mediastinum evaluated?
   C. How are distant metastases evaluated?
   D. Special case: how is small cell lung cancer evaluated?
   E. Special case: what is the appropriate radiologic follow-up?

Key Points

- Screening with chest radiographs does not decrease disease-specific lung cancer mortality (moderate evidence).
- CT scan is able to detect lung cancers at a smaller size. Screening with CT can reduce lung cancer mortality by 20% in a high risk population (strong evidence).
- CT and PET should be the primary tools for staging non-small cell lung cancer (NSCLC) and guiding invasive studies (strong evidence).

Definition and Pathophysiology

Malignant neoplasms of the pulmonary parenchyma can be loosely categorized as lung cancer. Simplistically stated, cancer in the lung occurs through a complex interaction of DNA damage, repair, and mutation (1, 2). Lung cancer includes a variety of histologic cell types. Squamous cell, large cell, and adenocarcinoma are categorized as non-small cell carcinoma

J.G. Ravenel (✉)
Department of Radiology, Medical University of South Carolina,
94 Jonathan Lucas St. MSC 323, Charleston, SC 29425, USA
e-mail: ravenejg@musc.edu

based on their common staging and treatment regimens. Small cell carcinoma is distinctly more aggressive and is treated differently from the other cell types.

Epidemiology

Lung cancer remains a preeminent public health concern, with over 221,000 cases diagnosed annually and over 157,000 deaths per year in the USA (3). Perhaps even more daunting is the fact that over one million people worldwide will succumb to the disease (4). Lung cancer is the leading cause of cancer-specific mortality, outpacing breast, prostate, colon, and ovarian cancer combined. Regardless of histologic subtype, smoking is the presumed causative agent in over 85% of cases (5). Although smoking cessation reduces the risk of developing lung cancer, up to 50% of newly diagnosed lung cancers occur in former smokers (6). Other occupational and environmental exposures can contribute to the risk and development of lung cancer, including arsenic, nickel, chromium, and asbestos (1). Radiation makes up the primary environmental source of lung cancer. Radon, of primary concern to uranium miners, is an ubiquitous environmental source (50–100 times lower than uranium mines) of high-LET (linear energy transfer) radiation (7, 8). The relationship with low-level radiation is less clear. Intermittent lower dose radiation given to tuberculosis patients showed that the risk, if any, was small (9).

Overall Cost to Society

Tobacco smoke, the major risk for development of lung cancer, is estimated to result in costs over $157 billion in health related economic losses (10) and constitutes approximately 6–8% of personal health care expenditures in the USA (11). The estimated annual cost for the treatment of lung cancer is approximately $21,000 per patient, but rises to approximately $47,000 for those who do not survive 1 year (12, 13). Conservatively, this results in an annual cost of treating lung cancer in the United States of $3.6 billion per year.

Goals

The goal of screening is to detect serious disease at a preclinical stage where treatment for the disease is more effective when administered early (14). At this level, lung cancer appears to be an ideal candidate for screening. There is a well-defined high-risk population, and when detected by symptoms the disease is advanced in over 80% of cases. Furthermore, treatment is more efficacious at an earlier stage as measured by 5-year survival (15). The goal of staging is to define the extent of disease and help select the optimum course of treatment. As such, staging has both therapeutic and prognostic implications.

Methodology

A Medline search was performed using PubMed (National Library of Medicine, Bethesda, Maryland) for original research publications discussing the diagnostic performance and effectiveness of imaging strategies in lung cancer screening. The search covered the years 1966 to 2010 and included the following search terms: (1) *lung cancer screening*, (2) *lung cancer* and *computed tomography*, and (3) *lung cancer* and *chest X-ray*. Additional articles were identified by reviewing the reference lists of relevant papers. This review was limited to human studies and the English-language literature. For lung cancer staging, the authors built on a recent meta-analysis of the literature authored by one of the chapter's coauthors (G.A.S.) (16, 17). This study included a full review of the literature from January 1991 to July 2001. Articles prior to 1991 were excluded due to marked improvements in imaging technology. To ensure that more recent articles were included, a search was performed using PubMed using the following terms: (1) *lung cancer* and *computed tomography*, (2) *lung cancer* and *positron emission tomography* (PET), (3) *lung cancer* and *magnetic resonance imaging* (MRI), and (4) *lung cancer staging* for the period 1 July 2001, to December 2010. The authors performed an initial review of the titles and abstracts of the identified articles followed by review of the full text in articles that were relevant.

I. Is There a Role for Imaging in Lung Cancer Screening?

Summary of Evidence: Screening for lung cancer with chest radiographs has not been shown to reduce lung cancer mortality. The addition of sputum cytology does not increase the yield of screening. The National Screening Trial has shown a lung cancer mortality reduction of 20% in high risk individuals compared with screening chest radiographs.

Supporting Evidence

A. What Is the Role of Chest X-Ray?

Radiographic screening for lung cancer dates back to the 1950s (Table 6.1). The Philadelphia Pulmonary Neoplasm Research Project performed periodic photofluorography screening on over 6,000 male volunteers, with disappointing results. Although survival was slightly better in the screen-detected cancers versus symptom-detected cancers, screen-detected cancers had the same outcome regardless of the time from the previous negative study (Fig. 6.1) (18). At about the same time, the North London study randomized over 50,000 men, ages 40–64, to biannual chest X-rays over 3 years or chest X-rays at the beginning and end of the 3-year period. More cancers were detected in the study group (101 vs. 77), and the 5-year survival rate was better (15% vs. 6%), although this was not statistically significant (19). The study also suffered from problems with randomization, as there were statistically more ex-smokers in the screened group and more participants aged 60–64 in the control group (20).

Case–control series of chest radiographs for lung cancer screening have been performed in Japan owing to the large amount of available data from tuberculosis control programs. The first trial reported from Osaka estimated a 28% reduction in mortality and better survival for those in the screen-detected group compared to those in the Osaka Cancer Registry (21). Four more recent case–control series show an estimated mortality reduction between 30 and 60% (22–25). Pooling the data of these four Prefectures resulted in an estimated mortality reduction of 44% (26).

Two European nonrandomized trials of chest radiograph screening have been performed. In Varese, Italy, 2,444 heavy smokers were screened annually for 3 years; 16 cancers were detected during the prevalence screen, 31% stage I, and 7 cancers were detected during the two incidence screens, 71% stage I (27). The Turku Study in Finland studied 93 men out of 33,000 who had lung cancer detected on a one-time screen and compared them to those detected by symptoms or serendipitously noted on chest radiograph performed for other purposes. Screen-detected cases tended to be of an earlier stage and thus resectable (37% vs. 19%), and 5-year survival was better in the screen-detected group (19% vs. 10%) (28).

Taken all together, the nonrandomized studies performed in Europe and Japan would seemingly give credence to an advantage for screened populations. As pointed out previously, however, the biases present in the design of these studies make it impossible to definitively attribute the apparent benefit to screening. Furthermore, there are likely differences in the populations studied when compared to the US population. In Japan, lung cancer in females is a disease of nonsmokers, and female smoking-related cases were excluded to facilitate matching controls (22, 25). A high proportion of male never-smokers were present in the Miyagi screening study. Furthermore, peripheral adenocarcinoma occurs in a higher percentage of cases in Japan, and thus the efficacy of screening seen in Japan may not translate to US populations (25).

Including the previously mentioned North London study, a total of six randomized controlled trials and one nonrandomized trial of chest radiograph lung cancer screening have been performed. In all of these studies, the control group underwent some form of screening, though less frequently than the intervention arm. The Kaiser Foundation trial, though not specifically performed for lung cancer, randomized over 10,000 participants aged 35–54 into an intervention group that was encouraged to participate in a multiphasic health checkup, including chest X-ray, and a control group that was not. Seventeen percent of participants in both groups were smokers. All-cause mortality was not significantly different between groups (29). The Erfurt, Germany, study was a nonrandomized trial with 41,000 males in the intervention group, who underwent biannual chest X-rays and 102,000 males in the control group, who had chest X-rays every 18 months. The intervention group had a higher rate of cancers detected (9% vs. 6.5%), a higher resection rate (28% vs. 19%), and better 5- and 10-year survival. However, there was no difference in lung cancer or all-cause mortality (30).

Under the auspices of the National Cancer Institute (NCI), three separate screening trials were performed in the US during the 1970s (31). Two of these studies, the Johns Hopkins study (32) and the Memorial Sloan-Kettering (33) study, enrolled over 10,000 males each into an intervention group that received annual chest X-rays and sputum cytology every 4 months, and a control group that received only an annual chest X-ray. While there was a slight benefit to sputum cytology at the prevalence screen, all-cause mortality was the same in both groups (34–36). The results led to the conclusion that sputum cytology does not significantly improve the yield of chest X-ray screening.

The Czech Study on Lung Cancer Screening had a rather unique design. At the initial screen, all participants received a chest X-ray and sputum analysis. After 19 prevalence cases were excluded, 6,345 were randomized to either semiannual chest X-rays and sputum analysis for 3 years or a chest X-ray and sputum analysis at the end of the 3-year period. Both groups then received annual chest X-rays at 1-year intervals from years 4 through 6. The first reported results were promising, with 48% diagnosed at stage I or II and 27% undergoing curative resections in the intervention arm (37). The number of stage III cancers in each arm was similar (17 vs. 15). At follow-up, however, despite the fact that the lung cancer in the screened group was of earlier stage, almost three times as likely to be resectable, and had a better 5-year survival from time of diagnosis, there were more lung cancer deaths in the intervention arm, all-cause mortality was greater in the intervention arm, and smoking-related deaths were greater in the interventional arm (38). Conclusions did not change at extended follow-up (39).

The Mayo Lung Project randomized 10,933 participants into an intervention arm of chest X-ray and sputum cytology every 4 months and a control arm of "usual care" for 6 years (40). Ninety-one prevalence cancers were detected with over 50% postsurgical stage I or II and

5-year survival of 40%. Prevalence cases tended to be of a more well-differentiated histology (41) and complete resection could be performed in twice as many screening participants compared to a previous cohort of over 1,700 patients. By the end of the trial, 206 lung cancers had been detected in the screening arm and 160 in the control arm. Although screen-detected cancers were more resectable (54% vs. 30%), there was no stage shift and no statistically significant difference between the groups in lung cancer mortality (42, 43). With follow-up out to 20 years, no benefit could be detected in the screened group (44).

The results of the Mayo Lung Project remain controversial. Contamination of the control group was considered substantial. Over 73% of subjects received a chest radiograph in the last 2 years of the study, and 30% of the cancers in the control group were discovered on chest radiographs performed for reasons other than suspicion of lung cancer (43). The majority of these ostensibly "screen" cancers in the control group were resectable. Overdiagnosis bias is one of the proposed reasons for the excess cancers in the screen group, although this hypothesis, particularly as it applies to lung cancer, remains controversial (45–47). It has also been suggested that the Mayo Lung Project was underpowered and thus had only a 20% chance of showing a mortality benefit should it have existed (48). Although it was also suggested that there was heterogeneity between the groups that affected mortality (49), reappraisal of the populations in the study showed no difference in age at entry, cigarette smoking history, exposure to nontobacco lung carcinogens, and comorbid pulmonary diseases (50). Regardless of the controversy, it is important to realize that to date, lung cancer screening with chest radiographs has not been shown to reduce lung cancer mortality. There is one ongoing larger randomized control trial of lung cancer screening with chest radiograph as part of the Prostate, Lung, Colorectal, and Ovarian Cancer Screening Trial (51).

B. What Is the Role of Computed Tomography?

Early experience of a total of nine trials of nonrandomized screening, three in Japan, three in Europe, and three in the USA, enrolling a total of 20,116 individuals for prevalence screens (52–60). Several of these studies have reported annual incidence data, and thus far 25,406 incidence screens have been reported (55, 57, 61–63) (Table 6.2). It is important to realize that the superiority of CT for the detection of abnormalities is not in question; however, CT identifies many smaller, "indeterminate" nodules, the majority of which will eventually turn out to be benign, but represent a diagnostic dilemma at the time of screening. The rate of false-positive exams must be taken into consideration in the context of lung cancer screening.

The most extensive experience has been seen in Japan where the three trials, Anti-Lung Cancer Association (ALCA) (55), Hitachi Employee's Health Insurance Group (Hitachi) (57), and Matsumoto Research Center (Matsumoto) (52, 61), have reported on 15,050 participants. These studies utilized 10-mm collimation for the computed tomography (CT) scans. Two studies, ALCA and Matsumoto, included sputum cytology in the screening regimen and screening was performed at 6-month intervals in ALCA. A total of 72 lung cancers were detected during the prevalence screen (0.5%), 57 of which were stage IA (79.2%). At the same time, non-calcified nodules were present in 2,564 (17%, range 5–26%) individuals. A total of 7,891 follow-up examinations have been reported in the ALCA study with 19 additional cancers detected, 15 of which were stage IA (78.9%). One incidence screen has been reported in the Hitachi study in 5,568 individuals with four additional detected lung cancers, three stage IA. In total, 8,303 incidence screens have been reported over 2 years in the Matsumoto study with a total of 37 cancers detected, 32 of which were stage IA (86.5%). A major consideration in the Japanese trials is that screening was made available at a younger age, usually 40, and that smoking history was not a requirement for participation (nonsmokers accounted for 14% of the ALCA study, 38% of the Hitachi study, and 53% of the Matsumoto study). Thus it is unclear that these results can be generalized to usual screening cohorts.

Three European trials were reported in the literature. In Germany, 817 asymptomatic volunteers over the age of 40 with at least a 20-pack-a-year smoking history underwent screening. At the prevalence screen 43% were found to have at least one noncalcified nodule, and 11 patients had malignancy including

seven stage IA (one participant had two squamous cell carcinomas considered to be synchronous primary lesion) (60). One video-assisted thoracotomy surgery was performed for benign disease. In Finland, 602 workers with asbestos exposure (mean 26 years) and smoking history underwent screening. The prevalence screen detected 111 cases with at least 1 nodule by consensus review (18%) and 5 lung cancers (all at least stage IIA). The authors also provided the number of follow-up procedures required; 54 repeat CT, 15 bronchoscopy, 6 image-guided fine-needle aspiration and 9 thoracotomy/thoracoscopy (only 1 for malignant disease) (53). Finally, the first 2 years of screening of 1,035 subjects in Italy have been reported. All were 50 years old or older and had at least a 20-pack-a-year smoking history. The study is scheduled to perform annual screening for 5 years. Twenty percent had indeterminate nodules at baseline screening. Twenty-two lung cancers have been detected, 11 during the prevalence screen (6 stage IA) and 11 during the incidence screen (10 stage IA) (56).

Three studies in the US have published results. A small study designed to test the feasibility of a randomized controlled trial showed that almost 80% of subjects would be willing to be randomized to either observation or chest CT (59). Of the initial 92 randomized to CT, 30 had noncalcified nodules (32.6%). One stage I and one stage IV lung cancer were detected. The Mayo Clinic evaluated 1,520 individuals 50 and older with at least a 20-pack-a-year smoking history (54, 62). Sputum cytology was also performed. Noncalcified nodules were found in 69% of participants. Over 3 years, 40 cancers were detected in the population: 26 prevalence, 10 incidence, 2 interval (symptom detected between screening exams), and 2 by sputum cytology alone. Twenty-two cancers were stage 1A, 17 prevalence and 5 incidence. There were four limited-stage small cell carcinomas. The first US CT screening study, the Early Lung Cancer Action Project (ELCAP), enrolled 1,000 symptom-free individuals 60 and older with at least a 10-pack-a-year smoking history (64). The prevalence screen revealed 233 noncalcified nodules and 27 lung cancers, 23 stage I. During incidence screens, seven additional lung cancers were identified by screening, five stage I, and two by symptoms, both advanced (63).

Over the next 6 years, data from non-randomized trials continued to suggest a possible benefit. The largest reported experience was the International Early Lung Cancer Action project (IELCAP), reporting on over 31,000 prevalence screens and over 27,000 annual screens. From these subjects, they found 85% with clinical stage I cancer resulting in a 10 year survival of 88% for the stage I group. The percentage of stage I cancers as well as survival were much higher than traditionally reported for lung cancer (65). In a related study, the authors found a statistically significant relationship between tumor size and tumor stage at smaller sizes. This trend was most pronounced with solid nodules (66). At the same time, competing evidence against CT screening was derived by modeling risk. Bach et al. (67) compared lung cancer diagnosis in three non-randomized trials with a previously validated model of lung cancer risk. By screening, there were 144 lung cancer cases diagnosed compared to 45 expected, 109 resections performed compared to 11 expected without a decline in either advanced lung cancers or lung cancer deaths.

There is a growing body of literature from RCTs in Europe. Data from the Lung Screening Study, a randomized-controlled feasibility study for the National Lung Screening Trial, showed, as expected, that CT detected more lung cancers overall and more Stage I lung cancers than chest radiographs, but also detected more late stage lung cancers (68). Although not powered to detect a mortality benefit and the number of late stage cancers detected was not statistically significant from zero, the data suggest that the necessary stage-shift away from late stage lung cancers may not be present. In Europe, the findings are similar. Reported studies from France and Italy (69, 70) show the same trend with more lung cancer diagnoses and early stage lung cancers, but no decrease in late stage lung cancers in the CT arm. Early mortality data from the DANTE trail in Italy also show no difference in lung cancer and all cause mortality between arms but with a p value that did not reach statistical significance (70).

Late in 2010, the Data Monitoring Safety Board for the National Lung Screening Trial decided on the early release of the mortality data. This was based on the fact that 442 lung cancer deaths occurred in the chest radiograph arm compared with 354 in the CT arm for a 20.3% reduction in lung cancer specific mortality, providing a scientific basis for CT screening (71). Prior to widespread adoption, however, a further understanding of risks associated with incidental findings and costs will be needed. Given that the data reveal that it requires 300 subjects screened to prevent one lung cancer death while indeterminate (and ultimately non-cancerous) nodules will be detected in up to 1 in 5 subjects (71), these factors are non-trivial from a policy standpoint.

Will Computed Tomography Screening Be Cost-Effective?

The ultimate fate of CT screening for lung cancer rests with the presence or absence of mortality benefit as well as the magnitude of benefit. Even if a benefit is detected, screening may be cost-prohibitive for the population as a whole. In the absence of long-term results, particularly as it relates to efficacy and morbidity associated with evaluation of nodules eventually deemed benign, cost-effectiveness is largely speculative as determined by cost-efficacy analysis. Two analyses have been wildly optimistic, suggesting that lung cancer screening may cost less than $10,000 per life year saved (72, 73). This becomes more apparent when compared with other well-accepted intervention screening strategies such as mammography, hypertension screening in 60-year-olds, and screening donated blood for HIV, which all result in a cost per life year saved of approximately $20,000 (74). In general, these studies have not accounted well for follow-up of indeterminate nodules and the possible harms of the diagnostic algorithms on benign disease. Two studies try to account for these factors. In one study, assuming 50% of cancers detected were localized and accounting for a full range of diagnostic workup and scenarios presumes a cost per life year saved ranging from $33,000 to $48,000 (75). The least optimistic model, assuming a stage-shift of 50%, used data from previous trials to account for follow-up procedures, benign biopsies, and nonadherence. Under these circumstances the cost per life year saved was calculated as $116,000 for current smokers, $558,600 for quitting smokers, and $2,322,700 for former smokers (76). Thus, the cost-effectiveness of lung cancer screening will have a great effect on its implementation and should eventually be directly ascertained from data collected during the national Lung Screening Trial (77).

II. How Should Lung Cancer Be Staged?

Summary of Evidence: Current staging of lung cancer usually consists of complementary anatomic and physiologic imaging by CT and PET (Fig. 6.2). MRI is useful for evaluating local extension of superior sulcus tumors into the brachial plexus. It may also be used for imaging the central nervous system and occasionally to image the liver and adrenal glands. Bone scintigraphy may be used to assess for osseous metastases. Histologic subtypes including squamous cell, adenocarcinoma, and large cell carcinoma are categorized as NSCLC due to the similar treatment and prognosis based on stage. Small cell carcinoma, the fourth major subtype, is staged separately.

Supporting Evidence: Staging of lung cancer is critical for choosing the appropriate treatment and for assessing overall prognosis. Staging is categorized by the tumor, node, metastasis (TNM) system as set forth in the American Joint Committee on Cancer, 7th Edition (78), and takes into account features of the primary tumor as well as dissemination to the mediastinum and distant organs (Tables 6.3 and 6.4).

A. How Is the Primary Tumor Evaluated?

Computed tomography is the preferred modality for initially establishing the diagnosis of lung cancer and providing initial staging information, as it is widely available, more sensitive than chest radiograph, rapid to perform, and guides further workup. The use of intravenous contrast is largely based on physician preference, as few studies have been performed to assess interpretive difference. Those that have been performed do not show clear superiority of enhanced over unenhanced scans (79–81). The evaluation of T stage is often straightforward with CT. Difficulty may arise in the evaluation of invasion into the chest wall and

mediastinum. Rib erosion, bone destruction, or tumor adjacent to mediastinal structures provides reliable evidence of invasion. Without these features, proximity and secondary signs (>3 cm of contact with the pleural surface, pleural thickening, absent fat planes, and obtuse angle of tumor with the chest wall) are only moderately helpful in predicting invasion (82–85), and localized chest pain is a more specific finding (82). MRI is slightly more successful at detecting chest wall invasion (86–88) owing to better spatial resolution particularly in the lung apex (Table 6.5). Using dynamic cine evaluation of the tumor during breathing provides reliable exclusion of parietal pleura invasion, although false-positive results still occur (89–91).

B. How Is the Mediastinum Evaluated?

Because size is the determining factor for the interpretation of mediastinal adenopathy, usually 1 cm in short axis, CT is an imperfect tool for categorization of mediastinal disease. Thirty-five studies performed between 1991 and 2006 pooling 5111 patients (prevalence of adenopathy (28%) gives a sensitivity and specificity of 51/86% for mediastinal disease (92).

While MRI staging is feasible, it is not widely utilized due to cost and availability. It has been suggested that MR is better at detecting hilar lymph nodes, although the clinical utility of this is unclear (93, 94). The few studies performed suggest that unenhanced MRI is at best equivalent to CT (95, 96), although gadolinium or new iron oxide-contrast agents may ultimately increase the utility of MRI (95, 97).

Forty-four studies performed between 1994 and 2006 pooling 2865 patients (prevalence of adenopathy 29%) gives a sensitivity and specificity of 74/85% for mediastinal disease (92). A similar sensitivity and specificity (85 and 90%) were found in a second meta-analysis (98). This study also showed that the value of PET was dependent on CT findings. In the setting of a positive CT scan, sensitivity approached 100%, whereas specificity fell to 78%. When the CT did not reveal adenopathy, PET was 82% sensitive and 93% specific (98). Most recently, five studies, each with over 100 patients, have presented a less optimistic view of PET for staging the mediastinum, with sensitivity ranging from 61 to 94% and specificity from 77 to 84% (99–103). More importantly, in two of these studies the false-negative rate of PET in the mediastinum was over 10% (99, 100). While PET clearly has better test characteristics than CT for staging the mediastinum, it is far from perfect. However, it may not be fair to judge the value of PET in staging lung cancer based on the accuracy in the mediastinum alone. The utility of PET lies in its ability to upstage or downstage patients with lung cancer based on its ability to detect previously unsuspected disease in the lung, mediastinum, or extrathoracic disease. Two studies have now shown that stand-alone PET avoids unnecessary thoracotomy in approximately 20% of cases (99, 104).

Fusion of images either obtained at different times or on a dedicated PET/CT scanner increases the sensitivity of PET alone by 5–8% without a change in specificity for lymph nodes and more accurate overall stage evaluation (105–107). The addition of PET/CT to the staging regimen in surgical candidates has also been shown in RCTs to reduce the number of futile thoracotomies (108, 109).

C.   How Are Distant Metastases Evaluated?

Pleural Effusion

Malignant pleural effusions by definition have tumor cells in the pleural space and almost always exudative (3–10% will be transudative) (110). However, the mere presence of pleural fluid cannot be used as de facto evidence of pleural metastases. Effusions may be paramalignant due to central venous or lymphatic obstruction, due to post-obstructive atelectasis/pneumonitis or due to causes unrelated to the tumor (cardiac, hepatic, renal disease, etc.) (111). Effusions in this category are not therefore indicative of metastatic disease. Thus, sampling of the fluid is mandatory prior to labeling a patient as having a malignant pleural effusion and therefore non-resectable. CT suggests a high likelihood of malignant effusion when the parietal pleural thickness is >1cm, there is circumferential thickening, pleural nodules or mediastinal pleural involvement (110). In these cases pleural biopsy should be strongly considered when pleural fluid cytology is negative. 18F-FDG PET has been shown to be quite accurate (>90%) in the confirmation of metastatic pleural disease in two series (112, 113).

Liver Metastasis

In the setting of negative clinical exam including normal liver function tests, the yield of CT for liver metastasis is less than 5% (17, 114). Furthermore, the liver is rarely the sole site of metastatic disease at the time of diagnosis, occurring in approximately 3% of cases (115, 116). Therefore, the majority of isolated liver lesions encountered during the workup of NSCLC will be benign hemangiomas or cysts. As most chest CT scans cover the majority of the liver, dedicated hepatic imaging is generally not indicated. In equivocal cases MR imaging may be best for problem solving. 18F-FDG PET has not been formally evaluated for imaging of liver metastasis related to lung cancer; however, experience in other malignancies suggests that 18F-FDG PET can accurately detect liver metastases by demonstrating focal uptake greater than the background of the liver (117).

Adrenal Metastasis

Incidental adrenal lesions are frequently encountered in the general population and thus encountered in up to 10% of lung cancer patients (118). The likelihood of metastasis is to some extent related to cancer stage, with benign adenomas predominating in stage I disease and metastases predominating in late-stage disease (114, 119–121). With CT, lesions can be assumed to be benign if <10 Hounsfield units (HU) on unenhanced images (122), or <60% washout of contrast is observed with 15-min delayed contrast-enhanced images (123–125). MR imaging with in-phase and out-of- phase sequences is an alternative to CT. Signal dropout on out-of-phase imaging can be used to reliably confirm a benign adrenal lesion (126). Unfortunately, MR is of limited utility in lipid poor lesions (unenhanced CT attenuation values > 10) (127, 128). 18F-FDG PET has been shown to reliably differentiate benign and malignant adrenal lesions, even those indeterminate at CT and MR, with a sensitivity and specificity of 94–100% and 74–91% in a total of four studies (129–132). It should be noted that benign nodules can be FDG avid and therefore malignancy should be confirmed when the adrenal is the only potential site of metastatic disease.

Bone Metastasis

The majority of patients with bone metastases are either symptomatic or have an elevated alkaline phosphatase (133). Since fewer than 5% of lung cancer patients have occult bone metastases at presentation (134), routine radiologic evaluation is not warranted in asymptomatic individuals. The sensitivity of a thorough clinical exam ranges from 79 to 100% (17, 133, 135, 136). While bone scintigraphy is quite sensitive for the detection of osseous metastases, the false-positive rate approaches 40%. PET also has the ability to detect bone metastases with a similar sensitivity to scintigraphy, but with a much higher specificity and NPV (137–139).

Cerebral Metastasis

In the setting of a normal central nervous system exam, the yield of cerebral imaging ranges from 0 to 10% (140–146). Asymptomatic cerebral metastases are most frequently associated with adenocarcinoma and large-cell carcinoma histologic subtypes (146, 147). Potentially operable tumors >3 cm in size are those most likely to benefit from routine cerebral imaging (148), but cerebral imaging is not routinely necessary for T1 tumors (145, 149). Both CT and MRI with contrast are accurate for the detection of cerebral lesions. Although MRI is slightly more sensitive (150), this may not be clinically meaningful and thus far has not been shown to more accurately stage lung cancer than CT alone. PET has rather poor sensitivity and is not suitable for excluding cerebral metastases (151) because the brain utilizes glucose at a high rate, thus obscuring metastatic uptake if present.

D. Special Case: How Is Small Cell Lung Cancer Evaluated?

Summary of Evidence: Small cell lung cancer (SCLC) is an aggressive neoplasm of neuroendocrine cell origin with a distinct biologic behavior and is therefore grouped separately from NSCLC. Based on analysis of resected small cell carcinomas, there is sufficient prognostic variability using the TNM system to warrant replacing the previous staging system (152), although on a practical basis the two-stage system developed by the Veterans Administration Lung Cancer Study Group (153) is usually sufficient to guide therapeutic decision making. Limited-stage disease historically includes disease confined to the chest and supraclavicular nodes that can be contained within a single, tolerable

radiation port. Under the TNM approach, this means that Stage I-III is encompassed under the old "limited disease" while extensive disease is equivalent to Stage IV disease. Staging strategies for SCLC are similar to NSCLC. Due to the high incidence of brain metastases, routine imaging of the central nervous system is warranted.

Supporting Evidence: Bone is considered to be the most common site of metastatic disease overall (35% of cases), and therefore bone scintigraphy should be part of the initial staging evaluation (154). In patients with extensive-stage disease, up to 60% have metastatic disease in the abdomen at the time of diagnosis (155, 156). This frequency warrants routine staging of the abdomen with CT scan or MRI. Cerebral metastases may be present in up to 10% of individuals at the time of diagnosis (157, 158). One small study looked at the efficacy of whole-body MRI as an alternative to CT and bone scintigraphy and found it to be equivalent (159). Fluorodeoxyglucose-PET has the potential to provide definitive whole-body staging in SCLC; however, experience at this time is limited. Three studies with a total of 59 exams in 53 patients showed agreement of PET with conventional staging in 43 of 59 cases and resulted in upstaging from limited to extensive disease in 9 cases (15%) (160–162). Moreover, PET/CT can improve the target delineation for radiation therapy in limited disease, changing field configuration in up to 25% as well as allow for more targeted irradiation of nodes with a lower rate of toxicity and low rate of local failure (163–164).

E. Special Case: What Is the Appropriate Radiologic Follow-Up?

Summary of Evidence: Two issues arise during the follow-up of lung cancer: measurement of tumors to document response to therapy and what routine follow-up tests are warranted after the completion of first-line therapy. Long-axis unidimensional measurements are appropriate for following lesions with CT or MRI. To the extent possible, the same scanning technique and interpreter should follow an individual case. Fluorodeoxyglucose-PET may eventually provide additional data by following metabolic response via standard uptake value (SUV) determination. After definitive therapy, routine imaging evaluations are not necessary.

Supporting Evidence: Originally, tumor response in clinical trials was guided by the World Health Organization (WHO) and required bidimensional measurements. Several studies have looked at the use of unidimensional long axis measurements [Response Evaluation Criteria in Solid Tumors (RECIST) Group] compared to bidimensional and volumetric measures of response. The RECIST criteria have been shown to be equivalent to WHO criteria and volumetric measurements in the classification of response to therapy (165–169). Evaluating 1,221 lung cancer patients in clinical trials, a 31% response rate was documented by using both RECIST and WHO criteria with only one disagreement between stable disease and partial response (168). While the criterion used does not seem to have an impact on response evaluation, two studies have looked at the effect of reader variability. Inter- and intraobserver variation for initial tumor size is 10–15% and 5%, respectively (170, 171). The impact on disease progression and response is affected to a greater degree. Using RECIST criteria, inter- and intraobserver variability for progressive disease ranged from 21 to 48% (average, 30%) and 3–15% (average, 9%), respectively. Response was affected to a lesser degree, interobserver 3–27% (average, 15%) and intraobserver 0–6% (average, 4%) (170).

Automated volumetric imaging has the potential advantage of eliminating measurement variability through improved precision (172, 173). As a practical matter, patient motion, respiration and relationships with adjacent structures further degrade the accuracy of volumetric change to a much greater extent then the precision of the technique (174). While studies comparing volumetry with RECIST have generally been favorable to volume assessment (175–177), in a study evaluating two dimensional measurements and semi-automated volume measurements on scans obtained the same day (no growth) showed similar degrees of variability (up to 20%) in size across all measurements (178). Additionally, most studies only account for the volume of pulmonary lesions that can be adequately segmented and do not include all sites of tumor as called for by RECIST. Thus, volumetry may not be an improvement over standard 2D measurements or an adequate tumor biomarker for therapeutic trials.

Regardless, all anatomic response measurements are limited in scope particularly in the setting of targeted therapies that may:

1. Prolong survival without change in tumor size; 2. Mischaracterize increased size due to tumor bleeding or edema (response to drug) as progression; or 3. Fail to characterize new tumor tissue in a complex mass (179). The rationale for using metabolic response criteria is based on the concept that metabolic changes are likely to precede anatomic changes. In addition, FDG-PET may provide more accurate information in anatomically complex regions, previously radiated tissues and in assessment of response to targeted therapies. Generalizability of results is difficult owing to different image acquisition techniques, measurement technique, response criteria and the difficulty in quantifying response in low SUV tumors (180). In practice, it has been generically a decrease in SUV that is associated with enhanced survival and overall improved prognosis (181–183). Ultimately, the utility of a metabolic response approach will require agreed upon criteria that can be reproduced across many sites. Two such methodologies have been proposed (186, 187).

Induction chemotherapy may be employed in selected patients with mediastinal disease in order to render patients resectable for cure. Because of the inherent difficulties of repeat mediastinoscopy, PET has been evaluated as a means of re-staging the mediastinum in 130 patients in four separate studies (188–191). Two reports, which included a total of 49 patients, had a combined accuracy of 95% (188, 191). This experience, however, has not been reproducible, with two other studies showing an accuracy of 50%. When compared directly to CT for all lymph nodes, accuracy was better for PET in one (189) and CT in the other (190). PET response, however, does correlate to some degree with survival as those with follow-up SUV less than 2.5 or decreased over 20% have improved time to disease progression and overall survival (185, 192).

Imaging following treatment with curative intent is of unclear value. Although the major professional societies include surveillance chest radiograph as part of follow-up recommendations (193–195), the hard evidence for this practice is difficult to find (196, 197). One prospective study of 192 patients with aggressive follow-up showed better 3-year survival for asymptomatic recurrence detection (31% vs. 13%) and that 43% of asymptomatic recurrences could be treated surgically (198). Similar to the screened population setting, lead and length time bias make the relevance of the survival data unclear. Two retrospective studies separately came to the conclusion that strict follow-up had little effect on mortality (199, 200). In the absence of good evidence, the ACCP guidelines suggest imaging and physical exam at 6 month intervals for two years and annually from then on, but were unable to come to consensus whether chest radiograph or CT was the preferred imaging modality (201).

Suggested Imaging Protocols

Low-Dose Screening Computed Tomography

Collimation: 1.25–2.5 mm

Reconstruction interval: 2 mm

Technique: 120 kVp/20–50 mA s

Extent: Scan from lung apices through posterior costophrenic sulcus

Breath hold: full inspiration

Reconstruction algorithm: standard or detail

Contrast: none

Chest Computed Tomography for Lung Cancer Staging

Collimation: 5 mm

Technique: 120 kVp/100–150 mA s

Extent: scan from lung apices through adrenal glands

Breath hold: full inspiration

Reconstruction algorithm: standard

Contrast (optional): ~100 cc nonionic contrast; injection rate = 2.5 cc/s; 30-s prescan delay

Take Home Tables and Figures

Tables 6.1–6.5 and Fig. 6.1–6.2 serve to highlight key recommendations and supporting evidence.

Table 6.1. Results of chest X-ray randomized control trials

Study site	Study arm	Sample size	No. of baseline screening cancers	No. of repeat screening cancers	Lung cancer mortality per 10,000 person-year
London 1960–1964	All	55,034	51	177	2.2
	Intervention	29,723	31	101	2.1
	Control	25,311	20	76	2.4
Mayo 1971–1983	All	10,933	91	366	NR
	Intervention	4,618[a]	NA	206	3.2
	Control	4,593[a]	NA	160	3.0
Czechoslovakia 1976–1980	All	6,364	18	66	NR
	Intervention	3,172[a]	NA	39	3.6
	Control	3,174[a]	NA	27	2.6
Memorial Sloan-Kettering Cancer Center 1974–1982	All	10,040	53	235	NR
	Intervention	4,968	30	114	2.7[b]
	Control	5,072	23	121	2.7[b]
Johns Hopkins 1973–1982	All	10,386	79	396[c]	
	Intervention	5,226	39	194	3.4[b]
	Control	5,161	40	202	3.8[b]

Reprinted with kind permission of Springer Science+Business Media from Ravenel JG, Silvestri GA. Imaging of Lung Cancer. In Medina LS, Blackmore DD (eds): *Evidence-Based Imaging: Optimizing Imaging in Patient Care.* New York: Springer Science+Business Media, 2006.

NA not available, *NR* not reported.

[a]Randomization subsequent to baseline screen. Sample size of the study arms do not equal number of total enrollees.

[b]Randomization prior to baseline screen. Total number of deaths may include prevalence cases.

[c]Includes 379 cancer detected during screening period and 17 cancers detected after the end of screening.

Table 6.2. Results of CT Screening Trials (202–214)

Study site	Date of publication	Baseline screen				Annual repeat screening			
		No. of patients screened	No. of abnormal results (% of total)	No. of malignancies detected (% of total)	Detected malignancies, stage 1 (%)	No. of patients screened	No. of newly identified abnormal results (% of total)	No. of detected malignancies (% of total)	Detected malignancies, stage 1 (%)
Cornell University, United States (ELCAP)	1999, 2001	1,000	233 (23)	27 (2.70)	81	1,184	63 (5)	7 (0.59)	85
Muenster University, Germany	2001	919	NR	17 (1.85)	76	NR	NR	2 (NR)	100
Matsumoto Research Center	2001	5,483	676 (12)	22 (0.40)	100	8,303	518 (6)	34 (0.41)	86
Hitachi Health Care Center	2001	8,546	NR	35 (0.41)	97	7,434	NR	7 (0.09)	100
Helsinki, Finland	2002	602	111 (18)	5 (0.8)	0	NR	NR	NR	NR
Anti-Lung Cancer Association	2002	1,611	186 (11.5)	14 (0.87)	77	7,891	721 (9.1)	22 (0.28)	82
Milan, Italy	2003	1,035	199 (19)	11 (1.1)	55	996	99 (10)	11	91
Mayo Clinic, United States	2005	1,520	782 (51)	31 (2.0)	58	5,609 (est)	847 (15)	35 (0.20)	49
Pamplona, Spain	2005	911	291 (32)	12 (1.3)	86	424	NR	2 (0.4)	100
Samsung Korea	2005	6,406	2,255 (35)	11 (0.2)	27	4,526 (est)	NR	12 (0.2)	83
LSS	2005	1,660	332 (20)	30 (1.8)	53	1,398	361 (26)	8 (0.6)	25
Dublin, Ireland	2006	449	93	2 (0.4)	50	922	NR	3 (0.3)	33
I-ELCAP	2006	31,567	4,186 (13)	405 (1.3)	86	27,456	1,460 (5)	74 (0.3)	86
Finland	2007	633	86 (14)	5 (0.8)	40	NR	NR	NR	NR
France	2007	336	152 (45)	8 (2.4)	38	NR	NR	NR	NR
Pittsburgh, US	2008	3,642	1,477 (41)	53 (1.5)	60	3,423	1,450[‡] (42)	27	33
DANTE Milan, Italy	2008, 2009	1,276	199 (16)	28 (2.2)	57	2,336 (est)	52 (6.5)	32	66
Denmark	2009	2,052	331 (16)	17 (0.8)	53	NR	NR	NR	NR
ITALUNG Florence, Italy	2009	1,613	426 (30)	20 (1.2)	55	NR	NR	NR	NR
Toronto, Canada	2009	3,352	600 (18)	44 (1.3)	73	2,686	NR (9–14)	21	48

Bold = CT Arm of RCT.

NR = Not Reported.

‡ = New or Changed Nodules.

Table 6.3. Staging of Lung Cancer-TNM Descriptors (215)

Site	Name	Comment
Primary lesion	TX	Primary tumor cannot be assessed or tumor detected by sputum or bronchial washings, but not visualized
	T0	No evidence of primary tumor
	Tis	Carcinoma in situ
	T1	Tumor < 3 cm surrounded by lung or visceral pleura without invasion proximal to lobar bronchus a) ≤ 2 cm b) > 2 cm but ≤ 3 cm
	T2	Tumors > 3 cm and ≤ 7 cm; any tumor invading main bronchi but > 2 cm from the carina; invasion of visceral pleura; obstructive pneumonitis extending to hila but does not involve entire lung a) > 3 cm but ≤ 5 cm b) > 5 cm but ≤ 7 cm
	T3	Tumor > 7 cm or of any size that directly invades chest wall, diaphragm, mediastinal pleura, or parietal pericardium; or involves main bronchus within 2 cm of carina, but does not involve carina; or results in obstructive atelectasis or pneumonitis of entire lung; or separate tumor nodule(s) in same lobe
	T4	Tumor invades any of the following: mediastinum, heart great vessels, trachea, esophagus, vertebral body or carina; malignant ipsilateral pleural or pericardial effusion; satellite tumor nodule within ipsilateral different lobe
Lymph nodes	N0	No regional lymph node metastases
	N1	Spread to ipsilateral peribronchial or hilar nodes
	N2	Spread to ipsilateral mediastinal or subcarinal nodes
	N3	Spread to contralateral mediastinal or hilar nodes; scalene nodes; supraclavicular nodes
Distant disease	M0	No distant metastases
	M1	Distant metastases a) Separate tumor nodule in contralateral lung, pleural nodules, malignant pleural or pericardial effusion b) Distant Metastases

Table 6.4. Stage of NSCLC based on TNM classification (215)

0	Carcinoma in situ
1A	T1N0M0
1B	T2aN0M0
2A	T2bN0M0 T1N1M0 T2aN1M0
2B	T2bN1M0 T3N0M0
3A	T3N1M0 T1–3N2M0 T4N0–1M0
3B	T4N2M0 Any N3
4	Any M1

Table 6.5. Suggested imaging studies for staging lung cancer

Non-small cell lung cancer	Small-cell lung cancer
CT of chest	CT of chest/abdomen
Whole-body PET/CT	Whole Body PET/CT
	MRI brain (optional; see text)

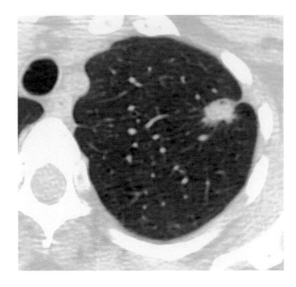

Figure 6.1. Typical CT screen detected lung cancer. Spiculated nodule present in left upper lobe measuring just over 1 cm. Surgery revealed T1N0 adenocarcinoma. (Reprinted with kind permission of Springer Science+Business Media from Ravenel JG, Silvestri GA. Imaging of Lung Cancer. In Medina LS, Blackmore DD (eds): *Evidence-Based Imaging: Optimizing Imaging in Patient Care.* New York: Springer Science+Business Media, 2006.)

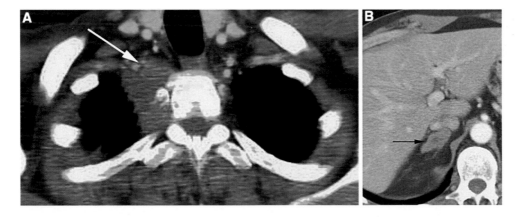

Figure 6.2. Staging lung cancer with CT and positron emission tomography (PET). (**A**) Contrast-enhanced CT reveals right apical mass with invasion of chest wall (*arrow*), T3 tumor. (**B**) Abnormal thickening of right adrenal gland (*arrow*) with lobular contours and central low attenuation suspicious for metastasis. (**C**) Fluorodeoxyglucose (FDG)-PET confirms primary neoplasm and adrenal metastasis (*arrow*). (Reprinted with kind permission of Springer Science+Business Media from Ravenel JG, Silvestri GA. Imaging of Lung Cancer. In Medina LS, Blackmore DD (eds): *Evidence-Based Imaging: Optimizing Imaging in Patient Care.* New York: Springer Science+Business Media, 2006.)

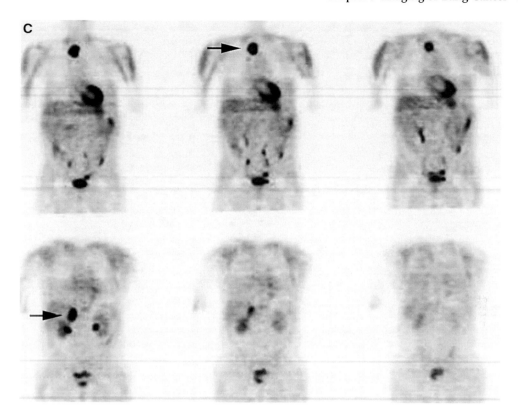

Figure 6.2. *continued*

Future Research

- Can biomarker analysis provide a better target population for screening?
- Does PET with SUV provide better or improved prognostic information than the current staging system?
- Can imaging be utilized noninvasively to detect microscopic metastases?
- Can imaging of biomarkers be utilized to select the most appropriate treatment regimen and aid in the delivery of novel treatments?

References

1. Alberg AJ, Samet JM. Chest 2003;123(suppl 1): 21S–49S.
2. Hecht SS. J Natl Cancer Inst 1999;91(14): 1194–1210.
3. Jemal A, Siegel R, Xu J, Ward E. CA Cancer J Clin 2010;60(5):277–300.
4. Carney DN. N Engl J Med 2002;346(2):126–128.
5. Wingo PA, Ries LA, Giovino GA et al. J Natl Cancer Inst 1999;91(8):675–690.
6. Tong L, Spitz MR, Fueger JJ, Amos CA. Cancer. 1996;78(5):1004–1010.
7. Lubin JH, Boice JD Jr, Edling C et al. J Natl Cancer Inst 1995;87(11):817–827.
8. Lubin JH, Boice JD Jr. J Natl Cancer Inst 1997;89(1):49–57.
9. Howe GR. Radiat Res 1995;142(3):295–304.
10. Fellows JL, Trosclair A, Adams EK, Rivera CC. MMWR 2002;51(14):300–303.
11. Warner KE, Hodgson TA, Carroll CE. Tob Control 1999;8(3):290–300.
12. Penberthy L, Retchin SM, McDonald MK et al. Health Care Manag Sci 1999;2(3):149–160.
13. Hillner BE, McDonald MK, Desch CE et al. J Clin Oncol 1998;16(4):1420–1424.
14. Herman CR, Gill HK, Eng J, Fajardo LL. AJR Am J Roentgenol 2002;179(4):825–831.
15. Mountain C. Chest 1997;111:1710–1717.
16. Silvestri GA, Tanoue LT, Margolis ML, Barker J, Detterbeck F. Chest 2003;123(suppl 1): 147S–156S.

17. Toloza EM, Harpole L, McCrory DC. Chest 2003;123(suppl 1):137S–146S.
18. Boucot KR, Weiss W. JAMA 1973;224(10): 1361–1365.
19. Brett GZ. Br Med J 1969;4:260–262.
20. Manser RL, Irving LB, Stone C, Byrnes G, Abramson M, Campbell D. Screening for lung cancer. Cochrane Database Syst Rev 2001;(3):1–20.
21. Sobue T, Suzuki T, Naruke T. Jpn J Cancer Res 1992;83(5):424–430.
22. Tsukada H, Kurita Y, Yokoyama A et al. Br J Cancer 2001;85(9):1326–1331.
23. Sagawa M, Tsubono Y, Saito Y et al. Cancer 2001;92(3):588–594.
24. Nishii K, Ueoka H, Kiura K et al. Lung Cancer 2001;34(3):325–332.
25. Nakayama T, Baba T, Suzuki T, Sagawa M, Kaneko M. Eur J Cancer 2002;38(10):1380–1387.
26. Sagawa M, Nakayama T, Tsukada H et al. Lung Cancer 2003;41(1):29–36.
27. Dominioni L, Imperatori A, Rovera F, Ochetti A, Paolucci M, Dionigi G. Cancer 2000;89(suppl 11): 2345–2348.
28. Salomaa ER. Cancer 2000;89(suppl 11): 2387–2391.
29. Friedman GD, Collen MF, Fireman BH. J Chronic Dis 1986;39(6):453–463.
30. Wilde J. Eur Respir J 1989;2(7):656–662.
31. Berlin NI, Buncher CR, Fontana RS, Frost JK, Melamed MR. Am Rev Respir Dis 1984;130(4): 545–549.
32. Frost JK, Ball WC Jr, Levin ML et al. Am Rev Respir Dis 1984;130(4):549–554.
33. Flehinger BJ, Melamed MR, Zaman MB, Heelan RT, Perchick WB, Martini N. Am Rev Respir Dis 1984;130(4):555–560.
34. Melamed MR, Flehinger BJ, Zaman MB, Heelan RT, Perchick WA, Martini N. Chest 1984;86(1): 44–53.
35. Melamed MR. Cancer 2000;89(suppl 11): 2356–2362.
36. Berlin NI. Cancer 2000;89(suppl 11):2349–2351.
37. Kubik A, Polak J. Cancer 1986;57(12):2427–2437.
38. Kubik A, Parkin D, Khlat M, Erban J, Polak J, Adamec M. Int J Cancer 1990;45:26–33.
39. Kubik AK, Parkin DM, Zatloukal P. Cancer 2000;89(suppl 11):2363–2368.
40. Fontana RS, Sanderson DR, Woolner LB et al. Clin Notes Respir Dis 1976;15(3):13–14.
41. Fontana R, Sanderson D, Taylor W et al. Am Rev Respir Dis 1984;130:561–565.
42. Fontana RS. Cancer 2000;89(suppl 11):2352–2355.
43. Fontana RS, Sanderson DR, Woolner LB et al. Cancer 1991;67(suppl 4):1155–1164.
44. Marcus P, Bergstralh E, Fagerstrom R et al. J Natl Cancer Inst 2000;92:1308–1316.
45. Grannis FW Jr. Chest 2001;119(2):322–323.
46. Strauss G. J Clin Oncol 2002;20:1973–1983.
47. Strauss GM, Gleason RE, Sugarbaker DJ. Chest 1995;107(suppl 6):270S–279S.
48. Flehinger BJ, Kimmel M, Polyak T, Melamed MR. Cancer 1993;72(5):1573–1580.
49. Strauss GM, Gleason RE, Sugarbaker DJ. Chest 1997;111(3):754–768.
50. Marcus PM, Prorok PC. J Med Screen 1999;6(1):47–49.
51. Prorok PC, Andriole GL, Bresalier RS et al. Control Clin Trials 2000;21(suppl 6):273S–309S.
52. Sone S, Takashima S, Li F et al. Lancet 1998;351(9111):1242–1245.
53. Tiitola M, Kivisaari L, Huuskonen MS et al. Lung Cancer 2002;35(1):17–22.
54. Swensen S, Jett J, Sloan J et al. Am J Respir Crit Care Med 2002;165:508–513.
55. Sobue T, Moriyama N, Kaneko M et al. J Clin Oncol 2002;20(4):911–920.
56. Pastorino U, Bellomi M, Landoni C et al. Lancet 2003;362(9384):593–597.
57. Nawa T, Nakagawa T, Kusano S, Kawasaki Y, Sugawara Y, Nakata H. Chest 2002;122(1):15–20.
58. Henschke CI. Cancer 2000;89(suppl 11):2474–2482.
59. Garg K, Keith RL, Byers T et al. Radiology 2002;225(2):506–510.
60. Diederich S, Wormanns D, Semik M et al. Radiology 2002;222:773–781.
61. Sone S, Li F, Yang ZG et al. Br J Cancer 2001;84(1):25–32.
62. Swensen S, Jett J, Hartman T et al. Radiology 2003;226:756–761.
63. Henschke CI, Naidich DP, Yankelevitz DF et al. Cancer 2001;92(1):153–159.
64. Henschke C, McCauley D, Yankelevitz D et al. Lancet 1999;354:99–105.
65. Henschke CI, Yankelevitz DF, Libby DM, Pasmantier MW, Smith JP, Miettinen OS. N Engl J Med 2006;355(17):1763–1771.
66. Henschke CI, Yankelevitz DF, Miettinen OS. Arch Intern Med 2006;166(3):321–325.
67. Bach PB, Jett JR, Pastorino U, Tockman MS, Swensen SJ, Begg CB. Jama 2007;297(9):953–961.
68. Gohagan J, Marcus P, Fagerstrom R, Pinsky P, Kramer B, Prorok P. Chest 2004;126(1):114–121.
69. Blanchon T, Brechot JM, Grenier PA, et al. Lung Cancer 2007;58(1):50–58.
70. Infante M, Cavuto S, Lutman FR, et al. Am J Respir Crit Care Med 2009;180(5):445–453.
71. http://www.cancer.gov/images/DSMB-NLST/pdf. Accessed 1/05, 2011.
72. Miettinen OS. Can Med Assoc J 2000;162(10): 1431–1436.
73. Wisnivesky JP, Mushlin AI, Sicherman N, Henschke C. Chest 2003;124(2):614–621.
74. Tengs TO, Adams ME, Pliskin JS et al. Risk Anal 1995;15(3):369–390.
75. Chirikos T, Hazelton T, Tockman M, Clark R. Chest 2002;121:1507–1514.
76. Mahadevia PJ, Fleisher LA, Frick KD, Eng J, Goodman SN, Powe NR. JAMA 2003;289(3): 313–322.

77. Radiology 2010;258(1):243–253.

78. Rami-Porta R, Ball D, Crowley J, et al. J Thorac Oncol 2007;2(7):593–602.

79. Haramati LB, Cartagena AM, Austin JH. J Comput Assist Tomogr 1995;19(3):375–378.

80. Cascade PN, Gross BH, Kazerooni EA et al. AJR 1998;170(4):927–931.

81. Patz EJ, Erasmus J, McAdams H et al. Radiology 1999;212:56–60.

82. Glazer HS, Duncan-Meyer J, Aronberg DJ, Moran JF, Levitt RG, Sagel SS. Radiology 1985;157(1): 191–194.

83. Glazer HS, Kaiser LR, Anderson DJ et al. Radiology 1989;173(1):37–42.

84. Pearlberg JL, Sandler MA, Beute GH, Lewis JW Jr, Madrazo BL. J Comput Assist Tomogr 1987;11(2):290–293.

85. Pennes DR, Glazer GM, Wimbish KJ, Gross BH, Long RW, Orringer MB. AJR 1985;144(3): 507–511.

86. Heelan R, Demas B, Caravelli J et al. Radiology 1989;170:637–641.

87. Padovani B, Mouroux J, Seksik L et al. Radiology 1993;187(1):33–38.

88. Haggar AM, Pearlberg JL, Froelich JW et al. AJR 1987;148(6):1075–1078.

89. Kodalli N, Erzen C, Yuksel M. Clin Imaging 1999;23(4):227–235.

90. Sakai S, Murayama S, Murakami J, Hashiguchi N, Masuda K. J Comput Assist Tomogr 1997;21(4):595–600.

91. Shiotani S, Sugimura K, Sugihara M et al. Radiat Med 2000;20:697–713.

92. Silvestri GA, Gould MK, Margolis ML, et al. Chest 2007;132(3S):178S–201S.

93. Hasegawa I, Eguchi K, Kohda E et al. Eur J Radiol 2003;45(2):129–134.

94. Boiselle PM, Patz EF Jr, Vining DJ, Weissleder R, Shepard JA, McLoud TC. Radiographics 1998;18(5):1061–1069.

95. Crisci R, Di Cesare E, Lupattelli L, Coloni GF. Eur J Cardiothorac Surg 1997;11:214–217.

96. Glazer GM. Chest 1989;96(suppl 1):44S–47S.

97. Kernstine KH, Stanford W, Mullan BF et al. Ann Thorac Surg 1999;68(3):1022–1028.

98. Gould MK, Kuschner WG, Rydzak CE et al. Ann Intern Med 2003;139(11):879–892.

99. Reed CE, Harpole DH, Posther KE et al. J Thorac Cardiovasc Surg 2003;126(6):1943–1951.

100. Gonzalez-Stawinski GV, Lemaire A, Merchant F et al. J Thorac Cardiovasc Surg 2003;126(6): 1900–1905.

101. Cerfolio RJ, Ojha B, Bryant AS, Bass CS, Bartalucci AA, Mountz JM. Ann Thorac Surg 2003;76(3):861–866.

102. Graeter TP, Hellwig D, Hoffmann K, Ukena D, Kirsch CM, Schafers HJ. Ann Thorac Surg 2003;75(1):231–235; discussion 235–236.

103. Kernstine KH, McLaughlin KA, Menda Y et al. Ann Thorac Surg 2002;73(2):394–401; discussion 401–392.

104. van Tinteren H, Hoekstra OS, Smit EF et al. Lancet 2002;359(9315):1388–1393.

105. Antoch G, Stattaus J, Nemat AT et al. Radiology 2003;229(2):526–533.

106. Hany TF, Steinert HC, Goerres GW, Buck A, von Schulthess GK. Radiology 2002;225(2):575–581.

107. Lardinois D, Weder W, Hany TF et al. N Engl J Med 2003;348(25):2500–2507.

108. Fischer B, Lassen U, Mortensen J, et al. N Engl J Med 2009;361(1):32–39.

109. Maziak DE, Darlin GE, Inculet RI, et al. Ann Intern Med 2009;151(4):221–228, W-248.

110. Heffner JE, Klein JS. Mayo Clin Proc 2008;83(2):235–250.

111. Am J Respir Crit Care Med 2000;162(5): 1987–2001.

112. Erasmus JJ, McAdams HP, Rossi SE, Goodman PC, Coleman RE, Patz EF. AJR Am J Roentgenol 2000;175(1):245–249.

113. Gupta NC, Rogers JS, Graeber GM, et al. Chest 2002;122(6):1918–1924.

114. Silvestri G, Littenberg B, Colice G. Am J Respir Crit Care Med 1995;152:225–230.

115. Kagohashi K, Satoh H, Ishikawa H, Ohtsuka M, Sekizawa K. Med Oncol 2003;20(1):25–28.

116. Hillers T, Sauve M, Guyatt G. Thorax 1994;49: 14–19.

117. Delbeke D, Martin WH, Sandler MP, Chapman WC, Wright JK, Jr, Pinson CW. Arch Surg 1998;133(5):510–515; discussion 515–516.

118. Oliver T Jr, Bernardino M, Miller J, Mansour K, Greene D, Davis W. Radiology 1984;153: 217–218.

119. Pearlberg JL, Sandler MA, Beute GH et al. Radiology 1985;157:187–190.

120. Heavey LR, Glazer GM, Gross BH, Francis IR, Orringer MB. AJR 1986;146(2):285–290.

121. Eggesbo HB, Hansen G. Acta Radiol 1996;37: 343–347.

122. Boland GW, Lee MJ, Gazelle GS, Halpern EF, McNicholas MM, Mueller PR. AJR 1998;171(1): 201–204.

123. Caoili EM, Korobkin M, Francis IR, Cohan RH, Dunnick NR. AJR 2000;175(5):1411–1415.

124. Caoili EM, Korobkin M, Francis IR et al. Radiology 2002;222(3):629–633.

125. Korobkin M, Brodeur FJ, Francis IR, Quint LE, Dunnick NR, Londy F. AJR 1998;170(3): 747–752.

126. Heinz-Peer G, Honigschnabi S, Schneider B et al. AJR 1999;173:15–22.

127. Korobkin M, Giordano TJ, Brodeur FJ, et al. Radiology 1996;200(3):743–747.

128. Outwater EK, Siegelman ES, Huang AB, Birnbaum BA. Radiology 1996;749–752.

129. Erasmus JJ, Patz EF Jr, McAdams HP et al. AJR 1997;168(5):1357–1360.

130. Gupta NC, Graeber GM, Tamim WJ, Rogers JS, Irisari L, Bishop HA. Clin Lung Cancer 2001;3(1):59–64.

131. Vikram R, Yeung HD, Macapinlac HA, Iyer RB. AJR Am J Roentgenol 2008;191(5):1545–1551.

132. Yun M, Kim W, Alnafisi N, Lacorte L, Jang S, Alavi A. J Nucl Med 2001;42(12):1795–1799.
133. Salvatierra A, Baamonde C, Llamas JM et al. Chest 1990;97:1052–1058.
134. Little AG, Stitik FP. Chest 1990;97(6):1431–1438.
135. Tornyos K, Garcia O, Karr B et al. Clin Nucl Med 1991;16:107–109.
136. Michel F, Soler M, Imhof E et al. Thorax 1991;46:469–473.
137. Hsia TC, Shen YY, Yen RF, Kao CH, Changlai SP. Neoplasma 2002;49(4):267–271.
138. Bury T, Barreto A, Daenen F, Barthelemy N, Ghaye B, Rigo P. Eur J Nucl Med 1998;25(9):1244–1247.
139. Gayed I, Vu T, Johnson M, Macapinlac H, Podoloff D. Mol Imaging Biol 2003;5(1):26–31.
140. Cole FH Jr, Thomas JE, Wilcox AB, Halford HH 3rd. Ann Thorac Surg 1994;57(4):838–840.
141. Colice G, Birkmeyer J, Black W, Littenberg B, Silvestri G. Chest 1995;108:1264–1271.
142. Butler AR, Leo JS, Lin JP et al. Radiology 1979;131:339–401.
143. Ferrigno D, Buccheri G. Chest 1994;106:1025–1029.
144. Jacobs L, Kinkel WR, Vincent RG. Arch Neurol 1977;77:690–693.
145. Kormas P, Bradshaw J, Jeyasingham K. Thorax 1992;47:106–108.
146. Mintz BJ, Turhim S, Alexander S et al. Chest 1984;86:850–853.
147. Hooper RG, Tenholder MF, Underwood et al. Chest 1984;85:774–777.
148. Earnest F, Ryu J, Miller G et al. Radiology 1999;211:137–145.
149. Cole JFH, Thomas JE, Wilcox AB et al. Ann Thorac Surg 1994;57:838–840.
150. Davis PC, Hudgins PA, Peterman SB et al. AJR 1991;156:1039–1046.
151. Rohren EM, Provenzale JM, Barboriak DP, Coleman RE. Radiology 2003;226(1):181–187.
152. Vallieres E, Shepherd FA, Crowley J, et al. J Thorac Oncol 2009;4(9):1049–1059.
153. Osterlind K, Ihde DC, Ettinger DS et al. Cancer Treat Rep 1983;67(1):3–9.
154. Adjei AA, Marks RS, Bonner JA. Mayo Clin Proc 1999;74(8):809–816.
155. Whitley NO, Mirvis SE. Crit Rev Diagn Imaging 1989;29(2):103–116.
156. Mirvis SE, Whitley NO, Aisner J, Moody M, Whitacre M, Whitley JE. AJR 1987;148(5): 845–847.
157. Hirsch FR, Paulson OB, Hansen HH, Larsen SO. Cancer 1983;51(3):529–533.
158. Giannone L, Johnson DH, Hande KR, Greco FA. Ann Intern Med 1987;106(3):386–389.
159. Jelinek JS, Redmond J 3 rd, Perry JJ et al. Radiology 1990;177(3):837–842.
160. Hauber HP, Bohuslavizki KH, Lund CH, Fritscher-Ravens A, Meyer A, Pforte A. Chest 2001;119(3):950–954.
161. Chin R Jr, McCain TW, Miller AA et al. Lung Cancer 2002;37(1):1–6.
162. Schumacher T, Brink I, Mix M et al. Eur J Nucl Med 2001;28(4):483–488.
163. van Loon J, Grutters J, Wanders R, et al. Eur J Cancer 2009;45(4):588–595.
164. van Loon J, Offermann C, Bosmans G, et al. Radiother Oncol 2008;87(1):49–54.
165. Sohaib SA, Turner B, Hanson JA, Farquharson M, Oliver RT, Reznek RH. Br J Radiol 2000;73(875):1178–1184.
166. Watanabe H, Yamamoto S, Kunitoh H et al. Cancer Sci 2003;94(11):1015–1020.
167. Werner-Wasik M, Xiao Y, Pequignot E, Curran WJ, Hauck W. Int J Radiat Oncol Biol Phys 2001;51(1):56–61.
168. Therasse P, Arbuck SG, Eisenhauer EA et al. J Natl Cancer Inst 2000;92(3):205–216.
169. James K, Eisenhauer E, Christian M et al. J Natl Cancer Inst 1999;91(6):523–528.
170. Erasmus JJ, Gladish GW, Broemeling L et al. J Clin Oncol 2003;21(13):2574–2582.
171. Hopper KD, Kasales CJ, Van Slyke MA, Schwartz TA, TenHave TR, Jozefiak JA. AJR 1996;167(4): 851–854.
172. Petrou M, Quint LE, Nan B, Baker LH. AJR Am J Rentgenol 2007;188(2):306–312.
173. Revel MP, Lefort C, Bissery A, et al. radiology 2004;231(2):459–466.
174. Gavrielides MS, Kinnard LM, Myers KJ, Petrick N. Radiology 2009;251(1):26–37.
175. Marten K, Auer F, Schmidt S, Kohl G, Rummeny EJ, Engelke C. Eur Radiol 2006;16(4):781–790.
176. Tran LN, Brown MS, Goldin JG, et al. Acad Radiol 2004;11(12):1355–1360.
177. Zhao B, Schwartz LH, Moskowitz CS, Ginsberg MS, Rizvi NA, Kris MG. Radiology 2006;241(3): 892–898.
178. Zhao B, james LP, Moskowitz CS, et al. Radiology 2009;252(1):263–272.
179. Shanker LK, Van den Abbeele A, yap J, Benjamin R, Scheutze S, Fitzgerald TJ. Clin Cancer Res 2009;15(6):1891–1897.
180. Hicks RJ. J Nucl Med 2009;50 Suppl1:31S–42S.
181. de Geus-OeiLF, van der Heijden HF, Visser EP, et al. J Nucl Med 2007;48(10):1592–1598.
182. Mac Manus MP, Hicks RJ, Matthews JP, et al. J Clin Oncol 2003;21(7):1285–1292.
183. Mac Manus MP, Hicks RJ, Matthews JP, Wirth A, Rischin D, Ball DL. Lung Cancer 2005;49(1): 95–108.
184. Nahmias C, Hanna WT, Wahl LM, Long MJ, Hubner KF, Townsend DW. J Nucl Med 2007;48(5):744–751.
185. Weber WA, petersen V, Schmidt B, et al. J Clin Oncol 2003;21(14):2651–2657.
186. Wahl RL, jacene H, Kasamon Y, Lodge MA. J Nucl Med 2009;50 Suppl1:122S–150S.

187. Young H, baum R, Cremerius U, et al. Eur J Cancer 1999;35(13):1773–1782.
188. Cerfolio RJ, Ojha B, Mukherjee S, Pask AH, Bass CS, Katholi CR. J Thorac Cardiovasc Surg 2003;125(4):938–944.
189. Akhurst T, Downey RJ, Ginsberg MS et al. Ann Thorac Surg 2002;73(1):259–264; discussion 264–256.
190. Port JL, Kent MS, Korst RJ, Keresztes R, Levin MA, Altorki NK. Ann Thorac Surg 2004;77(1): 254–259.
191. Vansteenkiste JF, Stroobants SG, De Leyn PR, Dupont PJ, Verbeken EK. Ann Oncol 1998;9(11): 1193–1198.
192. Patz EF Jr, Connolly J, Herndon J. AJR 2000; 174(3):769–774.
193. Association of Community Cancer Centers. Oncology Patient Management Guidelines, Version 3.0. Rockville, MD: Association of Community Cancer Centers, 2000.
194. National Comprehensive Cancer Network. Practice Guidelines for Non-small Cell Lung Cancer. Rockledge, PA: National Comprehensive Cancer Network, 2000.
195. American College of Radiology. Follow-up of Non-small Cell Lung Cancer: Appropriateness Criteria. Reston, VA: American College of Radiology, 1999.
196. Smith TJ. Semin Oncol 2003;30(3):361–368.
197. Colice GL, Rubins J, Unger M. Chest 2003;123(suppl 1):272S–283S.
198. Westeel V, Choma D, Clement F et al. Ann Thorac Surg 2000;70(4):1185–1190.
199. Walsh GL, O'Connor M, Willis KM et al. Ann Thorac Surg 1995;60(6):1563–1570; discussion 1570–1562.
200. Younes RN, Gross JL, Deheinzelin D. Chest 1999;115(6):1494–1499.
201. Rubins J, Unger M, Colice GL. Chest 2007;132(3Suppl):355S–367S.
202. Sobue T, Moriyama N, Kaneko M, et al. J Clin Oncol 2002;20:911–920.
203. Diederich S, Thomas M, Semik M, et al. Eur Radiol 2004;14(4):691–702.
204. Bastarrika G, Garcia-Velloso MJ, Lozano MD, et al. Am J Respir Crit Care Med 2005;171(12): 1378–1383.
205. Chong S, lee KS, Chung MJ, et al. J Korean Med Sci 2005;20(3):402–408.
206. Gohagan JK, Marcus PM, Fagerstrom RM, et al. Lung Cancer 2005;47(1):9–15.
207. MacRedmond R, McVey G, Lee M, et al. Thorax 2006;61(1):54–56.
208. Vierikko T, Jarvenpaa R, Autti T, et al. Eur Respir J 2007;29(1):78 84.
209. Infante M, Lutman FR, Cavuto S, et al. Lung Cancer 2008;59(3):355–363.
210. Wilson DO, Weissfeld JL, Fuhrman CR, et al. Am J Respir Crit Care Med 2008;178(9): 956 961.
211. Lopes Pegna A, Picozzi G, Mascalchi M, et al. Lung Cancer 2009;64(1):34–40.
212. Menezes RJ, Roberts HC, Paul NS, et al. Lung Cancer 2009;67(2):177–83.
213. Pedersen JH, Ashraf H, Dirksen A, et al. J Thorac Oncol 2009;4(5):608–614.
214. Ravenel JG. Updates in Lung cancer: Role of Imaging in Screening, Staging and Restaging Lung Cancer. In ARRS Categorical Course: Practical Approaches to Common Clinical Conditions. 2009.
215. Goldstraw P (ed). Based on International Association for the Study of Lung Cancer. Staging Handbook in Thoracic Oncology. Orange Park Florida: Editorial Rx Press, 2009

7

Imaging-Based Screening for Colorectal Cancer

James M. A. Slattery, Lucy E. Modahl, and Michael E. Zalis

Issues

I. Who should undergo colorectal screening?
  A. Fecal occult blood testing
  B. Sigmoidoscopy
  C. Combined sigmoidoscopy and FOBT
  D. Colonoscopy
II. What imaging-based screening methods are available, and how do they compare with FOBT, sigmoidoscopy, and colonoscopy?
  A. Double-contrast barium enema
  B. Computed tomographic colonography
  C. Special case: patients with increased risk of CRC
  D. Special case: patients with high risk of CRC
III. What is the role of imaging in staging colorectal carcinoma?
IV. Applicability to children
V. Cost-effectiveness
VI. What imaging-based screening developments are on the horizon that may improve compliance with coloretal screening?

Key Points

- Screening reduces colorectal cancer (CRC) incidence and mortality (strong evidence).
- All major strategies for CRC screening have favorable cost-effectiveness ratios compared to no screening (moderate evidence).
- Available evidence does not support choosing one test over another (moderate evidence).
- Increased compliance with CRC screening is critical to reduce CRC incidence and mortality (moderate evidence).

M.E. Zalis (✉)
Department of Radiology, Massachusetts General Hospital, 55 Fruit Street, Boston, MA 02114, USA
e-mail: mzalis@mgh.harvard.edu

L.S. Medina et al. (eds.), *Evidence-Based Imaging: Improving the Quality of Imaging in Patient Care, Revised Edition,*
DOI 10.1007/978-1-4419-7777-9_7, © Springer Science+Business Media, LLC 2011

Definition and Pathophysiology

The consensus now holds that in the vast majority of sporadic cases, CRC arises within a precursor lesion, the adenomatous polyp (1, 2). The adenoma–carcinoma sequence hypothesis is supported by indirect evidence from several sources. Both CRC and polyps have a similar anatomic distribution. The mean age of onset of polyps predates the mean age of onset of carcinoma by several years, and cancer rarely develops in the absence of polyps (3). Patients with one or more large adenomatous polyps (≥1 cm) are at increased risk of developing CRC (4, 5), most of which develop at the site of the polyp, if left in place (5). In addition, patients with genetic predisposition to colonic polyp formation are at greatly increased risk of CRC (6). Finally, several studies have shown that polypectomy significantly reduces the incidence of CRC (7–9). Importantly for imaging-based screening, the risk of a polyp harboring a carcinoma is related directly to the size of the lesion: in polyps less than 1 cm in size, the risk is estimated to be <1%; in polyps measuring 1–2 cm, the risk increases to 10%; and in polyps larger than 2 cm, the risk is 25% or more (10).

Initiation of CRC is thought to require only two mutations in the adenomatous polyposis coli (*APC*) gene (a tumor suppressor gene). *APC* mutations are seen in about 60% of sporadic CRC (11). The germline *APC* gene is mutated in familial adenomatous polyposis (FAP) coli (12). Progression from premalignant polyp to invasive carcinoma is the result of further mutations in other genes, including *K-ras*, *DCC*, and *p53*.

Epidemiology

CRC remains the second most common cause of cancer-related death in the USA, with an estimated annual incidence of 150,000 (13). Mortality rates from CRC are equal in both sexes, with approximately 60,000 individuals in the USA succumbing to this disease annually, which accounts for approximately 10% of cancer deaths. The lifetime risk of developing CRC is approximately 6%, while the estimated lifetime risk of CRC-related death is approximately 2.6%. The 5-year survival rate is 90% for early-stage CRC localized to the colon or rectum, 66% if there is regional spread, and 10% if there are distant metastases (13). Only 38% of CRC is diagnosed before it has spread beyond the bowel (13). The overall 5-year survival has increased from 50% in 1974 to 62% in 1999 (13). Risk factors for CRC include FAP, hereditary nonpolyposis colorectal cancer (HNPCC), family history of CRC in a first-degree relative before age 60, personal history of CRC, age, diet high in animal fat, chronic inflammatory bowel disease, obesity, physical inactivity, diabetes, smoking, and alcohol.

Overall Cost to Society

Treatment of colorectal carcinoma is estimated to cost between $5.5 and $6.5 billion per year in the USA, and between $14 and $22 billion worldwide. All currently available screening strategies are estimated to cost less than $40,000 per year of life saved, comparable to other screening programs utilized in the USA, such as screening mammography in women over age 50 (14).

Goals

In general, screening for any disease can be justified in the following circumstances: (a) the disease is prevalent and is associated with clinically significant morbidity and mortality; (b) screening tests are available, acceptable, feasible, and sufficiently accurate for the detection of early disease; (c) earlier diagnosis and treatment is associated with improved prognosis; and (d) the sum of the benefits associated with screening outweighs the sum of the potential harms and costs. CRC screening fulfills each of these criteria. The goal of image-based screening is to detect premalignant adenomatous polyps in an average risk population, thereby enabling removal prior to the development of invasive CRC. There is growing consensus that the target lesion is the advanced adenoma, a polyp containing high-grade cellular dysplasia, the vast majority of which are >1 cm in size (15).

Methodology

We reviewed listings and articles available by Medline (PubMed, National Library of Medicine, Bethesda, Maryland) related to CRC, colon cancer screening strategies, and cost-effectiveness of colon cancer screening. The search covered the period 1966 to January 2004, and employed search strategies including the terms *colon cancer, colon cancer screening, barium enema, CT colonography, virtual colonoscopy,* and *colonoscopy.* The authors performed preliminary evaluation of abstracts resulting from the on-line search and followed this with analysis of full articles; analysis was limited to articles and material relating to human subjects and published in English.

I. Who Should Undergo Colorectal Screening?

Summary of Evidence: In a person with average risk for CRC, the most significant risk factor for developing CRC is age. Over 90% of CRC occurs over the age of 50. Average-risk individuals are those who are deemed not to have an increased or high risk for colorectal carcinoma. Individuals at increased or high risk are those who have a personal or family history of FAP syndrome, hereditary nonpolyposis CRC, adenomatous polyps, or CRC, or a personal history of inflammatory bowel disease, colonic polyps, or CRC. Methods to detect polyps and colon cancer include fecal occult blood testing (FOBT), flexible sigmoidoscopy, and colonoscopy. Imaging-based screening methods are double-contrast barium enema (DCBE), and more recently computed tomographic colonography (CTC). Published randomized controlled trials (RCTs) and case-control studies have demonstrated that FOBT and sigmoidoscopy can reduce CRC incidence and mortality. To date, there are no RCTs evaluating sigmoidoscopy, DCBE, or colonoscopy in average risk screening populations. Recent data suggest that CTC has performance characteristics equivalent to conventional colonoscopy for detection of polyps, when adequately trained radiologists employing state-of-the-art technique perform it. The American Cancer Society currently recommends that all adults aged 50 or older with average risk of CRC follow one of the following screening schedules: FOBT every year; flexible sigmoidoscopy every 5 years; annual FOBT and flexible sigmoidoscopy every 5 years (preferred to either alone); DCBE every 5 years; colonoscopy every 10 years.

In persons with increased risk of CRC, screening may be more frequent and start at an earlier age (see Special Case: Patients with Increased Risk of CRC, below).

Supporting Evidence

A. Fecal Occult Blood Testing

The strongest evidence for CRC screening efficacy comes from trials using FOBTs. The FOBT is used to detect blood in the stool and is a guaiac-based test for peroxidase activity. Three RCTs have demonstrated that FOBT when followed by colonoscopy can reduce CRC mortality (7, 16, 17) (strong evidence). The largest of these is the Minnesota Trial (7), which has reported a mortality reduction of 33% at 13 years of follow-up, based on annual FOBT with hydration and 21% at 18 years of follow-up based on biennial testing. The two European studies have examined biennial testing without rehydration and have reported mortality reductions at 7.8 (16) and 10 years (17) of 15 and 18%, respectively. FOBT, while inexpensive and well tolerated, has limitations. One-time testing has sensitivity for cancer detection of only 33–50% (7, 18). Specificity ranges from 90 to 98% (7, 16, 17). This means that up to 10% of all patients screening will have a false-positive result. In fact, only 5–10% of positive reactions are due to cancer (19). The diagnostic performance for detection of asymptomatic polyps is poor, the majority of patients with adenomas testing negative (20, 21). Furthermore, FOBT offers no precise anatomic localization of lesions. Current guidelines suggest yearly FOBT testing with colonoscopic follow-up for patients with a positive test.

B. Sigmoidoscopy

Evidence of mortality reduction for sigmoidoscopy is derived from case-control studies (8, 22, 23) and a cohort study (24). One study estimated that sigmoidoscopy reduced rectal cancer mortality by approximately 70% (22). However, a rigid sigmoidoscope was used and therefore, on the basis of strict technique-linked criterion, the results are not applicable to flexible sigmoidoscopy (moderate evidence). In another case-control study (23), approximately two-thirds of the procedures were performed with a flexible sigmoidoscope. However, only 27 patients had fatal distal cancer and some were at higher risk for CRC (limited evidence). In a case-control study by Muller and Sonnenberg (8), the study population was symptomatic (moderate evidence). A cohort study of 25,000 asymptomatic men and women followed from 1986 to 1994 showed that sigmoidoscopy reduced the overall risk of colorectal carcinoma by 40% (24) (moderate evidence). Sigmoidoscopy has several limitations. Total colon exam recommended by several expert panels, including the American Cancer Society (25), is not accomplished. Flexible sigmoidoscopy allows examination of only about 60 cm of the colon and detects only 60% of colon cancers, while lesions in the transverse and right colon are not at all detected by this technique (26). Approximately 30% of patients with colon cancer have disease proximal to the splenic flexure without evidence of neoplasia distal to the splenic flexure, which will not be detected at sigmoidoscopy (27). A screening study of 2,000 patients (28), demonstrated that 62% of patients with advanced proximal neoplasia had either no distal lesions or only hyperplastic polyps, which currently do not warrant colonoscopy. Clearly, sigmoidoscopy is inadequate in this setting.

C. Combined Sigmoidoscopy and FOBT

The evidence base for combining FOBT with sigmoidoscopy is limited, but it is likely that the combination of both screening methods is more effective than either method of screening alone for several reasons. Both strategies have been demonstrated to reduce deaths from CRC individually. A study of biennial FOBT (29) reported a reduction in mortality from CRC of 8% when lesions were located in the sigmoid/rectum and 28% when located elsewhere in the colon. This suggests that FOBT is less sensitive for the detection of distal colorectal lesions. Based on this evidence, the authors recommended a prospective RCT to evaluate the possible benefit of combining FOBT with sigmoidoscopy by increasing cancer detection in the distal colon (limited evidence). A recent study (30) demonstrated that by combining a one-time FOBT with sigmoidoscopy, the detection rate for

advanced neoplasia increased to 76 from 70% with sigmoidoscopy alone (limited evidence).

D. Colonoscopy

At present, video-assisted colonoscopy is the clinical gold standard for polyp detection. Current recommendations suggest colonoscopy once every 10 years. To date, there are no studies evaluating whether screening colonoscopy alone reduces the incidence or mortality from CRC in patients at average risk. However, colonoscopy was the primary method of diagnostic follow-up used in three fecal occult blood trials (7, 16, 17). Direct identification of cancer was actually responsible for the mortality reduction (moderate evidence). Two cohort studies have demonstrated the efficacy of colonoscopy and polypectomy in reducing the incidence of CRC (9, 31) (moderate evidence). In the National Polyp Study (9) in which the screening population underwent colonoscopic polypectomy at the time of entry and during surveillance, researchers determined a 76–90% decrease in cancer incidence compared with that expected on the basis of historical controls, suggesting a strong correlation between adenoma removal and cancer reduction (moderate evidence). The Italian multicenter study (31) reported a two-thirds risk reduction for colorectal carcinoma following colonoscopic removal of an adenoma (moderate evidence). In addition, indirect evidence from studies demonstrating that sigmoidoscopy reduces CRC mortality points toward the effectiveness of colonoscopy. A recent randomized trial examining screening sigmoidoscopy with follow-up colonoscopy for those patients with polyps versus no screening has demonstrated a significant reduction in CRC incidence in the screened group (32) (moderate evidence). Despite being widely accepted as the gold standard for interrogation of the large bowel, colonoscopy has limitations. There is a risk of approximately 0.2% for serious bleeding or perforation during the screening exam, the risk being greatest if polypectomy is performed (33). In addition, it has been estimated that the cost of colonoscopic screening in adults over age 50 could reach $3.5 billion per year, in part due to the conscious sedation required to perform the exam (34). The diagnostic performance of colonoscopy has been estimated by evaluation of interobserver variability for detection of polyps (35). The overall miss rate for adenomas was 24%. The miss rate was 27% for adenomas ≥5 mm, 13% for adenomas 6–9 mm, and 6% for adenomas ≥10 mm. Right colon adenomas were missed more often (27%) than left colon adenomas (21%), but the difference was not significant.

II. What Imaging-Based Screening Methods Are Available, and How Do They Compare with FOBT, Sigmoidoscopy, and Colonoscopy?

Summary of Evidence: Until recently the DCBE was the only imaging-based study for CRC screening. Evidence for the use of DCBE in the average-risk screening population is limited. Over the past decade CTC has rapidly developed and is becoming a realistic option for CRC screening. Recent data suggest that properly performed CTC rivals colonoscopy for lesion detection in the average-risk screening population.

Supporting Evidence

A. Double Contrast Barium Enema

The efficacy of DCBE as a screening test has not been evaluated in a randomized trial. The strongest support for DCBE is based on the observation that treatment of early cancer in asymptomatic individuals lowers disease-specific mortality, and the removal of adenomatous polyps reduces cancer incidence. The National Polyp Study reported a reduction in cancer incidence after adenoma removal (9). The relative contribution of initial polypectomy and surveillance to this effect cannot be determined. However, initial polypectomy is likely to have been the major contributing factor in incidence reduction given the size and nature of lesions at entry and the relatively short follow-up time in this study. Approximately one-third of patients with polyps entered the study after receiving positive results on barium enema (36) (limited evidence). Several studies have looked at the sensitivity of DCBE in polyp detection. A meta-analysis (37) demonstrated a sensitivity of 70% or greater for polyps of 5 mm or more in size (range 30–96%). A retrospective review (38) of 2,193 consecutive CRCs demonstrated DCBE sensitivity for cancer detection to be 85 versus 95% for colonoscopy. More recently, as part of the National Polyp study, Winawer and colleagues (39) undertook colonic surveillance of patients' postpolypectomy using both colonoscopy and DCBE. The DCBE was performed first and the endoscopist was blinded to its result. Detection rates of DCBE for polyps of 1.0 cm and greater was 48%, with an overall detection rate for adenomas of only 39%. Although this study has raised doubts about the justification of using DCBE for CRC screening, the results relate to a symptomatic population and are therefore not applicable to the average risk population. In addition, only 23 patients with polyps greater than 1.0 cm were included, which seems a small number on which to base conclusions regarding the effectiveness of DCBE in polyp detection (limited evidence). DCBE is currently not recommended by the American College of Gastroenterologists as a primary screening strategy in average-risk patients.

B. Computed Tomographic Colonography

CTC is a rapidly evolving technique for total colon examination and is the only imaging alternative developed since the barium enema with the potential for CRC screening. First described in 1994, CTC utilizes high-resolution helical CT data in combination with advanced graphical software to generate two-dimensional (2D) and three-dimensional (3D) endoluminal views of the colon. The endoluminal images, which may be viewed dynamically and interactively, simulate what is seen at conventional colonoscopy. Volumetric data are acquired with the patient in both the prone and supine positions. While limited only to detection, CTC offers several potential advantages: it presents minimal risk to patients, has a short procedure time of approximately 15 min, can be performed in patients with distal occluding lesions, and affords more precise lesion localization than colonoscopy. It is performed using a low X-ray dose technique that results in approximately 15% absorbed dose reduction compared to DCBE (40). It also is well tolerated, with less discomfort reported for the exam than for either colonoscopy or DCBE (41, 42). With over 2,000 cases reported in the literature, there are no reports of serious morbidity or mortality associated with CTC. Conscious sedation is not required, limiting cost and time for the patient. In addition, as the entire abdomen and pelvis are visualized, this method has the potential to simultaneously detect and stage malignant lesions in a single sitting; however, this capability has not yet been fully validated in a clinical trial. The diagnosis of extracolonic pathology is also possible (43, 44). Moderately significant findings such as gallstones, as well as highly significant findings such as renal cell carcinoma, large abdominal aortic aneurysms, and liver and adrenal masses can be identified. This may prove advantageous if the cost-effectiveness of CTC is not affected by the diagnostic workup of these lesions.

The performance characteristics of CT colonography in polyp detection have been assessed in several published studies. Results have been encouraging in symptomatic cohorts and in populations with an increased incidence of polyps (45–47) (limited evidence). The sensitivity of CTC for detection of polyps measuring 10 mm or more compares favorably with the gold standard of colonoscopy, ranging from 90 to 93%. Reported sensitivity in populations with a lower prevalence of polyps has until recently been relatively poor (48, 49). However, at least one of these studies (48) was performed with essentially naive CTC readers and limited evaluation software. Recently the first large cohort evaluation (50) in 1,200 individuals from an average-risk population comparing CTC to colonoscopy has been completed (moderate evidence). Using a combination of digital subtraction bowel cleansing (see below) and traditional cathartic preparation, CTC was performed prior to colonoscopy. The results of the CTC were disclosed when colonoscopic examination of a colon segment was complete, thereby allowing unblinded colonoscopic reevaluation of each bowel segment. The final unblinded colonoscopy was used as the reference standard. The sensitivity of CTC for adenomatous polyps was 93.8% for polyps at least 10 mm in diameter, 93.9% for polyps at least 8 mm in diameter, and 88.7% for polyps at least 6 mm in diameter. The sensitivity of optical colonoscopy for detection of adenomatous polyps was 87.5, 91.5, and 92.3% for the three sizes of polyps, respectively. The specificity of CTC

for adenomatous polyps was 96.0% for polyps at least 10 mm in diameter and 92.2% for polyps at least 8 mm in diameter. Setting the threshold polyp size for colonoscopic referral at 8 mm results in 13.5% of patients who undergo screening being referred for colonoscopic evaluation. This reduces to 7.5% if a threshold polyp size of 10 mm is chosen. Interestingly, the frequency of extracolonic findings was less than half that reported in higher-risk populations, which may have implications for cost-effectiveness in the future.

The excellent performance data for CTC reported in this trial are at odds with other published series (48, 49). The authors suggest that the discrepancy in results, while probably multifactorial, is primarily attributable to the use of 3D display, which aids polyp conspicuity and duration of visualization. Previous studies have primarily used 2D image interpretation. Further studies are required to clarify the factors that contributed to the high performance observed in this study and to ensure reproducibility of these data. Despite great advances in CTC, however, the current implementation of the technique is subject to three important limitations. First, the cost of CTC remains a significant hurdle to its implementation as a mainstream screening modality. If the cost of CTC reflects standard contrast-enhanced abdominal and pelvic CT rather than a special reduced cost for CTC, then it is doubtful that it will be adopted as a first-line screening tool. Second, in its current form, CTC requires full cathartic bowel preparation. This has been identified as a barrier to improved screening compliance. Future developments in fecal tagging techniques (see below) may help to address this problem. Finally, although the interpretation time for a CTC study has decreased as better technology and more expertise become available, the mean time required in the Bethesda study was still almost 20 min. Strategies to streamline study interpretation need to be addressed if CTC is to cope with the huge population eligible for CRC screening.

C. Special Case: Patients with Increased Risk of CRC

Summary of Evidence: People at increased risk of CRC include those with a family history of CRC or adenomatous polyps, and those with a personal history of adenomatous polyps, CTC, or inflammatory bowel disease.

Supporting Evidence

Family History of CRC or Adenomatous Polyps

Colon cancer screening recommendations based on familial risk are derived from the known effectiveness of available screening strategies and the observed colon cancer risk in relatives of patients with large-bowel malignancy and relatives of patients diagnosed with adenomas at a young age (≤60 years). The lifetime risk for CRC in the general population is 6%. Estimates of risk of CRC in close relatives of individuals with adenomatous polyps are still evolving. A meta-analysis (51) examined all studies that assessed familial risk of colon cancers and adenomatous polyps (27 studies) since 1966 (moderate evidence). The relative risk of colon cancer when a first-degree relative was affected with large-bowel malignancy was 2.4. Increased risk was found when the relative was affected with either colon or rectal cancers, but was greater for colon. If more than one relative was affected, the risk increased to 4.2. The risk was 3.8 for relatives if colon cancer was diagnosed before age 45 years, 2.2 if it was diagnosed between ages 45 and 59 years, and 1.8 if the cancer was diagnosed at >59 years. The relative risk for colon cancer if the first-degree relative had an adenomatous polyp was 1.9. People with a first-degree relative (parent, sibling, or child) with colon cancer or adenomatous polyps diagnosed at age >60 years or two first-degree relatives diagnosed with CRC at any age are recommended to have screening colonoscopy starting at age 40 or 10 years younger than the earliest diagnosis in their family, whichever comes first, and repeated every 5 years (52). People with a first-degree relative with colon cancer or adenomatous polyp diagnosed at age ≥60 years or two second-degree relatives (grandparent, aunt, or uncle) with CRC are recommended to undergo screening as average risk persons, but beginning at age 40 years. People with one second-degree relative or third-degree relative (great-grandparent or cousin) with CRC should be screened as average risk persons.

History of Adenomatous Polyps: Several studies have demonstrated that colonoscopic polypectomy and surveillance reduces subsequent CRC incidence (9, 31). The rate of developing advanced adenomas after polypectomy is low after several years of follow-up, suggesting that the initial colonoscopy and polypectomy offers the major benefit and that surveillance may only benefit those at highest risk. The National Polyp Study (53) found that the rate of adenoma detection 3 years after the initial adenoma resection was 32–42%. Recurrent adenomas were mostly small, tubular adenomas with low-grade dysplasia and therefore were of negligible immediate clinical significance. Only 3.3% of patients in each follow-up group had advanced adenomas (>1 cm, or with villous tissue or high-grade dysplasia) after 3 years of follow-up (moderate evidence). Another long-term follow-up study (4) of 1,618 postpolypectomy patients also found no increased risk for cancer in patients undergoing resection of single small (<1 cm) tubular adenomas, but an increased risk of 3.6 times in those with index adenomas that were large (≥1 cm) or contained villous tissue, and 6.6 times in patients with multiple adenomas on their original examinations compared with the known rates in the local community. In patients found to have a colorectal adenoma, the prevalence of synchronous polyps is 30–50% (54–56). Some of these polyps, especially those measuring <1 cm in diameter, will be missed on the initial colonoscopy (57, 58). Metachronous adenomas are reported in 20–50% of patients, depending on the follow-up surveillance interval used (59–63). Thus, the purpose of postpolypectomy colonoscopic surveillance is twofold. First, previously missed adenomas can be detected and removed. Second, the patient's tendency to form new adenomas with advanced pathology can be assessed.

In the National Polyp Study, colonoscopy performed 3 years after initial colonoscopic removal of adenomatous polyps detected advanced adenomas as effectively as follow-up colonoscopy performed after both 1 and 3 years. At 3 years, only 3.3% of patients in each group had advanced adenomas. On this basis, an interval of at least 3 years before follow-up colonoscopy after resection of newly diagnosed adenomatous polyps was recommended. Further analysis of these data as well as data from more recent studies suggest that it is possible to further stratify risk of recurrent advanced adenomas based on baseline features of each case (63–65). Patients with a relatively high risk of developing advanced adenomas during follow-up include those with multiple adenomas (more than two), large adenomas (≥1 cm), or a first-degree relative with CRC. Patients with a low risk of metachronous advanced adenomas include those with only one or two small adenomas (<1 cm) and no family history of CRC. Surveillance should be of greatest intensity in those most likely to benefit and reduced in those least likely to benefit so as to avoid complications associated with unnecessary removal of small polyps. Surveillance can be accomplished by well-performed CTC or colonoscopy.

History of CRC: Aside from recurrence of the original cancer, the incidence of CRC is increased after the first occurrence (66). Adenomatous polyps again precede these subsequent cancers. Although colonoscopy can detect recurrent colon cancer, anastomotic recurrences occur in only about 2% of colon cancers and are generally accompanied by surgically incurable disease (67). In an RCT performed in 325 patients with curative resections of CRC (68), the value of colonoscopy was confined to detection of metachronous adenomas and not recurrent intraluminal cancer (moderate evidence). Patients with a colon cancer that has been resected with curative intent should have a complete structural colon examination around the time of initial diagnosis to rule out synchronous neoplasms. This exam can be performed by either colonoscopy or CTC; CTC has proven especially effective in the setting of a colorectal mass that prevents passage of the colonoscope, as only air insufflation is required for evaluation (69). Thus, if the colon is obstructed preoperatively, CTC should be performed. It offers the advantage that extracolonic structures can be assessed simultaneously. If this does not reveal synchronous lesions, subsequent surveillance by colonoscopy or CTC should be offered after 3 years, and then, if normal, every 5 years.

Inflammatory Bowel Disease: There is extensive experience with DCBE for evaluation of inflammatory bowel disease and its complications, including CRC (70, 71). Inflammatory polyps project above the level of the surrounding mucosa. Pseudopolyposis is seen when extensive ulceration of the mucosa down to the submucosa results in scattered circumscribed islands of relatively normal mucosal remnants. Postinflammatory polyps reflect a nonspecific healing of undermined mucosal and submucosal remnants and ulcers, and are mostly multiple. They have no malignant potential. Patients with extensive long-standing ulcerative colitis or Crohn's disease have an increased risk for the development of CRC (72). Importantly, cancers that develop in patients with inflammatory bowel disease differ from more typical CRCs in that they generally develop not from adenomatous polyps but rather from areas of high-grade dysplasia (73). Dysplasia is a precancerous histologic finding, and the risk of colon cancer increases with the degree of mucosal dysplasia. Dysplasia may be found in a radiographically normal-appearing mucosa, or it may be accompanied by a slightly raised mucosal lesion, a so-called dysplasia-associated lesion or mass and as a consequence radiographically detectable. Because differentiation of adenocarcinoma and dysplasia from inflammatory or postinflammatory polyps is sometimes difficult or impossible on double-contrast enema, endoscopy and biopsy are necessary for making a final diagnosis. Therefore, regular colonoscopy and mucosal biopsy is recommended for both. There are no RCTs of surveillance colonoscopy in patients with chronic ulcerative colitis or Crohn's colitis. A case-control study has found better survival in ulcerative colitis patients in surveillance programs (74) (moderate evidence). Commonly colonoscopy is performed every 1–2 years after 8 years of disease. Patients with high-grade dysplasia or multifocal low-grade dysplasia in flat mucosa should be advised to undergo colectomy. While CTC could potentially permit evaluation of the colon, it has not been formally evaluated in this setting.

D. Special Case: Patients with High Risk of CRC

Summary of Evidence: Essentially, there are two broad categories of hereditary CRC-distal or proximal-based on the predominant location of disease. CRCs involving the distal colon are more likely to have mutations in the adenomatous polyposis coli (*APC*), *p53*, and *K-ras* genes, and behave more aggressively (75); proximal CRCs are more likely to possess microsatellite instability (genomic regions in which short DNA sequences or a single nucleotide is repeated), harbor mutations in the mismatch-repair genes, and behave less aggressively, as in HNPCC (75). FAP and most sporadic cases may be considered a paradigm for the first, or distal, class of CRCs, whereas hereditary nonpolyposis CRC more clearly represents the second, or proximal, class (75). Familial CRC is a major public health problem by virtue of its relatively high frequency. Some 15–20% of all CRCs are familial. Among these, FAP accounts for less than 1%; HNPCC, also called Lynch syndrome, accounts for approximately 5–8% of all CRC patients.

Supporting Evidence

Familial Adenomatous Polyposis
Familial adenomatous polyposis is an autosomal-dominant disease caused by mutations in the adenomatous polyposis coli (*APC*) gene. The associated risk of CRC approaches 100%. The average age of adenoma development in FAP is 16 years, and the average age of colon cancer is 39 years. Most affected patients develop >100 colorectal adenomas, and persons with more than 100 adenomas have FAP by definition. Attenuated APC (AAPC) is a variant of FAP and is associated with a variable number of adenomas, usually 20–100, a tendency toward right-sided colonic adenomas, and an age onset of CRC that is approximately 10 years later than for FAP. The CRC mortality rate is lower in FAP patients who choose to be screened compared with those who present with symptoms (76) (moderate evidence). Colonoscopy should be used in those with AAPC, beginning in the late teens or early 20s, depending on the age of polyp expression in the family, while sigmoidoscopy is adequate screening for most FAP patients as numerous polyps almost invariably involve the sigmoid and rectum. People who have a genetic diagnosis of FAP, or are at risk of having FAP but genetic testing has not been performed or is not feasible, should have annual sigmoidoscopy, beginning at age 10–12 years, to determine if they are expressing the genetic abnormality.

HNPCC: HNPCC, also referred to as the Lynch syndrome, is the most common form of hereditary CRC. Multiple generations are affected with CRC at an early age (mean, approximately 45 years) with a predominance of right-sided CRC (approximately 70% proximal to the splenic flexure). There is an excess of synchronous CRC (multiple CRCs at or within 6 months after surgical resection for CRC) and metachronous CRC (CRC occurring more than 6 months after surgery). In addition, there is an excess of extracolonic cancers, namely carcinoma of the endometrium (second only to CRC in frequency), ovary, stomach, small bowel, pancreas, hepatobiliary tract, brain, and upper uroepithelial tract (77). A recent study suggests that HNPCC accounts for between 0.86 and 2.0% of colon cancer cases (78). Criteria for the diagnosis of HNPCC (the Amsterdam criteria) have been devised (79). The criteria are as follows: at least three relatives with an HNPCC-associated cancer (CRC and cancer of the endometrium, small bowel, ureter, or renal pelvis) plus all of the following: (a) one affected patient is a first-degree relative of the other two; (b) two or more successive generations affected; (c) one or more affected relative received CRC diagnosis at age <50 years; (d) FAP excluded in any case of CRC; and (e) tumors verified by pathologic examination.

The efficacy of surveillance for CRC in families with HNPCC was evaluated in a controlled clinical trial extending over a 15-year period (80). The study concluded that screening for CRC at 3-year intervals more than halves the risk of CRC, prevents deaths from CRC, and decreases the overall mortality rate by about 65% in such families (moderate evidence). The incidence of CRC in the screened group was 6%, suggesting that a shorter screening interval may be appropriate. The age to begin screening in HNPCC is based on the observation that the average age of colon cancer diagnosis is 44 years, and cancers before the age of 25 years are very unusual.

III. What Is the Role of Imaging in Staging Colorectal Carcinoma?

Depth of invasion (T stage) and nodal involvement (N stage) are both important features for prognosis. A reliable preoperative test that can accurately stage tumor invasion into the colorectal wall (T) and regional lymph involvement (N) is essential to assess these prognostic indicators and to correctly assign patients to an appropriate treatment strategy. Both transrectal ultrasonography (US) and magnetic resonance imaging (MRI) with endorectal coils are considered superior to conventional CT in the preoperative assessment of tumor depth in the rectal wall. In a meta-analysis of 90 published series, comparing endorectal US, CT, and MRI (81), MRI and US demonstrated equal sensitivity for detection of muscularis propria invasion. However, US specificity (86%) was significantly higher than that of MRI (69%). For perirectal tissue invasion, sensitivity of US (90%) was significantly higher than that of CT (79%) and MRI (82%); specificities were comparable. For adjacent organ invasion and lymph node involvement, estimates for US, CT, and MRI were comparable. US showed better diagnostic accuracy than that of CT and MRI for perirectal tissue invasion. Analysis of lymph node involvement showed no differences in accuracy (moderate evidence). Although endorectal US is very accurate for staging of superficial rectal cancer, it has several limitations including operator dependency, limitation to tumors located 8–10 cm from the anal verge when using a rigid probe, and inability to assess stenosing lesions. In addition, endorectal US fails to detect lymph nodes that are outside the range of the transducer and cannot discriminate between lymph nodes inside or outside the mesorectal fascia, since the fascia is not depicted at endorectal US – an important factor in determining the spread of T3 tumors considered for total mesorectal excision. This limitation does not apply to MRI with external coils, as the mesorectal fascia is clearly depicted. To improve the sensitivity values of MRI for lymph node detection, newer techniques, such as use of new lymph node-specific MRI contrast agents, may provide a more sensitive MRI method to detect lymph node involvement (82, 83).

In the past, CT has been limited in differentiating and distinguishing the different layers of the rectal wall, demonstrating the mesorectal fascia, and depicting tumor invasion in surrounding pelvic structures due to poor spatial and contrast resolution. A recent study evaluated the role of CTC in local staging of CRC (84). The imaging protocol included contrast enhancement with 1-mm reconstruction intervals for arterial phase imaging. Overall accuracy for T and N staging was 73 and 59%, respectively. In this study the N staging accuracy increased to 80% with the use of multiplanar reconstruction. Improving CT spatial and contrast resolution combined with the use of arterial phase imaging and multiplanar reconstruction for bowel wall assessment may lead to increased diagnostic accuracy of local CRC staging.

IV. Applicability to Children

In general, CRC screening does not apply to children. However, if there is a family history of FAP, then screening beginning at puberty is recommended. Colectomy is advocated if genetic testing is positive.

V. Cost-Effectiveness

Evidence from several studies suggests that screening for, detecting, and removing CRC and precancerous polyps can reduce CRC incidence and related mortality. Accordingly, analyses have demonstrated that screening for CRC by any method is cost-effective when compared with no screening. The incremental cost-effectiveness ratio (ICER) for commonly considered strategies lies between $10,000 and $25,000 per life year saved (85), which compares favorably with other cancer screening strategies such as annual mammography for women aged 55–64 years ($132,000 per life year saved, in 1,998 dollars) (86). However, because different models and modeling assumptions were used and because different strategies were compared, the studies vary widely in their recommended strategies and in their estimates of cost-effectiveness ratios. Some studies advocate annual FOBT combined with a sigmoidoscopy every 5 years (87, 88), while others advocate a colonoscopy every 10 years (89, 90). McMahon and colleagues (91) compared and reanalyzed the results of three often-cited cost-effectiveness analyses of CRC screening in average-risk populations. The study found that in average-risk individuals, screening with DCBE examination every 3 years, or every 5 years with annual FOBT, had an ICER of less than $55,600 per life year saved. However,

DCBE examination screening every 3 years plus annual FOBT had an ICER of more than $100,000 per life year saved. Colonoscopic screening had an ICER of more than $100,000 per life year saved, was dominated by other screening strategies, and offered less benefit than did DCBE examination screening. However, this analysis assumed a greater sensitivity for DCBE for polyp detection than that determined by Winawer and colleagues (39), thereby introducing a possible bias into their competitive choice analysis; CTC was not included in the analysis.

A further study compared cost-effectiveness of CTC to colonoscopy and to no screening, and CTC was found to be cost-effective compared to no screening but not cost-effective compared to colonoscopy (92). The author concluded that CTC must be 54% less expensive than conventional colonoscopy and be performed at 10-year intervals to have equal cost-effectiveness to conventional colonoscopy. This analysis was based on preliminary CTC results and may be overly pessimistic, especially given the more recent evidence from Pickhardt and colleagues (50). Clearly, these data demonstrated that sensitivity of CTC for clinically significant lesions is equal to if not better than colonoscopy. In addition, the competitive choice analysis of Sonnenberg (92) did not include the use of CTC for surveillance postpolypectomy. Given the performance of CTC for detection of polyps and relatively low likelihood of average risk individuals developing significant adenomas following colonoscopic resection (39), this omission may have biased the results of their analysis.

VI. What Imaging-Based Screening Developments Are on the Horizon that May Improve Compliance with Colorectal Screening?

Despite the observed prevalence of polyps and the modification of risk obtained through screening, by current estimates only 15–19% of individuals eligible for screening actually undergo colon evaluation of any kind (93). A recent study found that although 80% of the doctors advised screening for CRC to their patients over the age of 50, only about 50% of eligible patients studied had their stool tested

for blood and about 30% had a sigmoidoscopy or colonoscopy (94). The perceived discomfort and inconvenience associated with bowel purgation has been identified as a barrier to screening (95, 96). Hence, methods to improve patient tolerance may lead to improved compliance with colon cancer screening. Currently, CTC requires a full cathartic bowel preparation, as do sigmoidoscopy and colonoscopy. At present, electronic bowel cleansing using a digital subtraction technique is being developed (97–101). This "prepless" colonography requires the patient to ingest a tagging agent such as barium sulfate or nonionic iodinated contrast to tag solid stool and luminal fluid. The bowel contents are thus uniformly opacified allowing subsequent digital subtraction from the image; soft tissue elements such as polyps are unaffected. This method potentially obviates bowel catharsis, a major factor in poor compliance with CRC screening. Fecal tagging was successfully used in conjunction with catharsis in a screening setting by Pickhardt and coworkers (98). Data, beyond pilot data, to validate this noncathartic technique is not yet available, but this technique may lead to better patient compliance in the future (102).

Computer-assisted detection (CAD) algorithms are also being developed to aid lesion detection (103, 104). Yoshida and colleagues (103) detected 89% of polyps (16 of 18) with 2.5 false-positive findings per patient. Such a CAD system has the potential to reduce the time of interpretation and may improve render performance. These developments, if rigorously validated in clinical trials, may make CT colonography a more easily tolerated, cost-effective alternative for CRC screening.

Take Home Tables and Figures (Tables 7.1–7.3)

Tables 7.1–7.3 and Fig. 7.1–7.4 serve to highlight key recommendations and supporting evidence.

Imaging Case Studies

The following cases (Figs. 7.1–7.4) highlight the advantages and limitations of colonoscopy and CTC.

Case 1: False-Negative CTC (Fig. 7.1)

Case 2: False-Positive CTC (Fig. 7.2)

Case 3: True-Positive CTC and Colonoscopy (Fig. 7.3)

Case 4: True-Positive CTC and False-Negative Colonoscopy (Fig. 7.4)

Suggested Imaging Protocol for Asymptomatic Screening Patients

The following protocol pertains to a General Electric 16-slice CT scanner:

- Indication: structural evaluation of the colon in patients without colon symptoms or completion CTC if the patient presented to colonoscopy for asymptomatic screening, and no polyps, strictures, or masses found
- Bowel preparation: standard catharsis and air insufflation (patient or technician controlled)
- Collimation 2.5 mm, kVp 140, mA 70, sec 0.6
- Pitch 1.3, table speed 13.75 mm/rotation, reconstruction interval 1.25 mm
- Prone and supine series
- No intravenous contrast

Table 7.1. Computed tomographic colonography (CTC) results to date: Sensitivity

Hospital (reference)	Polyp size		
	>10 mm	>5–10 mm	0–5 mm
University of California at San Francisco (46)	72% (all sizes)		
Boston University (47)	97%	97%	92%
Mayo Clinic (48)	98% (387/394)	95% (358/378)	
New York University (45)	98% (all sizes)		
Bethesda Naval (50)	96% (1,137/1,185)	92% (1,061/1,151)	n/a

n/a not available.

Reprinted with kind permission of Springer Science+Business Media from Slattery JMA, Modahl LE, Zalis ME. Imaging-Based Screening for Colorectal Cancer. In Medina LS, Blackmore DD (eds): *Evidence-Based Imaging: Optimizing Imaging in Patient Care.* New York: Springer Science+Business Media, 2006.

Table 7.2. CTC results to date: specificity

Hospital (reference)	Polyp size			No. of patients
	>10 mm	>5–10 mm	0–5 mm	
University of California at San Francisco (46)	94% (64/68)	82% (72/78)	66% (95/142)	300
Boston University (47)	91% (20/22)	82% (33/40)	55% (29/53)	100
Mayo Clinic (48)	73% (27/37)	57% (36/63)	n/a	703
New York University (45)	93% (13/14)	70% (19/27)	12% (11/91)	105
Bethesda Naval (50)	92% (47/51)	92% (88/95)	n/a	1,233

n/a not available.

Reprinted with kind permission of Springer Science+Business Media from Slattery JMA, Modahl LE, Zalis ME. Imaging-Based Screening for Colorectal Cancer. In Medina LS, Blackmore DD (eds): *Evidence-Based Imaging: Optimizing Imaging in Patient Care.* New York: Springer Science+Business Media, 2006.

Table 7.3. Sensitivity and specificity of other modalities

Modality	Sensitivity (reference)	Specificity (reference)
FOBT	30–50% (one-time testing) (7, 18)	90–98% (7)
DCBE	30–96% (all lesions) (37)	85–90%
Colonoscopy	94% (lesions ≥1 cm) (35)	100%

FOBT fecal occult blood testing, *DCBE* double contrast barium enema.
Reprinted with kind permission of Springer Science+Business Media from Slattery JMA, Modahl LE, Zalis ME. Imaging-Based Screening for Colorectal Cancer. In Medina LS, Blackmore DD (eds): *Evidence-Based Imaging: Optimizing Imaging in Patient Care.* New York: Springer Science+Business Media, 2006.

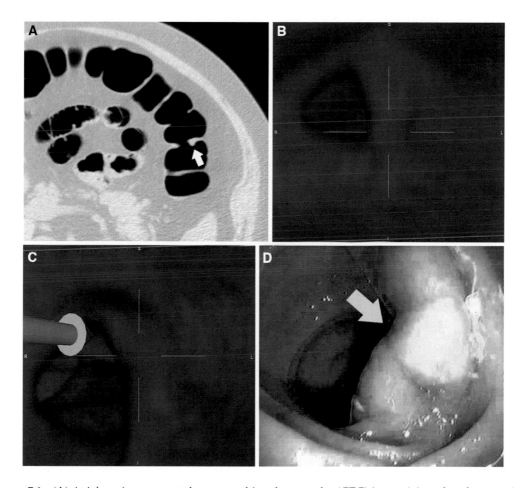

Figure 7.1. (**A**) Axial supine computed tomographic colonography (CTC) image (viewed on lung settings) demonstrates a prominent haustral fold in the transverse colon. This was interpreted as being within normal limits. (**B, C**) Three-dimensional reconstruction does not reveal a significant lesion. (**D**) Endoscopic view of the transverse colon in the same region (*arrow*) reveals a 20-mm sessile lesion. Biopsy confirmed a tubular adenoma. (Reprinted with kind permission of Springer Science+Business Media from Slattery JMA, Modahl LE, Zalis ME. Imaging-Based Screening for Colorectal Cancer. In Medina LS, Blackmore DD (eds): *Evidence-Based Imaging: Optimizing Imaging in Patient Care.* New York: Springer Science+Business Media, 2006.)

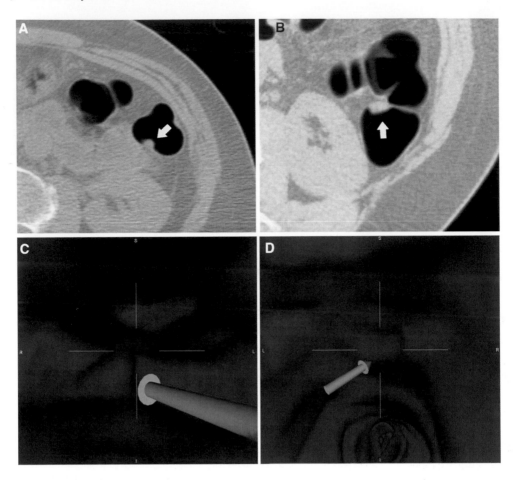

Figure 7.2. (**A, B**) Axial supine and prone CTC images (viewed on lung settings) reveal a polypoid lesion (*arrow*) in the region of the splenic flexure. (**C, D**) Three-dimensional reconstruction of region in A and B support the presence of a polypoid mass in the splenic flexure. Subsequent colonoscopy was normal. (Reprinted with kind permission of Springer Science+Business Media from Slattery JMA, Modahl LE, Zalis ME. Imaging-Based Screening for Colorectal Cancer. In Medina LS, Blackmore DD (eds): *Evidence-Based Imaging: Optimizing Imaging in Patient Care*. New York: Springer Science+Business Media, 2006.)

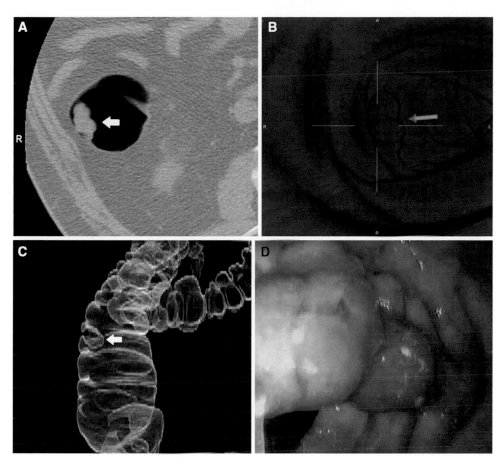

Figure 7.3. (**A**) Axial supine CTC image (viewed on lung settings) reveals a polypoid mass in the ascending colon. (**B, C**) Three-dimensional (3D) reconstruction of the region renders an endolumial view of the lesion (**B**). Digitally subtracted 3D image of the ascending colon provides a lesion projection similar to double contrast barium enema (**C**). (**D**) Endoscopy reveals a 15-mm polyp. Biopsy confirmed a tubulovillous adenoma. (Reprinted with kind permission of Springer Science+Business Media from Slattery JMA, Modahl LE, Zalis ME. Imaging-Based Screening for Colorectal Cancer. In Medina LS, Blackmore DD (eds): *Evidence-Based Imaging: Optimizing Imaging in Patient Care*. New York: Springer Science+Business Media, 2006.)

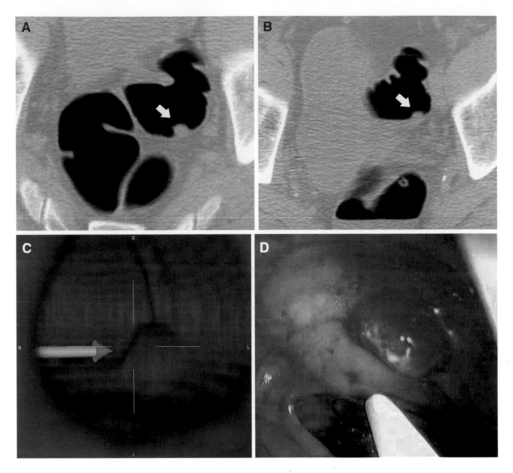

Figure 7.4. Axial supine (**A**) and prone (**B**) CTC images (viewed on lung settings) reveals a polypoid mass in the sigmoid colon. (**C**) Three-dimensional endoluminal reconstruction supports the findings on axial imaging. (**D**) Colonoscopy performed on the same day as the CTC in a trial protocol was negative. Repeat sigmoidoscopy was advised based on the CTC findings. This revealed a 10-mm invasive carcinoma in the sigmoid colon. (Reprinted with kind permission of Springer Science+Business Media from Slattery JMA, Modahl LE, Zalis ME. Imaging-Based Screening for Colorectal Cancer. In Medina LS, Blackmore DD (eds): *Evidence-Based Imaging: Optimizing Imaging in Patient Care*. New York: Springer Science+Business Media, 2006.)

Future Areas of Research

- Further clinical trials of CTC in average-risk populations
- CTC using digital subtraction bowel cleansing
- Computer-assisted polyp detection

References

1. Hill MJ, Morson BC, Bussey HJ. Lancet 1978;1:245–247.
2. Morson BC. Clin Radiol 1984;35:425–431.
3. Winawer SJ, Zauber AG, Diaz B. Gastrointest Endosc 1987;33:167.
4. Atkin WS, Morson BC, Cuzick J. N Engl J Med 1992;326:658–662.
5. Stryker SJ, Wolff BG, Culp CE, Libbe SD, Ilstrup DM, MacCarty RL. Gastroenterology 1987;93:1009–1013.
6. Burt RW, Bishop DT, Cannon LA, Dowdle MA, Lee RG, Skolnick MH. N Engl J Med 1985;312:1540–1544.
7. Mandel JS, Bond JH, Church TR et al. N Engl J Med 1993;328:1365–1371.
8. Muller AD, Sonnenberg A. Ann Intern Med 1995;123:904–910.
9. Winawer SJ, Zauber AG, Ho MN et al. N Engl J Med 1993;329:1977–1981.

10. Muto T, Bussey HJ, Morson BC. Cancer 1975;36: 2251–2270.
11. Powell SM, Zilz N, Beazer-Barclay Y et al. Nature 1992;359:235–237.
12. Nagase H, Nakamura Y. Hum Mutat 1993;2: 425–434.
13. Jemal A, Tiwari RC, Murray T et al. CA Cancer J Clin 2004;54:8–29.
14. Redaelli A, Cranor CW, Okano GJ, Reese PR. Pharmacoeconomics 2003;21:1213–1238.
15. Bond JH. Semin Gastrointest Dis 2000;11: 176–184.
16. Hardcastle JD, Chamberlain JO, Robinson MH et al. Lancet 1996;348:1472–1477.
17. Kronborg O, Fenger C, Olsen J, Jorgensen OD, Sondergaard O. Lancet 1996;348:1467–1471.
18. Ahlquist DA, Wieand HS, Moertel CG et al. JAMA 1993;269:1262–1267.
19. Simon JB. Gastroenterologist 1998;6:66–78.
20. Rex DK, Lehman GA, Ulbright TM et al. Am J Gastroenterol 1993;88:825–831.
21. Lieberman DA, Smith FW. Am J Gastroenterol 1991;86:946–951.
22. Selby JV, Friedman GD, Quesenberry CP Jr, Weiss NS. N Engl J Med 1992;326:653–657.
23. Newcomb PA, Norfleet RG, Storer BE, Surawicz TS, Marcus PM. J Natl Cancer Inst 1992;84: 1572–1575.
24. Kavanagh AM, Giovannucci EL, Fuchs CS, Colditz GA. Cancer Causes Control 1998;9: 455–462.
25. Dachman AH, Kuniyoshi JK, Boyle CM et al. AJR Am J Roentgenol 1998;171:989–995.
26. Maglinte DD, Keller KJ, Miller RE, Chernish SM. Radiology 1983;147:669–672.
27. Rex DK, Chak A, Vasudeva R et al. Gastrointest Endosc 1999;49:727–730.
28. Imperiale TF, Wagner DR, Lin CY, Larkin GN, Rogge JD. N Engl J Med 2000;343:169–174.
29. Jorgensen OD, Kronborg O, Fenger C. Gut 2002;50:29–32.
30. Lieberman DA, Weiss DG, Veterans Affairs Cooperative Study Group 380. N Engl J Med 2001;345:555–560.
31. Citarda F, Tomaselli G, Capocaccia R, Barcherini S, Crespi M, Italian Multicentre Study Group. Gut 2001;48:812–815.
32. Thiis-Evensen E, Hoff GS, Sauar J, Langmark F, Majak BM, Vatn MH. Scand J Gastroenterol 1999;34:414–420.
33. Winawer SJ, Fletcher RH, Miller L et al. Gastroenterology 1997;112:594–642.
34. Ransohoff DF, Lang CA. N Engl J Med 1991;325: 37–41.
35. Rex DK, Cutler CS, Lemmel GT et al. Gastroenterology 1997;112:24–28.
36. Winawer SJ, Zauber AG, O'Brien MJ et al. Cancer 1992;70:1236–1245.
37. Glick S, Wagner JL, Johnson CD. AJR Am J Roentgenol 1998;170:629–636.
38. Rex DK, Rahmani EY, Haseman JH, Lemmel GT, Kaster S, Buckley JS. Gastroenterology 1997;112: 17–23.
39. Winawer SJ, Stewart ET, Zauber AG et al. N Engl J Med 2000;342:1766–1772.
40. Johnson CD, Dachman AH. Radiology 2000;216:331–341.
41. Taylor SA, Halligan S, Saunders BP, Bassett P, Vance M, Bartram CI. AJR Am J Roentgenol 2003;181:913–921.
42. Svensson MH, Svensson E, Lasson A, Hellstrom M. Radiology 2002;222:337–345.
43. Hara AK, Johnson CD, MacCarty RL, Welch TJ. Radiology 2000;215:353–357.
44. Gluecker TM, Johnson CD, Wilson LA et al. Gastroenterology 2003;124:911–916.
45. Macari M, Bini EJ, Xue X et al. Radiology 2002;224:383–392.
46. Yee J, Akerkar GA, Hung RK, Steinauer-Gebauer AM, Wall SD, McQuaid KR. Radiology 2001; 219:685–692.
47. Fenlon HM, Nunes DP, Schroy PC 3rd, Barish MA, Clarke PD, Ferrucci JT. N Engl J Med 1999; 341:1496–1503.
48. Johnson CD, Harmsen WS, Wilson LA et al. Gastroenterology 2003;125:311–319.
49. Cotton PB, Durkalski VL, Pineau BC et al. JAMA 2004;291:1713–1719.
50. Pickhardt PJ, Choi JR, Hwang I et al. N Engl J Med 2003;349:2191–2200.
51. Johns LE, Houlston RS. Am J Gastroenterol 2001;96:2992–3003.
52. Fuchs CS, Giovannucci EL, Colditz GA, Hunter DJ, Speizer FE, Willett WC. N Engl J Med 1994;331:1669–1674.
53. Winawer SJ, Zauber AG, O'Brien MJ et al. N Engl J Med 1993;328:901–906.
54. Winawer SJ, O'Brien MJ, Waye JD et al. Bull WHO 1990;68:789–795.
55. Rex DK, Smith JJ, Ulbright TM, Lehman GA. Gastroenterology 1992;102:317–319.
56. Morson BC, Konishi F. Gastrointest Radiol 1982;7:275–281.
57. Gilbertsen VA, Williams SE, Schuman L, McHugh R. Surg Gynecol Obstet 1979;149:877–878.
58. de Roos A, Hermans J, Shaw PC, Kroon H. Radiology 1985;154:11–13.
59. Henry LG, Condon RE, Schulte WJ, Aprahamian C, DeCosse JJ. Ann Surg 1975;182:511–515.
60. Kirsner JB, Rider JA, Moeller HC, Palmer WL, Gold SS. Gastroenterology 1960;39:178–182.
61. Waye JD, Braunfeld S. Endoscopy 1982;14:79–81.
62. Matek W, Guggenmoos-Holzmann I, Demling L. Endoscopy 1985;17:175–181.
63. Winawer SJ. Gastrointest Endosc 1999;49: S63–S66.
64. Noshirwani KC, van Stolk RU, Rybicki LA, Beck GJ. Gastrointest Endosc 2000;51:433–437.

65. van Stolk RU, Beck GJ, Baron JA, Haile R, Summers R. Gastroenterology 1998;115:13–18.
66. Cali RL, Pitsch RM, Thorson AG et al. Dis Colon Rectum 1993;36:388–393.
67. Jahn H, Joergensen OD, Kronborg O, Fenger C. Dis Colon Rectum 1992;35:253–256.
68. Schoemaker D, Black R, Giles L, Toouli J. Gastroenterology 1998;114:7–14.
69. Morrin MM, Farrell RJ, Raptopoulos V, McGee JB, Bleday R, Kruskal JB. Dis Colon Rectum 2000;43:303–311.
70. Carucci LR, Levine MS. Gastroenterol Clin North Am 2002;31:93–117, ix.
71. Hooyman JR, MacCarty RL, Carpenter HA, Schroeder KW, Carlson HC. AJR Am J Roentgenol 1987;149:47–51.
72. Gillen CD, Walmsley RS, Prior P, Andrews HA, Allan RN. Gut 1994;35:1590–1592.
73. Lennard-Jones JE, Melville DM, Morson BC, Ritchie JK, Williams CB. Gut 1990;31:800–806.
74. Choi PM, Nugent FW, Schoetz DJ Jr, Silverman ML, Haggitt RC. Gastroenterology 1993;105:418–424.
75. Lynch HT, de la Chapelle A. J Med Genet 1999;36:801–818.
76. Heiskanen I, Luostarinen T, Jarvinen HJ. Scand J Gastroenterol 2000;35:1284–1287.
77. Lynch HT, de la Chapelle A. N Engl J Med 2003;348:919–932.
78. Samowitz WS, Curtin K, Lin HH et al. Gastroenterology 2001;121:830–838.
79. Vasen HF, Watson P, Mecklin JP, Lynch HT. Gastroenterology 1999;116:1453–1456.
80. Jarvinen HJ, Aarnio M, Mustonen H et al. Gastroenterology 2000;118:829–834.
81. Bipat S, Glas AS, Slors FJ, Zwinderman AH, Bossuyt PM, Stoker J. Radiology 2004;232:773–783.
82. Harisinghani MG, Saini S, Weissleder R et al. AJR Am J Roentgenol 1999;172:1347–1351.
83. McCauley TR, Rifkin MD, Ledet CA. J Magn Reson Imaging 2002;15:492–497.
84. Filippone A, Ambrosini R, Fuschi M, Marinelli T, Genovesi D, Bonomo L. Radiology 2004;231:83–90.
85. Pignone M, Saha S, Hoerger T, Mandelblatt J. Ann Intern Med 2002;137:96–104.
86. Tengs TO, Adams ME, Pliskin JS et al. Risk Anal 1995;15:369–390.
87. Vijan S, Hwang EW, Hofer TP, Hayward RA. Am J Med 2001;111:593–601.
88. Frazier AL, Colditz GA, Fuchs CS, Kuntz KM. JAMA 2000;284:1954–1961.
89. Khandker RK, Dulski JD, Kilpatrick JB, Ellis RP, Mitchell JB, Baine WB. Int J Technol Assess Health Care 2000;16:799–810.
90. Sonnenberg A, Delco F, Inadomi JM. Ann Intern Med 2000;133:573–584.
91. McMahon PM, Bosch JL, Gleason S, Halpern EF, Lester JS, Gazelle GS. Radiology 2001;219:44–50.
92. Sonnenberg A, Delco F, Bauerfeind P. Am J Gastroenterol 1999;94:2268–2274.
93. Brown ML, Potosky AL, Thompson GB, Kessler LG. Prev Med 1990;19:562–574.
94. Hawley ST, Vernon SW, Levin B, Vallejo B. Cancer Epidemiol Biomarkers Prev 2004;13:314–319.
95. Wardle J, Sutton S, Williamson S et al. Prev Med 2000;31:323–334.
96. Ristvedt SL, McFarland EG, Weinstock LB, Thyssen EP. Am J Gastroenterol 2003;98:578–585.
97. Zalis ME, Hahn PF. AJR Am J Roentgenol 2001;176:646–648.
98. Pickhardt PJ, Choi JH. AJR Am J Roentgenol 2003;181:799–805.
99. Lefere PA, Gryspeerdt SS, Dewyspelaere J, Baekelandt M, Van Holsbeeck BG. Radiology 2002;224:393–403.
100. Chen D, Liang Z, Wax MR, Li L, Li B, Kaufman AE. IEEE Trans Med Imaging 2000;19:1220–1226.
101. Callstrom MR, Johnson CD, Fletcher JG et al. Radiology 2001;219:693–698.
102. Zalis ME, Perumpillichira J, Del Frate C, Hahn PF. Radiology 2003;226:911–917.
103. Yoshida H, Masutani Y, MacEneaney P, Rubin DT, Dachman AH. Radiology 2002;222:327–336.
104. Summers RM, Johnson CD, Pusanik LM, Malley JD, Youssef AM, Reed JE. Radiology 2001;219:51–59.

8

Imaging of Brain Cancer

Soonmee Cha

Issues

   I. Who should undergo imaging to exclude brain cancer in adult individual?

II A. Who should undergo imaging to exclude brain cancer in pediatric age group?

II B. What imaging is appropriate in high-risk pediatric subjects?

  III. What is the appropriate imaging in subjects at risk for brain cancer?

  IV. What is the role of proton magnetic resonance spectroscopy in the diagnosis and follow-up of brain neoplasms?

   V. Can imaging be used to differentiate post-treatment necrosis from residual/recurrent Tumor?

  VI. What is the added value of functional MRI in the surgical planning of patients with suspected brain neoplasm or focal brain lesions?

 VII. What is the cost-effectiveness of imaging in patients with suspected primary brain and disease?

Key Points

- Brain imaging is necessary for optimal localization, characterization, and management of brain cancer prior to surgery in patients with suspected or confirmed brain tumors (strong evidence).
- Due to its superior soft tissue contrast, multiplanar capability and biosafety, magnetic resonance imaging (MRI) with and without gadolinium-based intravenous contrast material is the preferred method for brain cancer imaging when compared to computed tomography (moderate evidence).

S. Cha (✉)
Department of Radiology and Biomedical Imaging, University of California San Francisco Medical Center, 350 Parnassus Avenue, Suite 307, San Francisco, CA 94117, USA
e-mail: Soonmee.Cha@ucsf.edu

L.S. Medina et al. (eds.), *Evidence-Based Imaging: Improving the Quality of Imaging in Patient Care, Revised Edition,*   **127**
DOI 10.1007/978-1-4419-7777-9_8, © Springer Science+Business Media, LLC 2011

- No adequate data exist on the role of imaging in monitoring brain cancer response to therapy and differentiating between tumor recurrence and therapy related changes (insufficient evidence).
- No adequate data exist on the role of nonanatomic, physiology-based imaging, such as proton MR spectroscopy, perfusion and diffusion MRI, and nuclear medicine imaging (SPECT and PET) in monitoring treatment response or in predicting prognosis and outcome in patients with brain cancer (insufficient evidence).
- Human studies conducted on the use of Magnetic resonance spectroscopy (MRS) for brain tumors demonstrate that this noninvasive method is technically feasible and suggest potential benefits for some of the proposed indications. However, there is a paucity of high quality direct evidence demonstrating the impact on diagnostic thinking and therapeutic decision making.
- There is added value of fMRI in the surgical planning of patients with suspected brain cancer or focal brain lesion (moderate evidence).

Definition and Pathophysiology

The term brain cancer, or more commonly referred to as brain tumor, is used here to describe all primary and secondary neoplasms of the brain and its covering, including the leptomeninges, dura, skull, and scalp. Brain cancer is comprised of a variety of central nervous system tumors with a wide range of histopathology, molecular/genetic profile, clinical spectrum, treatment possibilities, and patient prognosis and outcome. The pathophysiology of brain cancer is complex and dependent on various factors, such as histology, molecular and chromosomal aberration, tumor related protein expression, primary versus secondary origin, and host factors (1–4).

Unique Challenges of Brain Cancer

When compared to systemic cancers (e.g., lung, breast, colon), brain cancer is unique in several different ways. First, the brain is covered by a tough, fibrous tissue dura mater and a bony skull that protects the inner contents. This rigid covering allows very little, if any, increase in volume of the inner content and, therefore, brain tumor cells adapt to grow in a more infiltrative rather than expansive pattern. This growth pattern limits the disruption to the underlying cytoarchitecture. Second, the brain capillaries have a unique barrier known as the blood–brain barrier (BBB), which limits the

entrance of systemic circulation into the central nervous system. Cancer cells can hide behind the protective barrier of BBB, migrate with minimal disruption to the structural and physiologic milieu of the brain, and escape imaging detection since intravenous contrast agent becomes visible when there is BBB disruption, allowing the agent to leak into the interstitial space (5–9).

Epidemiology

Adult Brain Cancer

Primary malignant or benign brain cancers were estimated to be newly diagnosed in about 35,519 Americans in 2001 (CBTRUS, 2000). Primary brain cancers are among the top 10 causes of cancer-related deaths (American Cancer Society, 1998). Nearly 13,000 people die from these cancers each year in the USA (CBTRUS, 2000). About 11–12 per 100,000 persons in the USA are diagnosed with a primary brain cancer each year, and 6–7 per 100,000 are diagnosed with a primary malignant brain cancer. Almost 1 in every 1,300 children will develop some form of primary brain cancer before age 20 years (CBTRUS, 1998). Between 1991 and 1995, 23% of childhood cancers were brain cancers, and about one fourth of childhood cancers deaths were from a malignant brain tumor.

The epidemiologic study of brain cancer is challenging and complex due to number of factors unique to this disease. First, primary and secondary brain cancers are vastly different diseases that clearly need to be differentiated and categorized, which is an inherently difficult task. Second, histopathologic classification of brain cancer is complicated due to the heterogeneity of the tumors at virtually all levels of structural and functional organization such as differential growth rate, metastatic potential, sensitivity irradiation and chemotherapy, and genetic liability. Third, several brain cancer types have benign and malignant variants with a continuous spectrum of biologic aggressiveness. It is therefore difficult to assess the full spectrum of the disease at presentation (10).

The most common primary brain cancers are tumors of neuroepithelial origin, which include astrocytoma, oligodendroglioma, mixed glioma (oligoastrocytoma), ependymoma, choroids plexus tumors, neuroepithelial tumors of uncertain origin, neuronal and mixed neuronal-glial tumors, pineal tumors, and embryonal tumors. The most common type of primary brain tumor that involves the covering of the brain (as opposed to the substance) is meningioma, which accounts for more than 20% of all brain tumors (11). The most common type of primary brain cancer in adults is glioblastoma multiforme (GBM). In adults, brain metastases far outnumber primary neoplasms owing to high incidence of systemic cancer (e.g., lung and breast carcinoma).

The incidence rate of all primary benign and malignant brain tumors based on the Central Brain Tumor Registry of the United States (12) is 14 cases per 100,000 person-years (5.7 per 100,000 person-years for benign tumors and 7.7 person-years for malignant tumors). The rate is higher in males (14.2 per 100,000 person-years) than females (13.9 per 100,000 person-years). According to the Surveillance, Epidemiology, and End Results (SEER), the 5-year relative survival rate following the diagnosis of a primary malignant brain tumor (excluding lymphoma) is 32.7% for males and 31.6% for females. The prevalence rate for all primary brain tumors based on CBTRUS is 130.8 per 100,000 and the estimated number of people living with a diagnosis of primary brain tumors was 359,000 persons. Two-, five-, and ten-year observed and relative survival rates for each specific type of malignant brain tumor, according to the SEER report from 1973 to 1996, showed that GBM has the poorest prognosis. More detailed information on the brain cancer

survival data is available at the Central Brain Tumor Registry of US website (http://www.cbtrus.org/2001/table2001_12.htm).

In terms of brain metastases, the exact annual incidence remains unknown due to a lack of dedicated national cancer registry, but is estimated to be 97,800–170,000 new cases each year in the USA. The most common types of primary cancer causing brain metastasis are cancers of the lung, breast, unknown primary, melanoma, and colon.

Pediatric Brain Cancer

The epidemiologic studies of brain cancer suggest that the incidence of pediatric brain cancer is rising but the actual details remain unclear. There are two fundamental problems that might explain the difficulty in elucidating epidemiological changes in pediatric brain cancer. First, the definition and histopathological criteria for each type of primary pediatric brain cancer remain inconsistent and variable. Second, there is a lack of true brain cancer registry that is critical for monitoring incidence and epidemiology. Rather, data from nine registries have been compiled since 1973 by the National Cancer Institute as the SEER program and extrapolated to represent national data. These data demonstrate an overall incidence of pediatric central nervous system cancer to be 3.5 per 100,000 children less than 15 years of age. Pediatric central nervous system cancers account for about 15–20% of all childhood cancers and the peak age is 5–8 years old. There is no definitive evidence to suggest any gender or race predilection for pediatric brain tumors. An additional source of epidemiologic information is a report from the Central Brain Tumor Registry of the United States (12), a nonprofit agency organized for the purpose of collecting and publishing epidemiologic data for brain tumors (CBTRUS, 2002). Syndromes associated with central nervous system tumors are Neurofibromatosis type 1 and 2, Tuberous sclerosis type 1 and 2, von Hippel–Lindau syndrome, Li–Fraumeni syndrome, Nevoid basal cell carcinoma, Turcot's syndrome, Gorlin syndrome, Ataxia-telangiectasia syndrome, Gardner's syndrome, and Down syndrome (13). The molecular genetics of pediatric brain tumors may provide valuable insights into the etiology and biology of these tumors but the specific genetic alterations for tumor development in a majority of patients remain elusive.

The most common primary pediatric brain cancers are astrocytomas, which account for approximately 50% of all pediatric CNS tumors (14). Pediatric astrocytomas can arise within the optic pathway (15–25%), cerebral hemisphere (12%), spine (10–12%), and brain stem (12%) (15). Contrary to adult primary brain cancer, which is more common in supratentorial brain, more than half of all pediatric brain cancers occurs in infratentorial brain. The most common infratentorial pediatric brain cancer is medulloblastoma/primary neuroectodermal tumor (PNET) (30–35%), closely followed by pilocytic astrocytoma (20–35%), brain stem gliomas (25%), ependymoma (10%), and other miscellaneous types (5%) (15). The long-term survival rate for the two most common types of pediatric brain cancers, namely pilocytic astrocytoma and medulloblastoma, differ substantially in that medulloblastoma tends to have poorer survival especially when it occurs in children younger than 3 years of age or those with metastatic disease at the time of initial diagnosis (15).

Overall Cost to Society

Brain cancer is a rare neoplasm but affects people of all ages (10). It is more common in the pediatric population and tends to cause high morbidity and mortality (15). The overall cost to society in dollar amount is difficult to estimate and may not be as high as other, more common systemic cancers. The cost of treating brain cancer in the USA is difficult to determine, but can be estimated to be far greater than four billion dollars per year based on 359,000 estimated number of people living with brain cancer (12) and $11,365.23 per patient for initial cost of surgical treatment. There are very few articles in medical literature that address the cost-effectiveness or overall cost to society in relation to imaging of brain cancer. One of the few articles that discusses the actual monetary cost to society is a 1998 article by Latif et al. (16) from Great Britain. The team measured the mean costs of medical care for 157 patients with brain cancer in British Pounds. Based on this study, the average cost of imaging was less than 3% of the total, whereas radiotherapy was responsible for greater than 50% of the total

cost. The relative contribution of imaging in this study appears low, however, and what is not known from this report is what kind and how often imaging was done in these patients with brain cancer during their hospital stay and as out-patients. In addition, the vastly different health care reimbursement structure in Britain and the US makes interpretation difficult.

Goals

The goals of imaging in patients, pediatric or adult age group, with suspected brain cancer are (1) diagnosis at acute presentation, (2) preoperative or treatment planning to further characterize brain abnormality, and (3) posttreatment evaluation for residual disease and therapy related changes. The role of imaging is critically dependent upon the clinical context that the study is being ordered (17). The initial diagnosis of brain cancer is often made on a CT scan in an emergency room setting when a patient presents with an acute clinical symptoms such as seizure or focal neurologic deficit. Once a brain abnormality is detected on the initial scan, MRI with contrast agent is obtained to further characterize the lesion and the remainder of the brain and to serve as a part of preoperative planning for a definitive histologic diagnosis. If the nature of the brain lesion is still in question after a comprehensive imaging, further imaging with advanced techniques such as diffusion, perfusion, or proton spectroscopic imaging may be warranted to differentiate brain cancer from tumor-mimicking lesions such as infarcts, abscesses, or demyelinating lesions (18–20). In the immediate postoperative imaging, the most important imaging objectives are to (a) determine the amount of residual or recurrent disease, (b) assess early postoperative complications such as hemorrhage, contusion, or other brain injury, and (c) determine delay treatment complications such as radiation necrosis and treatment leukoencephalopathy.

Methodology

A MEDLINE search was performed using PubMed (National Library of Medicine, Bethesda, Maryland) for original research publications discussing the diagnostic performance and effectiveness of imaging strategies in brain cancer. Systematic literature review was performed from 1966 through January 2010. Keywords included are (1) brain cancer, (2) brain tumor, (3) glioma, (4) diagnostic imaging, and (5) neurosurgery. In addition, the following three cancer databases were reviewed:

1. The SEER program maintained by the National Cancer Institute (http://www.seer.cancer.gov) for incidence, survival, and mortality rates, classified by tumor histology, brain topography, age, race, and gender. SEER is population-based reference standard for cancer data and collects incidence and follow-up data on malignant brain cancer only.

2. The Central Brain Tumor Registry of the United States (12) (http://www.cbtrus.org) collects incidence data on all primary brain tumors from 11 collaborating state registries; however, follow-up data are not available.

3. The National Cancer Data Base (NCDB) (http://www.facs.org/cancer/ncdb) serves as a comprehensive clinical surveillance resource for cancer care in the USA. While not population-based, the NCDB identifies newly diagnosed cases and conducts follow-up on all primary brain tumors from hospitals accredited by the American College of Surgeons. The NCDB is the largest of the three databases and also contains more complete information regarding treatment of tumors than SEER or CBTRUS databases.

I. Who Should Undergo Imaging to Exclude Brain Cancer in Adult Individual?

Summary of Evidence: The scientific evidence on this topic is limited. No strong evidence studies are available. Most of the available literature is classified as limited and moderate evidence. First, the three most common clinical symptoms of brain cancer are headache, seizure, and focal weakness – all of which are neither unique nor specific for the presence of brain cancer (see Chap. 14 on seizures and Chap. 15 on headaches). Second, the clinical manifestation of brain cancer

is heavily dependent on the topography of the lesion. For example, lesions in the motor cortex may have more acute presentation whereas more insidious onset of cognitive or personality changes are commonly associated with prefrontal cortex tumors (21, 22).

Despite the aforementioned nonspecific clinical presentation of subjects with brain cancer, a summary of the guidelines is shown in Table 8.1. A relatively acute onset of any one of these symptoms that progresses over time should strongly warrant a brain imaging. Newton et al. (23) cite a consensus among neurologists that the most specific clinical feature of a brain cancer versus other brain mass lesions is not one particular individual symptom or sign but, rather, progression over time.

Supporting Evidence: It remains difficult, however, to narrow down the criteria for the "suspected" clinical symptomatology of brain cancer. In a retrospective study of 653 patients with supratentorial brain cancer, Salcman (24) found that the three most common clinical features of brain cancer were headache (70%), seizure (54%), cognitive or personality change (52%), focal weakness (43%), nausea or vomiting (31%), speech disturbances (27%), alteration of consciousness (25%), sensory abnormalities (14%), and visual disturbances (8%) (moderate evidence). Similarly, Snyder et al. (25) studied 101 patients who were admitted through an emergency room and discharged with a diagnosis of brain cancer (moderate evidence). They found that the three most frequent clinical features were headache (55%), cognitive or personality changes (50%), ataxia (40%), focal weakness (36%), nausea or vomiting (36%), papilledema (27%), cranial nerve palsy (25%), seizure (24%), visual disturbance (20%), speech disturbance (20%), sensory abnormalities (18%), and positive Babinski's sign (17%). No combination of these factors has been shown to reliably differentiate brain cancer from other benign causes.

IIA. Who Should Undergo Imaging to Exclude Brain Cancer in Pediatric Age Group?

Summary of Evidence: Determination of which children with clinical suspicion of brain cancer should undergo imaging is a complex issue for a number of reasons. As in adults, the three most common clinical symptoms of brain cancer are headache, seizure, and focal weakness – all of which are neither unique nor specific for the presence of brain cancer. Hence, it is difficult to perform a prospective study based on these clinical symptoms to determine whether or not imaging is indicated. Second, as discussed earlier, the clinical manifestation of brain cancer is heavily dependent on the topography of the lesion. Third, neurocognitive dysfunction may not necessarily be due to a mass lesion within the brain, but can also be the secondary effects of systemic disease, chemical or hormonal imbalance, toxic exposure, drug or radiation therapy, or nonorganic neurodegenerative disorder (21, 22).

Despite the aforementioned nonspecific clinical presentation of subjects with brain cancer, there are guidelines one can use to determine who should undergo imaging (Table 8.1).

A relatively acute onset of any one of these symptoms that progresses over time should strongly warrant brain imaging, preferably with MRI (strong evidence). See also Chaps. 14 and 15 on seizures and headaches.

Supporting Evidence: It remains difficult, in children as well as adults, to define criteria for "suspected" brain cancer. It should be noted that there is marked difference between adult and pediatric subjects with suspected brain cancer in terms of epidemiology, clinical presentation, tomography of the lesion, histologic tissue type, metastatic potential, and prognosis (26). Headache, posterior fossa symptoms such as nausea and vomiting, ataxia, and cranial nerve symptoms predominate in children due to the fact that the overwhelming majority of pediatric brain cancers occur infratentorially (15). Table 8.1 lists various clinical symptoms that are associated with pediatric brain cancer.

The two most common types of pediatric brain cancer are medulloblastoma and juvenile pilocytic astrocytoma (JPA), both of which commonly occur in the posterior fossa. Medulloblastomas and other small round blue cell tumors (pineoblastoma and primitive neuroectodermal tumor) have high propensity to spread along the leptomeningeal route within the central nervous system (13). JPAs are also commonly seen in supratentorial brain, especially near the hypothalamic region (26, 27). Prognosis differs vastly depending on the tissue

histology and metastatic potential since medulloblastoma and other small cell tumors tend to have aggressive biology and poor outcome whereas JPAs tend to have more favorable long-term prognosis (1, 10, 15).

Non-migraine, nonchronic headache in a child should raise a high suspicion for an intracranial mass lesion, especially if there are any additional posterior fossa or visual symptoms, and imaging should be conducted without delay. (See details in Chap. 15 on headaches transpose).

IIB. What Imaging Is Appropriate in High-Risk Pediatric Subjects?

Summary of Evidence: In the high-risk children suspected of having brain cancer, MRI without and with gadolinium-based contrast agent is the imaging modality of choice (Table 8.2). There is no evidence to suggest that the addition of other diagnostic tests, such as CT, catheter angiography, or PET scan, improves either the cost effectiveness or the outcome in the high-risk group at initial presentation (Table 8.2) (strong evidence).

Supporting Evidence: There is strong evidence to suggest that MRI is the diagnostic imaging test of choice in high-risk subjects suspected of having brain cancer (17, 28, 29) (Table 8.2). For example, superiority of MRI over CT in detection of brain cancer has been supported by an animal study done by Whelan et al (30). However, since CT scanners are more widely available and easily performed than MR scanners, especially in an emergency department setting, it is commonly performed even though CT is inferior to MR in lesion detection and characterization. Table 8.3 lists advantages and limitations of CT and MRI in the evaluation of children with suspected brain cancer.

Unenhanced CT is good for assessing acute intracranial hemorrhage, midline shift/mass effect, or hydrocephalus. CT, however, is not ideal for detecting subtle parenchymal abnormality (17). As seen in Fig. 8.1, in comparing an unenhanced CT and an enhanced MRI, a rather large abnormality can be quite subtle to detect on the CT study due to its inferior soft tissue contrast, whereas the lesion is clearly visible in the MRI. However, CT does have advantage in depicting calcium much better than MRI as can be seen in Fig. 8.1. Contrast-enhanced CT offers improved sensitivity, but the addition of iodinated contrast agent is not without risk of anaphylactic reaction (truly the risk is very low for nonionic low osmolar contrast in children – moderate to severe reactions are less than 1:10,000). As shown in Fig. 8.2, MRI is superior to CT in its ability to depict brain cancer in multiple planes with greater soft tissue resolution and without the use ionizing radiation. It is important to note that the addition of MRI contrast agent, gadolinium, is necessary to fully characterize the extent of disease, especially to assess leptomeningeal spread of disease (Fig. 8.2D–F) (Table 8.2). Table 8.4 lists suggested MR imaging protocol for a pediatric subject suspected of having brain cancer. Imaging strategy in pediatric brain cancer subjects should be tailored to the need of clinical management and treatment decisions.

Nuclear Medicine Imaging Tests

There has been tremendous progress in research involving various brain radiotracers, which provide the valuable functional and metabolic pathophysiology of brain cancer. Yet the question remains as to how best to incorporate radiotracer imaging methods into diagnosis and management of patients with brain cancer. The most widely used radiotracer imaging method in brain cancer imaging is [201]Thalium single photon emission computed tomography (SPECT) (Table 8.2). Although very useful, it has a limited role in initial diagnosis or predicting the degree of brain cancer malignancy. Positron emission tomography (PET) using ^{18}F-2-fluoro-2-deoxy-d-glucose (FDG) radiotracer can be useful in differentiating recurrent brain cancer from radiation necrosis but similar to SPECT, its ability as an independent diagnostic and prognostic value above that of MR imaging and histology remains debated (31) (Table 8.2).

In pediatric patients with brain cancer, it is important to assess whether imaging of the entire craniospinal axis is warranted to detect any drop metastases and staging (Table 8.2). This is especially true for children with aggressive neoplasm with high propensity for tumor spread along the cerebrospinal fluid route such as medulloblastoma/PNET and ependymoma.

In pediatric patients with suspected brain metastatic disease, MRI is the imaging test of choice, especially when leptomeningeal spread of disease is considered. CT is indicated when there is suspected calvarial metastasis. Surveillance imaging with MRI is a cost-effective way of monitoring disease stability or symptomatic progression in pediatric patients with brain cancer (32).

III. What Is the Appropriate Imaging in Subjects at Risk for Brain Cancer?

Summary of Evidence: The sensitivity and specificity of MRI is higher than CT for brain neoplasms (moderate evidence). Therefore, in high-risk subjects suspected of having brain cancer MRI with and without gadolinium-based contrast agent is the imaging modality of choice to further characterize the lesion. Table 8.3 lists advantages and limitations of CT and MRI in the evaluation of subjects with suspected brain cancer.

There is no strong evidence to suggest that the addition of other diagnostic tests, such as MR spectroscopy, perfusion MR, PET, or SPECT improves either the cost effectiveness or the outcome in the high-risk group at initial presentation.

Supporting Evidence: Medina et al. (28) found in a retrospective study of 315 pediatric patients that overall MR imaging was more sensitive and specific than CT in detecting intracranial space-occupying lesions (92 and 99%, respectively, for MR imaging versus 81 and 92%, respectively, for CT). However, no difference in sensitivity and specificity was found in the surgical space-occupying lesions (28). Table 8.3 lists sensitivity and specificity of MRI and CT for brain cancer as outlined by Hutter et al. (33). Figures 8.2 and 8.3 illustrate limitations and advantages of MRI and CT.

There has been a tremendous progress in research involving various brain radiotracers, which provide the valuable functional and metabolic pathophysiology of brain cancer. Yet the question remains as to how best to incorporate radiotracer imaging methods into diagnosis and management of patients with brain cancer. The most widely used radiotracer imaging method in brain cancer imaging is [201]Thalium SPECT. Although very purposeful, it has a limited role in initial diagnosis or predicting the degree of brain cancer malignancy. PET using FDG radiotracer can be useful in differentiating recurrent brain cancer from radiation necrosis but similar to SPECT, its ability as an independent diagnostic and prognostic value above that of MR imaging and histology remains debated (31). There is limited evidence behind perfusion MR in tumor diagnosis and grading despite several articles proposing its useful role. Similar to proton MR spectroscopy (see issue III), perfusion MR imaging remains an investigational tool at this time pending stronger evidence proving its effect on health outcomes of patients with brain cancer.

Special Case: Neuroimaging Differentiation of Post-treatment Necrosis from Residual Tumor

Imaging differentiation of treatment necrosis and residual/recurrent tumor is challenging because they both can appear similar and also can coexist in a single given lesion. Hence the traditional anatomy based imaging methods have a limited role in the accurate differentiation between the two entities. Nuclear medicine imaging techniques such as SPECT and PET provide functional information on tissue metabolism and oxygen consumption and thus offer theoretical advantage over anatomic imaging in differentiation tissue necrosis and active tumor. Multiple studies demonstrate that SPECT is more sensitive and specific than is PET in differentiating tumor recurrence from radiation necrosis (33) (Table 8.3). There is also insufficient evidence of the role of MR spectroscopy in this topic (see Issue III).

Special Case: Neuroimaging Modality in Patients with Suspected Brain Metastatic Disease

Brain metastases are far more common than primary brain cancer in adults owing to higher prevalence of systemic cancers and their propensity to metastasize (34–36). Focal neurologic symptoms in a patient with history of systemic cancer should raise a high suspicion for intracranial metastasis and prompt imaging. The preferred neuroimaging modality in patients with suspected brain metastatic disease is MRI with single dose (0.1 mmole/kg body weight) of gadolinium-based contrast agent. Most studies described in the literature suggest that contrast-enhanced MR imaging is superior to contrast-enhanced CT in the detection of brain metastatic disease, especially if the lesions are less than 2 cm (moderate evidence).

Davis and colleagues (moderate evidence) (37) studied comparative imaging studies in 23 patients comparing contrast-enhanced MRI with double dose-delayed CT. Contrast-enhanced MRI demonstrated more than 67 definite or typical brain metastases. The double dose-delayed CT revealed only 37 metastatic lesions. The authors concluded that MR imaging with enhancement is superior to double dose-delayed CT scan for detecting brain metastasis, anatomic localization, and number of lesions. Golfieri and colleagues (38) reported similar findings (moderate evidence). They studied 44 patients with small cell carcinoma to detect cerebral metastases. All patients were studied with contrast-enhanced CT scan and gadolinium-enhanced MR imaging. Of all patients, 43% had cerebral metastases. Both contrast-enhanced CT and gadolinium-enhanced MR imaging detected lesions greater than 2 cm. For lesions less than 2 cm, 9% were detected only by gadolinium-enhanced T1-weighted images. The authors concluded that gadolinium-enhanced T1-weighted images remain the most accurate technique in the assessment of cerebral metastases. Sze and colleagues (39) performed prospective and retrospective studies in 75 patients (moderate evidence). In 49 patients, MR imaging and contrast-enhanced CT were equivalent. In 26 patients, however, results were discordant, with neither CT nor MR imaging being consistently superior. MR imaging demonstrated more metastases in 9 of these 26 patients. Contrast-enhanced CT, however, better depicted lesions in 8 of 26 patients.

There are several reports on using triple dose of contrast agent to increase sensitivity of lesion detection (40, 41). In another study by Sze et al. (42), however, have found that routine triple-dose contrast agent administration in all cases of suspected brain metastasis was not helpful, could lead to increasing number of false-positive results, and concluded that the use of triple-dose contrast material is beneficial in selected cases with equivocal findings or solitary metastasis. Their study was based on 92 consecutive patients with negative or equivocal findings or a solitary metastasis on single-dose contrast-enhanced MR images underwent triple-dose studies.

Special Case: How Can Tumor Be Differentiated from Tumor-Mimicking Lesions?

There are several intracranial disease processes that can mimic brain cancer and pose a diagnostic dilemma on both clinical presentation and conventional MRI (19, 43–47), such as infarcts, radiation necrosis, demyelinating plaques, abscesses, hematomas, and encephalitis. On imaging, any one of these lesions and brain cancer can both demonstrate contrast enhancement, perilesional edema, varying degrees of mass effect, and central necrosis.

There are numerous reports in the literature of misdiagnosis and mismanagement of these subjects who were erroneously thought to have brain cancer and, in some cases, went on to surgical resection for histopathologic confirmation (18, 46, 48). Surgery is clearly contraindicated in these subjects and can lead to unnecessary increase in morbidity and mortality. A large acute demyelinating plaque, in particular, is notorious for mimicking an aggressive brain cancer (46, 49–52). Due to presence of mitotic figures and atypical astrocytes, this uncertainty occurs not only on clinical presentation and imaging, but also on histopathological examination (46). The consequence of unnecessary surgery in subjects with tumor-mimicking lesions can be quite grave and hence every effort should be made to differentiate them from brain cancer. Anatomic imaging of the brain suffers from nonspecificity and its inability to differentiate tumor from tumor-mimicking lesions (18). Recent developments in nonanatomic, physiology based MRI methods, such as diffusion/perfusion MRI and proton spectroscopic imaging, promise to provide information not readily available from structural MRI and improve diagnostic accuracy (53, 54).

Diffusion-weighted MRI has been shown to be particularly helpful in differentiating cystic/necrotic neoplasm from brain abscess by demonstrating marked reduced diffusion within an abscess. Chang et al. (55) compared diffusion-weighted imaging (DWI) and conventional

anatomic MRI to distinguish brain abscesses from cystic or necrotic brain tumors in 11 patients with brain abscesses and 15 with cystic or necrotic brain gliomas or metastases. They found that postcontrast T1WIs yielded a sensitivity of 60%, a specificity of 27%, a positive predictive value (PPV) of 53%, and a negative predictive value (NPV) of 33% in the diagnosis of necrotic tumors. DWI yielded a sensitivity of 93%, a specificity of 91%, a PPV of 93%, and a NPV of 91%. Based on the analysis of receiver operating characteristic curves, they found clear advantage of DWI as a diagnostic tool in detecting abscess when compared to postcontrast T1-weighted images. Figure 8.4 illustrates the value of DWI in differentiating pyogenic abscess and high-grade brain tumor.

Table 8.5 lists neurological diseases that can mimic brain cancer both on clinical grounds and on imaging. By using DWI, acute infarct and abscess could readily be distinguished from brain cancer since reduced diffusion seen with the first two entities (55–59). Highly cellular brain cancer can have reduced diffusion but not to the same degree as acute infarct or abscess (60).

IV. What Is the Role of Proton Magnetic Resonance Spectroscopy in the Diagnosis and Follow-Up of Brain Neoplasms?

Summary of Evidence: The Blue Cross Blue Shield Association (BCBSA) Medical Advisory Panel concluded that the MRS in the evaluation of suspected brain cancer did not meet the Technology Evaluation Center (TEC) criteria as a diagnostic test; hence further studies in a prospectively defined population is needed. A similar conclusion was obtained by the systematic literature review done by Hollingworth et al. (61). However, the study highlighted two important findings in the literature (1) one large study demonstrating a statistically significant increase in diagnostic accuracy for indeterminate brain lesions from 55%, based on MR imaging, to 71% after analysis of ¹H-MR spectroscopy (61) and (2) several studies have found that ¹H-MR spectroscopy is highly accurate for distinguishing high- and low-grade gliomas, though the incremental benefit of ¹H-MR spectroscopy in this setting is less clear (61). Figure 8.5 shows a prominent lactate peak seen on a single voxel MRS of a right frontal anaplastic astrocytoma.

Supporting Evidence: No systematic review of MRS has been done only for pediatric patients with brain neoplasms. The systematic reviews available include adult and pediatric patients. The BCBSA Medical Advisory Panel made the following judgments about whether ¹H-MRS for evaluation of suspected brain tumors meets the BCBSA TEC criteria based on the available evidence (62). The Advisory Panel reviewed seven published studies that included a total of up to 271 subjects (63–69). These seven studies were selected for inclusion in the review of evidence because (1) the sample size was at least 10; (2) criteria for a positive test were specified; (3) there was a method to confirm ¹H-MRS diagnosis; and (4) the report provided sufficient data to calculate diagnostic test performance (sensitivity and specificity). The reviewers specifically addressed whether ¹H-MRS for evaluation of suspected brain tumors meets the following five TEC criteria:

1. The technology must have approval from the appropriate governmental regulatory bodies.
2. The scientific evidence must permit conclusions concerning the effect of the technology on health outcomes.
3. The technology must improve the net health outcomes.
4. The technology must be as beneficial as any established alternatives.
5. The improvement must be attainable outside the investigational settings.

With the exception of the first criterion, the reviewers concluded that the available evidence on ¹H-MRS in the evaluation of brain neoplasm was insufficient. The TEC also concluded that the overall body of evidence does not provide strong and consistent evidence regarding the diagnostic test characteristics of MRS in determining the presence or absence of brain neoplasm, both for differentiation of recurrent/residual tumor versus delayed radiation necrosis (69) or for diagnosis of brain tumor versus other nontumor diagnosis (63, 64, 66–68). Assessment of the health benefit of MRS in avoiding brain biopsy was evaluated two studies (63, 68), but the results were limited by study

limitations. Therefore, human studies conducted on the use of MRS for brain tumors demonstrate that this noninvasive method is technically feasible and suggest potential benefits for some of the proposed indications. However, there is a paucity of high quality direct evidence demonstrating the impact on diagnostic thinking and therapeutic decision making.

The systematic review by Hollingworth et al. showed no articles evaluated patient health or cost-effectiveness (61). Methodologic quality was mixed; most used histopathology as the reference standard, but did not specify blinded interpretation of histopathology (61). One large study demonstrated a statistically significant increase in diagnostic accuracy for indeterminate brain lesions from 55%, based on MR imaging, to 71% after analysis of ¹H-MR spectroscopy (61). Several studies have found that ¹H-MR spectroscopy is highly accurate for distinguishing high- and low-grade gliomas, though the incremental benefit of ¹H-MR spectroscopy in this setting is less clear. Interpretation for the other clinical subgroups is limited by the small number of studies (61).

V. Can Imaging Be Used to Differentiate Post-treatment Necrosis from Residual/Recurrent Tumor?

Summary of Evidence: No adequate data exist on the role of imaging in monitoring pediatric brain cancer response to therapy and differentiating between tumor recurrence and therapy related changes (insufficient evidence).

Supporting Evidence: Imaging differentiation of posttreatment necrosis and residual/recurrent tumor is challenging because they can appear similar and can coexist in a single given lesion. Hence the traditional anatomy-based imaging methods have a limited role in the accurate differentiation of the two entities. Nuclear medicine imaging techniques such as SPECT and FDG PET have been proposed as a diagnostic alternative, particularly when coregistered with MRI to provide functional information on tissue metabolism and oxygen consumption and thus offer a theoretical advantage over anatomic imaging in differentiating tissue necrosis and active tumor. Chao et al. (70) studied 47 patients with brain tumors treated with stereotactic radiosurgery and followed with FDG PET. For all tumor types, the sensitivity of FDG PET for diagnosing tumor was 75% and the specificity was 81%. For brain metastasis without MRI coregistration, FDG PET had a sensitivity of 65% and a specificity of 80%. For brain metastasis with MRI coregistration, FDG PET had a sensitivity of 86% and specificity of 80%. MRI coregistration appears to improve the sensitivity of FDG PET, making it a useful modality to distinguish between radiation necrosis and recurrent brain metastasis (70). Khan et al. (71) studied the value of SPECT versus PET in 19 patients with evidence of tumor recurrence of CT or MR images using both 201TI SPECT and FDG PET imaging and were unable to detect a statistically significant difference in sensitivity or specificity between the two scans. They found both techniques to be sensitive for tumor recurrence for lesions 1.6 cm or larger and concluded that SPECT, given its greater availability, simplicity, ease of interpretation, and lower cost is a better method of choice (71). However, there is insufficient data to determine whether SPECT, PET, or any other imaging modality can confidently discriminate tumor recurrence from treatment effect.

VI. What Is the Added Value of Functional MRI in the Surgical Planning of Patients with Suspected Brain Neoplasm or Focal Brain Lesions?

Summary of Evidence: The addition of fMRI in the surgical planning of patients with suspected brain neoplasm or focal brain lesions can influence diagnostic and therapeutic decision making (moderate evidence).

Supporting Evidence: fMRI is a noninvasive tool to assess brain function and has been around since the early 1990s, largely as a research tool with limited clinical availability and application. Over the past several years, however, fMRI has crossed over to the clinical realm and is gaining more acceptance as a useful clinical tool. The growing use of fMRI in clinical areas include mapping of critical or eloquent areas such as the motor cortex in patients undergoing brain surgery, early identification of psychiatric

disorder, and measurement of the effect of therapies on neurodegenerative and neurodevelopmental disorders. Figure 8.6 shows the location of motor cortex activation in relation to a frontal brain tumor that can be useful in surgical planning of the tumor. Medina et al. (72) evaluated the effect of adding fMRI on diagnostic work-up and treatment planning in 53 patients with seizure disorders who are candidates for surgical treatment. They found that fMRI results influenced diagnostic and therapeutic decision making. Specifically, the fMRI results indicated language dominance changed, confidence level in identification of critical brain function areas increased, patient and family counseling were altered, and intraoperative mapping and surgical approach were altered (72).

VII. What Is the Cost-Effectiveness of Imaging in Patients with Suspected Primary Brain and Disease?

Summary of Evidence: Routine brain CT in all patients with lung cancer has a cost-effectiveness ratio of $69,815 per QALY. However, the cost per QALY is highly sensitive to variations in the negative predictive value of a clinical evaluation, as well as to the cost of CT. CEA of patients with headache suspected of having a brain neoplasm are presented in Chap. 15 on headaches.

Supporting Evidence: In a study from the surgical literature, Colice et al. (73) compared the cost-effectiveness of two strategies for detecting brain metastases by CT in lung cancer patients (1) routine CT for all patients irrespective of clinical (neurologic, hematologic) evidence of metastases (CT first) and (2) CT for only those patients in whom clinical symptoms developed (CT deferred). For a hypothetical cohort of patients, it was assumed that all primary lung carcinomas were potentially resectable. If no brain metastasis were detected by CT, the primary lung tumor would be resected. Brain metastasis as detected by CT would disqualify the patient for resection of the primary lung tumor. Costs were taken from the payer's perspective and based on prevailing Medicare payments. The rates of false-positive and false-negative findings were also considered in the calculation of the effectiveness of CT. The cost of the CT-first strategy was $11,108 and the cost for the CT-deferred strategy $10,915; however, the CT-first strategy increased life expectancy by merely 1.1 days. Its cost-effectiveness ratio was calculated to be $69,815 per QALY. The cost per QALY is highly sensitive to variations in the negative predictive value of a clinical evaluation, as well as to the cost of CT. This study is instructive, because it highlights the importance of considering false-positive and false-negative findings and performing sensitivity analysis. For a detailed discussion of the specifics of the decision-analytic model and sensitivity analysis, the reader is referred to the article by Hutter et al. and Colice et al. (33, 73).

Take Home Tables and Figures (Figs. 8.1–8.6; Tables 8.1–8.5)

Tables 8.1–8.5 and Fig. 8.1–8.6 serve to highlight key recommendations and supporting evidence.

Table 8.1. Clinical symptoms suggestive of a brain cancer

- Non-migraine, nonchronic headache of moderate to severe degree (see Chap. 15)
- Partial complex seizure (Chap. 14)
- Focal neurological deficit
- Speech disturbance
- Cognitive or personality change
- Visual disturbance
- Altered consciousness
- Sensory abnormalities
- Gait problem or ataxia
- Nausea and vomiting without other gastrointestinal illness
- Papilledema
- Cranial nerve palsy

Reprinted with kind permission of Springer Science+Business Media from Cha S. In Medina LS, Blackmore CC (eds.): *Evidence-Based Imaging: Optimizing Imaging in Patient Care.* New York: Springer Science+Business Media, 2006.

Table 8.2. Sensitivity and specificity of brain tumor imaging

Type of brain cancer	Imaging modality	Sensitivity (%)	Specificity (%)
Primary brain cancer	MRI with contrast	Gold standard	–
	CT with contrast	87	79
Primary brain cancer in children [Medina et al. (28)]	MRI	92	99
	CT	81	92
Brain metastasis	MRI with single dose contrast	93–100	–
	MRI without contrast	36	–
	^{201}Tl SPECT	70	–
	^{18}FDG PET	82	38
Recurrent tumor versus treatment-related necrosis	^{201}Tl SPECT	92	88
	^{18}FDG PET		
	MRI with co-registration	86	80
	MRI without co-registration	65	80

Source: Adapted from Hutter et al. (33), with permission from Elsevier.

Table 8.3. Advantages and limitations of computed tomography (CT) and magnetic resonance imaging (MRI)

	Advantages	Limitations
Computed tomography	• Widely available • Short imaging time • Lower cost • Excellent for detection of acute hemorrhage or bony abnormality	• Inferior soft tissue resolution • Prone to artifact in posterior fossa • Ionizing radiation • Risk of allergy to iodinated contrast agent
Magnetic resonance imaging	• Multi-planar capability • Superior soft tissue resolution • No ionizing radiation • Safer contrast agent (gadolinium-based) profile	• Higher cost • Not as widely available • Suboptimal for detection of acute hemorrhage or bony/calcific abnormality

Reprinted with kind permission of Springer Science+Business Media from Cha S. In Medina LS, Blackmore CC (eds.): *Evidence-Based Imaging: Optimizing Imaging in Patient Care.* New York: Springer Science+Business Media, 2006.

Table 8.4. MR imaging protocol for a subject with suspected brain cancer

- 3D localizer
- Axial and sagittal precontrast T1-weighted imaging
- Diffusion-weighted imaging
- Axial fluid-attenuated inversion recovery (FLAIR)
- Axial T2-weighted imaging
- Axial, coronal, and sagittal postcontrast T1-weighted imaging
- Optional: Dynamic contrast-enhanced perfusion MR imaging Proton MR spectroscopic imaging
- Consider doing gadolinium enhanced MRI of entire spine to rule out metastatic disease

Reprinted with kind permission of Springer Science+Business Media from Cha S. In Medina LS, Blackmore CC (eds.): *Evidence-Based Imaging: Optimizing Imaging in Patient Care.* New York: Springer Science+Business Media, 2006.

Table 8.5. Brain cancer mimicking lesions

- Infarct
- Radiation necrosis
- Abscess
- Demyelinating plaque
- Subacute hematoma
- Encephalitis

Reprinted with kind permission of Springer Science+Business Media from Cha S. In Medina LS, Blackmore CC (eds.): *Evidence-Based Imaging: Optimizing Imaging in Patient Care.* New York: Springer Science+Business Media, 2006.

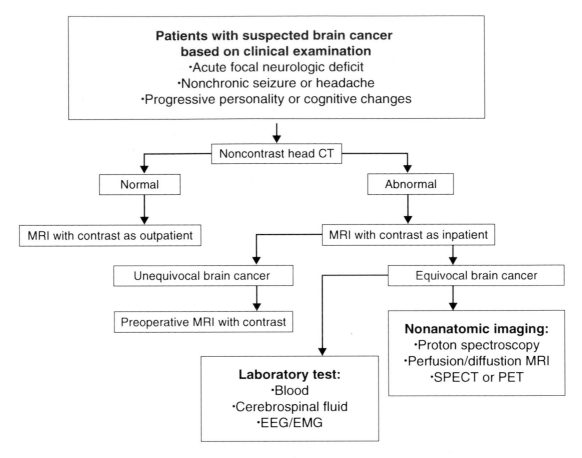

Figure 8.1. Decision flow chart to study patients with suspected brain cancer. In patients with presenting with acute neurologic event such as seizure or focal deficit, noncontrast head CT examination should be done expeditiously to exclude any life-threatening conditions such as hemorrhage or herniation. (Reprinted with kind permission of Springer Science+Business Media from Cha S. In Medina LS, Blackmore CC (eds.): *Evidence-Based Imaging: Optimizing Imaging in Patient Care.* New York: Springer Science+Business Media, 2006.)

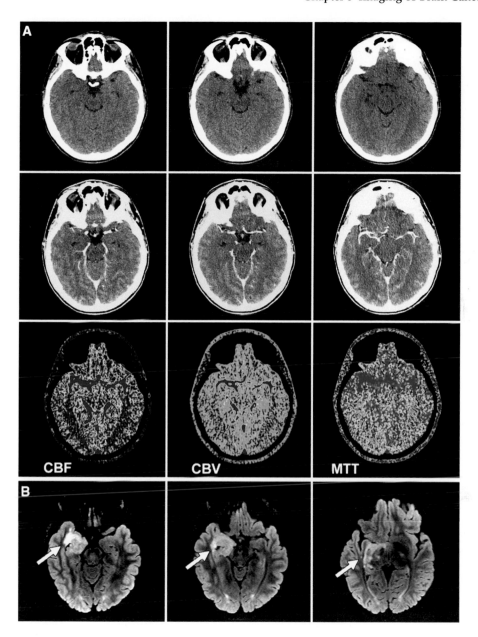

Figure 8.2. Seventeen-year-old girl with left sided weakness with clinical suspicion for acute stroke. (**A**) Unenhanced CT images (*top row*), enhanced CT images (*middle row*), and perfusion maps (*bottom row*) through the level of temporal lobe and basal ganglia demonstrate no obvious mass lesion. (**B**) Axial fluid-attenuated inversion recovery (FLAIR) MR images done 3 days after the CT clearly show large extent of abnormality (*white arrows*) involving most of the right medial temporal extending superiorly to basal ganglia and thalamus. Dysembryoblastic neuroepithelial tumor was at surgery

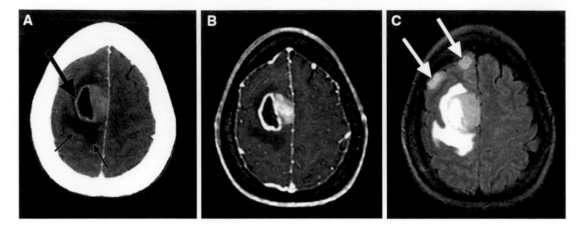

Figure 8.3. Forty-two-year-old woman with difficulty in balancing and left sided weakness and a pathologic diagnosis of GBM. (**A**) Contrast-enhanced CT image demonstrates an enhancing solid and necrotic mass (*large black arrow*) within the right superior frontal gyrus associated with surrounding low density (*small arrows*). (**B**) Contrast-enhanced T1-weighted MR image performed on the same day as the CT study shows similar finding. (**C**) FLAIR MR image clearly demonstrates two additional foci of cortically based signal abnormality (*white arrows*) that were found to be infiltrating glioma on histopathology. (Reprinted with kind permission of Springer Science+Business Media from Cha S. In Medina LS, Blackmore CC (eds.): *Evidence-Based Imaging: Optimizing Imaging in Patient Care.* New York: Springer Science+Business Media, 2006.)

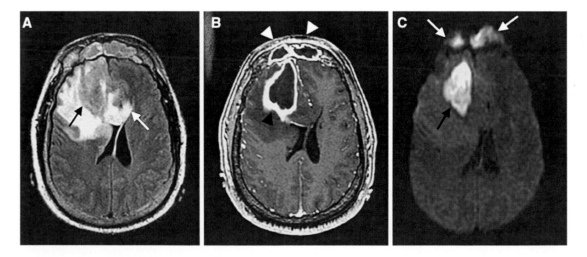

Figure 8.4. Fifty-three-year-old man with right frontal abscess with irregular enhancement with central necrosis simulating a brain cancer. (**A**) FLAIR MR image demonstrates a large mass lesion (*black arrow*) with extensive surrounding edema that crosses the corpus callosum (*white arrow*). (**B**) Contrast-enhanced T1-weighted MR image shows thick rim enhancement (*black open arrow*) and central necrosis associated with the mass. Similar pattern of abnormality is noted within the frontal sinuses (*open white arrows*). (**C**) Diffusion-weighted MR image depicts marked reduced diffusion within the frontal lesion (*black arrow*) and the frontal sinus lesion (*white arrows*), both of which were proven to be a bacterial abscess at histopathology. (Reprinted with kind permission of Springer Science+Business Media from Cha S. In Medina LS, Blackmore CC (eds.): *Evidence-Based Imaging: Optimizing Imaging in Patient Care.* New York: Springer Science+Business Media, 2006.)

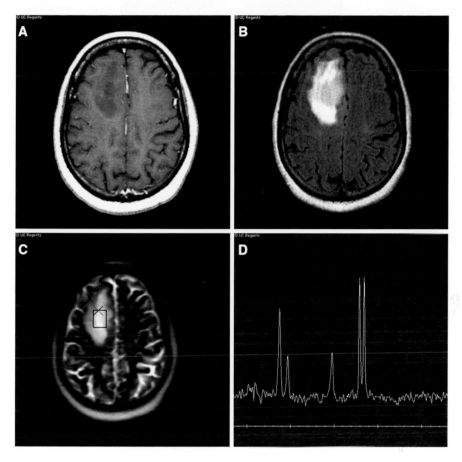

Figure 8.5. Single voxel MR spectroscopy in a 59-year-old woman right frontal grade III anaplastic astrocytoma. (**A**) Axial post-contrast T1-weighted image shows a nonenhancing right frontal mass. (**B**) Axial FLAIR image clearly demonstrates a hyperintense mass. (**C**) A screen save image from single voxel MRS shows a box overlaid on an axial T2-weighted image showing the mass. (**D**) A single voxel MRS using echo time of 288 ms demonstrates a prominent doublet lactate peak at 1.3 ppm suggestive of an aggressive tumor

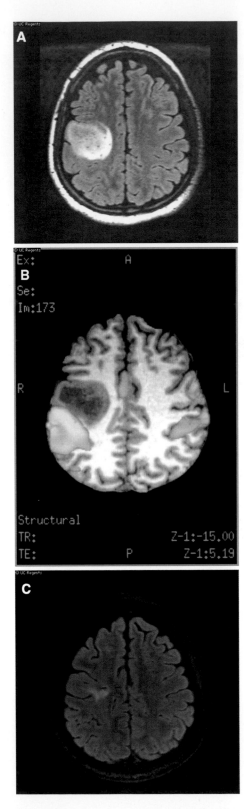

Figure 8.6. Functional MR imaging (fMRI) of motor activation in a 22-year-old man with right frontal grade II astrocytoma located near the motor cortex. (**A**) Axial FLAIR image shows a mass near the right motor cortex. (**B**) fMRI color map demonstrates the motor cortex to be located immediately posterior and not within the right frontal low grade tumor. (**C**) Postoperative axial FLAIR image shows minimal residual signal abnormality at the resection site anterior to normal appearing motor cortex

Future Research

- Rigorous technology assessment of noninvasive imaging modalities such as MRS, diffusion and perfusion MRI, fMRI, PET, and SPECT.
- Assessment of the effects of imaging on the patient outcome and costs of diagnosis and management.
- Rigorous cost-effectiveness analysis of competing imaging modalities.
- Development and clinical validation of physiologic MRI to assess biologic and molecular features of pediatric brain cancer.
- Identification and validation of noninvasive imaging biomarkers of tumor activity during and after therapy.
- Development and clinical validation of physiologic MRI to assess biologic and molecular features of pediatric brain cancer.
- National database dedicated to epidemiology of adult and pediatric brain cancer.

References

1. Burger PC, Vogel FS. In Burger PC, Vogel FS (eds.): Surgical Pathology of the Central Nervous System and Its Coverings. New York: Wiley, 1982;223–266.
2. Burger PC et al. Cancer 1985;56:1106–1111.
3. Kleihues P, Sobin LH. Cancer 2000;88(12):2887.
4. Kleihues P, Ohgaki H. Toxicol Pathol 2000;28(1):164–170.
5. Go KG. Adv Tech Stand Neurosurg 1997;23:47–142.
6. Sato S et al. Acta Neurochir Suppl 1994;60:116–118.
7. Stewart PA et al. J Neurosurg 1987;67(5):697–705.
8. Stewart PA et al. Microvasc Res 1987;33(2):270–282.
9. Abbott NJ et al. Adv Drug Deliv Rev 1999;37(1–3):253–277.
10. DeAngelis LM. N Engl J Med 2001;344(2):114–123.
11. Longstreth WT Jr et al. Cancer 1993;72(3):639–648.
12. CBTRUS. Statistical Report: Primary Brain Tumors in the United States, 1998–2002. Chicago, IL: Central Brain Tumor Registry of the United States, 2005.
13. Becker LE. Neuroimaging Clin N Am 1999;9(4):671–690.
14. Rickert CH, Probst-Cousin S, Gullotta F. Childs Nerv Syst 1997;13(10):507–513.
15. Pollack IF. Semin Surg Oncol 1999;16(2):73–90.
16. Latif AZ et al. Br J Neurosurg 1998;12(2):118–122.
17. Ricci PE. Neuroimaging Clin N Am 1999;9(4):651–669.
18. Cha S et al. AJNR Am J Neuroradiol 2001;22(6):1109–1116.
19. Kepes JJ. Ann Neurol 1993;33(1):18–27.
20. De Stefano N et al. Ann Neurol 1998;44(2):273–278.
21. Porter RJ et al. Br J Psychiatry 2003;182:214–220.
22. Meyers CA. Oncology (Hunting) 2000;14(1):75–9;discussion 79,81–2,85.
23. Newton HB et al. Ann Pharmacother 1999;33(7–8):816–32.
24. Salcman M. In Wilkins R, Rengachary S (eds.): Neurosurgery. New York: McGraw-Hill, 1985;579–590.
25. Snyder H et al. J Emerg Med 1993;11(3):253–258.
26. Miltenburg D, Louw DF, Sutherland GR. Can J Neurol Sci, 1996;23(2):118–122.
27. Davis FG, McCarthy BJ. Curr Opin Neurol 2000;13(6):635–640.
28. Medina LS et al. Radiology 1997;202(3):819–824.
29. Medina LS, Kuntz KM, Pomeroy S. Pediatrics 2001;108(2):255–263.
30. Whelan HT et al. Pediatr Neurol 1988;4(5):279–283.
31. Benard F, Romsa J, Hustinx R. Semin Nucl Med 2003;33(2):148–162.
32. Kovanlikaya A et al. Eur J Radiol 2003;47(3):188–192.
33. Hutter A et al. Neuroimaging Clin N Am 2003;13(2):237–250,x–xi.
34. Walker AE, Robins M, Weinfeld FD. Neurology 1985;35(2):219–226.
35. Wingo PA, Tong T, Bolden S. CA Cancer J Clin 1995;45:8–30.
36. Patchell RA. Neurol Clin 1991;9:817–827.
37. Davis PC et al. AJNR Am J Neuroradiol 1991;12(2):293–300.
38. Golfieri R et al. Radiol Med (Torino) 1991;82(1–2):27–34.
39. Sze G et al. Radiology 1988;168(1):187–194.
40. Kuhn MJ et al. Comput Med Imaging Graph 1994;18(5):391–399.
41. Yuh WT et al. AJNR Am J Neuroradiol 1995;16(2):373–380.
42. Sze G et al. AJNR Am J Neuroradiol 1998;19(5):821–828.
43. Morgenstern LB, Frankowski RF. J Neurooncol 1999;44(1):47–52.
44. Barcikowska M et al. Folia Neuropathol 1995;33(1):55–57.
45. Kim YJ et al. AJR Am J Roentgenol 1998;171(6):1487–1490.

46. Zagzag D et al. Am J Surg Pathol 1993;17(6): 537–545.
47. Itto H et al. No To Shinkei 1972;24(4):455–458.
48. Babu R et al. J Neurooncol 1993;17(1):37–42.
49. Dagher AP, Smirniotopoulos J. Neuroradiology 1996;38(6):560–565.
50. Giang DW et al. Neuroradiology 1992;34(2): 150–154.
51. Kurihara N et al. Clin Imaging 1996;20(3): 171–177.
52. Prockop LD, Heinz ER. Arch Neurol 1965;13(5): 559–564.
53. Schaefer PW, Grant PE, Gonzalez RG. Radiology 2000;217(2):331–345.
54. Cha S et al. Radiology 2002;223(1):11–29.
55. Chang SC et al. Clin Imaging 2002;26(4): 227–236.
56. Castillo M, Mukherji SK. Semin Ultrasound CT MR 2000;21(6):405–416.
57. Ebisu T et al. Magn Reson Imaging 1996;14(9):1113–1116.
58. Laing AD, Mitchell PJ, Wallace D. Australas Radiol 1999;43(1):16–19.
59. Tsuruda JS et al. AJNR Am J Neuroradiol 1990;11(5):925–931;discussion 932–934.
60. Okamoto K et al. Eur Radiol 2000;10(8): 1342–1350.
61. Hollingworth W et al. AJNR Am J Neuroradiol 2006;27:1404–1411.
62. Technology Evaluation Center. TEC Bull (Online) 2003;20(1):23–26.
63. Adamson AJ et al. Radiology 1998;209(1): 73–78.
64. Rand SD et al. AJNR Am J Neuroradiol 1997;18(9):1695–1704.
65. Shukla-Dave A. et al. Magn Reson Imaging 2001;19(1):103–110.
66. Kimura T et al. NMR Biomed 2001;14(6):339–349.
67. Wilken B et al. Pediatr Neurol 2000;23(1): 22–31.
68. Lin A, Bluml S, Mamelak AN. J Neurooncol 1999;45(1):69–81.
69. Taylor JS et al. Int J Radiat Oncol Biol Phys 1996;36(5):1251–1261.
70. Chao ST et al. Int J Cancer 2001;96:191–197.
71. Khan D et al. AJR Am J Roentgenol 1994;163: 1459–1465.
72. Medina LS et al. Radiology 2005;236:247–253.
73. Colice GL et al. Chest 1995;108(5):1264–1271.

9

Imaging in the Evaluation of Patients with Prostate Cancer

Jeffrey H. Newhouse

I. Is transrectal ultrasound valuable as a prostate cancer screening tool?
II. Is transrectal ultrasound useful to guide prostate biopsy?
III. Is imaging accurate for staging prostate cancer?
   A. Ultrasound
   B. Computed tomography scan
   C. Magnetic resonance imaging
   D. Magnetic resonance spectroscopic imaging
   E. Positron emission tomography
IV. How accurate is bone scan for detecting metastatic prostate cancer?
   A. Special case: which patients should undergo imaging after initial treatment to look for metastatic disease?
	Issues

■ Ultrasound probably aids in the effectiveness of biopsy for diagnosis, although imaging is not of proven value in screening (moderate evidence). ■ Skeletal scintigraphy and computed tomography (CT) play a crucial role in assessing metastatic disease; they can be eliminated, however, in patients whose tumor volume, Gleason score, and prostate-specific antigen (PSA) are relatively low (strong evidence). ■ Magnetic resonance imaging (MRI) is the most accurate of the imaging techniques in local staging, but its relative expense and persistent false-positive and false-negative rates for locally invasive disease suggest that it should be interpreted along with all additional available data, and reserved for patients in whom other data leave treatment choices ambiguous (strong evidence).	**Key Points**

J.H. Newhouse (✉)
Department of Radiology, Columbia University College of Physicians and Surgeons, 177 Fort Washington Avenue, Milstein Building, Third Floor, New York, NY 10032, USA
e-mail: jhn2@columbia.edu

■ Assessment of metastatic tumor burden by bone scan and CT are of prognostic value. After initial therapy, monitoring disease is primarily done with serial PSA determinations; imaging for recurrence should be limited to patients whose PSA levels clearly indicate recurrent or progressive disease and in whom imaging results have the potential to affect treatment (limited evidence).

Definition and Pathophysiology

Although there are a number of histologic varieties of prostate malignancies, overwhelmingly, the most common is adenocarcinoma. Etiologic factors are not known in detail, but it is clearly an androgen-dependent disease in most cases; it is almost unheard of in chronically anorchid patients. Age is the most important risk factor; the disease is very rare in men under 40 years, but in men over 70 years, histologic evidence of intraprostatic adenocarcinoma can be found in at least half the population. A family history of the disease is a risk factor. Black men are more prone to develop the tumor, and it is more likely to be biologically malignant among them. There are probably environmental factors as well, but these are less well established.

Epidemiology

Prostate cancer is the most common internal malignancy of American men, and the second most common cause of death. In 2004, 230,110 new cases and 29,900 deaths were expected (1).

Overall Cost to Society

Although the low ratio of annual deaths to new cases reflects the fact that most histologic cases are not of clinical importance, the high absolute numbers of deaths and the 9-year average loss of life that each prostate cancer death causes suggest that the cost to society is huge. Most patients who die of prostate cancer are under treatment for years, and patients whose cancer is cured usually require major surgery or radiotherapy. The exact cost to society in the USA for prostate cancer is not clear, but if the cost of screening and treatment are added to the indirect cost of income loss and diversion of other resources, a very approximate figure of $10 billion a year would not be an excessive estimate.

Goals

The goals of imaging in prostate cancer are (1) to guide biopsy of the peripheral zone, (2) to stage prostate cancer accurately, and (3) to detect metastatic or recurrent cancer.

Methodology

The Ovid search engine was used to query the Medline database from 1966 to May 2004 for all searches. In all cases, the searches were limited to human investigations. No language limitations were imposed, but for articles published in languages other than English, only the abstracts were reviewed. Multiple individual searches were conducted. In each, the phrase *prostate and (cancer or carcinoma)* limited the basic scope. Each search was also limited to the radiologic literature by the phrase *radiology, or radiography, or ultrasound, or sonography, or CT, or computed tomography, or MRI, or magnetic resonance imaging, or scan, or scintigraphy, or PET, or positron emission tomography.* Individual searches were then limited by using the phrases *screen or screening, diagnosis, stage or staging,* or *recurrence or (monitor or monitoring)* as appropriate.

I. Is Transrectal Ultrasound Valuable as a Prostate Cancer Screening Tool?

Summary of Evidence: Transrectal ultrasound (TRUS) lacks the sensitivity and specificity that would be required to recommend it as a stand-alone screen. If it is used in combination with digital rectal examination (DRE) and PSA, the additionally discovered tumors are very few and a normal TRUS cannot obviate biopsy, which might otherwise be indicated by an abnormal DRE or PSA (insufficient evidence for using TRUS alone).

Supporting Evidence: Transabdominal sonography of the prostate gland provides insufficient resolution of prostatic tissue to be of value in searching for prostate cancer. High-frequency transrectal probes provide better spatial resolution, and since their introduction, there has been continued interest in the role of sonography in screening for prostate cancer (2–7).

The peripheral zone for most prostate glands appears relatively uniform in echogenicity, and the classic appearance of a focus of tumor in it is a relatively hypoechoic region (7). The central portions of the gland are more heterogeneous in appearance, especially in patients with benign prostatic hypertrophy; for this reason, and because only a minority of tumors is initially found in the central gland, tumors are primarily sought in the peripheral zone. Unfortunately, not all tumors are relatively hypoechoic; some are hyperechoic, some are isoechoic, and some are of mixed echogenicity (8, 9). Focal benign abnormalities of the peripheral zone of the prostate, including prostatitis, focal hypertrophy, hemorrhage, and even prostatic intraepithelial neoplasia make differential diagnosis a problem. In some cases, the echogenicity of the tumor cannot be distinguished from that of the background tissue and only distortion of the prostatic capsule may provide a clue that a neoplasm exists. Given all of this, it has become apparent that TRUS is neither highly sensitive nor highly specific in the detection of prostate cancer (10–15).

Although current practice in the United States is not to employ TRUS frequently as a standalone screen for prostate cancer, finding a consensus in the literature is not easy. When the technique was introduced, investigators were enthusiastic about it, citing relatively high sensitivity and specificity values, and even a few relatively modern series purport to show high accuracy (2, 6, 7). But most current literature suggests relatively low sensitivity and specificity and does not recommend use of TRUS as a screen (1, 8, 9, 13–16). The reasons for diminishing enthusiasm are probably several: In the earliest years of TRUS investigation, the only

competing screening modality was DRE, with which TRUS compared relatively favorably (5, 17), but nearly two decades ago PSA was introduced, which in most series proved to be more accurate and cheaper than TRUS (8, 16, 18, 19). At the same time, the criteria for defining screening populations and statistics for assessing the efficacy of the test have become more stringent. There are probably several reasons for the widely varying claims regarding the efficacy of TRUS as well, including the considerable subjectivity of analysis of findings on the TRUS images, varying practices with regard to blinding TRUS practitioners to results of other screening modalities, and the considerable lack of standardization and characterization of tested populations.

As recently as 2002, some authors claimed sensitivities of TRUS ranging from 74 to 94% (2). But other studies have looked more closely at the sensitivity of TRUS and found considerably lower numbers. For example, a series of patients with prostate cancer diagnosed only on one side of the prostate, in whom TRUS was followed by prostatectomy and careful pathologic examination of the entire prostate, found a sensitivity of 52%, specificity of 68%, positive predictive values (PPV) of 54%, and negative predictive value (NPV) of 66% (15). Another group found that among patients with normal PSA and DRE, if TRUS was positive, only 9% of biopsied patients had tumor (8). Another investigator found that under the same circumstances the PPV for TRUS was 7% and that biopsies would have to be performed on 18 TRUS-positive patients to detect one tumor (11). Flanigan et al. (13) found a PPV for TRUS of 18% in patients with abnormal PSA or DRE; Cooner et al. (20) found that when DRE and PSA were normal, the PPV of TRUS was 9% (21). Babaian et al. (18) found that using a combination of DRE and PSA, a significantly higher PPV could be found than with a combination of TRUS and PSA. If TRUS is performed in addition to DRE, slightly more tumors are found than if DRE is used alone (3, 17, 21).

There have been technical advantages that have been applied in hopes of improving the performance of TRUS. Color Doppler imaging (22) improves the sensitivity from that of conventional gray-scale imaging, as does Doppler flow imaging, using intravascular ultrasound contrast agent (23). Still, these techniques have not made the quantum leap that would be necessary to propel TRUS into a widely used screening role. Also, TRUS costs considerably more than DRE or PSA, which diminishes its cost-effectiveness further (17, 18, 24), as does the lower patient compliance with TRUS than with DRE and PSA (17).

Ultrasound does play a limited role in screening for prostate cancer by refining the use of serum PSA, which is another test with less-than-ideal sensitivity and specificity (23). The ratio of PSA to prostate volume, usually determined by TRUS and termed PSA density, has been found in some series to be a more accurate test than a single PSA determination (24–30). Transrectal ultrasound facilitates volume assessment of the peripheral zone, where most prostate cancer arises; using this volume to calculate PSA density may increase accuracy (31). The PSA density may help predict whether extracapsular disease will be found at surgery and longer-term prognosis (32, 33).

II. Is Transrectal Ultrasound Useful to Guide Prostate Biopsy?

Summary of Evidence: Transrectal ultrasound appears to be useful to guide systematic biopsies into the peripheral zone, and increase diagnostic yield if focal abnormalities (especially those demonstrated by flow-sensitive techniques) are biopsied, hence justifying its continued use as a biopsy guide (limited evidence).

Supporting Evidence: Intraprostatic carcinoma can be diagnosed only histologically, and, as screening becomes more widespread and as fewer prostate resections are performed for voiding symptoms, an ever-higher percentage of prostate cancers are diagnosed by prostate biopsy. Originally, prostate biopsy was performed using digital guidance, but with the advent of TRUS, an increasing number of biopsies have been performed using this method as guidance. Early after the invention of TRUS, it became apparent that certain prostates contained local abnormalities in echogenicity, which, at least sometimes, indicated foci of carcinoma. The commonest appearance was that of a local region of diminished echogenicity; with time, it became apparent that some prostate carcinomas presented as hyperechoic regions, some as discrete areas with echogenicity

roughly equal to the surrounding tissue, and many were not visible at all (34). The last observation led to the realization that to biopsy only sonographically abnormal regions of the prostate would cause many cancers to be missed; with experience, it also became apparent that many focally abnormal regions were found by biopsy not to harbor neoplasm (35, 36).

Given these findings, systematic biopsy of specific regions of the prostate, whether or not they were seen to obtain focal abnormalities, became commonplace. Originally, relatively few biopsies were performed: four or six biopsies, equally divided between the right and left sides and at different zones in the craniocaudad direction, were used. Since then, a number of studies have shown that increasing the number of biopsies to 6, 8, 10, or even 12 cores leads to an increased likelihood of recovering cancer (37–42). Since many cancers could not be visualized, and their locations cannot be exactly predicted, the phenomenon appeared stochastic: that is, assuming random distribution of prostate cancers, the more biopsies were done, the more likely cancer was to be found. This observation could call into question the necessity for performing TRUS during biopsy at all; indeed, at least one publication suggested that the performance of multiple segmental biopsies in a systematic pattern was more important than the method used to guide the biopsy needle (43).

Nevertheless, many authors continue to feel that visualization of the prostate by TRUS during biopsy leads to an increased yield. Several studies have shown that if, in addition to systematic biopsies, foci of ultrasound abnormality are also biopsied, an increased number of carcinomas are detected (44–46). These papers tend not to be controlled for the possibility that the extra biopsies might yield an increased number of prostate cancers simply because they involved a greater number of needle passes (the stochastic model) rather than because specific areas were biopsied. But there appears to be evidence that TRUS really can maximize the number of prostate cancers detected. First of all, since most carcinomas appear in the peripheral zone of the prostate, and since the peripheral zone can more accurately be localized with TRUS, using TRUS to biopsy the peripheral zone has led to an increased yield of carcinoma (39). In addition, statistical analysis of the likelihood of finding tumor with any given needle track has found that a sample from a region seen to be abnormal by TRUS is more likely to contain tumor than a sample obtained elsewhere. Technical enhancements of ultrasound also appear to be of assistance. The use of power Doppler ultrasound to assess the level of local tissue blood flow has shown that biopsies from sites of high blood flow are more likely to contain carcinoma than are biopsies from other sites (47). Enhanced visualization of flow permitted by simultaneous use of Doppler ultrasound and the intravenous infusion of an ultrasound contrast agent has also led to an increased yield (48).

In summary, the initial hopes that TRUS-guided biopsy of regions in the prostate that demonstrate focal ultrasound abnormality would be a technique of high sensitivity and specificity and that might permit a small number of biopsies have not been supported; to fail to biopsy systematically the various parts of the prostate leads to an unacceptable number of false-negative biopsy sessions. Nevertheless, TRUS still appears to be useful: its ability to guide systematic biopsies into the peripheral zone and the increase in diagnostic yield if focal abnormalities (especially those demonstrated by flow-sensitive techniques) are biopsied justify its continued use as a biopsy guide.

III. Is Imaging Accurate for Staging Prostate Cancer?

Summary of Evidence: MRI is the most accurate of the imaging techniques in local staging, but its relative expense and persistent false-positive and false-negative rates for locally invasive disease suggest that it should be interpreted along with all additional available data, and reserved for patients in whom other data leave treatment choices ambiguous. Due to the higher accuracy of MRI in revealing the local extent of disease, computed tomography (CT) has been largely abandoned as an initial test for evaluating local disease (strong evidence).

Supporting Evidence

A. Ultrasound

The early literature regarding ultrasound of the prostate claimed a startlingly high accuracy for local staging (49), despite the fact that the images

were transabdominal rather than transrectal, fine detail could not be observed, and that later investigation (50) showed that the ultrasound features identified as the capsule of the prostate correlated poorly with the anatomic capsule. Currently, transabdominal probes are not used for local staging of prostate cancer. It is not surprising that ultrasound was found to be relatively poor in evaluating lymph node metastases (51), given the technical difficulties in visualizing normal or slightly enlarged nodes, and the frequency with which tumor-bearing nodes are not enlarged.

The development of high-frequency TRUS probes was expected to produce more accurate results with regard to whether the tumor had transgressed the capsule or invaded the neurovascular bundles or seminal vesicles. But even the best probes produce images that turn out to be much less than 100% accurate in evaluating these features. The last decade and a half has seen continued controversy with regard to whether even transrectal probe images are sufficiently accurate to be used in stage-dependent therapeutic decisions.

A number of investigators remain relatively enthusiastic, stating that the sensitivity, specificity, PPV, NPV, and accuracy for identifying locally invasive disease are sufficiently high to be trustworthy for local staging (52–54). Others, realizing that very high accuracy is necessary to choose among therapies with significantly different side effects, have investigated ultrasound-guided biopsy of seminal vesicles and regions near the neurovascular bundles to confirm or help to exclude tumor invasion (55, 56). Other investigators, citing a variety of figures, are convinced that TRUS is simply too inaccurate to trust for therapeutic planning (57–64).

Prior to the advent of imaging, only DRE provided direct information regarding local stage, and the inability to palpate all parts of the prostate and seminal vesicles, or to feel microscopic disease, limited the accuracy of this examination. The combination of stage estimation by both DRE and TRUS, however, with appropriate weighting for each, may lead to an overall increase in accuracy of staging (54, 65). All other things being equal, the higher the PSA level, the higher the local stage is likely to be, but this single parameter does not permit exact establishment of local stage any more than DRE or TRUS can; but the combination of PSA levels and TRUS findings permits a more accurate determination of local stage.

The modality that continues to be used for the local staging of prostate cancer is MRI, which, when performed using an intrarectal coil, has the potential for high spatial resolution images of the prostate and adjacent structures. An early comparison of TRUS and MRI purported to demonstrate that TRUS was more accurate than MRI in evaluating capsular invasion but that MRI outperformed TRUS for invasion of the seminal vesicles (52). Later publications comparing the two suggest that MRI may be more sensitive but less specific in evaluating capsular invasion (66).

There are characteristics of intraprostatic tumor other than direct visualization of sites of extraglandular invasion that are correlated with the likelihood of invasive disease; in general, the larger the intraprostatic tumor is, the more likely it is to have escaped the bounds of the gland and the more likely it is to be histologically undifferentiated. These features can be used during TRUS analysis to predict likelihood of invasion; in particular, tumor volume, tumor diameter, and the area of the surface of the tumor that directly abuts the capsule are directly correlated with likelihood of invasion (67, 68). Even the degree to which the tumor is visible at all may be important in this regard (69). Other publications, however, fail to find any correlation between sonographic visibility of the tumors and stage (70, 71).

In keeping with the general tendency of many neoplasms to have high blood flow and vessel density correlate positively with degree of biologic malignancy, power Doppler assessment of the amount of flow within the tumor and visibility of the supplying vessels have been found, at least by a few investigators, to correlate with invasiveness, stage, grade, and tendency to recur after initial therapy (72–74). Reconstructed three-dimensional images of multiplanar data have also been found to increase slightly the likelihood that ultrasound will correctly predict stage (75).

In summary, it is probably fair to say that the literature to date does not support the capacity of TRUS to perform local staging of prostate cancer with great accuracy. The inability to detect microscopic portions of tumor, discrepancies between real anatomic and ultrasound findings, and the invisibility of certain tumors all suggest that the few publications that claim high accuracy for ultrasound are not likely to stand up to rigorous scrutiny or reproducibility.

The main roles of staging ultrasound in prostate cancer are likely to be complementary in some cases in which other staging data are conflicting, and as a guide for biopsy of juxtaprostatic structures.

B. Computed Tomography Scan

In patients with newly diagnosed prostate cancer, management decisions depend critically on anatomic stage. In brief, among patients for whom treatment is necessary at all, those in whom disease is confined within the prostatic capsule may be treated with surgery or radiotherapy, those whose tumor remains local but has transgressed the capsule or invaded the seminal vesicle can be treated with radiotherapy, and those who have demonstrated metastatic disease or whose local stage and grade strongly suggest that metastases are present are treated with orchiectomy or anti-androgen therapy.

Early in the development of CT, when it became apparent that the prostate, seminal vesicle, and bladder could be demonstrated, there was considerable hope that local tumor extent could be established by this technique. Asymmetry in prostate shape, invasion of periprostatic fat, and obliteration of the angle between the seminal vesicle and bladder were signs thought to hold promise for indicating local extracapsular tumor extension. Early investigations involving a comparatively small series concluded that these signs were indeed reliable and that CT was quite accurate in detecting and excluding local extracapsular disease (76). It might be expected that, as scanning technology improved and anatomic detail could be seen better, accuracy of demonstrating disease extent should improve. Unfortunately, microscopic invasion of structures immediately outside the capsule is crucial, and microscopic changes cannot be detected by CT at all; high accuracy has never been possible (77). A careful study with appropriate blinding of observers yielded a sensitivity of only 50% in predicting intracapsular disease; errors were found in analysis of seminal vesicle images and other regions immediately surrounding the prostate (78). Since CT can demonstrate only morphologic changes of the seminal vesicles, and since tumor may invade these structures without changing their gross configuration, CT frequently misses such invasion; MRI, which is discussed later, may demonstrate similar abnormalities and thus be more sensitive (79). A larger study of CT, in which CT interpretation results were compared with surgical–pathologic findings, showed the accuracy of CT was only 24% for capsular extension and 59% for seminal vesicle invasion (80). Due to these discouraging results, and to the higher accuracy of MRI in revealing the local extent of disease, CT has been largely abandoned as an initial test for evaluating local disease.

Computed tomography may still have a role, however, in evaluating lymphatic metastases. Metastases may enlarge nodes, and since CT can evaluate nodal size well, it has become the primary modality for searching for nodal disease. It is well recognized that patients may have metastatic nodal disease from prostate cancer in which individual nodal deposits are sufficiently small that the overall node size is not enlarged, so that the sensitivity of the CT is considerably less than 100%. The studies of false-negative rates for CT in detecting nodal metastasis have reported sensitivities of only 0–7% (76, 81, 82). Careful dissection studies (83) have confirmed that this is due to the relatively small size of many tumor-bearing nodes. Large nodes are felt to be a more accurate CT sign of metastatic disease than small ones are of disease without metastases; still, enlarged nodes (77, 83) may occasionally be found in patients without metastatic disease. The occasional false-positive case notwithstanding, definitely enlarged nodes seen on CT are usually regarded as reliable evidence of metastatic disease, especially if local tumor volume and grade suggest that metastases are likely, and if the location of the enlarged nodes is compatible with metastatic prostate cancer. This disease tends to spread to and enlarge nodes in the pelvic retroperitoneum before causing enlargement of nodes in the abdomen or elsewhere (84).

It has been well known for a long time that clinical stage, PSA, and Gleason score are independent predictors of the likelihood that metastases will be found in surgically resected lymph nodes. It seemed logical that these factors might be useful in predicting which CT scans are likely to show enlarged nodes, and, indeed, all three factors have been found to be independent predictors of CT-demonstrated lymphadenopathy (85). Of these, a high Gleason score seems to confer the highest risk (85). These findings have been substantiated by

another study (86), and still others (87, 88) corroborate the importance of PSA; all studies suggest that in patients with an initial PSA below 20, a positive CT scan is extremely unlikely. These findings have primarily been interpreted as indicators that for these patients at low risk, CT need not be performed; they may also be useful for radiologists confronted with CT scans with marginal nodal findings; in these cases, investigation of the PSA and Gleason score may aid in reaching radiologic decisions.

C. Magnetic Resonance Imaging

Early in the development of body MRI it became apparent that the prostate could be visualized, and even that the zones within it could be distinguished. Although little success was met in screening for prostate cancer, a series of publications investigated the technique as a staging technique for recently diagnosed prostate cancer. Most of these relied on external coils (89–93), which continued to be used in a later series as well (94). Staging of the local extent of disease, rather than detecting metastatic disease, was the task at hand, and the external coil was not highly accurate. Accuracy percents tended to be in the low 60 s, and many studies found no improvement over simply using PSA or DRE. A few investigators managed to achieve higher accuracy with body coil MRI (95, 96), finding that MRI was superior to sonography and CT for evaluating seminal vesicle invasion (95) and achieving high specificities in predicting capsular penetration (80%) and seminal vesicle invasion (86%) with a moderately high sensitivity for capsular penetration (62%) (96).

With the introduction of the intrarectal surface coil, the higher spatial resolution that the technique permitted improved accuracy of staging (92, 97–102). Various levels of sensitivity, specificity, PPV, and NPV have been reported; overall staging accuracy ranges from 62 to 84%. Even with the rectal coil techniques, however, not all authors were enthusiastic (103, 104). Ekici et al. (103) found endorectal coil MRI no better than TRUS for staging.

Detection of metastatic disease in pelvic and abdominal lymph nodes by body coil MRI suffers from the same problem as CT, which is that size is the only parameter that can be accurately measured, and that tumor is often found in nonenlarged nodes. In one study, sensitivity of MRI for tumor in nodes was only 27% (81). In attempts to continue to use endorectal MRI to improve staging, many authors have developed staging schemes that combine the results of PSA, PSA density, Gleason score, percentage of tumor-bearing cores in a biopsy series, and age, along with MRI, and have found various combinations that work better than individual ones. Statistics presented in support of the combinations use a variety of outcome parameters, but do not permit gross comparisons of the studies, however (105–111). A combination of using highly trained observers and a computer system, without addition of non-MRI data, achieved an accuracy of 87% (112).

Most studies reporting interpretation of MRI rely most heavily on T2-weighted images. In these images, the peripheral zone of the prostate, where most tumors appear and from which extracapsular extension occurs, appears bright, and tumor tissue is relatively of low intensity. A line felt to represent the prostatic capsule can usually be identified, and the seminal vesicles are visible by virtue of having comparatively dark walls and bright luminal fluid. When there is gross invasion of a large segment of tumor from the confines of the capsule, the low-intensity tumor can be seen to extend directly into periprostatic fat or the seminal vesicles; signs of more subtle invasion have included bulges of various configurations in the capsule, irregularity of the capsule, and thickening of the walls of the seminal vesicles. In T1-weighted images, all the portions of the prostate and seminal vesicles are of approximately the same medium-low intensity, and the capsule is not clearly visualized, so these images are less helpful in staging; they may be valuable, however, when looking for extracapsular tumor that invades the neurovascular bundles. Several publications describe evaluation of enhanced T1-weighted images using gadolinium chelates (113–116), some of which (112–116) use a dynamic technique. This technique has failed to improve consistently the accuracy of staging, but it is claimed to show enhanced delineation of the prostate capsule (113, 114), a weak correlation between tumor permeability and MR stage (115), and accuracies of 84–97% in detecting specific features of extracapsular extension (116). A novel use of an MR contrast agent was reported for investigating nodes (30); administration of nanoparticles permitted identification of nonenlarged nodes (117) with focal regions of tumor and permitted 100% sensitivity in identifying patients with nodal metastases.

Investigators have also presented data regarding the ability of MRI findings to predict posttherapy PSA failures (105, 108, 110, 118, 119) and positive margins in surgical specimens (120). MRI in combination with other data permitted improvements of these prediction rates, but, as in evaluations of its ability to predict exact stage, did not achieve accuracies of 100%. Given the inability of MRI to achieve very high degrees of accuracy among all patients undergoing initial evaluation for prostate cancer, attempts have been made to find some groups in which MRI might be particularly useful. One of these investigations found that if MRI were limited to a subgroup of those with a Gleason score of 5–7 and a PSA higher than 10–20 ng/mL, increased accuracy for both extracapsular extension and seminal vesicle invasion could be achieved (106). Another study investigated only the ability of MRI to detect enlarged nodes, and suggested that the examination could be withheld from patients with a serum PSA of less than 20 ng/mL (121).

In summary, MRI probably permits better local staging than older techniques in certain subgroups of patients, but with considerably less than 100% accuracy; the inability to detect microscopic invasion remains an important limitation, as does the inability to detect disease in nonenlarged lymph nodes with standard techniques. These facts have led to only cautious and scattered acceptance of the technique. Currently, it is probably wise to restrict its use to a subgroup of patients – those whose physical examination, PSA, Gleason score, results of standard workup for metastatic disease, and personal preferences leave them on the cusp of choosing surgery or local radiotherapy. When interpreting examinations in these patients, it should be remembered that diagnosis or exclusion of microscopic invasion cannot be performed with accuracy, but that visualization of gross tumor extension beyond the capsule or into the seminal vesicle is a relatively specific sign of invasive disease.

D. Magnetic Resonance Spectroscopic Imaging

In addition to high spatial resolution imaging by proton MRI, technology for spatially resolved spectroscopy of the prostate has been under development for some years. This usually involves a high-field magnet (at least 1.5 T) and an intrarectal coil. Proton spectroscopic data can be acquired from a three-dimensional array of voxels. These voxels are about two orders of magnitude larger than the voxels used for proton imaging, but can be superimposed on proton MRI maps to permit reasonably accurate spatial identification of the intraprostatic region supplying specific spectra.

Spectral analysis relies on the fact that normal prostate tissue and the tissue of benign prostatic hypertrophy secrete relatively large amounts of citrate; prostate adenocarcinoma elaborates much less citrate, but produces a relatively elevated amount of choline; the ratios between the spectral peaks for these molecules are used to distinguish voxels containing neoplasm from those that do not (122, 123).

Currently, the potential uses for magnetic resonance spectroscopic imaging (MRSI) of the prostate might be original diagnosis, biopsy guidance, local staging, and evaluation of recurrent following local therapy.

With regard to diagnosis, several studies have shown that MRSI analysis of small groups of patients containing those without tumor and those with tumor can identify and localize tumors with reasonable, if less than perfect, sensitivity and specificity (124–127). But no sufficiently large or sufficiently well-controlled investigation has addressed whether MRSI is effective in screening for disease in a large sample reflecting either the population at large or those at increased risk because of an elevated PSA. And given that many prostate tumors are considerably smaller than the MRSI voxels, it is unlikely that sensitivity can ever be very high until considerable improvements in spatial resolution can be made.

Series have been published to investigate whether patients whose prostate biopsies have been negative, even though their elevated PSA levels suggest tumor, might be aided by using MRSI to guide further attempts at biopsy. The data show that biopsies using information from MRI and MRSI converts some of these patients from being false negative (for the original biopsy) to true positive for the MR-guided biopsies, but there are few data to show that adding MRSI information to the MRI information is of significant benefit in guiding these biopsies (128). Furthermore, the studies lack controls to investigate the possibility that the subsequent biopsies might have retrieved tumor tissue even without MR guidance. For patients who have had hormonal therapy (129) or who have had intraprostatic hemorrhage from a recent biopsy, localization of tumor by MRI can be difficult; MRSI may permit tumor identification in these circumstances (130), however, so if MRI-guided biopsy ever becomes widespread, MRSI may be of benefit.

There are also series that investigate whether MRSI might improve the accuracy of MRI for prostate staging (129, 131). In one, the addition of MRSI data to MRI data enabled inexperienced readers to become as accurate as experienced readers were with MRI alone, but, for experienced readers, MRSI data did not improve accuracy. However, MRSI may help in assessing overall tumor volume, which is also a factor in staging. But whether this information actually changes treatment decisions for the better has yet to be investigated.

The feasibility of using MRSI to localize prostate cancer in aiding placement of radioactive seeds for brachytherapy and adjusting local doses for external beam therapy has been established (132, 133). But whether this capacity actually improves outcomes, either in terms of disease control or complication reduction is not yet known. In patients who have had local therapy to destroy prostate tumors – in particular, cryotherapy – MRSI is likely to be better in detecting local tumor recurrence than MRI (134, 135). This has the potential for indicating salvage therapy in patients who do not have disseminated disease, but whether these management choices, aided by MRI, benefit patient outcome, also remains to be determined.

In summary, there seems to be little doubt that MRSI can with reasonable accuracy detect foci of intraprostatic tumor, at least when the tumor nodules are not small, and the technique holds promise for diagnosis, staging, prognosis, radiotherapy planning, and determining the need for salvage therapy. But series of sufficient size and sufficiently rigorous design to determine whether any of these functions will be of clinical benefit remain for the future (insufficient evidence).

E. Positron Emission Tomography

There has been considerable investigation of the role of 18-fluorodeoxyglucose positron emission tomography (FDG-PET) scanning in patients with prostate cancer (136–148).

Although carbon-11 acetate (136, 139, 141, 149–151) and carbon-11 choline (140, 149–155) have been found to have certain advantages over FDG, FDG is the most available and most frequently used.

There are no data supporting the use of PET scanning as a screen for detecting prostate cancer.

When used in patients with known prostate cancer in order to test its sensitivity, FDG-PET has yielded extremely disparate results, with reported sensitivities ranging from 19 to 83% (142, 144, 149). Sensitivity is probably higher among patients with higher histologic grades (144). No authors suggest that, among patients with palpable prostate nodules or elevated PSA values, FDG-PET can substitute for biopsy diagnosis of prostate cancer, or to identify a subset of patients with marginal findings who ought to undergo biopsy.

In patients undergoing initial staging of prostate cancer, FDG-PET has been assessed in a number of series (142, 144, 146, 148). The sensitivity for disease in lymph nodes has been reported as ranging from 0 to 67%, and in bones from 57 to 75%. This performance does not support utilization of FDG-PET for routine clinical staging.

In evaluating patients who have undergone therapy and who are at risk for recurrence, FDG-PET has also been tested (136, 138, 139, 143). Sensitivities for detecting recurrence have been reported from 9 to 75%, and are, not surprisingly, better in patients whose PSA levels and PSA velocities are higher (143). Sensitivity appears to be higher for nodal disease than skeletal disease (136); specificity, accuracy, PPV, and NPV have been found to be 100, 83, 100, and 67% in one publication (138). Although some of these figures appear impressive, the reported NPV and the range of reported sensitivities do not constitute strong evidence for routine use of FDG-PET.

IV. How Accurate Is Bone Scan for Detecting Metastatic Prostate Cancer?

Summary of Evidence: Radionuclide bone scan should be performed to evaluate for possible skeletal metastases in subjects with a PSA value of ten or more (strong evidence).

Supporting Evidence: During the evaluation of patients with recently diagnosed prostate cancer, assessment of metastatic disease is crucial. Prostate cancer frequently metastasizes to bones and pelvic nodes; either may occur first. For skeletal metastases, the standard imaging technique is a radionuclide bone scan. Although this is not a terribly expensive test, the number of patients with initial diagnoses of prostate cancer each year is very large; if it were possible to stratify these patients into those with significant or negligible risk of skeletal metastases so that many might not have to undergo bone scanning, savings would be considerable.

The simplest and most frequently cited parameter for assessing metastatic potential is PSA. A large number of investigations have found that when the PSA value is less than 10 ng/mL, the rate of positive bone scans is so low that the scan may be omitted (121, 156–162). Others have suggested a higher threshold – less than 20 ng/mL (88, 163–167). Given that the occasional poorly differentiated prostate cancer may produce very little PSA, and given the difficulty of establishing absolute biologic thresholds, it is not surprising that, on rare occasion, a patient with a very low PSA may still have a positive bone scan; at least some authors suggest that, no matter what the PSA, an initial scan should be obtained as a baseline.

Other characteristics of individual tumors are, not surprisingly, also related to the likelihood of metastatic disease; those that indicate likelihood of metastasis independent of PSA levels have been proposed to be used in conjunction with PSA in determining which patients should undergo bone scanning. Bone alkaline phosphate levels (168–170) have been found useful in this regard; indeed, at least one group found alkaline phosphate levels alone to be better determinants of a threshold than PSA (171). Gleason score and clinical stage have also been found to be independent risk factors for positive scans (172), although not by all investigators (173).

The false-negative rate for bone scans is not accurately known, although it is certainly true that in patients with high PSA levels there may be skeletal disease even in the face of a normal bone scan (161). The false-positive rate for bone scans is not well known either; in most cases, foci of increased activity due to fracture, Paget's disease, and degenerative spondylitis may be demonstrated to be false-positive indicators of metastatic disease by their characteristic pattern and by follow-up examinations with radiography and CT.

A. Special Case: Which Patients Should Undergo Imaging After Initial Treatment to Look for Metastatic Disease?

Follow-up imaging after initial treatment of prostate cancer should be instituted depending on the likelihood that it will aid in future therapeutic decisions. Metastatic disease is usually treated by maneuvers intended to reduce the effect of testosterone upon the tumors, including surgical orchiectomy and drugs that block the release or action of testosterone. Occasionally, salvage therapy is tried – that is, prostatectomy after initial radiotherapy or local radiotherapy after prostatectomy – if it is felt that disease has recurred locally after the initial treatment and that distant metastases are not likely. After initial treatment, serial PSA determinations are the usual surveillance mechanism to detect recurrent disease. When PSA levels begin to rise, there may still be a question of whether therapy should be initiated if the patient is asymptomatic and disease cannot be identified in any other way.

After primary local radiotherapy or prostatectomy, serial PSA determinations are usually used since it is felt that progressive elevation of PSA is more sensitive than any imaging technique and can detect recurrent disease at an earlier stage; most authorities suggest, therefore, that in the absence of PSA elevations, no imaging is necessary (174–180). There are a few publications which suggest that on rare occasion, bone scans may detect recurrent disease prior to PSA (181); given that a small percentage of poorly differentiated tumor may not produce much PSA, this should not be entirely surprising. Other investigators feel that bone alkaline phosphate determinations may indicate recurrent disease and the need for imaging prior to PSA elevations (182).

Salvage therapy requires both proof that there is local recurrent tumor, and, to whatever degree possible, that there is no metastatic disease. Local tumor proof usually requires biopsy, which may be digitally guided if a nodule is palpable, but ultrasound has also been shown to demonstrate residual tumor (183, 184), as has MRI (185) and even MR spectroscopy (134). Computed tomography is ineffective at this task (186). With

regard to distant metastases, a clearly positive bone scan or CT is usually felt to be accurate. There are undoubtedly false positives, but little work is available to quantify this problem, and there are undoubtedly false-negative imaging examinations in patients with recurrent distant disease. In general, after primary local therapy, patients whose lowest posttherapy PSA is relatively high, and in whom subsequent rises in PSA happen quickly after therapy and proceed with a high velocity, are more likely to have distant recurrences, and vice versa.

Positron emission tomography scanning has been tried to search for recurrent disease; FDG-PET has found to be only moderately sensitive and may fail to demonstrate small bone metastases (148, 187–189). Carbon-11 acetate may be more sensitive (136, 139, 152).

In patients who have metastatic disease, imaging may be useful. The number and intensity of metastases demonstrated by bone scan (190) mimics the amount of disease as indicated by tumor markers, and tumor burden as demonstrated by bone scans is of prognostic value (191, 192). Tumor volume in nodes as measured by CT also may be used for prognosis (193); when evaluating patients for recurrent disease by CT, enlarged nodes almost always appear in the pelvis first, unless the patient has had a lymphadenectomy, in which case the first enlarged nodes may be found in the upper abdomen (194).

Take Home Figures

Figure 9.1–9.3 is a flow chart for evaluating and treating patients suspected of having prostate cancer.

Imaging Case Studies

These cases highlight the advantages and limitations of imaging in patients with prostate cancer.

Case 1

A 65-year-old man's prostate biopsy is positive for adenocarcinoma. His Gleason score is 6 and his PSA is 7.1. A bone scan was performed despite

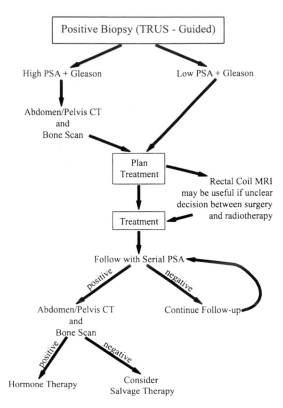

```
Positive Biopsy (TRUS - Guided)
```

High PSA + Gleason   Low PSA + Gleason

Abdomen/Pelvis CT
and
Bone Scan

Plan
Treatment
→ Rectal Coil MRI
may be useful if unclear
decision between surgery
Treatment ← and radiotherapy

Follow with Serial PSA

positive   *negative*

Abdomen/Pelvis CT
and   Continue Follow-up
Bone Scan

positive   *negative*

Hormone Therapy   Consider
Salvage Therapy

Figure 9.1. Flow chart of imaging evaluation of subjects with prostate cancer. (Reprinted with kind permission of Springer Science+Business Media from Newhouse JH. Imaging in the Evaluation of Patients with Prostate Cancer. In Medina LS, Blackmore CC (eds): *Evidence-Based Imaging: Optimizing Imaging in Patient Care.* New York: Springer Science+Business Media, 2006.)

the published data suggesting that he has a very low probability of having a true positive result for metastatic disease. Focal regions of increased activity in sites that are common locations for metastatic prostate cancer were identified. Computed tomography revealed that the changes were all due to degenerative disease, however, corroborating the predictive value of the PSA and Gleason data, and illustrating the value of these numbers in analyzing images (Fig. 9.2).

Case 2

A 59-year-old man's prostate cancer was recently diagnosed by biopsy. Computed tomography and bone scan showed no evidence of metastases. His Gleason score is 9 and his PSA is 21, which suggest that he is likely to have disseminated disease, and would probably have recurrent disease after prostatectomy. He continued to request radical surgery, stating that he had heard that surgery was his only chance for cure. Magnetic resonance imaging revealed gross tumor invasion of the seminal vesicles (the low-intensity regions replacing the bright lumina of the seminal vesicles), which both increased the likelihood of disseminated disease to the level at which surgery was felt to be inappropriate, precluded effective treatment by brachytherapy, and provided guidance for designing conformal external-beam radiotherapy (Fig. 9.3).

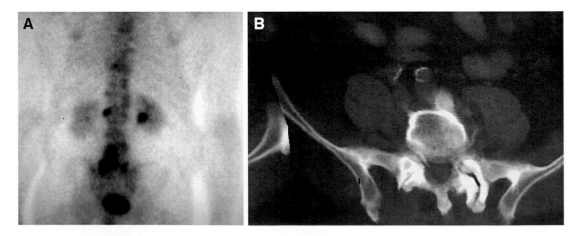

Figure 9.2. Case 1. (**A**) A 65-year-old man with prostate cancer recently diagnosed by biopsy. The Gleason score is 6 and his PSA is 5. Active foci originally interpreted as metastases despite the unlikelihood given the Gleason and PSA. (**B**) CT reveals abnormality to be degenerative spondylitis. (Reprinted with kind permission of Springer Science+Business Media from Newhouse JH. Imaging in the Evaluation of Patients with Prostate Cancer. In Medina LS, Blackmore CC (eds): *Evidence-Based Imaging: Optimizing Imaging in Patient Care.* New York: Springer Science+Business Media, 2006.)

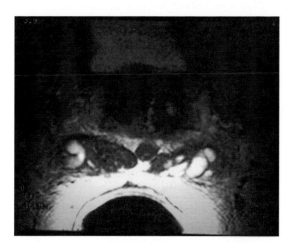

Figure 9.3. Case 2. A 59-year-old man with recently diagnosed prostate cancer, Gleason score 9, and PSA 21. T2-weighted MRI reveals low-intensity tumor invading the seminal vesicle lumen, primarily on the *right* (*arrows*). (Reprinted with kind permission of Springer Science+Business Media from Newhouse JH. Imaging in the Evaluation of Patients with Prostate Cancer. In Medina LS, Blackmore CC (eds): *Evidence-Based Imaging: Optimizing Imaging in Patient Care.* New York: Springer Science+Business Media, 2006.)

Imaging Protocols Based on the Evidence

Transrectal Ultrasound

Diagnostic images of the prostate should be recorded in planes both sagittal and transverse to the apex-to-base axis of the gland. Images are obtained at 6–9 MHz. Transverse images should be obtained at approximately 5-mm intervals; for large glands it may be necessary to angle the probe left and right to image the two sides of the gland independently. With the probe imaging in the sagittal plane, the mid-sagittal view should be accompanied by views produced with the probe angled to each side. There is no standard for the angle between successive views; obviously, the larger the gland the more images need to be obtained.

Although color Doppler and contrast-enhanced imaging have been described, they are not universally applied.

Computed Tomography

Evaluation of prostate cancer patients by CT involves a limited focus, which is to determine whether metastases are seen in lymph nodes or bones. Most patients have simultaneous skeletal scintigraphy, so that limiting the range of CT to the abdomen and pelvis – or even to the pelvis alone – is not likely to reduce sensitivity significantly.

Since node size is critical, a slice thickness that does not cause partial-volume averaging of structures as small as 1 cm in diameter is crucial; slices no thicker than 5 mm are ideal. Oral and intravenous contrasts are ideal, but not absolutely necessary. Inspection of the skeleton using bone windows is crucial.

Magnetic Resonance Imaging

Staging prostate cancer by MRI involves evaluation of the extent of any local extracapsular extent of tumor and detection of lymphatic disease that may have enlarged pelvic lymph nodes. The standard examination is limited to the prostate and periprostatic regions and pelvis; abdominal imaging is usually not routine.

Most imaging has been performed with 1.5-T magnets, with either a body coil or wraparound phased array pelvic coils. A series of T1-weighted spin–echo transverse images is performed, no thicker than 5 mm with the gap no greater than 1 mm. The TR should be several hundred milliseconds and the TE should be as short as the scanner permits.

Focused imaging of the prostate should be performed with an intrarectal coil, coupled with a body coil or wraparound pelvic coil. Imaging includes transverse T1-weighted spin–echo and T2-weighted fast spin–echo images of the prostate and seminal vesicles with T2-weighted sagittal and coronal series. Paramagnetic contrast agents are not routinely utilized. The reference axis for these images may be either the long axis of the entire body or the long axis of the prostate gland. The TR should be 4,000 or 5,000 ms, and effective TE from 90 to 110 ms. Slices should be no more than 4 mm thick, and slice gap should not exceed 1 mm.

Radionuclide Bone Scan

The protocol for scanning patients with prostate cancer is no different from that appropriate for scanning adults for other malignancies that metastasize to the skeleton; 20 mCi of technetium

99m (Tc-99m) ethylene hydroxydiphosphonate (HDP) or Tc-99m methylene diphosphonate (MDP) are administered with scanning 2.5–3 h after injection. The patient should drink sufficient fluid that he can void immediately before scanning, since the isotope accumulates in the bladder and may obscure pelvic metastases.

If planar scanning is performed, both anterior and posterior views should be obtained. A parallel-hole collimator should be used. A scan speed of 10–15 cm/min usually provides adequate recorded activity. If single photon emission computed tomography (SPECT) scanning is performed, a dual- or triple-head camera can be used; a 128 × 128 matrix with 30 s per frame and 360-degree acquisition should provide good images.

Positron Emission Tomography Scan

Although compounds currently under investigation may prove to be more effective than 18 F-FDG, this isotope continues to be the most frequently employed one for oncologic imaging; 10 mCi is an appropriate dose. It is important that the patient's blood glucose level not be elevated. Patients should fast for 4–6 h prior to the procedure so that blood glucose does not exceed 160 mg/dL; the level should be checked before administering the isotope intravenously. Sixty minutes should elapse before beginning the scan, during which time the patient must continue to fast. The patient should empty his bladder immediately before the scan begins.

Future Research

- Can any imaging technique – especially metabolism-dependent modalities like magnetic resonance spectroscopy (MRS) and PET – be used to determine which cases of prostate cancer safely may be managed by watchful waiting?
- Which clinical or serologic thresholds should be used to indicate imaging in detection and characterization of recurrent disease after initial therapy, and which modalities should be used?
- Can the initial research that suggests that superparamagnetic agents and lymph node imaging by MRI can detect tumor in normal-sized nodes be replicated?

References

1. Jemal A, Tiwari RC, Murray T et al. CA Cancer J Clin 2004;54:8–29.
2. Ciatto S, Bonardi R, Lombardi C et al. Tumori 2002;88(4):281–283.
3. Cupp MR, Oesterling JE. Mayo Clin Proc 1993;68(3):297–306.
4. Mandell MJ, Hopper KD, Jarowenko MV et al. Crit Rev Diagn Imaging 1991;32(4):273–300.
5. Lee F, Littrup PJ, Torp-Pedersen ST et al. Radiology 1988;168(2):389–394.
6. Lee F, Gray JM, McLeary RD et al. Radiology 1986;158(1):91–95.
7. Lee F, Gray JM, Mc Leary RD et al. Prostate 1985;7(2):117–129.
8. Ellis WJ, Chelner MP, Preston SD et al. J Urol 1994;152(5 pt 1):1520–1525.
9. Shinohara K, Wheeler TM, Scardino PT et al. J Urol 1989;142(1):76–82.
10. Ciatto S, Bonardi R, Lombardi C et al. Int J Biol Markers 2001;16(3):179–182.
11. Rietergen JB, Kranse R, Kirkels WJ et al. Br J Urol 1997;79(Suppl 2):57–63.
12. Ciatto S, Bonardi R, Gervasi G et al. Radiol Med 2002;103(3):219–224.
13. Flanigan RC, Catalona WJ, Richie JP et al. J Urol 1994;152(5 pt a):1506–1509.
14. Chancellor MB, Van Appledorn CA. Urology 1993;41(6):590–593.
15. Carter HB, Hamper UM, Sheth S et al. J Urol 1989;142(4):1008–1010.
16. Gustafsson O, Carlsson P, Norming U et al. Prostate 1995;26(6):299–309.
17. Norming U, Gustafsson O, Nyman CR. Acta Oncol 1991;30(2):277–279.
18. Ciatto S, Bonardi R, Mazzotta A et al. Tumori 1995;81(4):225–229.
19. Babaian RJ, Dinney CP, Ramirez EI et al. Urology 1993;41(5):421–425.
20. Cooner WH, Mosley BR, Rutrherfor CL Jr et al. J Urol 1990;143:1146.
21. Yamamoto T, Ito K, Ohi M et al. Urology 2001;58(6):994–998.
22. Kuligowska E, Barish MA, Fenlon HM et al. Radiology 2001;220(3):757–764.
23. Halpern EJ, Rosenberg M, Gomella LG. Radiology 2001;219(1):219–225.
24. Palken M, Cobb OE, Simons CE. J Urol 1991;145(1):86–90, discussion 90–92.

25. Benson MC, Whang IS et al. J Urol 1992;147(3 pt 2):815–816.
26. Bazinet M, Meshref AW et al. Comments. Urology 1994;44(1):150–151; 43(1):44–51, discussion 51–52.
27. Bretton PR, Evans WP et al. Cancer 1994;74(11):2991–2995.
28. Kochanska-Dziurowic AA, Mielniczuk MR et al. Comment. Br J Urol 1998;82(6):933; 81(6):834–838.
29. Men S, Cakar B et al. J Exp Clin Cancer Res 2001;20(4):473–480.
30. Catalona WJ, Richie JP et al. J Urol 1994;152(6 pt 1):2046–2048; 152(6 pt 1):2031–2036.
31. Zlotta AR, Djavan B et al. Comment. J Urol 1997;157(4):1335–1336; 157(4):1315–1321.
32. Horiguchi A, Nakashima J et al. Prostate 2003; 56(1):23–29.
33. Freedland SJ, Kane CJ et al. J Urol 2003;169(3):969–973.
34. Turkeri L, Tarcan T, Biren T. Int J Urol 1996;3(6):459–461.
35. Leibowitz CB, Staub PG. Australas Radiol 1996;40(3):240–243.
36. Hammerer P, Huland H. J Urol 1994;151(1):99–102.
37. de la Taille A, Antiphon P, Salomon L et al. Urology 2003;61(6):1181–1186.
38. Kojima M, Hayakawa T, Saito T et al. Int J Urol 2001;8(6):301–307.
39. Ravery V, Goldblatt L, Royer B et al. J Urol 2000;164(2):393–396.
40. Presti JC Jr, Chang JJ, Bhargava V et al. J Urol 2000;163(1):163–167.
41. Babaian RJ, Toi A, Kamoi K, Troncoso P et al. J Urol 2000;163(1):152–157.
42. Chen ME, Troncoso P, Johnston DA et al. J Urol 1997;158(6):2168–2175.
43. Lippman HR, Ghiatas AA, Sarosdy MF. J Urol 1992;147(3 pt 2):827–829.
44. Park SJ, Miyake H, Hara I et al. Int J Urol 2003;10(2):68–71.
45. Fleshner NE, O'Sullivan M, Premdass C et al. Urology 1999;53(2):356–358.
46. Melchior SW, Brawer MK. J Clin Ultrasound 1996;24(8):463–471.
47. Franco OE, Arima K, Yanagawa M. Br J Urol Int 2000;85(9):1049–1052.
48. Frauscher F, Klauser A, Volgger H et al. J Urol 2002;1767(4):1648–1652.
49. Abu-Yousef MM, Narayana AS. Radiology 1985;156(1):175–180.
50. Young MP, Jones DR, Griffiths GJ et al. Eur Urol 1993;24(4):479–482.
51. Magnusson A, Fritjofsson A, Norlen BJ, Wicklund H. Scand J Urol Nephrol 1988;22(1):7–10.
52. Friedman AC, Seidmon EJ, Radecki RD, Lev-Toaff A, Caroline DF. Urology 1988;31(6):530–537.
53. Perrapato SD, Carothers GG, Maatman TJ, Soechtig CE. Urology 1989;33(2):103–105.
54. Ohori M, Egawa S, Shinohara K, Wheeler TM, Scardino PT. Br J Urol 1994;74(1):72–79.
55. Okihara K, Kamoi K, Lane RB et al. J Clin Ultrasound 2002;30(3):123–131.
56. Deliveliotis CH, Varkarakis J, Trakas N et al. Int Urol Nephrol 1999;31(1):83–87.
57. Liebross RH, Pollack A, Lankford SP et al. Cancer, 1999;85(7):1577–1585.
58. Smith JA Jr, Scardino PT, Resnick MI et al. J Urol 1997;157(3):902–906.
59. Colombo T, Schips L, Augustin H et al. Minerva Urol Nefrol 1999;51(1):1–4.
60. Huchboni RA, Boner JA, Debatin JF et al. Clin Radiol 1995;50(9):593–600.
61. Rorvik J, Halvorsen OJ, Servoll E, Haukaas S. Br J Urol 1994;73(1);65–69.
62. Hamper UM, Sheth S, Walsch PC, Holtz PM, Epstein JI. AJR 1990;155(5):1015–1019.
63. Andriole GL, Coplen DE, Mikkelsen DJ, Catalona WJ. J Urol 1989;142(5):1259–1261.
64. Vijverberg PL, Giessen MC, Kurth KH, Dabhoiwala NF, de Reijke TM, van den Tweel JG. Eur J Surg Oncol 1992;18(5):449–455.
65. Wolf JS Jr, Shinohara K, Narayan P. Br J Urol 1992;70(5):534–541.
66. Presti JC Jr, Hricak H, Narayan PA, Shinohara K, White S, Carroll PR. AJR 1996;166(1):103–108.
67. Gerber GS, Goldberg R, Chodak GW. Urology 1992;40(4):311–316.
68. Ukimura O, Troncoso P, Ramirez EI, Babaian RJ. J Urol 1998;159(4):1251–1259.
69. Augustin H, Graefen M, Palisaar J et al. J Clin Oncol 2003;21(15):2860–2868.
70. Sanders H, el-Galley R. World J Urol 1997;15(6):336–338.
71. Werner-Wasik M, Whittington R, Malkowicz SB et al. Urology 1997;50(3):385–389.
72. Cornud F, Hamida K, Flam T et al. AJR 2003;175(4):1161–1168.
73. Sauvain JL, Palascak P, Bourscheid D et al. Eur Urol 2003;44(1):21–30.
74. Ismail M, Petersen RO, Alexander AA, Newschaffer C, Gomella LG. Urology 1997;50(6):906–912.
75. Garg S, Flortling B, Chadwick D, Robinson MC, Hamdy FC. J Urol 1999;162(4):1318–1321.
76. Giri PG, Walsh JW, Hazra TA, Texter JH, Koontz WW. Int J Radiat Oncol Biol Phys 1982; 8(2):283–287.
77. Sawczuk IS, deVere White R, Gold RP, Olsson CA. Urology 1983;21(1):81–84.
78. Platt JF, Bree RL, Schwab RE. AJR 1987;149(2):315–318.
79. Friedman AC, Seidmon EJ, Radecki PD, Lev-Toaff A, Caroline DF. Urology 1988;31(6):530–537.
80. Engeler CE, Wasserman, NF, Zhang G. Urology 1992;40(4):346–350.
81. Borley N, Fabrin K, Sriprasad S et al. Scand J Urol Nephrol, 2003;37(5):382–386.

82. Magnusson A, Fritjorfsson A, Norlen BJ, Wicklund H. Scand J Urol Nephrol 1988;22(1): 7–10.
83. Tiguert R, Gheiler EL, Tefilli MV et al. Urology 1999;53(2):367–371.
84. Burcombe RJ, Ostler PJ, Ayoub AW, Hoskin PJ. Clin Oncol 2000;12(1):32–35.
85. Lee N, Newhouse JH, Olsson CA et al. Urology 1999;54(3):490–494.
86. Spencer JA, Chng WJ, Hudson E, Boon AP, Whelan P. Br J Radiol 1998;7(851):1130–1135.
87. Huncharek M, Muscat J. Abdom Imaging 1996;21(4):364–367.
88. Levran Z, Gonzalez JA, Diokno AC, Jafri SZ, Steinert BW. Br J Urol 1995;75(6):778–781.
89. Rifkin MD, Zerhouni EA, Gatsonis CA et al. N Engl J Med 1990;323(10):621–626.
90. Tempany CM, Rahmouni AD, Epstein JI et al. Radiology 1991;181(1):107–112.
91. Schiebler ML, Yankaskas BC, Tempany C et al. Invest Radiol 1992;27(8):575–577.
92. Tempany CM, Zhou X, Zerhouni EA et al. Radiology 1994;192(1):47–54.
93. Mukamel E, de Kernion JB, Hannah J et al. J Urol (Paris) 1988;94(8):381–388.
94. Tuzel E, Sevinc M, Obuz F et al. Urol Int 1998;61(4):227–231.
95. Friedman AC, Seidmon EJ, Radecki PD et al. Urology 1988;31(6):530–537.
96. Rorvik J, Halvorsen OJ, Albrektsen G et al. Clin Radiol 1999;54(3):164–169.
97. Jager GJ, Barentsz JO, de la Rosette JJ et al. Radiologe 1994;34(3):129–133.
98. Cornud F, Belin X, Flam T et al. Br J Urol 1996;77(6):843–850.
99. Bartolozzi C, Menchi I, Lencioni R et al. Eur Radiol 1996;6(3):339–345.
100. Bates TS, Gillatt DA, Cavanagh PM et al. Br J Urol 1997;79(6):927–932.
101. Sheu MH, Wang JH, Chen KK et al. Chung Hua I Hsueh Tsa Chih 1998;61(5):243–252.
102. Rorvik J, Halvorsen OJ, Albrektsen G et al. Eur Radiol 1999;9(1):29–34.
103. Ekici S, Ozen H, Agildere M et al. Br J Urol Int 1999;83(7):796–800.
104. May F, Treumann T, Dettmar P et al. Br J Urol Int 2001;87(1):66–69.
105. D'Amico A, Altschuler M, Whittington R et al. Clin Perform Qual Health Care 1993;1(4):219–222.
106. D'Amico AV, Whittington R, Schnall M et al. Cancer 1995;75(9):2368–2372.
107. Huchboni RA, Boner JA, Debatin JF et al. Clin Radiol 1995;50(9):593–600.
108. Damico AV, Whittington R, Malkowicz SB et al. Urology 1997;49(3A suppl):23–30.
109. Getty DJ, Seltzer SE, Tempany CM et al. Radiology 1997;204(2):471–479.
110. D'Amico AV, Whittington R, Malkowicz SB. Urology 2000;55(4):572–577.
111. Horiguchi A, Nakashima J, Horiguch Y et al. Prostate 2003;56(1):23–29.
112. Seltzer SE, Getty DJ, Tempany CM et al. Radiology 1997;202(1):219–226.
113. Huchboni RA, Boner JA, Lutolf UM, et al. J Comput Assist Tomogr 1995;19(2):232–237.
114. Brown G, Macvicar DA, Ayton V et al. Clin Radiol 1995;50(9):601–606.
115. Padhani AR, Gapinski CJ, Macvicar DA et al. Clin Radiol 2000;55(2):99–109.
116. Ogura K, Maekawa S, Okubo K et al. Urology 2001;57(4):721–726.
117. Harisinghani MG, Barentsz J, Hahn PF et al. N Engl J Med 2003;348(25):2491–2499.
118. Cheng GC, Chen MH, Whittington R et al. Int J Radiat Oncol Biol Phys 2003;55(1):64–70.
119. D'Amico AV, Whittington R, Malkowicz B et al. J Urol 2000;164(3 pt 1):759–763.
120. Soulie M, Aziza R, Escourrou G et al. Urology 2001;58(2):228–232.
121. Huncharek M, Muscat J. Cancer Invest 1995; 13(1):31–35.
122. Kurhanewicz J, Vigneron DB, Nelson SJ et al. Urology 1995;45(3):459–466.
123. Narayan P, Jajodia P, Kurhanewicz J et al. J Urol 1991;146(1):66–74.
124. Hasumi M, Suzuki K, Taketomi A et al. Anticancer Res 2003;23(5b):4223–4227.
125. Hasumi M, Suzuki K, Oya N et al. Anticancer Res 2002;22(2B):1205–1208.
126. Garcia-Segura JM, Sanchez-Chapado M, Ibarburen C et al. Magn Reson Imaging 1999; 17(5):755–765.
127. Heerschap A, Jag GJ, van der Graaf M et al. Anticancer Res 1997;17(3A):1455–1460.
128. Yuen JS, Thng CH, Tan PH et al. J Urol 2004; 171(4):1482–1486.
129. Scheidler J, Srivastava A, Males RG. Radiology 2001;221(2):380–390.
130. Kaji Y, Kurhanewicz J, Hricak H et al. Radiology 1998;206(3):785–790.
131. Yu KK, Scheidler J, Hricak H et al. Radiology 1999;213(2):481–488.
132. Pouliot J, Kim Y, Lessard E et al. Int J Radiat Oncol Biol Phys 2004;59(4):1196–1207.
133. Zaider M, Zelefsky MJ, Lee EK et al. Int J Radiat Oncol Biol Phys 2000;47(4):1085–1096.
134. Parivar F, Hricak H, Shinohara K et al. Urology 1996;48(4):594–599.
135. Kurhanewicz J, Vigneron DB, Hricak H et al. Radiology 1996;200(2):489–496.
136. Fricke E, Machtens S, Hofmann M et al. Eur J Nucl Med Mol Imaging 2003;30(4):607–611.
137. Sung J, Espiritu JI, Segall GM et al. BJU Int 2003;92(1):24–27.
138. Chang CH, Wu HC, Tsai JJ et al. Urol Int 2003;70(4):311–315.
139. Oyama N, Miller TR, Dehdashti F et al. J Nucl Med 2003;44(4):549–555.

140. Picchio M, Messa C, Landoni C et al. J Urol 2003;169(4):1337–1340.
141. de Jong IJ, Pruim J, Elsinga PH et al. Eur Urol 2002;42(1):18–23.
142. Oyama N, Akino H, Kanamaru H et al. J Nucl Med 2002;43(2):181–186.
143. Seltzer MA, Barbaric Z, Belldegrun A et al. J Urol 1999;162(4):1322–1328.
144. Oyama N, Akino H, Zusuki Y et al. Jpn J Clin Oncol 1999;29(12):623–629.
145. Sanz G, Robles JE, Gimenez M et al. BJU Int 1999;84(9):1028–1031.
146. Heicappell R, Muller-Mattheis V, Reinhardt M et al. Eur Urol 1999;36(6):582–587.
147. Yeh SD, Imbriasco M, Larson SM et al. Nucl Med Biol 1996;23(6):693–697.
148. Shreve PD, Grossman HB, Gross MD et al. Radiology 1996;199(3):751–756.
149. Effert PJ, Bares R, Handt S et al. J Urol 1996;155(3):994–998.
150. Kotzerke J, Volkmer BG, Glatting G et al. Nuklearmedizin 2003;42(1).25–30.
151. Kato T, Tsukamoto E, Kuge Y et al. Eur J Nucl Med Mol Imaging 2002;29(11):1492–1495.
152. Kotzerke J, Volkmer BG, Neumaier B et al. Eur J Nucl Med Mol Imaging 2002;29(10):1380–1384.
153. deJong IJ, Pruim J, Elsinga PH et al. Eur Urol 2003;44(1):32–38, discussion 38–39.
154. deJong IJ, Pruim J, Elsinga PH et al. J Nucl Med 2003;44(3):331–335.
155. Kotzerke J, Prang J, Neumaier B et al. Eur J Nucl Med 2000;27(9):1415–1419.
156. Lin K, Szabo Z, Chin BB, Civelek AC. Clin Nucl Med 1999;24(8):579–582.
157. Ataus S, Citci A, Alici B, et al. Int Urol Nephrol 1999;31(4):481–489.
158. Wolff JM, Bares R, Jung PK, Buell U, Jakse G. Urol Int 1996;56(3):169–173.
159. Gleave ME, Coupland D, Drachenberg D et al. Urology 1996;47(5):708–712.
160. Sassine AM, Schulman C. Eur Urol 1993;23(3):348–351.
161. Pantelides ML, Bowman SP, George NJ. Br J Urol 1992;70(3):299–303.
162. Woff JM, Zimny M, Borchers H et al. Eur Urol 1998;33(4):376–381.
163. O'Sullivan JM, Norman AR, Cook GJ, Fisher C, Dearnaley DP. BJU Int 2003;92(7):685–689.
164. Rydh A, Tomic R, Tavelin B, Hietala SO, Damber JE. Scand J Urol Nephrol 1999;33(2):89–93.
165. Spencer JA, Chng WJ, Hudson E, Boon AP, Whelen P. Br J Radiol 1998;71(851):1130–1135.
166. Stokkel MP, Zwinderman AH, Zwartendijk J, Pauwels EK, Van Eck-Smith BL. Int J Biol Markers 1998;13(2):70–76.
167. Kemp PM, Maguire GA, Bird NJ. Br J Urol 1997;79(4):611–614.
168. Lorente JA, Valenzuela H, Morote J, Gelabert A. Eur J Nucl Med 1999;26(6):625–632.
169. Morote J, Lorenta JA, Encabo G. Cancer 1996;78(11):2374–2378.
170. Lorente JA, Morote J, Raventos C, Encabo G, Valenzuela H. J Urol 1996;155(4):1348–1351.
171. Wymenga LF, Boomsma JH, Groenier K, Piers DA, Mensink HJ. BJU Int 2001;88(3):226–230.
172. Lee N, Fawaaz R, Olsson CA et al. Int J Radiat Oncol Biol Phys 2000;48(5):1443–1446.
173. Vijayakumar V, Vijayakumar S, Quadri, SF, Blend MJ. Am J Clin Oncol 1994;17(5):432–436.
174. Colberg JW, Ornstein DK et al. J Urol 1999;161(2):520–523.
175. Lorente JA, Morote J, Raventos C et al. J Urol 1996;155(4):1348–1351.
176. Oommen R, Geethanjali FS, Gopalakrishnan G et al. Br J Radiol 1994;67(797):469–471.
177. Mulders PF, Fernandez del Moral P, Theeuwes AG et al. Eur Urol 1992;21(1):2–5.
178. Corrie D, Timmons JH, Bauman JM et al. Cancer 1988;61(12):2453–2454.
179. Huben RP, Schellhammer PF. J Urol 1982;128(3):510–522.
180. Yap BK, Choo R, Deboer G et al. Br J Urol Int 2003;91(7):613–617.
181. Kagan AR, Steckel RJ. Med Pediatr Oncol 1993;21(5):327–332.
182. Murphy GP, Troychak MJ, Cobb OE et al. Prostate 1997;33(2):141–146.
183. Salomon CG, Flisak ME, Olson MC et al. Radiology 1993;189(3):713–719.
184. Wasserman NF, Kapoor DA, Hildebrandt WC et al. Radiology 1992;185(2):367–372.
185. Silverman JM, Krebs TL. AJR 1997;168(2):379–385.
186. Older RA, Lippert MC, Gay SB et al. Acad Radiol 1995;2(6):470–474.
187. Jadvar H, Pinski JK, Conti PS. Oncol Rep 2003;10(5):1485–1488.
188. Salminen E, Hogg A, Binns D et al. Acta Oncol 2002;41(5):425–429.
189. Hofer C, Laubenbacher C, Block T et al. Eur Urol 1999;36(1):31–35.
190. Koizumi K, Uchiyama G, Komatsu H. Ann Nucl Med 1994;8(4):225–230.
191. Sabbatini P, Larson SM, Kremer A et al. J Clin Oncol 1999;17:948–957.
192. Soloway MS, Hardeman SW, Hichen D et al. Cancer 1988;61:195–202.
193. Cheng L, Bergstralh EJ, Cheville JC et al. Am J Surg Pathol 1998;22(12):1491–1500.
194. Spencer JA, Golding SJ. Clin Radiol 1994;49(6):404–407.

Part III

Neuroimaging

10

Neuroimaging in Alzheimer Disease

Kejal Kantarci and Clifford R. Jack

I. How accurate are the clinical criteria for the diagnosis of Alzheimer disease?
II. Does neuroimaging increase the diagnostic accuracy of Alzheimer disease in the clinical setting?
  A. Structural neuroimaging
    1. Special case: volumetric measurements
  B. Functional neuroimaging
  C. Other magnetic resonance techniques
III. Can neuroimaging identify individuals at elevated risk for Alzheimer disease and predict its future development?
  A. Prodromal Alzheimer disease, or mild cognitive impairment
  B. Asymptomatic apolipoprotein E ε4 carriers
IV. Is neuroimaging cost-effective for the clinical evaluation of Alzheimer disease?
V. Can neuroimaging measure disease progression and therapeutic efficacy in Alzheimer disease?

Issues

Key Points

- By differentiating potentially treatable causes, structural imaging with either computed tomography (CT) or magnetic resonance imaging (MRI) influences patient management during the initial evaluation of dementia (strong evidence).
- No evidence exists on the choice of either CT or MRI for the initial evaluation of dementia (insufficient evidence).

K. Kantarci (✉)
Division of Neuroradiology, Mayo Clinic, 200 First St. SW, Rochester, MN 55902, USA
e-mail: kantarci.kejal@mayo.edu

L.S. Medina et al. (eds.), *Evidence-Based Imaging: Improving the Quality of Imaging in Patient Care, Revised Edition,*   **167**
DOI 10.1007/978-1-4419-7777-9_10, © Springer Science+Business Media, LLC 2011

- Diagnostic accuracy of positron emission tomography (PET) and single photon emission computed tomography (SPECT) to distinguish patients with Alzheimer disease (AD) from normal is not higher than that for clinical evaluation (moderate evidence).
- Hippocampal atrophy on MRI-based volumetry and regional decrease in cerebral perfusion on SPECT correlates with the pathologic stage in AD (moderate evidence).
- PET, SPECT, and dynamic susceptibility contrast-enhanced MRI are not cost-effective for the diagnostic workup of AD with the assumed minimal effectiveness of the drug donepezil hydrochloride (moderate evidence).
- Use of PET in early dementia can increase the accuracy of clinical diagnosis without adding to the overall costs of the evaluation (moderate evidence).
- Longitudinal decrease in MRI-based hippocampal volumes, N-acetylaspartate (NAA) levels on ^{1}H magnetic resonance spectroscopy (MRS), glucose metabolism on PET, and cerebral blood flow on SPECT is associated with the rate of cognitive decline in patients with AD (moderate evidence).
- The validity of imaging techniques as surrogate markers for therapeutic efficacy in AD has not been tested in a positive disease-modifying drug trial (insufficient evidence).

Definition and Pathophysiology

Alzheimer disease (AD) is a progressive neurodegenerative dementia. The pathologic hallmarks of AD are accumulation of neurofibrillary tangles and senile plaques. The neurofibrillary pathology, which is associated with cognitive dysfunction, neuron and synapse loss, involves the limbic cortex early in the disease course, and extends to the neocortex as the disease progresses. In addition to the histopathologic changes, there is a gradual loss of cholinergic innervation in AD, which has been the basis for cholinesterase inhibitor therapy.

Epidemiology

Alzheimer disease is the most common cause of dementing illnesses. The prevalence of AD increases with age, and the disease is becoming a significant health problem as the aging population increases in size (1, 2). In the USA, the prevalence of AD was 2.32 million in 1997, and it is projected that 8.64 million people will have the disease by 2047 (3, 4).

Overall Cost to Society

The average lifetime cost per patient is estimated to be $174,000. The cost to US society of AD has been estimated at $100 billion per year (5).

Goals

The goals of imaging are to (1) exclude a potentially reversible cause of dementia in subjects with possible AD, (2) identify subjects at risk for AD, (3) quantify the stage of disease to enable tracking of treatment response, and (4) identify subjects who may respond to therapy. Although no currently available treatments have been proven to stabilize or reverse the neurodegenerative process, a number of putative disease modifying agents are now in development with early clinical trials (6, 7). The primary targets of such interventions are people who are at risk or who are at the mild to moderate stages of the disease. Imaging markers that can accurately discriminate individuals at risk, and are sensitive to disease onset and progression are needed for trials involving disease-modifying therapies.

Methodology

A literature search was conducted using Medline. The search included articles published from January 1966 through February 2004. The main search term was *Alzheimer* or *Alzheimer's disease*. Other terms combined with the main topic were *clinical diagnosis, clinical criteria, neuroimaging, MRI, MR spectroscopy, PET, SPECT,* and *cost-effectiveness*. The search yielded 3,284 articles. Animal studies, non-English-language articles, and articles published before 1980 were excluded, and only articles relevant to our search questions were included for review.

I. How Accurate Are the Clinical Criteria for the Diagnosis of Alzheimer Disease?

Summary of Evidence: There is strong evidence that the *Diagnostic and Statistical Manual of Mental Disorders*, 3rd edition revised (DSM-IIIR) and the National Institute of Neurologic, Communicative Disorders, and Stroke–Alzheimer Disease and Related Disorders Association NINCDS-ADRDA criteria are reliable for the diagnosis of dementia and AD (strong evidence). There are, however, limitations to the data supporting clinical criteria for the diagnosis of AD. Diagnostic accuracy of clinical criteria may vary with the extent of the disease and the skills of the clinician. Clinical criteria for AD need to be validated by clinicians with different levels of expertise and at different clinical settings if such criteria will have widespread use to identify patients for therapeutic interventions (insufficient evidence).

Supporting Evidence: The clinical diagnosis of AD in a living person is labeled either possible or probable AD. Definite diagnosis of AD requires tissue examination, through biopsy or autopsy, of the brain. Histopathologic hallmarks of the disease are neurofibrillary tangles and senile plaques, which show marked heterogeneity in the pathologic progression of AD, and are also encountered to a lesser extent in elderly individuals with normal cognition (8–12). Thus the boundary between the histopathologic changes in elderly individuals considered to be cognitively normal and

patients with AD is quantitative, not qualitative. The most recent recommendations for postmortem diagnosis of AD by the work group sponsored by the National Institute on Aging and the Reagan Research Institute of the Alzheimer's Association (13) defines AD as a clinicopathological entity, emphasizing the importance of clinical impression for pathologic diagnosis.

The diagnostic accuracy of clinical criteria is assessed by using the pathologic diagnosis as a standard. A shortcoming of this approach is that clinical and pathologic findings do not correlate perfectly. For example, some clinically demented patients do not meet the pathologic criteria for AD or any other dementing illness. Similarly, some patients who are clinically normal have extensive pathologic changes of AD. However, from a practical standpoint, by taking pathologic diagnosis as a gold standard, it is possible to assess the diagnostic accuracy of clinical or neuroimaging criteria for the diagnosis of AD. The two commonly used clinical criteria that were subject to assessment for the diagnosis of dementia and AD are the DSM-IIIR (14) and the NINCDS-ADRDA criteria (15).

When both the DSM-IIIR and NINCDS-ADRDA criteria are applied to the diagnosis, clinical-pathologic correlation ranges from 75 to 90% in studies involving a broad spectrum of patients (16–18) (strong evidence). The disagreement between clinical and pathologic diagnosis in 10–25% of the cases provides the motivation to develop neuroimaging markers that can accurately identify the effects of AD pathology even in the presymptomatic phase.

The sensitivity of the DSM-IIIR and NINCDS-ADRDA criteria for the diagnosis of AD ranges from 76 to 98% and the specificity from 61 to 84% (19–23), providing strong evidence that the accuracy of the two commonly used clinical criteria for identifying pathologically diagnosed AD is good, but show marked variability across academic centers. When community-based and clinic-based patients were evaluated by the same physicians, both the sensitivity and specificity of the clinical diagnosis were lower for the community – than for the clinic-based cohorts (92 and 79% for community vs. 98 and 84% for clinic) (19) (strong evidence).

Interrater agreement on the diagnosis of dementia and AD with the DSM-IIIR and NINCDS-ADRDA criteria has been good

[$\kappa = 0.54$–0.81 for DSM-IIIR (24, 25), and $\kappa = 0.51$–0.72 for NINCDS-ADRDA criteria (26, 27) in population-based studies (strong evidence)].

II. Does Neuroimaging Increase the Diagnostic Accuracy of Alzheimer Disease in the Clinical Setting?

A. Structural Neuroimaging

Summary of Evidence: The traditional use of structural neuroimaging to differentiate potentially reversible or modifiable causes of dementia such as brain tumors, subdural hematoma, normal pressure hydrocephalus, and vascular dementia from AD is widely accepted (28). There is strong evidence that structural imaging influences patient management during the initial evaluation of dementia. There is moderate evidence that the diagnostic precision of structural neuroimaging is higher with volume measurements than visual evaluation, especially in mildly demented cases, but the figures are still comparable to clinical evaluation.

Supporting Evidence: Besides the potential causes of dementia mentioned above, structural neuroimaging can also identify anatomic changes that occur due to the pathologic involvement in AD (29). Neurofibrillary pathology, which correlates with neuron loss and cognitive decline in patients with AD, follows a hierarchical topologic progression course in the brain (10, 30–32). It initially involves the anteromedial temporal lobe and limbic cortex. As the disease progresses it spreads over to the neocortex (30). The macroscopic result of this pathologic involvement is atrophy, which is related to the decrease in neuron density (33). For this reason, the search for anatomic imaging markers of AD has targeted the anteromedial temporal lobe, particularly the hippocampus and entorhinal cortex, which are involved earliest and most severely with the neurofibrillary pathology and atrophy in AD.

Visual evaluation or measurements of the anteromedial temporal lobe width with computed tomography (CT) detected 80–95% of the pathologically confirmed AD cases (23, 34). However, the accuracy declined to 57% when only mild AD cases with low pretest probability were quota studied, and the clinical diagnosis with the NINCDS-ADRDA criteria was more accurate than CT measurements for identifying AD patients at pathologically early stages of the disease (strong evidence) (35).

One study with a pathologically confirmed cohort (34) revealed that structural neuroimaging can help to identify vascular dementia or vascular component of AD (mixed dementia) by increasing the sensitivity of the clinical evaluation from 6 to 59%, and management of the vascular component may in turn slow down cognitive decline (strong evidence).

1. Special Case: Volumetric Measurements

A reliable and reproducible method for quantifying medial temporal lobe atrophy is MRI-based volume measurements of the hippocampus and the entorhinal cortex (29, 36). Antemortem hippocampal atrophy was not found to be specific for AD in a pathologically confirmed cohort; however, hippocampal volumes on MRI correlated well with the pathologic stage of the disease ($r = -0.63$; $p = 0.001$) (37). Structural neuroimaging changed the clinical diagnosis in 19–28% of the cases, and changed patient management in 15% (38) (strong evidence).

Visual evaluation of the anteromedial temporal lobe for atrophy on MRI to differentiate patients with AD from normal subjects had a sensitivity of 83–85% and a specificity of 96–98% in clinically confirmed cohorts (38, 39). Although visual evaluation of the temporal lobe accurately distinguishes AD patients in experienced hands, evidence is lacking on the precision of visual evaluation at different clinical settings. Diagnostic accuracy of this technique for distinguishing AD patients from normal has been 79–94% in clinically confirmed cohorts (40, 41), being comparable in mildly and moderately demented cases (42). Routine use of volumetry techniques for the diagnosis of AD may be time-consuming and cumbersome in a clinical setting. However, the intimate correlation between pathologic involvement and hippocampal volumes is encouraging for the use of hippocampal volumetry as an imaging marker for disease progression (moderate evidence).

By differentiating potentially treatable causes, structural imaging with either CT or MRI influences patient management during the initial evaluation of dementia (strong evidence). Evidence is lacking for the choice of either CT or MRI. Computed tomography may be appropriate when a brain tumor or subdural hematoma is suspected, and MRI may be the modality of choice for vascular dementia because of its superior sensitivity to vascular changes. The decision should be based on clinical impression at this time (insufficient evidence).

B. Functional Neuroimaging

Summary of Evidence: SPECT and PET are the two widely investigated functional neuroimaging techniques in AD. Measurements of regional glucose metabolism with PET, and regional perfusion measurements with SPECT indicate a metabolic decline and a decrease in blood flow in the temporal and parietal lobes of patients with AD relative to normal elderly. There is moderate evidence that the diagnostic accuracy of either SPECT or PET is not higher than the clinical criteria in AD. Nonetheless, both functional imaging techniques appear promising for differentiating other dementia syndromes (frontotemporal dementia and dementia with Lewy bodies) from AD due to differences in regional functional involvement.

Supporting Evidence: With visual evaluation of SPECT images for temporoparietal hypoperfusion, the sensitivity for distinguishing AD patients from normal differed from 42 to 79% at a specificity of 86 to 90%, being lower in patients with mild AD than in patients with severe AD in both clinically and pathologically confirmed cases (43–45), and not superior to the clinical diagnosis based on NINCDS-ADRDA criteria (46) (strong evidence). The regional decrease in cerebral perfusion with SPECT correlated with the neurofibrillary pathology staging of AD (47) (strong evidence); SPECT increased the accuracy of clinical evaluation for identifying AD pathology, but cases with other types of dementia were not included (48) (moderate evidence).

The sensitivity and specificity of the temporoparietal metabolic decline on PET for differentiating patients with pathologically confirmed AD from normal subjects was 63% and 82%, respectively, similar to the sensitivity (63%), but lower than the specificity (100%) of clinical diagnosis in the same cohort (49) (strong evidence). On the other hand, occipital hypometabolism on PET distinguished pathologically confirmed patients with dementia with Lewy bodies from AD patients with a comparable specificity (80%) and higher sensitivity (90%) than clinical evaluation (strong evidence) (50, 51).

Visual evaluation of SPECT images for temporoparietal hypoperfusion distinguished clinically confirmed AD patients from those with frontotemporal dementia by correctly classifying 74% of AD patients with decreased blood flow in the parietal lobes and 81% of frontotemporal dementia patients with decreased blood flow in the frontal lobes (52) (moderate evidence).

Visual interpretation of PET images for temporoparietal glucose metabolism was reliable (κ=0.42–0.61) (53), and PET was more useful than SPECT for differentiating clinically confirmed patients with AD from normal elderly (54). With automated data analysis methods, PET could distinguish clinically confirmed AD cases from normal with a sensitivity of 93–93% specificity (55) (moderate evidence).

C. Other Magnetic Resonance Techniques

Summary of Evidence: Due to the ease of integrating an extra pulse sequence into the standard structural MRI exam, and the advantage of obtaining metabolic or functional information different from that of the anatomic MRI, other magnetic resonance (MR) techniques have also been investigated for the diagnosis of AD. The utility of these MR techniques remains to be confirmed with the standard of histopathology (moderate evidence).

Supporting Evidence: One of the most extensively studied MR techniques for the diagnosis of AD is ^{1}H MR spectroscopy (^{1}H MRS), which provides biochemical information from hydrogen proton–containing metabolites in the brain (Fig. 10.1). A decrease in the ratio of the neuronal metabolite NAA to the metabolite myo-inositol (MI) distinguished AD patients from normal with a sensitivity of 83% and specificity of 98% in a clinically confirmed cohort (56). A decrease in NAA levels on ^{1}H MRS of the frontal lobe also distinguished clinically diagnosed patients with frontotemporal dementia from patients with AD with an accuracy of 84% (57) (moderate evidence). Another functional imaging technique, dynamic susceptibility MRI, has been proposed as an alternative to SPECT for the quantitation of temporoparietal hypoperfusion in AD, and the sensitivity and specificity of this technique have been comparable to those of SPECT (58) (moderate evidence).

The diagnostic accuracy of other quantitative MRI techniques, such as diffusion-weighted MRI (DWI) and magnetization transfer MRI to distinguish AD patients from normal elderly in clinically confirmed cohorts, was lower than that of clinical evaluation (59, 60), and evidence is lacking on the diagnostic accuracy of either functional MRI or phosphorus (^{31}P) MRS in AD (insufficient evidence).

III. Can Neuroimaging Identify Individuals at Elevated Risk for Alzheimer Disease and Predict Its Future Development?

A. Prodromal Alzheimer Disease, or Mild Cognitive Impairment

Summary of Evidence: There is moderate evidence that quantitative MR techniques and PET are sensitive to the structural and functional changes in patients with amnestic mild cognitive impairment (MCI). Magnetic resonance-based evaluation of the hippocampal volumes is associated with the rate of future development of AD in individuals with MCI based on clinically confirmed cases, and PET can predict subsequent clinical behavior in cognitively normal elderly.

Supporting Evidence: Risk groups for AD are composed of individuals identified through either clinical examination or family history and genetic testing who have a greater probability of developing AD than members of the general population, and in whom the relevant exposures are absent. The rationale for identifying imaging criteria for those at elevated risk comes from recent advances in disease-modifying therapies. Individuals with elevated probability of developing AD are the primary targets of these treatment trials aimed at preventing or delaying the neurodegenerative process. Thus, biomarkers that can accurately distinguish individuals at risk and predict if and when they will develop AD are required in

order to utilize these interventions before the neurodegenerative disease advances and irreversible damage occurs.

Aging is a risk factor for AD, and elderly individuals who develop AD pass through a transitional phase of a decline in memory function before meeting the clinical criteria for AD (61). This early symptomatic or prodromal phase has several clinical definitions some of which are MCI, age-associated memory impairment, clinical dementia rating score of 0.5, cognitive impairment, or minimal impairment. While the clinical criteria for each syndrome show similarities, they are subtly different. Longitudinal studies show that individuals with MCI, specifically amnestic MCI are at a higher risk of developing AD than normal elderly (62). Patients with MCI have the earliest features of AD pathology with neuron loss and atrophy in the anteromedial temporal lobe, specifically the entorhinal cortex, which is involved in memory processing (63). There is strong evidence that there is an association between pathologic involvement and cognitive impairment in the evolution of AD (8, 10, 11). Hence patients with MCI reside between normal aging and AD, both in the pathologic and in the cognitive continuum (Fig. 10.2) (strong evidence).

In concordance with the pathologic evolution of AD, MR-based volumetry identified smaller hippocampal and entorhinal cortex volumes in patients with MCI than in normal elderly (36, 64) (Fig. 10.3). Among several regions in the temporal lobe, reduced hippocampal volumes on MRI and hippocampal glucose metabolism on PET were the best discriminator of patients with MCI from normal elderly (65). Hippocampal volumes were also comparable to entorhinal cortex volumes for distinguishing patients with MCI (36, 65), elderly individuals with mild memory problems, and very mild AD (66, 67) from normal (moderate evidence). Other quantitative MRI techniques, such as DWI and magnetization transfer MRI measurements, have also revealed that the diffusivity of water is increased and magnetization transfer ratios are decreased in the hippocampi of patients with MCI relative to normals, both of which indicate an increase in free water, presumably due to hippocampal neuronal damage (59, 68) (moderate evidence).

Because all patients with MCI do not develop AD at a similar rate, markers that can predict the rate of development of AD have important implications for assessing the effectiveness of therapies aimed at preventing or delaying development of AD in patients with MCI. Premorbid hippocampal and parahippocampal volumes (69), visual ranking of hippocampal atrophy (70, 71), and measurements of entorhinal cortex volume (67) were associated with future development of AD in patients with mild memory difficulties and MCI. PET (72–74) and SPECT (75–77) have also been shown to predict subsequent development of MCI and AD in clinically determined normal elderly individuals, people with memory impairment, MCI, and questionable AD (moderate evidence).

Two ¹H MRS studies revealed that MI/creatine (Cr) levels are higher in both MCI and AD patients than in normal elderly. Furthermore, NAA/Cr levels were lower in AD, but not in MCI patients, than in normal elderly in the posterior cingulate gyri of clinically confirmed cases (78, 79) (Fig. 10.4). Similar findings were encountered from neocortical regions in mild AD patients (80), which suggest that MI/Cr levels increase before a significant decrease in the neuronal metabolite NAA/Cr (moderate evidence).

The finding of an early increase in MI/Cr in MCI is encouraging because NAA/Cr is a marker for neuronal integrity. Thus an increase in MI/Cr levels in patients with MCI may predict future development of AD before substantial neuronal damage occurs. This hypothesis remains to be tested with longitudinal studies on these individuals (insufficient evidence).

No study has yet investigated the pathologic correlates of neuroimaging findings in patients with MCI (insufficient evidence).

B. Asymptomatic Apolipoprotein E ε4 Carriers

Summary of Evidence: The most recognized susceptibility gene in sporadic AD is Apolipoprotein E (ApoE) ε4 allele, which has been shown to influence age of onset (81) and amyloid plaque burden (82) in AD. Posterior cingulate gyrus hypometabolism, and the rate of decline in glucose metabolism on PET, is associated with ApoE genotype in people with normal cognition (moderate evidence).

Supporting Evidence: While some studies showed that ApoE genotype does not have any influence on hippocampal volumes (83, 84), others found an association between ApoE genotype and medial temporal lobe atrophy (85, 86). The dissociation between hippocampal volumes and ApoE genotype may increase the accuracy of both markers for predicting development of AD in the elderly, when combined in prediction models. Posterior cingulate gyrus hypometabolism, and the rate of decline in glucose metabolism on PET on the other hand, is associated with ApoE genotype in people with normal cognition (87–89) (moderate evidence).

Evidence is lacking on the predictive value of PET for development of AD in carriers versus noncarriers of the ApoE ε4 allele, which requires further investigation with longitudinal studies. No studies were identified on the neuroimaging correlates of ApoE genotype in pathologically confirmed cohorts (insufficient evidence).

IV. Is Neuroimaging Cost-Effective for the Clinical Evaluation of Alzheimer Disease?

Summary of Evidence: Current treatment options for AD may reduce the social and economic costs of the disease by slowing the rate of cognitive decline, improving the quality of life, and delaying nursing home placement. Neuroimaging may contribute to identification of individuals with early AD who may benefit from such therapies. Use of PET in early dementia can increase the accuracy of clinical diagnosis without adding to the overall costs of the evaluation (moderate evidence). However, the cost-effectiveness analysis revealed that the addition of SPECT, dynamic susceptibility contrast-enhanced MRI, and PET to the diagnostic workup of AD was not cost-effective considering the currently available treatment options (moderate evidence).

Supporting Evidence: One study indicated that PET increases the diagnostic accuracy for early AD, reducing the rate of false-negative and false-positive diagnoses and avoiding unnecessary treatment costs and late interventions, without increasing the costs of evaluation and management of AD (90). On the other hand, the cost-effectiveness analysis of SPECT, dynamic susceptibility contrast-enhanced MRI (91), and PET (92, 93) for the diagnosis of AD revealed that the addition of functional neuroimaging to the diagnostic workup of AD in an AD clinic is not cost-effective considering the assumed effectiveness of the drug donepezil hydrochloride (moderate evidence).

The cost-effectiveness of a diagnostic modality is directly related to the effectiveness of the therapy for the condition being diagnosed. Thus, cost-effectiveness studies on the diagnostic procedures in AD should be viewed in the context of minimal effectiveness of currently available treatment options. The outcome of cost-effectiveness analyses of diagnostic modalities in AD could change dramatically when more effective therapies become available. No study investigated the cost-effectiveness of neuroimaging in clinical decision making in pathologically confirmed cohorts (insufficient evidence).

V. Can Neuroimaging Measure Disease Progression and Therapeutic Efficacy in Alzheimer Disease?

Summary of Evidence: Recent advances in treatments aimed at inhibiting the pathologic process of AD created a need for biologic markers that can accurately measure the effectiveness of therapeutic interventions. Neuropsychologic measures of memory and cognitive function can monitor the symptomatic progression in patients with AD. Yet, monitoring biologic progression is only possible with markers closely related to the neurodegenerative pathology. The usefulness of neuroimaging as a surrogate for therapeutic efficacy in AD remains to be tested in trials with large cohorts and positive therapeutic outcomes. Currently, there is insufficient evidence that neuroimaging can be a surrogate for therapeutic efficacy in AD (insufficient evidence).

Supporting Evidence: Magnetic resonance (MR)-based hippocampal volumetry and regional perfusion on SPECT correlate with the stage of pathologic involvement in AD (37, 47) (strong evidence). Serial measurements of whole brain volumes using the boundary shift integral method on MRI (94–96) and MR-based hippocampal volumetry (97, 98) revealed that the rate of atrophy is associated with cognitive

decline in patients with AD over time. Serial MR measures of the rate of atrophy in AD may be a valuable surrogate in drug trials. Serial brain to ventricular volume ratio measurements on MRI indicate that to detect a 20% excess rate of atrophy with 90% power in AD in 6 months, 135 subjects would be required in each arm of a randomized placebo-controlled trial, and for 30% excess rate of atrophy, 61 subjects would be required (99) (moderate evidence).

Magnetic resonance-based volume measurements of the whole brain and the hippocampus are valid macroscopic measures of ongoing atrophy in AD. Functional imaging techniques, on the other hand, provide markers related to the neurodegenerative pathology at the microscopic level. Longitudinal decrease of the neuronal metabolite NAA on ^{1}H MRS (100, 101), regional glucose metabolism on PET (102), and cerebral blood flow on SPECT (103, 104) are associated with the cognitive decline in AD (moderate evidence).

Although it is possible to monitor AD pathology once it is established, irreversible damage characterized by neuron and synapse loss in the anteromedial temporal lobe starts earlier (8–12). The effectiveness of disease-modifying treatments is expected to be greatest on those patients who are at the very early stages of pathologic involvement but have not yet met the current clinical criteria for AD. For these treatment trials, the most crucial stage for monitoring pathologic progression is the prodromal phase, such as MCI (62). The rate of hippocampal volume loss measured with serial MRI exams in patients with MCI and normal elderly individuals correlates with cognitive decline, as these individuals progress in the cognitive continuum from normal to MCI and to AD (105) (moderate evidence). Similarly, the decrease in whole brain volumes (106) and cerebral metabolism on PET (107) is associated with cognitive decline in patients under the genetic risk of developing AD, although the outcome of these risk groups is not known at this time (moderate evidence).

Clinical rating scales and neuropsychological tests are regarded as the gold standard for assessing disease progression and therapeutic efficacy in AD. However, imaging markers may be more accurate in measuring pathologic progression. Estimated sample sizes required to power an effective therapeutic trial (25–50% reduction in rate of deterioration over 1 year) in

MCI indicate that the required sample sizes are substantially smaller for MRI volumetry than commonly used cognitive tests or clinical rating scales at the early stages of disease progression (108). These data support the use of MRI along with clinical and psychometric measures as surrogate markers of disease progression in AD therapeutic trials (moderate evidence).

Take Home Tables (Tables 10.1 and 10.2)

Tables 10.1–10.2 and Fig. 10.1–10.4 serve to highlight key recommendations and supporting evidence.

Suggested Protocols

Computed Tomography Imaging

- *CT without contrast:* Axial 5- to 10-mm images should be used to assess for cerebral hemorrhage, mass effect, normal pressure hydrocephalus or calcifications.
- *CT with contrast:* Axial 5- to 10-mm enhanced images should be used in patients with suspected neoplasm, infection, or other focal intracranial lesion. If indicated, CT angiography can be performed as part of the enhanced CT.

Magnetic Resonance Imaging

- A scout image is acquired to ensure symmetric positioning of the brain within the field of view.

- Sagittal T1-weighted spin-echo sequence (TR/TE = 500/20) is used for standard diagnostic purposes and measuring intracranial volume where applicable.
- Coronal three-dimensional volumetric acquisition is used with 124 partitions and 1.6-mm slice thickness (TR/TE/flip angle = 23/6/25).
- Axial double spin echo (TR/TE = 2200/30 and 80) or axial fast FLAIR (fluid-attenuated inversion recovery) sequences (TR/TE/TI = 16000/140/2600) are used for standard diagnostic purposes and assessment of cerebrovascular disease.
- In patients with suspected neoplasm, infection, or focal intracranial lesions, gadolinium-enhanced T1-weighted conventional spin-echo (TR/TE = 500/20) images should be acquired in at least two planes.

Fluorodeoxyglucose-PET and SPECT Imaging

- Standard brain fluorodeoxyglucose (FDG)-PET and SPECT protocols can be used.
- The intravenously injection of the radiopharmaceutical should take place in a controlled environment with minimal sensory input (dimly lit room with minimal ambient noise).
- The dose of radiopharmaceuticals [FDG for PET, technetium-99m (Tc-99m) ECD (bicisate) or Tc-99m HMPAO (exametazime) for SPECT] may differ between scanners.

Table 10.1. Sensitivity and specificity of neuroimaging techniques in distinguishing Alzheimer disease (AD) from normal elderly

Source	No. of controls	No. of AD patients	Neuroimaging modality	Sensitivity (%)	Specificity (%)
Jack et al. (42)	126	94	MRI (hippocampal volumes)	CDR 0.5 : 78 CDR 1 : 84 CDR 2 : 87	80
O'Brien et al. (38)	40	77	MRI (visual evaluation)	83	80
Laasko et al. (41)	42	55	MRI (hippocampal volumes)	82–90	86–98
Wahlund et al. (39)	66	41	MRI (visual evaluation + MMSE scores)	95	96
Xu et al. (36)	30	30	MRI (hippocampal volumes)	83	80
Herholtz et al. (55)	110	395	PET (automated analysis)	93	93
Silverman et al. (109)[a]	97	18	PET (visual evaluation)	94	73
Claus et al. (43)	60	48	SPECT (visual evaluation)	42–79[b]	90
Shonk et al. (56)	65	32	^{1}H MRS (myoinositol/N-acetylaspartate)	83	98
Kantarci et al. (110)	61	22	^{1}H MRS (N-acetylaspartate/myoinositol)	82	80

CDR clinical dementia rating scale, *MMSE* mini-mental status examination, *MRI* magnetic resonance imaging, *MRS* magnetic resonance spectroscopy, *PET* positron emission tomography, *SPECT* single photon emission computed tomography.

[a]The diagnoses were pathologically confirmed.

[b]Mild to severe AD. Reprinted with kind permission of Springer Science+Business Media from Kantarci K, Jack, Jr, CR. Neuroimaging in Alzheimer Disease. In Medina LS, Blackmore CC (eds.): *Evidence-Based Imaging: Optimizing Imaging in Patient Care.* New York: Springer Science+Business Media, 2006.

Table 10.2. Suggested diagnostic evaluation for suspected dementia or mild cognitive impairment (MCI)

Detailed clinical evaluation
Structural imaging with CT or MRI
PET and SPECT if the diagnosis is still uncertain

Reprinted with kind permission of Springer Science+Business Media from Kantarci K, Jack, Jr, CR. Neuroimaging in Alzheimer Disease. In Medina LS, Blackmore CC (eds.): *Evidence-Based Imaging: Optimizing Imaging in Patient Care.* New York: Springer Science+Business Media, 2006.

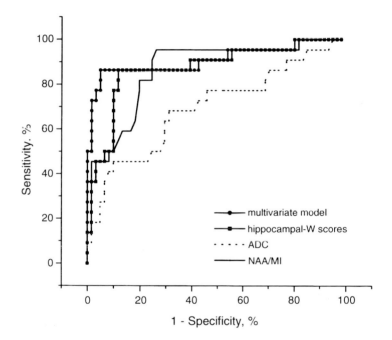

Figure 10.1. Receiver operating characteristic (ROC) plots of magnetic resonance (MR) measurements in distinguishing patients with a clinical diagnosis of Alzheimer disease (AD) from cognitively normal elderly. MRI-based hippocampal volumetry (W scores), hippocampal apparent diffusion coefficients (ADC) on diffusion weighted MRI, *N*-acetylaspartate/myoinositol (NAA/MI) on ^{1}H MR spectroscopy, and the multivariate model derived from these three MR measurements were plotted. While the multivariate model is slightly more accurate in distinguishing AD from normal, there is no significant difference between the hippocampal W scores and NAA/MI in distinguishing the two groups. The hippocampal ADC, on the other hand, is less accurate than hippocampal W scores and NAA/MI. (Source: Kantarci et al. (110), with permission from S. Karger AG, Base.)

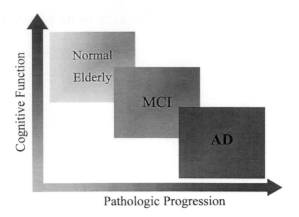

Figure 10.2. In the cognitive continuum, people with mild cognitive impairment (MCI) reside at a transitional clinical state between cognitively normal elderly, and people with AD. People with MCI are also at an intermediate stage between asymptomatic elderly individuals with early pathologic involvement of AD to people with established AD. (Reprinted with kind permission of Springer Science+Business Media from Kantarci K, Jack, Jr, CR. Neuroimaging in Alzheimer Disease. In Medina LS, Blackmore CC (eds): *Evidence-Based Imaging: Optimizing Imaging in Patient Care.* New York: Springer Science+Business Media, 2006.)

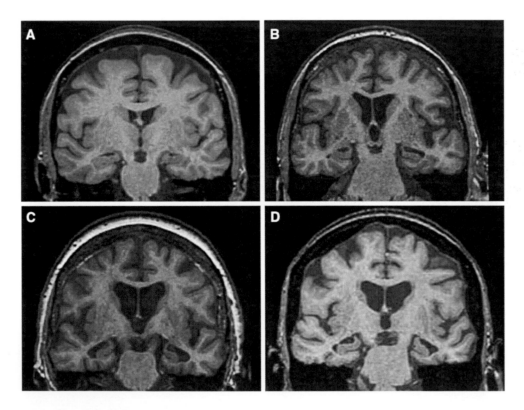

Figure 10.3. T1-weighted three-dimensional spoiled gradient echo images at the level of hippocampal heads in a 76-year-old cognitively normal subject (**A**), a 77-year-old patient with MCI (**B**), a 75-year-old patient with AD (**C**), and a 95-year-old cognitively normal subject (**D**). Patients with AD, MCI, and the 95-year-old cognitively normal subject have brain atrophy, which is marked in the hippocampi and the temporal lobes in the MCI and AD subject, compared to the younger normal subject. Atrophy is more severe in the AD subject than in the MCI subject. In this case, the age-adjusted regional and global volume measurements would be useful in differentiating atrophy due to normal aging from atrophy due to AD pathology. (Reprinted with kind permission of Springer Science+Business Media from Kantarci K, Jack, Jr, CR. Neuroimaging in Alzheimer Disease. In Medina LS, Blackmore CC (eds.): *Evidence-Based Imaging: Optimizing Imaging in Patient Care.* New York: Springer Science+Business Media, 2006.)

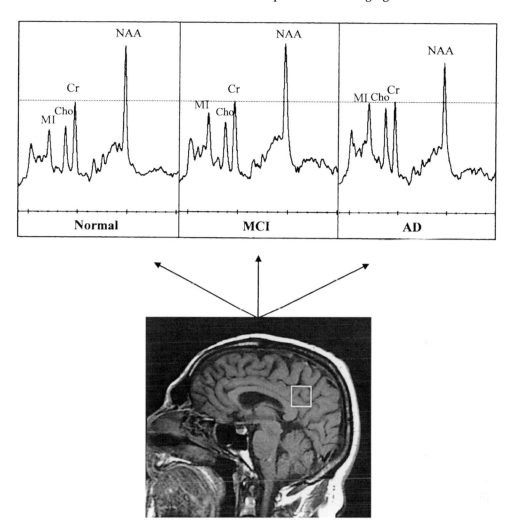

Figure 10.4. Examples of ^{1}H MR spectra obtained from the posterior cingulate volume of interest (VOI) with an echo time of 30 ms in an 81-year-old cognitively normal subject, a 77-year-old patient with MCI, and a 79-year-old patient with AD. The VOI is placed on a midsagittal T1-weighted localizing image, which includes right and left posterior cingulate gyri and inferior precunei. The ^{1}H MR spectra are scaled to the creatine (Cr) peak (dashed line). Cr peak is found to be stable in AD and is commonly used as an internal reference for quantitation of other metabolite peaks. Myoinositol (MI)/Cr ratio is higher in the patient with MCI than the normal subject. Choline (Cho)/Cr and MI/Cr ratio is higher, and N-acetylaspartate (NAA)/Cr ratio is lower in the patient with AD than in both the patient with MCI and the normal subject. (Reprinted with kind permission of Springer Science+Business Media from Kantarci K, Jack, Jr, CR. Neuroimaging in Alzheimer Disease. In Medina LS, Blackmore CC (eds.): *Evidence-Based Imaging: Optimizing Imaging in Patient Care.* New York: Springer Science+Business Media, 2006.)

Future Research Areas

- Validating the clinical criteria for AD by clinicians with different levels of expertise and at different clinical settings.
- Determining the choice of either CT or MRI for the initial evaluation of dementia in large-scale clinical trials.
- Validating the usefulness of PET, SPECT, and MR techniques for the diagnosis of AD with autopsy confirmation in large-scale clinical trials.
- Determining the cost-effectiveness of neuroimaging techniques as effective treatments become available for AD.
- Determining the usefulness of neuroimaging as a surrogate for therapeutic efficacy in trials with positive therapeutic outcomes.

References

1. Kokmen E, Beard CM, O'Brien PC et al. Neurology 1993;43:1887–1892.
2. Beard CM, Kokmen E, O'Brien PC et al. Neurology 1995;45:75–79.
3. Advisory Panel on Alzheimer Disease and Related Dementias: Acute and Long-Term Care Services. NIH publication 96–4136. Washington, DC: U.S. Department of Health and Human Services, 1996.
4. Brookmeyer R, Gray S, Kawas C. Am J Public Health 1998;88(9):1337–1342.
5. 2001–2002 Alzheimer Disease Progress Report. National Institutes of Health publication No. 03–5333, July 2003, p. 2.
6. Knapp MJ, Knopman DS, Solomon PR et al. JAMA 1994;271(13):985–991.
7. Rogers SL, Farlow MR, Doody RS et al. Neurology 1998;50(1):136–145.
8. Price JL, Morris JC. Ann Neurol 1999;45:358–368.
9. Schmitt FA, Davis DG, Wekstein DR, Smith CD et al. Neurology 2000;55:370–376.
10. Grober E, Dickson D, Sliwinski MJ et al. Neurobiol Aging 1999;20(6):573–579.
11. Delacourte A, David JP, Sergeant N et al. Neurology 1999;52:1158–1165.
12. Morris JC, Storandt M, McKeel DW Jr et al. Neurology 1996;46:707–719.
13. The National Institute on Aging, and Reagan Institute Working Group on Diagnostic Criteria for the Neuropathological Assessment of Alzheimer Disease. Neurobiol Aging 1997;18(4):S1–S2.
14. American Psychiatric Association. Diagnostic and Statistical Manual of Mental Disorders, 3rd ed., revised. DSM-IIIR. Washington, DC: APA, 1987.
15. Mc Khann GM, Drachman D, Folstein M et al. Neurology 1984;34:939–944.
16. Lim A, Tsuang D, Kukull W et al. J Am Geriatr Soc 1999;47(5):564–569.
17. Victoroff J, Mack WJ, Lyness SA et al. Am J Psychiatry 1995;152(10):1476–1484.
18. Galasko D, Hansen LA, Katzman R. Arch Neurol 1994;51(9):888–895.
19. Massoud F, Devi G, Stern Y et al. Arch Neurol 1999;56(11):1368–1373.
20. Blacker D, Albert MS, Bassett SS et al. Arch Neurol 1994;51(12):1198–1204.
21. Kukull WA, Larson EB, Reifler BV et al. Neurology 1990;40(9):1364–1369.
22. Massoud F, Devi G, Moroney JT. J Am Geriatr Soc 2000;48:1204–1210.
23. Jobst KA, Barnetson LP, Shepstone BJ. Int Psychogeriatr 1998;10(3):271–302.
24. Fratiglioni L, Grut M, Forsell Y et al. Arch Neurol 1992;49(9):927–932.
25. Graham JE, Rockwood K, Beattie BL et al. Neuroepidemiology 1996;15(5):246–256.
26. Blacker D, Albert MS, Bassett SS et al. Arch Neurol 1994;51(12):1198–204.
27. Baldereschi M, Amato MP, Nencini P et al. Neurology 1994;44(2):239–242.
28. Knopman DS, DeKosky ST, Cummings JL et al. Neurology 2001;56:1143–1153.
29. Jack CR Jr, Petersen RC, O'Brien PC et al. Neurology 1992;42:183–188.
30. Braak H, Braak E. Acta Neuropathol (Berl) 1991;82:239–259.
31. Gomez-Isla T, Hollister R, West H et al. Ann Neurol 1997;41:17–24.
32. Arriagata PV, Growdon JH, Hedley-Whyte ET et al. Neurology 1992;42:631–639.
33. Bobinski M, de Leon MJ, Wegiel J et al. Neuroscience 2000;95(3):721–725.
34. Chui H, Qian Z. Neurology 1997;49(4):925–935.
35. Nagy Z, Hindley NJ, Braak H. Dementia Geriatr Cogn Disord 1999;10(2):109–114.
36. Xu Y, Jack CR Jr, O'Brien PC et al. Neurology 2000;54:1760–1767.
37. Jack CR Jr, Dickson DW, Parisi JE et al. Neurology 2002;58:750–757.
38. O'Brien JT, Desmond P, Ames D, Schweitzer I, Chiu E, Tress B. Psychol Med 1997;27(6):1267–1275.
39. Wahlund LO, Julin P, Johansson SE et al. J Neurol Neurosurg Psychiatry 2000;69(5): 630–635.
40. Juottonen K, Laasko MP, Insausti R et al. Neurobiol Aging 1998;19(1):15–22.
41. Laasko MP, Soininen H, Partanen K et al. Neurobiol Aging 1998;19(1):23–3.
42. Jack CR, Petersen RC, Xu Y et al. Neurology 1997;49:786–794.

43. Claus JJ, van Harskamp F, Breteler MM. Neurology 1994;44(3 pt 1):454–461.
44. Van Gool WA, Walstra GJ, Teunisse S et al. J Neurol 1995;242(2):401–405.
45. Bonte FJ, Weiner MF, Bigio EH et al. Radiology 1997;202(3):793–797.
46. Mattman A, Feldman H, Forster B et al. Can J Neurol Sci 1997;24(1):22–28.
47. Bradley KM, O'Sullivan VT, Soper ND et al. Brain 2002;125(8):1772–1781.
48. Jagust W, Thisted R, Devous MD et al. Neurology 2001;56:950–956.
49. Hoffman JM, Welsh-Bohmer KA, Hanson MW et al. J Nucl Med 2000;41(11):1920–1928.
50. Minoshima S, Foster NL, Sima AA et al. Ann Neurol 2001;50(3):358–365.
51. McKeith IG, Ballard CG, Perry RH et al. Neurology 2000;54:1050–1058.
52. Pickut BA, Saerens J, Marien P et al. J Nucl Med 1997;38(6):929–934.
53. Hoffman JM, Hanson MW, Welsh KA et al. Invest Radiol 1996;31(6):316–322.
54. Messa C, Perani D, Lucignani G et al. J Nucl Med 1994;35(2):210–216.
55. Herholz K, Salmon E, Perani D et al. Neuroimage 2002;17:302–316.
56. Shonk TK, Moats RA, Gifford PG et al. Radiology 1995;195:65–72.
57. Ernst T, Chang L, Melchor R et al. Radiology 1997;203:829–836.
58. Harris GJ, Lewis RF, Satlin A et al. AJNR 1998;19(9):1727–1732.
59. Kantarci K, Jack CR, Xu YC et al. Radiology 2001;219:101–107.
60. Hanyu H, Asano T, Iwamoto T et al. AJNR 2000;21:1235–1242.
61. Petersen RC, Smith GE, Ivnik RJ et al. Neurology 1994;44:867–872.
62. Petersen RC, Smith GE, Waring SC et al. Arch Neurol 1999;56:303–308.
63. Kordower JH, Chu Y, Stebbins GT et al. Ann Neurol 2001;49:202–213.
64. Du AT, Schuff N, Amend D et al. J Neurol Neurosurg Psychiatry 2001;71(4):431–432.
65. De Santi S, de Leon MJ, Rusinek H et al. Neurobiol Aging 2001;22(4):529–539.
66. Dickerson BC, Goncharova I, Sullivan MP et al. Neurobiol Aging 2001;22(5):747–754.
67. Killany RJ, Gomez-Isla T, Moss M et al. Ann Neurol 2000;47:430–439.
68. Kabani NJ, Sled JG, Shuper A et al. Magn Reson Med 2002;47:143–148.
69. Jack CR, Petersen RC, Xu Y et al. Neurology 1999;52:1397–1403.
70. Visser PJ, Scheltens P, Verhey FR et al. J Neurol 1999;246(6):477–485.
71. de Leon MJ, Golomb J, George AE et al. AJNR 1993;14:897–906.
72. de Leon MJ, Convit A, Wolf AT et al. Proc Natl Acad Sci 2001;286:2120–2127.
73. Chetelat G, Desgranges B, de la Sayette V, Viader F, Eustache F, Baron JC. Neurology 2003;60:1374–1377.
74. Drzezga A, Lautenschlager N, Siebner H et al. Eur J Nucl Med Mol Imaging 2003;30(8):1104–1113.
75. Huang C, Wahlund LO, Svensson L, Winblad B, Julin P. BMC Neurology 2002;2(1):9.
76. Tanaka M, Fukuyama H, Yamauchi H et al. J Neuroimaging 2002;12(2):112–118.
77. Johnson KA, Jones K, Holman BL et al. Neurology 1998;50:1563–1571.
78. Kantarci K, Jack CR, Xu YC et al. Neurology 2000;55(2):210–217.
79. Catani M, Cherubini A, Howard R. Neuroreport 2001;12(11):2315–2317.
80. Huang W, Alexander GE, Chang L et al. Neurology 2001;57:626–632.
81. Tsai MS, Tangalos E, Petersen R et al. Am J Human Genet 1994;54:643–649.
82. Gomez-Isla T, West HL, Rebeck GW et al. Ann Neurol 1996;39:62–70.
83. Jack CR, Petersen RC, Xu Y et al. Ann Neurol 1998;43:303–310.
84. Barber R, Gholkar A, Scheltens P et al. Arch Neurol 1999;56(8):961–965.
85. Geroldi C, Pihlajamaki M, Laasko MP et al. Neurology 1999;53:1825–1832.
86. Lehtovirta M, Soininen H, Laasko MP et al. J Neurol Neurosurg Psychiatry 1996;60:644–649.
87. Small GW, Mazziotta JC, Collins MT et al. JAMA 1995;273:942–947.
88. Reiman EM, Caselli RJ, Yun LS et al. N Engl J Med 1996;334:752–758.
89. Small GW, Ercoli LM, Silverman DH et al. Proc Natl Acad Sci 2000;97(11):6037–6042.
90. Silverman DH, Gambhir SS, Huang HW. J Nucl Med 2002;43(2):253–266.
91. McMahon PM, Araki SS, Neumann PJ et al. Radiology 2000;217:58–68.
92. McMahon PM, Araki SS, Sandberg EA, Neumann PJ, Gazelle GS. Radiology 2003;228: 515–522.
93. Kulasingam SL, Samsa GP, Zarin DA et al. Value Health 2003;6(5):542–550.
94. Freeborough PA, Fox NC. IEEE Trans Med Imaging 1997;15:623–629.
95. Fox NC, Cousens S, Scahill R et al. Arch Neurol 2000;57(3):339–344.
96. Fox NC, Warrington EK, Rossor MN. Lancet 1999;353:2125.
97. Jack CR, Petersen RC, Xu Y et al. Neurology 1998;51:993–999.
98. Laasko MP, Lehtovirta M, Partanen K et al. Biol Psychiatry 2000;47(6):557–561.
99. Bradley KM, Bydder GM, Budge MM et al. Br J Radiol 2002;75(894):506–513.
100. Adalsteinsson E, Sullivan EV, Kleinhans N et al. Lancet 2000;355:1696–1697.

101. Jessen F, Block W, Träber F et al. Neurology 2001;57(5):930–932.
102. Smith GS, de Leon MJ, George AE et al. Arch Neurol 1992;49:1142–1150.
103. Brown DR, Hunter R, Wyper DJ et al. J Psychiatr Res 1996;30(2):109–126.
104. Shih WJ, Ashford WJ, Coupal JJ et al. Clin Nucl Med 1999;24(10):773–777.
105. Jack CR, Petersen RC, Xu Y et al. Neurology 2000;55:484–489.
106. Fox NC, Crum WF, Scahill RI et al. Lancet 2001;358:201–205.
107. Reiman EM, Caselli RJ, Chen K et al. Proc Natl Acad Sci 2001;98:3334–3339.
108. Jack CR, Shiung MM, Gunter JL et al. Neurology 2004;62:591–600.
109. Silverman DHS, Small GW, Chang CY et al. JAMA 2001;286(17):2120–2127.
110. Kantarci K, Xu YC, Shiung MM et al. Dementia Geriatr Cogn Disord 2002;14(4):198–207.

11

Neuroimaging in Acute Ischemic Stroke

Katie D. Vo, Weili Lin, and Jin-Moo Lee

Issues

   I. What is the imaging modality of choice for the detection of intra-cranial hemorrhage?
     A. Computed tomography
     B. Magnetic resonance imaging
  II. What are the imaging modalities of choice for the identification of brain ischemia and the exclusion of stroke mimics?
     A. Computed tomography
     B. Magnetic resonance imaging
 III. What imaging modality should be used for the determination of tissue viability: the ischemic penumbra?
     A. Magnetic resonance imaging
     B. Computed tomography
     C. Positron emission tomography
     D. Single photon emission computed tomography (SPECT)
 IV. What is the role of noninvasive intracranial vascular imaging?
     A. Computed tomography angiography
     B. Magnetic resonance angiography
  V. What is the role of acute neuroimaging in pediatric stroke?

Key Points

- Noncontrast computed tomography (CT) is currently accepted as the gold standard for the detection of intracranial hemorrhage, though rigorous data is lacking (limited evidence) Magnetic resonance imaging (MRI) is equivalent to CT in the detection of intracranial hemorrhage (strong evidence), but its role in the evaluation of thrombolytic candidates has not been studied.

K.D. Vo (✉)
Mallinckrodt Institute of Radiology, Washington University School of Medicine, St. Louis, MO 63110, USA
e-mail: vok@wustl.edu

L.S. Medina et al. (eds.), *Evidence-Based Imaging: Improving the Quality of Imaging in Patient Care, Revised Edition,*
DOI 10.1007/978-1-4419-7777-9_11, © Springer Science+Business Media, LLC 2011

- Noncontrast CT of the head should be performed in all patients who are candidates for thrombolytic therapy to exclude intracerebral hemorrhage (strong evidence).
- Magnetic resonance (MR) (diffusion-weighted imaging) is superior to CT for detection of cerebral ischemia within the first 24 h of symptom onset (moderate evidence); however, some argue that identification of ischemia merely confirms a clinical diagnosis and does not necessarily influence acute clinical decision making, or outcome.
- Advanced functional imaging such as MR perfusion, MR spectroscopy, CT perfusion, xenon CT, SPECT, and PET show promise in improving patient selection and individualizing therapeutic time windows (limited evidence), but the data are inadequate for routine use in the current management of stroke patients.

Definition and Pathophysiology

This chapter focuses on imaging within the first few hours of stroke onset, where issues relating to the decision to administer thrombolytics are of paramount importance. *Stroke* is a clinical term that describes an acute neurologic deficit due to a sudden disruption of blood supply to the brain. Stroke is caused by either an occlusion of an artery (ischemic stroke or cerebral ischemia/infarction) or rupture of an artery leading to bleeding into or around the brain (hemorrhagic stroke or intracranial hemorrhage). The vast majority of strokes are ischemic (88%), whereas 9% are intracerebral hemorrhages, and 3% are subarachnoid hemorrhages (1). Ischemic stroke can be divided into several subtypes based on etiology: small-vessel strokes (40%), large-vessel atherothrombotic strokes (20%), cardioembolic strokes (20%), and strokes from unknown etiologies (20%) (2). Risk factors for stroke include age, male gender, race (African American), previous history of stroke, diabetes, hypertension, heart disease, smoking, and alcohol. Treatment of ischemic stroke can be divided into acute therapies, consisting of thrombolysis with tissue plasminogen activator (tPA) and management of secondary complications (edema, herniation, and hemorrhage); and preventative therapies, aimed at reducing the risk of recurrent stroke.

Epidemiology

It is estimated that approximately 731,000 new or recurrent strokes occur annually, and that a new stroke occurs every 45 s in United States (1, 3).

This number is expected to increase as the population ages. The third leading cause of mortality after heart disease and cancer, stroke, results in approximately 160,000 deaths per year, leaving 4.6 million stroke survivors in the United States. Fifteen to 30% of stroke survivors are permanently disabled or require institutional care, making it the leading cause of severe long-term disability and the leading diagnosis from hospital to long-term care (1, 4, 5).

Overall Cost to Society

The estimated direct and indirect costs of stroke are $53.6 billion in 2004, with 62% of the cost related directly to medical expenditures (1). Acute inpatient hospital costs account for 70% of the first-year post-stroke cost; the contribution of diagnostic tests during the initial hospitalization accounts for 19% of total hospital costs (6). These diagnostic tests included MR or CT (91% of patients), echocardiogram (81%), noninvasive carotid artery evaluation (48%), angiography (20%), and electroencephalography (6%).

Goals

The primary goal of neuroimaging in patients presenting with acute neurologic deficits is to differentiate between ischemic and hemorrhagic stroke, and to exclude other diagnoses that may mimic stroke. Other emerging goals in acute stroke patients are to determine if brain tissue is viable and thereby amenable to interventional therapies, and to determine the localization of vascular occlusion.

Methodology

A comprehensive Medline search (United States National Library of Medicine database) for original articles published between 1966 and July 2004 using the Ovid and Pubmed search engines was performed using a combination of the following key terms: *ischemic stroke, hemorrhage, diagnostic imaging, CT, MR, PET, SPECT, angiography, gadolinium, circle of Willis, carotid artery, brain, technology assessment, evidence-based medicine,* and *cost.* The search was limited to English-language articles and human studies. The abstracts were reviewed and selected based on well-designed methodology, clinical trials, outcomes, and diagnostic accuracy. Additional relevant articles were selected from the references of reviewed articles and published guidelines.

I. What Is the Imaging Modality of Choice for the Detection of Intracranial Hemorrhage?

Summary of Evidence: Computed tomography (CT) is widely accepted as the gold standard for imaging intracerebral hemorrhage; however, it has not been rigorously examined in prospective studies, and thus the precise sensitivity and specificity is unknown (limited evidence). For the evaluation of thrombolytic candidates (exclusion of intracerebral hemorrhage), however, CT is clearly the modality of choice based on strong evidence (level I) from randomized controlled trials (7, 8). By many measures MR is at least as sensitive as CT in the detection of intracerebral hemorrhage, and it is suspected to be more sensitive during the subacute and chronic phases. A recent study indicates that the sensitivity and accuracy of MR in detecting intraparenchymal hemorrhage is equivalent to CT even in the hyperacute setting (within 6 h of ictus) (strong evidence) (9).

Supporting Evidence

A. Computed Tomography

It is essential that an imaging study reliably distinguish intracerebral hemorrhage from ischemic stroke because of the divergent management of these two conditions. This is especially critical for patients who present within 3 h of symptom onset under consideration for thrombolytic therapy. Noncontrast CT is currently the modality of choice for detection of acute intracerebral hemorrhage. Acute hemorrhage appears hyperdense for several days due to the high protein concentration of hemoglobin and retraction of clot, but becomes progressively isodense and then hypodense over a period of weeks to months from breakdown and clearing of the hematoma by macrophages. Rarely acute hemorrhage can be isodense in severely anemic patients with a hematocrit of less than 20% or 10 g/dL (10, 11). Although it has been well accepted that CT can identify intraparenchymal hemorrhage with very high sensitivity, surprisingly few studies have been conducted to support this (12, 13). In 1974, shortly after the introduction of the EMI scanner, Paxton and Ambrose (14) diagnosed 66 patients with intracerebral hemorrhages with this novel modality; the study was observational, lacking autopsy confirmation, and thus accuracy was not determined (insufficient evidence). Subsequently, in an autopsy series of 79 patients, EMI did not detect four out of 17 patients with hemorrhages – all were brainstem hemorrhages (limited evidence) (15). There is little doubt that the sensitivity of current third-generation CT scanners for the detection of intracerebral hemorrhage is far superior to the first-generation scanners; however, it is of interest that the precise sensitivity and specificity of this well-accepted modality is unknown, and the level of evidence supporting its use is limited (level III).

Four studies evaluating third-generation CT scanners in patients with nontraumatic subarachnoid hemorrhage identified by CT or cerebrospinal fluid (CSF) have been reported (16–19). The overall sensitivity of CT was 91–92%, but was dependent on the time interval between symptom onset and scan time. Sensitivity was 100% (80/80) for patients imaged within 12 h, 93% (134/144) within 24 h, and 84% (31/37) after 24 h (level III) (18, 19). These numbers were confirmed by two other studies that demonstrated a sensitivity of 98% (117/119) for scans obtained within 12 h, 95% (1,313/1,378) within 24 h, 91% (1,247/1,378) between 24 and 48 h, and 74% after 48 h (1,017/1,378) (moderate evidence) (16, 17). These studies relied on a diagnosis made by CT, or by blood detected in CSF in the absence of CT findings. No studies with autopsy confirmation have been reported.

Therefore, although CT is commonly regarded as the modality of choice for imaging intracranial hemorrhage, the precise sensitivity and specificity is unknown and is dependent on time after onset, concentration of hemoglobin, and size and location of the hemorrhage (limited evidence).

B. Magnetic Resonance Imaging

Like CT, the appearance and detectability of hemorrhage on MRI depends on the age of blood and the location of the hemorrhage (intraparenchymal or subarachnoid). In addition, the strength of the magnetic field and type of MR sequence influences its sensitivity (20). As the hematoma ages, oxyhemoglobin in blood breaks down sequentially into several paramagnetic products: first deoxyhemoglobin, then methemoglobin, and finally hemosiderin. Iron in hemoglobin is shielded from surrounding water molecules when oxygen is bound, resulting in a molecule (oxyhemoglobin) with diamagnetic properties. As a result, the MR signal is similar to that of normal brain parenchyma, making it difficult to detect on any MR sequence, including susceptibility weighted sequences (echoplanar imaging [EPI] T2* or gradient echo). In contrast, iron exposed to surrounding water molecules in the form of deoxyhemoglobin creates signal loss, making it easy to identify on susceptibility-weighted and T2-weighted (T2W) sequences (21, 22). Thus the earliest detection of hemorrhage depends on the conversion of oxyhemoglobin to deoxyhemoglobin, which was believed to occur after the first 12–24 h (20, 23). However, this early assumption has been questioned with reports of intraparenchymal hemorrhage detected by MRI within 6 h, and as early as 23 min from symptom onset (24–26). One of the studies prospectively demonstrated that MRI detected all nine patients with CT-confirmed intracerebral hemorrhage (ICH), suggesting the potential of MRI for the hyperacute evaluation of stroke (limited evidence) (24–26). More recently, a blinded study comparing MRI (diffusion-, T2-, and T2*-weighted images) to CT for the evaluation of ICH within 6 h of onset demonstrated that ICH was diagnosed with 100% sensitivity and 100% accuracy by expert readers using MRI; CT-detected ICH was used as the gold standard (strong evidence) (9).

Data regarding the detection of acute subarachnoid and intraventricular hemorrhage using MRI is limited. While it is possible that the conversion of blood to deoxyhemoglobin occurs much earlier than expected in hypoxic tissue, this transition may not occur until much later in the oxygen-rich environment of the CSF (20, 27). Thus the susceptibility-weighted sequence may not be sensitive enough to detect subarachnoid blood in the hyperacute stage. This problem is further compounded by severe susceptibility artifacts at the skull base, limiting detection in this area. The use of the fluid-attenuated inversion recovery (FLAIR) sequence has been advocated to overcome this problem. Increased protein content in bloody CSF appears hyperintense on FLAIR and can be readily detected. Three case-control series using FLAIR in patients with CT-documented subarachnoid or intraventricular hemorrhage demonstrated a sensitivity of 92–100% and specificity of 100% compared to CT and was superior to CT during the subacute to chronic stages (limited evidence) (28–30). Hyperintense signal in the CSF on FLAIR can be seen in areas associated with prominent CSF pulsation artifacts (i.e., third and fourth ventricles and basal cisterns) and in other conditions that elevate protein in the CSF such as meningitis or after gadolinium administration (level III) (31–33); however, these conditions are not usually confused with clinical presentations suggestive of subarachnoid hemorrhage.

At later time points in hematoma evolution (subacute to chronic phase) when the clot demonstrates nonspecific isodense to hypodense appearance on CT, MRI has been shown to have a higher sensitivity and specificity than CT (limited evidence) (28, 34, 35). The heightened sensitivity of MRI susceptibility-weighted sequences to microbleeds that are not otherwise detected on CT makes interpretation of hyperacute scans difficult, especially when faced with decisions regarding thrombolysis (Fig. 11.1). Patient outcome regarding the use of thrombolytic treatment in this subgroup of patients with microbleeds is not known; however, in one series of 41 patients who had MRI prior to intra-arterial tPA, 1 of 5 patients with microbleeds on MRI developed major symptomatic hemorrhage compared to 3 of 36 without (36), raising the possibility that the presence of microbleeds may predict the subsequent development of symptomatic hemorrhage following tPA treatment. As this finding was not statistically significant, a larger study is required for confirmation.

II. What Are the Imaging Modalities of Choice for the Identification of Brain Ischemia and the Exclusion of Stroke Mimics?

Summary of Evidence: Based on moderate evidence (level II), MRI (diffusion-weighted imaging) is superior to CT for positive identification of ischemic stroke within the first 24 h of symptom onset, allowing exclusion of stroke mimics. However, some argue that despite its superiority, positive identification merely confirms a clinical diagnosis and does not necessarily influence acute clinical decision making or outcome.

Supporting Evidence

A. Computed Tomography

Computed tomography images are frequently normal during the acute phase of ischemia and therefore the diagnosis of ischemic stroke is contingent upon the exclusion of stroke mimics, which include postictal state, systemic infection, brain tumor, toxic-metabolic conditions, positional vertigo, cardiac disease, syncope, trauma, subdural hematoma, herpes encephalitis, dementia, demyelinating disease, cervical spine fracture, conversion disorder, hypertensive encephalopathy, myasthenia gravis, and Parkinson disease (37). Based purely on history and physical examination alone without confirmation by CT, stroke mimics can account for 13–19% of cases initially diagnosed with stroke (37, 38). Sensitivity of diagnosis improves when noncontrast CT is used but still 5% of cases are misdiagnosed as stroke, with ultimate diagnoses including paresthesias or numbness of unknown cause, seizure,

complicated migraine, peripheral neuropathy, cranial neuropathy, psychogenic paralysis, and others (39).

An alternative approach to excluding stroke mimics, which may account for the presenting neurologic deficit, is to directly visualize ischemic changes in the hyperacute scan. Increased scrutiny of hyperacute CT scans, especially following the early thrombolytic trials, suggests that some patients with large areas of ischemia may demonstrate subtle early signs of infarction, even if imaged within 3 h after symptom onset. These early CT signs include parenchymal hypodensity, loss of the insular ribbon (40), obscuration of the lentiform nucleus (41), loss of gray–white matter differentiation, blurring of the margins of the basal ganglia, subtle effacement of the cortical sulci, and local mass effect (Fig. 11.2). It was previously believed that these signs of infarction were not present on CT until 24 h after stroke onset; however, early changes were found in 31% of CTs performed within 3 h of ischemic stroke (moderate evidence) (42). In addition, early CT signs were found in 81% of patients with CTs performed within 5 h of middle cerebral artery (MCA) stroke onset (demonstrated angiographically) (moderate evidence) (43). Early CT signs, however, can be very subtle and difficult to detect even among very experienced readers (moderate evidence) (44–46). Moreover, the presence of these early ischemic changes in only 31% of hyperacute strokes precludes its reliability as a positive sign of ischemia.

Early CT signs of infarction, especially involving more than 33% of the MCA distribution, have been reported to be associated with severe stroke, increased risk of hemorrhagic transformation (46–49), and poor outcome (50). Because of these associations, several trials involving thrombolytic therapy including the European Cooperative Acute Stroke Study (ECASS) excluded patients with early CT signs in an attempt to avoid treatment of patients at risk for hemorrhagic transformation (8, 46, 51, 52). Although ECASS failed to demonstrate efficacy of intravenous tPA administered within 6 h of stroke onset, a marginal treatment benefit was observed in the target population (post-hoc analysis), excluding patients with early CT signs that were inappropriately enrolled in the trial (46). The National Institute of Neurological Disorders and Stroke (NINDS) tPA stroke trial (7), which did demonstrate efficacy, did not exclude patients with early CT signs, and retrospective analysis of the data showed that early CT signs were associated with stroke severity but not with increased risk of adverse outcome after tPA treatment (42). Thus, based on current data, early CT signs should not be used to exclude patients who are otherwise eligible for thrombolytic treatment within 3 h of stroke onset (strong and moderate evidence) (7, 42).

B. Magnetic Resonance Imaging

Unlike CT and conventional MR, new functional MR techniques such as diffusion-weighted imaging (DWI) allow detection of the earliest physiologic changes of cerebral ischemia. DWI, a sequence sensitive to the random brownian motion of water, is capable of demonstrating changes within minutes of ischemia in rodent stroke models (53–55). Moreover, the sequence is sensitive, detecting lesions as small as 4 mm in diameter (56). Although the in vivo mechanism of signal alteration observed in DWI after acute ischemia is unclear, it is believed that ischemia-induced energy depletion increases the influx of water from the extracellular to the intracellular space, thereby restricting water motion, resulting in a bright signal on DW images (57, 58). DWI has become widely employed for clinical applications due to improvements in gradient capability, and it is now possible to acquire DW images free from artifacts with an echo planar approach. Because DW images are affected by T1 and T2 contrast, stroke lesions becomes progressively brighter due to concurrent increases in brain water content, leading to the added contribution of hyperintense T2W signal known as "T2 shine-through." To differentiate between true restricted diffusion and T2 shine-through, bright lesions on DWI should always be confirmed with apparent diffusion coefficient (ADC) maps, which exclusively measure diffusion. For stroke lesions in adults, although there is wide individual variability, ADC signal remains decreased for 4 days, pseudo-normalizes at 5–10 days, and increases thereafter (56). This temporal evolution of DWI signal allows one to determine the age of a stroke.

The high sensitivity and specificity of DWI for the detection of ischemia make it an ideal sequence for positive identification of hyperacute stroke, thereby excluding stroke mimics. Two studies evaluating DWI for the detection of ischemia within 6 h of stroke onset reported an 88–100% sensitivity and 95–100% specificity with a positive predictive value (PPV) of 98.5% and negative predictive value (NPV) of 69.5%, using final clinical diagnosis as the gold standard (moderate and limited evidence) (59, 60). In another study, 50 patients were randomized to DWI or CT within 6 h of stroke onset, and subsequently received the other imaging modality with a mean delay of 30 min. Sensitivity and specificity of infarct detection among blinded expert readers was significantly better when based on DWI (91 and 95%, respectively) compared to CT (61 and 65%) (moderate evidence) (61). The presence of restricted diffusion is highly correlated with ischemia, but its absence does not rule out ischemia: false negatives have been reported in transient ischemic attacks and small subcortical infarctions (moderate evidence) (60, 62–64). False-positive DWI signals have been reported in brain abscesses (65), herpes encephalitis (66, 67), Creutzfeldt-Jakob disease (68), highly cellular tumors such as lymphoma or meningioma (69), epidermoid cysts (70), seizures (71), and hypoglycemia (72) (limited evidence). However, the clinical history and the appearance of these lesions on conventional MR should allow for exclusion of these stroke mimics. Within the first 8 h of onset, the stroke lesion should be seen only on DWI, and its presence on conventional MR sequences suggests an older stroke or a nonstroke lesion. The DWI images, therefore, should not be interpreted alone but in conjunction with conventional MR sequences and within the proper clinical context.

Acute DWI lesion volume has been correlated with long-term clinical outcome, using various assessment scales including the National Institutes of Health Stroke Scale (NIHSS), the Canadian Neurologic Scale, the Barthel Index, and the Rankin Scale (moderate evidence) (73–77). This correlation was stronger for strokes involving the cortex and weaker for subcortical strokes (73, 74), which is likely explained by a discordance between infarct size and severity of neurologic deficit for small subcortical strokes.

In addition to DWI, MR perfusion-weighted imaging (PWI) approaches have been employed to depict brain regions of hypoperfusion. They involve the repeated and rapid acquisition of images prior to and following the injection of contrast agent using a two-dimensional (2D) gradient echo or spin echo EPI sequence (78, 79). Signal changes induced by the first passage of contrast in the brain can be used to obtain estimates of a variety of hemodynamic parameters, including cerebral blood flow (CBF), cerebral blood volume (CBV), and mean transit time (MTT, the mean time for the bolus of contrast agent to pass through each pixel) (79–81). These parameters are often reported as relative values since accurate measurement of the input function cannot be determined. However, absolute quantification of CBF has also been reported (82). Thus, hypoperfused brain tissue resulting from ischemia demonstrates signal changes in perfusion-weighted images, and may provide information regarding regional hemodynamic status during acute ischemia (insufficient evidence).

III. What Imaging Modality Should Be Used for the Determination of Tissue Viability: The Ischemic Penumbra?

Summary of Evidence: Determination of tissue viability using functional imaging has tremendous potential to individualize therapy and extend the therapeutic time window for some. Several imaging modalities, including MRI, CT, PET, and SPECT, have been examined in this role. Operational hurdles may limit the use of some of these modalities in the acute setting of stroke (e.g., PET and SPECT), while others such as MRI show promise (limited evidence). Rigorous testing in large randomized controlled trials that can clearly demonstrate that reestablishment of perfusion to regions "at risk" prevents progression to infarction and is needed prior to their use in routine clinical decision making.

Supporting Evidence

A. Magnetic Resonance Imaging

The combination of DWI and PWI techniques holds promise in identifying brain tissue at risk for infarction. It has been postulated that brain tissue dies over a period of minutes to hours following arterial occlusion. Initially, a core of tissue dies within minutes, but there is surrounding brain tissue that is dysfunctional but viable, comprising the ischemic penumbra. If blood flow is not restored in a timely manner, the brain tissue at risk dies, completing the infarct (83). The temporal profile of signal changes seen on DWI and PWI follows a pattern that is strikingly similar to the theoretical construct of the penumbra described above. On MR, images obtained within hours of stroke onset, the DWI lesion is often smaller than the area of perfusion defect (on PWI), and smaller than the final infarct (defined by T2W images obtained weeks later). If the arterial occlusion persists, the DWI lesion grows until it eventually matches the initial perfusion defect, which is often similar in size and location to the final infarct (chronic T2W lesion) (Fig. 11.3) (limited evidence) (84, 85). The area of normal DWI signal but abnormal PWI signal is known as the diffusion–perfusion mismatch and has been postulated to represent the ischemic penumbra. Diffusion–perfusion mismatch has been reported to be present in 49% of stroke patients during the hyperacute period (0–6 h) (limited evidence) (86). Growth of the DWI lesion over time has been documented in a randomized trial testing the efficacy of the neuroprotective agent citicoline. Mean lesion volume in the placebo group was increased by 180% from the initial DWI scan (obtained within 24 h of stroke onset) to the final T2W scan obtained 12 weeks later. Interestingly, lesion volume grew only 34% in the citicoline-treated group, suggesting a treatment effect (moderate evidence) (87). However, efficacy of the agent was not definitively demonstrated using clinical outcomes (88). The ultimate test of the hypothesis that mismatch represents "penumbra," will come from studies that correlate initial mismatch with salvaged tissue after effective treatment. One small prospective series of ten patients demonstrated that patients with successful recanalization after intra-arterial thrombolysis showed larger areas of mismatch that were salvaged compared to patients who were not successfully recanalized (limited evidence) (89).

The promise of diffusion–perfusion mismatch is that it will provide an image of ischemic brain tissue that is salvageable, and thereby individualize therapeutic time windows for acute treatments. The growth of the lesion to the final infarct volume may not occur until hours or even days later in some individuals (limited evidence) (84, 85), suggesting that tissue may be salvaged beyond the 3-h window in some. One of the assumptions underlying the hypothesis that diffusion–perfusion mismatch represents salvageable tissue is that the acute DWI lesion represents irreversibly injured tissue. However, it has been known for some time that DWI lesions are reversible after transient ischemia in animal stroke models (90, 91), and reversible lesions in humans have been reported following a transient ischemic attack (TIA) (92) or after reperfusion (93). These data suggest that at least some brain tissue within the DWI lesion may represent reversibly injured tissue.

Additional new experimental MR techniques such as proton MR spectroscopy (MRS) and T2 Blood Oxygen Level Dependent (BOLD) and 2D multiecho gradient echo/spin echo have also been explored for the identification of salvageable tissue (94, 95). Magnetic resonance spectroscopy is an MR technique that measures the metabolic and biochemical changes within the brain tissues. The two metabolites that are commonly measured following ischemia are lactate and N-acetylaspartate (NAA). Lactate signal is not detected in normal brain, but is elevated within minutes of ischemia in animal models, remaining elevated for days to weeks (96). The lactate signal can normalize with immediate reperfusion (97). N-acetylaspartate, found exclusively in neurons, decreases more gradually over a period of hours after stroke onset in animal stroke models (98). It has been suggested that an elevation in lactate with a normal or mild reduction in NAA during the acute period of ischemia may represent the ischemic penumbra (94), though this has not been examined in a large population of stroke patients. The cerebral metabolic rate of oxygen consumption ($CMRO_2$) has been measured in acute stroke patients using MRI, and a threshold value has been proposed to define irreversibly injured brain tissue (level III) (82). Though preliminary, these results appear to be in agreement with data obtained using PET (see below) (99, 100). Measurement of $CMRO_2$ has theoretical advantages over other measures (e.g., CBF, CBV), as the threshold value for irreversible injury is not likely to be time-dependent (101). Clearly research into the identification of viable ischemic brain tissue is at a preliminary stage. However, such techniques may be important for future acute stroke management. These new imaging approaches will require extensive validation and assessment in well-designed clinical trials.

B. Computed Tomography

In addition to anatomic information, CT is capable of providing some physiologic information, accomplished with either intravenous injection of nonionic contrast or inhalation of xenon gas. Like PWI, perfusion parameters can be obtained by tracking a bolus of contrast or inhaled xenon gas in blood vessels and brain parenchyma with sequential CT imaging. Using spiral CT technology, the study can be completed in 6 min.

Stable xenon (Xe) has been employed as a means to obtain quantitative estimates of CBF in vivo. Xenon, an inert gas with an atomic number similar to iodine, can attenuate X-rays like contrast material. However, unlike CT contrast, the gas is freely diffusable and can cross the blood–brain barrier. Sequential imaging permits the tracking of progressive accumulation and washout of the gas in brain tissue, reflected by changes in Hounsfield units over time, and quantitative CBF and CBV maps can be calculated (102). The quantitative CBF value from xenon-enhanced CT has been shown to be highly accurate compared with radioactive microsphere and iodoantipyrine techniques under different physiologic conditions and wide range of CBF rates in baboons (correlation coefficient $r = 0.67$–0.92, $p < 0.01$ and <0.001) (103, 104). The major advantage of the xenon CT is that it allows absolute quantification of the CBF, which may help to define a threshold value from reversible to irreversible cerebral injury. Low CBF (<15 mL/100 g/min) correlated with early CT signs of infarction, proximal M1 occlusion, severe edema, and life-threatening herniation. Very low CBF values (<7 mL/100 g/min) predicted irreversibly injured tissue (105, 106). In addition, xenon CT has been shown to be effective in obtaining cerebral vascular reserve (CVR) in patients with occlusive disease (107). Poor CVR has been shown to be a risk factor for stroke in patients with high-grade carotid stenosis or occlusion (108). However, to ensure a sufficient signal-to-noise ratio for Xe-CT perfusion, a high concentration of Xe is needed, which itself may cause respiratory depression, cerebral vasodilation, and thus confound the measurements of CBF (109).

In addition to inhalation xenon gas, bolus nonionic contrast can also be used to generate a CT perfusion map. Rapid repeated serial images of the brain are acquired during the first-pass passage of intravenous contrast to generate relative CBF, CBV, and MTT. The CT perfusion maps obtained within 6 h of stroke onset in patients with MCA occlusion had significantly higher sensitivity for the detection of stroke lesion volume compared to noncontrast CT, and the perfusion volume correlated with clinical outcome (limited evidence) (105, 110). Cerebral blood flow maps generated by CT perfusion in 70 acute stroke patients predicted the extent of cerebral infarction with a sensitivity of 93% and a specificity of 98% (limited evidence) (111). A major limitation to this technique is that only relative CBF map can be obtained, thus precluding exact determination of the transition from ischemia to infarction.

C. Positron Emission Tomography

Positron emission tomography imaging has provided fundamental information on the pathophysiology of human cerebral ischemia. Quantitative measurements of cerebral perfusion and metabolic parameters can be obtained, namely CBF, CBV, MTT, oxygen extraction fraction (OEF), and $CMRO_2$, using multiple tracers and serial arterial blood samplings. Based on the values of these hemodynamic parameters, four distinct successive pathophysiologic phases of ischemic stroke have been identified: autoregulation, oligemia, ischemia, and irreversible injury (112). Oligemia (low CBF, elevated OEF with normal $CMRO_2$) and ischemia (low CBF, elevated OEF but decreased $CMRO_2$) are sometimes termed misery perfusion, and have been postulated to represent the ischemic penumbra (113). During misery perfusion, a decline in $CMRO_2$ heralds the beginning of a transition from reversible to irreversible injury. Irreversible injury is reflected in tissue with $CMRO_2$ below 1.4 mL/100 g/min (99, 100). In three serial observational studies of acute ischemic stroke, elevation of OEF in the setting of low CBF has been suggested to be the marker of tissue viability in ischemic tissue (level II) (114–116). The CBF in ischemic tissue with elevated OEF is between 7 and 17 mL/100 g/min. Elevated OEF has been observed to persist up to 48 h after stroke onset (115). Progression to irreversible injury is reflected in decreased OEF (114, 115). Furthermore, in a prospective blinded longitudinal cohort study of 81 patients with carotid occlusion, elevated OEF was found to be an independent predictor for subsequent stroke and potentially defining a subgroup of patients who may benefit from revascularization (moderate evidence) (117). However, confirmation of tissue viability in the region of elevated OEF is best accomplished by large randomized controlled trials, which clearly demonstrate that reestablishment of perfusion to this region prevents progression to infarction. Such studies have not been done and are difficult to implement since PET is limited to major medical centers and requires considerable expertise and time. Moreover, the requirement for intra-arterial line placement precludes its use for evaluating thrombolytic candidates. Despite these hurdles one study assessed PET after thrombolysis in 12 ischemic stroke patients within 3 h of symptoms onset (118). Due to the above-mentioned hurdles, only relative CBF was obtained prior to and following intravenous thrombolysis (118). In all patients, early reperfusion of severely ischemic tissue (<12 mL/110 g/min in gray matter) predicted better clinical outcome and limited infarction.

D. Single Photon Emission Computed Tomography (SPECT)

The most commonly used radiopharmaceutical agent for SPECT perfusion study is technetium-99m pertechnetate hexamethylpropylene amine oxime (99m Tc-HMPAO). This lipophilic substance readily crosses the blood–brain barrier and interacts with intracellular glutathione, which prevents it from diffusing back. However, due to technical problems including incomplete first-pass extraction from blood, incomplete binding to glutathione leading to back diffusion, and metabolism within the brain, absolute quantification of the CBF cannot be determined. However, SPECT technology is much more accessible than PET and is more readily available. In a multicenter prospective trial with 99mTc-bicisate (99mTc-ECD, an agent with better brain-to-background contrast) of 128 patients with ischemic stroke and 42 controls, SPECT had a sensitivity of 86% and specificity of 98% for localization of stroke compared with final clinical, diagnostic, and laboratory studies (119). The sensitivity decreased to 58% for lacunar stroke (119). Perfusion studies with HMPAO-SPECT in early ischemic stroke demonstrated that patients with severe hypoperfusion on admission had poor outcome at 1 month (120).

Furthermore, reperfusion of ischemic tissue with 65–85% reduction of regional CBF (rCBF) compared to the contralateral hemisphere decreased the final infarct volume but had no affect on regions with reduction greater than 85% (121).

IV. What Is the Role of Noninvasive Intracranial Vascular Imaging?

Summary of Evidence: With the development of different delivery approaches for thrombolysis in acute ischemic stroke, there is a new demand for noninvasive vascular imaging modalities. While some data are available comparing magnetic resonance angiography (MRA) and computed tomography angiography (CTA) to digital substraction angiography (DSA) (moderate and limited evidence), strong evidence in support of the use of such approaches for available therapies is lacking. Prospective studies examining clinical outcome after the use of screening vascular imaging approaches to triage therapy are needed.

Supporting Evidence

A. Computed Tomography Angiography

One advantage of CTA is that it can be performed immediately following the prerequisite noncontrast CT for all stroke patients. Using spiral CT, the entire examination can be completed in 5 min with 100 cc of nonionic intravenous contrast, with an additional 10 min required for image reconstruction. The sensitivity and specificity of CTA for trunk occlusions of the circle of Willis are 83–100% and 99–100%, respectively, compared to DSA in several case series (limited evidence) (122–126). Few studies have examined the sensitivity of CTA for distal occlusions. In one study the reliability in assessing MCA branch occlusion was significantly lower (123).

B. Magnetic Resonance Angiography

In addition to tissue evaluation, MR is capable of noninvasively assessing the intracranial vascular status of stroke patients using MRA. One of the most commonly used MRA techniques is

the 2D or 3D time-of-flight technique. Stationary background tissue is suppressed while fresh flowing intravascular blood has bright signal. The source images are postprocessed using a maximal intensity projection (MIP) to display a 3D image of the blood vessel. However, the sensitivity and specificity of MRA are somewhat limited when compared to DSA. In a prospective nonconsecutive study of 50 patients, MRA had a sensitivity of 100% and a specificity of 95% for occlusion and 89% sensitivity and specificity for stenosis of the intracranial vessels compared to DSA (limited evidence) (127). In another study of 131 patients with 32 intracranial steno-occlusive lesions, MRA had a sensitivity of 85% and specificity of 96% for internal carotid artery (ICA) pathology, and for MCA lesions, 88% sensitivity and 97% specificity (moderate evidence) (128). A recent comparison of MRA and DSA in 24 children presenting with cerebral infarction demonstrated that all lesions detected on DSA were present on MRA; however, distal vascular lesions and the degree of stenosis were more accurately detected with DSA (moderate evidence) (129). In another study, DSA and MRA were compared to surgical and histologic findings of specimens removed during endarterectomy; MRA was 89% and DSA was 93% in agreement with histologic specimens in determining the degree of stenosis, and plaque morphology was in agreement in 91% of cases for MRA and 94% for DSA (130).

These findings are not surprising given the known technical limitations associated with MRA. First, the ability of MRA to accurately depict the vessel lumen is limited due to the fact that complete or partial signal voids in regions of high or turbulent flow normally occur (spin dephasing), leading to an overestimation of the extent of stenosis. Second, the inability to acquire high-resolution images due to limited signal-to-noise ratios and loss of contrast between blood and brain parenchyma for slow-flowing spins (spin saturation) makes it difficult for MRA to depict distal and small vessels. Therefore, while MRA is able to provide images of the cerebral vasculature noninvasively, cautious interpretation of lumen definition is warranted. Although contrast-enhanced MRA of the extracranial arteries appears to be better at defining the degree of stenosis than the time-of-flight MRA technique (131, 132), assessment of the intracranial vessels with contrast is limited due to venous contamination. However, while it may be possible to overcome this limitation with new technical development including ultrafast imaging techniques and better timing of the arrival of contrast, data regarding its accuracy has not yet been defined (133). Whether MRA can provide screening for future thrombolytic/ interventional approaches remains to be seen.

V. What Is the Role of Acute Neuroimaging in Pediatric Stroke?

Summary of Evidence: Due to the low incidence of stroke in the pediatric population, few studies are available regarding risk factors, recurrence, and outcome. Moreover, the efficacy of acute therapies has not been examined in this population, limiting the utility of acute neuroimaging in pediatric stroke for early therapeutic decision making.

Supporting Evidence: In contrast to stroke in the adult population, pediatric stroke is an uncommon disorder with a very different pathophysiology. The overall incidence of ischemic stroke is 2–13 per 100,000 children, with the highest rate occurring in the perinatal period (26.4 per 100,000 infants less than 30 days old) (134). The incidence of ischemic stroke has increased over the past two decades, probably due to better population-based studies (the Canadian Pediatric Stroke Registry), more sensitive imaging techniques (fetal MR, DWI), and an increased survival of immature neonates due to improved treatment modalities (extracorporeal membrane oxygenation). The etiologies of ischemic stroke in children are due to nonatherosclerotic causes such as congenital heart disease, sickle cell anemia, coagulation disorders, arterial dissection, varicella zoster infection, inherited metabolic disorders, and moyamoya, and is found to be idiopathic in one third of the cases (134, 135).

To date, there are no randomized clinical trials for the treatment of acute ischemic stroke in the pediatric population. Indeed, there is only one published randomized controlled trial for stroke prevention [the Stroke Prevention Trial (STOP) in Sickle Cell Anemia], which showed that blood transfusions greatly reduced the risk of stroke in children with sickle cell anemia who have peak mean blood flow velocities greater than 200 cm/s measured by transcranial Doppler ultrasonography in the ICA or proximal MCA (strong evidence) (136). Though there is no Food and Drug Administration (FDA)-approved treatment for children with acute ischemic stroke, several case reports have documented the use of intravenous tPA in this setting (insufficient evidence) (137–139).

The lack of proven therapeutic interventions for acute pediatric stroke limits the utility of acute neuroimaging for early therapeutic decision making. However, the diagnosis and differentiation of stroke subtypes may still be important for preventative measures. This is true especially in neonates and infants, where neurologic deficits may be subtle and difficult to ascertain. In this regard, MRI (with T1W, T2W, FLAIR, as well as DWI) may be superior to CT in the early identification of ischemic lesions and exclusion of stroke mimics (extrapolated from adult data).

Take Home Table

Table 11.1 summarizes sensitivity, specificity, and strength of evidence of neuroimaging in acute intraparenchymal hemorrhage, acute subarachnoid hemorrhage, and acute ischemic infarction.

Acute Imaging Protocols Based on the Evidence

Head CT: indicated for all patients presenting with acute focal deficits
Noncontrast examination
Sequential or spiral CT with 5-mm slice thickness from the skull base to the vertex
Head MR: indicated if stroke is in doubt
Axial DWI (EPI) with ADC map, GRE, or ep T2*, FLAIR, T1W
Optional sequences (insufficient evidence for routine clinical practice):
MRA of the circle of Willis (3D TOF technique)
PWI (EPI FLASH, 12 slices per measurement for 40 measurements, with 10- to 15-s injection delay, injection rate of 5 cc/s with single or double bolus of gadolinium, followed by a 20-cc saline flush)
Axial T1W postcontrast

Table 11.1. Diagnostic performance for patients presenting with acute neurological deficits

	Sensitivity (%)	Specificity (%)	References	Evidence
Acute intraparenchymal hemorrhage (<6 h)				
CT	100[a]	100[a]		[a]
MRI	100	100	(61)	Strong
Acute subarachnoid hemorrhage (<12 h)				
CT	98–100		(16, 17)	Moderate
MRI (FLAIR)	92–100	100	(28–30)	Limited
Acute ischemic infarction (<6 h)				
CT	61	65	(9)	Moderate
MRI	91	95	(9)	Moderate

Reprinted with kind permission of Springer Science+Business Media from Vo KD, Lin W, Lee J-W. Neuroimaging in Acute Ischemic Stroke. In Medina LS, Blackmore CC (eds): *Evidence-Based Imaging: Optimizing Imaging in Patient Care.* New York: Springer Science+Business Media, 2006.

[a]Although the exact sensitivity or specificity of CT for detecting intraparenchymal hemorrhage is unknown (limited evidence), it serves as the gold standard for detection in comparison to other modalities.

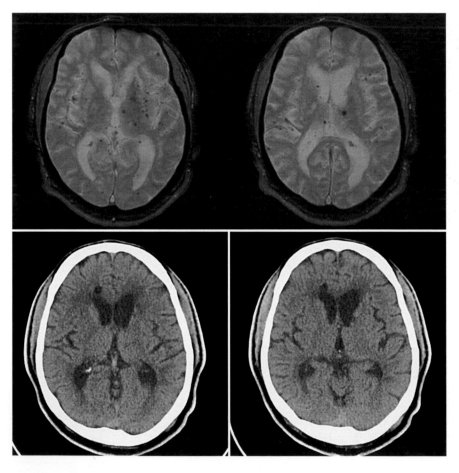

Figure 11.1. Microhemorrhages. *Top row*: Two sequential magnetic resonance (MR) images of T2* sequence show innumerable small low signal lesions scattered throughout both cerebral hemispheres compatible with microhemorrhages. *Bottom row*: Noncontrast axial computed tomography (CT) at the same anatomic levels does not show the microhemorrhages. (Reprinted with kind permission of Springer Science+Business Media from Vo KD, Lin W, Lee J-W. Neuroimaging in Acute Ischemic Stroke. In Medina LS, Blackmore CC (eds): *Evidence-Based Imaging: Optimizing Imaging in Patient Care.* New York: Springer Science+Business Media, 2006.)

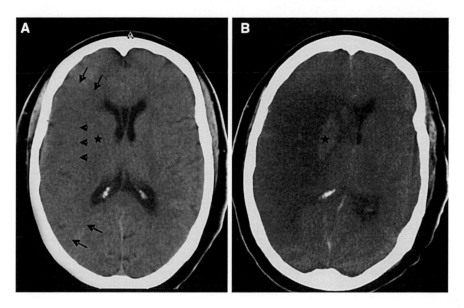

Figure 11.2. Early CT signs of infarction. (**A**) Noncontrast axial CT performed at 2 h after stroke onset shows a large low-attenuated area involving the entire right MCA distribution (bounded by *arrows*) with associated effacement of the sulci and sylvian fissure. There is obscuration the right lentiform nucleus (*asterisk*) and loss of the insular ribbon (*arrowhead*). (**B**) Follow-up noncontrast axial image 4 days later confirms the infarction in the same vascular distribution. There is hemorrhagic conversion (*asterisk*) in the basal ganglia with mass effect and subfalcine herniation. (Reprinted with kind permission of Springer Science+Business Media from Vo KD, Lin W, Lee J-W. Neuroimaging in Acute Ischemic Stroke. In Medina LS, Blackmore CC (eds): *Evidence-Based Imaging: Optimizing Imaging in Patient Care.* New York: Springer Science+Business Media, 2006.)

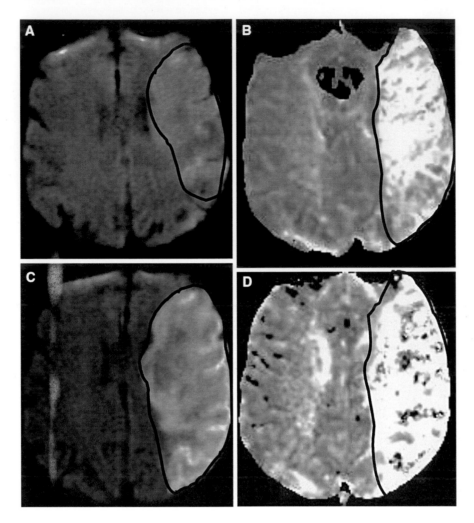

Figure 11.3. Evolution of the right middle cerebral distribution infarction on magnetic resonance imaging (MRI). (**A, B**) MRI at 3 h after stroke onset shows an area of restricted diffusion on diffusion-weighted imaging (DWI) (**A**) with a larger area of perfusion defect on perfusion-weighted imaging (PWI) (**B**). The area of normal DWI but abnormal PWI represents an area of diffusion–perfusion mismatch. (**C, D**) Follow-up MRI at 3 days postictus shows interval enlargement of the DWI lesion (**C**) to the same size as the initial perfusion deficit (**B**). There is now a matched diffusion–perfusion (**C, D**). (Reprinted with kind permission of Springer Science+Business Media from Vo KD, Lin W, Lee J-W. Neuroimaging in Acute Ischemic Stroke. In Medina LS, Blackmore CC (eds): *Evidence-Based Imaging: Optimizing Imaging in Patient Care.* New York: Springer Science+Business Media, 2006.)

Areas of Future Research

- Use of neuroimaging to select patients for acute therapies:
  - Imaging the ischemic penumbra to extend the empirically determined therapeutic windows for certain individuals
  - Predict individuals at high risk for hemorrhagic conversion
  - As more therapies are made available, neuroimaging has the potential to help determine which modality might be most efficacious (e.g., imaging large vessel occlusions for use of intra-arterial thrombolysis or clot retrieval).

- Use of neuroimaging to predict outcome:
  - Useful for prognostic purposes, or for discharge planning
  - Useful as a surrogate measure of outcome in clinical trials

References

1. American Heart Association. 2004 Heart Disease and Stroke Statistics Update. Dallas: AHA, 2004.
2. Bogousslavsky J, Van Melle G, Regli F. Stroke 1988;19(9):1083–1092.
3. Broderick J et al. Stroke 1998;29(2):415–421.
4. Centers for Disease Control, MMWR, 2001:50(7).
5. Sacco RL et al. Am J Epidemiol 1998;147(3): 259–268.
6. Diringer MN et al. Stroke 1999;30(4):724–728.
7. NINDS. N Engl J Med 1995;333(24):1581–1587.
8. Furlan A et al. JAMA 1999;282(21):2003–2011.
9. Fiebach JB et al. Stroke 2004;35(2):502–506.
10. New PF, Aronow S. Radiology 1976;121(3 pt 1): 635–640.
11. Smith WP Jr, Batnitzky S, Rengachary SS. AJR Am J Roentgenol 1981;136(3):543–546.
12. Culebras A et al. Stroke 1997;28(7):1480–1497.
13. Beauchamp NJ Jr et al. Radiology 1999;212(2): 307–324.
14. Paxton R, Ambrose J. Br J Radiol 1974;47(561): 530–565.
15. Jacobs L, Kinkel WR, Heffner RR Jr. Neurology 1976;26(12):1111–1118.
16. Adams HP Jr et al. Neurology 1983;33(8): 981–988.
17. van der Wee N et al. J Neurol Neurosurg Psychiatry 1995;58(3):357–359.
18. Sames TA et al. Acad Emerg Med 1996;3(1): 16–20.
19. Sidman R, Connolly E, Lemke T. Acad Emerg Med 1996;3(9):827–831.
20. Bradley WG Jr. Radiology 1993;189(1):15–26.
21. Gomori JM et al. Radiology 1985;157(1):87–93.
22. Edelman RR et al. AJNR Am J Neuroradiol 1986;7(5):751–756.
23. Thulborn K, Atlas SW. In: Atlas SW (ed.): Magnetic Resonance Imaging of the Brain and Spine. New York: Raven Press, 1991;175–222.
24. Schellinger PD et al. Stroke 1999;30(4):765–768.
25. Patel MR, Edelman RR, Warach S. Stroke 1996;27(12):2321–2324.
26. Linfante I et al. Stroke 1999;30(11):2263–2267.
27. Bradley WG Jr, Schmidt PG. Radiology 1985;156(1):99–103.
28. Noguchi K et al. Radiology 1997;203(1):257–262.
29. Noguchi K et al. Radiology 1995;196(3):773–777.
30. Bakshi R et al. AJNR Am J Neuroradiol 1999; 20(4):629–636.
31. Bakshi R et al. AJNR Am J Neuroradiol 2000;21(3): 503–508.
32. Dechambre SD et al. Neuroradiology 2000;42(8):608–611.
33. Melhem ER, Jara H, Eustace S. AJR Am J Roentgenol 1997;169(3):859–862.
34. Ogawa T et al. AJR Am J Roentgenol 1995;165(5): 1257–1262.
35. Hesselink JR et al. Acta Radiol Suppl 1986;369:46–48.
36. Kidwell CS et al. Stroke 2002;33(1):95–98.
37. Libman RB et al. Arch Neurol 1995;52(11): 1119–1122.
38. Norris JW, Hachinski VC. Lancet 1982;1(8267): 328–331.
39. Kothari RU et al. Stroke 1995;26(12):2238–2241.
40. Truwit CL et al. Radiology 1990;176(3):801–806.
41. Tomura N et al. Radiology 1988;168(2):463–467.
42. Patel SC et al. JAMA 2001;286(22):2830–2838.
43. von Kummer R et al. AJNR Am J Neuroradiol 1994;15(1):9–15; discussion 16–18.
44. Schriger DL et al. JAMA 1998;279(16):1293–1297.
45. Grotta JC et al. Stroke 1999;30(8):1528–1533.
46. Hacke W et al. JAMA 1995;274(13):1017–1025.
47. Toni D et al. Neurology 1996;46(2):341–345.
48. Larrue V et al. Stroke 1997;28(5):957–960.
49. Larrue V et al. Stroke 2001;32(2):438–441.
50. von Kummer R et al. Radiology 1997;205(2): 327–333.
51. Hacke W et al. Lancet 1998;352(9136):1245–1251.
52. Clark WM et al. JAMA 1999;282(21):2019–2026.
53. Kucharczyk J et al. Magn Reson Med 1991;19(2): 311–315.
54. Reith W et al. Neurology 1995;45(1):172–177.
55. Mintorovitch J et al. Magn Reson Med 1991;18(1): 39–50.
56. Warach S et al. Ann Neurol 1995;37(2):231–241.
57. Moseley ME et al. Magn Reson Med 1990;14(2): 330–346.
58. Hoehn-Berlage M et al. J Cereb Blood Flow Metab 1995;15(6):1002–1011.
59. Gonzalez RG et al. Radiology 1999;210(1): 155–162.
60. Lovblad KO et al. AJNR Am J Neuroradiol 1998;19(6):1061–1066.
61. Fiebach JB et al. Stroke 2002;33(9):2206–2210.
62. Marks MP et al. Radiology 1996;199(2):403–408.
63. Kidwell CS et al. Stroke 1999;30(6):1174–1180.
64. Ay H et al. Neurology 1999;52(9):1784–1792.
65. Ebisu T et al. Magn Reson Imaging 1996;14(9): 1113–1116.
66. Ohta K et al. J Neurol 1999;246(8):736–738.
67. Sener RN. Comput Med Imaging Graph 2001;25(5): 391–397.
68. Bahn MM et al. Arch Neurol 1997;54(11): 1411–1415.
69. Gauvain KM et al. AJR Am J Roentgenol 2001; 177(2):449–454.
70. Chen S et al. AJNR Am J Neuroradiol 2001; 22(6):1089–1096.
71. Chu K et al. Arch Neurol 2001;58(6):993–998.
72. Hasegawa Y et al. Stroke 1996;27(9):1648–1655; discussion 1655–1656.
73. Lovblad KO et al. Ann Neurol 1997;42(2): 164–170.
74. Schwamm LH et al. Stroke 1998;29(11):2268–2276.

75. Barber PA et al. Neurology 1998;51(2):418–426.
76. Tong DC et al. Neurology 1998;50(4):864–870.
77. van Everdingen KJ et al. Stroke 1998;29(9):1783–1790.
78. Villringer A et al. Magn Reson Med 1988;6(2):164–174.
79. Rosen BR et al. Magn Reson Med 1991;19(2):285–292.
80. Rosen BR et al. Magn Reson Med 1990;14(2):249–265.
81. Ostergaard L et al. Magn Reson Med 1996;36(5):726–736.
82. Lin W et al. J Magn Reson Imaging 2001;14(6):659–667.
83. Astrup J, Siesjo BK, Symon L. Stroke 1981;12(6):723–725.
84. Baird AE et al. Ann Neurol 1997;41(5):581–589.
85. Beaulieu C et al. Ann Neurol 1999;46(4):568–578.
86. Perkins CJ et al. Stroke 2001;32(12):2774–2781.
87. Warach S et al. Ann Neurol 2000;48(5):713–722.
88. Clark WM et al. Neurology 2001;57(9):1595–1602.
89. Uno M et al. Neurosurgery 2002;50(1):28–34; discussion 34–35.
90. Minematsu K et al. Stroke 1992;23(9):1304–1310; discussion 1310–1311.
91. Hasegawa Y et al. Neurology 1994;44(8):1484–1490.
92. Kidwell CS et al. Ann Neurol 2000;47(4):462–469.
93. Fiehler J et al. Stroke 2002;33(1):79–86.
94. Barker PB et al. Radiology 1994;192(3):723–732.
95. Grohn OH, Kauppinen RA. NMR Biomed 2001;14(7–8):432–440.
96. Decanniere C et al. Magn Reson Med 1995;34(3):343–352.
97. Bizzi A et al. Magn Reson Imaging 1996;14(6):581–592.
98. Sager TN, Laursen H, Hansen AJ. J Cereb Blood Flow Metab 1995;15(4):639–646.
99. Powers WJ et al. J Cereb Blood Flow Metab 1985;5(4):600–608.
100. Touzani O et al. Brain Res 1997;767(1):17–25.
101. Baron JC. Cerebrovasc Dis 1999;9(4):193–201.
102. Gur D et al. Science 1982;215(4537):1267–1268.
103. Wolfson SK Jr et al. Stroke 1990;21(5):751–757.
104. DeWitt DS et al. Stroke 1989;20(12):1716–1723.
105. Firlik AD et al. Stroke 1997;28(11):2208–2213.
106. Firlik AD et al. J Neurosurg 1998;89(2):243–249.
107. Pindzola RR et al. Stroke 2001;32(8):1811–1817.
108. Webster MW et al. J Vasc Surg 1995;21(2):338–344; discussion 344–345.
109. Plougmann J et al. J Neurosurg 1994;81(6):822–828.
110. Lev MH et al. Stroke 2001;32(9):2021–2028.
111. Mayer TE et al. AJNR Am J Neuroradiol 2000;21(8):1441–1449.
112. Baron JC et al. J Cereb Blood Flow Metab 1989;9(6):723–742.
113. Baron JC et al. Stroke 1981;12(4):454–459.
114. Wise RJ et al. Brain 1983;106(pt 1):197–222.
115. Heiss WD et al. J Cereb Blood Flow Metab 1992;12(2):193–203.
116. Furlan M et al. Ann Neurol 1996;40(2):216–226.
117. Grubb RL Jr et al. JAMA 1998;280(12):1055–1060.
118. Heiss WD et al. J Cereb Blood Flow Metab 1998;18(12):1298–1307.
119. Brass LM et al. J Cereb Blood Flow Metab 1994;149(suppl 1):S91–S98.
120. Giubilei F et al. Stroke 1990;21(6):895–900.
121. Sasaki O et al. AJNR Am J Neuroradiol 1996;17(9):1661–1668.
122. Katz DA et al. Radiology 1995;195(2):445–449.
123. Knauth M et al. AJNR Am J Neuroradiol 1997;18(6):1001–1010.
124. Shrier DA et al. AJNR Am J Neuroradiol 1997;18(6):1011–1020.
125. Wildermuth S et al. Stroke 1998;29(5):935–938.
126. Verro P et al. Stroke 2002;33(1):276–278.
127. Stock KW et al. Radiology 1995;195(2):451–456.
128. Korogi Y et al. Radiology 1994;193(1):187–193.
129. Husson B et al. Stroke 2002;33(5):1280–1285.
130. Liberopoulos K et al. Int Angiol 1996;15(2):131–137.
131. Cloft HJ et al. Magn Reson Imaging 1996;14(6):593–600.
132. Willig DS et al. Radiology 1998;208(2):447–451.
133. Okumura A et al. Neurol Res 2001;23(7):767–771.
134. Lynch JK et al. Pediatrics 2002;109(1):116–123.
135. Kirkham FJ et al. J Child Neurol 2000;15(5):299–307.
136. Adams RJ et al. N Engl J Med 1998;339(1):5–11.
137. Gruber A et al. Neurology 2000;54(8):1684–1686.
138. Carlson MD et al. Neurology 2001;57(1):157–158.
139. Thirumalai SS, Shubin RA. J Child Neurol 2000;15(8):558.

12

Pediatric Sickle Cell Disease and Stroke

Jaroslaw Krejza, Maciej Swiat, Maciej Tomaszewski, and Elias R. Melhem

Issues

I. What is the role of neuroimaging in acute stroke in children with sickle cell disease?

II. What is the role of neuroimaging in children with sickle cell disease at risk of their first stroke?

III. What is the role of neuroimaging in prevention of recurrent ischemic stroke in children with sickle cell disease?

IV. Are there neuroimaging criteria that indicate that blood transfusions can be safely halted?

V. What is the role of neuroimaging in hemorrhagic stroke in children with SCD?

Key Points

■ Implementation of the Stroke Prevention Trial in Sickle Cell Anemia (STOP) primary prevention strategy that uses transcranial Doppler (TCD) screening resulted in lower rates in stroke admissions in California (limited evidence).

■ Presence of silent infarcts on magnetic resonance (MR) scans in asymptomatic children with SCD is associated with higher risk for future stroke (limited evidence).

■ The risk of first stroke can be substantially reduced by chronic transfusions in asymptomatic children with SCD and hemoglobin (Hb) SS, in whom intracranial arterial mean velocities are over 200 cm/s on TCD examination (strong evidence).

J. Krejza (✉)
Department of Radiology, Hospital of the University of Pennsylvania, Philadelphia, PA 19104, USA
e-mail: jaroslaw.krejza@uphs.upenn.edu

L.S. Medina et al. (eds.), *Evidence-Based Imaging: Improving the Quality of Imaging in Patient Care, Revised Edition,*
DOI 10.1007/978-1-4419-7777-9_12, © Springer Science+Business Media, LLC 2011

- Management of children with SCD and acute stroke requires immediate non-contrast computed tomography (CT) to exclude intracranial hemorrhage (moderate–strong evidence).
- Children with symptoms of stroke and negative CT for hemorrhage require urgent MRI/diffusion-weighted imaging (DWI)/ MR angiography (MRA) to assess the degree and extent of brain structural abnormalities and positron emission tomography (PET)/single photon emission CT (SPECT) or MRS to determine the degree of ischemia (moderate evidence).
- Presence of intracranial arterial stenosis and new lesions on MR imaging in patients with stroke history is associated with high risk for recurrent stroke (limited evidence).
- There are no specific neuroimaging findings which can suggest that blood transfusions be safely halted in children with SCD (strong evidence).
- No data were found that evaluate the cost-effectiveness of the different neuroimaging modalities in the evaluation of symptomatic and asymptomatic patients with SCD and suspected stroke (limited evidence).

Definition, Pathophysiology, and Clinical Presentation

Sickle cell disease is a family of recessively inherited disorders of Hb. People who inherit only one sickle gene (HbS) are sickle cell carriers. Sickle cell anemia (SCA) is the most severe form of SCD developing when two sickle genes are inherited (homozygotic HbSS). Clinically significant SCD also arises when people inherit the sickle gene from one parent and another variant Hb gene from the second parent such as HbC (SC) or beta thalassemia gene (Sβ^+ or Sβ^0). Sickle Hb (HbS), particularly when not carrying oxygen, polymerizes to gel-like consistency, the red blood cell (RBC) becomes more rigid and deformed to less pliable sickle shape (1, 2). The ability of RBC to adopt a new shape becomes the only important factor determining their transit through microcirculation as the viscosity of blood is abnormally increased primarily due to a loss of normal RBCs' deformability (3, 4). Sickle RBCs are much more vulnerable to mechanical stress during passage through the vasculature, resulting in hemolytic anemia. There is also accumulating evidence that activated white blood cells change their rheological properties contributing to SCD pathophysiology (5, 6). Chronically elevated levels of biologic mediators and acute reactants and ongoing activation of the coagulation system associated with persistence of inflammation in sickle

subjects, even when they are in "steady state," further increase plasma viscosity and RBC aggregation (4, 7, 8). The viscosity of the oxygenated sickle blood is about 1.5-fold than that of normal at equal shear rates, but is increased to 10-fold than that of normal blood in the deoxygenated state (9).

There is a wide range of values for all RBC indices in chronic SCA (10). The reduction in volume of RBC restricts the oxygen-carrying capacity of Hb, leading to chronic Hb desaturation (11). Children with HbSS are more vulnerable to frequent episodes of pain, chest crisis, stroke (12–15), and delayed growth (16) than those with HbSC or HbSβ^0 thalassemia, who usually have less-severe neurological complications in later life. There is ongoing controversy as to whether stroke is more common in those with sickle cell trait than in the general population.

Stroke is a major cause of morbidity in SCD typically defined as a cerebral vascular accident (CVA) of sudden onset with focal neurological deficit persisting over 24 h, developed either spontaneously or in the context of an acute illness such as infection (17). There is a high risk of CVA recurrence – particularly for patients presenting spontaneously – that is reduced but not eliminated by regular blood transfusion (17, 18).

Both ischemic and hemorrhagic strokes may be encountered as well as common subclinical strokes called "silent infarcts." The typical areas of infarction are the frontal and parietal lobes, particularly in boundary zones of territories supplied by the internal carotid (ICA) and middle (MCA) and anterior (ACA) cerebral arteries, whereas the posterior circulation is affected much less frequently. Large-vessel vasculopathy and vaso-occlusion at the microvascular level, which enhances rheological insult, appear to be the dominant mechanisms of stroke in SCD. Not all patients who die after developing neurological symptoms have large-vessel disease, however. In addition to the typical small necrotic lesions in the border between the cortex and the subcortical white matter, acute demyelination and venous sinus thrombosis have also been documented on MRI (19, 20).

There is a broad spectrum of acute presentation with CVA and other neurological complications in patients with SCD (21–23). Besides clinical stroke, patients with SCD also can have transient ischemic attacks with symptoms and signs resolving within 24 h (21–23), although many of these individuals are found to have had recent cerebral infarction or atrophy on imaging (12). The insidious onset of "soft neurological signs," such as difficulty in tapping quickly, is usually associated with cerebral infarction (24, 25). In addition, seizures (26), coma (27) and headache (28) are common presentations of stroke and CVA in children with SCD. Altered mental status – with or without reduced level of consciousness, headache, seizures, visual loss, or focal signs can occur in numerous contexts, including infection, shunted hydrocephalus (29), acute chest syndrome (ACS) (30, 31), aplastic anemia secondary to parvovirus (32), after surgery (28, 33), transfusion (34), immunosuppression (35, 36), and apparently spontaneously (37). In one large series of 538 patients with ACS, 3% of children had neurological symptoms at presentation, and such symptoms developed in a further 7–10% in association with ACS (30). These patients are classified clinically as having had a CVA (12), although there is a wide differential of focal and generalized vascular and nonvascular pathologies – often distinguished using acute magnetic resonance techniques (37) – with important management implications (26, 29, 34, 38–41). Sixty-seven percent of those who have had an initial stroke and are not transfused will develop another, most likely within 36 months (42). With each episode, the child is usually left with more residual neurological deficit including some degree of mental retardation.

Epidemiology of SCD

SCD is one of the most prevalent genetic disorders and primarily affects people originating from sub-Saharan Africa, the Middle East, the Mediterranean, the Indian subcontinent, the Caribbean and South America, and their descendants in other parts of the world, and immigrants from the above countries (43–50). The incidence of SCA in the African American population is 0.2–0.3%; that of SS trait is 9–11%; and that of SC disease is 3% (48, 51–54). The sickle gene is present in about 20% of the indigenous black population in Africa (50, 55, 56). Approximately 80,000 African Americans in the USA have SCD. About 1 in 12 African Americans and 1 in 100 Hispanic Americans are carriers of the disease (57). This prevalence has remained constant primarily because the trait provides partial protection against malarial infection from *Plasmodium falciparum* (50, 58, 59). When RBCs containing HbS are deoxygenated, malarial parasites within these cells are destroyed. The parasites by themselves lower the pH causing the cells to sickle faster. Such protection has become irrelevant in the USA where malaria is no longer endemic.

Epidemiology of Stroke

Overall prevalence of stroke in all forms of SCD is 4%, and in those with SCA is 5%. First stroke occurs in all age groups, except for children under 1 year of age. The annual incidence of first stroke is approximately 0.6 per 100 patient-years or 600/100,000/year in SCA children. However, the highest incidence occurs in the first decade of life with rates of 1.02 per 100 patient-years in SCA patients 2–5 years of age and 0.8 in those 6–9 years of age (12). The cumulative risk of first stroke in SCA patients is 11% by the age of 20 years, 15% by age 30, and 24% by age 45 (12). The combined incidence of hemorrhagic and ischemic strokes in a general sample of American children 14 years of age was reported as 3.3 per 100,000 yearly or 0.0033 per 100 patient-years (60). The types of stroke differ between adults and children with SCD. Infarctive strokes are relatively more common in children than in adults while the reverse is true for hemorrhagic stroke. The Cooperative Study of Sickle Cell Disease (CSSCD) report 9.6% of first strokes in SCD patients under age 20 were hemorrhagic, while 52% of all strokes in those over 20 years of age were hemorrhagic (12). When compared with their peers, children with SCD have a 220-fold increase in stroke risk and a 410-fold increase in cerebral infarction.

In the CSSCD, stroke occurred less frequently in the other common genotypes of SCD. Age-adjusted prevalence rates of stroke at study entry were 2.43% for SB0 thalassemia (SCD-Sβ^0), 1.29% for SCD-Sβ^+, and 0.84% for SCD-SC. About 21% of SCD-SC patients who had a stroke were less than 10 years old compared to those with SCD-SS (31% under age 10).

Risk of Stroke

Clinically apparent stroke represents the most significant and recurrent threat to the SCD patient population. When compared with their peers, children with SCD have a 220-fold increase in stroke risk and a 410-fold increase in cerebral infarction; 11% of patients will have a clinically apparent stroke by age 20 years; and 24% by age 45 years (12). The risk of first symptomatic stroke is highest during the first decade of life, with an incidence of 1.02% per year between the ages of 2 and 5 years. Moreover, 17–35% of SCD children without a compatible history of a cerebrovascular event have "silent" infarctions detectable with MRI (41, 61, 62). Children with silent infarcts are at higher risk for further ischemia than are SCD children with a normal MRI (41, 61, 62). The CSSCD amassed clinical data from October 1978 through September 1988 on a cohort of 4,082 patients with SCD from 23 clinical centers across the USA (12). Subjects were followed for an average duration of 5.2 ± 2.0 years. The overall incidence of first stroke was 0.46 per 100 patient-years, the age-adjusted incidence of first CVA was 0.61% per 100 patient-years. The incidence and prevalence of CVA is given in Table 12.1.

Epidemiology of Recurrent Stroke

Stroke in SCD has a high tendency to recur. In untransfused patients there is a 67% recurrence rate with 70% of the recurrent strokes occurring within the first 3 years following the initial stroke (42). The high risk of CVA recurrence can be reduced but not eliminated by chronic blood transfusion (17, 18). Estimated risk of stroke of children with SCD receiving blood transfusion therapy for at least 5 years after initial stroke is 2.2 per 100 patient-years (17). There is no sufficient evidence to state that hydroxyurea therapy reduces the risk of stroke (63, 64); however, data from nonrandomized clinical series suggest that hydroxyurea might be an alternative to transfusion for primary stroke prevention (insufficient evidence) (65). Chance of stroke recurrence in SCD patients is given in Table 12.2.

Epidemiology of Silent Infarcts Diagnosed by MRI

Children with silent infarcts are at higher risk for further ischemia than are SCD children with a normal MRI (41, 59, 60). About 17–35% of SCD children without a compatible history of a CVA have "silent" infarctions (17, 41, 66), and up to 25% have silent infarction by adolescence, typically between the ACA and MCA or between MCA and Posterior Cerebral Artery territories (41, 67, 68). There is evidence of white matter damage in these border zones, even in those having normal T2-weighted MRI (69) and no neurological symptoms (24, 25). These patients, however, might have had subtle transient ischemic attacks, headaches, or seizures (68). Cognitive difficulties (70, 71), which commonly affect attention (70) and executive function (72), are common in SCD, sometimes from infancy (72); they can be progressive (73) and are associated with brain abnormalities on MRI (69, 70, 73, 74).

Overall Cost to Society

SCD affects about 72,000 African Americans (54). Nationally, total health-care costs for SCD exceeded $0.9 billion in 1995 (data provided by NHLBI). This estimated cost does not include direct and indirect non-health-related costs, patient's and family member's time lost from school, lost workdays and reduced productivity of the patient, lost earnings of unpaid caregivers, transportation expenses, and income lost from premature death. Moreover, pain, disruption of family life, and stress on the patient and family are not included in the estimate. In 2007 dollars, the total cost may exceed $1.5 billion, which makes SCD one of the most costly genetic disorders in the USA. During the years 1989–1993, there were on average 75,000 hospitalizations per year of patients with SCD for a total direct cost of $475 million per year (in 1996 dollars) (75). Government paid 66% of the cost of hospitalizations. Thus, research into interventions that prevent complications or result in better outpatient management of patients with SCD is important and has great potential for cost savings.

Cost of Screening

STOP research findings and NHLBI recommendations pose challenges to the health-care system. The time on transfusions necessary to decrease the stroke risk for patients with SCD remains unclear. As recommended by NHLBI, every child between the ages of 2 and 16 (approximately half of 72,000 people with SCD) should undergo two TCD studies a year. Estimated TCD exams cost $21.6 million ($300/TCD) a year, while estimated recommended transfusions cost about $154 million (76, 77).

Cost-Effectiveness Analysis

No data exist concerning cost-effectiveness of assessing the risk of first stroke, of neuroimaging in acute stroke, or of predicting stroke outcome in children with SCD.

Goals

The goal of neuroimaging such as CT, MR, PET, SPECT, and TCD in acute stroke is to document whether the stroke is ischemic or hemorrhagic, to assess the extent of parenchymal abnormalities, and to determine the presence of cerebrovascular changes. However, initiation of neuroprotective therapy, including exchange transfusion therapy to minimize secondary brain damage and neutralize "ischemic cascade," should not be delayed by arrangement for imaging studies. CT without contrast is the primary imaging modality for the assessment of acute stroke because of its 24/7 availability, ease of accessibility, and ability to exclude hemorrhagic

causes. MRI and MRA are recommended for better assessment of extent of infarction and demonstration of cerebrovascular abnormalities. In the case of hemorrhagic stroke, the goal is to identify with conventional angiography an arteriovenous malformation or aneurysm(s) amenable to surgery or catheter intervention. Exchange transfusion prior to invasive angiography is recommended.

The ultimate goal is to preserve brain function in children with SCD. A secondary goal is to prevent the progression of preclinical ischemia to permanent neuronal loss with disability. The first step is to identify young children at high risk of stroke before development of focal neurological deficits. The preferred imaging is dependent upon the neuroradiologist and the institution, but typically is large-vessel velocity measurements with TCD ultrasound confirmed by conventional MRI or quantitative MRI and MRA (Fig. 12.1). This should be followed by preventive therapy in those with evidence of parenchymal and/or cerebrovascular changes. In patients with neurological symptoms and negative MRI/MRA findings PET or SPECT is recommended.

Methodology

We conducted a systematic review of the literature using a database search of MEDLINE (PubMed, National Library of Medicine, Bethesda, MD) and of Web of Science® (Institute of Scientific Information, Philadelphia, PA) to identify studies dealing with SCD and stroke and relevant to neuroimaging. The search covered years 1990–2007, using the following key terms: (1) *sickle cell disease* and (2) *stroke*, and one of the following: *exp cerebral ischemia, cerebral infarction, cerebrovascular disorders or cerebrovascular accidents, epidemiology, cost, ultrasound, TCD or transcranial Doppler sonography, TCCS or transcranial color-coded sonography, TCCD or transcranial color-coded duplex sonography, MRI or magnetic resonance imaging, MRA or magnetic resonance angiography, angiography, DSA, or digital contrast angiography, CT or computed tomography, PET or positron emission tomography, and SPECT or single photon emission computerized tomography.* There was one randomized controlled trial, no meta-analyses, and no cost analysis of neuroimaging diagnostic options.

We expanded our retrieval to include also clinical trials, cohort studies, multicenter studies, comparative studies, case–control studies, and case reports having more than five subjects for the key question of the age-specific natural history of ischemic stroke. Reviews, letters, hospital bulletins, and single case reports were excluded.

I. What Is the Role of Neuroimaging in Acute Stroke in Children with Sickle Cell Disease?

Summary of Evidence: CT without contrast is the best tool to exclude hemorrhagic stroke in children as well as adults. There is need for a research study, however, to determine whether anatomical MR can replace CT (78, 79). Patients without hemorrhagic stroke should then undergo MRI with DWI and MRA to detect an infarct(s), determine location and extent of ischemic lesions, and presence of large-vessel occlusion/narrowing as soon as possible, the best on emergency basis. Vascular imaging of the neck vasculature with CT or MR angiography to exclude arterial dissection (80) and venous thrombosis should be undertaken within 48 h of presentation with arterial ischemic stroke. MRI and MR angiography become preferable due to noninvasive nature, and no requirement to administer iodinated IV contrast. MR venogram must be specially requested if cerebral venous thrombosis is suspected (81). Imaging from the aortic arch to the intracranial vasculature should be performed in all children with arterial ischemic stroke. TCD is not useful in acute stroke (limited evidence) (82–84).

Symptomatic children with negative CT and MR studies should be followed subacutely by PET or SPECT to identify loss of cerebral neuronal metabolic function.

Supporting Evidence

CT

Noncontrast CT provides sufficient information to make decisions about emergency management in hyperacute stroke, i.e., <6 h after onset of symptoms (moderate evidence) (85–88).

Unenhanced CT has 57% sensitivity and 100% specificity for acute stroke detection (89). The sensitivity can be improved up to 80% by use of variable window width and center level settings or 10-point topographic scoring system (90). The utility of CTA in acute adult stroke relies on demonstrating occlusion or significant arterial narrowings within intracranial vessels and on evaluating the carotid and vertebral arteries in the neck. The sensitivity of CTA was determined to be 88.5–98% in these aspects (91, 92). The utility of CTA in SCD children with stroke has not been determined.

MRI

MRI with DWI provides additional useful information on presence of ischemic stroke (moderate evidence) and visualization of silent cerebral infarcts (moderate evidence) (93–95). DWI determines ischemic regions that later progress to infarction and the volume of acute infarct correlates well with clinical outcome. Based on adults data DWI was reported to have had high sensitivity and specificity of 88–100 and 86–100%, respectively (96–98). DWI is superior to conventional MRI and CT in demonstrating ischemic stroke during the first 24 h after presentation (moderate evidence) (79, 99–101). The pattern of ischemic changes in the brain can be indicative but not specific for a particular stroke etiology (insufficient evidence) (102, 103).

MRA

Like CT angiography, MRA is useful for detecting intravascular occlusion due to a thrombus and for evaluating the carotid bifurcation in patients with acute stroke. Kandeel and colleagues reported that MRA is 85% accurate when compared to DSA (103). In a study of 22 SCD patients, MRA abnormality in a long segment (6 mm) with reduced distal flow correlated with subclinical infarction, while short focal areas of abnormal MRA most commonly in branching regions showed no associated MRI infarction (104).

More recent data from adults showed that MRA has 70–86% sensitivity for detection of intracranial stenosis compared to DSA, while sensitivity of CTA is higher up 98% (91, 92, 105).

Although CTA has better sensitivity than MRA, the advantage of MRA in SCD is that, unlike CTA, it does not require contrast agent, which can be toxic and can exacerbate symptoms in acute stroke (106). MR spectroscopy allows distinguishing an ischemic lesion from other nonischemic changes, but utility of MRS in hyperacute stroke is limited in children with SCD.

Angiography

Digital subtraction angiography (DSA) is not included in standard acute stroke imaging protocol in children with SCD (107). DSA is accurate in detecting intracranial vascular abnormalities (AVM, aneurysm, dissection, and occlusion) and quantifying arterial narrowing (moderate evidence), but is invasive and carries a risk of stroke (108–110). MR and CT angiography are not as accurate as DSA in evaluating vasculature (limited evidence) (103, 111–114), but DSA is performed when endovascular therapy is anticipated.

Nuclear Medicine (PET, SPECT)

PET and SPECT are indicated if CT and MR are negative in patients with clinical stroke to detect the functional activity of the cerebral tissues by using radioactive tracers to indicate glucose metabolism of 2-deoxy-2-[^{18}F]fluoro-D-glucose and evaluate microvascular perfusion ([^{15}O]H$_2$O) (limited evidence) (115, 116). PET studies (115, 117, 118) that have been done in patients with SCD have shown a variety of abnormalities including hypometabolism in frontal areas of the brain and areas of low perfusion that appear normal on MRI. The study of Powars et al. (116) suggested that few patients with SCD have normal PET studies, and areas of hypometabolism in brain regions with normal MR appearance are not uncommon (no sufficient evidence). The authors suggest that PET could be used to select patients for treatment as four patients showed improvement in metabolism and perfusion with transfusion treatment. The most powerful predictor of ischemia in other applications of PET is an increased oxygen extraction fraction, but this application and metabolism measurements remain to be established in children with SCD.

II. What Is the Role of Neuroimaging in Children with Sickle Cell Disease at Risk of Their First Stroke?

Summary of Evidence: TCD is currently the most commonly used screening method to identify children with SCD who are at high risk for first stroke. In the STOP (119) – a multicenter, randomized trial of standard care versus transfusion therapy to prevent first stroke in 130 children with SCD – the TCD ultrasonography was employed to identify patients with high risk at stroke based on mean flow velocity measurements in terminal segment of ICA and MCA. Patients with velocities over 200 cm/s, consistent with cerebral arterial narrowing, and at high risk of first-time stroke, were enrolled. Those treated with chronic blood transfusions (to keep the hemoglobin above 30%) had 92% lower stroke rate. Based on this trial and its follow-up study (120), the NHLBI recommends TCD screening in children starting at 2 years of age and continue annually if TCD is normal and every 4 months if TCD shows velocity over 170 cm/s but less than 200 cm/s. Asymptomatic children with abnormal TCD results should be retested within 2–4 weeks to confirm abnormality, while transfusion is recommended in symptomatic children and abnormal velocities, as patients with TIA whose symptoms are recognized and reported and with confirmed abnormality on neuroimaging are treated as having had a stroke.

There have been no randomized trials testing preventive treatment after the first stroke. However, a number of case series and a more recent review have reported that the risk of reduction appears to be substantial, reducing at least the recurrence in the first few years from over 50 to around 10% (121–123) (limited evidence).

The stroke risk may vary substantially among children with SCD who have abnormal TCD results, because high velocity can be consistent with arterial narrowing as well as hyperemic high blood flow (124). Although there are no data to stratify the risk of stroke based on presence of narrowing or hyperemia, in both situations higher risk of stroke seems to correlate with increased TCD velocities. The risk of ischemic stroke is also higher in children with silent infarctions on MRI and cerebrovascular disease on MRA.

Supporting Evidence: The use of TCD is currently the most commonly used screening method to identify children at high risk of both first and recurrent stroke (strong evidence) (119, 120, 125). TCD is a safe, noninvasive, well-tolerated, relatively low-cost procedure in which the velocity of blood flow can be measured in intracranial arteries using an ultrasound probe placed over the temporal bone (126, 127). In comparison with conventional angiography, TCD flow velocity measurements showed a sensitivity of 90% and specificity of 100% for the diagnosis of arterial narrowing greater than or equal to 50% lumen diameter reduction (moderate evidence) (108, 113). The STOP trial showed associations between stroke risk and TCD mean velocities in the MCA or terminal ICA (Table 12.3).

The NHLBI issued a clinical alert recommending TCD screening for cerebrovascular disease every 6 months on all children with SCD between the ages of 2 and 16 and consideration of chronic transfusions in those with two abnormal TCD test results (128). The timing of repeated TCDs is not clearly defined. If TCD is normal annual testing is proposed while every 4 months if TCD is marginal. Children with abnormal TCD results should be retested within 2–4 weeks (limited evidence) (77, 120, 129, 130).

Fullerton et al. (131) evaluated administrative data in California comparing the rates of hospital admissions for the first stroke in children with SCD between the early 1990s (before STOP) and from 1998 to 2000 (after STOP) and found sharp reduction in first stroke admissions (limited evidence). Further reports from STOP I and II trials (129) and two ongoing clinical trials in children with SCD – one testing other approaches to screening, silent infarct documented by MRI (SILENT Cerebral Infarct Multi-Center Clinical Trial) (132), and the other testing hydroxyurea compared with transfusion for secondary stroke prevention (Stroke With Transfusions Changing to Hydroxyurea Trial) (133) – may show improved outcomes in the future.

Imaging TCD has become a widely employed in practice because it allows accurate identification of intracranial arteries in color and placement of a sample volume in a site of arterial segment, where the velocity is the highest. Also imaging TCD allows determination of the angle of insonation and correction of velocity measurements for the error related to more than zero angles. However, there are no data to support that angle-corrected flow velocity measurements are better than uncorrected ones in risk assessment in children with SCD. There are several articles suggesting that imaging TCD flow velocity measurements obtained without correction for the angle of insonation can be used to identify children at high risk for stroke instead of conventional TCD (limited to moderate evidence) (84, 125, 134–138).

Elevation of cerebral blood flow velocities on TCD may precede abnormal findings in MRA (139, 140). MRA is more costly and children under 3 years may require general anesthesia; however, MRA can confirm the presence and extent of cerebrovascular disease in those with elevated TCD velocities (limited evidence) (103, 104, 141).

Risk of Symptomatic Stroke in Children with Silent Infarct on MRI

Data from the CSSCD showed that silent infarction seen on MRI was associated with an increased risk of symptomatic stroke (1.03 per 100 patient-years) and progression of silent infarction (7.06 per 100 patient-years) (moderate evidence) (41, 62, 68). The Silent Cerebral Infarct Multi-Center Clinical Trial, in which estimated number of 204 children with silent infarction seen on MRI will be randomized to chronic blood transfusions or observation, is currently enrolling patients and will report after 2012 (142).

III. What Is the Role of Neuroimaging in Prevention of Recurrent Ischemic Stroke in Children with Sickle Cell Disease?

Summary of Evidence: Recurrent stroke is observed in children with SCD despite proper regimen of transfusion therapy. Arterial stenosis is the main risk factor for recurrent stroke. Elevated cerebral artery mean velocities (>200 cm/s) on TCD and new lesions on MRI or MRA indicate higher risk of recurrent stroke. SCD children should be monitored after first stroke episode with TCD and MRI/MRA although no randomized or controlled data are available to optimize frequency of follow-up.

Supporting Evidence: Two studies found a high risk of stroke recurrence in children who had arterial abnormalities on conventional angiography (limited evidence) (121, 123). Moyamoya syndrome is characterized by chronic progressive narrowing of proximal segments of intracranial arteries with the characteristic distal collateral network on angiography.

It is a risk factor for stroke recurrence even in those children undergoing regular transfusion (limited evidence) (143, 144). Serial MRI scans in these individuals with preexisting cerebral damage might show new lesions as well as extension of existing abnormality (145). Some studies show this risk to be reduced after extracranial–intracranial bypass or indirect revascularization (146, 147) (limited evidence). Further studies of these procedures are needed as some researchers have not found progression (148), and the cerebrovascular disease can stabilize as demonstrated on both MRA (149) and TCD (limited evidence) (77).

IV. Are There Neuroimaging Criteria That Indicate That Blood Transfusions Can Be Safely Halted?

Summary of Evidence: : Limited data on discontinuation of blood transfusion suggest that halting transfusions increases the risk of stroke. A decision analytic model suggests follow-up of SCD children during transfusion therapy with annual TCD until age 10 years. The model also suggests transfusions until 18 years in children with high risk of stroke. The main risk of prolonged blood transfusions is iron overload which can result in organ failure and death.

Supporting Evidence: The STOP II trial followed the children in STOP I and showed that discontinuation of transfusions led to recurrence of TCD abnormalities and development of new stroke events (moderate evidence) (142, 150). However, only the baseline TCD results were used to determine stroke risk against follow-up observations. Transfusion therapy converts approximately 60% of patients to normal TCD results (150, 151) (moderate evidence). Similar findings were observed on MRA examinations (77) (limited evidence). The STOP II trial concluded that transfusions should not be stopped once TCD results were normal (moderate evidence) (150).

However, 20% of children who discontinued transfusion therapy did not develop abnormal

TCD or stroke. Mazumdar et al. performed a decision analysis model to compare various stroke prevention strategies for a hypothetical cohort of 2-year-old children (152), such as (1) annual TCD ultrasonography screening until age 16 years with children at high risk for stroke receiving monthly transfusion for life; (2) annual TCD ultrasonography until age 16 years with transfusions until age 18 years; (3) biannual TCD ultrasonography until age 16 years with transfusions until age 18 years; (4) annual TCD ultrasonography until age 10 years with transfusion until age 18 years; (5) one-time screening at age 2 years with transfusion until age 18 years; and (6) no intervention.

The optimal stroke prevention strategy was projected to be annual TCD ultrasonography screening until age 10 years with transfusion for children at high risk until age 18 years. Better adherence to chelation therapy would improve life expectancy in all intervention strategies with fewer deaths from iron overload in comparison to other more intensive strategies (152) (limited evidence).

V. What Is the Role of Neuroimaging in Hemorrhagic Stroke in Children with SCD?

Summary of Evidence: : Infarctive strokes are relatively more common in children than in adults with SCD while reverse is true for hemorrhagic stroke (12). Primary hemorrhagic stroke is much more devastating and in majority of patients is fatal (12). High leukocyte count and low steady-state Hb concentration were identified to be the main risk factors of hemorrhagic stroke in SCD patients (12). Other potential risk factors are hypertension, treatment with corticoids, previous ischemic stroke, or hypertransfusion (36). CT without contrast is still the first line examination in diagnosing hemorrhagic stroke. In acute intraparenchymal hemorrhage (ICH) the accuracy of MRI examination seems to be similar to accuracy of CT, especially when gradient echo sequences are used (78, 79); however, in patients with subarachnoid hemorrhage, (SAH) CT is superior (153). TCD seems to be ineffective in predicting hemorrhagic stroke (120). The role of TCD in pediatric SAH is unclear though in adults it is used to detect and monitor vasospasm. In cases with ICH, DSA is advisable to rule out lesions that should be treated with surgery. In cases with SAH, DSA is used to detect ruptured cerebral aneurysms. Hydration and reduction of HbS to less than 30% prior to DSA is the usual method of preparation, and there have been few reports of stroke complications since this practice was initiated.

It is not known if transfusion prevents recurrent hemorrhage. Patients with any form of intracranial bleeding, excepting subdural from trauma, need evaluation for a surgically correctable aneurysm even if the bleeding appears to be primarily intracerebral. If there is no aneurysm then transfusion for at least a year is often recommended, but it is not clear if this helps. Recurrent hemorrhage is less common than recurrent ischemic stroke, partly because more of the first events are fatal.

Supporting Evidence: The CSSCD showed about 9.6% of first strokes in SCD-SS patients less than 20 years old were hemorrhagic, compared to 52% of first strokes in those over 20 years old (12). There is nearly a 250-fold increase in the risk of hemorrhagic stroke compared with children under age 20 years (23). In CSSCD study almost all fatal cases (24%) were due to hemorrhagic stroke. However, in the first published series the mortality rate associated with hemorrhagic stroke was over 50% (154), similar to the rate (40%) reported by Strouse et al. (34). Typical clinical presentation of hemorrhagic stroke in SCD includes focal neurological deficits, severe headache, nuchal rigidity, and coma.

The CSSCD study showed that risk of hemorrhagic stroke increases along with decreasing steady-state Hb concentration (RR 1.61 per 1 g/dL decrease) and increasing steady leukocyte count (1.94 per 5×10^9/L increase) (limited evidence) (12). Associations with hypertension, recent blood transfusions, treatment with corticosteroids, previous ischemic stroke, moyamoya, cerebral aneurysms, or acute chest syndrome (ACS) were also reported (insufficient evidence) (34, 39, 143, 155–158).

CT is being used as an initial imaging study. In emergency setting, noncontrast CT is adequate and the most cost-effective strategy in diagnosing acute hemorrhagic stroke (moderate evidence) (159). In acute ICH the accuracy of MRI is similar to accuracy of CT, especially with the use of gradient echo sequences (78, 79)

(strong evidence). MRI is better than CT in evaluations of chronic hemorrhage (78, 79) (strong evidence). MRI, however, is not feasible in up to 20% acute stroke patients due to contraindications to MRI, impaired consciousness, hemodynamic compromise, vomiting, or agitation, and lack of cooperation (160). To obtain successful MRI results patients often need general anesthesia.

CT should be used if subarachnoid hemorrhage is suspected (153) (insufficient evidence). DSA is used to identify the source of bleeding (161, 162) (limited evidence), but most children require general anesthesia. DSA is invasive, however, and carries risk of stroke (163, 164). CTA and MRA are less accurate than DSA in depicting intracranial vascular anatomy, especially in visualization of tertiary branches and small cerebral arteries (161). The additional advantage of DSA is the potential to initiate therapy such as endovascular coiling of aneurysms and embolization of AVMs. TCD is not effective in predicting hemorrhagic stroke (120); however, TCD can be used to detect and monitor intracranial vasospasm in patients with SAH (165) (limited evidence).

Take Home Figures and Tables

Figure 12.1 shows a decision tree about the role of neuroimaging in the primary prevention against stroke and management of children with sickle cell disease (SCD) with neurological symptoms.

Table 12.1 shows incidence of first stroke and prevalence of CVA in the population of children with SCD. Table 12.2 shows risk of recurrent stroke in SCD patients. Table 12.3 shows risk for stroke in SCD patients in accordance with initial TCD velocities.

Imaging Case Studies

Case 1

Figure 12.2 presents brain images of an 11-year-old girl with SCD without neurological deficits.

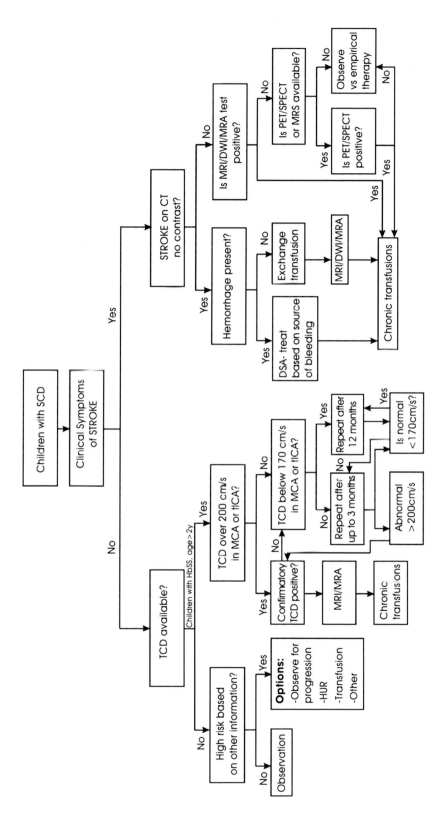

Figure 12.1. Decision tree shows the role of neuroimaging in primary prevention against stroke and management of *children* with sickle cell disease (SCD) with neurological symptoms. *TCD* transcranial Doppler sonography, *MRI* magnetic resonance imaging, *MRA* MR angiography, *DWI* diffusion weighted imaging, *PET* positron emission tomography, *SPECT* single photon emission computed tomography, *DSA* digital subtraction angiography, *HUR* hydroxyurea, *MCA* middle cerebral artery, and *ICA* internal carotid artery. Note: optimal frequency of rescreening with TCD is not established; younger children with velocity closer to 200 cm/s should be rescreened more frequently. (Reprinted with kind permission of Springer Science+Business Media from Krejza J, Swiat M, Tomaszewski M, Melhem ER. In Medina LS, Applegate KE, Blackmore CC (eds.): *Evidence-Based Imaging in Pediatrics: Optimizing Imaging in Pediatric Patient Care*. New York: Springer Science+Business Media, 2010.)

Table 12.1. Incidence (in %) of first stroke and prevalence of CVA in the population of children with sickle cell disease

	Hb SS	Hb SC	Hb S-β^+	Hb S-β^0	Total
Overall incidence	0.61	0.17	0.11	0.10	0.46
Age-adjusted incidence	0.61	0.15	0.09	0.08	
Overall prevalence	4.07	0.80	1.48	1.56	3.75
Age-adjusted prevalence	4.01	0.84	1.29	2.43	

Data from Ohene-Frempong et al. (12).
Reprinted with kind permission of Springer Science+Business Media from Krejza J, Swiat M, Tomaszewski M, Melhem ER. In Medina LS, Applegate KE, Blackmore CC (eds.): *Evidence-Based Imaging in Pediatrics: Optimizing Imaging in Pediatric Patient Care.* New York: Springer Science+Business Media, 2010.

Table 12.2. Risk of recurrent stroke in SCD patients in accordance with initial event

Initial event	Events per 100 patient-years
Symptomatic stroke	
Before age 20	6.4
After age 20	1.6
Silent infarct	0.54

Data from Ohene-Frempong et al. (12) and Balkaran et al. (40).
Reprinted with kind permission of Springer Science+Business Media from Krejza J, Swiat M, Tomaszewski M, Melhem ER. In Medina LS, Applegate KE, Blackmore CC (eds.): *Evidence-Based Imaging in Pediatrics: Optimizing Imaging in Pediatric Patient Care.* New York: Springer Science+Business Media, 2010.

Table 12.3. Risk of stroke in SCD patients in accordance with initial TCD mean velocities

TCD velocity (cm/s)	Stroke risk (%)
>200	40
>170	7
<170	2

Data from STOP trial results from Adams et al. (120).
Reprinted with kind permission of Springer Science+Business Media from Krejza J, Swiat M, Tomaszewski M, Melhem ER. In Medina LS, Applegate KE, Blackmore CC (eds.): *Evidence-Based Imaging in Pediatrics: Optimizing Imaging in Pediatric Patient Care.* New York: Springer Science+Business Media, 2010.

Suggested Imaging Protocol for Sickle Cell Disease and Stroke

Shown in Fig. 12.1.

Future Research

- Is TCD useful to assess the risk of stroke among children with hemoglobin SC and β-thalassemia?

- Is advanced MRI helpful to better select SCD patients for chronic transfusions?
- Is advanced MRI useful in secondary stroke prediction?
- Is neuroimaging useful to identify children in whom chronic transfusions can be safely stopped?
- Is there a role for PET-CT for better identification of ischemia in children with SCD?

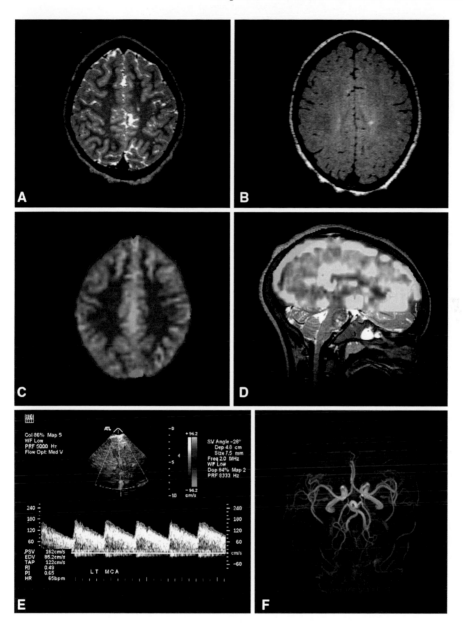

Figure 12.2. Brain images of an 11-year-old female with sickle cell disease (genotype HbSS) without neuro-logical deficits. (**A**) Axial T2-weighted image with small silent lesion located in left parietal region. (**B**) Axial flair image showing the same lesion in left parietal lesion. (**C**) Axial slice of CBF map obtained using arterial spin labeling perfusion MRI coregistered to T1-weighted image. (**D**) Sagittal projection of the CBF map registered to T2-weighted volumetric image; note the high CBF signal in sagittal sinus. (**E**) Image from transcranial color-coded Doppler study of the middle cerebral artery with velocity measurements and angle correction. (**F**) Axial projection of the 3D reconstruction of time-of-flight MRA. (Reprinted with kind permission of Springer Science+Business Media from Krejza J, Swiat M, Tomaszewski M, Melhem ER. In Medina LS, Applegate KE, Blackmore CC (eds.): *Evidence-Based Imaging in Pediatrics: Optimizing Imaging in Pediatric Patient Care.* New York: Springer Science+Business Media, 2010.)

References

1. Pavlakis SG, Kingsley PB, Bialer MG. J Child Neurol 2000;15:308–315.
2. Prohovnik I, Pavlakis SG, Piomelli S, Bello J, Mohr JP, Hilal S et al. Neurology 1989;39: 344–348.
3. Lipowsky H, Cram L, Justice W, Eppihimer M. Microvasc Res 1993;46:43–64.
4. Lipowsky H. Microcirculation 2005;12:5–15.
5. Zhao Y, Chien S, Skalak R, Lipowsky H. Ann Biomed Eng 2001;29:360–372.
6. Dong C, Cao J, Struble E, Lipowsky H. Ann Biomed Eng 1999;27:298–312.
7. Mulivor A, Lipowsky H. Am J Physiol Heart Circ Physiol 2004;286:H1672–H1680.
8. Hebbel RP, Osarogiagbon R, Kaul D. Microcirculation 2004;11:129–151.
9. Kaul DK, Fabry ME, Nagel RL. Blood Rev 1996; 10:29–44.
10. Serjeant GR. Br J Haematol 2001;112:3–18.
11. Stuart MJ, Setty BNY. Pediatr Pathol Mol Med 2001;20:27–46.
12. Ohene-Frempong K, Weiner SJ, Sleeper LA, Miller ST, Embury S, Moohr JW et al. Cooperative study sickle cell D. Blood 1998;91:288–294.
13. Embury SH. Microcirculation 2004;11:101–113.
14. Miller ST, Sleeper LA, Pegelow CH, Enos LE, Wang WC, Weiner SJ et al. New Engl J Med 2000;342:83–89.
15. Wethers DL. Am Fam Physician 2000;62: 1309–1314.
16. Stevens M, Maude G, Beckford M, Grandison Y, Mason K, Taylor B et al. Blood 1986;67:411–414.
17. Scothorn DJ, Price C, Schwartz D, Terrill C, Buchanan GR, Shurney W et al. J Pediatr 2002;140:348–354.
18. Hulbert ML, Scothorn DJ, Panepinto JA, Scott JP, Buchanan GR, Sarnaik S et al. J Pediatr 2006;149:710–712.
19. Garcia J, Anderson M. Crit Rev Neurobiol 1989;4:303–324.
20. Di Roio C, Jourdan C, Terrier A, Artru F. Ann Fr Anesth Reanim 1997;16:967–969.
21. Ganesan V, Prengler M, McShane M, Wade A, Kirkham F. Ann Neurol 2003;53:167–173.
22. Kirkham FJ, Prengler M, Hewes DKM, Ganesan V. J Child Neurol 2000;15:299–307.
23. Earley CJ, Kittner SJ, Feeser BR, Gardner J, Epstein A, Wozniak MA et al. Neurology 1998;51:169–176.
24. Melek I, Akgul F, Duman T, Yalcin F, Gali E. Tohoku J Exp Med 2006;209:135–140.
25. Mercuri E, Faundez J, Roberts I, Flora S, Bouza H, Cowan F et al. Eur J Pediatr 1995;154: 150–156.
26. Prengler M, Pavlakis SG, Boyd S, Connelly A, Calamante F, Chong WK et al. Ann Neurol 2005;58:290–302.
27. Huttenlocher P, Moohr J, Johns L, Brown F. Pediatrics 1984;73:615–621.
28. Kirkham FJ, Calamante F, Bynevelt M, Gadian DG, Evans JPM, Cox TC et al. Ann Neurol 2001;49:477–485.
29. Kirkham FJ, Hewes DKM, Prengler M, Wade A, Lane R et al. Lancet 2001;357:1656–1659.
30. Vichinsky E, Neumayr L, Earles A, Williams R, Lennette E, Dean D et al. N Engl J Med 2000;342:1855–1865.
31. Lee KH, McKie VC, Sekul EA, Adams RJ, Nichols FT. J Pediatr Hematol Oncol 2002;24: 585–588.
32. Wierenga KJJ, Serjeant BE, Serjeant GR. J Pediatr 2001;139:438–442.
33. Makani J, Meda E, Rwezaula S, Mwamtemi K, Thein SL, Williams T et al. Blood 2006;108:26B.
34. Strouse JJ, Hulbert ML, DeBaun MR, Jordan LC, Casella JF. Pediatrics 2006;118:1916–1924.
35. Coley S, Porter D, Calamante F, Chong W, Connelly A. AJNR Am J Neuroradiol 1999;20:1507–1510.
36. Horton D, Ferriero D, Mentzer W. Pediatr Neurol 1995;12:77–80.
37. Gadian D, Calamante F, Kirkham F, Bynevelt M, Johnson C, Porter D et al. J Child Neurol 2000;15:279–283.
38. Sébire G, Tabarki B, Saunders D, Leroy I, Liesner R, Saint-Martin C et al. Brain 2005;128: 477–489.
39. Powars D, Adams R, Nichols F, Milner P, Charache S, Sarnaik S. J Assoc Acad Minor Phys 1990;1:79–82.
40. Balkaran B, Char G, Morris J, Thomas P, Serjeant B, Serjeant G. J Pediatr 1992;120:360–366.
41. Pegelow C, Macklin E, Moser F, Wang W, Bello J, Miller S et al. Blood 2002;99:3014–3018.
42. Jeffries BF, Lipper MH, Kishore PR. Surg Neurol 1980;14:291–295.
43. Aluoch J, Jacobs P. S Afr Med J 1996;86: 982–983.
44. Al-Riyami A, Ebrahim G. J Trop Pediatr 2003;49(Suppl 1):i1–i20.
45. De D. Br J Nurs 2005;14:447–450.
46. Balgir R. J Assoc Physicians India 1996;44: 25–28.
47. Fattoum S. Tunis Med 2006;84:687–696.
48. Hamdallah M, Bhatia A. Lancet 1995;346: 707–708.
49. Kamble M, Chatruvedi P. Indian Pediatr 2000;37:391–396.
50. Williams T, Mwangi T, Wambua S, Alexander N, Kortok M, Snow R et al. J Infect Dis 2005;192:178–186.
51. Petrakis N, Wiesenfeld S, Sams B, Collen M, Cutler J, Siegelaub A. N Engl J Med 1970;282: 767–770.
52. Scott R. N Engl J Med 1970;282:164–165.
53. Boyle EJ, Thompson C, Tyroler H. Arch Environ Health 1968;17:891–898.

54. Nietert P, Silverstein M, Abboud M. Pharmacoeconomics 2002;20:357–366.
55. Hicks E, Miller G, Horton R. Am J Public Health 1978;68:1135–1137.
56. Ashley-Koch A, Yang Q, Olney R. Am J Epidemiol 2000;151:839–845.
57. National Human Genome Research Institute. Learning about SCD. http://www.genome.gov/10001219 [last accessed July 30, 2008].
58. Das L. Indian J Malariol 2000;37:34–38.
59. Rodríguez-Ojea Menéndez A, García de la Osa M. Rev Cubana Med Trop 1992;44:62–65.
60. deVeber G, Roach ES, Riela AR, Wiznitzer M. Semin Pediatr Neurol 2000;7:309–317.
61. Steen R, Emudianughe T, Hankins G, Wynn L, Wang W, Xiong X et al. Radiology 2003;228:216 225.
62. Miller S, Macklin E, Pegelow C, Kinney T, Sleeper L, Bello J et al. J Pediatr 2001;139:385–390.
63. Charache S, Terrin ML, Moore RD, Dover GJ, Barton FB, Eckert SV et al. N Engl J Med 1995;332:1317–1322.
64. Hankins JS, Ware RE, Rogers ZR, Wynn LW, Lane PA, Scott JP et al. Blood 2005;106:2269–2275.
65. Gulbis B, Haberman D, Dufour D, Christophe C, Vermylen C, Kagambega F et al. Blood 2005;105:2685–2690.
66. Moser F, Miller S, Bello J, Pegelow C, Zimmerman R, Wang W et al. AJNR Am J Neuroradiol 1996;17:965–972.
67. Bernaudin F, Verlhac S, Fréard F, Roudot-Thoraval F, Benkerrou M, Thuret I et al. J Child Neurol 2000;15:333–343.
68. Kinney T, Sleeper L, Wang W, Zimmerman R, Pegelow C, Ohene-Frempong K et al. Pediatrics 1999;103:640–645.
69. Baldeweg T, Hogan A, Saunders D, Telfer P, Gadian D, Vargha-Khadem F et al. Ann Neurol 2006;59:662–672.
70. DeBaun M, Schatz J, Siegel M, Koby M, Craft S, Resar L et al. Neurology 1998;50:1678–1682.
71. Watkins K, Hewes D, Connelly A, Kendall B, Kingsley D, Evans J et al. Dev Med Child Neurol 1998;40:536–543.
72. Hogan A, Kirkham F, Prengler M, Telfer P, Lane R, Vargha-Khadem F et al. Br J Haematol 2006;132:99–107.
73. Wang W, Enos L, Gallagher D, Thompson R, Guarini L, Vichinsky E et al. J Pediatr 2001;139:391–397.
74. Schatz J, Buzan R. J Int Neuropsychol Soc 2006;12:24–33.
75. Davis H, Moore RJ, Gergen P. Public Health Rep 1997;112:40–43.
76. Wayne A, Schoenike S, Pegelow C. Blood 2000;96:2369–2372.
77. Bernaudin F, Verlhac S, Coïc L, Lesprit E, Brugières P et al. Pediatr Radiol 2005;35:242–248.
78. Kidwell C, Chalela J, Saver J, Starkman S, Hill M, Demchuk A et al. JAMA 2004;292:1823–1830.
79. Fiebach J, Schellinger P, Gass A, Kucinski T, Siebler M, Villringer A et al. Stroke 2004;35:502–506.
80. Mokri B, Sundt TM Jr, Houser OW, Piepgras DG. Ann Neurol 1986;19:126–138.
81. de Bruijn SF, Stam J. Stroke 1999;30:481–483.
82. Adams R, Nichols F, McKie V, McKie K, Milner P et al. Neurology 1988;38:1012–1017.
83. Brambilla D, Miller S, Adams R. Pediatr Blood Cancer 2007;49:318–322.
84. Seibert J, Miller S, Kirby R, Becton D, James C, Glasier C et al. Radiology 1993;189:457–466.
85. Switzer J, Hess D, Nichols F, Adams R. Lancet Neurol 2006;5(6).501–512.
86. Kirkham F. Nat Clin Pract Neurol 2007;3:264–278.
87. Unit CEE. Stroke in Childhood: Clinical Guidelines for Diagnosis, Management and Rehabilitation. http://www.rcplondon.ac.uk/pubs/books/childstroke/childstroke_guidelines.pdf. London: Royal College of Physicians [online November 2004].
88. Winrow N, Melhem E. Neuroimaging Clin N Am 2003;13:185–196.
89. Lev MH, Farkas J, Gemmete JJ et al. Radiology 1999;213:150–155.
90. Lin K, Rapalino O, Law M, Babb JS, Siller KA, Pramanik BK. AJNR Am J Neuroradiol 2008;29:931–936.
91. Katz DA, Marks MP, Napel SA, Bracci PM, Roberts SL. Radiology 1995;195:445–449.
92. Bash S, Villablanca JP, Jahan R, Duckwiler G, Tillis M, Kidwell C et al. AJNR Am J Neuroradiol 2005;26:1012–1021.
93. Beyer J, Platt A, Kinney T, Treadwell M. J Soc Pediatr Nurs 1999;4(2):61–73.
94. Pavlakis S, Bello J, Prohovnik I, Sutton M, Ince C, Mohr J et al. Ann Neurol 1988;23:125–130.
95. DeBaun M, Glauser T, Siegel M, Borders J, Lee B. J Pediatr Hematol Oncol 1995;17:29–33.
96. Marks MP, de Crespigny A, Lentz D, Enzmann DR, Albers GW et al. Radiology 1996;199:403–408.
97. González RG, Schaefer PW, Buonanno FS, Schwamm LH, Budzik RF, Rordorf G et al. Radiology 1999;210:155–162.
98. Lövblad KO, Laubach HJ, Baird AE, Curtin F, Schlaug G, Edelman RR et al. AJNR Am J Neuroradiol 1998;19:1061–1066.
99. Mullins M, Schaefer P, Sorensen A, Halpern E, Ay H, He J et al. Radiology. 2002;224:353–360.
100. Lansberg M, Albers G, Beaulieu C, Marks M. Neurology 2000;54(8):1557–1561.
101. Lansberg M, Norbash A, Marks M, Tong D, Moseley M, Albers G. Arch Neurol 2000;57:1311–1316.

102. Rovira A, Grivé E, Alvarez-Sabin J. Eur Radiol 2005;15:416–426.
103. Kandeel AY, Zimmerman RA, Ohene-Frempong K. Neuroradiology 1996;38:409–416.
104. Gillams AR, McMahon L, Weinberg G, Carter AP. Pediatr Radiol 1998;28:283–287.
105. Korogi Y, Takahashi M, Nakagawa T et al. AJNR Am J Neuroradiol 1997;18:135–143.
106. Kielpinska K, Walecki J, Giedrojc J, Turowska A, Kordecki K. Acad Radiol 2002;9:283–289.
107. Srinivasan A, Goyal M, Al Azri F, Lum C. Radiographics 2006;26:S75–S95.
108. Adams R, Nichols F, Figueroa R, McKie V, Lott T. Stroke 1992;23:1073–1077.
109. Dawkins A, Evans A, Wattam J, Romanowski C, Connolly D et al. Neuroradiology 2007;49: 753–759.
110. Rao K, Lee M. Radiology 1983;147:600–601.
111. Coley S, Wild J, Wilkinson I, Griffiths P. Neuroradiology 2003;45:843–850.
112. Qureshi N, Lubin B, Walters M. Expert Opin Biol Ther 2006;6:1087–1098.
113. Verlhac S, Bernaudin F, Tortrat D, Brugieres P, Mage K, Gaston A. Pediatr Radiol 1995;25(Suppl 1): S14–S19.
114. Chooi W, Woodhouse N, Coley S, Griffiths P. AJNR Am J Neuroradiol 2004;25:1251–1255.
115. Reed W, Jagust W, Al-Mateen M, Vichinsky E. Am J Hematol 1999;60:268–272.
116. Powars D, Conti P, Wong W, Groncy P, Hyman C, Smith E et al. Blood 1999;93:71–79.
117. Rodgers GP, Clark CM, Larson SM, Rapoport SI, Nienhuis AW et al. Arch Neurol 1988;45: 78–82.
118. Herold S, Brozovic M, Gibbs J, Lammertsma AA, Leenders KL, Carr D et al. Stroke 1986;17:692–698.
119. Adams R, McKie V, Hsu L, Files B, Vichinsky E, Pegelow C et al. N Engl J Med 1998;339:5–11.
120. Adams R, Brambilla D, Granger S, Gallagher D, Vichinsky E, Abboud M et al. Blood 2004;103:3689–3694.
121. Russell M, Goldberg H, Hodson A, Kim H, Halus J, Reivich M et al. Blood 1984;63:162–169.
122. Pegelow CH, Adams RJ, McKie V, Abboud M, Berman B, Miller ST et al. J Pediatr 1995;126: 896–899.
123. Wilimas J, Goff J, Anderson HJ, Langston J, Thompson E. J Pediatr 1980;96:205–208.
124. Ausavarungnirun P, Sabio H, Kim J, Tegeler CH. J Neuroimaging 2006;16:311–317.
125. Adams R, Pavlakis S, Roach E. Ann Neurol 2003;54:559–563.
126. Krejza J, Rudzinski W, Pawlak M, Tomaszewski M, Ichord R, Kwiatkowski J et al. AJNR Am J Neuroradiol 2007;28:1613–1618.
127. Adams R. J Pediatr Hematol Oncol 1996;18:331–334.
128. National Heart, Lung, and Blood Institute. Clinical alert: periodic transfusions lower stroke risk in children with sickle cell anemia. http:// www.nim.nih.gov/databases/alerts/sickle97. html.
129. Lee M, Piomelli S, Granger S, Miller S, Harkness S, Brambilla D et al. Blood 2006;108:847–852.
130. Bulas D. Pediatr Radiol 2005;35:235–241.
131. Fullerton H, Adams R, Zhao S, Johnston S. Blood 2004;104:336–339.
132. Trial. http://www.clinicaltrials.gov/ct/show/ NCT00072761.CgWsSCIM-CC.
133. http://www.clinicaltrials.gov/ct/show/ NCT00122980.CgWsSwTCtHS.
134. Jones A, Seibert J, Nichols F, Kinder D, Cox K, Luden J et al. Pediatr Radiol 2001;31:461–469.
135. Malouf AJ, Hamrick-Turner J, Doherty M, Dhillon G, Iyer R, Smith M. Radiology 2001;219:359–365.
136. McCarville M, Li C, Xiong X, Wang W. AJR Am J Roentgenol 2004;183:1117–1122.
137. Riebel T, Kebelmann-Betzing C, Götze R, Overberg U. Eur Radiol 2003;13:563–570.
138. Lowe L, Bulas D. Pediatr Radiol 2005;35:54–65.
139. Abboud M, Cure J, Granger S, Gallagher D, Hsu L, Wang W et al. Blood 2004;103:2822–2826.
140. Wang W, Gallagher D, Pegelow C, Wright E, Vichinsky E, Abboud M et al. J Pediatr Hematol Oncol 2000;22:335–339.
141. Wiznitzer M, Ruggieri P, Masaryk T, Ross J, Modic M, Berman B. J Pediatr 1990;117: 551–555.
142. Kirkham F, Lerner N, Noetzel M, DeBaun M, Datta A, Rees D et al. Pediatr Neurol 2006;34:450–458.
143. Dobson S, Holden K, Nietert P, Cure J, Laver J, Disco D et al. Blood 2002;99:3144–3150.
144. Ganesan V, Prengler M, Wade A, Kirkham F. Circulation 2006;114:2170–2177.
145. Woodard P, Helton K, Khan R, Hale G, Phipps S, Wang W et al. Br J Haematol 2005;129:550–552.
146. Kirkham F, DeBaun M. Curr Treat Options Neurol 2004;6:357–375.
147. Fryer R, Anderson R, Chiriboga C, Feldstein N. Pediatr Neurol 2003;29:124–130.
148. Walters M, Storb R, Patience M, Leisenring W, Taylor T, Sanders J et al. Blood 2000;95: 1918–1924.
149. Steen R, Helton K, Horwitz E, Benaim E, Thompson S, Bowman L et al. Ann Neurol 2001;49:222–229.
150. Adams R, Brambilla D. N Engl J Med 2005;353:2769–2778.
151. Minniti C, Gidvani V, Bulas D, Brown W, Vezina G, Driscoll M. J Pediatr Hematol Oncol 2004;26:626–630.
152. Mazumdar M, Heeney M, Sox C, Lieu T. Pediatrics 2007;120:e1107–e1116.
153. Adams HP Jr, del Zoppo G, Alberts MJ, Bhatt DL, Brass L, Furlan A et al.; American Heart Association; American Stroke Association Stroke Council; Clinical Cardiology Council;

Cardiovascular Radiology and Intervention Council; Atherosclerotic Peripheral Vascular Disease and Quality of Care Outcomes in Research Interdisciplinary Working Groups. Stroke 2007;38:1655–1711.

154. Powars D, Wilson B, Imbus C, Pegelow C, Allen J. Am J Med 1978;65:461–471.

155. Diggs LW, Brookoff D. South Med J 1993;86:377–379.

156. Royal JE, Seeler RA. Lancet 1978;2(8101):1207.

157. Stockman JA, Nigro MA, Mishkin MM, Oski FA. N Engl J Med 1972;287:846–849.

158. Henderson JN, Noetzel MJ, McKinstry RC, White DA, Armstrong M et al. Blood 2003;101:415–419.

159. Wardlaw JM, Keir SL, Seymour J, Lewis S, Sandercock PA, Dennis MS et al. Health Technol Assess 2004;8(iii, ix–x):1–180.

160. Singer OC, Sitzer M, du Mesnil de Rochemont R, Neumann-Haefelin T. Neurology 2004;62:1848–1849.

161. Wardlaw JM, White PM. Brain 2000;123:205–221.

162. Chappell ET, Moure FC, Good MC. Neurosurgery 2003;52:624–631.

163. Willinsky RA, Taylor SM, TerBrugge K et al. Radiology 2003;227:522–528.

164. Burger IM et al. Stroke 2006;37:2535–2539.

165. Lysakowski C, Walder B, Costanza MC, Tramèr MR. Stroke 2001;32:2292–2298.

13

Neuroimaging for Traumatic Brain Injury

Karen A. Tong, Udochuckwu E. Oyoyo, Barbara A. Holshouser, Stephen Ashwal,
and L. Santiago Medina

Issues

I. Which patients with head injury should undergo imaging in the acute setting?
II. What is the sensitivity and specificity of imaging for injury requiring immediate treatment/surgery?
III. What is the overall sensitivity and specificity of imaging in the diagnosis and prognosis of patients with head trauma?
IV. What are considerations for imaging of children with head trauma?
V. What is the role of advanced imaging (functional MRI, MR spectroscopy, Diffusion Imaging, SPECT, and PET) in TBI?

Key Points

- Head injury is not a homogeneous phenomenon and has a complex clinical course. There are different mechanisms, varying severity, diversity of injuries, secondary injuries, and effects of age or underlying disease.
- Classifications of injury and outcomes are inconsistent. Differences in diagnostic procedures and practice patterns prevent direct comparison of population-based studies.
- There are a variety of imaging methods that measure different aspects of injury (Table 13.1), but there is no one all-encompassing imaging method.
- CT is the mainstay of imaging in the acute period. The majority of evidence relates to the use of CT for detecting injuries that may require immediate treatment or surgery. Speed, availability, ease of

K.A. Tong (✉)
Department of Radiology, Loma Linda University Medical Center, 11234 Anderson Street,
Schuman Pavilion, Room B623, Loma Linda, CA 92354, USA
e-mail: ktong@llu.edu

L.S. Medina et al. (eds.), *Evidence-Based Imaging: Improving the Quality of Imaging in Patient Care, Revised Edition*,
DOI 10.1007/978-1-4419-7777-9_13, © Springer Science+Business Media, LLC 2011

exam, and lesser expense of CT studies remain important factors for using this modality in the acute setting. Sensitivity of detection also increases with repeat scans in the acute period (strong evidence).

- The sensitivity and specificity of MRI for brain injury is generally superior to CT, although most studies have been retrospective and few direct comparisons have been performed in the recent decade. CT is clearly superior to MRI for the detection of fractures. MRI outperforms CT in detection of most other lesions (limited to moderate evidence), particularly diffuse axonal injury (DAI). MRI allows more detailed analysis of injuries, including metabolic and physiologic measures, but further evidence-based research is needed.
- Accurate prognostic information is important for determining management, but there are different needs for different populations. In severe TBI, information is important for acute patient management, long-term rehabilitation, and family counseling. In mild or moderate TBI, patients with subtle impairments may benefit from counseling and education.
- Prediction rules such as the CHALICE prediction rule (Table 13.2) and the CATCH decision rule (Table 13.3) have the potential to improve and standardize the care of pediatric patients with head injuries (moderate evidence). In addition, minimizing the use of CT in children with very low risk of clinically important TBI may reduce the risk of radiation-induced malignancies.
- Calvarial plain radiographs have a poor sensitivity for identifying pediatric patients with intracranial pathology (moderate to strong evidence) and hence, are not recommended unless for highly selected patients with suspected nonaccidental trauma.
- It is safe to discharge children with TBI, to home, after a negative CT study (moderate to strong evidence).

Definition and Pathophysiology

Head trauma is difficult to study because it is a heterogeneous entity that encompasses many different types of injuries that may occur together (Table 13.4). Definitions of age groups, injuries, and outcomes are also variable. Classification of injury severity is usually defined by the Glasgow Coma Scale (GCS) score, a scale ranging from 3 to 15, which is often grouped into mild, moderate, or severe categories. There is inconsistency in timing of measurement, with some investigators using "initial or field GCS" while others use "post-resuscitation GCS." Grouping of GCS scores also vary. There is no universal definition of mild or minor head injury (1), as some use GCS scores of 13–15 (2), while others use 14–15 (2), and others use only 15 (2, 3). Variable definitions result in inconsistencies in imaging recommendations (1). Moderate TBI is generally defined by GCS of 9–12. Severe TBI is defined by GCS of 3–8.

Classification and measures of outcome are even more variable. The most commonly used outcome measure is the Glasgow Outcome Scale (GOS) (4). It is an overall measure based on degree of independence and ability to participate in normal activities; with five categories: (5) good recovery, (4) moderate disability, (3) severe disability, (2) vegetative state (VS), and (1) death. The GOS is often dichotomized, although grouping is variable. A subsequent modification, the Extended GOS (5), has eight categories: (8) good recovery, (7) good recovery with minor physical or mental deficits, (6) moderate disability, able to return to work with some adjustments or, (5) works at lower level of performance, (4) severe disability, dependent on others for some activities, (3) completely dependent on others, (2) VS, and (1) death. Less common outcome scales include: the Differential Outcome Scale (DOS) (6), the Rappaport Disability Rating Scale (DRS) (7), the Disability Score (DS) (8), the Functional Independent

Measure (FIM) instrument (9), the Supervision Rating Scale (10), and the Functional Status Examination (11, 12).

Timing of outcome measurement also varies. Some investigators measure outcomes at discharge, 3, 6, or 12 months (or more) after injury. This may be problematic because outcomes often improve with time. However, there is moderate to strong evidence that 6 months is an appropriate time point to measure outcomes for clinical trials (13). Neuropsychological assessment is the most sensitive measure of outcome, although this is difficult to perform in severely injured patients, resulting in selection bias. There is a wide variety of psychometric scales for various components of cognitive function such as intellect, orientation, attention, language, speech, information processing, motor reaction time, memory, learning, visuoconstructive ability, verbal fluency, mental flexibility, executive control, and personality.

Epidemiology in USA

The prevalence of TBI is difficult to determine, because many less severely injured patients are not hospitalized and cases with multiple injuries may not be included. In addition, the number of people with TBI who are not seen in an emergency department or who receive no care is unknown. It is estimated that 1.7 million people per year sustain a TBI (14). About 1.365 million (nearly 80%) are treated and released from an emergency department. Most of these injuries are concussions or other forms of mild TBI (15). However, approximately 52,000 people with TBI die, and about 275,000 are hospitalized. In addition, TBI contributes to a third (30.5%) of all injury-related deaths in the US. Children aged 0–4 years, adolescents aged 15–19 years, and adults aged 65 years and older are most likely to sustain a TBI; in all age groups, TBI rates are higher for males than females. Almost half a million (473,947) ED visits per year for TBI are by children aged 0–14 years. Falls are a leading cause of TBI (35.2%), particularly for children aged 0–4 years and adults aged 75 years and older. Motor vehicle accidents account for 17.3% of TBI, but is the leading cause of TBI-related death, particularly in adults aged 20–24 years (16).

Overall Cost to Society

Over the last 30 years, there has been a progressive and significant reduction in severe TBI mortality, from 50% to less than 25% (16), probably from multiple factors including improvements in medical care, use of evidence-based guidelines, and injury-prevention efforts. An estimated 5.3 million US residents live with permanent TBI-related disabilities (17). Direct costs are estimated at $48.3 billion/year (18). In 2000, total direct and indirect costs of TBI were estimated at $60 billion/year (19). There are little data on costs of TBI related solely to imaging. There has been one small study (limited evidence) that determined that 60% of patients were found to have additional lesions on MRI, but because none of these additional findings changed management, MRI resulted in a nonvalue-added benefit incremental increase of $1,891 per patient and a $3,152 incremental increase in charges to detect each patient with a lesion not identified on CT (20).

Goals

- To detect the presence of injuries that may require immediate surgical or procedural intervention.
- To detect the presence of injuries that may benefit from early medical therapy.
- To determine the prognosis of patients to tailor rehabilitative therapy or help with family counseling.

Methodology

A search of the Medline/PubMed electronic database (National Library of Medicine, Bethesda, MD) was performed using keywords including: (1) head injury, head trauma, brain injury, brain trauma, traumatic brain injury, or TBI, and (2) CT, computed tomography, computerized tomography, MR, magnetic resonance, spectroscopy, diffusion, diffusion tensor, functional magnetic, functional MR*, T2*, FLAIR, GRE, gradient-echo. A systematic literature review was performed through March 2010. Limits included: English language, abstracts, and human subjects. A search of the National Guideline Clearinghouse at www.guideline.gov was also performed using key words including: (1) head injury, head trauma, brain injury and (2) parameter, guideline.

I. Which Patients with Head Injury Should Undergo Imaging in the Acute Setting?

Summary of Evidence: The need for acute imaging is generally based on the severity of injury. It is agreed that severe TBI (based on GCS score) indicates the need for urgent CT imaging to determine the presence of lesions that may require surgical intervention (strong evidence). There is greater variability concerning recommendations for imaging of patients with mild or moderate TBI, or in pediatric TBI patients, although there are several recent guidelines (strong evidence) summarized in Take Home Tables 13.2, 13.3, and 13.5.

Supporting Evidence: There are several clinical prediction rules (strong evidence) for evaluating mild/minor head injury in adults, based on prospective studies. The Canadian Head CT Rule (21) was developed from prospective analysis of 3,121 patients with GCS scores of 13–15. CT scan was recommended if a patient had any of the following: GCS score <15 after 2 h, suspected open or depressed skull fracture, any sign of basal skull fracture, episode(s) of vomiting, age greater than 65 (associated with high risk for neurosurgical intervention), amnesia for the period occurring 30 min or more before impact, or if injury was due to a dangerous mechanism, such as being struck by or ejected from a motor vehicle (associated with a medium risk for brain injury on CT). Another guideline by Haydel and colleagues was developed after prospective analysis of 520 patients in the first phase, and 909 patients in the second phase. After recursive partitioning of variables in the first phase, seven variables were tested in the second phase, including headache, vomiting, age over 60 years, drug or alcohol intoxication, short-term memory

deficits, physical evidence of trauma above the clavicles, and seizures. All patients with positive CT scans had at least one variable, resulting in 100% sensitivity (22). An older guideline by Madden and colleagues prospectively analyzed 51 clinical variables in 540 patients in the first phase, and ten remaining variables in 273 patients in the second phase. The resulting sensitivity and negative predictive value were 96 and 94%, respectively (23).

A guideline, "Practice management guidelines for the management of mild traumatic brain injury" developed by the Eastern Association for the Surgery of Trauma (EAST) Practice Management Guidelines Work Group (2001) (2), was based on Level II evidence from several studies (three retrospective and one uncontrolled prospective). They reported that 3–17% of patients with mild injuries had significant CT findings, although they noted that there was no uniform agreement as to what constitutes a "positive" CT scan in different studies. They also reported that a patient with a normal head CT had 0–3% probability for neurologic deterioration. Therefore, if a patient had a GCS of 15 and no neurologic/cognitive abnormalities it was recommended that the patient be discharged. CT was recommended for all patients with transient neurologic deficits.

One guideline for severe TBI, "Management and Prognosis of Severe Traumatic Brain Injury," was jointly developed by the Brain Trauma Foundation (BTF), American Association of Neurological Surgeons (AANS) Joint Section on Neurotrauma and Critical Care, and was also approved by the American Society of Neuroradiology, the American Academy of Neurology, the American College of Surgeons, the American College of Emergency Physicians, the Society for Critical Care Medicine, and the American Academy of Physical Medicine and Rehabilitation (24, 25). An extensive review of previous CT literature supported the need for CT in the acute period. CT was reported to be abnormal in 90% of patients with severe head injury. CT is included as a necessary step in the algorithm of initial management. A more recent 3rd edition of "Guidelines for the Management of Severe Traumatic Brain Injury" (2007) does include the same CT information as the 2000 edition.

II. What Is the Sensitivity and Specificity of Imaging for Injury Requiring Immediate Treatment/ Surgery?

Summary of Evidence: CT is the mainstay of imaging in the acute period. The majority of evidence relates to the use of CT for detecting injuries that may require immediate treatment or surgery. Speed, availability, and lesser expense of CT studies remain important factors for using this modality in the acute setting. Sensitivity of detection also increases with repeat scans in the acute period (strong evidence).

Supporting Evidence: The incidence of injury-related abnormalities on CT is related to the severity of injury. After minor head injury, the incidence is approximately 6% (26) and increases up to 15% in the elderly population (27); those with GCS 13 or 14 have higher frequency of abnormalities than those with GCS 15 (28). The incidence of CT abnormalities in moderate head injury (with GCS of 9–13) has been reported to be 61% (29). The sensitivity of CT for detecting abnormalities after severe TBI (GCS below 9) varies from 68 to 94%, while normal scans range from approximately 7 to 12% (30). Several studies have shown that timing of CT studies also affects the sensitivity. Oertel and colleagues (strong evidence) prospectively studied 142 patients with moderate or severe injury, who had undergone more than one CT scan within the first 24 h, and found that the initial CT scan did not detect the full extent of hemorrhagic injuries in almost 50% of patients, particularly if scanned within the first 2 h (31). Likelihood of progressive hemorrhagic injury, that potentially required surgical intervention was greatest for parenchymal hemorrhagic contusions (51%), followed by epidural hematoma (EDH) (22%), subarachnoid hemorrhage (SAH) (17%), and subdural hemorrhage (SDH) (11%). Servedei and colleagues (strong evidence) prospectively studied 897 patients with more than one CT scan, and found that 16% of patients with diffuse brain injury demonstrated significant evolution of injury. This was more frequent in those with midline shift, often evolving to mass lesions (31). Similar results have been seen in retrospective studies

(32). Therefore, it may be useful to perform repeat CT scans in the acute period, particularly after moderate and severe injury, although the timing has not been clearly determined.

III. What Is the Overall Sensitivity and Specificity of Imaging in the Diagnosis and Prognosis of Patients with Head Trauma?

Summary of Evidence: The overall sensitivity and specificity of MRI for brain injury is generally superior to CT, although most studies have been retrospective and very few head-to-head comparisons have been performed in the recent decade. CT is clearly superior to MRI for the detection of fractures. MRI outperforms CT in detection of most other lesions (limited to moderate evidence), particularly DAI. Because different sequences vary in ability to detect certain lesions, it is often difficult to compare results. MRI allows more detailed analysis of injuries, including metabolic and physiologic measures, but further evidence-based research is needed.

There are fewer pediatric studies regarding the use of imaging and outcome predictions.

Supporting Evidence: Early research on CT predictors was performed with older technology that was less sensitive to the presence of injuries. Some studies analyzed the first scans while others analyzed the worst scans. Many studies used a crude categorization system, with limited information regarding the degree of abnormalities. Others have attempted to assess outcome prediction using more detailed classification schemes. Accordingly, there has been variability in the reported predictors and success at prediction.

MRI has higher sensitivity than CT, though most comparison studies were performed in the late 1980s and early 1990s (with older-generation or lower-field scanners). Orrison and colleagues (moderate evidence) retrospectively studied 107 patients with MRI and CT within 48 h and showed MRI had an overall sensitivity of 97% compared to 63% for CT, even when a low field MRI scanner was used, with better sensitivity for contusion, shearing injury, subdural and EDH (33). Ogawa and colleagues (moderate evidence) detected more lesions with conventional MRI than CT with the exception of subdural and SAHs, in a prospective study of 155 patients, although they were studied at variable time points (34). Other studies (moderate evidence), showed better detection of non-hemorrhagic contusions and shearing injuries (35), and of brainstem lesions (36), using MRI.

Some lesions, such as DAI, are clearly better detected with MRI, and have been reported in up to 30% of patients with mild head injury with normal CT (37) (limited evidence). However, sensitivity depends on the sequence, field strength, and type of lesion. *Gradient echo (GRE)* sequences are best for detecting hemorrhagic DAI, although the proportion of hemorrhagic versus nonhemorrhagic DAI is not truly known. An early report (limited evidence) suggested that less than 20% of DAI lesions were visibly hemorrhagic (38), but this is likely to be erroneously low, due to poor sensitivity of the imaging methods available at that time. Scheid and colleagues (moderate evidence) prospectively studied 66 patients using high field (3.0T) MRI and found that T2*-weighted GRE sequences detected significantly more lesions than conventional T1- or T2-weighted sequences (39). Tong and colleagues studied a new susceptibility-weighted imaging (SWI) sequence (at 1.5T) that is a modified GRE sequence, and have shown significantly better detection of small hemorrhagic shearing lesions compared to conventional GRE (40) (limited evidence).

The *fluid attenuated inversion recovery (FLAIR)* sequence is useful for detecting SAH, SDH, contusions, nonhemorrhagic DAI, and perisulcal lesions, but there are few studies comparing the sensitivity of FLAIR to other sequences. One study (limited to moderate evidence) found that FLAIR sequences were significantly more sensitive than spin echo (SE) sequences ($p < 0.01$) in detection of all lesions studied within 1–36 days (0.5T), particularly in those who had DAI-type lesions (41).

Diffusion-weighted imaging (DWI) has also recently been shown to improve the detection of nonhemorrhagic shearing lesions, although there are only a few small studies describing sensitivity. A small study (insufficient evidence) of patients scanned within 48 h found that DWI identified an additional 16% of shearing lesions that were not seen on conventional MRI. The majority of DWI-positive lesions (65%) had decreased diffusion (42). Another descriptive study (limited evidence) characterized several different types and patterns of DWI lesions, although there was no comparison with other MRI sequences or analysis of diffusion changes over time (43). A recent study (limited evidence) found a strong correlation between apparent diffusion coefficient (ADC) histograms and GCS score (44). There are even less data on the sensitivity of *diffusion tensor imaging (DTI)*. A few small studies (insufficient or limited evidence) have shown decreased anisotropy in brain parenchyma of TBI patients (45–47).

There are various studies demonstrating the use of specific imaging findings or patterns for outcome prediction. These are discussed in the sections that follow.

Imaging Classification Schemes

Several classification schemes have now been used to predict clinical outcomes. The earliest and most widely studied scheme, often named the "Marshall CT classification," is based on CT findings in the Trauma Coma Databank (TCDB), developed by Marshall and colleagues (48); it is based on the status of cisterns, midline shift and mass lesions. Six categories include (a) Diffuse injury I (normal): no visible intracranial pathology; (b) Diffuse injury II (small lesions): cisterns are present, midline shift <5 mm, and no lesions greater than 25 cc; (c) Diffuse injury III (swelling): cisterns are compressed, midline shift <5 mm, and no lesions greater than 25 cc; (d) Diffuse injury IV (shift): midline shift of >5 mm, no lesions greater than 25 cc; (e) any surgically evacuated lesion; and (f) any nonevacuated mass lesion greater than 25 cc. The TCDB classification was developed in severely injured patients (GCS <8) and initially compared to discharge outcomes although it has more recently been validated using 3 and 6 month GOS (49). It is reasonably good at predicting mortality, but it may not be as applicable to mild/moderately injured patients and has been criticized as poorly predictive of functional recovery (50). The TCDB classification has been variously modified, often to include the type, number (32, 51), or location of lesions (52). In the BTF/AANS guideline (25), an extensive review of the previous CT literature (strong evidence) showed that the TCDB CT classification scheme strongly correlated with outcome.

Maas and colleagues subsequently developed a more discriminative six-point CT score, deemed the "Rotterdam Classification Scheme," in which certain individual CT characteristics of the Marshall CT classification were emphasized, and other findings were added. The scoring was based on four main features: (a) status of basal cisterns (normal, compressed, or absent), (b) degree of midline shift (normal, shift less than 5 mm, or greater than 5 mm), (c) presence of traumatic subarachnoid or intraventricular hemorrhage, and (d) presence of different types of mass lesions (epidural vs. SDH). This prognostic scoring system was tested in a large study population of moderate and severely injured patients involved in the International and North American Tirilazad trials. They showed that this combination of individual CT indicators had a better prediction and discrimination of long-term outcome than the Marshall CT classification system alone (strong evidence) (53).

Normal Scans

Extensive review (strong evidence) shows that normal CT scans in severe TBI patients are predictive of favorable outcome (61–78.5% positive predictive value) (30). In a more recent study (moderate evidence), normal CT scans in moderate/severe TBI patients were associated with better neuropsychological performance at 6 months (54).

Brain Swelling

Brain swelling is a subjective finding and more difficult to evaluate as an outcome predictor. Partly compressed ventricles and cisterns are not as reliably measured as obliterated ventricle and cisterns (55). Marshall and colleagues (strong evidence) studied the TCDB classification in 746 patients and reported that brain swelling on CT (categorized by Diffuse injury III) was predictive of mortality, and that survivors showed a trend of worse GOS associated with increasing grade of diffuse injury (48). Compressed basal cisterns have been associated with a threefold risk of raised ICP, and two- to threefold increase in mortality (25). However, brain swelling on CT does not appear to correlate with neuropsychological outcomes (56) (moderate evidence).

Midline Shift

Midline shift is felt to be less important than other CT parameters for predicting mortality or GOS (25). However, some investigators have shown that midline shift may be predictive of worse outcomes based on rehabilitation measures such as greater need for assistance with ambulation, activities of daily living (ADLs), and supervision at rehabilitation discharge (57).

Hemorrhage

The presence of hemorrhage has different prognostic significance depending on extent and location of blood. Traumatic SAH is a significant independent prognostic indicator (25, 58) (strong evidence), associated with a twofold increase in mortality, and a 70% positive predictive value for unfavorable outcome (25). Mortality is higher and outcome is worse with acute subdural hematoma compared to extradural hematoma (25). Hematoma volume correlates with outcome and has a 78–79% positive predictive value for an unfavorable outcome (25). Another study (moderate evidence) found that patients with combined SDH + ICH on CT had poor outcome even after surgery compared to EDH or ICH alone (59). A small study (limited evidence) also found that IVH in all four ventricles was significantly associated with poor outcome (60).

Number, Size, and Depth of Lesions

Some investigators have attempted to evaluate the predictive ability of number, size, depth, or location of lesions. Van der Naalt and colleagues (moderate evidence) studied 67 patients with mild/moderate TBI and found that the outcome (1 year extended GOS or DOS) was related to number, size, and depth of lesions on CT (6). Kido and colleagues (moderate evidence) found GOS was correlated with the size of intracranial lesions (independent of compartment or brain region) on CT (61). A small MRI study (limited evidence) suggested that size, depth, and multiplicity of lesions correlated with neurobehavioral outcomes (62).

Location of lesions is partly related to mechanism of injury and is associated with different outcomes. The most available evidence is related to brainstem injuries. Firsching and colleagues (moderate evidence) studied 102 patients in coma with MRI in the first 8 days and found that mortality was 100% with lesions in the bilateral pons (52). Kampfl and colleagues (moderate evidence) studied 80 patients and also showed that lesion location could predict recovery from post-traumatic VS by 12 months, whereas clinical variables such as initial GCS, age, and pupillary abnormalities were poor predictors. Logistic regression showed that corpus callosum and dorsolateral brainstem injuries were predictive of nonrecovery. This information is helpful in that almost half of the patients with initial VS may recover within 1 year (63). The association between extent or location of injuries and neuropsychological recovery has been, up to now, less studied, with only a few studies (limited evidence) that suggest that location of injury may be associated with specific neuropsychological impairments (62, 64).

Diffuse Axonal Injury

It has been repeatedly demonstrated that CT and MR findings are poor predictors of functional outcome of TBI patients, probably because DAI is frequently not detected (7). Because CT clearly underestimates DAI, this can lead to inaccurate prediction of outcome. CT studies, many of which were performed with older generation CT scanners, predominantly report that DAI is associated with mortality (limited evidence) (65) or poor outcome (moderate evidence) (66, 67). However, it has been shown that patients with mild or moderate injuries can also have DAI (37), that is better detected with newer generation CT scanners or MRI, and therefore better outcomes than previously realized. Severe DAI can transform young productive individuals into dependent patients requiring institutionalized care; milder DAI can result in neuropsychiatric problems, cognitive deficits including memory loss, concentration difficulties, decreased attention span, intellectual decline, headaches, and seizures (68). The improved ability to detect DAI on CT even in milder injuries has also allowed comparison with neuropsychological outcome. Wallesch and colleagues (moderate evidence) studied 60 patients with mild or moderate injuries, who underwent neuropsychological assessment 18–45 weeks later. Patients with DAI identified on CT had relatively transient deficits of

psychomotor speed, verbal short-term memory and frontal lobe cognitive functions, whereas patients with frontal contusions had persistent behavior alterations (69).

MRI studies also suggest an association between TBI severity and depth of axonal injury as well as outcomes. However, most MRI studies evaluating prognosis after DAI have consisted of small sample sizes. Small studies (limited to moderate evidence) have demonstrated that patients in VS are more likely to have DAI lesions in the corpus callosum and dorsolateral brainstem (70), compared to patients with mild TBI who were more likely to have lesions in the subcortical white matter without involvement of the corpus callosum or brainstem (66). The presence of hemorrhage in DAI lesions may also affect prognosis, although results depend on the MRI sequence. One study of patients in VS (moderate evidence) found more nonhemorrhagic DAI lesions than hemorrhagic lesions, although only T1- and T2-weighted sequences were used (70). In contrast, another study (limited evidence) showed that hemorrhage in DAI lesions (detected by GRE) was associated with poor outcomes (6 month GOS), and that isolated nonhemorrhagic DAI lesions were not associated with poor outcome (71). There is also disagreement over whether the degree of hemorrhage correlates with outcomes, although this may be partly due to differences in outcome measures. One study (moderate evidence) found that the number of lesions (hypointense or hyperintense) detected by T2*-weighted GRE images, correlated with duration of coma and 3 month GOS (72). However, another study (moderate evidence) (MRI sequence not specified) found no correlation between hemorrhagic lesion volume and neuropsychological outcome measures obtained more than 6 months after injury (73). A more recent prospective study (moderate evidence) of 66 patients imaged with T2*-weighted GRE at 3.0 T found no correlation between the total amount of microhemorrhages and patient outcomes measured by GOS. However, these patients were imaged in the chronic phase (39).

Combinations of Imaging Abnormalities and Progressive Brain Injury

Some studies have shown that combinations of imaging abnormalities are predictive of outcome, although not necessarily in agreement.

Fearnside and colleagues (strong evidence) prospectively studied 315 patients and found three CT findings to be highly predictive of mortality – cerebral edema, intraventricular blood, and midline shift. Three other CT findings were highly predictive of poor outcome in survivors – SAH, intracerebral hematoma, or intracerebral contusion (74). In contrast, Lanoo and colleagues (moderate evidence) retrospectively reviewed 115 patients, and found that subarachnoid, intracerebral, and SDH were predictive of mortality, but not significantly related to morbidity (75). Wardlaw and colleagues (moderate evidence) retrospectively reviewed 414 patients and developed a simple rating system of "overall appearance" of CT findings. They reported that "massive" injuries and SAH could predict poor prognosis (1 year GOS) (50).

Measures of Atrophy

Quantification of the atrophy of various brain structures/regions (such as corpus callosum, hippocampus, and ventricles) has also been studied with respect to predicting outcome, but is time-consuming, and often requires experienced raters and specialized software. Blatter and colleagues (moderate evidence) studied 123 patients with moderate to severe TBI compared to 198 healthy volunteers using MRI volumetric analysis of total brain volume, total ventricular volume, and subarachnoid CSF volume. TBI patients, particularly if studied later, had the greatest decrease in brain volume, suggesting that progressive brain atrophy in TBI patients occurs at a rate greater than with normal aging (76). However, because atrophy takes time to develop, it cannot be used acutely as an early predictor of outcome. Blatter and colleagues also showed that correlations with cognitive outcomes did not become significant until after 70 days (76). One study of late CT scans (moderate evidence) of Vietnam War veterans with penetrating or closed head injuries found that total brain volume loss and enlargement of the third ventricle were significantly related to cognitive abnormalities and return to work (77). Another study (moderate evidence) showed that frontotemporal atrophy on late MRI was predictive of 1-year outcome (measured by extended GOS or DOS) (6). In an MRI study (moderate evidence) of late MRI findings and neuropsychological outcome, hippocampal

atrophy was correlated with verbal memory function, whereas temporal horn enlargement was correlated with intellectual outcome (78).

Combinations of Clinical and Imaging Findings

Numerous studies have attempted to analyze combinations of clinical and imaging findings to determine the best approach to predicting outcome. The diversity of TBI makes this a difficult although worthy task. There is agreement that there is no one single variable that can predict outcome after TBI. In fact, there is often disagreement between studies regarding the predictive value of certain clinical variables, including GCS. Ideally, a combined clinical and imaging approach to outcome prediction would likely be most accurate. Ratanalert and colleagues (moderate evidence) studied 300 patients and reported that logistic regression showed that age, status of basal cisterns on initial CT, GCS at 24 h, and electrolyte derangement strongly correlated with a 6-month GOS score (79). Ono and colleagues (moderate evidence) retrospectively studied 272 patients who were first divided into CT categories according to the TCDB classification and found that within certain groups, additional variables such as age and GCS score were helpful predictors of outcome (51). Schaan and colleagues (moderate evidence) studied the utility of creating a single score based on a weighted scale of clinical variables and CT findings including pupillary reaction, hemiparesis, brainstem signs, contusion, SDH, EDH, and cerebral edema. In their retrospective study of 554 patients, they divided the range of scores into three severity groups and found that there were significant differences in mortality and GOS scores between groups, suggesting that this approach had predictive value (80).

IV. What Are Considerations for Imaging of Children with Head Trauma?

Summary of Evidence: Pediatric TBI patients are known to have different biophysical features, risks, mechanisms, and outcomes after injury. There are also differences between infants and older children, although this remains controversial. Categorization of pediatric age groups is variable and measures of injury or outcomes are inconsistent. The GCS and GOS have been used for pediatric studies, sometimes with modifications (81–83), or with variable dichotomization (81, 84). For infants and toddlers, some investigators have used a Children's Coma Scale (CCS) (85). There are several pediatric adaptations of the GOS, such as the King's Outcome Scale for Childhood Head Injury (KOSCHI) (86), the Pediatric Cerebral Performance Category Score (PCPCS), or the Pediatric Overall Performance Category Score (POPCS) (87).

A highly sensitive clinical decision rule, the CHALICE rule (Table 13.2), has been derived for the identification of children over 2½ years of age, who should undergo CT imaging after head trauma of any severity (moderate evidence). The authors of the decision rule also showed that calvarial plain radiographs have a poor sensitivity for identifying pediatric patients with intracranial pathology (moderate to strong evidence) and hence are not recommended unless for highly selected patients with suspected nonaccidental trauma (88). A recommended decision tree for children with acute head injury is shown in Fig. 13.1. Two other prediction rules have been developed for children with mild head injury (moderate to strong evidence) (89, 90). These rules have the potential to improve and standardize the care of pediatric patients with head injuries.

Supporting Evidence: The CHALICE (Children's Head injury ALgorithm for the prediction of Important Clinical Events) study, conducted by Dunning and colleagues, was a large prospective multicenter diagnostic cohort study of 22,772 children over the age of 2.5 years, with head injury of any severity in the UK (88) (moderate evidence). All children who had a clinically significant head injury (death = 15, need for neurosurgical intervention = 137, or abnormality on a CT study = 281) were identified. Multivariate recursive partitioning on 40 clinical variables was performed in order to create a highly sensitive rule for predicting significant intracranial pathology. Abnormalities on CT included intracranial hematomas of any size, cerebral contusion, diffuse cerebral edema, and depressed skull fractures. Simple or nondepressed skull fractures alone were not considered to be significant predictors of intracranial

injury (88). The CHALICE rule was derived (Table 13.2) with a sensitivity of 98% (95% confidence interval (CI) 96–100%) and a specificity of 87% (95 CI 86–87%) for the prediction of clinically significant head injury, and requires a CT imaging rate of 14%. Prospective validation of this rule with new cohorts is ongoing.

Two recent studies have been performed to develop rules for use of CT in children with mild head injury. The larger of the two studies was performed by Kuppermann and colleagues (89), who conducted a large multicenter prospective study in North America, in which 42,412 pediatric patients (younger than 18 years old) with GCS scores of 14–15 were divided into those younger than 2 years of age and those 2 years or older. Given increasing awareness of radiation-induced malignancy, the investigators sought to identify children at very low risk of clinically important TBI, for whom CT might be unnecessary. They developed prediction rules for clinically important TBI – defined as death from TBI, neurosurgery, intubation >24 h, or hospital admission ≥2 nights. In the validation population of children under 2 years of age, there was a negative predictive value for clinically important TBI of 100% (95% CI 99.7–100) and sensitivity of 100% (95% CI of 86.3–100) if there was normal mental status, no scalp hematoma (except frontal), no loss of consciousness or LOC of less than 5 s, non-severe injury mechanism, no palpable skull fracture, and acting normally according to the parents. In the validation population of children 2 years or older, there was a negative predictive value of 99.95% (95% CI of 99.81–99.99) and sensitivity of 96.8% (95% CI of 89.0–99.6) if there was normal mental status, no LOC, no vomiting, non-severe injury mechanism, no signs of basilar skull fracture, and no severe headache. Neurosurgery events were not missed in either age group.

A more recent prospective multicenter cohort study was performed in Canada, which resulted in the development of the CATCH (Canadian Assessment of Tomography for Childhood Head injury) rule (Table 13.3) (90). The investigators enrolled 3,866 pediatric patients (aged 0–16 years) with GCS of 13–15, and performed recursive partitioning to find the best combination of predictor variables that were highly sensitive (with maximal specificity) for detecting neurologic injury and presence of brain injury on CT. Four high-risk factors were identified as being 100.0% sensitive (95% CI of 86.2–100.0) for predicting the need for neurologic intervention and would result in 30.2% of patients undergoing CT; these risk factors included failure to reach GCS score of 15 within 2 h, suspicion of open skull fracture, and worsening headache and irritability. Three medium-risk factors were identified as being 98.1% sensitive (95% CI of 94.6–99.4) for predicting brain injury by CT and would result in 50.2% of patients undergoing CT: these risk factors included large boggy hematoma of the scalp, signs of basal skull fracture, and dangerous mechanism of injury.

Oman and colleagues studied the test performance of the eight-variable NEXUS II decision instrument to detect the presence of clinically import intracranial injury (ICI) in 1,666 pediatric patients with blunt head trauma and who had CT. The decision instrument utilized seven variables and correctly identified 136/138 cases (98.6% sensitivity) and classified 230 as low risk (99.1% NPV, 230/232; 15.1% specificity, 230/1,528). Findings showed that significant ICI is extremely unlikely in any child who does not exhibit at least one of the following high-risk criteria: (1) evidence of significant skull fracture (diastatic, depressed, open, or basilar); (2) altered level of consciousness; (3) neurologic deficit; (4) persistent vomiting; (5) presence of scalp hematoma; (6) abnormal behavior; and (7) coagulopathy (moderate to strong evidence) (91).

Palchak and colleagues derived a rule on 2,043 pediatric patients under 18 years who had head trauma and positive findings on history or clinical examination such as loss of consciousness, memory loss, headache, or emesis (92). Of the nine predictive variables studied, abnormal mental status, clinical findings of calvarial fracture, history of emesis, scalp hematoma in children 2 years of age or less, and cephalagia were identified in 96 of 98 patients with a positive intracranial lesion on CT (98% sensitivity, 95% CI 93–100%) (moderate evidence). Since then, they have tested the decision rule against clinician judgment, and found that application of the rule to the study population would have required 24.7% (289/1,168) fewer CT scans. The decision rule had 98.9% sensitivity (88/89) vs. 94.4% (84/89) for clinician judgment. Specificity of the rule was 26.7% (288/1,079) vs. 30.5% (329/1,079) for judgment. The decision rule classified children as being at very low risk of ICI if none of the following findings were present: abnormal mental status, clinical signs of skull fracture, a history of vomiting, scalp

hematoma (in children <2 years), and headache (strong evidence) (93).

Greenes and Shutzman (94) performed a prospective study on 608 patients under 2 years of age in a single hospital setting (moderate evidence). Their study demonstrated that pediatric patients with suspected nonaccidental trauma, lethargy or a major scalp hematoma had an increased risk of significant intracranial injury. This study found that loss of consciousness, seizures, or emesis alone was not an adequate predictor of intracranial injury, and furthermore, the absence of clinical symptoms or signs did not fully exclude the possibility of having positive intracranial pathology (94). They allocated patients into four risk groups, with CT imaging recommended in the highest risk group of children who vomited more than three times or had loss of consciousness, lethargy, a high-risk mechanism or considerable bruising (94). This study and the CHALICE study showed that it was safe to discharge children with a negative CT study (88, 94).

Haydel and Shembekar (95) evaluated the adult New Orleans criteria (22) in children under age 5 years. They studied 175 children with GCS of 15 at a single institution. They concluded that the 14 positive CT scans could be identified with this adult predictive rule (95). The Canadian CT rule for children was proposed by the UK National Institute of Clinical Excellence before the CHALICE study was published (88). The CHALICE group assessed the diagnostic performance of this rule in children (96) to detect intracranial injury and found a sensitivity of 94% (95% CI 91–97%), specificity of 89% (95% CI 89–90%), and a CT ordering rate of 12% (88).

Boran and Colleagues (97) studied 421 children with GCS of 15 and without any focal neurological deficit (moderate evidence). Intracranial lesion was noted in 37 cases (8.8%). The clinical parameters associated with an increased incidence of intracranial pathology were post-traumatic seizures and loss of consciousness. However, when patients with these predictive parameters were subtracted, intracranial lesions were still identified in 4.1% of the cases, and 1.8% required neurosurgical operation. Boran and Colleagues also found a low sensitivity of plain radiographs of 43.2% and specificity of 93% 97. The CHALICE study (88) and other studies (98) support the recommendation of not performing skull radiographs except for highly selected patients who may have had a nonaccidental injury. Calvarial plain radiographs have a poor sensitivity for identifying pediatric patients with intracranial pathology (moderate to strong evidence) (88).

The literature on repeat CT scans in pediatric patients seems to differ from adult studies, in that the yield of new clinically significant lesions is low in routine repeat studies (moderate evidence). In addition, because of the long-term effects of CT radiation exposure the decision to order a CT scan also should be weighed against the risk of long-term radiation exposure. Hollingworth and colleagues studied the prevalence of worsening brain injury on repeat CT, predictors of worsening CT findings, and the frequency of neurosurgical intervention after the repeat CT; in 521 pediatric patients with moderate or severe TBI. For severe TBI, the multivariate adjusted OR for worsening or new second CT findings was 2.4. Children with moderate or severe TBI, especially if they had ICI, were more likely to have deteriorating CT (43%; 107/248) and 10% (11/107) required surgery. Of those with stable CT (57%, 141/248) only 3% (4/141) required surgery. In most surgical patients, repeat CT was preceded by rapid decline in neurologic status or elevated ICP (99). Figg and colleagues performed a retrospective study in severely injured children and demonstrated that most second scans showed no change (53%). Some showed improvement (34%), and even less showed worsening (13%). Only five (4.3%) patients had a surgical intervention based on the results of the second CT scan, but all five scans were ordered based on a clinical indicator (increased intracranial pressure or worsening neurologic status), and not on routine follow-up (100) (moderate evidence). Similar findings were reported by Tabori and colleagues (limited evidence) (101). Therefore repeat CT scans may be considered when there is evidence of neurologic deterioration or increasing intracranial pressure. Routine repeat CT scans are not recommended.

There is less literature on imaging and prediction of outcome from head injury in pediatric subjects, compared to adults. Importantly, within the pediatric population, age may be a confounding variable or effect modifier for outcomes. Levin and colleagues (moderate evidence) studied 103 children at one of the original four centers participating in the TCDB and found heterogeneity in 6-month outcomes based on age. Worst outcomes were found in the 0- to 4-year-old patients and best outcomes were found in the 5- to 10-year-old patients, while adolescents had intermediate outcomes. They suggested that studies involving severe TBI in children should analyze age-defined subgroups rather than pooling a wide range of pediatric ages (102).

Many studies have consisted of relatively small sample sizes and used varying outcome, possibly accounting for conflicting reports regarding outcomes related to TBI in children. There have been several studies evaluating CT in predicting outcome in children with variable results. Suresh and colleagues (moderate evidence) studied 340 children and compared CT findings to discharge GOS outcomes. They found that poor outcome (death) occurred in 16% of their patients. In addition progressively worse outcomes were found with: fractures, EDH, contusion, diffuse head injury, and acute SDH (84). Hirsch and colleagues (moderate evidence) studied 248 children after severe TBI and compared initial CT findings to the level of consciousness (measured by a modified GCS score) at 1 year after injury. They found that children with normal CT, or isolated SDH or EDH were least impaired, while children with diffuse edema had the most impairment. Those with parenchymal hemorrhage, ventricular hemorrhage, or focal edema had intermediate outcomes (103). A study of 82 children (moderate evidence) found that unfavorable prognosis (using a three-category Lidcombe impairment scale) was more likely to occur after shearing injury or intracerebral/subdural hematomas, whereas a better outcome was more likely in patients with EDH (104). Another study of 74 children (moderate evidence) found that the presence of traumatic SAH on CT was an independent predictor of poorer discharge outcome ($p < 0.001$), but did not find that DAI or diffuse swelling was associated with outcome. After stepwise logistic regression analysis, CT findings did not have prognostic significance compared to other variables such as GCS and the oculocephalic reflex (82). Another study (moderate evidence) compared 59 children and 59 adults and found that a CT finding of absent ventricles/cisterns was associated with a slightly lower frequency of poor outcome (6 month GOS) in children, suggesting that diffuse swelling may be more benign in children than adults unless there was a severe primary injury or a secondary hypotensive insult (55).

Bonnier and colleagues studied 50 children with severe TBI before 4 years of age (moderate evidence) (105). TBI severity (initial GCS or coma duration) was significantly associated with subcortical lesions. A greater deterioration in intellectual quotient over time was noted in patients with subcortical lesions. Sigmund and colleagues studied 40 children with TBI using CT and MRI (moderate evidence) (106). T2-weighted, FLAIR, and susceptibility-weighted MRI findings showed no significant difference in lesion volume between normal and mild outcome groups, but did indicate significant differences between normal and poor, and between mild and poor outcome groups. CT revealed no significant differences in lesion volume between any groups. The findings suggest that these MRI sequence findings provide a more accurate assessment of injury severity and detection of outcome-influencing lesions than does CT in pediatric DAI patients (moderate evidence).

There have been some studies specifically evaluating MRI for outcome prediction in children with TBI. Prasad and colleagues (moderate evidence) prospectively studied 60 children with acute CT and MRI. Hierarchical multiple regression indicated that the number of lesions, as well as certain clinical variables such as GCS (modified for children) and duration of coma, were predictive of outcomes up to 1 year (modified GOS) (81). Several investigators have studied the correlation between depth-of-lesion and outcomes, with varying results. Levin and colleagues (moderate evidence) studied 169 children prospectively as well as 82 patients retrospectively with MRI at variable time points, and showed a correlation between depth of brain lesions and functional outcome (107). Grados and colleagues (moderate evidence) studied 106 children with a SPGR (T1-weighted) MRI sequence obtained 3 months after TBI, and classified lesions into a depth-of-lesion model. They found that depth and number of lesions predicted outcome, although correlation was better with discharge outcomes than 1-year outcomes (108). Blackman and colleagues (moderate evidence) studied 92 children in the rehabilitation setting (using variable imaging modalities) and used a depth-of-lesion classification (based on the Grados model) to study neuropsychological outcomes. They found that this classification had limited usefulness. Although patients with deeper lesions tended to have longer stays in rehabilitation, they were able to "catch up" after sufficient time had elapsed (109).

In a study of acute hemorrhagic DAI lesions (moderate evidence) on MRI, Tong and colleagues studied 40 children and found that the degree and location of hemorrhagic lesions correlated with GCS, duration of coma, and outcomes at 6–12 months after injury (110). Children with normal outcomes or mild disability ($n = 30$) at 6–12 months had, on average, fewer hemorrhagic lesions ($p = 0.003$) and lower volume ($p = 0.003$) of lesions than those who were moderately or severely disabled or in a vegetative state. In a subgroup of these patients, Babikian and colleagues studied 18 children and adolescents 1–4 years after injury using SWI (limited evidence). Negative correlations between lesion number and volume with neuropsychologic functioning were shown (111).

Some have also studied volumetric changes after TBI in children. Levin and colleagues (moderate evidence) showed that in children, as in adults, corpus callosum area (measured on subacute MR) correlated with functional outcome. They found that the size of the corpus callosum decreased after severe TBI in contrast to mild/moderately injured children who showed growth of the corpus callosum on follow up studies (112). Wilde and colleagues studied 16 children with DAI and 16 individually matched uninjured children (limited evidence) (113), using morphologic measurements on MRI. Analysis demonstrated significant volume loss in the hippocampus, amygdala, and globus pallidus in the TBI group. They also found that a significant group difference was found in cerebellar white matter volume with children in the TBI group (limited evidence) (114).

V. What Is the Role of Advanced Imaging (Functional MRI, MR Spectroscopy, Diffusion Imaging, SPECT, and PET) in TBI?

Summary of Evidence: There is moderate evidence that MR spectroscopic changes can help predict outcome after TBI. SPECT hypoperfusion abnormalities may be an indicator of a worse outcome in children (moderate evidence).Brain PET metabolic abnormalities may also predict outcome (limited to moderate evidence). Data about functional MRI (fMRI), MR perfusion, and DTI are limited. Large studies are required with these advanced imaging modalities to determine the role and outcome after TBI.

Supporting Evidence: Table 13.1 describes briefly the current imaging methods of TBI including principle, advantages/limitations, and use.

DWI has also recently been shown to improve the detection of nonhemorrhagic shearing lesions, although there are only a few small studies describing sensitivity. A small study (insufficient evidence) of patients scanned within 48 h, found that DWI identified an additional 16% of shearing lesions that were not seen on conventional MRI. The majority of DWI-positive lesions (65%) had decreased diffusion (42). Another descriptive study (limited evidence) characterized several different types and patterns of DWI lesions, although there was no comparison with other MRI sequences or analysis of diffusion changes over time (43). Schaefer and colleagues studied 26 patients (age range 4–72 years) with closed head injury (limited evidence) (115). This study demonstrated strongest correlation between signal-intensity abnormality volume on DWI and modified Rankin score ($r = 0.772$, $P < 0.001$). Total lesion number also correlated well with the modified Rankin score (115).

A few investigators have studied the role of *DTI*. Wozniak and colleagues studied 14 children with TBI and 14 controls aged 10–18 years who had DTI studies and neurocognitive evaluations at 6–12 months (116). The TBI group had lower fractional anisotropy (FA) in three white matter regions: inferior frontal, superior frontal, and supracallosal (limited evidence). Supracallosal FA correlated with motor speed and behavior ratings. Parent-reported executive deficits were inversely correlated with FA. Levin and colleagues studied the use of DTI in 32 children with moderate to severe TBI, compared to 36 children with orthopedic injury (OI). They found that fractional anisotropy and ADC values

differentiated the groups, and that both cognitive and functional outcome measures were related to the DTI findings. Dissociations were present wherein the relation of fractional anisotropy to cognitive performance differed between the TBI and OI groups. A DTI composite measure of white matter integrity was related to global outcome in the children with TBI (moderate evidence) (117).

Magnetic resonance spectroscopy (MRS) can detect subtle cellular abnormalities that may more accurately estimate the extent of brain injury, particularly DAI, compared to conventional MRI. Investigators have compared MRS findings from noncontused brain with various measures of clinical neurological outcome such as GOS or DRS scores and found a general trend of reduced NAA corresponding to poor outcome (limited evidence) (118–121). However, results are difficult to compare since varied anatomical areas were studied and results were often acquired over a wide range of times after injury. It is uncertain whether the timing of MRS measurement affects outcome prediction. Subacute MRS studies have suggested that decreased NAA correlates with poor outcomes. There have been few acute MRS studies evaluating outcome prediction. In a prospective MRS study (122) of 42 severely injured adults (limited to moderate evidence), Shutter and colleagues measured quantitative metabolite changes as soon as possible (mean of 7 days) after injury, in normal appearing GM and WM. In contrast to other studies, they found no correlation between NAA-derived metabolites and outcomes at 6–12 months, possibly because their MRS studies were performed earlier than others. However, glutamine/glutamate (Glx) and Cho were significantly elevated in occipital GM and parietal WM in patients with poor 6–12 month outcomes and these two variables predicted outcome at 6–12 months with 89% accuracy. A combination of Glx and Cho ratios with the motor component of the GCS score provided the highest predictive accuracy (97%). It may be that elevated Glx and Cho are more sensitive indicators of injury and predictors of poor outcome when spectroscopy is obtained early after injury. This may be a reflection of early excitotoxic injury (i.e., elevated Glx) and of injury associated with membrane disruption secondary to DAI (i.e., increased Cho). An example of spectra from parietal and occipital

GM in a TBI patient with poor outcome is shown in Case Study 2.

There have been few published results comparing data from multivoxel MR spectroscopy (MRSI) to clinical outcomes. Holshouser and colleagues studied MRSI (limited to moderate evidence) in 42 patients with severe TBI, obtained through the corpus callosum and surrounding GM and WM. MRSI showed significant decreases in NAA/Cre and increases in Cho/Cre ratios in areas of visibly injured and normal-appearing brain. Averaged ratios from all regions were able to differentiate between patients with mild, moderate, and severe/vegetative neurologic outcomes as measured with the GOS at 6 months compared to control values. The results suggest that decreased NAA-derived ratios and increased Cho/Cre ratios, detected by MRSI, are associated with worse outcomes (123).

There are a few MRS studies in children. Makaroff and colleagues studied 11 children with TBI (limited evidence) (124). Four children demonstrated elevated lactate and diminished NAA within several regions, indicating global ischemic injury. All four children had seizures, abnormal neurological examination, and required admission to the PICU. In four other children, lactate was detected at least in one region, indicating a focal ischemic injury. Two children had seizures and two had abnormal neurological examination. The remaining three children had no evidence of elevated lactate. Clinically, no seizures were demonstrated and no PICU admission was required. Holshouser and colleagues performed MRS in 40 children with TBI 1–16 days after injury (moderate evidence) (125). Neurologic outcome was evaluated at 6–12 months after TBI. A logistic regression model demonstrated a significant decrease in the NAA/creatine and increase in the choline/creatine ratios in normal-appearing ($P<0.05$) and visibly injured brain ($P<0.001$). In normal appearing brain, NAA/creatine decreased more in patients with poor outcomes (1.32 ± -0.54) than in those with good outcomes (1.61 ± -0.50). Babikian and colleagues studied 20 children and adolescents and demonstrated a moderate to strong correlation between decreased NAA and worse cognitive scores (limited evidence) (126). Ashwal and colleagues in 38 children with TBI demonstrated that the occipital

glutamate/glutamine in the short echo MRS was significantly increased in TBI when compared with controls (limited evidence) (127). No difference was seen in this ratio between children with good versus poor outcome. They also demonstrated that occipital gray matter myoinositol was increased in these children with TBI (4.30 ± 0.73) compared with controls (3.53 ± 0.48; $P=0.003$). In addition, those with poor outcomes 6–12 months after injury had higher myoinositol levels (4.78 ± 0.68) than those with good outcomes (4.15 ± 0.69; $p=0.05$) (moderate evidence) (128) indicating that myoinositol elevation after pediatric TBI is associated with a poor neurologic outcome. The reasons for the increased myoinositol may be due to astrogliosis or a disturbance in osmotic function. In this same group of children, Ashwal and colleagues (moderate evidence) also demonstrated significant decreases in NAA-derived ratios and elevation of Cho/Cre measured in occipital GM within 13 days of neurological insult. These metabolite changes correlated with poor neurological outcome at 6–12 months after injury ($n=52$) (129). In a subgroup of these patients ($n=24$), neuropsychological evaluations were performed at 3–5 years after neurological insult. It was found that these metabolite changes strongly correlated with below average functioning in multiple areas including full scale IQ, memory, sensorimotor and attention/executive functioning (130).

Single photon emission computed tomography can measure regional cerebral blood flow (CBF) and assess localized perfusion deficits that may correlate with cognitive deficits even in the absence of structural abnormalities. However, SPECT has low spatial and temporal resolution, does not permit imaging of transient cognitive events, and interpretation is often highly subjective. In addition, results of studies vary, possibly related to the severity of injury or timing of studies. SPECT studies generally show patchy perfusion deficits, often in areas with no visible injury on CT. One of the largest studies, although retrospective, was performed by Abdel-Dayem and colleagues (moderate evidence) who reviewed SPECT findings in 228 subjects with mild or moderate TBI. They found focal areas of hypoperfusion in 77% of patients. However, there was no comparison to CT or MRI (131).

Stamatakis and colleagues (moderate evidence) studied 61 patients with SPECT and MRI, within 2–18 days after injury, and found that SPECT detected more extensive abnormality than MRI in acute and follow-up studies (132). A small study (limited evidence) of patients with persistent post-concussion syndrome after mild TBI found that SPECT showed abnormalities in 53% of patients whereas MRI and CT only showed abnormalities in 9 and 5% respectively (133). A more recent study by Gowda and colleagues (134) studied 28 children and 64 adults with SPECT using technetium Tc99m ethyl cysteinate dimer within 72 h of the traumatic brain injury. The most common abnormality was hypoperfusion of the temporal lobe in children and the frontal lobe in adults (moderate evidence). A significantly higher number of perfusion abnormalities were seen in patients with posttraumatic amnesia ($p = 0.03$), loss of consciousness ($p = 0.02$), and post-concussion syndrome ($p = 0.01$) than in patients without these symptoms. CT findings were abnormal in 31 (34%) versus SPECT in 58 (63%). Difference between the SPECT and CT detection rate was statistically significant ($P < 0.05$). The largest study with patient outcomes was performed by Jacobs and colleagues (moderate to strong evidence) who prospectively studied 136 patients with mild injury, within 4 weeks of injury. SPECT had a high sensitivity and negative predictive value. A normal scan reliably excluded clinical sequelae of mild injury (135). A small study (limited evidence) of patients with severe TBI and diffuse brain injury, showed that total CBF values initially increased above normal in the first 1–3 days and then decreased below normal in the subacute period of 14–42 days. The early CBF increase has been postulated to reflect vasodilatation due to high tissue CO_2 and lactic acidosis. They found that the initial elevation and subsequent drop in blood flow was more marked in the poor-outcome group (136). However, another small study (limited evidence) of patients with a spectrum of injury, studied within 3 weeks of brain injury, found that focal zones of hyperemia in normal-appearing brain was associated with slightly better outcomes than patients without hyperemia (93). SPECT findings have also been compared with neuropsychological outcomes, although studies have consisted of small sample sizes, and have found varying results (133, 137).

Positron emission tomography can measure regional glucose and oxygen utilization, CBF at rest, and CBF changes related to performances of different tasks. Spatial and temporal resolution is also limited, although better than SPECT. However, PET is not widely available. A few PET studies have reported various areas of decreased glucose utilization, even without visible injury. Bergsneider and colleagues (limited to moderate evidence) prospectively studied 56 patients with mild to severe TBI, evaluated with 18F fluorodeoxyglucose (FDG)-PET within 2–39 days of injury, 14 of which had subsequent follow-up studies. They describe in this and previous reports that TBI patients demonstrate a triphasic pattern of glucose metabolism changes that consist of early hyperglycolysis, followed by metabolic depression, and subsequent metabolic recovery (after several weeks). These patients recovered metabolically, with similar patterns of changes in glucose metabolism suggesting that FDG-PET cannot estimate degree of functional recovery (138). Wu and colleagues (139) performed a study evaluating the gray matter and white matter with PET. Fourteen TBI patients and 19 normal volunteers were studied with a quantitative FDG-PET, a quantitative $H_2^{15}O$-PET and MRI acutely following TBI. The gray to white matter ratios for both FDG uptake rate and changes of glucose metabolic rate were significantly decreased in TBI patients ($P < 0.001$). The changes of glucose metabolic rate decreased significantly in gray matter ($P < 0.001$) but not in white matter ($P > 0.1$). The glucose to white matter ratios of changes in glucose metabolic rate correlated with the initial Glasgow Coma Score (GCS) of TBI patients with $r = 0.64$. The patients with higher changes of glucose metabolic rate (>1.54) showed good recovery a year after TBI. A more recent study by Lupi and colleagues evaluated PET in 58 consecutive patients (age range 14–69 years) with brain injury (44 with TBI) and demonstrated relative hypermetabolic cerebellar vermis as a common finding in an injured brain regardless of the nature of the trauma (140).

There are few small studies evaluating sensitivity of *Xenon CT* and even fewer describing the sensitivity of fMRI or MR perfusion. Newsome and colleagues studied eight children with moderate to severe TBI and eight matched, uninjured control children with fMRI using an

N-back task to test effects of TBI on working memory performance and brain activation (limited evidence) (141). Two patterns in TBI patients were seen. Patients whose criterion performance was reached at lower memory loads than control children demonstrated less extensive frontal and extrafrontal brain activation than controls. Patients who performed the same, highest (3-back) memory load as controls demonstrated more frontal and extrafrontal activation than controls. This is a small series and further longitudinal studies are needed.

MR Perfusion can also provide a measure of tissue perfusion similar to results found using PET or SPECT methods of CBF determination. However there have been little data in the literature regarding its use in predicting outcome after TBI. To date there is one small study (insufficient evidence) that showed that patients who had reduced regional cerebral blood volume in areas of contusions had poorer outcome. A subset of these patients that had reduced regional cerebral blood volume in normal-appearing white matter had significantly poorer outcomes (142). *fMRI* can provide noninvasive, serial mapping of brain activation, such as with memory tasks. This form of imaging can potentially assess the neurophysiological basis of cognitive impairment, with better spatial and temporal resolution than SPECT or PET. However, it is susceptible to motion artifact and requires extremely cooperative subjects, and therefore is more successful in mildly injured than moderate or severely injured patients. There have only been a few small studies (insufficient evidence) attempting to correlate fMRI with outcomes (143, 144).

Take Home Data

Table 13.2 shows suggested guidelines for acute neuroimaging in children with severe TBI. Table 13.3 shows suggested guidelines for acute neuroimaging in children with mild TBI.

Table 13.4 shows a list of possible types of head injuries, excluding penetrating or missile injuries, or nonaccidental trauma. Table 13.5 shows suggested guidelines for acute CT imaging in adult patients with mild TBI, modified from the Canadian Head CT Rule (21), EAST guidelines (2), and the Neurotraumatology Committee of the World Federation of Neurosurgical Societies (32).

Imaging Case Studies

Cases presented below highlight advantages and limitations of the different neuroimaging modalities.

Study 1: Example of MR Imaging for TBI

This case study illustrates imaging findings of DAI in a 10-year-old male struck by a car (Fig. 13.2).

Study 2: Example of MR Spectroscopy

This case study illustrates metabolite changes in single voxel short echo time proton spectra (TE = 20 ms) from a 28-year-old male admitted to hospital with severe TBI (GCS of 4) following a motor vehicle accident, compared to a normal 27-year-old control subject (Fig. 13.3).

Suggested Protocols for Acute TBI Imaging

- CT: axial 5 mm images in standard and bone algorithms; viewed with brain, intermediate and bone windows.
- MR: T1-weighted, T2-weighted, FLAIR, T2*-weighted GRE or SWI, DWI

Table 13.1. Current imaging methods of traumatic brain injury (TBI)

Modality	Principle and advantages/limitations	Use in TBI	Potential correlation with outcome
CT	Based on X-rays, measures tissue density; rapid, inexpensive, and widespread	Detects hemorrhage and "surgical lesions"	Short term outcome – mortality versus survival
Xenon CT perfusion	Inhalation of stable xenon gas which acts as a freely diffusible tracer; requires additional equipment and software that is available only in a few centers	Detects disturbances in CBF due to injury, edema, or infarction	Long term outcome – global or neuropsychological
MRI	Uses RF pulses in magnetic field to distinguish tissues, employs many different techniques; currently has highest spatial resolution; complex and expensive	Detection of various injuries and sensitivity varies with different techniques	Long term outcome – global or neuropsychological
MRI – FLAIR	Suppresses CSF signal	Detection of edematous lesions, particularly near ventricles and cortex; as well as extra-axial blood	Long term outcome – global or neuropsychological
MRI – T2* GRE	Accentuates blooming effect, such as blood products	Detection of small parenchymal hemorrhages	Long term outcome – global or neuropsychological
MRI – DWI	Distinguishes water mobility in tissue	Detection of recent tissue infarction or traumatic cell death	Long term outcome – global or neuropsychological
MRI – DTI	Based on DWI, maps degree and direction of major fiber bundles; requires special software	Detects impaired connectivity of white matter tracts, even in normal-appearing tissue	Long term outcome – global or neuropsychological
MRI – MT	Suppression of "background" brain tissue containing protein-bound H_2O, enhances contrast between water and lipid-containing tissue	May detect microscopic neuronal dysfunction, even in normal-appearing tissue	Long term outcome – global or neuropsychological
MRI – MRS	Analyzes chemical composition of brain tissue; requires special software	Metabolite patterns indicate neuronal dysfunction or axonal injury, even in normal-appearing tissue	Long term outcome – global or neuropsychological
MR volumetry	Measures volumes of various brain structures or regions; time-consuming, requires special software	Detects atrophy of injured tissue and can quantitate progression over time	Long term outcome – global or neuropsychological

fMRI	Measures small changes in blood flow related to brain activation; requires cooperative patients	Detects impairment or redistribution of areas of brain activation	Long term outcome – neuropsychological
MR perfusion (global, non fMRI)	Measures tissue perfusion using contrast or noncontrast methods; better temporal resolution than PET, SPECT; not as well studied	Detects disturbances in CBF due to injury, edema, or infarction	Long term outcome – global or neuropsychological
SPECT	Photon emitting radioisotopes used to measure CBF	Detects disturbances in CBF due to injury, edema, or infarction	Long term outcome – global or neuropsychological
PET	Positron emitting radioisotopes act as freely diffusible tracers, used to measure CBF, metabolic rate (glucose metabolism or oxygen consumption) or response to cognitive tasks; available only in a few centers	Detects disturbances in CBF due to injury, edema, or infarction	Long term outcome – global or neuropsychological

Reprinted with kind permission of Springer Science+Business Media from Tong KA, Oyoyo U, Holshouser BA, Ashwal S. Neuroimaging for traumatic brain injury. In Medina LS, Blackmore CC (eds.): *Evidence-Based Imaging: Optimizing Imaging in Patient Care*. New York: Springer Science+Business Media, 2006.
CT computed tomography, *MRI* magnetic resonance imaging, *FLAIR* fluid attenuated inversion recovery, *GRE* gradient recalled echo, *DWI* diffusion weighted imaging, *DTI* diffusion tensor imaging, *MT* magnetization transfer, *MRS* magnetic resonance spectroscopy, *fMRI* functional magnetic resonance imaging, *SPECT* single photon emission computed tomography, *PET* positron emission tomography, and *CBF* cerebral blood flow.

Table 13.2. The children's head injury algorithm for the prediction of important clinical events (CHALICE) rule

A computed tomography scan is required if *any* of the following criteria are present.

History
- Witnessed loss of consciousness of >5 min duration
- History of amnesia (either antegrade or retrograde) of >5 min duration
- Abnormal drowsiness (defined as drowsiness in excess of that expected by the examining doctor)
- ≥3 vomits after head injury (a vomit is defined as a single discrete episode of vomiting)
- Suspicion of non-accidental injury (NAI, defined as any suspicion of NAI by the examining doctor)
- Seizure after head injury in a patient who has no history of epilepsy

Examination
- Glasgow Coma Score (GCS) <14, or GCS <15 if <1 year old
- Suspicion of penetrating or depressed skull injury or tense fontanelle
- Signs of a basal skull fracture (defined as evidence of blood or cerebrospinal fluid from ear or nose, panda eyes, Battles sign, haemotympanum, facial crepitus or serious facial injury)
- Positive focal neurology (defined as an focal neurology, including motor, sensory, coordination or reflex abnormality)
- Presence of bruise, swelling or laceration >5 cm if <1 year old

Mechanism
- High-speed road traffic accident either as pedestrian, cyclist or occupant (defined as accident with speed >40 m/h)
- Fall of >3 m in height
- High-speed injury from a projectile or an object
If none of the above variables are present, the patient is at low risk of intracranial pathology.

Reprinted with permission by BJ Publishing Group LTD from Dunning et al. (88).

Table 13.3. Canadian Assessment of Tomography for Childhood Head injury: the CATCH rule

CT of the head is required for children with minor head injury[a] if any one of the following findings are present:

High risk (need for neurologic intervention)
1. Glasgow Coma Scale score <15 at 2 h after injury
2. Suspected open or depressed skull fracture
3. History of worsening headache
4. Irritability on examination

Medium risk (brain injury on CT scan)
1. Any sign of basal skull fracture (e.g. hemotympanum, "raccoon" eyes, otorrhea or rhinorrhea of the cerebrospinal fluid, Battle's sign)
2. Large, boggy hematoma of the scalp
3. Dangerous mechanism of injury (e.g. motor vehicle crash, fall from elevation ≥3 ft or 5 stairs, fall from bicycle with no helmet)

Reprinted with permission from Osmond et al. (90).
CT computed tomography.
[a]Minor head injury is defined as injury within the past 24 h associated with witnessed loss of consciousness, definite amnesia, witnessed disorientation, persistent vomiting (more than one episode), or persistent irritability (in a child under 2 years of age) in a patient with a Glasgow Coma Scale score of 13–15.

Table 13.4. Types of head injury (excluding penetrating/missile injuries and nonaccidental trauma)

Primary injuries
- Peripheral, non-intracranial
  - Scalp or soft tissue injury
  - Facial or calvarial fractures
- Extra-axial
  - Extradural or Epidural hemorrhage
  - Subdural hemorrhage
  - Traumatic subdural effusion or "hygroma"
  - Subarachnoid hemorrhage
  - Intraventricular hemorrhage
- Parenchymal
  - Contusion
    (a) Hemorrhagic
    (b) Nonhemorrhagic
    (c) Both
  - Shearing injury or "diffuse axonal injury"
    (a) Hemorrhagic
    (b) Nonhemorrhagic
    (c) Both
- Vascular
  - Arterial dissection/laceration/occlusion
  - Dural venous sinus laceration/occlusion
  - Carotid-cavernous fistula

Secondary injuries
- Cerebral edema
- Focal infarction
- Diffuse hypoxic-ischemic injury
- Hydrocephalus
- Infection

Reprinted with kind permission of Springer Science+Business Media from Tong KA, Oyoyo U, Holshouser BA, Ashwal S. Neuroimaging for traumatic brain injury. In Medina LS, Blackmore CC (eds.): *Evidence-Based Imaging: Optimizing Imaging in Patient Care.* New York: Springer Science+Business Media, 2006.

Table 13.5. Suggested guidelines for acute neuroimaging in adult patients with mild TBI (GCS 13–15)

If GCS 13–15, CT recommended if have any one of the following:
- High risk
  - GCS remains <15 at 2 h after injury
  - Suspected open or depressed skull fracture
  - Any clinical sign of basal skull fracture
  - Two or more episodes of vomiting
  - Aged 65 years or older
- Medium risk
  - Possible loss of consciousness
  - Amnesia for period before impact, of at least 30 min time span
  - Dangerous mechanism (pedestrian versus motor vehicle, ejected from motor vehicle, or fall from greater than 3 feet or 5 stairs)
  - Any transient neurologic deficit
  - Headache and vomiting

If GCS of 15, patient can be discharged home without CT scan if:
- Low risk
  - GCS remains 15
  - No loss of consciousness or amnesia
  - No neurologic/cognitive abnormalities
  - No headache, vomiting

Sources: Data from the Canadian Head CT Rule (21), EAST guidelines (2), and the Neurotraumatology Committee of the World Federation of Neurosurgical Societies (32).
Reprinted with kind permission of Springer Science+Business Media from Tong KA, Oyoyo U, Holshouser BA, Ashwal S. Neuroimaging for traumatic brain injury. In Medina LS, Blackmore CC (eds.): *Evidence-Based Imaging: Optimizing Imaging in Patient Care.* New York: Springer Science+Business Media, 2006.
CT computed tomography, *TBI* traumatic brain injury, *GCS* Glasgow coma scale.

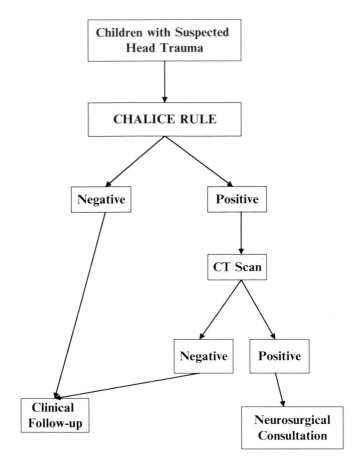

Figure 13.1. Recommended decision tree for children with acute head injury. (Reprinted with kind permission of Springer Science+Business Media from Tong KA, Oyoyo UE, Holshouser BA, Ashwal S, Medina SA. Evidence-based neuroimaging for traumatic brain injury in children. In Medina LS, Applegate KE, Blackmore CC (eds.): *Evidence-Based Imaging in Pediatrics: Optimizing Imaging in Pediatric Patient Care*. New York: Springer Science+Business Media, 2010.)

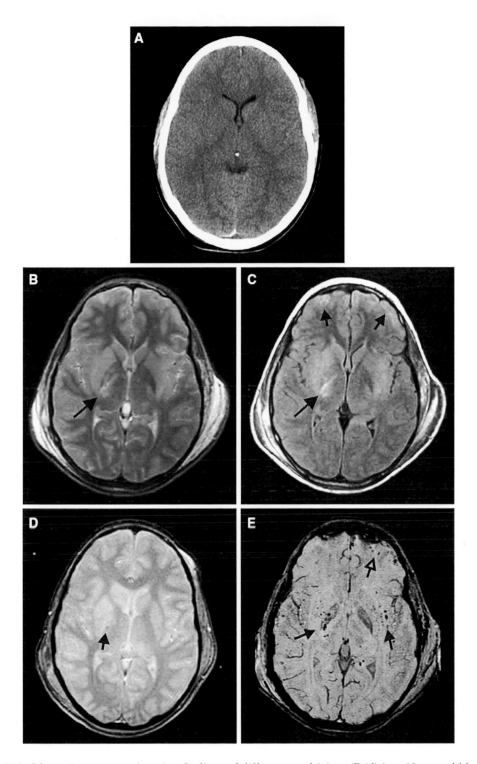

Figure 13.2. Magnetic resonance imaging findings of diffuse axonal injury (DAI) in a 10-year-old boy who was struck by a car. He had an initial GCS score of 3, was in a coma for 11 days, and had an elevated ICP. (**A**) His admission CT scan was normal. (**B**) An MRI was obtained 2 days after injury. Subtle hyperintense signal is seen in the right basal ganglia and posterior limb of the internal capsule (*arrow*), on the T2-weighted images. (**C**) The FLAIR sequence accentuates the edema in those areas (*long arrow*), as well as along the periphery of the frontal lobes (*short arrows*). (**D**) The standard T2*-GRE sequence shows a subtle punctuate hypointense focus in the right internal capsule (*arrow*). (**E**) The susceptibility-weighted imaging (SWI) technique (a modified T2*-GRE sequence) shows multiple tiny hemorrhagic foci within the bilateral basal ganglia and capsular white matter (*closed arrows*) as well as within the left frontal contusion (*open arrow*). (Reprinted with kind permission of Springer Science+Business Media from Tong KA, Oyoyo U, Holshouser BA, Ashwal S. Neuroimaging for traumatic brain injury. In Medina LS, Blackmore CC (eds.): *Evidence-Based Imaging: Optimizing Imaging in Patient Care*. New York: Springer Science+Business Media, 2006.)

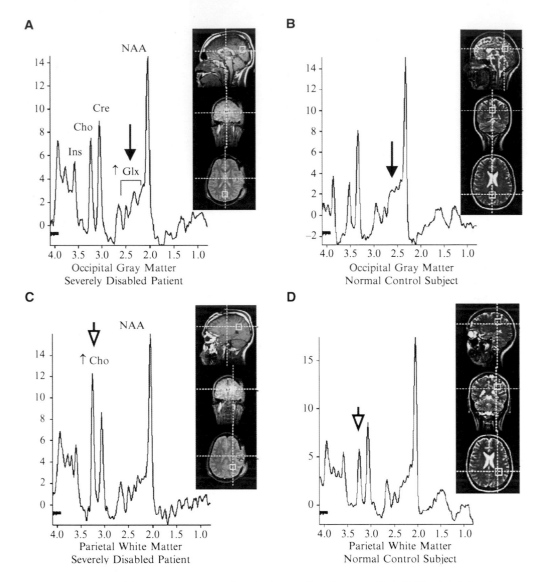

Figure 13.3. A 28-year-old man was admitted to the hospital with severe TBI (GCS of 4) following a motor vehicle accident. (**A**) Single voxel short-echo magnetic resonance spectroscopy taken from occipital gray matter shows increased glutamate/glutamine (Glx) compared to the control spectrum (**B**) (*arrows*). (**C**) Image taken from parietooccipital white matter shows increased choline (Cho, *arrowheads*) compared to the control spectrum (**D**). Evaluation at 6 months after the injury revealed severe disabilities (GOS of 3) in this patient. (Reprinted with kind permission of Springer Science+Business Media from Tong KA, Oyoyo U, Holshouser BA, Ashwal S. Neuroimaging for traumatic brain injury. In Medina LS, Blackmore CC (eds.): *Evidence-Based Imaging: Optimizing Imaging in Patient Care*. New York: Springer Science+Business Media, 2006.)

Future Research

- Clinical trials have been disappointing in TBI research, perhaps due to different mechanisms of injury included in trials, but also probably due to nonuniformity in classification of injuries and outcomes. There is a need for a consistent, widely accepted classification of information to facilitate comparisons of different groups of patients and institutions. The vast amount of clinical and imaging data can yield elaborate approaches, but this must be balanced with practicality in clinical situation. The system should be simple, relevant, reliable, and acceptable to clinicians in routine practice.
- Promising pediatric head trauma prediction rules need to be validated in actual practice.
- More research is needed, and ultimately a multimodal prognostic index for a wide range of disability probably needs to be developed.
- The link between imaging findings, neurobehavioral deficits and outcome requires further research, particularly after mild TBI.
- Larger, prospective studies are needed to evaluate the sensitivity, specificity, predictive accuracy, and cost-effectiveness of various neuroimaging methods in TBI.

References

1. Servadei F, Teasdale G, Merry G [on behalf of the Neurotraumatology Committee of the World Federation of Neurosurgical Societies]. J Neurotrauma 2001;18:657–664.
2. Cushman JG, Agarwal N, Fabian TC et al. J Trauma 2001;51:1016–1026.
3. Iverson GL, Lovell MR, Smith S, Franzen MD. Brain Inj 2000;14:1057–1061.
4. Jennett B, Bond M. Lancet 1975;1:480–484.
5. Jennett B, Snoek J, Bond MR, Brooks N. J Neurol Neurosurg Psychiatry 1981;44:285–293.
6. van der Naalt J, van Zomeren AH, Sluiter WJ, Minderhoud JM. J Neurol Neurosurg Psychiatry 1999;66:207–213.
7. Rappaport M, Hall KM, Hopkins K, Belleza BS, Cope DN. Arch Phys Med Rehabil 1982;63: 118–123.
8. Schwab K, Grafman J, Salazar AM, Kraft J. Neurology 1993;43:95–103.
9. Guide for the Uniform Data Set for Medical Rehabilitation (Including the FIM™ Instrument), Version 5.1. Buffalo, NY: State Univ New York, 1997.
10. Boake C. Arch Phys Med Rehabil 1996;77: 765–772.
11. Dikmen S, Machamer J, Miller B, Doctor J, Temkin N. J Neurotrauma 2001;18:127–140.
12. Temkin NR, Machamer JE, Dikmen SS. J Neurotrauma 2003;20:229–241.
13. Choi SC, Barnes TY, Bullock R, Germanson TA, Marmarou A, Young HF. J Neurosurg 1994;81:169–173.
14. Faul M, Xu L, Wald MM, Coronado VG. Traumatic Brain Injury in the United States: Emergency Department Visits, Hospitalizations and Deaths 2002-2006. Atlanta, GA: Centers for Disease Control and Prevention, National Center for Injury Prevention and Control, 2010.
15. Centers for Disease Control and Prevention, National Center for Injury Prevention and Control. Report to Congress on Mild Traumatic Brain Injury in the United States: Steps to Prevent a Serious Public Health Problem. Atlanta, GA: CDC, National Center for Injury Prevention and Control, 2003.
16. Lu J, Marmarou A, Choi S et al. Acta Neurochir 2005;95(suppl):281–285.
17. Adekoya N, Thurman DJ, White DD, Webb KW. MMWR Surveill Summ 2002;51(SS10):1–16.
18. Agency for Healthcare Research and Quality, Evidence Report: Number 2; Rehabilitation for Traumatic Brain Injury, 1999.
19. Finkelstein E, Corso P, Miller T et al. The Incidence and Economic Burden of Injuries in the United States. New York: Oxford University Press, 2006.
20. Fiser SM, Johnson SB, Fortune JB. Am Surg 1998;64:1088–1093.
21. Stiell IG, Wells FA, Vandemheen K, Clement C, Lesiuk H et al. Lancet 2001;357:1391–1396.
22. Haydel MJ, Preston CA, Mills TJ et al. N Engl J Med 2000;343:100–105.
23. Madden C, Witzke DB, Sanders AB, Valente J, Fritz M. Acad Emerg Med 1995;2:248–253.
24. Brain Trauma Foundation, Inc, American Association of Neurological Surgeons. Part I: Guidelines for the Management of Severe Traumatic Brain Injury. New York, NY: Brain Trauma Foundation, Inc., 2000.
25. Brain Trauma Foundation, Inc, American Association of Neurological Surgeons. Part II: Early Indicators of Prognosis in Severe Traumatic Brain Injury. New York, NY: Brain Trauma Foundation, Inc., 2000.
26. Eng J, Chanmugam A. Neuroimaging Clin N Am 2003;13:273–282.
27. Mack LR, Chan SB, Silva JC, Hogan TM. J Emerg Med 2003;24:157–162.
28. McAllister TW, Sparling MB, Flashman LA, Saykin AJ. J Clin Exp Neuropsychol 2001;23: 775–791.

29. Fearnside M, McDougall P. Aust N Z J Surg 1998;68:58–64.
30. The Brain Trauma Foundation. The American Association of Neurological Surgeons. The Joint Section on Neurotrauma and Critical Care. J Neurotrauma 2000;17:597–627.
31. Oertel M, Kelly DF, McArthur D et al. J Neurosurg 2002;96:109–116.
32. Servadei F, Murray GD, Penny K et al. European Brain Injury Consortium. Neurosurgery 2000;46:70–75.
33. Orrison WW, Gentry LR, Stimac GK, Tarrell RM, Espinosa MC, Cobb LC. Am J Neuroradiol 1994;15:351–356.
34. Ogawa T, Sekino H, Uzura M et al. Acta Neurochir 1992;suppl:8–10.
35. Hadley DM, Teasdale GM, Jenkins A et al. Clin Radiol 1988;39:131–139.
36. Gentry LR, Godersky JC, Thompson B, Dunn VD. AJR Am J Roentgenol 1988;150:673–682.
37. Mittl RL Jr, Grossman RI, Hiehle JF et al. Am J Neuroradiol 1994;15:1583–1589.
38. Gentry LR, Godersky JC, Thompson B. AJR Am J Roentgenol 1988;150:663–672.
39. Scheid R, Preul C, Gruber O, Wiggins C, von Cramon DY. Am J Neuroradiol 2003;24:1049–1056.
40. Tong K, Ashwal S, Holshouser B et al. Radiology 2003;227:332–339.
41. Ashikaga R, Araki Y, Ishida O. Neuroradiology 1997;39:239–242.
42. Huisman TAGM, Sorensen AG. J Comput Assist Tomogr 2003;27:5–11.
43. Hergan K, Schaefer PW, Sorensen AG, Gonzalez RG, Huisman TAGM. Eur Radiol 2002;12:2536–2541.
44. Shanmuganathan K, Gullapalli RP, Mirvis SE, Roys S, Murthy P. AJNR Am J Neuroradiol 2004;25:539–544.
45. Ptak T, Sheridan RL, Rhea JT et al. AJR Am J Roentgenol 2003;181:1401–1407.
46. Arfenakis K, Haughton VM, Carew JD et al. AJNR Am J Neuroradiol 2002;23:794–802.
47. Jones DK, Dardis R, Ervine M et al. Neurosurgery 2000;47:306–314.
48. Marshall LF, Marshall SB, Klauber M et al. J Neurotrauma 1992;9(suppl 1):287–292.
49. Vos PE, van Voskuilen AC, Beems T, Krabbe PF, Vogels OJ. J Neurotrauma 2001;18:649–655.
50. Wardlaw JM, Easton VJ, Statham P. J Neurol Neurosurg Psychiatry 2002;72:188–192.
51. Ono J, Yamaura A, Kubota M, Okimura Y, Isobe K. J Clin Neurosci 2001;8:120–123.
52. Firsching R, Woischneck D, Klein S, Reissberg S, Dohring W, Peters B. Acta Neurochir 2001; 143:263–271.
53. Maas AIR, Hukkelhoven CWPM, Marshall LF, Steyerberg EW. Neurosurgery 2005;57:1173–1182.
54. Mataro M, Poca MA, Sahuquillo J et al. J Neurotrauma 2001;18:869–879.
55. Lang DA, Teasdale GM, Macpherson P, Lawrence A. J Neurosurg 1994;80:675–680.
56. Levin HS, Gary HEJ, Eisenberg HM et al. J Neurosurg 1990;73:699–709.
57. Englander J, Cifu DX, Wright JM, Black K. Arch Phys Med Rehabil 2003;84:214–220.
58. Servadei F, Murray GD, Teasdale GM et al. Neurosurgery 2002;50:261–267.
59. Caroli M, Locatelli M, Campanella R, Balbi S, Martinelli F, Arienta C. Surg Neurol 2001;56:82–88.
60. LeRoux PD, Haglund MM, Newell DW, Grady MS, Winn HR. Neurosurgery 1992;31:678–684.
61. Kido DK, Cox C, Hamill RW, Rothenberg BM, Woolf PD. Radiology 1992;182:777–781.
62. Godersky JC, Gentry LR, Tranel D, Dyste GN, Danks KR. Acta Neurochir Suppl 1990;51:311–314.
63. Kampfl A, Schmutzhard E, Franz G et al. Lancet 1998;351:1763–1767.
64. Wilson JTL, Hadley DM, Wiedmann KD, Teasdale GM. J Neurol Neurosurg Psychiatry 1995;59: 328–331.
65. Tomei G, Sganzerla E, Spagnoli D et al. J Neurosurg Sci 1991;35:61–75.
66. Cordobes F, Lobato RD, Rivas JJ et al. Acta Neurochir 1986;81:27–35.
67. Wang HD, Duan GS, Zhang J, Zhou DB. Chin Med J 1998;111:59–62.
68. Parizel PM, Ozsarlak O, Van Goethem JW et al. Eur Radiol 1998;8:960–965.
69. Wallesch C-W, Curio N, Kutz S, Jost S, Bartels C, Synowitz H. Brain Inj 2001;15:401–412.
70. Kampfl A, Franz G, Aichner F et al. J Neurosurg 1998;88:809–816.
71. Paterakis K, Karantanas H, Komnos A, Volikas Z. J Trauma 2000;49:1071–1075.
72. Yanagawa Y, Tsushima Y, Tokumaru A et al. J Trauma 2000;49:272–277.
73. Kurth SM, Bigler ED, Blatter DD. Brain Inj 1994;8:489–500.
74. Fearnside MR, Cook RJ, McDougall P, McNeil RJ. Br J Neurosurg 1993;7:267–279.
75. Lannoo E, Van Rietvelde F, Colardyn F et al. J Neurotrauma 2000;17:403–414.
76. Blatter DD, Bigler ED, Gale SD et al. Am J Neuroradiol 1997;18:1–10.
77. Groswasser Z, Reider-Groswasser II, Schwab K et al. Brain Inj 2002;16:681–690.
78. Bigler ED, Blatter DD, Anderson CV et al. Am J Neuroradiol 1997;18:11–23.
79. Ratanalert S, Chompikul J, Hirunpat S, Pheunpathom N. Br J Neurosurg 2002;16:487–493.
80. Schaan M, Jaksche H, Boszczyk B. J Trauma 2002;52:667–674.
81. Prasad MR, Ewing-Cobbs L, Swank PR, Kramer L. Pediatr Neurosurg 2002;36:64–74.
82. Pillai S, Praharaj SS, Mohanty A, Sastry Kolluri VR. Pediatr Neurosurg 2001;34:98–103.
83. Sganzerla EP, Tomei G, Guerra P et al. Childs Nerv Syst 1989;5:168–171.
84. Suresh HS, Praharaj SS, Indira Devi B, Shukla D, Sastry Kolluri VR. Neurol India 2003;51:16–18.
85. Raimondi AJ, Hirschauer J. Childs Brain 1984; 11:12–35.

86. Crouchman M, Rossiter L, Colaco T, Forsyth R. Arch Dis Child 2001;84:120–124.
87. Fiser DH. J Pediatr 1992;121:69–74.
88. Dunning J, Daly JP, Lomas JP et al. Arch Dis Child 2006;91:885–891.
89. Kuppermann N, Holmes JF, Dayan PS et al. Lancet 2009;374:1160–1170.
90. Osmond MH, Klassen TP, Wells GA et al. CMAJ 2010;182(4):341–348.
91. Oman JA, Cooper RJ et al. Pediatrics 2006;117(2):e238–e246.
92. Palchak M, Holmes J, Vance C et al. Ann Emerg Med 2003;42(4):492–506.
93. Palchak MJ, Holmes JF et al. Pediatr Emerg Care 2009;25(2):61–65.
94. Greenes DS, Schutzman SA. Pediatrics 1999; 104:861–867.
95. Haydel MJ, Shembekar AD. Ann Emerg Med 2003;42:507–514.
96. Dunning J, Daly JP, Malhotra R et al. Arch Dis Child 2004;89:763–767.
97. Boran B, Boran P, Barut N. Pediatr Neurosurg 2006;42:203–207.
98. Lloyd DA, Carty H, Patterson M et al. Lancet 1997;349:821–824.
99. Hollingworth W, Vavilala MS et al. Pediatr Crit Care Med 2007;8(4):348–356.
100. Figg RE, Stouffer CW, Vander Kolk WE, Connors RH. Pediatr Surg Int 2006;22:215–218.
101. Tabori U, Kornecki A et al. Crit Care Med 2000;28(3):840–844.
102. Levin HS, Aldrich EF, Saydjari C et al. Neurosurgery 1992;31.435–443.
103. Hirsch W, Schobess A, Eichler G, Zumkeller W, Teichler H, Schluter A. Paediatr Anaesth 2002;12:337–344.
104. Tomberg T, Rink U, Pikkoja E, Tikk A. Acta Neurochir 1996;138:543–548.
105. Bonnier C, Marique P, Van Hout A et al. J Child Neurol 2007;22:519–529.
106. Sigmund GA, Tong KA, Nickerson JP et al. Pediatr Neurol 2007;36:217–226.
107. Levin HS, Mendelsohn D, Lilly MA et al. Neurosurgery 1997;40:432–440.
108. Grados MA, Slomine BS, Gerring JP, Vasa R, Bryan N, Denckla MB. J Neurol Neurosurg Psychiatry 2001;70:350–358.
109. Blackman JA, Rice SA, Matsumoto JA et al. J Head Trauma Rehabil 2003;18:493–503.
110. Tong K, Ashwal S, Holshouser BA et al. Ann Neurol 2004;56:36–50.
111. Babikian T, Freier MC, Tong K et al. Pediatr Neurol 2005;33:184–194.
112. Levin HS, Benavidez DA, Verger-Maestre K et al. Neurology 2000;54:647–653.
113. Wilde EA, Bigler ED, Haider JM et al. J Child Neurol 2006;21:769–776.
114. Spanos GK, Wilde EA, Bigler ED et al. AJNR Am J Neuroradiol 2007;28:537–542.
115. Schaefer P, Huisman T, Thierry AGM et al. Radiology 2004;233:58–66.
116. Wozniak JR, Krach L, Ward E. Archives of Clinical Neuropsychology 2007;22(5): 555–568.
117. Levin HS, Wilde EA, Chu Z et al. J Head Trauma Rehabil 2008;23(4):197–208.
118. Ross BD, Ernst T, Kreis R et al. J Magn Reson Imaging 1998;8:829–840.
119. Cecil KM, Lenkinski RE, Meaney DF, McIntosh TK, Smith DH. J Neurochem 1998;70: 2038–2044.
120. Sinson G, Bagley LJ, Cecil KM et al., Grossman RI. Am J Neuroradiol 2001;22:143–151.
121. Garnett MR, Blamire AM, Corkill RG et al. Brain 2000;123:2046–2054.
122. Shutter L, Tong KA, Holshouser BA. J Neurotrauma 2004;21:1693–1705.
123. Holshouser BA, Tong KA, Ashwal S et al. J Magn Reson Imaging 2006;24:33–40.
124. Makaroff KL, Cecil KM. Care M et al. Pediatr Radiol 2005;35.668–676.
125. Holshouser BA, Tong K, Ashwal S et al. American Journal of Neuroradiology 2005;26: 1276–1285.
126. Babikian T, Freier MC, Ashwal S. J Magn Reson Imaging 2006;24:801–811.
127. Ashwal S, Holshouser B, Tong K et al. J Neurotrauma 2004;21:1539–1552.
128. Ashwal S, Holshouser BA, Tong K et al. Pediatr Res 2004;56:630–638.
129. Ashwal S, Holshouser BA, Shu SK et al. Pediatr Neurol 2000;23:114–125.
130. Brenner T, Freier MC, Holshouser BA, Burley T, Ashwal S. Pediatr Neurol 2003;28:104–114.
131. Abdel-Dayem HM, Abu-Judeh H, Kumar M et al. Clin Nucl Med 1998;23:309–317.
132. Stamatakis EA, Wilson JT, Hadley DM, Wyper DJ. J Nucl Med 2002;43:476–483.
133. Kant R, Smith-Seemiller L, Isaac G, Duffy J. Brain Inj 1997;11:115–124.
134. Gowda NK, Agrawal D, Bal C et al. AJNR Am J Neuroradiol 2006;27:447–451.
135. Jacobs A, Put E, Ingels M, Put T, Bossuyt A. J Nucl Med 1996;37:1605–1609.
136. Shiina G, Onuma T, Kameyama M et al. AJNR Am J Neuroradiol 1998;19:297–302.
137. Kesler SR, Adams HF, Bigler ED. Brain Inj 2000;14:851–857.
138. Bergsneider M, Hovda DA, McArthur D et al. J Head Trauma Rehabil 2001;16:135–148.
139. Wu HM, Huang SC, Hattori N. J Neurotrauma 2004;21:149–161.
140. Lupi A, Bertagnoni G, Salgarello M. Clin Nucl Med 2007;32:445–451.
141. Newsome MR, Scheibal RS, Hunter J et al. Neurocase 2007;13:16–24.
142. Garnett MR, Blamire AM, Corkill RG et al. J Neurotrauma 2001;18:585–593.
143. Christodoulou C, DeLuca J, Ricker JH et al. Neurology 2003;60:1793–1798.
144. McAllister TW, Saykin AJ, Flashman LA et al. Neurology 1999;53:1300–1308.

14

Neuroimaging of Seizures

Byron Bernal and Nolan Altman

Issues

  I. Is neuroimaging appropriate in patients with febrile seizures?
 II. What neuroimaging examinations do patients with acute nonfe-
     brile symptomatic seizures need?
III. What is the role of neuroimaging in patients with first unprovoked
     seizures?
 IV. What is the most appropriate study in the workup of patients with
     temporal lobe epilepsy of remote origin?
  V. When should functional imaging be performed in seizure patients
     and what is the study of choice?

Key Points

- The main goal of neuroimaging in seizures is to rule out focal lesions
  that could threaten the patient's life (i.e., neoplasm or other intracranial space-occupying lesion).
- The most important role of neuroimaging in epilepsy is to identify the
  structural substrate of the epileptogenic focus.
- Neuroimaging is not recommended for a simple febrile seizure
  (limited evidence).
- Computed tomography scan is the best imaging study in the evaluation of patients with acute nonfebrile symptomatic seizures because it
  detects important abnormalities, such as acute intracranial hemorrhage, that may require immediate medical or surgical treatment
  (limited evidence).
- Magnetic resonance imaging (MRI) is the neuroimaging study of choice
  in the workup of first unprovoked seizures (moderate evidence).

B. Bernal (✉)
Department of Radiology, Miami Children's Hospital, 3100 SW 62 Avenue, Miami, FL 33176, USA
e-mail: byron.bernal@mch.com

L.S. Medina et al. (eds.), *Evidence-Based Imaging: Improving the Quality of Imaging in Patient Care, Revised Edition*,   **245**
DOI 10.1007/978-1-4419-7777-9_14, © Springer Science+Business Media, LLC 2011

- Focal neurologic deficit is an important predictor of an abnormality in the neuroimaging examination (moderate evidence).
- Magnetic resonance (MR) evaluation should be performed in non-acute symptomatic seizure patients with confusion and postictal deficits (moderate evidence).
- MR should be performed in children with unexpected cognitive or motor delays or children under 1 year of age, with remote symptomatic seizures (moderate evidence).
- Patients with focal seizures, abnormal EEG, or generalized epilepsy should be imaged (moderate evidence).
- MRI is the imaging modality of choice in temporal lobe epilepsy (moderate evidence).
- Ictal single photon emission computed tomography (SPECT) is the best neuroimaging examination to localize seizure activity (moderate evidence).

Definitions

A seizure is a symptom; epilepsy is a disease. Seizures occur as the result of an electrical discharge in the brain. Epilepsy is a disease characterized by more than one seizure. The International League Against Epilepsy (1) has proposed a classification of the epileptic syndromes, epilepsies, and related seizure disorders. Five main parameters are considered: age, etiology (symptomatic, cryptogenic, or idiopathic), electroclinical features (generalized vs. partial), prognosis (benign vs. malignant), and response to treatment (responsive vs. refractory epilepsy).

Numerous categories are produced from the combination of these factors, which creates confusion in the classification of seizures and epilepsies not only for the general physician, but also for specialists. Based on clinical findings, seizures are usually divided into symptomatic and nonsymptomatic seizures. The term *symptomatic* indicates that the seizure is a symptom with an underlying cause. This may be systemic (e.g., hyponatremia, hypocalcemia) or localized (e.g., tumor, cortical dysplasia, abscess). Seizures are categorized as acute symptomatic or remote symptomatic, depending on how long the underlying cause predated the seizure. *Acute symptomatic seizures* occur as the result of a proximate precipitant, such as fever, electrolyte imbalance, drug intoxication, alcohol withdrawal, brain trauma, central nervous system (CNS) infection, or aggressive neoplasm. In *remote symptomatic seizures* the lesion is preexistent and the seizure is the main or only symptom (e.g., cortical dysplasia, ganglioglioma, hippocampal sclerosis (HS), scar, or gliosis). Nonsymptomatic seizures include cryptogenic and idiopathic seizures. In *cryptogenic seizures* (or epilepsy), no cause can be found, even though one is clinically suspected by focal electroencephalography (EEG) or lateralized neurologic examination. In *idiopathic generalized epilepsy* there are no focal clinical signs or clear macrostructural cause for the epilepsy. In these cases, a genetic factor is presumed to be present. The term *unprovoked seizures* is used for seizures in patients without history or abnormal neurologic examination. They may turn out to be cryptogenic, idiopathic, or remote symptomatic after the appropriate workup. Partial seizures have a focal origin demonstrated by clinical semiology or EEG. Partial seizures are divided into simple and complex, the latter affecting the patient's awareness.

Epidemiology

The prevalence of epilepsy in industrialized countries is between 5 and 10 cases per 1,000 persons (2); hence, epilepsy affects between 1.5 and 3.0 million in the USA. Higher prevalence of epilepsy has been reported in developing countries (3), with a few exceptions. The incidence of epilepsy is age dependent. It peaks at the extremes of life, ranging from 100 to 140 per 100,000 in neonates and infants, and about 140 cases per 100,000 persons in the elderly; 50% of cases occur under the age of 1 year or over 60 years of age (2). The incidence is lowest in early adulthood (25 per 100,000), followed by an increase during late adulthood (4). A different age-specific distribution is seen in developing countries, with a second peak in early adulthood (5, 6).

Specific Epidemiologic Data

Febrile seizures affect children between 6 months and 6 years of age. The cumulative incidence of febrile seizures is 2% in children (7). The two most important predictors for first episode of febrile seizures are age less than 1 year and family history of febrile seizures (8). The overall incidence of febrile seizures recurrence is 35% (9). The recurrence of seizures after a focal febrile seizure lasting more than 15 min (complex febrile seizure) is two- to fourfold compared to an initial simple febrile seizure (10).

Acute afebrile symptomatic seizures affect 31 of 100,000 people per year and accounts for 40% of all new-onset afebrile seizures. The incidence is highest in the neonatal period (100 per 100,000 inhabitants), with a second peak in patients older than 75 years (123 per 100,000).

The probability of recurrent seizures after an initial *unprovoked seizure* is 36% by 1 year of age, and increases yearly up to 56% by 5 years (11). The presence of neurodevelopmental abnormalities increases the probability of future unprovoked seizures (12). The recurrence of all types of seizures ranges between 24 and 67% (13). Of all patients with recurrent seizures, up to 20% may have an intractable epilepsy (14).

Overall Cost to Society

Murray et al. (15) analyzed the cost of neuroimaging in the US health care system in 1994 for adult refractory epilepsy. Computed tomography (CT) was used in 60% of new and in 5% of existing cases of epilepsy, whereas MRI was requested in 90% of new and 12% of existing cases (15). Cost was determined by multiplying the CT or MRI incidence rate of usage by the incidence of new-onset seizures and by the cost of the exam. The cost for an MRI of the brain in the USA is between $1,200 and $2,000 (16). Therefore, the CT and MRI workup expenses of new-onset seizures in the USA is between $28,000 and $84,000 per 100,000 inhabitants per year.

A French cohort study on medical costs of epilepsy in 1,942 patients (17) reported that neuroimaging studies accounted for 8% of the total health care costs for these patients.

Bronen et al. (18) have reported the economic impact of replacing CT with MRI for refractory epilepsy, based on the assumption that the higher sensitivity of MRI in lesion detection would result in reducing the costs of interoperative electrocorticography otherwise needed to localize the site of the epileptogenic focus. They found that in 29 of 117 patients the replacement of CT by MRI eliminated the need for surgical placement of intracranial electrodes with potential savings of $1,450,000 in 29 patients.

Goals

The main goal of the neuroimaging in seizures and epilepsy is to rule out focal lesions that could threaten the patient's life. Neuroimaging also allows the identification of the structural substrate of the epileptogenic focus. Neuroimaging may increase or decrease the pretest probability of having a particular etiology or confirm a clinical diagnosis.

Methodology

For each of the procedures, MRI, CT, SPECT, positron emission tomography (PET), magnetic resonance spectroscopy (MRS), and functional MRI (fMRI), a systematic review of the literature from January 1, 1982, to January 31, 2004, for abstracts in English and for human subjects only, was performed utilizing PubMed (National Library of Medicine, Bethesda, Maryland) with the following terms: *epilepsy, seizure, evidence-based review,* and *neuroimaging evidence*. Titles and abstracts were reviewed to determine the appropriateness of content. Articles were excluded if they studied fewer than 30 patients, lacked pathologic verification, had no standard of reference, or had no significant influence on clinical decision making. Articles about MRI using less than 1.5 T were also excluded. The specificity, sensitivity, likelihood ratios, probability, predictors, and techniques were summarized for each procedure.

Seizures were divided into two main categories – new-onset seizures and established epilepsy – with particular emphasis on partial types. Adult and childhood epilepsy were addressed as well as febrile and temporal lobe epilepsy due to their clinical and radiologic importance.

Each of the selected articles was reviewed, abstracted and classified by two reviewers. Of a total of 606 abstracts, 131 articles met inclusion criteria and the full text was reviewed in detail.

I. Is Neuroimaging Appropriate in Patients with Febrile Seizures?

Summary of Evidence: Neuroimaging is not recommended for a simple febrile seizure (limited evidence).

Supporting Evidence: No level I or II (strong or moderate evidence) articles were found. In a level III article (limited evidence), Offringa et al. (19) reported an evidence-based medicine study for the management of febrile seizures and the role of neuroimaging in regard to detection of meningitis. The overall prevalence of meningitis detected by CT/MRI scans was 1.2% of 2,100 cases of seizures associated with fever. This manuscript, as well as the study by the American Academy of Pediatricians (20) (limited evidence) suggests that CT and MRI are not recommended for a simple febrile seizure.

II. What Neuroimaging Examinations Do Patients with Acute Nonfebrile Symptomatic Seizures Need?

Acute nonfebrile symptomatic seizures occur in nonfebrile patients having neurologic findings pointing to an underlying abnormality. It excludes meningitis, encephalitis, abscess, and empyema.

Summary of Evidence: CT scan is the best imaging study in the evaluation of patients with acute symptomatology, as it is sensitive for finding abnormalities such as acute intracranial hemorrhage, which may require immediate medical or surgical treatment. It is also fast and readily available (limited evidence).

Supporting Evidence: No articles meeting the criteria for level I or II (strong or moderate evidence) were found. Several level III (limited evidence) studies were found as discussed. Eisner and colleagues (21) reported a study with 163 patients, who presented to the emergency room with first seizure (Table 14.1). All patients older than 6 years of age who had recent head trauma, focal neurologic deficit, or focal seizure activity underwent head CT. Of 19 patients, five (26%) had CT abnormalities, including one subdural hematoma, resulting in a change of medical care. Earnest and colleagues (22) found CT abnormalities in 6.2% of 259 patients with alcohol withdrawal seizures. In 3.9% medical management was changed because of the CT result. Reinus and colleagues (23) retrospectively evaluated the medical records of 115 consecutive patients who had seizures after acute trauma and underwent a noncontrast cranial CT. An abnormal neurologic examination predicted 95% (19 of 20) of the positive CT scans $p < 0.00004$.

Henneman et al. (24) conducted a retrospective study on 333 patients with new-onset seizures, not associated with acute head trauma, hypoglycemia from diabetic therapy, or alcohol or recreational drug use. Of the 325 patients studied with CT scans, 134 (41%) had clinically significant results.

Bradford and Kyriakedes (25) reported an evidence-based review (limited evidence) of diagnostic tests in this population. The authors report a diagnostic yield of 87% for CT. Predictors of abnormal CT scans in patients with new onset of seizures had the following risk factors: head trauma, abnormal neurologic findings, focal or multiple seizures (within a 24-h period), previous CNS disorders, and history of malignancy. The article concludes that there are supportive data to perform CT scanning in the evaluation of all first-time acute seizures of unknown etiology.

III. What Is the Role of Neuroimaging in Patients with First Unprovoked Seizures?

Summary of Evidence: MRI is the neuroimaging study of choice in the workup of first unprovoked seizures (moderate evidence). Neuroimaging is positive in 3–38% of cases.

The probability is higher in patients with partial seizures and focal neurological deficit (Fig. 14.1). Neuroimaging is advised in children under 1 year of age and in those with significant unexplained cognitive or motor impairment, or prolonged postictal deficit. Significant neuroimaging findings impacting medical care are found in up to 50% of adults and in 12% of children.

Supporting Evidence: No level I (strong evidence) studies were available (Table 14.2). One level II study (moderate evidence) was found describing a cohort study in which neuroimaging studies were performed in 218 of 411 children (26); CT was performed in 159 and MRI in 59 cases. The cohort was followed for a mean of 10 years and none of the patients had evidence of neoplasm (accepted as the reference standard); 21% of the 218 exams were abnormal. The most frequent diagnoses were encephalomalacia (16 cases) and cerebral dysgenesis (11 cases). Six children had gray-matter migration disorders, which were seen only on MRI. In this study, a higher number of MRIs (34%) than CT studies (22%) were abnormal. In four cases (1.8%) the results altered both the diagnosis and the acute management of the patient. Children in this study who had a neurologic deficit (56 vs. 12%, $p < 0.001$), or abnormal EEG and partial seizures ($p < 0.05$) were more likely to have abnormal imaging.

A level III (limited evidence) case series study of 300 adults and children with an unexplained first seizure was reported by King et al. (27) in 1998; 92% of these patients had neuroimaging. A total of 263 patients had MRI and 14 had only CT. Epileptogenic lesions were found in 38 patients (13%). Of these, 17 had neoplasms that changed the patient's medical care. MRI detected abnormalities in 17% of patients. CT was performed in 28 of the 38 cases, with lesions on MRI being concordant with MRI in only 12 cases. CT missed a cavernous angioma and eight tumors. MRI was done in 50 patients with generalized epilepsy and only one had a neoplasm causing partial epilepsy.

In pediatric studies, neuroimaging diagnostic performance was similar to that in the adult literature according to an evidence-based study by Hirtz et al. (28) (limited evidence). However, the overall effect of neuroimaging on medical management was less in children than in adults (28).

The role of CT in evaluating children with new-onset unprovoked seizure was analyzed in a retrospective (limited evidence) study by Maytal et al. (29). Of 66 patients, 21.2% had abnormal CT results. The seizure etiology was clinically determined to be cryptogenic in 33 patients. Two of these children (6%) had abnormal nonspecific CT findings that did not require intervention. No abnormal CT results were seen in 13 cases with complex febrile seizures.

In a level III (limited evidence) study of 408 adults, CT scanning found tumors in 3% of patients. These patients were more likely to have recurrent seizures (30). Other studies have shown a higher percentage of positive imaging results in this population. A total of 119 adult patients with new-onset seizure underwent CT of the brain. Focal structural brain lesions were found in 40 patients (34%; 95% confidence interval, 25–42%). In 50% of the patients, the imaging findings prompt an important change in therapeutic management. The major predictor for finding a focal lesion on CT was the presence of a focal neurologic deficit (sensitivity of 50%, specificity of 89%) (31). Another study evaluated 50 patients referred for CT from a group of 107 children with first unprovoked seizure. A total of 19 children had brain abnormalities on CT. Of these, six patients had significant changes in medical workup or treatment (32).

The Quality Standards Subcommittee of the America Academy of Neurology, the Child Neurology Society, and the American Epilepsy Society have published a special report on practice guidelines in the evaluation of first nonfebrile seizures in children (unprovoked seizure) based on evidence-based medicine (EBM) (28) (limited evidence). The selection criteria included some small sample studies that lack stringent EBM criteria. This review article included studies in adults and in children. Analysis of the results found a range of 0–7% of children had lesions on CT that changed management of epilepsy (i.e., tumors, hydrocephalus, arachnoid or porencephalic cysts, and cysticercosis). Focal lesions on CT were more common in adults (18–34%).

Overall, MRI found more lesions than CT, but did not always change medical management (i.e., atrophy, mesial temporal sclerosis, and brain dysgenesis). This report concluded that there is insufficient evidence to support the recommendation for routine neuroimaging after the first unprovoked seizure. Neuroimaging, however, may be indicated in cases of focal seizures associated with positive neurologic clinical findings. If a neuroimaging study is required, MR is the preferred modality. Emergency imaging with CT or MR should be performed in cases of long-lasting postictal focal deficit, or in those patients who remain confused several hours after the seizure. Nonurgent imaging studies with MRI should be considered in children less than 1 year of age, significant and unexplained cognitive or motor impairment, a partial seizure, EEG findings not consistent with benign partial epilepsy of childhood, and primary generalized epilepsy.

IV. What Is the Most Appropriate Study in the Workup of Patients with Temporal Lobe Epilepsy of Remote Origin?

Summary of Evidence: MRI is the imaging modality of choice in temporal lobe epilepsy (moderate evidence). The seizure focus may be lateralized by MR volumetric techniques. MR sensitivity reaches 97% for HS using FLAIR (fluid-attenuated inversion recovery) imaging. Loss of digitations of the hippocampal head has a sensitivity of 92% for HS. Quantitative measurement of hippocampal size has a higher sensitivity than qualitative inspection with 76 vs. 71%, respectively.

Supporting Evidence: No level I (strong evidence) studies are available (Table 14.3). There is one prospective cohort level II study (moderate evidence) of neuroimaging in temporal lobe epilepsy of childhood (33). Sixty-three children with new-onset temporal lobe epilepsy were included; MRI was performed in 58 (92%) and CT in 48 (76%). The MRI was abnormal in 23 children (36.5%) and included unilateral HS in 12, bilateral HS in one, temporal lobe tumor in eight, arachnoid cyst in one, and cortical dysplasia in one. CT was positive in 23% of cases, which included all tumors, but failed to detect cases of HS. CT demonstrated calcifications in the posterior area of the hippocampus in one case that was not detected on MR. This lesion was shown to be a small hamartoma pathologically. The authors proposed three groups to classify

partial seizures based on the relationship among neuroimaging findings, prior history, and age:

Group I: Developmental temporal lobe epilepsy (ten patients). Seizures begin in mid- to late childhood (mean age 8.2 years) and neurobehavioral problems are infrequent. This epilepsy is associated with tumors and malformations that are usually long-standing and nonprogressive cortical lesions such as gangliogliomas, dysembryoplastic neuroepithelial tumors, and pilocytic xanthochromic astrocytomas.

Group II: Temporal lobe epilepsy with HS (18 patients), included children with significant prior clinical history of neurologic insult, including complicated febrile seizures, hypoxic-ischemic encephalopathy, and meningitis.

Group III: Cryptogenic temporal lobe epilepsy (34 patients) in whom no etiology could be determined.

A level III study (limited evidence) by Kramer et al. (34) studied the predictive value of abnormal neurologic findings on the neuroimaging of 143 children with partial seizures. Fifty patients had neuroimaging abnormalities and 36 had abnormal clinical findings. The neurologic exam findings of hemiparesis, mental retardation, and neurocutaneous stigmata were risk factors in predicting abnormal neuroimaging findings. However, the abnormality detected on neurologic examination or the type of seizure was not a predictive parameter in determining tumor resectability as shown by neuroimaging.

A level III study (limited evidence) by Berg and coworkers (35) reported the neuroimaging findings in a group of 613 children with newly diagnosed temporal lobe epilepsy. A total of 359 patients had partial seizures. Of this group, 312 (86.9%) underwent imaging; 283 had MRI alone or with CT. Relevant abnormalities were found in 43 (13.8% of those imaged). The strongest predictor of abnormal imaging was an abnormal motor examination (odds ratio: 18.9; 95% confidence interval, 9.9–36.3%; and $p < 0.0001$).

The MR findings in 186 of 274 consecutive patients who underwent temporal lobectomy for intractable epilepsy were retrospectively reviewed (moderate evidence) (Table 14.4) (36).

This was a blinded study with pathology as the reference standard. MRI detected 121 hippocampal/amygdala abnormalities (sensitivity and specificity of 93 and 83%, respectively) and 60 other abnormalities in the remainder of the temporal lobe (sensitivity and specificity of 97 and 97%, respectively). Increased signal of the hippocampus on T2-weighted images had a sensitivity of 93% and specificity of 74% in predicting mesial temporal sclerosis (Fig. 14.2). Forty-two temporal tumors were detected with a sensitivity and specificity of 83 and 97%, respectively.

The sensitivity of CT and MRI in temporal lobe pathology was recently reported by Sinclair et al. (37) (limited evidence). Forty-two pediatric patients were studied. All patients underwent temporal lobectomy for intractable epilepsy, hence providing histopathology as the reference standard. MRI found abnormalities in 27 cases (64%) and CT scan in 12 of 39 cases (31%). MRI was clearly more sensitive than CT in the detection of pathology.

The MRI sensitivity in demonstrating the epileptogenic zone determined by EEG (a weak standard reference) was investigated in a level III study (limited evidence). The weakness of the reference standard is in part compensated by the number of cases. Pooled data of 809 patients, of whom 370 had temporal lobe abnormalities, were analyzed (38). The sensitivity of MR was 55% for temporal epileptogenic zones and 43% for extratemporal regions as determined by EEG.

Moore et al. (39) addressed the incidence of HS in normal subjects in a level III article (limited evidence). They studied 207 patients referred for hearing loss with high-resolution MR and found two cases of unsuspected HS. Retrospective chart review revealed that both patients had seizures. One of them had seizure onset 18 months prior to the MR study that was believed to be associated with hemorrhage from an arteriovenous malformation ipsilateral to the HS.

The most important neuroimaging findings in HS are small size (atrophy) and intense T2 signal of the hippocampus (Table 14.5). These signs have been quantified in a level III retrospective study (limited evidence) of 41 MRI of patients who underwent temporal lobectomy (40). The authors compared measurements of the left and right hippocampal formations and found them to have 76%

sensitivity and 100% specificity for correct seizure lateralization.

Watson et al. (41) performed a comparison among different types of epilepsy with volumetric measuring of the hippocampus in 110 patients with chronic epilepsy of whom 81 had partial seizures (limited evidence) and 17 had pathologically proven HS. All 17 patients with HS had reduced absolute hippocampal volumes, greater than 2 standard deviations (SD) below the mean of the control group. The degree of reduced hippocampal size correlates well with the severity of the HS. Hippocampal volumes were within normal range in all patients with generalized epilepsy, and in extratemporal and extrahippocampal temporal lesions.

Oppenheim et al. (42) proposed that the loss of digitations of the hippocampal head on MRI be considered a major criterion of HS along with signal abnormality and reduced volume. In a level III case-series study (limited evidence) of 193 patients with intractable epilepsy evaluated retrospectively for atrophy, 63 patients were diagnosed as having mesial temporal sclerosis based on T2 signal changes and loss of digitations of the hippocampal head; 24 of these patients underwent surgery and HS was confirmed in all of them. A control group of 60 patients with frontal seizures and normal MRI was also studied. The digitations of the hippocampal head were evaluated in the two groups. Digitations were not visible in 51 and poorly visible in eight of the 63 patients with mesial temporal sclerosis. Of 24 hippocampi in which HS was confirmed histologically, 22 had no MRI-visible digitations. In the control group digitations were sharply visible in 55 and poorly visible in five. The sensitivity and specificity of complete loss of hippocampal head digitations in HS was 92 and 100%, respectively.

Jack et al. (43) in a level II study (moderate evidence) compared the accuracy of FLAIR sequence with that of conventional dual spin–echo (SE) sequence in the identification of increased signal of HS. The study was blinded and controlled with a reference standard criterion of the histopathologic examination. A total of 36 patients were included. The sensitivity was 97% for FLAIR vs. 91% for SE in the diagnosis of HS.

The MRI findings as predictors of outcome of temporal lobectomy were assessed in a cohort (moderate evidence) study of 135 patients (44).

Sixty months after surgery, 69% of patients with neuroimaging lesions, 50% with HS, and 21% with normal MRIs had no postoperative seizures. Outcome was worse in those with normal MRI examinations.

V. When Should Functional Imaging Be Performed in Seizure Patients and What Is the Study of Choice?

Summary of Evidence: Functional neuroimaging can provide additional data in seizure patients (Table 14.6). The sensitivity of SPECT for localizing epileptogenic focus increases from interictal (44%) to ictal examinations (97%) (moderate evidence). The sensitivity is lower in cases of extratemporal partial epilepsy in which only the ictal exam is reliable (sensitivity of 92%). Subtraction techniques of the interictal from the ictal study may be helpful; however, the ictal study remains the preferred examination. PET is more sensitive than interictal SPECT in localizing temporal and extratemporal epilepsy, but far less sensitive than ictal SPECT for the localization of epileptogenic foci. More research is needed on MRS as a tool to lateralize the epilepsy focus. fMRI can help to lateralize language in the workup of patients for epilepsy surgery (limited evidence). fMRI has a sensitivity greater than 91% for language lateralization, when the intracarotid Amytal test (Wada test) is used as the reference standard (Table 14.7). fMRI influences the seizure team's diagnostic and therapeutic decision making (moderate evidence).

Supporting Evidence: No level I studies (strong evidence) were found. In the level II meta-analysis study (moderate evidence) reported by Spencer (38), ictal SPECT was performed in 108 patients. Eighty epileptogenic foci were localized by SPECT in the temporal lobe. In temporal lobe epilepsy the diagnostic sensitivity for ictal or postictal SPECT is 90% and the specificity of 73%. In extratemporal lobe epilepsy ictal SPECT sensitivity decreases to 81% and specificity increases to 93% when using EEG criteria as the standard of reference. False localization was found in 5% of cases. Interictal SPECT sensitivity and specificity were found to be significantly lower, at 66 and 68%, respectively, for temporal lobe, and at 60

and 93%, respectively, for extratemporal regions when compared to EEG. False localization was found in 10–25%. A later level II study (moderate evidence) by Devous et al. (45) presented a second meta-analysis of SPECT brain imaging in partial epilepsy (temporal and extratemporal). The pooled data were gathered from 624 interictal, 101 postictal, and 136 ictal cases. The vast majority of patients were adults. The reference standard was EEG or surgical outcome (162 cases). The results from this study showed that the sensitivity of technetium-99m labeled hexamethyl-propylene amine oxime (HMPAO) SPECT in localizing a temporal lobe epileptic focus increases from 44% in interictal studies to 75% in postictal studies and reaches 97% in ictal studies. False positives, when compared to surgical outcome, were 4.4% for interictal and 0% for postictal and ictal studies.

A level III study (limited evidence) by Newton et al. (46) of 177 patients with partial epilepsy showed similar results. In 119 patients with known unilateral temporal lobe epilepsy, correct localization by ictal SPECT was demonstrated in 97% of cases. Postictal SPECT was correct in 71% of cases and interictal SPECT in 48% of cases. In extratemporal epilepsy, the yield of ictal SPECT studies was 92% and that of postictal SPECT studies was 46%. The interictal SPECT was of little value in extratemporal epilepsy.

Lewis et al. (47) reported a small level III case series (limited evidence) of 38 patients with seizures not associated with HS using subtraction techniques of interictal SPECT from ictal SPECT. In 58% of the studies the subtraction images "contributed additional information" but were confusing in 9%.

In a level III study (limited evidence) of 312 patients pooled by Spencer (38), PET was compared to EEG for localization. A total of 205 patients had reduced temporal lobe metabolism of which 98% were concordant with EEG findings. Thirty-two patients had hypometabolism in an extratemporal location, which was concordant with EEG in 56% of cases. The abnormalities in 75 patients were not localized by PET, 36 of whom had temporal lobe EEG abnormalities. The diagnostic sensitivity for fluorodeoxyglucose (FDG)-PET was 84% (specificity of 86%) for temporal, and 33% (specificity of 95%) for extratemporal epilepsy, respectively.

A level III study (limited evidence) of single-voxel proton MRS was performed to lateralize seizures; MRS was compared with MRI and PET in a case series of 33 HS patients (48). Ratios <0.8 for N-acetylaspartate (NAA)/ choline (Cho), and 1.0 for NAA/creatine (Cr) were regarded as abnormal. The sensitivity of MRS and PET in lesion lateralization was 85% for both, using MRI as the reference standard. False lateralization rates for MRS and PET were 3 and 6%, respectively. The concordance between MRS and PET was 73%. These results did not influence medical decisions making.

fMRI is a new technique based on the ability to detect small amounts of paramagnetic susceptibility produced by blood-oxygen level changes linked to brain cortical activity. Although fMRI is still under investigation and is without Food and Drug Administration (FDA) approval, it has shown promise as an examination that might replace the more invasive and expensive Wada intracarotid amobarbital exam in the lateralization and location of language in patients who are candidates for epilepsy surgery.

Most fMRI papers are based on small samples. One level III case-series paper (limited evidence) (49) describes procedures and results of language dominance lateralization in 100 patients with partial epilepsy performing a covert word generation task. The reference standard was a bilateral Wada intracarotid amobarbital test (IAT) performed in all cases. The results impacted clinical decision making. There was 91% concordance between both tests. Divergent results between the tasks included two cases in which the IAT showed absence of lateralization. Discordance was much higher in cases of left-sided extratemporal epilepsy (25%). In another level III case-series paper (limited evidence), Gaillard et al. (50) described the findings of language lateralization in a group of 30 patients with temporal lobe epilepsy. They used IAT in 21 cases as the reference standard. Eighteen cases had temporal resection and further follow-up. There were no divergent results (i.e., methods pointing to the opposite side). One case showed bilateral fMRI activation and lateralized IAT. Two cases had bilateral IAT and left lateralized fMRI.

The Miami Children's Hospital Group, in a prospective study (moderate evidence), enrolled prospectively, 60 subjects to determine the role of fMRI in the diagnostic evaluation and surgical treatment of patients with seizure disorders. In 35 (58.3%) of the 60 patients, the seizure team thought that fMRI results altered patient and family counseling. In 38 (63.3%) of the 60 patients, fMRI avoided further studies including Wada test. In 31 (51.7%) and 25 (41.7%) of the 60 patients, fMRI altered intraoperative mapping plans and surgical approach plans, respectively. In five (8.3%) patients, a two-stage surgery with extraoperative direct electrical stimulation mapping was averted and resection could be accomplished in a one-stage surgery. In four (6.7%) patients, the extent of surgical resection was altered because eloquent areas were identified close to the seizure focus. The authors concluded that fMRI influences the seizure team's diagnostic and therapeutic decision making (51).

A recent study compared the costs of fMRI and IAT (Wada test) in the workup of language lateralization in patients who where candidates for epilepsy surgery (52). Two age-matched groups were studied prospectively. Twenty-one patients had fMRI and 18 IAT. Total direct costs of the Wada test ($1130.01 ± $138.40) and of fMRI ($301.82 ± $10.65) were significantly different ($p < 0.001$). The cost of the Wada test was 3.7 times higher than that of fMRI.

Take Home Figure

Figure 14.3 provides a decision-making algorithm for children and adults with seizure disorders.

Future Research

- To define better the different seizure risk groups so neuroimaging can be tailored appropriately.
- To determine the advantages, limitations, indications, and pitfalls of new imaging studies such as fMRI and MRS.
- To determine the impact that imaging has in the outcome of patients with seizure disorders.
- To perform formal cost-effectiveness analysis of the role of imaging in patients with seizure disorders.

Imaging Case Studies

CT and MRI images of a child with epilepsy and postural plagiocephaly

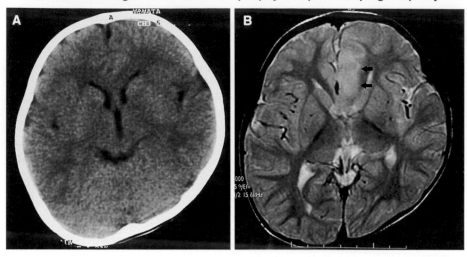

Figure 14.1. Computed tomography (CT) vs. magnetic resonance imaging (MRI) sensitivity in nonacute symptomatic seizure. This figure illustrates the higher sensitivity of MRI in the detection of cortical dysplasia. The transverse CT (**A**) is compared to the MRI (**B**) in a child with intractable epilepsy and postural plagio-cephaly. The region of cortical dysplasia in the left parasagittal frontal lobe is clearly seen only on the MRI exam by the loss of gray–white matter interface and the increased T2-weighted signal intensity. (Reprinted with kind permission of Springer Science+Business Media from Bernal B, Altman N. Neuroimaging of Seizures. In Medina LS, Blackmore CC (eds): *Evidence-Based Imaging: Optimizing Imaging in Patient Care.* New York: Springer Science+Business Media, 2006.)

MRI of a patient with complex partial seizures and left temporal EEG abnormalities

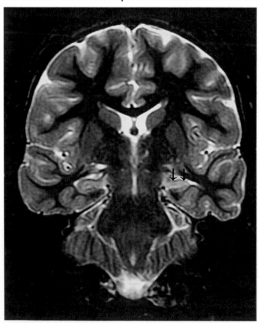

Figure 14.2. T2-inversion recovery MRI. The image corresponds to a patient with intractable epilepsy and EEG findings of left temporal origin. Coronal image at the level of the temporal lobes demonstrates left hip-pocampal sclerosis characterized by reduction in size, and increased signal intensity (*arrows*), compared to the normal right hippocampus. (Reprinted with kind permission of Springer Science+Business Media from Bernal B, Altman N. Neuroimaging of Seizures. In Medina LS, Blackmore CC (eds): *Evidence-Based Imaging: Optimizing Imaging in Patient Care.* New York: Springer Science+Business Media, 2006.)

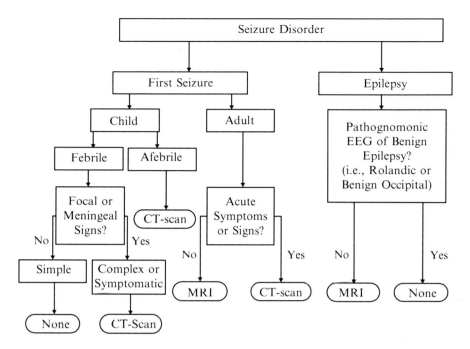

Figure 14.3. Algorithm for seizure disorders. (Reprinted with kind permission of Springer Science+Business Media from Bernal B, Altman N. Neuroimaging of Seizures. In Medina LS, Blackmore CC (eds): *Evidence-Based Imaging: Optimizing Imaging in Patient Care*. New York: Springer Science+Business Media, 2006.)

Table 14.1. Neuroimaging in acute symptomatic seizures (CT/MRI)

Author	No. of Patients	CT/MRI	% of positive	Comments
Eisner et al. (21)	163	19	25	Positive results in 3% of the total of patients
Earnest et al. (22)	259	259	6.2	Only patients with seizures after alcohol withdrawal were included; 3.9% of patients resulted in significant treatment changes
Reinus et al. (23)	115	?	36	Postacute head trauma (60 patients had previous seizure disorder)
Henneman et al. (24)	333	325	41	Seizures no associated with head trauma

Reprinted with kind permission of Springer Science+Business Media from Bernal B, Altman N. Neuroimaging of Seizures. In Medina LS, Blackmore CC (eds): *Evidence-Based Imaging: Optimizing Imaging in Patient Care*. New York: Springer Science+Business Media, 2006.

Table 14.2. Neuroimaging in first unprovoked seizure

Author	Patients	CT/MRI	% of positives	Comments
Shinnar et al. (26)	218	186/59	34/22	1.8% significant findings
King et al. (27)	300	263/14	17/8	
Hirtz et al. (28)	(EBM review)		18–34	In children: significant findings in less than 7%
Maytal et al. (29)	66	66/20	21	None with significant findings
Hopkins et al. (30)	408	408/0	?	3% tumors
Schoenenberger and Heim (31)	119	119/0	34	17% with significant findings
Garvey et al. (32)	50	50/0	17	12% with significant findings

Reprinted with kind permission of Springer Science+Business Media from Bernal B, Altman N. Neuroimaging of Seizures. In Medina LS, Blackmore CC (eds.): *Evidence-Based Imaging: Optimizing Imaging in Patient Care.* New York: Springer Science+Business Media, 2006.

Table 14.3. Neuroimaging in temporal lobe epilepsy (TLE) and other partial seizures

Author	Patients	CT/MRI	% of positives	Comments
Harvey et al. (33)	63	48/58	23/36.5	Study done with two magnets: 0.3 T and 1.5 T; etiologies: 13 HS, 8 tumors, 1 cortical dysplasia, 1 arachnoidal cyst, and 1 hamartoma
Kramer et al. (34)	143	117/42	(35)	Study in children and adolescents: 8 diffuse atrophy, 8 porencephalic cyst, 6 tumors, 6 neurocutaneous syndrome, 6 dysgenesis; neither an abnormality in the neurologic exam nor the type of seizure were predictors for finding a tumor
Lee et al. (36)	274	0/186	97	Patients with intractable TLE; 65% had HS, 32 had abnormalities in the rest of the temporal lobe; 42 tumors in pediatric patients
Berg et al. (35)	359	(312)	(13.8)	All pediatric patients; in 3 normal-CT cases the MRI was abnormal; the strongest predictor of abnormal imaging was abnormal motor examination
Sinclair et al. (37)	42	39/42	31/64	Patients with intractable partial epilepsy; postoperative findings: 13 tumors, 8 HS, 5 dual pathology, 4 cortical dysplasia, 4 tuberous sclerosis, 1 porencephalic cyst
Spencer (38)	809	?	43–55	370 Patients with temporal lobe abnormalities; the lowest percent for extratemporal lobe epilepsy

Note: The reported data in parenthesis are not divided due to lack of further information.
Reprinted with kind permission of Springer Science+Business Media from Bernal B, Altman N. Neuroimaging of Seizures. In Medina LS, Blackmore CC (eds): *Evidence-Based Imaging: Optimizing Imaging in Patient Care.* New York: Springer Science+Business Media, 2006.

Table 14.4. MRI sensitivity and specificity in temporal lobe epilepsy

Item	Sensitivity (%)	Specificity (%)	Reference
Hippocampal lesion	93	83	Lee et al. (36)
Nonhippocampal temporal lobe lesion	97	97	Lee et al. (36)
Global sensitivity for tumor detection	83	97	Lee et al. (36)
High T2 signal for hippocampal sclerosis	93	74	Lee et al. (36)
High FLAIR signal for hippocampal sclerosis	97	?	Jack et al. (43)

Reprinted with kind permission of Springer Science+Business Media from Bernal B, Altman N. Neuroimaging of Seizures. In Medina LS, Blackmore CC (eds): *Evidence-Based Imaging: Optimizing Imaging in Patient Care.* New York: Springer Science+Business Media, 2006.

Table 14.5. MRI sensitivity and specificity for hippocampal sclerosis

Author	Patients	Sensitivity	Specificity	Comments
Spencer (38)	153	71	?	Review
Moore et al. (39)	207	100	100	Study conducted in "normal volunteers"; 2 had HS and prior history of seizures in detail chart review
Jack et al. (40)	41	76	100	Quantitative volumetric measurement of the hippocampus
Oppenheim (42)	63	92	100	Based on loss of digitations in hippocampal head
Jack et al. (43)	36	97	?	FLAIR sequence was compared to SE (91% sensitivity)

Reprinted with kind permission of Springer Science+Business Media from Bernal B, Altman N. Neuroimaging of Seizures. In Medina LS, Blackmore CC (eds): *Evidence-Based Imaging: Optimizing Imaging in Patient Care.* New York: Springer Science+Business Media, 2006.

Table 14.6. Functional neuroimaging in epileptic focus detection

Author	Procedure	No. of patients	Ictal Sen/Spec	Postictal Sen/Spec	Interictal Sen/Spec	Comments
Spencer (38)	PET	312			84/86[a] 33/95[b]	
Spencer (38)	SPECT	80	90/73[a] 81/93[b]	90/73[a]	66/68[a] 60/93[b]	Compared to EEG False localization was found in 10–25%
Newton et al. (46)	SPECT	177	97/[a] 92/[a]	71/[a] 46/[b]	48/[a]	
Devous et al. (45)	SPECT	624	97/[a]	75/[a]	44/[a]	Compared to EEG and/ or surgical outcome

Sen sensitivity, *Spec* specificity.
Reprinted with kind permission of Springer Science+Business Media from Bernal B, Altman N. Neuroimaging of Seizures. In Medina LS, Blackmore CC (eds): *Evidence-Based Imaging: Optimizing Imaging in Patient Care.* New York: Springer Science+Business Media, 2006.
[a]In temporal lobe epilepsy.
[b]In extratemporal lobe epilepsy.

Table 14.7. Functional MRI in language lateralization for epilepsy Surgery

Author	Paradigm	No. of patients	Reference standard	Sensitivity (%)	Comments
Woermann et al. (49)	Word generation	100	Bilateral IAT	91	Cases with localization-related epilepsy; discordant categorization between fMR and IAT includes absence of IAT lateralization in 2 cases
Gaillard et al. (50)	Reading and naming	30 IAT	Bilateral	93	All cases temporal lobe epilepsy; no disagreement with reference standard

IAT intracarotid amobarbital test.
Reprinted with kind permission of Springer Science+Business Media from Bernal B, Altman N. Neuroimaging of Seizures. In Medina LS, Blackmore CC (eds): *Evidence-Based Imaging: Optimizing Imaging in Patient Care.* New York: Springer Science+Business Media, 2006.

References

1. Commission on Classification and Terminology of the International League Against Epilepsy. Epilepsia 1989;34:592–596.
2. Bell GS, Sander JW. Seizure 2001;10:306–316.
3. Senanayake N, Roman GC. Bull WHO 1993;71: 247–225.
4. Hauser WA, Annegers JF, Kurland LT. Epilepsia 1993;34:453–468.
5. Lavados J, Germain L, Morales A et al. Acta Neurol Scand 1992;85:249–256.
6. Rwiza HT, Kilonzo GP, Haule J et al. Epilepsia 1992;33:1051–1056.
7. Hauser WA, Annegers JF, Rocca WA. Mayo Clin Proc 1996;71:576–586.
8. Berg AT, Shinnar S, Hauser WA et al. J Pediatr 1990;116:329–337.
9. Knudsen FU. Arch Dis Child 1985;60:1045–1049.
10. Offringa M, Bossuyt PMM, Lubsen J et al. J Pediatr 1994;124:574–584.
11. Annegers JF, Shirts SB, Hauser WA et al. Epilepsia 1986;27:43–50.
12. Berg AT, Shinnar S. Neurology 1996;47:562–568.
13. Berg AT, Shinnar S. Neurology 1991;41: 965–972.
14. Shorvon SD. Epilepsia 1996;37(suppl 2):S1–S3.
15. Murray MI, Halpern MT, Leppik IE. Epilepsy Res 1996;23:139–148.
16. Ho SS, Kuzniecky RI. J Neuroimaging 1997;7: 236–241.
17. De Zelicourt M, Buteau L, Fagnani F et al. Seizure 2000;9:88–95.
18. Bronen RA, Fulbright RK, Spencer SS et al. Magn Reson Imaging 1997;15:857–862.
19. Offringa M, Moyer VA. West J Med 2001;175: 254–259.
20. American Academy of Pediatrics Provisional Committee on Quality Improvement, Subcommittee on Febrile Seizures. Pediatrics 1996;97:769–772; discussion 773–775.
21. Eisner RF, Turnbull TL, Howes DS et al. Ann Emerg Med 1986;15:33–39.
22. Earnest MP, Feldman H, Marx JA et al. Neurology 1988;38:1561–1565.
23. Reinus WR, Wippold FJ 2nd, Erickson KK. Ann Emerg Med 1993;22:1298–1303.
24. Henneman PL, DeRoos F, Lewis RJ. Ann Emerg Med 1994;24:1108–1114.
25. Bradford JC, Kyriakedes CG. Emerg Med Clin North Am 1999;17:203–220.
26. Shinnar S, O'Dell C, Mitnick R et al. Epilepsy Res 2001;43:261–269.
27. King MA, Newton MR, Jackson GD et al. Lancet 1998;352:1007–1011; comments 1855–1857.
28. Hirtz D, Ashwal S, Berg A et al. Neurology 2000;55:616–623.
29. Maytal J, Krauss JM, Novak G et al. Epilepsia 2000;41:950–954.
30. Hopkins A, Garman A, Clarke C. Lancet 1988;1: 721–726.
31. Schoenenberger RA, Heim SM. Br Med J 1994;309:986–989.
32. Garvey MA, Gaillard WD, Rusin JA et al. J Pediatr 1998;133:664–669.
33. Harvey AS, Berkovic SF, Wrennall JA et al. Neurology 1997;49:960–968.
34. Kramer U, Nevo Y, Reider-Groswasser I et al. Seizure 1998;7:115–118.
35. Berg A, Testa FM, Levy SR et al. Pediatrics 2000;106:527–532.

36. Lee DH, Gao F-Q, Rogers JM et al. AJNR Am J Neuroradiol 1998;19:19–27.
37. Sinclair DB, Wheatley M, Aronyk K et al. Pediatr Neurosurg 2001;35:239–246.
38. Spencer SS. Epilepsia 1994;35(suppl):S72–S89.
39. Moore KR, Swallow CE, Tsuruda JS. AJNR Am J Neuroradiol 1999;20:1609–1612.
40. Jack CR Jr, Sharbrough FW, Twomey CK et al. Radiology 1990;175:423–429.
41. Watson C, Cendes F, Fuerst D et al. Arch Neurol 1997;54:67–73.
42. Oppenheim C, Dormont D, Biondi A et al. AJNR Am J Neuroradiol 1998;19:457–463.
43. Jack CR Jr, Rydberg CH, Krecke KN et al. Radiology 1996;1996:367–373.
44. Berkovic SF, McIntosh AM, Kalnins RM et al. Neurology 1995;45:1358–1363.
45. Devous MD Sr, Thisted RA, Morgan GF et al. J Nucl Med 1998;39:285–293.
46. Newton MR, Berkovic SF, Austin MC et al. J Neurol Neurosurg Psychiatry 1995;59:26–30.
47. Lewis PJ, Siegel A, Siegel AM et al. J Nucl Med 2000;41:1619–1626.
48. Park S-W, Chang K-H, Kim H-D et al. AJNR Am J Neuroradiol 2001;22:625–631.
49. Woermann FG, Jokeit H, Luerding R et al. Neurology 2003;61:699–701.
50. Gaillard WD, Balsamo L, Xu B et al. Neurology 2002;59:256–265.
51. Medina LS, Bernal B, Dunoyer C et al. Radiology 2005;236:247–253.
52. Medina LS, Aguirre E, Bernal B, Altman NR. Radiology 2004;230:49–54.

15

Adults and Children with Headaches: Evidence-Based Role of Neuroimaging

L. Santiago Medina and Elza Vasconcellos

Issues

I. Which adults with new-onset headache should undergo neuroimaging?
II. What neuroimaging approach is most appropriate in high risk adults with new-onset of headache?
III. What is the role of neuroimaging in adults with migraine or chronic headaches?
IV. What is the recommended neuroimaging examination in adults with headache and known primary neoplasm suspected of having brain metastases?
V. When is neuroimaging appropriate in children with headache?
VI. What is the sensitivity and specificity of CT and MR imaging for space occupying lesions?
VII. What is the sensitivity and specificity of CT and MRI of imaging in patients with headache and subarachnoid hemorrhage suspected of having an intracranial aneurysm?
VIII. What is the role of advance imaging techniques in primary headache disorders?
IX. What is the cost-effectiveness of neuroimaging in patients with headache?

Issues

Key Points

- CT imaging remains the initial test of choice for: (1) new-onset of headache in high risk adults and (2) headache suggestive of subarachnoid hemorrhage (limited evidence).
- Neuroimaging is recommended in adults with nonacute headache and unexplained abnormal neurologic examination (moderate evidence).

L.S. Medina (✉)
Department of Radiology, Miami Children's Hospital, 3100 SW 62 Ave, Miami, FL 33155, USA
e-mail: smedina@post.harvard.edu

L.S. Medina et al. (eds.), *Evidence-Based Imaging: Improving the Quality of Imaging in Patient Care, Revised Edition,*
DOI 10.1007/978-1-4419-7777-9_15, © Springer Science+Business Media, LLC 2011

- In adults with headache and known primary neoplasm suspected of having brain metastatic disease, MR imaging with contrast is the neuroimaging study of choice (moderate evidence).
- Although most headaches in children are benign in nature, a small percentage is caused by serious diseases, such as brain neoplasm.
- Neuroimaging is recommended in children with headache and an abnormal neurologic examination or seizures (moderate evidence).
- Sensitivity and specificity of MR imaging are greater than CT for intracranial lesions. For intracranial surgical space-occupying lesions, however, there is no difference in diagnostic performance between MR imaging and CT (limited evidence).
- Conventional CT Angiography (CTA) and MR Angiography (MRA) have sensitivities greater than 85% for aneurysms greater than 5 mm. Multidetector CT (MDCT) sensitivity and specificity is greater than 90% for aneurysms greater than 4 mm (moderate evidence).
- MDCTA and Digital subtraction angiography (DSA) have similar sensitivities and specificities for aneurysms >4 mm (moderate evidence).
- Advance brain imaging may help differentiate the different types of primary headache disorders. Preliminary MRI studies in patients with migraine have demonstrated increased iron levels and increased fMRI activation in the midbrain. Positron emission tomography (PET) has demonstrated increase uptake in the hypothalamus and phosphorus MR Spectroscopy (MRS) has revealed mitochondrial dysfunction in those with cluster headaches (limited evidence).

Definition and Pathophysiology

Headaches can be divided into primary and secondary (Table 15.1). Primary causes include migraine, cluster, and tension-type headaches, while secondary etiologies include neoplasms, arteriovenous malformations, aneurysm, infection, trauma, and hydrocephalus. Diagnosis of primary headache disorders is based on clinical criteria as set forth by the International Headache Society (1). A detailed history and physical examination help distinguish between primary and secondary headaches. Neuroimaging should aid in the diagnosis of secondary headache disorders.

Secondary headaches in children are more likely to present as acute headache, sudden onset in an otherwise healthy child, or as a chronic progressive headache, with gradual increase in frequency and severity. Acute recurrent headaches in an otherwise healthy child most often represent migraine or episodic tension-type headaches (2). Sinus disease is a common cause of acute headache. See separate Sinus Disease Chapter.

Epidemiology

Adults

Headache is a very common symptom among adults, accounting for 18 million (4%) of the total outpatient visits in the United States each year (3). In any given year, more than 70% of the US population has a headache (4). An estimated 23.6 million people in the US have migraine headaches (5, 6).

In the elderly population, 15% of patients 65 years or older versus 1–2% of patients younger than 65 years presented with secondary headache disorders such as neoplasms, strokes and temporal arteritis (5, 7). Brain metastases are the most common intracranial tumors, far outnumbering primary brain neoplasms (8). Approximately 58% of primary brain neoplasms in adults are malignant (8). Common primary malignant neoplasms include astrocytomas and glioblastomas (8). Benign brain tumors account for 38% of primary brain neoplasm (8). Despite their "benign" name they may have aggressive characteristics causing significant morbidity and mortality (8). Meningioma is the most common type (8).

Children

Pediatric headache is a common health problem in children, with a significant headache reported in more than 75% by the age of 15 years (9). In approximately 50% of patients with migraines, the headache disorder starts before the age of 20 years (5). In the US, adolescent boys and girls have a headache prevalence of 56 and 74%, and a migraine prevalence of 3.8 and 6.6%, respectively (3). A small percentage of headaches in children are secondary in nature. A primary concern in children with headache is the possibility of a brain tumor (10, 11). Although brain tumors constitute the largest group of solid neoplasms in children and are second only to leukemia in overall frequency of childhood cancers, the annual incidence is low at 3 in 100,000 (11). Primary brain neoplasms are far more prevalent in children than they are in adults (12). They account for almost 20% of all cancers in children but only 1% of cancers in adults (5). Central nervous system (CNS) tumors are the second cause of cancer-related deaths in patients younger than 15 years (13).

Overall Cost to Society

Headache is the most common and one of the most disabling type of chronic pain among children and adolescent (14, 15). The incidence of migraine peaks in adolescence, but the prevalence of migraine continues to increase and is highest in the most productive years of life between the ages of 25 and 55 years (16, 17). The direct and indirect annual cost of migraine in the USA has been estimated at more than $5.6 billion (18). A recent US study showed that migraine families incur far higher direct and indirect healthcare costs (70% higher than non-migraine families) with most of the difference concentrated in outpatient costs (19). Of interest, in families that the sole migraineur was a child versus a parent the total healthcare costs per family were about $600 higher and almost $2,500 higher when both a parent and child were affected (19). Work absence days, short-term

disability, and workman's compensation days all were higher among migraine families than among families without a migraineur (19).

Goals

- To diagnose the secondary causes of headache (Table 15.1) so that appropriate treatment can be instituted.
- Exclude secondary etiologies of headache in patients with atypical primary headache disorders.
- Decrease the risk of brain herniation prior to lumbar puncture by excluding intracranial space occupying lesions.
- Differentiate between the types of primary headache disorders using advanced imaging techniques.

Methodology

MEDLINE search using Ovid (Wolters Kluwer US Corporation, New York, NY) and PubMed (National Library of Medicine, Bethesda, MD) was used. Systematic literature review was performed from 1966 through January 2009. Keywords included: (1) headache, (2) cephalgia, (3) diagnostic imaging, (4) clinical examination (5) practice guidelines and (6) surgery. The Cochrane Collaboration had no reviews of imaging for headache.

I. Which Adults with New-Onset Headache Should Undergo Neuroimaging?

Summary of Evidence: The most common causes of secondary headache in adults are brain neoplasms, aneurysms, arteriovenous malformations, intracranial infections, and sinus disease. Several history and physical examination findings may increase the yield of the diagnostic study discovering an intracranial space-occupying lesion in adults. Table 15.2 shows the scenarios that should warrant further diagnostic testing (limited evidence) (3, 5, 20).

The factors outlined in Table 15.2 increase the pretest probability of finding a secondary headache disorder.

II. What Neuroimaging Approach Is Most Appropriate in High Risk Adults with New-Onset of Headache?

Summary of Evidence: The data reviewed demonstrate that 11–21% of patients presenting with new-onset headache have serious intracranial pathology (moderate and limited evidence) (5, 21–25). CT examination studies have been the standard of care for the initial evaluation of new-onset headache because CT is faster, more readily available, less costly than MR imaging, and less invasive than lumbar puncture (5). In addition, CT has a higher sensitivity than MR imaging for subarachnoid hemorrhage (SAH) (21, 22). Unless further data becomes available that demonstrate higher sensitivity of MR imaging, CT study is recommended in the assessment of all patients who present with new-onset headache (limited evidence) (5). Lumbar puncture is recommended in those patients in which the CT scan is nondiagnostic and the clinical evaluation reveals abnormal neurologic findings, or in those patients in whom SAH is strongly suspected (limited evidence) (5). Figure 15.1 shows a suggested decision tree to evaluate adult patients with new-onset headache.

Supporting Evidence: Duarte and colleagues (23) studied 100 consecutive patients over a 1-year period (moderate evidence): Inclusion criteria included patients admitted to the neurology unit with recent onset of headache. Recent onset of headache was defined by the authors as persistent headache of less than 1 year's duration. All the patients studied had an unenhanced and enhanced CT. Lumbar puncture, MR imaging, and MR angiogram were performed in selected cases. Tumors were identified in 21% of the patients, which comprised 16% of the patients with a negative neurologic examination.

A smaller-scale prospective study examined the association of acute headache and SAH (limited evidence) (24). All patients were examined using state-of-the art-CT. Patients had a mean headache duration of approximately 72 h

(24). Of the 27 patients studied, 20 had a negative CT and four were diagnosed with SAH. Among the remaining three patients, one had a frontal meningioma, another had a hematoma associated with SAH, and the other had diffuse meningeal enhancement caused by bacterial meningitis. Lumbar puncture was performed in 19 of the patients with negative CT, yielding five additional cases of SAH. Hence, CT did not demonstrate SAH in 5 of 9 patients.

A retrospective study of 1,111 patients with acute headache who had CT evaluation revealed 120 (10.8%) abnormalities, including hemorrhage, infarct, or neoplasm (limited evidence) (25). All imaging studies were done at two teaching institutions over a 3-year period. There were statistical differences in the percentage of intracranial lesions based on the setting in which the CT was ordered. The inpatient rate (21.2%) was twice that of emergency patients (11.7%) and three times more than for outpatients (6.9%; $P < 0.005$). Of 155 CT studies performed for headache as the sole presenting symptom (13.9%), nine (5.8%) patients had acute intracranial abnormalities. One study in the outpatient setting that studied 1,284 patients with new headaches found no serious intracranial disease (limited evidence) (7). The difference in prevalence of disease between emergency patients, inpatients, and outpatients is probably related to patient selection bias.

III. What Is the Role of Neuroimaging in Adults with Migraine or Chronic Headaches?

Summary of Evidence: Most of the available literature (moderate and limited evidence) suggests that there is no need for neuroimaging in patients with migraine and normal neurologic examination. Neuroimaging is indicated in patients with nonacute headache and unexplained abnormal neurologic examination; or in patients with atypical features or headache that does not fulfill the definition of migraine.

Supporting Evidence: Evidence-based guidelines on the use of diagnostic imaging in patients presenting with migraine have been developed by a multispecialty group called the US Headache Consortium (26). Data were examined from 28 studies (moderate and limited evidence); six not blinded prospective and 22 retrospective studies. The specific recommendations from the US Headache Consortium were:

(1) Neuroimaging should be considered in patients with nonacute headache and unexplained abnormal findings on the neurologic examination; (2) Neuroimaging is not usually warranted in patients with migraine and normal findings on neurologic examination; (3) A lower threshold for CT or MRI may be applicable in patients with atypical features or with headache that do not fulfill the definition of migraine.

The study by Joseph and colleagues (limited evidence) (27) in 48 headache patients revealed five patients with neoplasms and one patient with an arteriovenous malformation. Of these patients, five had physical examination signs and one had headache on exertion. Weingarten and colleagues (limited evidence) (28) extrapolated data from 100,800 adult patients enrolled in a health maintenance organization and estimated that, in patients with chronic headache and a normal neurologic examination, the chance of finding abnormalities on CT requiring neurosurgical intervention were as low as 0.01% (1 in 10,000).

In 1994, the American Academy of Neurology provided a summary statement on the use of neuroimaging in patients with headache and a normal neurologic examination based on a review of the literature (moderate and limited evidence) (29). They concluded that routine imaging "in adult patients with recurrent headaches that have been defined as migraine – including those with visual aura – with no recent change in pattern, no history of seizures, and no other focal neurologic signs of symptoms. is not warranted" (5). This statement was based on a 1994 literature review by Frishberg (30) of 17 articles published between 1974 and 1991 that were limited to studies with more than 17 subjects per study (moderate evidence). All patients had normal neurologic examinations. Of 897 CT or MR imaging studies performed in patients with migraine, only three tumors and one arteriovenous malformation were noted, resulting in a yield of 0.4% (4 in 1,000). The summary statements mention, however, that "patients with atypical headache patterns, a history of seizure, or focal neurological signs or symptoms, CT or MRI may be indicated" (5, 29).

IV. What Is the Recommended Neuroimaging Examination in Adults with Headache and Known Primary Neoplasm Suspected of Having Brain Metastases?

Summary of Evidence: In patients older than 40 years, with known primary neoplasm, brain metastasis is a common cause of headache (31). Most studies described in the literature suggest that contrast-enhanced MR imaging is superior to contrast-enhanced CT in the detection of brain metastatic disease, especially if the lesions are less than 2 cm (moderate evidence). In patients with suspected metastases to the CNS, enhanced brain MR imaging is recommended.

Supporting Evidence: Davis and colleagues (moderate evidence) (32) studied comparative imaging studies in 23 patients comparing contrast-enhanced MR with double dose-delayed CT. Contrast-enhanced MR imaging demonstrated more than 67 definite or typical brain metastases. The double dose-delayed CT revealed only 37 metastatic lesions. The authors concluded that MR imaging with enhancement is superior to double dose-delayed CT scan for detecting brain metastasis, anatomic localization, and number of lesions.

Golfieri and colleagues (33) reported similar findings (moderate evidence). They studied 44 patients with small cell carcinoma to detect cerebral metastases. All patients were studied with contrast-enhanced CT scan and gadolinium-enhanced MR imaging. Of all patients, 43% had cerebral metastases. Both contrast-enhanced CT and gadolinium-enhanced MR imaging detected lesions greater than 2 cm. For lesions less than 2 cm, 9% were detected only by gadolinium-enhanced T1-weighted images. The authors concluded that gadolinium-enhanced T1-weighted images remain the most accurate technique in the assessment of cerebral metastases. Sze and colleagues (34) performed prospective and retrospective studies in 75 patients (moderate evidence). In 49 patients, MR imaging and contrast-enhanced CT were equivalent. In 26 patients, however, results were discordant, with neither CT nor MR imaging being consistently superior. MR imaging demonstrated more metastases in 9 of these 26 patients. Contrast-enhanced CT, however, better depicted lesions in 8 of 26 patients.

V. When Is Neuroimaging Appropriate in Children with Headache?

Summary of Evidence: Determination of the appropriateness of imaging is made based on the frequency, pattern, family history, and associated seizure or neurological findings (Table 15.3) (moderate evidence). These guidelines reinforce the primary importance of careful acquisition of the medical history and performance of a thorough examination, including a detailed neurologic examination (35). Among children at risk for brain lesions based on these signs and symptoms, neuroimaging with either MR imaging or CT is valuable in combination with close clinical follow up (Fig. 15.2).

Supporting Evidence: In 2002, the American Academy of Neurology and Child Neurology Society published evidence-based neuroimaging recommendations for children (36). Six studies (one prospective and five retrospective) met inclusion criteria (moderate evidence). Data on 605 of 1,275 children with recurrent headache who underwent neuroimaging found only 14 (2.3%) with nervous system lesions that required surgical treatment. All 14 children had definite abnormalities on neurologic examination. The recommendations from this study were as follows: (1) Neuroimaging should be considered in children with an abnormal neurologic examination or other physical findings that suggest CNS disease. Variables that predicted the presence of a space-occupying lesion included (a) headache of less than 1-month duration; (b) absence of family history of migraine; (c) gait abnormalities; and (d) occurrence of seizures; (2) Neuroimaging is not indicated in children with recurrent headaches and a normal neurologic examination; (3) Neuroimaging should be considered in children with recent onset of severe headache, change in the type of headache, or if there are associated features suggestive of neurologic dysfunction.

Medina and colleagues (35) performed a 4-year retrospective study of 315 children with no known underlying CNS disease who underwent brain imaging for a chief complaint of headache (moderate evidence). All patients underwent brain MR imaging; 69 patients also underwent brain CT. Clinical data were correlated with findings from MR imaging and CT, and the final diagnosis, using logistic regression. Thirteen (4%) of patients had surgical space-occupying lesions, including nine malignant neoplasms, three hemorrhagic vascular malformations, and one arachnoid cyst.

In this study, they identified seven independent multivariate predictors of a surgical lesion, the strongest of which were sleep-related headache (odds ratio 5.4, 95% CI: 1.7–17.5) and no family history of migraine (odds ratio 15.4, 95% CI: 5.8–41.0). Other predictors included vomiting, absence of visual symptoms, headache of less than 6 months' duration, confusion, and abnormal neurologic examination findings. The risk of surgical lesion increased with the increased number of these seven factors ($P < 0.0001$). No difference between MR imaging and CT was noted in detection of surgical space-occupying lesions, and there were no false-positive or false-negative surgical lesions detected with either modality on clinical follow-up.

In a study by Schwedt and colleagues of 241 pediatric patients with headache who had MRI or CT, 23 patients (9.5%) had findings requiring a change in management (37) (limited to moderate evidence). These included five sinus disease, four tumors, four old infarcts, three Chiari I, two Moyamoya, one intracranial vascular stenosis, one internal jugular vein occlusion, one arteriovenous malformation, one demyelinating disease, and one intracerebral hemorrhage. When sinus disease was excluded, three patients (1.2%) had normal neurologic symptoms and signs, and imaging findings that resulted in a change in management (limited to moderate evidence).

VI. What Is the Sensitivity and Specificity of CT and MR Imaging for Space Occupying Lesions?

Summary of Evidence: Sensitivity and specificity of MR imaging is greater than CT for intracranial lesions. For surgical intracranial space-occupying lesions, however, there is no difference between MR imaging and CT in diagnostic performance (moderate evidence). The use of intravenous contrast material after unenhanced CT of the brain in children did not change the diagnosis frequently (moderate evidence).

Supporting Evidence: Sensitivity and specificity of CT and MR imaging for intracranial lesions is shown in Table 15.4. Medina and colleagues (moderate evidence) (35) showed that the overall sensitivity and specificity with MR imaging (92 and 99%, respectively) were higher than with CT (81 and 92%, respectively). Comparison of patients who underwent both MR imaging and CT revealed no significant disagreement between the tests for surgical space-occupying lesions (McNemar test, $P = 0.75$). The US Headache Consortium evidence-based guidelines from systematic review of the literature similarly concluded that MR imaging may be more sensitive than CT in identifying clinically insignificant abnormalities, but MRI imaging may be no more sensitive than CT in identifying clinically significant pathology (26).

Recent study by Branson et al. in 353 children studied with unenhanced and enhanced CT demonstrated that unenhanced CT of developing brains has high sensitivity and specificity in the diagnosis of pathologic findings (38). Sensitivity, specificity, positive predictive value, and negative predictive value for unenhanced scans were 97, 89, 87, and 97%, respectively (38). The use of contrast material led to a change in the original normal or equivocal diagnosis to an abnormal diagnosis for only five (2.7%) of the 183 normal unenhanced scans. Therefore, the use of intravenous contrast material after unenhanced CT of the brain in children did not change the diagnosis frequently (38).

VII. What Is the Sensitivity and Specificity of CT and MRI of Imaging in Patients with Headache and Subarachnoid Hemorrhage Suspected of Having an Intracranial Aneurysm?

Summary of Evidence: In North America, 80–90% of nontraumatic SAH in older children and adults is caused by the rupture of nontraumatic cerebral aneurysms (39). CTA and MRA have sensitivities greater than 85% for aneurysms greater than 5 mm. Most recent studies with newer generations of multidetector CT, report sensitivity and specificity greater than 90% for aneurysms greater than 4 mm (Moderate Evidence). Studies that have compared sensitivity and specificity of CTA and DSA report similar sensitivities and specificities (moderate evidence). The sensitivity of CTA and MRA examinations drops significantly for aneurysms less than 5 mm.

Supporting Evidence: White et al. (40) searched the literature from 1988 through 1998 to find studies with ten or more subjects in which the conventional angiography results were compared with noninvasive imaging. They included 38 studies, which scored more than 50% on evaluation criteria by using intrinsically weighted standardized assessment to determine suitability for inclusion (moderate evidence). The rates of aneurysm accuracy for CTA and MRA were 89 and 90%, respectively. The study showed greater sensitivity for aneurysms larger than 3 mm than for aneurysms 3 mm or smaller for CTA (96 versus 61%) and for MRA (94 versus 38%).

White et al. (41) also performed a prospective blinded study in 142 patients who underwent intra-arterial DSA to detect aneurysms (moderate evidence). Results were compared with CTA and MRA. The accuracy rates per patient for the best observer were 87 and 85% for CTA and MRA, respectively. The accuracy rates for brain aneurysm for the best observer were 73 and 67% for CTA and MRA, respectively. The sensitivity for the detection of aneurysms 5 mm or larger was 94% for CTA and 86% for MRA. For aneurysms smaller than 5 mm, sensitivities for CTA and MRA were 57 and 35% respectively.

More recent studies using CTA have shown even higher sensitivity and specificity, which may reflect technological improvements. Uysal and colleagues using spiral CT in 32 cases with aneurysm size from 3 to 13 mm (42) reported sensitivity of 97 and specificity of 100% (limited evidence). Teksam and colleagues studied 100 consecutive patients with 113 aneurysm with MDCT (43), and reported sensitivity for detecting aneurysms of less than 4 mm, 4–10 mm, and greater than 10 mm on a per aneurysm basis of 84, 97 and 100%, respectively (moderate evidence). Overall specificity was 88%. Karamessini and colleagues using CTA with three-dimensional techniques in 82 consecutive patients (44), demonstrated sensitivity of 89% and specificity of 100% for CTA, and sensitivity of 88% and specificity of 98% of DSA when compared with the reference standard of surgical findings (Moderate Evidence). Therefore, CTA was equivalent to DSA. Tipper and colleagues with 16-row MDCT in 57 patients with 53 aneurysms (45), reported sensitivity and specificity of 96.2 and 100% for both CTA and DSA, respectively (moderate evidence). In this study, mean diameter of the aneurysm was 6.3 mm with a range of 1.9–28.1 mm (25). Study published by Taschner and colleagues (46) in 2007 in 27 consecutive patients with 24 aneurysms using a 16-row multisection CTA reported an overall sensitivity and specificity of 100 and 83%, respectively (limited evidence) . Study by Papke and colleagues comparing DSA with 16-row CTA in 87 patients (47), reported sensitivity and specificity of 98 and 100% for DSA and CTA, respectively (moderate evidence). Yoon and colleagues using 16-row multidetector CTA in 85 patients (48), had overall sensitivity and specificity of 92.5 and 93.3%, respectively (moderate evidence). For aneurysm less than 3 mm, however, sensitivity decreased for reader 1 and reader 2 to 74.1 and 77.8%, respectively (Yoon). More recent study done by Lubicz and colleagues (49) in 54 consecutive patients with 67 aneurysms using a 64-row multisection CTA reported an overall sensitivity and specificity of 94 and 90.2%, respectively (moderate evidence). For aneurysms less than 3 mm, CTA had a mean sensitivity of 70.4% (49).Intertechnique and interobserver agreements were good for aneurysm detection with a mean Kappa of 0.673 (49). Agid and colleagues (50) in 73 patients with 47 aneurysms using a 64-row multisection CTA reported an overall sensitivity and specificity of 98 and 98%, respectively (moderate evidence).

VIII. What Is the Role of Advance Imaging Techniques in Primary Headache Disorders?

Summary of Evidence: High resolution MR technique using transverse relaxation rates have demonstrated increased tissue iron levels in the brainstem (periaqueductal gray [PAG], red nucleus [RN] and subtantia nigra [SN]) in patients with headache disorders (limited evidence). Functional MR has demonstrated activation of the red nuclei and substantia nigra

in patients during spontaneous migraine episodes (limited evidence) (51, 52).

In cluster headache disorders, MR phosphorus spectroscopy (31P-MRS) has demonstrated brain mitochondrial dysfunction (limited evidence) (53, 54). PET has demonstrated strong activation in the hypothalamic gray matter in acute cluster headache attacks (limited evidence) (55). In contrast to migraine disorders, there is no brainstem activation during acute cluster headache episodes compared with the resting state (56). These initial studies suggest that, although primary headaches such as migraine and cluster headache may share a common pain pathway – the trigeminovascular innervation – their underlying pathogenesis differs significantly (53).

Supporting Evidence: The underlying pathophysiology of migraine disorders is not well understood (57). Conventional CT and MRI studies are usually normal with no evidence of a structural lesion. Studies have shown involvement of the nociceptive pathways in chronic daily headache and migraine (57). Study by Raskin and colleagues (58), revealed migraine-like headache in patients with electrodes implanted in the PAG matter. The ventral brainstem has also been identified to be involved in migraine disorders (58). Reports of multiple sclerosis plaque (59), and cavernous malformation (60), involving the PAG and causing migraine-like disorders have been reported. Imaging studies have been performed to study the iron homeostasis in the midbrain. High resolution MR techniques have been used to map the transverse relaxation rates R2 (1/T2), R2* (1/T2*) and R2' (R2*-R2) in the PAG, RN and SN (61). A positive correlation ($r = 0.80$; $P < 0.006$) was identified between the duration of illness and the increase in R2' (increased tissue iron levels) for patients with episodic migraine disorders and chronic daily headaches (61, 62) (limited evidence), Another study by Kruit and colleagues (63) in patients studied in a 1.5 T MR scanner, revealed higher iron concentrations in the RN and putamen in patient with migraines (limited to moderate evidence), Functional MR has demonstrated activation of the RN and SN in patients during spontaneous migraine episodes (limited evidence) (51, 52).

In cluster headaches, in-vivo MR phosphorus spectroscopy (31P-MRS) have demonstrated brain mitochondrial dysfunction characterized by reduced phosphocreatine levels, an increased ADP concentration, and a reduced phosphorylation potential (limited evidence) (53, 54). In a study of nine patients, PET demonstrated strong activation in the hypothalamic gray matter in acute cluster headache attacks (limited evidence) (55). In contrast to migraine disorders, there is no brainstem activation during acute cluster headache episodes compared with the resting state (56). These initial studies suggest that, although primary headaches such as migraine and cluster headache may share a common pain pathway – the trigeminovascular innervation – their underlying pathogenesis differs significantly (53).

IX. What Is the Cost-Effectiveness of Neuroimaging in Patients with Headache?

Summary of Evidence: No well-designed cost-effectiveness analysis (CEA) in adults could be found in the literature. A CEA study (64) assessed the clinical and economic consequences of three diagnostic strategies in the evaluation of children with headache suspected of having a brain tumor: MR imaging, CT followed by MR imaging for positive results (CT-MR imaging), and no neuroimaging with close clinical follow-up (64). This model suggests that MR imaging maximizes quality-adjusted life years (QALY) gained at a reasonable cost-effectiveness ratio in patients at high risk of having a brain tumor. Conversely, the strategy of no imaging with close clinical follow up is cost saving in low-risk children. Although the CT-MR imaging strategy maximizes QALY gained in the intermediate-risk patients, its additional cost per QALY gained is high. In children with headache, appropriate selection of patients and diagnostic imaging strategies may maximize quality-adjusted life expectancy and decrease costs of medical workup.

Supporting Evidence: A CEA in children with headaches has been published in Pediatrics (64). A decision-analytic Markov model and CEA were performed incorporating the risk group pretest probability, MR imaging and CT

sensitivity and specificity, tumor survival, progression rates, and cost per strategy. Outcomes were based on QALY gained and incremental cost per QALY gained.

The results were as follows: For low-risk children with chronic non-migraine-headaches of more than 6 months' duration as the sole symptom (pretest probability of brain tumor, 0.01% [1 in 10,000])-close clinical observation without neuroimaging was less costly and more effective than the two neuroimaging strategies. For the intermediate-risk children with migraine headache and normal neurologic examination (pretest probability of brain tumor, 0.4% [4 in 1,000]), CT-MR imaging was the most effective strategy but cost more than $1 million per QALY gained compared with no neuroimaging. This cost is not typically justified by health policy makers. For high-risk children with headache of less than 6 months' duration and other clinical predictors of a brain tumor, such as an abnormal neurologic examination (pretest probability of brain tumor, 4% [4 in 100]), the most effective strategy was MR imaging, with a cost-effectiveness ratio of $113,800 per QALY gained compared with no imaging.

The cost-effectiveness ratio in the high-risk children with headache, is in the comparable range of annual mammography for women aged 55–64 years at $110,000 per life-year saved (65), colonoscopy for colorectal cancer screening for persons older than 40 years at $90,000 per life year-saved, (65, 66) and annual cervical cancer screening for women beginning at age 20 years at $220,000 per life-year saved (65, 67). Therefore, this CEA model supports the use of MR imaging in high risk children.

Take Home Data

Table 15.1 shows common causes of primary and secondary headache. Table 15.2 summarizes clinical guidelines in adults with new-onset headache. Table 15.3 summarizes clinical guidelines in children with headache. Table 15.4 shows the sensitivity and specificity of CT and MRI imaging. Figure 15.1 provides the decision trees for diagnostic work-up of adults with headache. Figure 15.2 provides the decision tree for diagnostic work-up of children with headache.

Imaging Case Studies

Study 1: Colloid Cyst

Patient presented with headache and vomiting (Fig. 15.3).

Study 2: Chiari I

Patient presented with persistent headaches triggered by cough or exertion (Valsalva maneuver) (Fig. 15.4).

Study 3: Brain Stem Infiltrative Glial Neoplasm

The patient presented with ataxia and headaches (Fig. 15.5).

Suggested Protocols

CT Imaging

CT Without Contrast

Axial 5–10 mm nonspiral images should be used to assess for SAH, tumor hemorrhage or calcifications. In infants and toddlers axial 2.5–5 mm sections are recommended.

CT with Contrast

Axial 5–10 mm non spiral enhanced images should be used in patients with suspected neoplasm, infection or other focal intracranial lesion. If indicated, CTA can be performed as part of the enhanced CT. Contrast enhanced CTA should ideally be done in a multidetector CT angiogram with multiplanar and 3D reconstructions.

MR Imaging

Basic Brain MR protocol sequences include Sagittal T1-weighted conventional spin-echo (repetition time, 600 ms; echo time 11 ms [600/11]), axial proton density-weighted conventional or fast spin echo (2,000/15), axial T2-weighted conventional or fast spin-echo (3,200/85), axial FLAIR (fluid attenuation inversion recovery) spin echo (8,800/152, inversion time [TI] 2,200 ms), and coronal T2-weighted fast spin-echo (3,200/85) images. In patient with suspected neoplasm, infection or focal intracranial lesions gadolinium enhanced T1-weighted conventional spin-echo (600/11) images should be acquired in at least two planes. If MR angiogram is indicated, then 3D Time of Flight study of the circle of Willis should be performed. Consideration should be given to complementing the MRA with a multiphase dynamic contrast enhanced study to reduce potential flow artifacts and to assess arterial, capillary and venous phases.

Table 15.1. Common causes of primary and secondary headache

Primary headaches   • **Migraine**   • **Cluster**   • **Tension-type**

Secondary headaches
 • **Intracranial space occupying lesions**
   – **Neoplasm**
   – **Arteriovenous malformation**
   – **Abscess**
   – **Hematoma**
 • **Cerebrovascular disease**
   – **Intracranial aneurysms**
   – **Occlusive vascular disease**
 • **Infection**
   – **Acute Sinusitis**
   – **Meningitis**
   – **Encephalitis**
 • **Inflammation**
   – **Vasculitis**
   – **Acute disseminated encephalomyelitis**
 • **Increased intracranial pressure**
   – **Hydrocephalus**
   – **Idiopathic intracranial hypertension**
     (pseudotumor cerebri)

Reprinted with kind permission of Springer Science+Business Media from Medina LA, Shah A, Vasconcellos E. Adults and children with headache: evidence-based role of neuroimaging. In Medina LS, Blackmore CC (eds.): *Evidence-Based Imaging: Optimizing Imaging in Patient Care*. New York: Springer Science+Business Media, 2006.

Table 15.2. Suggested guidelines for neuroimaging in adult patients with new-onset headache

- "First or worst" headache
- Increased frequency and increased severity of headache
- New-onset headache after age 50
- New-onset headache with history of cancer or immunodeficiency
- Headache with fever, neck stiffness, and meningeal signs
- Headache with abnormal neurologic examination

Reprinted with kind permission of Springer Science+Business Media from Medina LS, Shah A, Vasconcellos E. Adults and children with headache: evidence-based role of neuroimaging. In Medina LS, Blackmore CC (eds.): *Evidence-Based Imaging: Optimizing Imaging in Patient Care.* New York: Springer Science+Business Media, 2006.

Table 15.3. Suggested guidelines for neuroimaging in pediatric patients with headache

- Persistent headaches of less than 6 months duration.
- Headache associated with abnormal neurologic examination.
- Headache associated with seizures.
- Recent onset of severe headache or change in the type of headache.
- Persistent headache without family history of migraine.
- Headaches that persistently awakens a child from sleep or occurs immediately on awakening
- Family or medical history of disorders that may predispose one to CNS lesions, and clinical or laboratory findings that suggest CNS involvement.

Reprinted with permission of the RSNA from Medina et al. (35).

Table 15.4. Diagnostic sensitivity and specificity of CT and MRI imaging

Variable	Baseline %	Range %	References
Diagnostic tests			
MR imaging			
Sensitivity	92	82–100	(35, 68, 69)
Specificity	99	81–100	(35, 69)
CT			
Sensitivity	81	65–100	(35, 68, 69)
Specificity	92	72–100	(35, 68, 69)

Adapted with kind permission of Springer Science+Business Media from Medina LS, Shah A, Vasconcellos E. Adults and children with headache: evidence-based role of neuroimaging. In Medina LS, Blackmore CC (eds.): *Evidence-Based Imaging: Optimizing Imaging in Patient Care.* New York: Springer Science+Business Media, 2006.

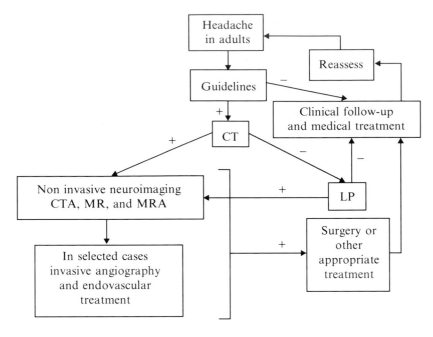

Figure 15.1. Decision tree for use in adults with new-onset headache. For those patients who meet any of the guidelines in Table 15.2, CT is suggested. For patients who do not meet these criteria or those with negative workup, clinical observation with periodic reassessment is recommended. If CT is positive, further workup with CT angiography or MR imaging plus MR angiography is recommended. In selected case, conventional angiography and endovascular treatment may be warranted. If CT is negative, lumbar puncture is advised. In patients with suspected metastatic brain disease, contrast-enhanced MR imaging is recommended. In patients with suspected intracranial aneurysm, further assessment with CT angiography or MR angiography is warranted. *CTA* CT angiography, *LP* lumbar puncture, *MRA* MR angiography, *MRI* MR imaging. (Source: Medina et al. (31), with permission from Elsevier.)

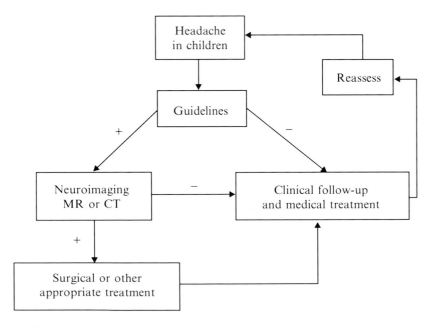

Figure 15.2. Decision tree for use in children with headache disorder. Neuroimaging is suggested for patients who meet any of the signs or symptoms in the guidelines (Table 15.3). For patients who do not meet these criteria or those with negative findings from imaging studies, clinical observation with periodic reassessment is recommended. (Source: Medina et al. (35), with permission from the Radiological Society of North America.)

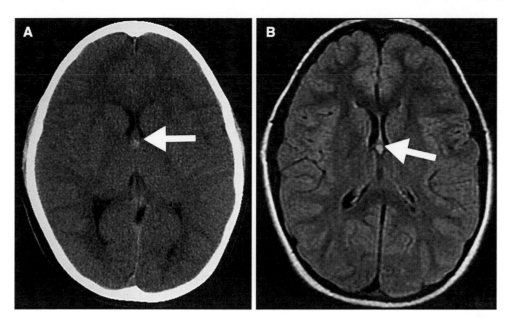

Figure 15.3. (**A**) Unenhanced CT shows a small focal lesion with increased density at the level of the foramen of Monro. (**B**) Axial Flair sequence reveals increased T2-weighted signal in the lesion. No hydrocephalus noted. Neuroimaging findings consistent with colloid cyst. (Reprinted with kind permission of Springer Science+Business Media from Medina LA, Shah A, Vasconcellos E. Adults and children with headache: evidence-based role of neuroimaging. In Medina LS, Blackmore CC (eds.): *Evidence-Based Imaging: Optimizing Imaging in Patient Care.* New York: Springer Science+Business Media, 2006.)

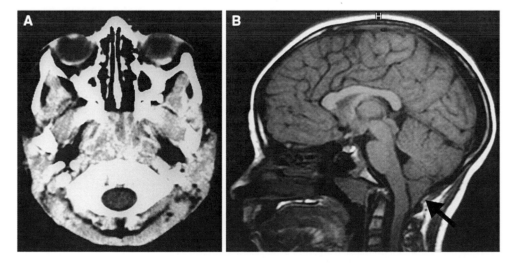

Figure 15.4. (**A**) Unenhanced CT at craniocervical junction was interpreted as unremarkable. (**B**) Sagittal MRI T1-weighted image reveals pointed cerebellar tonsils extending more than 5 mm below the foramen magnum consistent with Chiari I. No cervical cord hydrosyrinx noted. (Reprinted with kind permission of Springer Science+Business Media from Medina LA, Shah A, Vasconcellos E. Adults and children with headache: evidence-based role of neuroimaging. In Medina LS, Blackmore CC (eds.): *Evidence-Based Imaging: Optimizing Imaging in Patient Care.* New York: Springer Science+Business Media, 2006.)

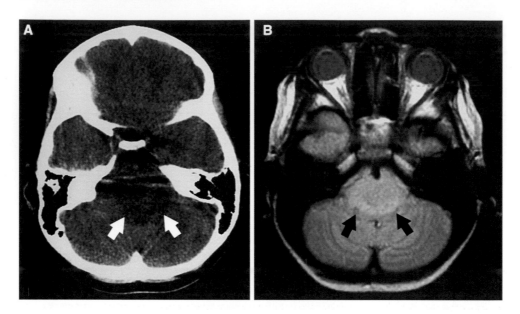

Figure 15.5. (**A**) Unenhanced CT through posterior fossa is limited by beam hardening artifact. A hypo-dense lesion is seen in the pons. (**B**) Axial proton density MR image better depicts the anatomy and extent of the lesion without artifact. (Reprinted with kind permission of Springer Science+Business Media from Medina LA, Shah A, Vasconcellos E. Adults and children with headache: evidence-based role of neuroimaging. In Medina LS, Blackmore CC (eds.): *Evidence-Based Imaging: Optimizing Imaging in Patient Care*. New York: Springer Science+Business Media, 2006.)

Future Research

- Large scale prospective studies to validate risk factors and prediction rules of significant intracranial lesions in children and adults with headache.
- Large diagnostic performance studies comparing the sensitivity, specificity and ROC curves of neuroimaging in adults and children with headache.
- CEA of neuroimaging in adults with headaches.

References

1. Headache Classification Subcommittee of the International Headache Society. Cephalalgia 2004;24(suppl 1):1–160.
2. Rothner AS. Pediatr Neurol 1995;2:109–118.
3. Linet MS, Stewart WF, Celentano DD et al. JAMA 1989;261:2211–2216.
4. Silberstein SD. Headache 1992;32:396–407.
5. Field AG, Wang E. Emerg Clin North Am 1999;17:127–152.
6. Stewart WF, Lipton RB, Celentano DD et al. JAMA 1992;267:64–69.
7. Hale WE, May FE, Marks RG et al. Headache 1987;27:272–276.
8. Hutter A, Schwetye K, Bierhals A, McKinstry RC. Clin N Am 2003;13:237–250.
9. Bille BS. Acta Paediatr 1962;51(suppl 136):1–151.
10. Honig PJ, Charney EB. Am J Dis Child 1982;136:121–124.
11. The Childhood Brain Tumor Consortium. J Neurooncol 1991;10:31–46.
12. Rorke L, Schut L. In McLaurin RL (ed.): Pediatric Neurosurgery, 2nd ed. Philadelphia: WB Saunders, 1989;335–337.
13. Silverberg E, Lubera J. Cancer 1986;36:9–23.
14. Roth-Isigkeit A, Thyen U, Stöven H, Schwarzenberger J, Schmucker P. Pediatrics 2005;115:e152–e162.
15. Peterson CC, Palermo DM. J Pediatr Psychol 2004;29:331–341.
16. Pryse-Phillips W, Findlay H, Tugwell P et al. Can J Neurol Sci 1992;19:333–339.
17. Lipton RB, Stewart WF. Neurology 1993;43:S6–S10.
18. de Lissovoy G, Lazarus SS. Neurology 1994;44(suppl):S56–S62.
19. Stang PE, Crown WH, Bizier R, Chatterton ML, White R. Am J Manag Care 2004;10:313–320.

20. Evans RW. Med Clin North Am 2001;85: 865–885.
21. Prager JM, Mikulis DJ. Med Clin North Am 1991;75:525–544.
22. Edelman RR, Warach S. N Engl J Med 1993;328:708–715.
23. Duarte J, Sempere AP, Delgado JA et al. Acta Neurol Scand 1996;94:67–70.
24. Lledo A, Calandre L, Martinez-menendez B et al. Headache 1994;34:172–174.
25. Kahn CEJ, Sanders GD, Lyons EA et al. Can Assoc Radiol J 1993;44:189–193.
26. Morey SS. Am Fam Physician 2000;62: 1699–1701.
27. Joseph R, Cook GE, Steiner TJ et al. Practitioner 1985;229:477–481.
28. Weingarten S, Kleinman M, Elperin L et al. Arch Intern Med 1992;152:2457–2462.
29. Quality Standards Subcommittee of the American Academy of Neurology. Neurology 1994;44: 1353–1354.
30. Frishberg BM. Neurology 1994;44:1191–1197.
31. Medina LS, D'Souza B, Vasconcellos E. Neuroimag Clin N Am 2003;13:225–235.
32. Davis PA, Hudgins PA, Peterman SB et al. AJNR Am J Neuroradiol 1991;12:293–300.
33. Golfieri R, Cherryman GR, Oliff JF et al. Radiol Med (Torino) 1991;82:27–34.
34. Sze G, Shin J, Krol G et al. Radiology 1988;168: 187–194.
35. Medina LS, Pinter JD, Zurakowski D et al. Radiology 1997;202:819–824.
36. Lewis D, Ashwal S, Dahl G et al. Neurology 2002;51:490–498.
37. Schwedt TJ, Guo Y, Rothner AD. Headache 2006;46(3):387–398.
38. Branson HM, Doria AS, Moineddin R, Shroff M. Radiology 2007;244:838–844.
39. Gentry LR, Gordersky JC, Thopson BH. Radiology 1989;171:177–187.
40. White PM, Wardlaw JM, Easton V. Radiology 2000;217:361–370.
41. White PM, Teasdale EM, Wardlaw JM et al. Radiology 2001;219:739–749.
42. Uysal E, Yanbuloglu B, Erturk M, Kilinc BM, Basak M. Diagn Interv Radiol 2005;11(2):77–82.
43. Teksam M, McKinney A, Asis M et al. AJNR Am J Neuroradiol 2004;25(9):1485–1492.
44. Karamessini MT, Kagadis GC, Petsas T et al. Eur J Radiol 2004;49(3):212–223.
45. Tipper G, U-King-Im JM, Price SJ, Trivedi RA et al. Clin Radiol 2005;60(5):565–572.
46. Taschner CA, Thines L, Lernout M et al. J Neuroradiol 2007;34(4):243–249.
47. Papke K, Kuhl CK, Fruth M et al. Radiology 2007;244(2):532–540.
48. Yoon DY, Lim KJ, Choi CS, Cho BM, Oh SM, Chang SK. AJNR Am J Neuroradiol 2007;28(1):60–67.
49. Lubicz B, Levivier M, Francois O et al. Am J Neuroradiol 2007;28(10):1949–1955.
50. Agid R, Lee SK, Willinsky RA, Farb RI, terBrugge KG. Neuroradiology 2006;48(11):787–794.
51. Welch KMA, Cao Y, Aurora SK et al. Neurology 1998;51:1465–1469.
52. Cao Y, Aurora SK, Vikingstad EM et al. Neurology 2002;59:72–78.
53. May A, Goadsby PJ. Curr Opin Neurol 1998; 11(3):199–203.
54. Montagna P, Lodi R, Cortelli P. Neurology 1997;48:113–118.
55. May A, Bahra A, Buchel C, Frackowiak RSJ, Goadsby PJ. Lancet 1998;351:275–278.
56. Weiller C, May A, Limmroth V, Juptner M, Kaube H, van Schayck R. Nat Med 1995;1:658–660.
57. Aurora SK. Curr Pain Headache Rep 2003;7: 209–211.
58. Raskin NH, Hosobuchi Y, Lamb S. Headache 1987;27:416–420.
59. Haas DC, Kent PF, Friedman DI. Headache 1993; 33:452–455.
60. Goadsby PJ. Cephalgia 2002;22:107–111.
61. Gelman N, Gorell JM, Barker PB et al. Radiology 1999;210:759–767.
62. Welch KMA, Nagesh V, Aurora SK, Gelman N. Headache 2001;41:629–637.
63. Kruit MC, van Buchem MA, Overbosch J et al. Cephalgia 2002;22:571.
64. Medina LS, Kuntz KM, Pomeroy SL. Pediatrics 2001;108:255–263.
65. Tengs T, Adams M, Pliskin J et al. Risk Anal 1995;15:369–390.
66. England W, Halls J, Hunt V. Med Decis Making 1989;9:3–13.
67. Eddy DM. Gynecol Oncol 1981;12(2 Part 2): S168–S187.
68. Haughton VM, Rimm AA, Sobocinski KA et al. Radiology 1986;160:751–755.
69. Orrison WJ, Stimac GK, Stevens EA et al. Radiology 1991;181:121–127.

16

Imaging Evaluation of Sinusitis: Impact on Health Outcome

Yoshimi Anzai

Issues

I. Is there a role for imaging in the initial diagnosis of acute bacterial sinusitis?
II. What is the diagnostic performance of sinus radiography and sinus CT in acute bacterial sinusitis? What diagnostic criteria should we use?
III. When are imaging studies indicated for the diagnosis and the management of patients with sinusitis?
IV. What is the most cost effective strategy for the diagnosis and the management of acute sinusitis?
V. What is the imaging role for patients with chronic sinusitis?
VI. Special situation: what is the role of imaging in immunocompromised patients?

Key Points

- The clinical signs and symptoms of acute bacterial sinusitis (ABS) overlap with that of nonspecific upper respiratory track viral infection (strong evidence).
- Children under the age of 6 years should not undergo sinus radiographs due to their limited sinus development (moderate evidence).
- Sinus radiographs are moderately sensitive to diagnose ABS compared with sinus puncture and culture (moderate evidence).
- Although a CT scan is frequently performed to assist diagnosis of sinusitis, no adequate data exists on the sensitivity and specificity of sinus CT for diagnosis of ABS (limited evidence).
- Definitive imaging criteria are presence of frothy air-fluid levels or complete sinus opacification, but do not include mucosal thickening (limited evidence).

Y. Anzai
Department of Radiology, University of Washington, 1959 NE Pacific Street, Seattle, WA 98195, USA
e-mail: anzai@u.washington.edu

L.S. Medina et al. (eds.), *Evidence-Based Imaging: Improving the Quality of Imaging in Patient Care, Revised Edition*,
DOI 10.1007/978-1-4419-7777-9_16, © Springer Science+Business Media, LLC 2011

- Despite relatively high sensitivity of CT or sinus radiography, imaging is not indicated in the initial diagnostic work up for acute uncomplicated sinusitis, due to cost and radiation dose (strong evidence).
- Imaging study is indicated for patients who fail to respond to medical management, or severe symptoms suspicious for complications related to acute sinusitis, or patients planning to undergo surgery (moderate evidence).
- The diagnosis of chronic sinusitis is based on clinical grounds. No gold standard exists to confirm clinical diagnosis. CT findings for chronic sinusitis often do not correlate with patients' clinical symptoms (limited evidence).
- Imaging (contrast enhanced CT or MR) is indicated in immunocompromised patients with acute progression of sinus infection with neurological symptoms in order to assess potential complications from acute sinusitis.

Definition and Pathophysiology

The term "*sinusitis*" technically refers to inflammation of the mucosal of the paranasal sinuses. Under normal circumstance, the paranasal sinuses are assumed to be sterile. However, the paranasal sinuses are continuous to nasal mucosa or nasopharynx that are heavily colonized with bacteria. These bacteria are present in low density and removed by the normal mucociliary function of the paranasal sinuses. Normal mucous secretions contain antibodies, and together with mucociliary clearance, work to clear bacterial from the paranasal sinuses. Thus, maintaining the mucociliary flow and an intact local mucosal surface are key host defenses against infection (1). Sinusitis is classified as acute, subacute, or chronic, based on the duration of the illness. Acute sinusitis refers to sinusitis symptoms lasting fewer than 4 weeks, and chronic sinusitis refers to sinusitis lasting more than 12 weeks. Subacute sinusitis falls in between these two.

The common predisposing events that set the stage for ABS is an acute viral upper respiratory infection that results in a viral rhinosinusitis (predisposes to approximately 80% of bacterial sinus infections) and allergic inflammation (that predisposes to 20% of bacterial infection). Once the mucosa of the paranasal sinuses swells due to either viral infection or allergy, it causes sinus ostia obstruction, thus interfering with normal mucociliary clearance. This leads to low pressure within the paranasal sinuses thus further exaggerate mucosal thickening and poor sinus clearance, resulting in acute bacterial sinus infection. *Streptococcus pneumoniae* and *Hemophilus influenzae* are two common organisms causing ABS. Since the widespread use of the heptavalent pneumococcal conjugate vaccine (PCV7) in 2004, pneumococcal strains have declined and thus *H. influenzae* has become a more prevalent organism (2, 3). Other organisms include *Moraxella catarrhalis*, other *Streptococcus* species, and *Staphylococcus*.

Epidemiology

Acute sinusitis is one of the most common diagnoses in primary care setting in the USA; affecting 31 million individuals diagnosed each year (4). Fourteen percent of Americans claim to have had a previous diagnosis of sinusitis (5). The prevalence of sinusitis has increased in the last decade due to increased air pollution and resistance to antibiotics. There is no gender difference in sinusitis prevalence. Sinusitis is more common in the Midwest and south of the country compared to the coasts. Acute sinusitis more often affects patients with a history of allergy or asthma. Other patients with high risk of developing acute sinusitis include individuals with defects in immunity (HIV, agammaglobulinemia), delayed or absent mucociliary activity (Kartagener's syndrome, cystic fibrosis), structural defects (cleft palate), and white blood cell functional abnormalities (chronic granulomatous disease, Wegener's granulomatosis) (6). Dental infections may cause 5–10% of all cases of maxillary sinusitis; the roots of the upper back teeth (second bicuspid, first and second molars) about the floor of the maxillary sinus.

Sinusitis affects all age groups. The prevalence of sinusitis among children is even higher than adults, and may be as high as 32% in young children (7–9). The average child has between 6 and 8 "cold" episodes annually and it is estimated that 5–10% of all upper respiratory infections are complicated by sinusitis. Children under the age of 6 years are the most likely to have ABS (10).

Acute maxillary sinusitis in adults is characterized with purulent nasal discharge, facial tenderness, headache or toothache, and fever. Children, however, may have less specific symptoms, such as a prolonged daytime cough lasting more than 10 days. The development of paranasal sinuses in children also contributes to diagnostic challenges. The maxillary and the ethmoid sinuses are present at birth. The sphenoid sinuses generally start to pneumatize by age 5 years, the frontal sinuses start to develop around age 7–8 years (10). Both frontal and sphenoid sinuses continue to develop until late adolescence. Sinus tenderness is not a typical sign observed in pediatric patients with acute sinusitis.

Diagnosis of chronic sinusitis is even more challenging. No gold standard, i.e., pathological diagnosis, exits for chronic sinusitis. Diagnostic workups and treatment is often driven by patients' symptoms.

Overall Cost to Society

Sinusitis has a significant economic impact on health care organizations. In 1992, Americans spent $200 million on prescription medications and more than $2 billion for over-the counter medications to treat sinusitis (11). There were 11 million doctor visits and 1.3 million outpatients visit due to sinusitis in 1999 (12). Approximately 500,000 sinus surgeries are performed each year. The study using data from AHCPR's 1987 National Medical Expenditure Survey (inflated to 1996 dollars) estimated overall health care expenditures attributable to sinusitis were $5.8 billion, mainly from ambulatory and emergency department services and 50,000 surgical procedures performed on paranasal sinuses (13). Approximately 31% ($1.8 billion) of the cost was attributed to treatment expenditures for children

12 years or younger (14). They concluded that sinusitis needed to be recognized as a serious, debilitating, costly disease that warrants precise diagnosis and effective specific therapy (15). This estimate of direct costs does not include indirect costs, such as expense of care of sick children, transportation costs, the value of work time lost, baby-sitting costs, ancillary medication costs, and expenditures for treatment of adverse effects. Clearly, sinusitis imposes a considerable economic burden for the patients and family. Therefore, improved diagnosis and the use of the most effective agents with the highest tolerability profile will improve outcomes and lower the overall cost of therapy.

It is important to keep in mind that the majority of "sinusitis" is caused by upper respiratory tract viral infection. The symptoms with acute viral sinusitis and allergic rhinitis overlap with that with ABS, leading to misdiagnosis. Consequently, ABS is overdiagnosed (in as many as 50–60% of cases), and therefore antibiotics are overprescribed in the primary care setting. Clinical studies showed that as many as 60% of patients with colds are prescribed antibiotics (16). The overprescription of antibiotics leads to a wide spread of antibiotic resistant infection. Antibiotic resistant infections are an increasing problem in hospitals in terms of the number of resistant organisms and their prevalence. Consequently, the costs of these infections are also increasing. Antibiotic resistance increases the costs of care in hospitals in various ways including increased length of stay, more admissions to intensive care unit, and more intensive resource use.

Goals

In patients presenting with acute sinusitis symptoms, the goal is to differentiate those with ABS who benefit from antibiotics from those with non-specific virus infection. Imaging is not indicated for the initial diagnostic workup for acute sinusitis, due to increasing cost and radiation for pediatric patients. Diagnosis and treatment decision, particularly prescribing antibiotics or not, is often made based on clinical examination for uncomplicated sinusitis.

Imaging is, however, indicated for patients who failed to respond to initial medical management. The goal of imaging at this setting is to exclude (or include) diagnosis of ABS, to assess potential causes of poor mechanical drainage of the paranasal sinuses, and complications such as orbital cellulitis or abscess formation (i.e., orbital subperiosteal abscess and anterior cranial fossa abscess).

The goal of sinus CT for chronic sinusitis is to provide objective information to support the clinical diagnosis, to provide detailed anatomy for surgical planning, and to predict which patients most benefit from endoscopic sinus surgery.

Methodology

The authors performed a MEDLINE search using PubMed (National Library of Medicine, Bethesda, MD) for data relevant to the diagnostic performance and accuracy of both clinical and radiographic examinations of patients with acute sinusitis. The diagnostic performance of clinical examination (history and physical exam) and clinical outcome was based on a systematic literature review performed in MEDLINE from January 1966 to May 2010. The clinical examination search strategy used the following statements: (1) acute rhinosinusitis, (2) ABS, (3) diagnosis, (4) clinical examination, (5) outcomes. The review of the current diagnostic imaging literature was done with MEDLINE covering from January 1966 to May 2010, the following key statements and words: (1) rhinosinusitis, (2) sinusitis, (3) radiograph, (4) CT, as well as combinations of these search strings. We excluded animal studies and non-English articles.

I. Is There a Role for Imaging in the Initial Diagnosis of Acute Bacterial Sinusitis?

Summary of Evidence: Diagnosis of acute sinusitis should be made on clinical criteria. Radiographic imaging study should not be obtained to diagnose acute sinusitis or to confirm clinical diagnosis of acute sinusitis, particularly in children who are below 6 years of age (17). Imaging as an initial diagnostic workup not only substantially increases the cost but also is potentially harmful from radiation exposure.

It is controversial if sinus radiography is needed as a confirmatory test of acute sinusitis in children older than 6 years with persistent and severe symptoms. Although sinus radiograph has lower cost and readily available, the ability to evaluate intracranial or intraorbital complications is limited. CT is a preferred imaging modality for diagositc work-ups for patients with recurrent or chronic sinusitis. The ACR (American College of Radiology) guidelines state that the diagnosis of uncomplicated acute sinusitis should be made on clinical grounds alone, and reserves the use of imaging for situations for medically refractory cases or worsening during the course of antibiotics treatment (18) (http://acsearch.acr.org/) (moderate evidence).

Supporting Evidence: Acute sinusitis is a common clinical condition. Diagnosis of acute sinusitis should be made on clinical criteria in patients who present with uncomplicated upper respiratory symptoms (strong recommendation) (13). Clinical guidelines and criteria have been developed to distinguish ABS from acute viral rhinosinusitis. For adult maxillary sinusitis, William's criteria are often used, which include: (1) maxillary toothache, (2) poor response to decongestants, (3) history of colored nasal discharge, (4) purulent nasal secretion on physical examination, and (5) abnormal transillumination result. On the other hand, Gonzales et al. reported that purulent nasal secretions alone predict neither bacterial infection nor benefit from antibiotic treatment (19). Transillumination is a useful technique in the hands of experienced personnel, but only negative findings are useful (limited evidence). The clinical diagnostic guidelines for ABS in children are (a) persistent symptoms include nasal or postnasal discharge (of any quality), daytime cough (which may be worse in night) and (b) symptoms lasting more than 10–14 days but less than 30 days (10). Severe symptoms include a temperature of at least 102°F, and purulent nasal discharge present concurrently for at least 3–4 consecutive days in a child who seems ill or toxic (10). Respiratory symptoms related to acute viral sinusitis may not have completely resolved by the tenth day, but almost always have peaked in severity and begun to improve. Therefore, persistence of respiratory symptoms without any signs of improvement suggests the presence of bacterial infection (13). Facial pain is rare and unreliable for children. If fever is present in uncomplicated viral infection, it is usually at earlier phase of illness and accompanied by other constitutional symptoms such as headache. Purulent nasal discharge does not appear for several days for uncomplicated viral infection. The concurrent presentation of fever and purulent nasal discharge for at least 3–4 consecutive days helps diagnose ABS (17).

Physical examination does not contribute to the diagnosis of ABS. Sinus aspiration is the gold standard for the diagnosis of ABS; but it is an invasive, time-consuming, and potentially painful procedure that should only be performed by a specialist (otolaryngologist) (20). Nasal swab and culture from the middle meatus is also reported but the correlation with nasal swab with sinus puncture remains weak. Endoscopic guided swab culture is more accurate to sample secretion from a sinus of interest. However this is usually performed by otolaryngologists, resulting in higher cost, and thus is not feasible for routine use.

Radiographic imaging should not be obtained for patients who meet clinical diagnostic criteria for ABS. The paranasal sinuses are still under development in younger children. Therefore, lack of aeration of the sinuses may be physiological rather than infection, limiting the accuracy of radiography (21).

In children younger than 6 years of age, clinical history correlates with sinus radiography in 88% of time (22), therefore radiography can be safely omitted for children under age 6 (strong consensus based on limited evidence).

For children over 6 years of age with persistent symptoms, the need for radiograph as a confirmatory test of acute sinusitis remains controversial. When an alternative diagnosis is considered, imaging might be useful. Normal radiographs or CT is powerful evidence that bacterial sinusitis is not the causes of the symptoms (23) (limited evidence). A practical guideline by AHRQ indicates that imaging study is not warranted when the likelihood of acute sinusitis is either high or low, but imaging is useful when a diagnosis is in doubt (limited evidence).

Sinus CT is indicated for patients with acute sinusitis symptoms in the following three conditions: (1) when complications related to sinusitis are suspected, (2) when symptoms persist without response to medical management, or (3) surgery is considered (strong recommendation based on moderate evidence). Complicated sinusitis is suspected when patients present with ptosis, cranial nerve palsies, facial and orbital swelling. Contrast enhanced CT of the sinuses and orbit is recommended when orbital cellulites or periosteal abscess as a complication of sinusitis is suspected (18, 24, 25). Contrast enhanced MRI is occasionally recommended when intracranial extension, such as epidural empyema or brain abscess is suspected (21, 26–29) (limited evidence).

II. What Is the Diagnostic Performance of Sinus Radiography and Sinus CT in Acute Bacterial Sinusitis? What Diagnostic Criteria Should We Use?

Summary of Evidence: Although the diagnosis of acute sinusitis should be made on clinical grounds, the accuracy of such clinical diagnosis is not well documented compared with the gold standard of direct sinus puncture. Compared with sinus radiography as the gold standard, clinical diagnosis has moderate accuracy (moderate level of evidence) (13). Summary Receiver Operating Characteristics (SROC) is used to represent the accuracy of a diagnostic test, where one is perfect accuracy and 0.5 is no better than the flip of a coin. The area under the curve (AUC) of clinical diagnosis compared with sinus radiograph is 0.74 (30). Compared with sinus puncture as the gold standard, sinus radiography offers moderate ability to diagnose acute sinusitis (SROC area 0.83) (moderate evidence) (31–35). No single study comparing CT or MR with sinus puncture to evaluate accuracy of CT or MR for acute sinusitis was found. Given CT and MRI's superior spatial and soft tissue resolution to radiography, both are likely more sensitive for detection of acute sinusitis, but specificity is questionable. Lack of definitive diagnostic criteria for sinus disease makes it difficult to interpret studies investigating specificity of sinus CT or MRI.

Sinus puncture performed by an otolaryngologist is the gold standard; however, it is rarely performed due to its invasiveness and cost. An inexpensive, simple, and accurate diagnostic test is needed to better differentiate patients who need antibiotics from those with nonspecific viral illness. Good, high-quality evidence for acute uncomplicated sinusitis in children is limited. Diagnostic modalities show poor concordance. More evidence is needed for defining the optimal treatment and diagnostic methods for this common condition (7) (insufficient evidence).

Supporting Evidence: The diagnosis of acute sinusitis is often made based on clinical grounds, but the accuracy of such clinical diagnosis is not well documented. Engles performed a meta-analysis of diagnostic tests for acute sinusitis that showed clinical history and physical examination had moderate ability to identify patients with positive radiography (SROC area 0.74) (34).

Using sinus opacity or the presence of an air-fluid level as the criterion for sinusitis, sinus radiography had sensitivity of 0.73 and specificity of 0.80. Compared with sinus puncture and aspiration as the gold standard, sinus radiography offers moderate ability to diagnose acute sinusitis (SROC area 0.83). Another systematic review performed by Varonen published concurrently with Engles study focused on adult patients suspected of acute maxillary sinusitis. They compared sinus radiography, ultrasound, and clinical examination with sinus puncture as the gold standard and concluded that sinus radiography was more accurate method for diagnosing acute sinusitis (SROC area of 0.82) than clinical examination. Clinical examination even by experienced physicians was less reliable (area under SROC is 0.75) (35). Using sinus puncture as the gold standard, Berg reported that clinical examination had a sensitivity of 66% and specificity of 79% in the setting of Emergency clinic (36). Sinus radiograph is more accurate than clinical examination for diagnosis of ABS. However, clinical application for sinus radiograph as an initial workup is not justified due to its costs and radiation exposure.

In Europe, A mode ultrasound is used to diagnose acute maxillary sinusitis in primary care setting with moderately strong accuracy (SROC area of 0.80) (31, 35, 37). Savolainen reported among 234 patients suspected of maxillary sinusitis that Ultrasound had a sensitivity of 81% and specificity of 72%, as compared with sinus puncture (38). Ultrasound waves are transmitted to the sinus then reflected back from the interface of two different media. A sinus cavity is filled with secretions results in an echo in the display screen. It is insensitive for mucosal thickening of the sinus (39).

Computed tomography (CT) provides superior assessment of all paranasal sinuses compared with sinus radiograph (40). However, CT has not been directly compared with sinus puncture for assessment of diagnostic accuracy (34, 35). Given the invasiveness of sinus puncture and need for otolaryngology referral (additional cost), sinus CT can be used as a proxy of sinus puncture. Sinus CT is considered more sensitive than sinus radiograph for diagnosis of acute sinusitis. A study comparing sinus plain radiograph and CT in 47 consecutive patients showed that sinus radiograph had a high specificity but markedly low sensitivity for disease in the ethmoid, frontal, and sphenoid sinuses (41). The sensitivity of sinus radiograph for maxillary sinus was 80% in this study. Another study enrolled 134 patients with suspected sinusitis who underwent a single Water's view of sinus and CT revealed that plain film has markedly low sensitivity for a disease outside of maxillary sinus. The sensitivity, specificity of Water's view compared with CT for maxillary sinus disease was 67.7% and 87.6%, respectively (42). They recommended the use of a low-dose, high resolution CT scan of the paranasal sinuses (moderate evidence). The problem is its lack of specificity data of sinus CT, compared with sinus puncture. A question is if CT scan overdiagnoses sinusitis.

Another reason that accuracy of sinus CT remains uncertain and controversial is lack of definitive diagnostic criteria. Diagnostic criteria of sinus radiography for acute sinusitis are complete opacification or sinus air fluid level. Diagnostic criteria for sinus CT are not well defined, but usually include mucosal thickening greater than 4 mm, any degree of sinus opacification, and any type of fluid level are considered positive for acute sinusitis. Mild mucoperiosteal thickening can be found on head CT in patients without any sinusitis related symptoms in up to 40% of individuals (43). Gwaltney reported that CT scan of 31 patients with self diagnosed common cold. They found that 87% of 31 patients had occlusion (or mucosal thickening) of ethmoid infundibulum, and 65% of patients had mucoal abnormality in maxillary sinuses (44). It is of paramount importance to define what CT finings constitute ABS.

The only specific CT finding to indicate acute sinusitis is a frothy, bubbly air fluid level, which indicates purulent secretion within the sinuses (21). Waterish smooth air fluid level may be nasal secretion without bacterial infection or clear secretion related to allergic rhinitis (45). Complete opacification of a sinus with bone thickening may indicate chronically obstructed sinus rather than acute sinusitis (46).

III. When Are Imaging Studies Indicated for the Diagnosis and the Management of Patients with Sinusitis?

Summary of Evidence: Imaging studies, such as sinus CT should be performed for patients who present with complications of ABS or who have very persistent or recurrent disease not responding to medical management. When patients do not respond to medical management, the patients may have mechanical obstruction that prevents restoration of mucociliary clearance, such as a polyp or structural anomalies of the nasal cavity and sinuses.

Sinusitis is a self-limiting disease with complete cure in most cases. However, serious complications still do occur in a small percentage (3.7–11%) of these patients with acute sinusitis (47). When patients with sinusitis symptoms present with orbital swelling, ptosis, visual changes, cranial nerve palsies, and mental status changes, contrast enhanced CT and/or MR is recommended to diagnose orbital cellulitis/abscess, epidural or subdural empyema, cavernous sinus thrombosis, and intracranial extension of infection (29).

When surgery is considered for patients with recurrent or medically refractory disease, details sinus CT is indicated to define the bony anatomy, including the osteomeatal complex, and correlated with patients' clinical symptoms (13, 48, 49) (limited evidence).

Supporting Evidence: Sinusitis is a common condition and in most cases a self-limited disease. Most cases of sinusitis resolve completely with appropriate antibiotic therapy. Patients with complicated acute sinusitis have severe symptoms, including high fever, intense headache that is above or behind the eye, periorbital

swelling, or pressure over the face. Complicated acute sinusitis results from a delay in initiating treatment, antibiotic resistant infection, and incomplete treatment. Immunocompromised patients, such as cystic fibrosis, often present with extensive sinus infection. The incidence of sinusitis related complications remain indeterminate as many literatures reporting sinusitis related complications were case series or case reports. A retrospective review from a single institution revealed that 5.3% of ENT emergencies were sinusitis complications. Among them, orbital complications were the most common (62%) followed by acute subdural empyema (23%) and meningitis (15%) (50). Among the transplant patients, patients with graft versus host disease (GVHD) were 4.3 times more likely than patients without GVHD to develop sinusitis post transplant (51).

These include intra-orbital complications, such as orbital cellulitis and subperiosteal abscess, cavernous sinus thrombosis, epidural empyema, meningitis, cerebritis, and brain abscess. Therefore, contrast enhanced CT or MR is indicated when patients with sinusitis symptoms present with orbital swelling, proptosis, visual changes, and cranial nerve palsies. (28, 52, 53). Clary investigated the accuracy of sinus CT for orbital abscess as compared with surgical exploration in 19 patients and reported that CT had a sensitivity of 93% and specificity of 67% (54).

With the advent of antibiotics, the incidence of orbital cellulitis has decreased. Approximately 3% of sinusitis progresses to orbital cellulitis (40). This can be divided into pre- and postseptal cellulitis. The septum is defined as the medial orbital periosteal reflection attaching to the medial eyelid at the tarsal plate. The majority of orbital cellulitis is due to either direct spread from ethmoid sinusitis through porous lamina papyracea or through the valveless anterior and posterior ethmoid veins (40). The periosteum of the medial orbital wall is loosely attached to the lamina papyracea; as such it often forms subperiosteal abscess or phlegmon. Clinically, these patients may present with deviation of the globe or proptosis. Cavernous sinus thrombosis results from infection of the midface, orbit, and sinonasal cavity. This may lead to cranial nerve paralysis and blindness. In the setting of orbital cellulitis, the presence of cranial nerve paralysis involving cranial nerve III, IV, V, and/or VI, raise the suspicion of cavernous sinus thrombosis. Contrast enhanced CT or MR show an engorged superior ophthalmic vein. Enhancing cavernous carotid artery may stand out from the surrounding thrombosed cavernous sinus (55–58).

Intracranial spread of sinus infection most commonly originates from frontal or sphenoid sinusitis (52, 59). Intracranial extension of infection is facilitated by the abundant valveless emissary venous plexus of the posterior frontal sinus, known as Behcet's plexus. Infection spreads through the sinus to dura, meninges, and parenchyma, resulting in epidural or subdural empyema, meningitis, cerebritis, and brain abscess (55). Contrast enhanced brain MR is recommended when intracranial spread of sinusitis is suspected (52, 55). One study comparing diagnostic accuracy of CT, MR, and clinical diagnosis for sinusitis related complications revealed that the diagnostic accuracy was 82% for clinical assessment compared with 91% for CT for orbital complications. For patients with intracranial complications, meningitis was the most common diagnosis, and MRI was more accurate (97%) in determining the diagnosis than CT (87%) or clinical findings (82%). Both CT and MR have improved the management and outcomes of patients who have sinusitis with complications (60).

Surgery of the sinuses or nasal passage may be considered for patients who do not respond to medical management for sinusitis, Sinus CT is the primary imaging test and provides detailed images of sinus anatomy in multiple planes. Attention should be paid to the status of osteomeatal complex, particularly the curvature and superior extension of the uncinate process. Patients with chronic sinusitis often received the maximum medical therapy before CT scan in order to evaluate the bony details. Thus, mucosal disease is often minimum for those patients. What we should look for is bony anatomy related to osteomeatal complex and also dangerous anatomical variations, such as dehiscent optic canal or carotid canal, low lying fovea ethmoidalis, or Onodi cells. These findings alert ENT surgeons prior to surgical intervention.

Sinus CT often reveals various common anatomical variations, such as nasal septum deviation or concha bullosa. A study evaluating anatomical variations of sinuses on CT revealed that 64.9% of 202 patients had anatomical variations. The significance of such anatomical variant remains uncertain, as these anatomical variations are often seen in patients without any sinusitis symptoms (61). A detailed sinus CT, instead of screening or limited sinus CT is recommended for patients with chronic sinusitis who undergo sinus surgery. The screening sinus CT for preoperative assessment was thought to be inadequate for operative planning (62).

IV. What Is the Most Cost Effective Strategy for the Diagnosis and the Management of Acute Sinusitis?

Summary of Evidence: The most cost-effective method to manage patients presented with mild to moderate symptoms of acute sinusitis is to use clinical guidelines and treat with first line antibiotic therapy (63). For patients with severe symptoms or high disease prevalence population, empirical antibiotic treatment is cost effective. This leads to many unnecessary antibiotic prescription that leads to antibiotics resistant infection.

Cost-effectiveness analysis (CEA) comparing four different management strategies (empirical antibiotics, no antibiotics, or clinical diagnosis or sinus CT based treatment) of adult acute sinusitis revealed that empirical antibiotic therapy is most cost effective from the societal perspective, as patients return to normal life more quickly, offsetting the upfront cost of antibiotics (64, 65). From the payer's perspective, clinical diagnosis based treatment was the most cost effective strategy (64). The effectiveness of antibiotic therapy in children remains controversial. The study results highly depend on the inclusion criteria of the study population. Antibiotic therapy was effective for patients with radiographically confirmed pediatric acute sinusitis, but little or no effect is seen when patients were selected based on clinical diagnosis (9). This is likely due to the fact that some of these patients had viral infection, therefore potentially diluting the effectiveness of antibiotic therapy.

Supporting Evidence: A diagnostic workup strategy for any disease should be directly connected to its management of the disease. Although sinusitis is a self-limiting disease in most cases, under-treating acute sinusitis may lead to rare but serious complications. Patients remain sick longer, thus requiring time away from work, loss of productivity, and over-the counter medications (65). Over-treating sinusitis may result in unnecessary costs and adverse effects from antibiotic therapy, such as allergic reaction or gastrointestinal disturbance, as well as future development of antibiotic resistant infection. Treating a viral illness with antibiotics lead to no benefit, but potential adverse drug effects. Accurate diagnosis by CT scan improves effectiveness of antibiotic therapy, by selecting patients who benefit from antibiotics. However, such additional benefit is too small to justify the additional cost of CT scan and the additional risks from radiation exposure, particularly in children.

The effectiveness of antibiotic therapy in children remains controversial. The results highly depend on the study inclusion criteria. Antibiotic therapy was found effective for patients with radiographically confirmed acute sinusitis. Patients treated with antibiotics recovered more quickly than those under placebo (22). On the third day of treatment, 83% of children receiving antibiotics were cured or improved compared with 51% of the children in the placebo group. However, little or no effective is seen in antibiotic treatment when patients were selected based on clinical diagnosis alone. A study by Garbutt challenged the notion that children having acute sinusitis based on clinical ground will benefit from antibiotic therapy. Since "sinusitis patients" defined by clinical diagnosis include children with viral infection, the effectiveness of antibiotics is diluted.

The American Academy of Pediatrics clinical practice guidelines for the management of sinusitis show that children with mild and moderate symptoms who do not attend daycare should receive the usual dose of amoxicillin (17). Those patients who (a) do not improve while receiving the usual dose of amoxicillin, or (b) have been recently been treated with antibiotics, or (c) have illness that is moderate to severe, or (d) attend daycare should receive high dose amoxicillin with clavulanate. Higher doses of amoxicillin are effective for *S. pneumoniae* species that are intermediate in resistance to penicillin and potassium clavulanate is effective against beta-lactamase producing *H. influenzae* and *M. catarrhalis*. The AAP guidelines make no recommendations about the use of antihistamines, decongestants, and intranasal steroids based on limited or controversial data (10).

V. What Is the Imaging Role for Patients with Chronic Sinusitis?

Summary of Evidence: Clinical diagnosis of chronic sinusitis is even more difficult than that of acute sinusitis. Patients with chronic sinusitis have relatively vague symptoms that overlap with viral upper respiratory infection, allergy, and migraine. Imaging plays an important role for excluding diagnosis or identifying anatomical causes leading to sinusitis. CT is a modality of choice as it provides anatomical roadmaps much better than plain radiography or Ultrasound. Although rare, for children suspected for serious complications, such as intracranial or orbital abscess, MR with contrast is recommended to assist surgical treatment planning.

Supporting Evidence: Chronic sinusitis is defined as sinusitis symptoms lasting more than 12 weeks. The diagnosis of chronic sinusitis is difficult because of relatively nonspecific signs and symptoms that overlap with viral upper respiratory infection and allergy. Children or adolescents with chronic headache are often misdiagnosed as sinus headache and receive sinus medication (66). Imaging plays a major role for making or excluding diagnosis or assessing the anatomy of sinuses leading to recurrent or chronic infection (67).

In terms of the choice of imaging for children with chronic sinusitis, sinus radiography was reported to overestimate abnormalities. In a study performed sinus radiography and CT in 34 children with chronic sinusitis, sinus radiography (waters and occipitomental views) overestimated ethmoid sinus disease in 24% and maxillary sinus disease in 56% (68). Sinus CT provides details anatomy as well as extent of disease better than sinus radiography and remains the imaging study of choice for patients with chronic sinusitis. CT scan is often performed in patients who remain symptomatic following multiple courses of antibiotics in order to diagnose or rule out presence of obstructive lesion interfering mucocillary clearance. Multi-institutional prospective dual cohort study comparing the severity of CT findings using Lund-MacKay staging system in 66 pediatric patients with chronic sinusitis and control showed that the AUC of CT is 0.923 ($p < 0.01$), indicating excellent diagnostic accuracy (69).

If sinus CT is completely normal in patients who are suspected of having chronic sinusitis, diagnosis can be generally excluded. When sinus CT shows a focal intranasal mass with unilateral sinus opacification, this may lead to evaluation by endoscopy for possible surgical resection. The problem lies, however, when sinus CT shows mild, nonspecific, diffuse mucosal thickening without correlation with clinical symptoms, in terms of facial pain, or tenderness, it is difficult to determine if sinusitis contributes to patients' clinical symptoms.

A study comparing CT scan findings of 60 children age 2–12 with chronic sinusitis with 50 control subjects who underwent CT scan for indications other than sinusitis found that mucoperiosteal thickening is highly prevalent findings seen in 60% of patients and 46% of control groups. Early stage (mild) mucoperiosteal thickening was present in the majority of children who had sinus CT (98% of control and 85% of children with chronic sinusitis) (70). Certain anatomical variations are thought to contribute causality of chronic sinusitis as these variations may interfere with sinus drainage pathways. These include, but not limited to, nasal septum deviation, concha bullosa, and Haller cells. Significance of anatomic variations in children is still controversial as these findings can be seen in asymptomatic subjects (71).

Medical management remains the cornerstone for children with chronic sinusitis. Indication for sinus surgery is controversial. No prospective randomized trial comparing medical management with surgery has been reported. The decision regarding the need for sinus surgery should not be solely based on imaging abnormalities. A study investigated the impact of sinus CT on therapeutic decision by otolaryngologists showed that the concordance between CT abnormality with patient's symptoms and obstruction of ostiomeatal complex are main predictors for favorable surgical treatment (72). Sinus surgery may be performed in children with nasal obstruction from polyposis or refractory sinusitis aggravating asthma (73). Outcome assessment for 308 children with chronic sinusitis after sinus surgery revealed that endoscopic sinus surgery improved outcomes in 2-year follow-up in the intermediate stages of chronic sinusitis (stage II and III out of stage I-IV) (74). Some study suggested use of IV antibiotics for children who have failed to respond to traditional oral antibiotics therapy (75).

VI. Special Situation: What Is the Role of Imaging in Immunocompromised Patients?

Summary of Evidence: Invasive fungal sinusitis (IFS) has been increasingly seen in patients with an immunocompromised status. The incidence has increased in accordance with increase use of antibiotics, steroids, chemotherapy, and radiation treatment. IFS is a difficult disease to treat. CT findings that are characteristics for IFS includes mucoperiosteal thickening associated with bone erosion or extra-sinus soft tissue invasion to orbit or retroantral fat pad. CT is helpful for planning of surgical debridement. However, diagnosis of IFS should not solely based on CT, as CT findings suggestive of IFS, bone erosion or extrasinus invasion, are often absent in an earlier course of disease (76). With a high clinical suspicion, rigid nasal endoscopy with biopsy is recommended for early diagnosis (76). Complete surgical resection and reversal of neutropenia are critical elements for improved outcomes.

Supporting Evidence: IFS is rare, but a life threatening disease in children with underlying immunocompromised disease. Incidence has been increasing in accordance with expansion of transplant medicine and advancement in antineoplastic medication for hematological malignancies. Common fungal organisms seen in immunocompromised patients include aspergillosis, mucormycosis, and zygomycosis. IFS often spreads directly to brain via vascular channels or is blood borne from pulmonary infection. Abscess formation along blood vessels often causes thrombosis of vessels leading to neurological deficit (77). Therefore when immunocompromised patients present with stroke type of symptoms, intracranial involvement of IFS is highly suspected.

IFS in immunocompromised children has a high mortality rate and requires early diagnosis and treatment.

Imaging study such as sinus CT plays important role in demonstrating the extent of disease, degree of bone destruction, orbital invasion, extra-sinus soft tissue invasion, and vascular encasement. When intracranial involvement is suspected, such as epidural abscess/phlegmon, cerebritis, or septic emboli, brain MR with and without contrast is essential to make a diagnosis and plan appropriate surgical management. MR allows differentiation of direct cerebral invasion from multiple brain abscess or septic emboli. Venous sinus thrombosis is also another serious complication that can be diagnosed with MR and MR venogram. Some of fungal disease has markedly low T2 signal mimicking well aerated sinuses on T2-weighted images. These lesions may appear slightly hyperdense on non-contrast CT examination. Contrast enhancement is useful in order to assess extrasinus extent of disease.

However, classic CT findings of IFS are often absent in *earlier* course of disease. Retrospective review of CT findings in 23 immunocompromised patients with confirmed IFS showed that many patients had mucoperiosteal thickening of sinuses (21/23), but bone erosion (8/23) or orbital invasion (6/23) were seen only in more advanced IFS. They found that disease was frequently unilateral (21/23). Thus, clinician should not rely solely on imaging to make a diagnosis of IFS. With a high index of suspicion, early nasal endoscopy and biopsy as well as initiation of antifungal therapy is critical to improve prognosis.

Treatment for IFS includes surgical debridement, followed by high dose antifungal treatment, and attempts to correct underlying immunocompromised state are essential for improved survival.

Take Home Tables

Table 16.1 gives the definition of ABS. Table 16.2 shows the clinical diagnostic criteria for ABS. Table 16.3 gives a summary of diagnostic performance of imaging and clinical examinations for diagnosing acute sinusitis and its complications.

Table 16.1. Definition of acute bacterial sinusitis (acute sinusitis)

Acute sinusitis:
Infection of the paranasal sinuses lasting less than 30 days that presents with either *persistent or severe symptoms.*
Persistent symptoms are those that last longer than 10–14 days. Sinusitis symptoms include nasal discharge, nasal congestion, maxillary or facial pain, or toothache. Such symptoms for children include nasal or postnasal discharge, daytime cough (which may be worse at night) or both.
Severe symptoms include a temperature of at least 102°F and purulent nasal discharge present concurrently for at least 3–4 consecutive days.

Adapted with kind permission of Springer Science+Business Media from Anzai Y, Paladin A. Diagnosis and Management of Acute and Chronic Sinusitis in Children. In Medina LS, Applegate KE, Blackmore CC (eds.): *Evidence-Based Imaging in Pediatrics: Optimizing Imaging in Pediatric Patient Care.* New York: Springer Science+Business Media, 2010.

Table 16.2. Acute bacterial sinusitis vs. viral upper respiratory infection: clinical signs and symptoms

	Acute bacterial sinusitis	Viral URI
Duration of illness	Longer than 10–14 days	Usually less than 5–7 days
Symptoms	Persistent or worsening after mild resolution (double sickening)	Improved or resolved by 10 days
Fever	Concurrent presentation of high fever and nasal discharge	Earlier in illness and later nasal discharge
Headache	Severe headache behind eyes	Mild headache
Facial pain	Unilateral pain But not reliable for small children	Mild or absent

Reprinted with kind permission of Springer Science+Business Media from Anzai Y, Paladin A. Diagnosis and Management of Acute and Chronic Sinusitis in Children. In Medina LS, Applegate KE, Blackmore CC (eds.): *Evidence-Based Imaging in Pediatrics: Optimizing Imaging in Pediatric Patient Care.* New York: Springer Science+Business Media, 2010.

Table 16.3. Summary table of diagnostic performance of imaging and clinical examinations for diagnosing acute sinusitis in children (only those using sinus puncture as gold standards)

	Sensitivity (95% CI)	Specificity (95% CI)	References
Physical exam only	0.66 (0.58–0.73)	0.79 (0.73–0.87)	(15, 34–36)
Radiographs	0.87 (0.85–0.88)	0.89 (0.85–0.91)	(32–35)
Ultrasound	0.85 (0.84–0.87)	0.82 (0.80–0.83)	(23, 26, 31, 37, 38)
CT: No study assessing accuracy of CT using sinus puncture as the gold standard.			
CT (orbital abscess)	0.93	0.67	5

Adapted with kind permission of Springer Science+Business Media from Anzai Y, Paladin A. Diagnosis and Management of Acute and Chronic Sinusitis in Children. In Medina LS, Applegate KE, Blackmore CC (eds.): *Evidence-Based Imaging in Pediatrics: Optimizing Imaging in Pediatric Patient Care.* New York: Springer Science+Business Media, 2010.

Imaging Case Studies

Figure 16.1 shows various imaging findings and suggested diagnosis. Figure 16.2 shows CT images for a patient with cavernous sinus thrombosis. Figure 16.3 shows CT images of a patient with allergic fungal sinusitis. Figure 16.4 shows CT images of a patient with epidural abscess secondary to sphenoid sinusitis and mucocele rupture.

Suggested Imaging Protocols for Children Clinically Suspected Acute Sinusitis

Sinus Radiographs

Sinus radiographic series has been rapidly replaced by the limited sinus CT for evaluation of sinusitis. However some pediatrician still order sinus radiograph, likely due to either lower costs or easier access to radiographs than CT. In order to visualize and assess all paranasal sinuses, at least three views of sinus are required. These include Waters' view, Caldwell view, and Lateral view. In children under age 6 years, the ACR (appropriateness criteria) states that radiographs of the paranasal sinuses are both not indicated and technically difficult to perform. For recurrent infection, some clinicians order a single Waters' view to evaluate the maxillary sinuses.

Low Dose Screening Sinus CT

Using low mA and low kVP is most widely used for assessment of sinus infection in our institution, when available, reducing radiation dose compared with the standard CT (78). Screening sinus CT demonstrates air fluid level or sinus opacification, as well as adjacent soft tissue abnormalities and mastoid and middle ear fluid collection.

MDCT allows rapid acquisition of axial images through paranasal sinuses with thin collimation (≤3 mm), in supine position using 100 mAs and 120 kVp. Reconstruction of these images in the coronal plane is routinely performed. No intravenous contrast is necessary unless there is a suspected complication such as orbital abscess or epidural empyema. No sedation is needed for these rapidly acquired CTs.

MRI

When MR is needed to assess intracranial complications, the following sequences should be included: Axial FLAIR, Axial Diffusion, Axial T2 FSE, pre and post contrast T1 multiplanar images. Fat suppression should be used for assessment of post contrast images in order to better visualize cavernous sinuses, orbital apex, skull base, as well as epidural and subdural spaces.

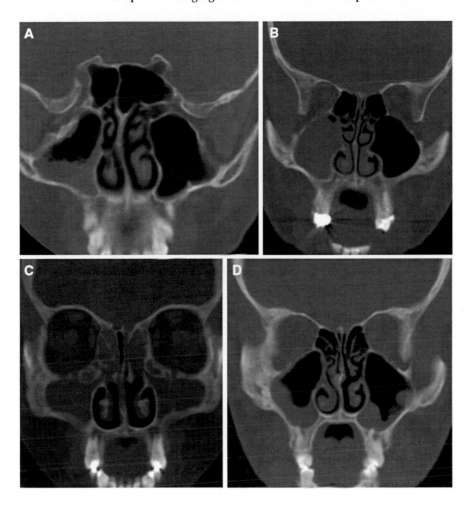

Figure 16.1. Various imaging findings and suggested diagnoses. (**A**) Air-fluid level in the right maxillary sinus: findings highly suspicious for acute bacterial sinusitis. (**B**) Near complete opacification of right maxillary sinus in a patient suspected of acute sinusitis. (**C**) Diffuse mucosal swelling and opacification of maxillary and ethmoid sinuses with thickening of bone walls in a patient with sinonasal polyposis. (**D**) Nonspecific mucosal swelling of maxillary sinus bilaterally. This could be viral infection, allergy, or common cold. (Reprinted with kind permission of Springer Science+Business Media from Anzai Y, Paladin A. Diagnosis and Management of Acute and Chronic Sinusitis in Children. In Medina LS, Applegate KE, Blackmore CC (eds.): *Evidence-Based Imaging in Pediatrics: Optimizing Imaging in Pediatric Patient Care.* New York: Springer Science+Business Media, 2010.)

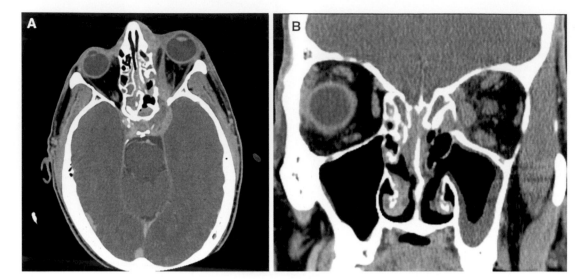

Figure 16.2. (**A**) A patient with fungal infection involving ethmoid sinuses complicated with left cavernous sinus thrombosis. (**B**) Coronal image show extension of infection to the medial left orbit associated with focal bone erosion. (Reprinted with kind permission of Springer Science+Business Media from Anzai Y, Paladin A. Diagnosis and Management of Acute and Chronic Sinusitis in Children. In Medina LS, Applegate KE, Blackmore CC (eds.): *Evidence-Based Imaging in Pediatrics: Optimizing Imaging in Pediatric Patient Care*. New York: Springer Science+Business Media, 2010.)

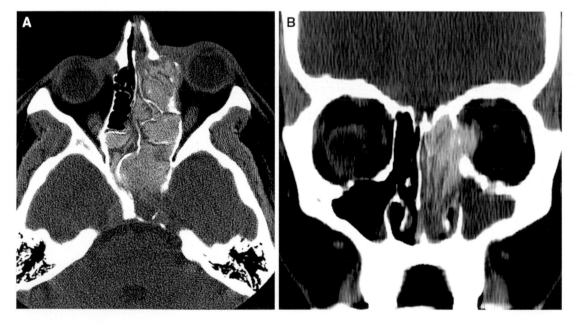

Figure 16.3. (**A**) A patient with allergic fungal infection involving the bilateral ethmoid sinuses with medial orbital extension. Notice the content of sinus opacification is markedly increased attenuation with low attenuation edematous mucosa. (Reprinted with kind permission of Springer Science+Business Media from Anzai Y, Neighbor, Jr. WE. Imaging Evaluation of Sinusitis: Impact on Health Outcome. In Medina LS, Blackmore CC (eds.): *Evidence-Based Imaging: Optimizing Imaging in Patient Care*. New York: Springer Science+Business Media, 2006.); (**B**) Coronal reformatted image of the same patient shows medical orbital extension with displacement of medical rectus muscle

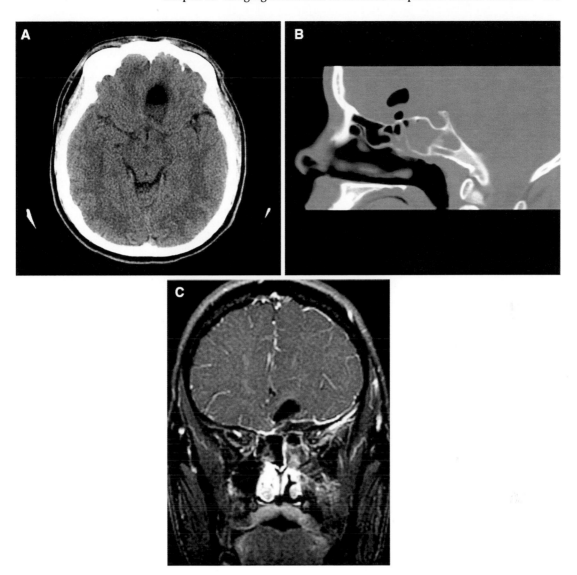

Figure 16.4. (**A**) A young patient presented with headache and mental status change. Non-contrast head CT shows focal air near the fluid collection in the base of left frontal lobe. (**B**) Sagittal reformatted image shows an expansive sphenoid sinus with adjacent pneumocephalus. (**C**) Contrast enhanced fat suppressed coronal image shows a focal epidural abscess adjacent to the left sphenoid sinus, underneath the air pocket. This patient was thought to have left sphenoid mucocele with intracranial ruptured, resulting in epidural abscess. (Reprinted with kind permission of Springer Science+Business Media from Anzai Y, Paladin A. Diagnosis and Management of Acute and Chronic Sinusitis in Children. In Medina LS, Applegate KE, Blackmore CC (eds.): *Evidence-Based Imaging in Pediatrics: Optimizing Imaging in Pediatric Patient Care*. New York: Springer Science+Business Media, 2010.)

Future Research

- Large clinical study correlating imaging and clinical findings with sinus aspiration and treatment outcomes.
- Develop noninvasive strategies to accurately diagnose acute sinusitis, particularly imaging that differentiates bacterial infection from viral infection or allergic inflammation.
- Determine better staging strategy using sinus CT for patients with chronic sinusitis.

References

1. Kennedy DW. Otolaryngol Head Neck Surg 1990;103:884–886.
2. Fletcher MA, Fritzell B. Vaccine 2007;25: 2507–2512.
3. Brook I. Int J Pediatr Otorhinolaryngol 2007;71: 1653–1661.
4. Lethbridge-Cejku M, Schiller JS, Bernadel L. Vital Health Stat 2004;10:1–151.
5. Willett LR, Carson JL, Williams JW, Jr. J Gen Intern Med 1994;9:38–45.
6. Senior BA, Kennedy DW, Tanabodee J, Kroger H, Hassab M, Lanza D. Laryngoscope 1998;108: 151–157.
7. Ioannidis JP, Lau J. Pediatrics 2001;108:E57. p 51–58
8. Clement PA, Bluestone CD, Gordts F, Lusk RP, Otten FW, Goossens H, et al. Int J Pediatr Otorhinolaryngol 1999;49:S95–S100.
9. Garbutt JM, Goldstein M, Gellman E, Shannon W, Littenberg B. Pediatrics 2001;107:619–625.
10. Ioannidis JP, Lau J. American Academy of Pediatrics. Subcommittee on Management of Sinusitis and Committee on Quality Improvement Pub Med Pediatrics 2001;108:798–808.
11. Collins JG. Vital Health Stat 1997;10:1–89.
12. NCHS. National Center for Health Statistics: Sinusitis. 2002.
13. Rosenfeld RM, Andes D, Bhattacharyya N, Cheung D, Eisenberg S, Ganiats TG, et al. Otolaryngol Head Neck Surg 2007;137:S1–S31.
14. Ray NF, Baraniuk JN, Thamer M, Rinehart CS, Gergen PJ, Kaliner M et al. J Allergy Clin Immunol 1999;103:408–414.
15. Lau J, Zucker D, Engles E, Balk E, Barza M, Terrin N et al. Diagnosis and treatment of Acute Bacterial Rhinosinusitis. Rockwille, MD: Agency for Health Care Policy and Research, 1999:1–38.
16. Brooks I, Gooch WM, 3rd, Jenkins SG, Pichichero ME, Reiner SA, Sher L et al. Ann Otol Rhinol Laryngol Suppl 2000;182:2–20.
17. Nash D, Wald E. Pediatr Rev 2001;22:111–117.
18. McAlister WH, Parker BR, Kushner DC, Babcock DS, Cohen HL, Gelfand MJ et al. Radiology 2000;215(suppl):811–818.
19. Gonzales R, Bartlett JG, Besser RE, Cooper RJ, Hickner JM, Hoffman JR et al. Ann Emerg Med 2001;37:690–697.
20. Wald ER. Am J Med Sci 1998;316:13–20.
21. Diament MJ. J Allergy Clin Immunol 1992;90: 442–444.
22. Wald ER, Chiponis D, Ledesma-Medina J. Pediatrics 1986;77:795–800.
23. Reider JM, Nashelsky J. J Fam Pract 2003;52:565–567; discussion 567
24. Kronemer KA, McAlister WH. Pediatr Radiol 1997;27:837–846.
25. Howe L, Jones NS. Clin Otolaryngol Allied Sci 2004;29:725–728.
26. Dessi P, Champsaur P, Paris J, Moulin G. Rev Laryngol Otol Rhinol (Bord) 1999;120:173–176.
27. Eufinger H, Machtens E. J Craniomaxillofac Surg 2001;29:111–117.
28. Eustis HS, Mafee MF, Walton C, Mondonca J. Radiol Clin North Am 1998;36:1165–1183, xi.
29. Mafee MF, Tran BH, Chapa AR. Clin Rev Allergy Immunol 2006;30:165–186.
30. Williams JW, Jr., Simel DL, Roberts L, Samsa GP. Ann Intern Med 1992;117:705–710.
31. Revonta M, Blokmanis A. Can Fam Physician 1994;40:1969–1972, 1975–1966.
32. van Buchem FL, Knottnerus JA, Schrijnemaekers VJ, Peeters MF. Lancet 1997;349:683–687.
33. Laine K, Maatta T, Varonen H, Makela M. Rhinology 1998;36:2–6.
34. Engels EA, Terrin N, Barza M, Lau J. J Clin Epidemiol 2000;53:852–862.
35. Varonen H, Makela M, Savolainen S, Laara E, Hilden J. J Clin Epidemiol 2000;53:940–948.
36. Berg O, Carenfelt C. Acta Otolaryngol 1988;105: 343–349.
37. Berg O, Carenfelt C. Laryngoscope 1985;95:851–853.
38. Savolainen S, Pietola M, Kiukaanniemi H, Lappalainen E, Salminen M, Mikkonen P. Acta Otolaryngol Suppl 1997;529:148–152.
39. Varonen H, Savolainen S, Kunnamo I, Heikkinen R, Revonta M. Rhinology 2003;41:37–43.
40. Som PM. Neuroradiology 1985;27:189–201.
41. Aalokken TM, Hagtvedt T, Dalen I, Kolbenstvedt A. Dentomaxillofac Radiol 2003;32:60–62.
42. Konen E, Faibel M, Kleinbaum Y, Wolf M, Lusky A, Hoffman C et al. Clin Radiol 2000;55:856–860.
43. Glasier CM, Ascher DP, Williams KD. AJNR Am J Neuroradiol 1986;7:861–864.
44. Gwaltney JM, Jr., Phillips CD, Miller RD, Riker DK. N Engl J Med 1994;330:25–30.
45. Berg O, Bergstedt H, Carenfelt C, Lind MG, Perols O. Ann Otol Rhinol Laryngol 1981;90:272–275.
46. April MM, Zinreich SJ, Baroody FM, Naclerio RM. Laryngoscope 1993;103:985–990.

47. Vazquez E, Creixell S, Carreno JC, Castellote A, Figueras C, Pumarola F et al. Curr Probl Diagn Radiol 2004;33:127–145.
48. Kennedy DW, Senior BA. Otolaryngol Clin North Am 1997;30:313–330.
49. Jiannetto DF, Pratt MF. Laryngoscope 1995;105: 924–927.
50. Ali A, Kurien M, Mathews SS, Mathew J. Singapore Med J 2005;46:540–544.
51. Thompson AM, Couch M, Zahurak ML, Johnson C, Vogelsang GB. Bone Marrow Transplant 2002;29:257–261.
52. Grundmann T, Weerda H. Laryngorhinootologie 1997;76:534–539.
53. Larson TL. Semin Ultrasound CT MR 1999;20: 379–390.
54. Clary RA, Cunningham MJ, Eavey RD. Ann Otol Rhinol Laryngol 1992;101:598–600.
55. Reid JR. Pediatr Radiol 2004;34:933–942.
56. Unlu HH, Aslan A, Goktan C, Egrilmez M. Auris Nasus Larynx 2002;29:69–71.
57. Nawashiro H, Shimizu A, Shima K, Chigasaki H, Kaji T, Doumoto E et al. Neurol Med Chir (Tokyo) 1996;36:808–811.
58. Rochat P, von Buchwald C, Wagner A. Rhinology 2001;39:173–175.
59. Fountas KN, Duwayri Y, Kapsalaki E, Dimopoulos VG, Johnston KW, Peppard SB, et al. South Med J 2004;97:279–282; quiz 283.
60. Younis RT, Anand VK, Davidson B. Laryngoscope 2002;112:224–229.
61. Bolger WE, Butzin CA, Parsons DS. Laryngoscope 1991;101:56–64.
62. Franzese CB, Stringer SP. Am J Rhinol 2004;18: 329–334.
63. Proposed rule. Fed Regist 1998;63:1659–1728.
64. Anzai Y, Jarvik JG, Sullivan SD, Hollingworth W. Am J Rhinol 2007;21:444–451.
65. Balk EM, Zucker DR, Engels EA, Wong JB, Williams JW, Jr., Lau J. J Gen Intern Med 2001;16:701–711.
66. Senbil N, Gurer YK, Uner C, Barut Y. J Headache Pain 2008;9:33–36.
67. Triulzi F, Zirpoli S. Pediatr Allergy Immunol 2007;18(suppl 18):46–49.
68. Lee HS, Majima Y, Sakakura Y, Inagaki M, Sugiyama Y, Nakamoto S. Nippon Jibiinkoka Gakkai Kaiho 1991;94:1250–1256.
69. Bhattacharyya N, Jones DT, Hill M, Shapiro NL. Arch Otolaryngol Head Neck Surg 2004;130: 1029–1032.
70. Cotter CS, Stringer S, Rust KR, Mancuso A. Int J Pediatr Otorhinolaryngol 1999;50:63–68.
71. Al-Qudah M. Int J Pediatr Otorhinolaryngol 2008;72:817–821.
72. Anzai Y, Weymuller EA, Jr., Yueh B, Maronian N, Jarvik JG. Arch Otolaryngol Head Neck Surg 2004;130:423–428.
73. Daele JJ. Acta Otorhinolaryngol Belg 1997;51: 285–304.
74. Lieu JE, Piccirillo JF, Lusk RP. Otolaryngol Head Neck Surg 2003;129:222–232.
75. Adappa ND, Coticchia JM. Am J Otolaryngol 2006;27:384–389.
76. DelGaudio JM, Swain RE, Jr., Kingdom TT, Muller S, Hudgins PA. Arch Otolaryngol Head Neck Surg 2003;129:236–240.
77. Nadkarni T, Goel A. J Postgrad Med 2005;51 (suppl 1):S37–41.
78. Hagtvedt T, Aalokken TM, Notthellen J, Kolbenstvedt A. Eur Radiol 2003;13: 976–980.

Part IV
Musculoskeletal Imaging

17

Imaging of Acute Hematogenous Osteomyelitis and Septic Arthritis in Children and Adults

John Y. Kim and Diego Jaramillo

Issues

  I. What are the clinical findings that raise the suspicion for acute hematogenous osteomyelitis and septic arthritis to direct further imaging?
 II. What is the diagnostic performance of the different imaging studies in acute hematogenous osteomyelitis and septic arthritis?
III. What is the natural history of osteomyelitis and septic arthritis, and what are the roles of medical therapy versus surgical treatment?
 IV. Is there a role for repeat imaging in the management?
  V. What is the diagnostic performance of imaging of osteomyelitis and septic arthritis in the adult?
 VI. What are the roles of the difference imaging modalities in the evaluation of acute osteomyelitis and septic arthritis?

Key Points

- The clinical presentation of acute osteomyelitis and septic arthritis can be nonspecific and sometimes confusing (moderate evidence).
- When signs and symptoms cannot be localized, bone scintigraphy is preferred over magnetic resonance imaging (MRI) (moderate evidence).
- When signs and symptoms can be localized, MRI is preferred (moderate to limited evidence).
- Ultrasound is the preferred imaging modality for evaluating joint effusions of the hip (moderate evidence).
- Magnetic resonance imaging is highly sensitive for the detection of osteomyelitis and its complications (abscess), but incurs added cost (moderate evidence).
- No data were found in the medical literature that evaluate the cost-effectiveness of the different imaging modalities in the evaluation of hematogenous osteomyelitis and septic joint (limited evidence).

J.Y. Kim (✉)
Department of Radiology, Texas Health Presbyterian Hospital of Plano, Plano, TX 75093, USA
e-mail: Johnny.young.kim@gmail.com

L.S. Medina et al. (eds.), *Evidence-Based Imaging: Improving the Quality of Imaging in Patient Care, Revised Edition*,   297
DOI 10.1007/978-1-4419-7777-9_17, © Springer Science+Business Media, LLC 2011

> ■ Overall, MRI is the imaging modality of choice to evaluate for osteo-myelitis and septic arthritis in the adult population, including the diabetic patient and intravenous drug users. The ability to localize symptoms and the inherent high spatial resolution allows exact anatomic detail that may be helpful for surgical planning (limited to moderate evidence).

Definition and Pathophysiology

Osteomyelitis is an infection of bone and bone marrow. Routes of infection include hematogenous spread, spread by contiguity, and direct infection by a penetrating wound (1). Hematogenous spread is the most common route in children, usually seeding the metaphyses of long bones due to sluggish blood flow patterns in this region (2, 3). It arises in the setting of bacteremia. In children, the capillaries in the metaphyses are the terminal branches of the nutrient artery. The capillaries form loops that end in large venous sinusoids where there is decreased blood flow. The inflammatory response to infection leads to increased intraosseous pressure and stasis of blood flow, causing thrombosis and eventual bone necrosis (4). In children <18 months of age, transphyseal vessels allow metaphyseal infections to cross the physis and infect the epiphyses and joints. The most common bones affected by acute hematogenous osteomyelitis (AHO) are the tibia and femur (3); the most common organism is *Staphylococcus aureus*.

Acute septic arthritis is a bacterial infection of a joint. Most cases arise from hematogenous spread or contiguous spread from adjacent osteomyelitis in the metaphysis or epiphysis (5–7). The most common organism is *S. aureus* (3). The prognosis worsens with increasing delay of treatment due to lytic enzymes that destroy the articular and epiphyseal cartilage. In addition, increased pressure within the joint capsule reduces blood flow to the epiphyses. This can lead to long-term disability resulting from growth disturbances, dislocations, and mala-lignment (8, 9).

There is evidence that acute osteomyelitis and septic arthritis are a spectrum of the same disease process (moderate evidence) (10). This hypothesis argues for a similar clinical approach and treatment for these two diseases.

The pattern of hematogenous spread of osteomyelitis and septic arthritis in the adult is different from the pediatric population. The unique vascular supply in the metaphysis normally seen in children is no longer present in adults, and most hematogenous infections arise in the diaphyseal marrow space, similar in pattern to hematogenous metastatic disease to the bone (11). Contiguous spread of infection from adjacent soft tissues is more prevalent in the adults than in children, although hematogenous spread is still more common (12). Contiguous infections can occur in trauma patients with open fractures, in bedridden patients with decubitus ulcers, and in patients with a diabetic foot. Localizing symptoms are more prevalent in the adult population as opposed to the pediatric population, allowing for more dedicated anatomic imaging with MRI, rather than a survey with radionuclide bone scanning.

Epidemiology

The annual incidence of osteomyelitis in children under 13 years of age is 1/5,000 (13). With boys slightly more often affected than girls, fast-growing long bones such as the tibia and femur are the most affected regions. Approximately 25% of cases affect the flat bones including the pelvis. Although a single bone is usually affected, polyostotic involvement has been reported in up to 6.8% of cases in infants and in 22% of neonates (4, 14, 15). The most common organisms are *S. aureus*, followed by β-hemolytic *Streptococcus*, *Streptococcus pneumoniae*, *Escherichia coli*, and *Pseudomonas aeruginosa* (3, 16). Clinical presentation can be confusing, and many laboratory findings such as elevated sedimentation rate may be sensitive but not specific. Serial blood cultures are only positive in 32–60% of cases (1, 17, 18). Infections in infants and neonates are usually clinically silent, and toddlers may present with limping, pseudoparalysis, or pain on passive movement (19).

Half of the cases of septic arthritis occur in children <3 years of age (20). Approximately, 53% are isolated cases of septic arthritis and 47% are cases of septic arthritis associated with osteomyelitis (21). Conversely, 30% of patients with osteomyelitis have adjacent septic arthritis (22). Boys are slightly more affected than girls (1.2:1), and the hip is the most affected joint (23). The most common symptoms are pain, fever, refusal to bear weight, and joint swelling. Most cases involve a single joint, although up to 15% of cases can affect multiple joints. Mortality rates of up to 7% have been reported (21). Similar organisms to those in osteomyelitis are found in septic arthritis, including *S. aureus* and *S. pneumoniae* (21, 24). The most common sequelae of septic arthritis include joint instability, joint function limitation, and limb shortening (25).

Overall Cost to Society

No data were found in the medical literature on the overall cost to society from the diagnosis, treatment, and complications of AHO or septic arthritis. Although there are several cost-effectiveness analyses evaluating the type, extent, and route of antibiotic administration in the treatment of osteomyelitis and septic arthritis, no cost-effectiveness data were found in the literature specifically incorporating imaging strategies in the management of AHO or septic arthritis.

Goals

In AHO and septic arthritis, the goal is early diagnosis and treatment to prevent the long-term sequelae of these diseases, which include growth disturbances, joint instability, chronic infection, malalignment, and limb deformity. The standard treatments include intravenous antibiotics and/or surgical debridement. Septic arthritis usually requires surgical therapy in order to decompress the intraarticular pressure. Surgical debridement may be necessary for osteomyelitis if frank pus can be aspirated from the bone, if there is necrotic bone present, or if there is failure to respond to antibiotic therapy (15, 26).

Methodology

The authors performed a Medline search using PubMed (National Library of Medicine, Bethesda, Maryland) for data relevant to the diagnostic performance and accuracy of both clinical and radiographic examination of patients with AHO and septic arthritis. The diagnostic performance of the clinical examination (history and physical exam) and surgical outcome was based on a systematic literature review performed for the years 1966–2004. The clinical examination search strategy used the following terms: (1) *acute hematogenous osteomyelitis*, (2) *septic arthritis*, (3) *pediatric*, (4) *children*, (5) *clinical examination*, (6) *epidemiology* or *physical examination* or *surgery*, and (7) *treatment* or *surgery*. The review of the diagnostic imaging literature was done for the same years. The search strategy used the following key words: (1) *acute hematogenous osteomyelitis*, (2) *septic arthritis*, (3) *magnetic resonance imaging* or *MRI*, (4) *bone scan*, (5) *ultrasound*, and (6) *imaging*, as well as combinations of these search strings. We excluded animal studies and non-English-language articles.

I. What Are the Clinical Findings that Raise the Suspicion for Acute Hematogenous Osteomyelitis and Septic Arthritis to Direct Further Imaging?

Summary of Evidence: The clinical presentation of AHO and septic arthritis can be confusing and nonspecific in the pediatric population. No single clinical finding in isolation leads to the diagnosis of osteomyelitis or septic arthritis. Repeat high-resolution imaging may be required to determine the need for surgical debridement, including extension into soft tissues or complications that are not amenable to systemic antibiotic therapy (limited evidence).

Supporting Evidence: Standard laboratory tests such as elevated sedimentation rate can be nonspecific or even normal (19) (limited evidence). Serial blood cultures are reported to be positive in 32–60% of cases (1, 17, 18) (moderate and limited evidence). Occasionally, direct aspiration of bone material may be needed for diagnosis.

These aspirations can yield positive cultures in 87% of cases (27) (limited evidence).

The clinical presentation in the pediatric age group can be nonspecific. Infection in the neonate and infant is usually clinically silent. Toddlers can present with limping, pseudoparalysis, or pain on passive movement (4, 28) (moderate to limited evidence).

Due to similarities in pathogenesis, there is also overlap in the clinical presentation of septic arthritis and osteomyelitis. Irritability, limping, or refusal to bear weight, along with elevated sedimentation rate or leukocytosis are the most common presentations (15, 23, 24, 29, 30) (moderate to limited evidence). Kocher et al. (30) proposed probabilities for the presence of septic arthritis in the hip in order to guide further imaging and joint aspiration based on four clinical variables. These four predictors were leukocytosis >12,000/mL, fever, inability to bear weight, and erythrocyte sedimentation rate (ESR) >40 mm/h. If none of these predictors were present, there was a 0.2% chance of septic arthritis. The predicted probability of septic arthritis with one predictor was 3, 40% with two predictors, 93.1% with three predictors, and 99.6% with four predictors. This constellation of clinical findings was most suggestive of osteomyelitis or septic arthritis and warranted further evaluation with imaging (moderate to limited evidence).

II. What Is the Diagnostic Performance of the Different Imaging Studies in Acute Hematogenous Osteomyelitis and Septic Arthritis?

Summary of Evidence: Although plain radiographs are neither sensitive nor specific, their low cost, ready availability, and ability to exclude other diseases that can produce similar symptoms (fractures, tumors) argue for their continued use as the initial evaluation (moderate to limited evidence) (31–35).

Several studies have shown that MRI and radionuclide bone scintigraphy have high sensitivity for detection of osteomyelitis (moderate evidence). Their relative merits have not been established. Bone scintigraphy has the advantage of whole-body imaging when symptoms cannot be localized, but has decreased specificity. This is especially true in the presence of superimposed disease processes such as a joint under pressure, or underlying bone diseases such as sickle cell or Gaucher's disease (moderate to limited evidence) (36–43).

Magnetic resonance imaging has the advantage of higher specificity and higher resolution to evaluate for soft tissue extension or complications, but has limited coverage of the body. This can be a disadvantage if symptoms cannot be localized or if there is polyostotic involvement (moderate to limited evidence).

Ultrasound is highly sensitive for the detection of a joint effusion, but not specific for the presence of infection. Based on the clinical predictors proposed by Kocher et al. (30), a decision to aspirate an effusion can be reliably made to exclude septic arthritis (moderate evidence) (44).

Supporting Evidence: Initial radiographs can detect deep soft tissue swelling and loss of soft tissue planes as early as 48 h after onset of symptoms, but bone destruction is usually not detectable until 7–10 days after onset of symptoms (45). At least 30% of bone destruction is required before osteomyelitis becomes radiographically apparent (2). The sensitivity and specificity of plain radiographs are 43–75% and 75–83%, respectively (limited evidence) (32, 46, 47). If bone destruction is detected, however, no further imaging may be necessary. In addition, radiographs can detect other pathologies such as fractures and tumors that can clinically mimic osteomyelitis (moderate to limited evidence) (31–35, 48).

The overall sensitivity and specificity for radionuclide bone scanning are 73–100% and 73–79% (moderate evidence) (36, 41, 49–53). In the neonate, however, the sensitivity of radionuclide bone scanning is decreased, ranging from 53 to 87% (54, 55). Advantages of bone scintigraphy include the ability to image the entire body, delayed imaging with a single administration of tracer, and less sedation requirements. The ability to image the entire skeleton is ideal if symptoms cannot be localized or if there is polyostotic disease (limited to weak evidence) (33, 51, 52, 56).

The sensitivity and specificity for MRI are 82–100% and 75–96% (moderate evidence) (33, 57–64). MRI has the advantage of both high sensitivity and specificity. It can also display high-resolution images and evaluate for complications such as abscesses, joint effusions, and soft tissue extension that would require surgical intervention (63, 65, 66). The disadvantages include slighter higher cost relative to bone scintigraphy; prolonged imaging times, which may require sedation; and limited coverage.

Ultrasound is highly sensitive for the evaluation of joint effusions and can detect as little as 5–10 cc of fluid within a joint (67). However, no ultrasound characteristics, including complexity of the fluid, the quantity of fluid, or adjacent hyperemia on color Doppler imaging, have been shown to be definitive in distinguishing septic arthritis from other noninfectious causes of joint effusions (68–71). Despite this limitation, the absence of fluid by ultrasound can be very helpful as septic arthritis is very unlikely in this setting (33, 71, 72). As outlined above, Kocher et al. (30) have provided clinical guidelines to direct joint aspiration. These include fever, the presence of elevated white count, an elevated sedimentation rate, and inability to bear weight (moderate evidence).

immediately. Patients are admitted for initiation of systemic antibiotic therapy. Average length of stay ranges from 3 to 7 days (16, 24, 74). Average course of systemic antibiotic therapy is approximately 11–14 days with an additional 4 weeks of outpatient oral antibiotic therapy (5, 7, 16, 75). Many of the clinical signs and symptoms improve within 48 h of initiation of systemic antibiotics, which is a reassuring sign. If there is no clinical improvement, further evaluation including imaging may be required to exclude complications not amenable to antibiotics alone, such as abscess collections, necrotic tissue, or extension into soft tissues.

Approximately 20–50% of all cases eventually require surgical intervention (28). Up to 10% of patients eventually have long-term sequelae, including growth disturbance, loss of function, malalignment, and deformity (8, 9, 16, 23, 28). Up to 6% of patients eventually have chronic osteomyelitis. There is evidence that a delay in initiation of therapy (>4 days after onset of symptoms), certain infecting organisms (methicillin-resistant *S. aureus*), and age of the patient (<6 months of age) are predictors of bad outcomes (moderate evidence) (3, 7, 16, 73).

III. What Is the Natural History of Osteomyelitis and Septic Arthritis, and What Are the Roles of Medical Therapy Versus Surgical Treatment?

Summary of Evidence: Most uncomplicated cases of osteomyelitis require hospitalization and the institution of systemic intravenous antibiotic therapy. If there is a delay of more than 4 days prior to institution of therapy, there is increased poor outcomes and long-term sequelae (moderate evidence). Approximately 5–10% of cases require surgical intervention after initial antibiotic therapy, and up to 20–50% of all cases eventually require some form of surgery, including reconstruction and repeat debridements.

Approximately 5–10% of all cases have long-term sequelae such as growth disturbance, loss of function, malalignment, and deformity. Approximately 6% of cases develop chronic osteomyelitis (73).

Supporting Evidence: Most cases of acute osteomyelitis and septic arthritis are treated with antibiotics. If frank pus is aspirated from a joint, surgical debridement is required

IV. Is There a Role for Repeat Imaging in the Management?

Summary of Evidence: Most patients respond clinically to systemic antibiotics within 48 h. If there is no clinical response to therapy, repeat imaging should be performed to exclude complications that would require surgical intervention such as abscess collections, extensive soft tissue extension, or necrotic tissue. The performance characteristics of MRI are ideal in this setting (moderate to limited evidence).

Supporting Evidence: Approximately 95–98% of patients respond clinically to antibiotic therapy alone (76). Children usually respond quickly to antibiotics, on average within 48 h. However, approximately 5–10% of patients eventually require surgical intervention (77, 78). These patients require high-resolution imaging to evaluate for surgical disease. The literature supports the use of MRI for evaluation of necrosis, abscess collections, and soft tissue extension (63–65, 79) (moderate evidence to limited evidence). This information can be helpful for the surgeon in planning the surgical approach and method of debridement. There are also some data in the literature suggesting that MRI should be the repeat imaging modality of choice if the site of infection is localized to the spine or pelvis. There is a higher incidence of abscess formation in these deep infections, which would require earlier surgical evaluation and treatment (33, 57, 63, 80).

V. What Is the Diagnostic Performance of Imaging of Osteomyelitis and Septic Arthritis in the Adult?

Summary of Evidence: Overall, MRI appears to be the imaging modality of choice to evaluate for osteomyelitis and septic arthritis in the adult population, including the diabetic patient and intravenous drug users. The ability to localize symptoms and inherent high spatial resolution allows exact anatomic detail that may be helpful for surgical planning (limited to moderate evidence).

Supporting Evidence: Osteomyelitis in the diabetic foot represents a diagnostic challenge both clinically and by imaging. The diabetic foot is prone to infection and suboptimal healing due to the decreased blood supply from diabetic vasculopathy, decreased immune response, and repetitive trauma and abnormal mechanics from diabetic neuropathy (81). Because of these abnormalities, there are baseline abnormal imaging findings of the bones and joints without superimposed infection.

Radiographically, the diabetic foot has many features mimicking infection, including destruction, debris, and subluxation. The diabetic foot can also have abnormal findings without osteomyelitis on three-phase radionuclide bone scan (82). There is some evidence of using both bone scan with methylene diphosphanate (MDP) as well as a white blood cell scan to map out specific areas of infection (82–85) (limited to moderate evidence). Although it has excellent sensitivity and specificity (92 and 97%, respectively), the technique is cumbersome and laborious (83). Its lower resolution relative to MRI also limits the imaging of anatomic detail for surgical planning (86, 87).

Magnetic resonance imaging has both high sensitivity and specificity for evaluating osteomyelitis in the diabetic foot (88–91). Sensitivity ranges from 88 to 92% and specificity ranges from 82 to 100% (85, 90, 92) (moderate evidence). However, the diagnosis is frequently not made based on specific imaging characteristics, but by the location of the abnormality. The neuropathic foot inherently contains signal abnormalities similar to osteomyelitis. Imaging diagnosis is made by identifying signal abnormalities in the bone contiguous and in direct contact with adjacent skin ulcers and known pressure points in the diabetic foot (87).

Hematogenous osteomyelitis and septic arthritis also occurs in intravenous drug users. Many of these infections arise initially in the soft tissues, such as the psoas muscle, with subsequent involvement into the spine or sacroiliac (SI) joint (93, 94). Septic arthritis with osteomyelitis is slightly more common in this population than osteomyelitis alone (95). The plain film is neither sensitive nor specific in commonly involved locations, such as the spine and SI joint. Computed tomography (CT) scan with intravenous contrast material has been shown to be very accurate in the identification of the soft tissue infections and abscesses, but not as accurate in the evaluation of the spinal osteomyelitis/discitis or sacroiliitis (96, 97) (limited to moderate evidence). MRI is superior in evaluating these structures due to its higher contrast, signal-to-noise ratio, and multiplanar imaging.

Ultrasound can still detect joint effusions, but can be technically more difficult due to the larger amount of soft tissue in adults compared to the pediatric population (98, 99). MRI is highly sensitive for the evaluation of septic arthritis (97, 100, 101). Hyperemia and synovitis can also be elucidated with the use of intravenous gadolinium, increasing the accuracy of septic arthritis (102).

VI. What Are the Roles of the Difference Imaging Modalities in the Evaluation of Acute Osteomyelitis and Septic Arthritis?

The decision tree in Fig. 17.1 outlines the role of each imaging modality in the evaluation of suspected osteomyelitis. Table 17.1 summarizes the diagnostic performance of the imaging studies for osteomyelitis in children and adults. The plain radiograph is the initial imaging evaluation due to its relative low cost, rapid acquisition, and ready availability. If there is frank evidence of osteomyelitis on the radiograph, immediate antibiotic therapy can be instituted and further imaging may not be necessary, as up to 80% of patients are successfully treated with antibiotics alone.

If the radiograph is negative for osteomyelitis, and there are no localizing symptoms clinically, radionuclide bone scintigraphy is the next imaging modality, based on its ability to provide whole-body imaging.

If there are localized symptoms, MRI would be a better choice due to higher resolution, more specificity, and ability to immediately evaluate complications.

Repeat imaging with MRI should be considered in all patients who do not improve clinically after 48 h of systemic antibiotic therapy, and to direct management of those who require surgical therapy. In addition, if immediate surgical therapy is planned, such as in cases of infections involving the spine or pelvis, earlier imaging with MRI may be of use.

If symptoms are referable to the hip, an ultrasound should be performed to rapidly evaluate for the presence of an effusion, and also to provide imaging-guided joint aspiration.

Table 17.1 presents the performance characteristics of imaging studies for osteomyelitis in children and adults.

Imaging Case Studies

Case 1

This case shows a young child with fever and limp (Fig. 17.2).

Case 2

This case shows a child with fever (Fig. 17.3).

Case 3

This case shows a teenager with right buttock pain and fever (Fig. 17.4).

Suggested Imaging Protocols

- Plain radiograph: At least two orthogonal views of the body part of interest should be obtained; views of the opposite limb may be useful for comparison to detect subtle changes. Imaging should be performed on all patients suspected of osteomyelitis or septic arthritis to evaluate for destruction, as well as to exclude other pathologies such as tumors or fractures.
- Radionuclide bone scintigraphy: Three-phase radionuclide bone scintigraphy with technetium 99m (Tc-99m)-labeled MDP should be obtained, with planar images during blood flow and soft tissue phases. Planar images of extremities and single photon emission computed tomography (SPECT) images of the axial skeleton during the bone phase should be obtained. This imaging should be used if symptoms are nonlocalizing or if there is a suspicion of polyostotic disease.
- Magnetic resonance imaging: Axial and coronal T1-spin echo, axial and sagittal T2-fast spin echo with fat saturation, coronal short-time inversion recovery, axial and coronal T1 two-dimensional spoiled gradient recalled with fat saturation before and after intravenous gadolinium should be obtained. Imaging should be performed if there are localizing symptoms or if the patient fails to respond to antibiotics within 48 h. Early evaluation with MRI also may be of use if immediate surgery is planned.
- Ultrasound: Linear transducer high-frequency probe (7–12 MHz) imaging should be obtained and compared with that for the opposite joint to assess symmetry. Color or power Doppler assesses for hyperemia. Imaging should be performed to evaluate for joint effusion and joint aspiration. It is most commonly used for the hip joint.

Take Home Tables and Figures

Fig. 17.1–17.4 and Tables 17.1 serve to highlight key recommendations and supporting evidence.

Table 17.1. Diagnostic performance characteristics of imaging studies for osteomyelitis in children and adults

	Sensitivity	Specificity
Plain radiograph (32, 46, 47)	43–75%	75–83%
Radionuclide scintigraphy (36, 41, 49–53)	73–100% (53–87% in infants)	73–79%
MRI (33, 57–64)	82–100%	75–96%

Reprinted with kind permission of Springer Science+Business Media from Kim JY, Jaramillo D. Imaging of Acute Hematogenous Osteomyelitis and Septic Arthritis in Children and Adults. In Medina LS, Blackmore CC (eds): *Evidence-Based Imaging: Optimizing Imaging in Patient Care*. New York: Springer Science+Business Media, 2006.

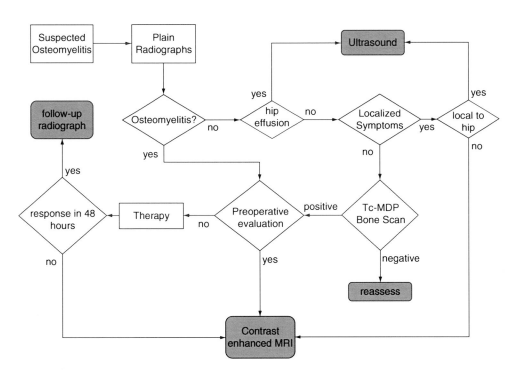

Figure 17.1. Algorithm for imaging suspected osteomyelitis or septic arthritis in the pediatric population. (Reprinted with kind permission of Springer Science+Business Media from Kim JY, Jaramillo D. Imaging of Acute Hematogenous Osteomyelitis and Septic Arthritis in Children and Adults. In Medina LS, Blackmore CC (eds): *Evidence-Based Imaging: Optimizing Imaging in Patient Care*. New York: Springer Science+Business Media, 2006.)

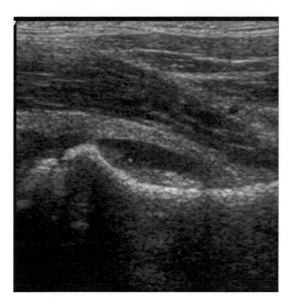

Figure 17.2. Ultrasound depicting hip effusion with synovitis. Frank pus was aspirated from the joint. (Reprinted with kind permission of Springer Science+Business Media from Kim JY, Jaramillo D. Imaging of Acute Hematogenous Osteomyelitis and Septic Arthritis in Children and Adults. In Medina LS, Blackmore CC (eds): *Evidence-Based Imaging: Optimizing Imaging in Patient Care*. New York: Springer Science+Business Media, 2006.)

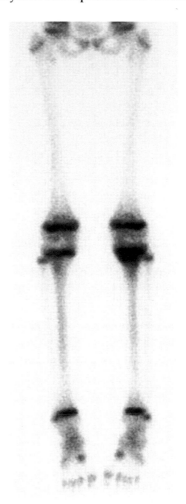

Figure 17.3. Radionuclide bone scan shows abnormal uptake in the proximal left tibial metaphysis that was found to be osteomyelitis. The imaging findings are not specific for osteomyelitis, because neoplasms and trauma could have a similar appearance. (Reprinted with kind permission of Springer Science+Business Media from Kim JY, Jaramillo D. Imaging of Acute Hematogenous Osteomyelitis and Septic Arthritis in Children and Adults. In Medina LS, Blackmore CC (eds): *Evidence-Based Imaging: Optimizing Imaging in Patient Care*. New York: Springer Science+Business Media, 2006.)

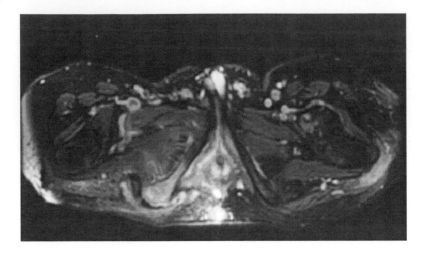

Figure 17.4. Axial MRI of the pelvis after administration of gadolinium shows abnormal enhancement of the right ischial tuberosity and surrounding soft tissues consistent with osteomyelitis. There is also enhancement around the left greater trochanter, consistent with trochanteric bursitis. (Reprinted with kind permission of Springer Science+Business Media from Kim JY, Jaramillo D. Imaging of Acute Hematogenous Osteomyelitis and Septic Arthritis in Children and Adults. In Medina LS, Blackmore CC (eds): *Evidence-Based Imaging: Optimizing Imaging in Patient Care*. New York: Springer Science+Business Media, 2006.)

Future Research

- Can the use of emerging whole-body imaging techniques in MRI obviate the need for radionuclide scintigraphy in the evaluation of osteomyelitis?
- Can MRI with gadolinium provide more information than ultrasound in the evaluation of septic arthritis?
- Can findings on imaging (plain film, MRI, and ultrasound) predict the likelihood of success of medical therapy alone, and provide early triage to surgical therapy?
- Does positron emission tomography have a role in the evaluation of osteomyelitis or septic arthritis?

References

1. Waldvogel FA, Medoff G, Swartz MN. N Engl J Med 1970;282(4):198–206.
2. Faden H, Grossi M. Am J Dis Child 1991; 145(1):65–69.
3. Kao HC et al. J Microbiol Immunol Infect 2003;36(4):260–265.
4. Oudjhane K, Azouz EM. Radiol Clin North Am 2001;39(2):251–266.
5. Barton LL, Dunkle LM, Habib FH. Am J Dis Child 1987;141(8):898–900.
6. Azouz EM, Greenspan A, Marton D. Skeletal Radiol 1993;22(1):17–23.
7. Welkon CJ et al. Pediatr Infect Dis 1986;5(6):669–676.
8. Choi IH et al. J Bone Joint Surg Am 1990;72(8): 1150–1165.
9. Betz RR et al. J Pediatr Orthop 1990;10(3): 365–372.
10. Alderson M et al. J Bone Joint Surg Br 1986;68(2):268–274.
11. Tice AD, Hoaglund PA, Shoultz DA. J Antimicrob Chemother 2003;51(5):1261–1268.
12. Jensen AG et al. J Infect 1997;34(2):113–118.
13. Sonnen GM, Henry NK. Pediatr Clin North Am 1996;43(4):933–947.
14. Asmar BI. Infect Dis Clin North Am 1992;6(1): 117–132.
15. Nelson JD. Infect Dis Clin North Am 1990;4(3): 513–522.
16. Karwowska A, Davies HD, Jadavji T. Pediatr Infect Dis J 1998;17(11):1021–1026.
17. Dormans JP, Drummond DS. J Am Acad Orthop Surg 1994;2(6):333–341.
18. Nixon GW. AJR Am J Roentgenol 1978;130(1): 123–129.
19. Restrepo SC, Gimenez CR, McCarthy K. Rheum Dis Clin North Am 2003;29(1):89–109.
20. Matan AJ, Smith JT. Orthopedics 1997;20(7): 630–635, quiz 636–637.
21. Caksen H et al. Pediatr Int 2000;42(5):534–540.

22. Perlman MH et al. J Pediatr Orthop 2000;20(1): 40–43.
23. Wang CL et al. J Microbiol Immunol Infect 2003;36(1):41–46.
24. Razak M, Nasiruddin J. Med J Malaysia 1998;53(suppl A):86–94.
25. Campagnaro JG et al. Chir Organi Mov 1992;77(3):233–245.
26. Dagan R. Pediatr Infect Dis J 1993;12(1):88–92.
27. Howard CB et al. J Bone Joint Surg Br 1994;76(2):311–314.
28. Razak M, Ismail MM, Omar A. Med J Malaysia 1998;53(suppl A):83–85.
29. Khachatourians AG et al. Clin Orthop 2003;409:186–194.
30. Kocher MS, Zurakowski D, Kasser JR. J Bone Joint Surg Am 1999;81(12):1662–1670.
31. Zucker MI, Yao L. West J Med 1992;156(3): 297–298.
32. Bonakdar-pour A, Gaines VD. Orthop Clin North Am 1983;14(1):21–37.
33. Jaramillo D et al. AJR Am J Roentgenol 1995;165(2):399 403.
34. Gold R. Pediatr Infect Dis J 1995;14(6):555.
35. Fordham L, Auringer ST, Frush DP. J Pediatr 1998;132(5):906–908.
36. Sullivan DC et al. Radiology 1980;135(3):731–736.
37. Wald ER, Mirro R, Gartner JC. Clin Pediatr (Phila) 1980;19(9):597–601.
38. Jones DC, Cady RB. J Bone Joint Surg Br 1981;63B(3):376–378.
39. Berkowitz ID, Wenzel W. Am J Dis Child 1980;134(9):828–830.
40. Handmaker H. Radiology 1980;135(3):787–789.
41. Barron BJ, Dhekne RD. Clin Nucl Med 1984;9(7): 392–393.
42. Park HM, Rothschild PA, Kernek CB. AJR Am J Roentgenol 1985;145(5):1079–1084.
43. Stark JE et al. Radiology 1991;179(3):731–733.
44. Klein DM et al. Clin Orthop 1997;338:153–159.
45. Capitanio MA, Kirkpatrick JA. Am J Roentgenol Radium Ther Nucl Med 1970;108(3):488–496.
46. Kaye JJ. Pediatr Ann 1976;5(1):11–31.
47. Keenan AM, Tindel NL, Alavi A. Arch Intern Med 1989;149(10):2262–2266.
48. Gold R. Pediatr Rev 1991;12(10):292–297.
49. Duszynski DO et al. Radiology 1975;117(2): 337–340.
50. Gelfand MJ, Silberstein EB. JAMA 1977;237(3): 245–247.
51. Hankins JH, Flowers WM Jr. J Miss State Med Assoc 1978;19(1):10–12.
52. Nelson HT, Taylor A. Eur J Nucl Med 1980;5(3):267–269.
53. Erasmie U, Hirsch G. Z Kinderchir 1981;32(4): 360–366.
54. Ash JM, Gilday DL. J Nucl Med 1980;21(5): 417–420.
55. Bressler EL, Conway JJ, Weiss SC. Radiology 1984;152(3):685–688.
56. Handmaker H, Leonards R. Semin Nucl Med 1976;6(1):95–105.
57. Modic MT et al. Radiol Clin North Am 1986;24(2):247–258.
58. Unger E et al. AJR Am J Roentgenol 1988; 150(3):605–610.
59. Morrison WB et al. Radiology 1993;189(1): 251–257.
60. Fletcher BD, Scoles PV, Nelson AD. Radiology 1984;150(1):57–60.
61. Berquist TH et al. Magn Reson Imaging 1985;3(3):219–230.
62. Dangman BC et al. Radiology 1992;182(3): 743–747.
63. Mazur JM et al. J Pediatr Orthop 1995;15(2): 144–147.
64. Umans H, Haramati N, Flusser G. Magn Reson Imaging 2000;18(3):255–262.
65. Connolly LP et al. J Nucl Med 2002;43(10): 1310–1316.
66. Lee SK et al. Radiology 1999;211(2):459–465.
67. Moss SG et al. Radiology 1998;208(1):43–48.
68. Chao HC et al. Acta Paediatr Taiwan 1999; 40(4):268–270.
69. Chao HC et al. J Ultrasound Med 1999;18(11): 729–734, quiz 735–736.
70. Strouse PJ, DiPietro MA, Adler RS. Radiology 1998;206(3):731–735.
71. Zawin JK et al. Radiology 1993;187(2):459–463.
72. Lim-Dunham JE, Ben-Ami TE, Yousefzadeh DK. Pediatr Radiol 1995;25(7):556–559.
73. Espersen F et al. Rev Infect Dis 1991;13(3):347–358.
74. Speiser JC et al. Semin Arthritis Rheum 1985;15(2):132–138.
75. Scott RJ et al. J Pediatr Orthop 1990;10(5). 649–652.
76. Le Saux N et al. BMC Infect Dis 2002;2(1):16.
77. Roine I et al. Clin Infect Dis 1997;24(5):849–853.
78. Dirschl DR. Orthop Rev 1994;23(4):305–312.
79. McAndrew PT, Clark C. Br Med J 1998; 316(7125):147.
80. Middleton MS. AJR Am J Roetgenol 1988;151(3): 612–613.
81. Snyder RJ et al. Ostomy Wound Manage 2001;47(1):18–22, 25–30, quiz 31–32.
82. Unal SN et al. Clin Nucl Med 2001;26(12): 1016–1021.
83. Poirier JY et al. Diabet Metab 2002;28(6 Pt 1): 485–490.
84. Crerand S et al. J Bone Joint Surg Br 1996;78(1): 51–55.
85. Cook TA et al. Br J Surg 1996;83(2):245–248.
86. Sella EJ, Grosser DM. Clin Podiatr Med Surg 2003;20(4):729–740.
87. Schweitzer ME, Morrison WB. Radiol Clin North Am 2004;42(1):61–71, vi.
88. Craig JG et al. Radiology 1997;203(3):849–855.
89. Marcus CD et al. Radiographics 1996;16(6): 1337–1348.

90. Morrison WB et al. Radiology 1995;196(2): 557–564.
91. Ledermann HP, Morrison WB, Schweitzer ME. Radiology 2002;223(3):747–755.
92. Croll SD et al. J Vasc Surg 1996;24(2):266–270.
93. Alcantara AL, Tucker RB, McCarroll KA. Infect Dis Clin North Am 2002;16(3):713–743, ix–x.
94. Kak V, Chandrasekar PH. Infect Dis Clin North Am 2002;16(3):681–695.
95. Chandrasekar PH, Narula AP. Rev Infect Dis 1986;8(6):904–911.
96. Bonham P. J Wound Ostomy Continence Nurs 2001;28(2):73–88.
97. Sturzenbecher A et al. Skeletal Radiol 2000;29(8):439–446.
98. Wingstrand H, Egund N, Forsberg L. J Bone Joint Surg Br 1987;69(2):254–256.
99. Zieger MM, Dorr U, Schulz RD. Skeletal Radiol 1987;16(8):607–611.
100. Karchevsky M et al. AJR Am J Roentgenol 2004;182(1):119–122.
101. Learch TJ, Farooki S. Clin Imaging 2000;24(4): 236–242.
102. Graif M et al. Skeletal Radiol 1999;28(11): 616–620.

18

Imaging for Knee and Shoulder Problems

William Hollingworth, Adrian K. Dixon, and John R. Jenner

Imaging of the Knee

I. What is the role of radiography in patients with an acute knee injury and possible fracture?
   A. Cost-effectiveness analysis
   B. Applicability to children
II. When should magnetic resonance imaging be used for patients with suspected meniscal or ligamentous knee injuries?
   A. Cost-effectiveness analysis
III. Is radiography useful in evaluating the osteoarthritic knee?
IV. Special case: Imaging of the painful prosthesis

Imaging of the Shoulder

V. When is radiography indicated for patients with acute shoulder pain?
VI. Which imaging modalities should be used in the diagnosis of soft tissue disorders of the shoulder?

Issues

■ Knee radiographs of the acutely injured knee in the emergency department are rarely useful for determining therapy except in patients aged 55 or older, or with isolated tenderness of patella, tenderness at the head of fibula, inability to flex the knee 90°, or the inability to bear weight both immediately and in the emergency department for four steps (strong evidence).
■ Magnetic resonance imaging (MRI) is an accurate and valuable diagnostic tool for confirming or excluding the presence of meniscal and cruciate ligamentous knee injuries (moderate evidence). If used

Key Points

W. Hollingworth (✉)
Health Economics, School of Social and Community Medicine, University of Bristol, Bristol BS8 2PS, UK
e-mail: William.hollingworth@bristol.ac.uk

L.S. Medina et al. (eds.), *Evidence-Based Imaging: Improving the Quality of Imaging in Patient Care, Revised Edition*, DOI 10.1007/978-1-4419-7777-9_18, © Springer Science+Business Media, LLC 2011

in selected patients, in whom arthroscopy is probable, but not inevitable, MRI can reduce the overall arthroscopy rate and the number of purely diagnostic arthroscopies (moderate evidence).

- There is currently insufficient evidence to demonstrate that the routine use of radiography in patients with suspected chronic osteoarthritic knee pain will alter management or the outcome of patients. However, radiography is required before making decisions regarding knee replacement surgery.
- The use of radiography to evaluate patients with suspected recurrent atraumatic shoulder dislocation is unnecessary in most cases (limited evidence). Furthermore, selective imaging strategies may be able to rationalize the number of prereduction or postreduction radiographs required in suspected first-time or traumatic shoulder dislocations (limited evidence).
- Ultrasound, MRI, and MR arthrography all have high specificity in the diagnosis of full-thickness rotator cuff tears. Therefore, in populations with a moderate prevalence of rotator cuff tears, a positive result on any one of these tests can confirm the diagnosis with a high degree of certainty (moderate evidence). Until further data are available, the choice between these tests will be largely dependent on physician preference and available resources.

Epidemiology

Approximately 0.3% of the US population seeks medical care for an acute knee injury each year. These injuries are most frequently seen in young males and are usually precipitated by sports (36%); twisting, bending, or stepping motions (27%); or falls (21%) (1). The annual incidence of traumatic anterior shoulder dislocation is less than 0.02%, most commonly observed in young males with sporting injuries (2, 3). Chronic knee and shoulder problems are much more prevalent. One community survey in the United Kingdom found that 19% of adults reported knee pain lasting more than 1 week in the previous month and 16% reported shoulder pain (4). Prevalence in both sexes rose steadily with age, reaching a plateau at about age 65 and was also positively associated with social deprivation. Although the prevalence is high, many people with knee or shoulder pain do not seek medical care (5).

Overall Cost to Society

In the year 2001, knee symptoms and injuries were the primary reason reported by the patients for 1.5 million (1.4%) of all emergency department visits in the USA (6). Furthermore, knee symptoms and injuries led to an estimated 861,000 (1.0%) hospital outpatient department visits and 13.8 million (1.6%) visits to office-based physicians (6, 7). Knee problems, therefore, are in the top 15 most frequent reasons for consulting a physician, second only to back pain among musculoskeletal problems. Medical care visits for shoulder problems are slightly less frequent. In total, shoulder symptoms and injury lead to 1.2 million (1.1%) emergency department visits, 425,000 (0.5%) outpatient visits and 8.9 million (1.0%) of office visits (6, 7).

For knee and shoulder problems seen in outpatient settings, imaging utilization varies greatly by specialty. A study conducted in the USA observed that orthopedic surgeons requested radiography in 80% of first knee pain consultations and 78% of first shoulder pain consultations, whereas rheumatologists utilized radiography in far fewer knee (45%) and shoulder (36%) cases (8). Orthopedic surgeons were also more likely to refer for MRI of the knee (20 versus 6%) and, to a lesser extent, of the shoulder (4 versus 2%). The direct cost of health care for musculoskeletal problems is about 1% of gross national product in several industrialized countries (9), although we found no convincing estimates of the total societal costs for knee and shoulder problems.

Goals

Among patients who seek medical attention for knee and shoulder problems, the clinician's task is to find the appropriate balance between physical examination, diagnostic imaging, and arthroscopic investigation to achieve accurate diagnosis and initiate cost-effective therapy.

Methodology

Our initial search strategy identified systematic literature reviews of knee and shoulder imaging studies. We searched the Medline database using the PubMed interface for abstracts published between January 1966 and March 2004 with the search words *knee* and *shoulder* and the PubMed designation of a systematic review (systematic [sb]). This strategy identified 203 shoulder and 442 knee abstracts. From this group, we selected several key articles reviewing the role of imaging (10–19). We then searched the articles cited by these systematic reviews to identify the relevant primary studies. For topics where no recent systematic review was available, we selected two seminal articles on the topic and searched for similar work using the related articles PubMed function. Where possible, we obtained and reviewed the full text of all relevant English-language articles identified.

I. What Is the Role of Radiography in Patients with an Acute Knee Injury and Possible Fracture?

Summary of Evidence: Acute knee trauma provides a common diagnostic quandary in accident and emergency departments. Fractures are present in 4–12% of patients presenting with knee injuries (20, 21), and yet radiography may be requested in excess of 70% of cases (22). Several guidelines are available to help clinicians target imaging in high-risk patients. There is strong evidence (level I) to suggest that the five criteria of the Ottawa knee rule (OKR) are highly sensitive at predicting fractures in adults and moderate evidence (level II) that this rule can be generalized to children older than 5 years of age. Further work is needed to evaluate the impact of the OKR on the cost-effectiveness of medical care.

Supporting Evidence: Several groups have developed clinical decision rules to guide knee radiography requests following trauma in order to save costs and prevent unnecessary radiation (23–26). These decision rules focus variously on patient age, injury mechanism, inability to ambulate, and other clinical signs such as fibula head tenderness. Table 18.1 provides details of four published decision rules. The optimal threshold for radiography requests depends on the trade-off between the clinical and possible legal consequences of a missed fracture compared to the time, cost, and radiation exposure of radiographs. In practice, all of the decision rules place great emphasis on sensitivity at the expense of specificity.

To date, the OKR (25, 27) has undergone the most extensive validation. Other decision rules may have greater specificity, but they have not yet been validated by independent investigators. The OKR suggests that radiography should be performed on the acutely injured knee when the patient has one or more of the following criteria: (1) age 55 years or older, (2) isolated tenderness of the patella (no other knee bone tenderness), (3) tenderness of the head of the fibula, (4) inability to flex the knee to 90°, or (5) inability to bear weight both immediately and in the emergency department for four steps. Initial assessment of the interobserver reliability of the OKR suggested excellent agreement between physicians (27); however, more recent work evaluating the agreement between nurses and physicians has been less impressive (20, 28, 29). These variable results emphasize the need for thorough training and support for clinicians before implementing the OKR.

A recent systematic review found 11 studies evaluating the diagnostic accuracy of the OKR (10). Six of these studies were suitable for inclusion in a meta-analysis, of which four were considered to be of high quality (i.e., consecutive enrollment, universal reference standard, and radiographic assessment of fracture blind to clinical findings). The mean sensitivity of the OKR in these studies was 98.5% and specificity was 48.6%. While this provides strong evidence (level I) that the OKR is sensitive at predicting fracture, it does not prove that it is a cost-effective method of organizing care.

Based on case series, several authors have speculated that adherence to the OKR would reduce the utilization of knee radiography in the emergency department by between 17 and 49% (25, 27, 30–35). However, these estimates rely on the assumption that clinicians would rigidly follow the OKR and would not be swayed by fears of missed diagnoses or patient expectations of imaging. Only one controlled trial has evaluated whether radiography utilization can be curtailed in practice following the introduction of the OKR (22). Stiell and colleagues (22) enrolled 3,907 patients with isolated knee trauma at four hospitals in a prospective, controlled, before-and-after study. In the hospitals where the OKR was introduced, the absolute rate of radiography requests fell by 20.5%. By comparison, there was a minimal (1%) reduction at the control hospitals; this disparity was statistically significant. Furthermore, patients who were not imaged spent less time in the emergency department and had lower follow-up costs than their counterparts who were referred for radiography. Therefore, there is moderate evidence (level II) that the OKR has a beneficial impact.

A. Cost-Effectiveness Analysis

The same research group has also developed a simple cost-benefit decision model comparing the OKR to usual practice (36). The reduced costs of imaging, follow-up care, and days off from work observed after the implementation of the OKR are balanced against the potential for increased malpractice costs. However, in the primary analysis, the model did not quantify any costs that might result from the delayed recovery of patients with fractures falsely diagnosed as normal. The authors conclude that the introduction of the OKR resulted in a modest ($34) saving per patient, but, due to the high volume of minor knee injuries, the total economic impact is large. Because of the high cost of litigation, especially in the US, these conclusions were dependent on the exact diagnostic sensitivity of the OKR. If the sensitivity of OKR falls more than 1% below that of usual practice, the conclusions are reversed. Until a broader body of research is available comparing the sensitivity and specificity of OKR to usual practice, we consider that there is limited evidence (level III) to support the hypothesis that the OKR is cost-effective in emergency departments.

In many cases plain radiography is all that is required to allow the clinician to proceed with conservative therapy. If a fracture is seen, there is increasing use of computed tomography (CT) or MRI to determine whether structures such as the tibial plateau are depressed to an extent that warrants surgical elevation. Because there are anecdotal accounts of CT and MRI identifying fractures when plain radiographs are normal, some clinicians seek reassurance from CT/MRI in equivocal cases. Different clinicians have different thresholds for this need for reassurance, and there is little evidence to help in making such decisions. Even when plain radiographs show subtle tibial plateau depression and CT in the coronal or sagittal plane shows 2- to 5-mm depression, clinicians vary in their subsequent management decisions; some may proceed with surgical elevation and some may not. The evidence that patients with a 4-mm depression do significantly better with surgery than without is also scant. However, with increasingly noninvasive techniques now on offer, there is a trend toward more imaging being used as a roadmap for intervention.

B. Applicability to Children

The diagnostic performance of the OKR may be altered in the skeletally immature knee due to open growth plates and secondary ossification centers resulting in different injury patterns (37). Additionally, tests such as weight bearing, which rely on considerable patient interaction, may not be as valid in the youngest children. Two case series have studied the applicability of the OKR to children (30, 32). In the largest study involving 750 children aged 2–16, Bulloch et al. (30) found that the OKR was 100% sensitive [95% confidence interval (CI), 94.9–100%] in predicting the 70 fractures observed and 43% specific (95% CI, 39.1–46.5%). Due to the small numbers of children in the youngest age category, these authors endorsed the OKR in children 5 years of age or over. In a smaller study conducted by Khine et al. (32), the OKR correctly predicted 12 of 13 fractures observed in 234 children aged 2–18 years. The one missed injury was a non-displaced fracture of the proximal tibia in an 8-year-old. In totality, the similarity between these two studies and evaluations conducted in adults provide reassurance that the OKR is valid in children (level II, moderate evidence). However, there is not yet sufficient evidence to demonstrate the cost-effectiveness of the OKR in children.

II. When Should Magnetic Resonance Imaging Be Used for Patients with Suspected Meniscal or Ligamentous Knee Injuries?

Summary of Evidence: Empirical work demonstrates that the utilization of knee MRI among Medicare and Medicaid enrollees increased rapidly by 140% in the early 1990s (38). There is limited evidence (level III) to support the theory that, for some patients, a composite clinical examination performed by an experienced musculoskeletal specialist can bypass the need for MRI by directly identifying patients with cruciate or meniscal injuries amenable to arthroscopic repair. However, there is also moderate evidence (level II) that MRI is a highly accurate method of diagnosing soft tissue knee injuries in patients where the clinical picture is not clear. If MRI is used in patients likely to undergo arthroscopy, there is moderate evidence (level II) indicating that it can substantially reduce the overall arthroscopy rate and limit the number of purely diagnostic arthroscopies without detriment to the patient's quality of life.

Supporting Evidence: The mechanism of injury, clinical history, and physical examination can provide important information on the likelihood of injuries to the menisci and ligaments of the knee. Indeed, some authorities have observed that, with sufficiently experienced clinicians, these methods have high diagnostic accuracy and might render the use of imaging unnecessary prior to arthroscopy in many cases (39, 40). Conversely, others have argued that MRI is an essential component of the presurgical assessment, which saves money and reduces referrals for purely diagnostic arthroscopy (41, 42).

Four systematic reviews have summarized the diagnostic accuracy of the physical examination for suspected injury to the cruciate ligaments and the menisci (11–14). Each review notes that most diagnostic accuracy studies interpret the reference standard, usually arthroscopy, without masking the surgeon to the findings of the physical examination and

that, as in many clinical studies, verification bias (patients with abnormal physical tests were more likely to undergo the reference standard) was often present. These biases tend to artificially enhance sensitivity estimates.

Two reviews (11, 12) included studies that reported data on composite clinical examinations without specifying the precise examination maneuvers that were used. In general, these composite examinations resulted in reasonable sensitivity and specificity for anterior cruciate ligament (82 and 94%, respectively), posterior cruciate ligament (91 and 98%), and meniscal (77 and 91%) injuries (12). However, it is very difficult to replicate or generalize these findings given the lack of detail about the individual components of the examination.

To date, the majority of studies have been conducted by musculoskeletal specialists skilled in physical examination techniques. Therefore, these methods may be less accurate if applied in primary care. Given the inevitable methodologic flaws in many of these studies, we conclude that there is limited evidence (level III) that the clinical examination can accurately select patients most likely to benefit from therapeutic arthroscopy. More high-quality studies of individual physical tests are urgently required.

The rise in MRI utilization is probably due to increased availability of equipment and reluctance on the part of physicians to rely solely on the clinical examination to determine treatment. Furthermore, some legal judgments have criticized surgeons for operating without full information about the extent of the lesion(s). However, overreliance on advanced imaging technology might be counterproductive if MRI is not sufficiently accurate. In particular, age-related degeneration of the menisci might lead to false-positive MRI findings and unnecessary surgery (43).

Demographic aspects also play a part: there may be much more reason for a professional athlete to undergo soft tissue imaging in the acute phase compared with a middle-aged sedentary person (Fig. 18.1). The advice for the athlete may be merely to train or not to train. Few surgeons relish intervening in the acute phase when there is a lot of hemorrhage still masking the operative field. Although MRI may show many unexpected lesions in the acute phase, the immediate clinical management of the patient rarely changes (44).

We identified four reviews summarizing the accuracy of MRI compared to arthroscopy for soft tissue knee injuries (11, 15, 16, 45). All reviewed a wealth of evidence, albeit from methodologically weak studies in many instances. The most recent review identified 29 studies conducted between 1991 and 2000 (15). Of these studies, only four (14%) had adequate blinding of the index test (MRI) when conducting arthroscopy, the reference standard. In addition only ten (34%) studies clearly avoided verification bias. The pooled weighted sensitivity and specificity estimates from this review are reported in Table 18.2. The results suggest that the sensitivity of MRI is consistently lower in lateral meniscal tears than medial meniscal and cruciate injuries; conversely, specificity is higher. One explanation for this finding is that radiologists may have a lower threshold for reporting medial meniscal tears as opposed to lateral tears. Overall, there is moderate evidence (level II) that MRI of the knee is a highly accurate method of diagnosing soft tissue knee injuries. In actuality the accuracy of MRI might be higher than the figures indicated in Table 18.2. It is recognized that, while arthroscopy is the only viable reference standard, in particular regions of the knee, such as the posterior horn of the medial meniscus, the arthroscopic diagnosis is imperfect, often relying on probing rather than direct visualization of lesions (Fig. 18.2) (46).

Several observational studies have gone beyond the intermediate outcome of diagnostic accuracy to examine whether MRI can decrease the rate of arthroscopy (42, 47–53). The estimated reduction in arthroscopy following MRI varies widely. This lack of consensus is not surprising given the range of primary and secondary care settings examined, and varying definitions of what constitutes a purely diagnostic arthroscopy. In perhaps the most detailed study, Vincken et al. (52) performed MRI on 430 consecutive patients who underwent a standardized physical examination performed by an orthopedic surgeon and met a priori criteria for arthroscopic surgery. The MRI results indicated that no arthroscopy was required in 209 (49%) patients. Of these patients with negative MRI findings, 93 were randomly selected and received immediate arthroscopy. Ninety-one percent (85/93) of arthroscopies subsequently performed in these patients were purely diagnostic (86%) or had a minor therapeutic procedure (5%) on a lesion that, according to the study protocol, did not require surgical intervention. The remaining 9% (8/93) of negative MRI findings were genuine false negatives overlooking clinically important lesions. Most patients (200/221) with positive MRI findings had subsequent arthroscopy; only 11% (21/200) of these had a purely diagnostic arthroscopy. Based on the large proportion of diagnostic arthroscopies that could have been avoided, these authors concluded that a combination of a clinical examination and MRI was useful in selecting patients for arthroscopy.

A. Cost-Effectiveness Analysis

Two small randomized trials have analyzed the impact of knee MRI on costs and patient quality of life. Both trials were conducted by the same research team (17). The first trial recruited patients attending orthopedic outpatient clinics for whom arthroscopy was contemplated; 118 patients were randomly allocated to MRI or no-MRI prior to the decision to perform arthroscopy. Over the 12 months after randomization, the proportion of patients receiving arthroscopy was statistically significantly lower among patients who were referred for MRI (41% MRI arm versus 71% in the no-MRI arm). This equated to a sizable reduction in surgery costs, but these savings were almost exactly canceled out by the additional costs of the MRI examination itself. This trial found no significant difference in patient quality of life 12 months after randomization, although interpretation is seriously limited by a low response rate.

The second randomized trial recruited patients from a specialist knee clinic assessing patients referred from a hospital emergency department. A total of 120 patients were recruited, all of whom received an MRI examination of the knee. However, in the no-MRI arm of the trial, the imaging results were withheld from patients and clinicians for at least 6 weeks. Unlike the first trial, the arthroscopy rate during 1 year of follow-up was low and was not significantly affected by the availability of MRI findings (30% MRI arm, 24% no-MRI arm). Therefore, in this setting, MRI did not prevent surgery and increased costs. Again, there was no statistically significant effect on patient quality of life at 12 months.

These two trials demonstrate the complexity of judging the cost-effectiveness of MRI for internal derangement of the knee. Routine MRI is not likely to be cost-effective in patients with a low prevalence of soft tissue injuries who are unlikely to receive arthroscopy; this situation might exist in primary care settings (11). Likewise, MRI may not be cost-effective in a subset of patients referred to musculoskeletal specialists who have clear-cut clinical signs of soft tissue injury with a very high probability of requiring therapeutic arthroscopy. However, there is moderate evidence (level II) that MRI can reduce the need for surgery, without increasing costs in many patients who have an intermediate probability of soft tissue injury. The exact threshold at which MRI becomes cost-effective depends on the relative costs of MRI and arthroscopy and the relative scarcity of imaging facilities and musculoskeletal specialists (54–56).

III. Is Radiography Useful in Evaluating the Osteoarthritic Knee?

Summary of Evidence: Radiography is frequently used to assess the extent of disease in the osteoarthritic knee. However, there is poor correlation between imaging findings and patient symptoms. Furthermore, there is currently insufficient evidence (level IV) to support the hypothesis that routine use of radiography in patients with chronic knee pain will improve patient management and quality of life.

Supporting Evidence: For patients with knee pain and locking, the plain radiograph is often regarded as the key investigation to establish the diagnosis and identify/exclude radiopaque loose bodies that may be amenable to arthroscopic removal (57). For patients with chronic knee pain without locking or restriction of movement, the role of radiography is poorly defined. More than 40% of adults aged 40–80 years have radiographic evidence of knee osteophytes or joint space narrowing despite reporting no knee pain within the last year (58). Furthermore, a substantial minority (≈35%) of adults in the same age range who do report persistent knee pain have no osteophytes or joint space narrowing on radiography (58), although this proportion diminishes in patients

with severely disabling pain (59). Longitudinal studies have also highlighted the weak correlation between radiographic and symptomatic changes over time (60). Therefore, basing management decisions purely on radiographic anomalies risks targeting treatment on innocuous anatomical factors that are not the cause of the patient's joint pain. Despite this, there is evidence that physicians place more emphasis on radiographic rather than clinical signs of osteoarthritis when deciding on the need for an orthopedic referral (61).

In one review of 1,153 knee radiographs requested by primary care physicians, most imaging reports (59%) described normal anatomy or degenerative changes (29%) (62). In 20% of patients radiography was used to bolster the case for, or against, referral to a specialist. Other important changes in therapy based on radiography findings were observed in only 3% of cases (62).

In the U.K., the Royal College of Radiologists guidelines recommend that radiography for knee pain without locking or restriction of movement is only indicated in specific circumstances, such as when considering surgery (63). Still, many primary care physicians feel that radiographs are necessary in order to reassure patients, to justify a specialist referral, or for other nondiagnostic reasons (59, 61). Therefore, continued use of radiography for patients with chronic knee pain seems inevitable. However, trial data have demonstrated that radiography requests can be reduced by regular educational messages reminding physicians of the limited value of radiography in this setting (64, 65).

IV. Special Case: Imaging of the Painful Prosthesis

The potentially infected knee prosthesis is a case where the evidence for the various imaging investigations is rather weak. The patient presents with pain and perhaps instability some months/years after a successful knee replacement. Plain radiography of the total extent of the prosthesis (including the femoral and tibial tips) is performed; interpretation is easier if these images can be compared with those obtained at the postoperative stage, if available; lucency around the stem of the prosthesis may be associated with loosening or infection. Despite software developments to reduce artifacts from the metallic prosthesis, neither CT nor MRI can offer much here. Skeletal scintigraphy can provide evidence of abnormal osteoblastic activity around the prosthesis, which should be more intense in relation to infection than loosening; some centers proceed to white cell scintigraphy, which may help in this distinction. Other centers use arthrography, which may provide a microbiologic sample if there is a large effusion. In any event, there is a wide range of sensitivities and specificities in these tests. Interpretation is also complex because the investigations are often spread out over several weeks. Furthermore there is frequently no gold standard, as the ultimate arbiter, the decision to perform revision surgery, is not undertaken lightly and is ultimately still based on clinical rather than radiologic grounds. At present, there is insufficient evidence (level IV) to recommend any particular imaging approach.

V. When Is Radiography Indicated for Patients with Acute Shoulder Pain?

Summary of Evidence: Conventional teaching advocates both pre- and postreduction radiographs for patients with clinically suspected shoulder dislocation, and survey data confirm that many hospitals follow this recommendation (66). However, more recent research has provided limited evidence (level III) that radiographs are not necessary in most patients with recurrent atraumatic dislocation. Furthermore, there is limited evidence (level III) that the prereduction radiograph may be omitted in traumatic joint dislocations provided that the clinician is confident of the diagnosis. An alternative approach that eliminates the postreduction radiograph in patients with prereduction radiographs demonstrating dislocation and no fracture is also supported by limited evidence (level III). Limited evidence also suggests that, in patients without obvious shoulder deformity, radiography should be targeted at those with bruising or joint swelling, or with a history of fall, pain at rest, or abnormal range of motion. However, more research is needed to validate these guidelines and to provide head-to-head comparisons of selective imaging strategies to demonstrate the relative feasibility and cost-effectiveness of implementation.

Supporting Evidence: Imaging is commonly requested following shoulder trauma. The questions posed differ according to the nature of the injury and the age of the patient. In the elderly, a fracture of the surgical neck of humerus is common after a fall. In the younger patient the clinician may be more worried about possible dislocation, especially in those with recurrent episodes where the chance of recurrent dislocation is high. It is in this precise group of young patients that ionizing radiation should be kept as low as reasonably achievable and requests for imaging kept to a minimum.

A retrospective study conducted in a North American medical center found that radiographs were performed in 59% of emergency department patients with shoulder pain (67). Twenty percent of these radiographs provided therapeutically important information (defined as glenohumeral dislocation, fracture, severe acromioclavicular joint separation, infection, or malignancy).

Hendey (68) has demonstrated that, for patients with suspected recurrent relatively atraumatic dislocation, physicians were certain of the dislocation in more than 90% of cases. In every case this preimaging confidence was justified by radiographic evidence of dislocation without fracture. After reduction of these atraumatic dislocations, physicians were also confident that relocation had been achieved in more than 90% of patients; again this was subsequently radiographically confirmed in all cases. Although this work requires validation, it does provide limited evidence (level III) that radiographs are not routinely indicated in this well-defined recurrent dislocation population.

Opinions differ for suspected traumatic or first-time dislocations. Some have suggested that many postreduction radiographs are not diagnostically or therapeutically useful when the prereduction radiograph demonstrates dislocation without fracture (68–70). In 53 patients with simple dislocation and clinically successful relocation, Hendey reported that all postreduction radiographs confirmed the reduction and found no unsuspected fractures. Others have argued that it is more practical to eliminate the prereduction radiograph when the physician is certain of the clinical diagnosis of dislocation (71). Omitting the prereduction radiograph enables prompt joint relocation, which would, in any case, be the preferred management even if Hill-Sachs lesions, Bankart lesions, or greater tuberosity fractures are later demonstrated on the postreduction radiograph. Shuster et al. (71) estimated that eliminating the prereduction radiograph would remove approximately 30 min from the delay between presentation and reduction.

Either of the strategies described above will significantly reduce radiograph utilization at centers that routinely image pre- and postreduction. There is currently insufficient evidence (level IV) to definitively choose between these selective imaging strategies; both have potential drawbacks. In high-energy injury mechanisms, omitting the prereduction radiograph risks an iatrogenic displacement of an unrecognized fracture of the humeral neck during the attempted reduction (72). Conversely, some physicians are reluctant to eliminate the postreduction radiograph for fear of missing a fracture not evident on initial imaging or overlooking a failed reduction (71).

In patients without obvious bone deformity on initial clinical examination, Fraenkel et al. (73) report that only 12% of shoulder radiographs are therapeutically informative (i.e., demonstrating acute fracture, severe acromioclavicular joint separation, dislocation, infection, or malignancy). In a prospective study involving 206 radiographs, they identified two higher-risk patient groups in which radiographs were most likely to be informative: (1) patients with bruising or joint swelling on examination; and (2) patients with a history of fall, pain at rest, or abnormal range of joint motion. In these two groups 32% of radiographs were therapeutically informative. Only one therapeutically informative radiograph, in a patient with a lytic lesion with known multiple myeloma, would have been missed by a strategy limiting radiography to these two groups. Therefore, the authors advise imaging for all patients with a history of cancer that might involve bone. This prediction rule requires external validation and currently provides no more than preliminary and limited evidence (level III) that some emergency department radiographs on painful shoulders could be avoided by careful patient selection.

VI. Which Imaging Modalities Should Be Used in the Diagnosis of Soft Tissue Disorders of the Shoulder?

Summary of Evidence: There is moderate evidence (level II) that both MRI and ultrasound have fairly high sensitivity (>85%) and specificity (>90%) in the diagnosis of full-thickness rotator cuff (RC) tears, and therefore a positive test result is likely to be useful for confirming tears in patients for whom surgery is being considered. The results of ultrasound studies were more variable perhaps reflecting the operator-dependent nature of the technique. The few studies conducted on the accuracy of MR arthrography (MRA) suggest that it may be more accurate than either MRI or ultrasound; however, more data are needed to reinforce the limited evidence (level III) to date. Until these data are available, the choice between ultrasound and MR techniques is likely to be primarily based on physician preference and the availability of imaging equipment and personnel. The sensitivity of all three of these minimally invasive tests for partial-thickness RC tears is relatively poor. This may be due in part to the poorly defined diagnostic criteria for these more subtle lesions. Several studies including a randomized trial have provided strong evidence (level I) that MRI can influence the management of patients with shoulder pain. However, there is insufficient evidence (level IV) demonstrating an eventual benefit to patient quality of life.

Supporting Evidence: Once a patient has developed chronic shoulder problems there are a large number of differential diagnoses, including impingement syndrome, partial- and full-thickness RC tears, acromioclavicular joint injuries, adhesive capsulitis, glenohumeral arthritis, glenohumeral instability, and other extrinsic conditions (74, 75). The delineation between these diagnoses is not always precise, as evidenced by the existence of multiple diagnostic criteria for categorizing chronic shoulder pain and relatively poor interrater reliability in making the diagnosis (76). Despite this complexity, it is thought that most shoulder problems evaluated in primary care stem from subacromial impingement of the RC tendons, leading to degenerative change and, eventually, partial- and full-thickness tears of the soft tissues, particularly in older patients (77, 78). Several tests and signs have been promoted in the literature that aim to help the clinician pinpoint the source of the shoulder pain (78). Some authors have claimed that the diagnostic accuracy of these clinical tests is equal to or better than ultrasound and MRI for many soft tissue injuries (75). Limited evidence (level III) indicates that, when performed by experienced clinicians, the composite clinical evaluation is sensitive in predicting RC tears and bursitis and can therefore accurately rule out these diagnoses in patients with negative test findings (79, 80). However, a recent systematic review concluded that too few studies had been conducted to enable any firm conclusions to be drawn about the value of any individual clinical tests (18).

If imaging is requested, there is a range of potential imaging options available, perhaps reflecting that no single investigation is perfect (Table 18.3). It might also reflect the fact that the choice of some treatment options remains controversial and not fully evaluated in terms of cost-effectiveness (77).

Conventional arthrography is falling out of favor but it still remains useful for identifying capsulitis (by showing increase of resistance on installation and lymphatic filling). It also provides unequivocal proof of a full-thickness RC tear (by showing direct extension of contrast medium into the subacromial space). However, the anatomical features of the tear are not well demonstrated. Hence the growing interest in alternative imaging techniques.

Ultrasound is a relatively inexpensive but highly operator dependent investigation that can potentially yield exquisite views of the distal RC. The systematic review by Dinnes et al. (18) identified 38 studies including a total of 2,435 patients where the accuracy of ultrasound for RC tears was compared to arthrography, arthroscopy, open surgery, or MRI. These studies were highly heterogeneous, both in the quality of the research design adopted and in their findings. The overall trends from these studies indicate that ultrasound has high specificity for all RC tears, but sensitivity was lower for both full- and particularly partial-thickness tears (Table 18.4). Therefore, in secondary care settings, a patient with positive ultrasound findings is very likely to truly have a RC tear

and could be considered a potential surgical candidate. However, ultrasound has several potential diagnostic pitfalls (81) and, unlike MRI, cannot provide an entire anatomical overview of the shoulder.

Magnetic resonance imaging can show most of the relevant anatomical features and can identify a large proportion of RC tears (Fig. 18.3). Indeed an MR roadmap of anatomical features is often required before a surgeon will contemplate surgery; the anatomy of the acromioclavicular joint is well demonstrated and most surgeons now require information about this area before performing decompression (e.g., acromioplasty – one of the commonest shoulder operations). The pooled results of 20 diagnostic accuracy studies indicate that MRI is not substantially more accurate than ultrasound in detecting RC tears (Table 18.4). In fact, a review of 14 studies focusing on partial-thickness tears indicated that the sensitivity of MRI is only 44%, lower than that of ultrasound (18). Few of these studies used fat-suppressed MRI techniques, which might have increased the diagnostic accuracy for partial-thickness tears.

Direct comparison of the intermodality diagnostic accuracy figures in Table 18.4 may be misleading as the table is based on studies of variable quality. The majority of five studies that conducted head-to-head comparisons of MRI and ultrasound against a common reference standard have concluded that MRI has equal or better accuracy than ultrasonography (82–86). However, taken in aggregate, data from these studies suggest that both the sensitivity and specificity of ultrasound and MRI are similar (18). It is important that imaging findings are closely correlated with the patient's symptoms when selecting management strategies; asymptomatic full-thickness RC tears may be present in one quarter of adults aged 60 or over (87).

One anatomical feature that MR does not demonstrate well is the glenoid labrum. The anatomy of this structure, along with the anterior extent of the anterior joint capsule, is crucial for the surgeon considering strength procedures for anterior instability. Estimates of the sensitivity of MRI without intra-articular contrast range from 55 to 90% (88–92). It has been claimed that MRA procedures (indirect or direct) can help clarify the detection of partial RC tears and labral tears (93–97). Nevertheless, it remains difficult, at best, to differentiate normal appearances of the labrum, anatomical variations thereof, and subtle tears (e.g., superior labrum anterior–posterior lesions). The few diagnostic accuracy studies that have been conducted have demonstrated that MRA is a highly sensitive and specific investigation for identifying full-thickness RC tears, but there is currently insufficient evidence (level IV) to support its accuracy for partial-thickness tears (Table 18.4). In some centers CT arthrography is used, especially where access to MR is limited. Although the bone texture is exquisitely demonstrated, CT gives little information about bone edema and the radiation dose has to be justified.

Most of the published literature evaluates the technical performance and diagnostic accuracy of imaging. Less is known concerning whether imaging is actually effective at influencing diagnosis, changing therapy, or improving patients' health. In a review of studies of shoulder MRI, Bearcroft and colleagues (98) found that less than 2% of publications (4/265) addressed the effectiveness of imaging. These studies have collectively demonstrated that MRI and MRA might change therapeutic plans in between 15 and 61% of patients imaged (98, 99). This wide range of therapeutic impact probably stems from differences in study methodology and case mix, whereby imaging has most influence in groups of patients with poorly defined symptoms and diagnoses. Furthermore, the presumption that imaging will lead to better treatment selection remains unproven. The sole randomized controlled trial comparing MRI with arthrography demonstrated that 52% of preimaging treatment plans changed following MRI compared to 66% of preimaging treatment plans in the arthrography group (100). However, this trial did not measure patient outcomes; therefore, it is impossible to judge the final benefit of these therapeutic changes. Therefore, we conclude that there is currently insufficient evidence (level IV) to demonstrate that any imaging modality will lead to improved health for patients with suspected soft tissue shoulder injuries.

Despite the limitations in knowledge expressed above, there are now quite robust guidelines designed to help the clinician though the maze of potential investigations (63). At present, there appears to be a split between European practice (18), which emphasizes the value of ultrasound as an inexpensive screening test before more sophisticated evaluation, and

North American practice (101), where there is greater reliance on MRI, MRA, and conventional arthrography. However, all of these recommendations are based primarily on consensus opinion.

Take Home Tables and Figures

Tables 18.1–18.4 and Fig. 18.1–18.3 serve to highlight key recommendations and supporting evidence.

Suggested Imaging Protocols

- Knee radiography: Anteroposterior (AP) and lateral views often suffice. Following trauma, the lateral is usually obtained as a "shoot-through" to see an effusion and a fluid/fluid level. Depending on the clinical question, tunnel views of the intercondylar notch and skyline views of the patella may be indicated.
- Magnetic resonance imaging of the knee: direct imaging in the three orthogonal planes is desirable. A sensible protocol might include a sagittally acquired 3D gradient echo data set, coronal T1- and T2-weighted images (or dual echo techniques) followed by a fat-suppressed T2-weighted axial series.
- Shoulder radiography: Conventional imaging includes an AP view of the glenohumeral joint, which includes the acromioclavicular joint and either an axial or an oblique view. The axial view may be difficult if the patient cannot fully abduct the arm.
- Ultrasound of the shoulder: This is very highly operator dependent. Increasing use is being made of high-frequency (e.g., 10–15 MHz) probes to provide optimal demonstration of tendons.
- Magnetic resonance imaging of the shoulder: Coronal oblique imaging along the plane of the supraspinatus tendon is a key sequence; it can be done by T1- and

T2-weighted imaging or by a dual echo technique. Axial views are essential to see the labrum; T1-weighted views provide good anatomical overview; fat-suppressed T2-weighted images can be very helpful. Many medical centers also use sagittal T1- and T2-weighted images routinely; they provide a good overview of the RC.

• Magnetic resonance arthrography of the shoulder: This can either be done directly [by instilling dilute gadolinium (Gd) diethylenetriamine pentaacetic acid (DTPA) into the shoulder joint] or indirectly (by giving Gd DTPA intravenously and obtaining images following exercise of the muscles around the joint). There is increasing use of direct MRA.

Table 18.1. Clinical decision rules for radiography of acute knee injury

Rule	Criteria for radiography	% Sensitivity (Ref.)	% Specificity (Ref.)	Validation studies
Ottawa knee rule (25)	• Age 55 or older; or • Isolated tenderness of patella (no other bone tenderness); or • Tenderness at head of fibula; or • Inability to flex 90 degrees; or • Inability to bear weight both immediately and in the emergency department for four steps	99 (10)	49 (10)	20–22, 27–35
Pittsburgh rule (24)	• Fall or blunt-trauma and age <12 or >50; or • Fall or blunt trauma and inability to walk four weight-bearing steps in emergency Department	99 (21)	60 (21)	21, 24, 26
Fagan and Davies (23)	Two or more of the following: • Age over 55 years • Effusion • Hemarthrosis • Not able to bear weight in the department (includes touch weight-bearing as non-weight bearing) • History of direct trauma to the knee • Point bony tenderness at the patella, tibial plateau, femoral condyles, or the head of Fibula	95 (23)	62 (23)	23
Weber et al. (26)	Patient does not need radiograph if: • Able to walk without limping • Twist injury without effusion	100 (26)	34 (26)	26

Reprinted with kind permission of Springer Science+Business Media from Hollingworth W, Dixon AK, Jenner JR. Imaging for Knee and Shoulder Problems. In Medina LS, Blackmore CC (eds): *Evidence-Based Imaging: Optimizing Imaging in Patient Care.* New York: Springer Science+Business Media, 2006.

Table 18.2. Diagnostic accuracy of MRI for soft tissue knee injuries

Lesion	Pooled weighted sensitivity[a]	Pooled weighted specificity[a]	Positive likelihood ratio	Negative likelihood ratio
Medial meniscal tear	93 (92–95)	88 (85–91)	7.75	0.08
Lateral meniscal tear	79 (74–84)	96 (95–97)	19.75	0.22
Anterior cruciate ligament complete tear	94 (92–97)	94 (93–96)	15.67	0.06
Posterior cruciate ligament complete tear	91 (83–99)	99 (99–100)	91.00	0.09

Source: Data extracted from the systematic review of Oei et al. (15).
Reprinted with kind permission of Springer Science+Business Media from Hollingworth W, Dixon AK, Jenner JR. Imaging for Knee and Shoulder Problems. In Medina LS, Blackmore CC (eds): *Evidence-Based Imaging: Optimizing Imaging in Patient Care*. New York: Springer Science+Business Media, 2006.
[a]Figures in parentheses represent the 95% confidence intervals.

Table 18.3. Some of the common radiologic investigations available for shoulder problems

Examination	Radiation	Cost
Plain radiograph AP/axial	+	+
Plain radiographs under fluoroscopy	+ +	+ +
Ultrasound	–	+
Arthrography under fluoroscopy	+ + +	+ +
CT	+ + +	+ +
CT arthrography	+ + +	+ + +
MRI	–	+ + +
MRI indirect arthrography	–	+ + + +
MRI direct arthrography	–	+ + + +

Reprinted with kind permission of Springer Science+Business Media from Hollingworth W, Dixon AK, Jenner JR. Imaging for Knee and Shoulder Problems. In Medina LS, Blackmore CC (eds): *Evidence-Based Imaging: Optimizing Imaging in Patient Care*. New York: Springer Science+Business Media, 2006.

Table 18.4. Diagnostic accuracy of ultrasound, MRI, and MRA for rotator cuff (RC) tears

Modality	Lesion	Pooled sensitivity[a]	Pooled specificity[a]	Pooled positive likelihood ratio	Pooled negative likelihood ratio
Ultrasound	Full-thickness RC tear	87 (84–89)[b]	96 (49–97)[b]	13.16	0.16[b]
	Partial-thickness RC tear	67 (61–73)[b]	94 (92–96)[b]	8.90[b]	0.36[b]
MRI	Full-thickness RC tear	89 (86–92)	93 (91–95)	10.63[b]	0.16
	Partial-thickness RC tear	44 (36–51)[b]	90 (87–92)[b]	3.99[b]	0.66[b]
MRA	Full-thickness RC tear	95 (82–98)	93 (84–97)	10.05[b]	0.11[b]
	Partial-thickness RC tear	62 (40–80)[b]	92 (83–97)	8.90[b]	0.43[b]

Source: Data extracted from the systematic review of Dinnes et al. (18) The likelihood ratio estimates cannot be derived directly from sensitivity and specificity estimates as Dinnes et al. separately pooled data from the source studies.
Reprinted with kind permission of Springer Science+Business Media from Hollingworth W, Dixon AK, Jenner JR. Imaging for Knee and Shoulder Problems. In Medina LS, Blackmore CC (eds): *Evidence-Based Imaging: Optimizing Imaging in Patient Care.* New York: Springer Science+Business Media, 2006.
[a]Figures in parentheses represent 95% confidence intervals.
[b]Authors report that significant heterogeneity existed between the results of the source publications.

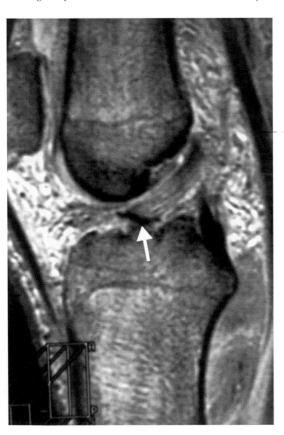

Figure 18.1. Three-dimensional (3D)-gradient echo MRI of a soccer player following recent trauma. The intact anterior cruciate ligament has pulled off a small rind of cortex from the proximal tibia (*arrow*). Prompt surgery allowed this avulsion fracture, well shown on this preoperative roadmap, to be pinned back promptly. This probably speeded up his return to top-class soccer. (Reprinted with kind permission of Springer Science+Business Media from Hollingworth W, Dixon AK, Jenner JR. Imaging for Knee and Shoulder Problems. In Medina LS, Blackmore CC (eds): *Evidence-Based Imaging: Optimizing Imaging in Patient Care.* New York: Springer Science+Business Media, 2006.)

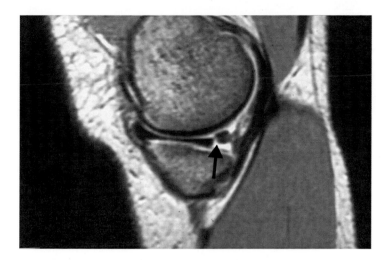

Figure 18.2. A patient with chronic symptoms in the posteromedial aspect of the knee. The 3D-gradient echo MRI shows a classical tear at the junction of the middle and posterior thirds of medial meniscus (*arrow*). Arthroscopy was initially negative. Continuing symptoms led to clinicoradiologic discussion; a second arthroscopy confirmed the tear. (*Source*: from Mackenzie et al. (46), with permission.)

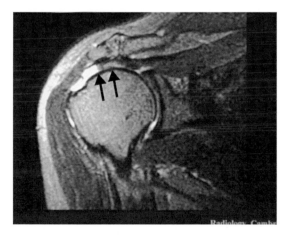

Figure 18.3. Magnetic resonance image of right shoulder. On this fat-suppressed T2-weighted MRI, the high signal intensity defect in the distal supraspinatus tendon provides convincing evidence of a full-thickness rotator cuff tear (*arrows*). The surgeon can readily assess the degree of retraction, which is essential information before considering repair. Although ultrasound could give some of this information, the full relationship of the damaged frayed tendon with the subacromial region is well demonstrated here. (Reprinted with kind permission of Springer Science+Business Media from Hollingworth W, Dixon AK, Jenner JR. Imaging for Knee and Shoulder Problems. In Medina LS, Blackmore CC (eds): *Evidence-Based Imaging: Optimizing Imaging in Patient Care*. New York: Springer Science+Business Media, 2006.)

Future Research

This chapter has summarized the available evidence on the appropriate roles of imaging in knee and shoulder problems. However, in areas where evidence is sparse or where the clinician is in doubt, a comprehensive history and clinical examination remain vital in determining the most appropriate investigation and whether or not imaging is likely to influence diagnosis and treatment. A good clinician should be prepared to disregard imaging guidelines if the patient presents with an unusual clinical picture. For example, a plain radiograph or skeletal scintigraphy, which would not normally be indicated, may reveal a previously unsuspected lesion such as malignancy and help achieve a timely diagnosis. Further research is needed to plug the gaps in the existing literature and to keep evidence up to date. In particular we believe that future research should focus on the following:

- Providing appropriate training for clinicians to implement the Ottawa knee rule while monitoring its impact on the cost-effectiveness of care.
- Defining diagnostic thresholds to ensure the cost-effective use of MRI for meniscal and ligamentous knee injuries in primary and specialist care settings.
- Validating the sensitivity, specificity, and therapeutic impact of clinical prediction rules for radiographic evaluation of patients with shoulder pain in the emergency department.
- Direct comparisons of the diagnostic accuracy of ultrasound, MRI, and MRA for the diagnosis of full- and partial-thickness RC tears.

References

1. Yawn BP, Amadio P, Harmsen WS, Hill J, Ilstrup D, Gabriel S. J Trauma 2000;48(4):716–723.
2. Simonet WT, Melton LJ 3rd, Cofield RH, Ilstrup DM. Clin Orthop 1984;186:186–191.
3. Kroner K, Lind T, Jensen J. Arch Orthop Trauma Surg 1989;108(5):288–290.
4. Urwin M, Symmons D, Allison T et al. Ann Rheum Dis 1998;57(11):649–655.
5. Picavet HS, Schouten JS. Pain 2003;102(1–2): 167–178.
6. National Center for Health Statistics. National Hospital Ambulatory Medical Care Survey: 2001. Hyattsville, MD, 2003.
7. National Center for Health Statistics. National Ambulatory Medical Care Survey: 2001. Hyattsville, MD, 2003.
8. Katz JN, Solomon DH, Schaffer JL, Horsky J, Burdick E, Bates DW. Am J Med 2000;108(1): 28–35.
9. Woolf AD, Pfleger B. Bull WHO 2003;81(9): 646–656.
10. Bachmann LM, Haberzeth S, Steurer J, ter Riet G. Ann Intern Med 2004;140(2):121–124.
11. Jackson JL, O'Malley PG, Kroenke K. Ann Intern Med 2003;139(7):575–588.
12. Solomon DH, Simel DL, Bates DW, Katz JN, Schaffer JL. JAMA 2001;286(13):1610–1620.
13. Scholten RJ, Deville WL, Opstelten W, Bijl D, van der Plas CG, Bouter LM. J Fam Pract 2001;50(11):938–944.
14. Scholten RJ, Opstelten W, van der Plas CG, Bijl D, Deville WL, Bouter LM. J Fam Pract 2003;52(9): 689–694.
15. Oei EH, Nikken JJ, Verstijnen AC, Ginai AZ, Myriam Hunink MG. Radiology 2003;226(3): 837–848.
16. Mackenzie R, Palmer CR, Lomas DJ, Dixon AK. Clin Radiol 1996;51(4):251–257.
17. Bryan S, Weatherburn G, Bungay H et al. Health Technol Assess 2001;5(27):1–95.
18. Dinnes J, Loveman E, McIntyre L, Waugh N. Health Technol Assess 2003;7(29):iii, 1–166.
19. Schulte-Altedorneburg G, Gebhard M, Wohlgemuth WA et al. Skeletal Radiol 2003;32(1):1–12.
20. Matteucci MJ, Roos JA. J Emerg Med 2003;24(2): 147–150.
21. Seaberg DC, Yealy DM, Lukens T, Auble T, Mathias S. Ann Emerg Med 1998;32(1):8–13.
22. Stiell IG, Wells GA, Hoag RH, Sivilotti ML, Cacciotti TF, Verbeek PR et al. JAMA 1997;278(23):2075–2079.
23. Fagan DJ, Davies S. Injury 2000;31(9):723–727.
24. Seaberg DC, Jackson R. Am J Emerg Med 1994;12(5):541–543.
25. Stiell IG, Greenberg GH, Wells GA et al. Ann Emerg Med 1995;26(4):405–413.
26. Weber JE, Jackson RE, Peacock WF, Swor RA, Carley R, Larkin GL. Ann Emerg Med 1995;26(4):429–433.
27. Stiell IG, Greenberg GH, Wells GA et al. JAMA 1996;275(8):611–615.
28. Szucs PA, Richman PB, Mandell M. Acad Emerg Med 2001;8(2):112–116.
29. Kec RM, Richman PB, Szucs PA, Mandell M, Eskin B. Acad Emerg Med 2003;10(2):146–150.
30. Bulloch B, Neto G, Plint A et al. Ann Emerg Med 2003;42(1):48–55.
31. Ketelslegers E, Collard X, Vande Berg B et al. Eur Radiol 2002;12(5):1218–220.

32. Khine H, Dorfman DH, Avner JR. Pediatr Emerg Care 2001;17(6):401–404.

33. Emparanza JI, Aginaga JR. Ann Emerg Med 2001;38(4):364–368.

34. Tigges S, Pitts S, Mukundan S Jr, Morrison D, Olson M, Shahriara A. AJR Am J Roentgenol 1999;172(4):1069–1071.

35. Richman PB, McCuskey CF, Nashed A et al. J Emerg Med 1997;15(4):459–463.

36. Nichol G, Stiell IG, Wells GA, Juergensen LS, Laupacis A. Ann Emerg Med 1999;34(4 pt 1): 438–447.

37. Tepper KB, Ireland ML. Instr Course Lect 2003;52:667–676.

38. Solomon DH, Katz JN, Carrino JA et al. Med Care 2003;41(5):687–692.

39. O'Shea KJ, Murphy KP, Heekin RD, Herzwurm PJ. Am J Sports Med 1996;24(2):164–167.

40. Miller GK. Arthroscopy 1996;12(4):406–413.

41. Suarez-Almazor ME, Kaul P, Kendall CJ, Saunders LD, Johnston DW. Int J Technol Assess Health Care 1999;15(2):392–405.

42. Carmichael IW, MacLeod AM, Travlos J. J Bone Joint Surg Br 1997;79(4):624–625.

43. Guten GN, Kohn HS, Zoltan DJ. WMJ 2002;101(1):35–38.

44. Odgaard F, Tuxoe J, Joergensen U et al. Scand J Med Sci Sports 2002;12(3):154–162.

45. Rappeport ED, Mehta S, Wieslander SB, Lausten GS, Thomsen HS. Acta Radiol 1996;37(5): 602–609.

46. Mackenzie R, Keene GS, Lomas DJ, Dixon AK. Br J Radiol 1995;68(814):1045–1051.

47. Bui-Mansfield LT, Youngberg RA, Warme W, Pitcher JD, Nguyen PL. AJR Am J Roentgenol 1997;168(4):913–918.

48. Chissell HR, Allum RL, Keightley A. Ann R Coll Surg Engl 1994;76(1):26–29.

49. Mackenzie R, Dixon AK, Keene GS, Hollingworth W, Lomas DJ, Villar RN. Clin Radiol 1996;51(4):245–250.

50. Ruwe PA, Wright J, Randall RL, Lynch JK, Jokl P, McCarthy S. Radiology 1992;183(2):335–339.

51. Rappeport ED, Wieslander SB, Stephensen S, Lausten GS, Thomsen HS. Acta Orthop Scand 1997;68(3):277–281.

52. Vincken PW, ter Braak BP, van Erkell AR et al. Radiology 2002;223(3):739–746.

53. Weinstabl R, Muellner T, Vecsei V, Kainberger F, Kramer M. World J Surg 1997;21(4):363–368.

54. Sherman PM, Penrod BJ, Lane MJ, Ward JA. Arthroscopy 2002;18(2):201–205.

55. Uppal A, Disler DG, Short WB, McCauley TR, Cooper JA. Radiology 1998;207(3):633–636.

56. Watura R, Lloyd DC, Chawda S. Br Med J 1995;311(7020):1614.

57. Bianchi S, Martinoli C. Radiol Clin North Am 1999;37(4):679–690.

58. Lanyon P, O'Reilly S, Jones A, Doherty M. Ann Rheum Dis 1998;57(10):595–601.

59. Peat G, Croft P, Hay E. Best Pract Res Clin Rheumatol 2001;15(4):527–544.

60. Dieppe PA, Cushnaghan J, Shepstone L. Osteoarthr Cartil 1997;5(2):87–97.

61. Bedson J, Jordan K, Croft P. Ann Rheum Dis 2003;62(5):450–454.

62. Morgan B, Mullick S, Harper WM, Finlay DB. Br J Radiol 1997;70:256–260.

63. RCR Working Party. Making the Best Use of a Department of Clinical Radiology: Guidelines for Doctors, 5th ed. London: Royal College of Radiologists, 2003.

64. Eccles M, Steen N, Grimshaw J et al. Lancet 2001;357(9266):1406–1409.

65. Ramsay CR, Eccles M, Grimshaw JM, Steen N. Clin Radiol 2003;58(4):319–321.

66. te Slaa RL, Wijffels MP, Marti RK. Eur J Emerg Med 2003;10(1):58–61.

67. Fraenkel L, Lavalley M, Felson D. Am J Emerg Med 1998;16(6):560–563.

68. Hendey GW. Ann Emerg Med 2000;36(2): 108–113.

69. Harvey RA, Trabulsy ME, Roe L. Am J Emerg Med 1992;10(2):149–151.

70. Hendey GW, Kinlaw K. Ann Emerg Med 1996;28(4):399–402.

71. Shuster M, Abu-Laban RB, Boyd J. Am J Emerg Med 1999;17(7):653–658.

72. Demirhan M, Akpinar S, Atalar AC, Akman S, Akalin Y. Injury 1998;29(7):525–528.

73. Fraenkel L, Shearer P, Mitchell P, LaValley M, Feldman J, Felson DT. J Rheumatol 2000;27(1): 200–204.

74. Steinfeld R, Valente RM, Stuart MJ. Mayo Clin Proc 1999;74(8):785–794

75. Brox JI. Best Pract Res Clin Rheumatol 2003;17(1):33–56.

76. de Winter AF, Jans MP, Scholten RJ, Deville W, van Schaardenburg D, Bouter LM. Ann Rheum Dis 1999;58(5):272–277.

77. Speed C, Hazleman B. Clin Evid 2003;9:1372–1387.

78. Stevenson JH, Trojian T. J Fam Pract 2002;51(7): 605–611.

79. Litaker D, Pioro M, El Bilbeisi H, Brems J. J Am Geriatr Soc 2000;48(12):1633–1637.

80. MacDonald PB, Clark P, Sutherland K. J Shoulder Elbow Surg 2000;9(4):299–301.

81. Allen GM, Wilson DJ. Eur J Ultrasound 2001;14(1):3–9.

82. Nelson MC, Leather GP, Nirschl RP, Pettrone FA, Freedman MT. J Bone Joint Surg Am 1991;73(5):707–716.

83. Burk DL Jr, Karasick D, Kurtz AB et al. AJR Am J Roentgenol 1989;153(1):87–92.

84. Hodler J, Terrier B, von Schulthess GK, Fuchs WA. Clin Radiol 1991;43(5):323–327.

85. Martin-Hervas C, Romero J, Navas-Acien A, Reboiras JJ, Munuera L. J Shoulder Elbow Surg 2001;10(5):410–415.

86. Swen WA, Jacobs JW, Algra PR et al. Arthritis Rheum 1999;42(10):2231–2238.
87. Sher JS, Uribe JW, Posada A, Murphy BJ, Zlatkin MB. J Bone Joint Surg Am 1995;77(1): 10–15.
88. Zlatkin MB, Hoffman C, Shellock FG. J Magn Reson Imaging 2004;19(5):623–631.
89. Tung GA, Entzian D, Green A, Brody JM. AJR Am J Roentgenol 2000;174(4):1107–1114.
90. Tuite MJ, Cirillo RL, De Smet AA, Orwin JF. Radiology 2000;215(3):841–845.
91. Shellock FG, Bert JM, Fritts HM, Gundry CR, Easton R, Crues JV 3rd. J Magn Reson Imaging 2001;14(6):763–770.
92. Gusmer PB, Potter HG, Schatz JA et al. Radiology 1996;200(2):519–524.
93. Waldt S, Burkart A, Lange P, Imhoff AB, Rummeny EJ, Woertler K. AJR Am J Roentgenol 2004;182(5):1271–1278.
94. Parmar H, Jhankaria B, Maheshwari M et al. J Postgrad Med 2002;48(4):270–273; discussion 273–274.
95. Herold T, Hente R, Zorger N et al. Rofo 2003;175(11):1508–1514.
96. Jee WH, McCauley TR, Katz LD, Matheny JM, Ruwe PA, Daigneault JP. Radiology 2001;218(1): 127–132.
97. Bencardino JT, Beltran J, Rosenberg ZS et al. Radiology 2000;214(1):267–271.
98. Bearcroft PW, Blanchard TK, Dixon AK, Constant CR. Skeletal Radiol 2000;29(12):673–679.
99. Zanetti M, Jost B, Lustenberger A, Hodler J. Acta Radiol 1999;40(3):296–302.
100. Blanchard TK, Bearcroft PW, Maibaum A, Hazelman BL, Sharma S, Dixon AK. Eur J Radiol 1999;30(1):5–10.
101. Oh CH, Schweitzer ME, Spettell CM. Skeletal Radiol 1999;28(12):670–678.

19

Pediatric Fractures of the Ankle

Martin H. Reed and G. Brian Black

Issues

I. What are the clinical indications for obtaining the ankle X-ray series following trauma in a child?
II. What is the diagnostic performance of computed tomography in the investigation of ankle fractures in children?
III. What is the diagnostic performance of magnetic resonance imaging in the investigation of ankle injuries in children?
IV. What is the diagnostic performance of ultrasound in the investigation of ankle injuries in children?

Key Points

■ Most ankle injuries in children do not require imaging (strong evidence)
■ A three-view radiographic series of the ankle is indicated only in children who (a) have pain near the malleoli and (b) have an inability to bear weight immediately after the injury and in the Emergency Department or (c) have bone tenderness at the posterior edge or the tip of either malleolus (strong evidence). There is insufficient evidence to guide use of evidence in children too young to provide reliable history and physical exam.
■ CT is useful for surgical planning in children with complex ankle fractures; MRI may also be used but may be less available and may require sedation.
■ MRI is the imaging modality of choice for evaluation of (a) ligamentous injuries, (b) occult injuries, such as talar dome fracture, and (c) possible premature physeal closure (limited evidence).
■ Ultrasound has no proven role in the imaging of acute ankle trauma in children (insufficient evidence).

M.H. Reed (✉)
Department of Diagnostic Imaging, Children's Hospital of Winnipeg,
University of Manitoba, Winnipeg, Manitoba, Canada, R3A 1S1
e-mail: mreed@hsc.mb.ca

L.S. Medina et al. (eds.), *Evidence-Based Imaging: Improving the Quality of Imaging in Patient Care, Revised Edition*,
DOI 10.1007/978-1-4419-7777-9_19, © Springer Science+Business Media, LLC 2011

Definition and Pathophysiology

For the purposes of this chapter, fractures of the ankle will be defined as fractures involving the metaphysis, the growth plate, or the epiphysis of the distal tibia and fibula. Prior to growth plate closure, Salter–Harris Types I–IV fractures of the distal tibia occur. The higher the SH number, the higher the risk of premature closure of the growth plate.

Type II fractures are most common (Fig. 19.1) (Table 19.1) (1). A characteristic fracture pattern, which is seen in adolescents, is the juvenile Tillaux fracture, a Salter–Harris Type III fracture of the lateral aspect of the distal tibia (2). An unusual growth plate injury that occurs in the distal tibia is the triplane fracture (3). This injury is characterized by a fracture line through the metaphysis in the coronal plane, which is visible on the lateral view, an extension of the fracture through the growth plate in the axial plane, and a further extension through the epiphysis in the sagittal plane best seen on the frontal view (Fig. 19.2). This fracture can be thought of as a combination of a Salter–Harris Type II and a Salter–Harris Type III fracture. Characteristically, this fracture occurs in adolescence also.

A Pilon fracture is an intraarticular fracture of the distal tibia with an associated articular disruption and usually other injuries. These fractures are rare in the pediatric age group, although they occasionally occur in adolescents. The prognosis in this age group may be better than in adults (insufficient evidence) (4).

Salter–Harris Type I fractures are thought to be the most common fractures involving the distal fibula, but these are difficult to diagnose radiologically because they are characteristically nondisplaced. Other growth plate injuries of the distal fibula are quite uncommon. Avulsion fractures of the tip of the lateral malleolus can occur (5).

Epidemiology

Ankle fractures are common in both children and adults. The incidence of ankle fractures in children in Britain ranges from 4.2 per 10,000 person-years (6) to 10.3 per 10,000 person-years (7). The incidence of ankle fractures in children increases year by year throughout childhood (6, 7). The incidence is higher in boys than girls, particularly in older children (6, 7). Ankle fractures comprise between 3 and 5% of all pediatric fractures and 15% of physeal injuries (6, 7).

Overall Cost to Society

There is no information about the overall societal cost of ankle fractures in children. There is also no information on the cost-effectiveness of the use of the Ottawa Ankle Rule in children, but Anis et al. estimated that the implementation of the Ottawa Ankle Rule for the radiography of ankles following trauma in adults would result in savings of between US $600,000 and US $3,000,000 per 100,000 patients in the United States and of CAN $700,000 per 100,000 patients in Canada (8).

Goals

The goals of imaging are to detect or exclude fractures accurately, to help to determine appropriate treatment, and to aid in surgical planning when necessary. In addition, imaging is essential for follow-up if there is clinical concern that premature physeal closure is occurring.

Methodology

A PubMed search was undertaken using the following terms: *ankle, tibia, fibula, epidemiology, cost, radiography, computed tomography, magnetic resonance imaging,* and *ultrasound.* Limits placed on all searches included the following: English language only, humans only, and all children (0–18 years). There was no date limit on the search. The searches were all completed in October 2008.

I. What Are the Clinical Indications for Obtaining the Ankle X-ray Series Following Trauma in a Child?

Summary of Evidence: A well-validated clinical prediction rule provides guidance for which children should undergo ankle radiography in the setting of acute trauma. Imaging is indicated only in children who meet the criteria of the pediatric modification of the Ottawa Ankle Rule (strong evidence). The criteria are the following:

Following an injury, radiography of the ankle is indicated only in children who have pain near the malleoli and at least one of the following:

(a) Inability to bear weight immediately after the injury and in the Emergency Department for four steps
(b) Bone tenderness at the posterior edge or the tip of either malleolus

Supporting Evidence: Ian Stiell and his group carried out a multicenter, prospective study using a multivariate analysis technique to establish the Ottawa Ankle Rule in adults. This rule identifies the symptoms and signs most likely to predict the presence of a fracture. Without these signs, a fracture is very unlikely (sensitivity 100%, specificity 40.1%) (9). Stiell and associates validated this rule with a prospective multicenter study involving 12,777 adults 18 years of age and older (10), and it has been independently validated by several other studies as well (11, 12).

The rule has also been validated with minor modifications for use in children: in the United States, in one study of 71 patients (sensitivity 100%, specificity 32%) (13) and in another study of 195 patients by Clark and Tanner (sensitivity 83%, specificity 50%) (14), in one Canadian study of 671 patients (sensitivity 100%, specificity 24%) (15), and in one English study of 432 patients (sensitivity 98.3%, specificity 46.9%) (16) (Table 19.2). The sensitivity of the rule was not quite as good in the series by Clark and Tanner (14) as it was in the other three studies. Five of thirty (17%) fractures would have been missed in that study using the Ottawa Ankle Rule, but the authors did not state why they were missed or what type of fractures were missed (14).

Boutis et al. proposed and assessed a more detailed decision rule, classifying the findings on physical examination into low and high risk. A low-risk clinical examination comprised isolated pain or tenderness with or without edema or ecchymosis in the region of the distal fibula below the level of the joint line and in the regions of the adjacent ligaments (17). Fractures in this region are always stable and are treated

on the basis of clinical findings rather than radiologic findings. Therefore, patients with low-risk findings may not need to be radiographed. Of the 381 children in the low-risk category in this two-center study, none had a high-risk fracture requiring surgery, whereas 54 of the 226 children in the high-risk category had fractures, 45 of which were high risk potentially requiring surgery (17). Using the rule that children with a low-risk examination do not need to be radiographed would have reduced the number of radiographs obtained by 62.8% compared to a reduction of only 12% using the Ottawa Ankle Rule (17). This guideline has not been validated by an independent prospective study (limited evidence).

II. What Is the Diagnostic Performance of Computed Tomography in the Investigation of Ankle Fractures in Children?

Summary of Evidence: Computed tomography is of value in the preoperative assessment of complex distal tibial epiphyseal fractures because it shows more accurately the degree of comminution and the severity of displacement than do ordinary X-rays (Fig. 19.2) (insufficient evidence). This examination would normally be ordered by an orthopedic surgeon.

Supporting Evidence: Brown et al. retrospectively studied 51 patients who had had CT scans to evaluate triplane fractures. This type of imaging showed the detailed anatomy of the fractures and the precise degree of displacement of the fragments (3). Cutler et al., in a study of 62 patients with distal tibial physeal fractures, showed that CT scans helped in more accurately positioning screws used for internal fixation (18).

Benefits of using CT for treatment planning include improved anatomic detail, especially of the articular surfaces, and improved visualization of bones that often are not well seen by radiography if there is overlying cast/splint material. Relative to radiography, CT has both higher cost and radiation exposure. The role of CT in other specific fracture types has not been adequately explored, although it may be useful in Pilon fracture treatment planning.

III. What Is the Diagnostic Performance of Magnetic Resonance Imaging in the Investigation of Ankle Injuries in Children?

Summary of Evidence: MRI detects more injuries, including injuries of the bone marrow, stress injuries, and ligamentous injuries, than do radiographs. However, there is no evidence that its routine use affects the acute management of ankle fractures in children (limited evidence). Like CT, it may be of value in providing more detailed assessment of the anatomy of complex fractures preoperatively (limited evidence). It is the imaging modality of choice for the assessment of premature physeal (growth plate) closure (limited evidence).

Supporting Evidence: Lohman et al. (19), in a prospective study of 60 children 7 years of age and older with ankle injuries who were all examined with X-rays and MRIs, found one false-negative and one false-positive fracture of the tibia on X-ray and 11 false-positive and 4 false-positive fractures of the fibula on radiographs. Twenty-two of the patients had bone bruises, mostly associated with ligamentous injuries, none of which was seen on radiographs. However, they concluded that routine MRI examination of children with mild ankle injuries was not indicated, although MRI was useful for showing the anatomy of complex fractures in detail (limited evidence). Seifert et al. (20) prospectively studied 22 patients, 10–16 years of age, with distal tibial fractures using X-ray and MRI. Ten of these cases were thought to require internal fixation based on the X-rays and 15 based on the MRIs because X-ray underestimated the degree of displacement of the fragments in five patients. They therefore recommended MRI in all Salter Type III and IV fractures and all triplane fractures of the distal tibia (limited evidence). They comment that CT can also be used, but they prefer MRI because it avoids radiation. Bone bruises or ligamentous damage were also shown in eight patients only by MRI, but these findings did not affect management of the patients.

MRI can also be used to evaluate premature closure of the distal tibial epiphysis following an acute ankle injury by accurately demonstrating the site and degree of the fusion. Ecklund and Jaramillo (21) studied 43 children with post-traumatic physeal bars of the distal tibia and Sailhan et al. (22) studied 14 patients, both in larger series of premature physeal fusion at a variety of sites. MRI visualized the sites and sizes of the physeal bridges well, and in Sailhan's series, the MRI findings correlated well with the surgical findings in eight patients (22) (limited evidence).

IV. What Is the Diagnostic Performance of Ultrasound in the Investigation of Ankle Injuries in Children?

Summary of Evidence: Ultrasound may be of value in detecting fractures not visible on X-rays in children following trauma (insufficient evidence). Sonography is also able to detect ankle joint effusions and in experienced hands, it can detect ligamentous or tendon injuries (insufficient evidence).

Supporting Evidence: Simanovsky et al. (23) prospectively studied 20 children aged 5–13 years who had no fractures seen on radiographs following ankle trauma. They found seven minor fractures in these patients with ultrasound, all of which were confirmed by follow-up radiographs (insufficient evidence). Two other studies assessed the accuracy of ultrasound in the diagnosis of fractures around the ankle, both including adults as well as children. Singh et al. studied 114 patients aged 10–80 years, 27 of whom had fractures detected by ultrasound. Twenty-three of these were visible on the initial X-rays and four were confirmed on follow-up X-rays (limited evidence) (24). In a study by Wang et al. of 268 patients (aged 8–63 years), 24 fractures were identified sonographically that had not been seen on the initial X-rays, although they were visible in retrospect (insufficient evidence) (25).

Take Home Tables

Table 19.1 presents the Salter–Harris classification of physeal fractures of the distal tibia. Tables 19.2 and 19.3 discuss the Ottawa Ankle Rule for children and its diagnostic performance.

Imaging Case Studies

Case 1

Figure 19.1 presents a case of a Salter Type II fracture in a 12-year-old boy.

Case 2

Figure 19.2 presents a case of a triplane fracture in a 14-year-old boy.

Suggested Imaging Protocol for Fractures of the Ankle

Radiographs

A three-view series of radiographs of the ankle (AP view, internal oblique or Mortise view, and lateral view) is the initial imaging study of choice following trauma in children. It is indicated only if the child presents with pain around the malleoli and if either of the following two signs is present:

(a) Inability to bear weight for four steps both immediately following the trauma and at the time of examination
(b) Bone tenderness at the posterior edge or the tip of the lateral or medial malleolus (Table 19.3)

CT and MRI

In cases of complex fractures of the distal tibia, CT or MRI may provide better details of the anatomy prior to surgery; MRI is useful for the assessment of premature physeal closure. The MDCT can be performed with low-dose technique to minimize radiation exposure.

Table 19.1. Physeal fractures of the distal tibia (Salter–Harris classification)

Type	Percentage (%)
Type I	6
Type II	46
Type III	25
Type IV	10
Miscellaneous	12

Reprinted with permission from MacNealy et al. (1).

Table 19.2. Diagnostic performance of the Ottawa Ankle Rule in children

Author	Patients (N)	Sensitivity (%)	Specificity (%)	Strength of evidence
Chande (13)	71	100	32	Moderate
Plint et al. (15)	670	100	24	Strong
Libetta et al. (16)	761	98.3	46.9	Strong
Clark et al. (14)	195	83	50	Moderate

Reprinted with kind permission of Springer Science+Business Media, from Reed MH, Black GB. Fractures of the Ankle. In Medina LS, Applegate KE, Blackmore CC (eds): *Evidence-Based Imaging in Pediatrics: Optimizing Imaging in Pediatric Patient Care.* New York: Springer Science+Business Media, 2010.

Table 19.3. The Ottawa Ankle Rule for children[a]

Following trauma, a child should receive ankle radiographs if

There is pain around the malleoli and either

(a) Inability to bear weight for four steps both immediately following the trauma and at the time of examination

(b) Bone tenderness at the posterior edge or the tip of the lateral or medial malleolus

Data from Chande (13), Clark and Tanner (14), Plint et al. (15), and Libetta et al. (16).

Reprinted with kind permission of Springer Science+Business Media, from Reed MH, Black GB. Fractures of the Ankle. In Medina LS, Applegate KE, Blackmore CC (eds): *Evidence-Based Imaging in Pediatrics: Optimizing Imaging in Pediatric Patient Care.* New York: Springer Science+Business Media, 2010.

[a]For children aged 2–16 who can verbalize pain.

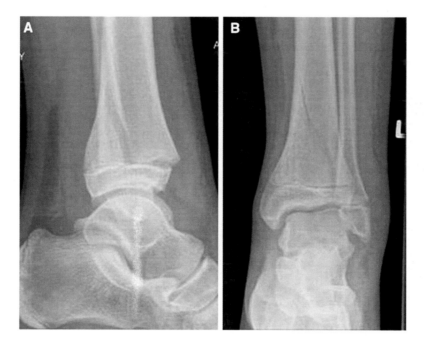

Figure 19.1. Salter Type II fracture in a 12-year-old boy. There is a fracture of the metaphysic of the distal tibia. (Reprinted with kind permission of Springer Science+Business Media from Reed MH, Black GB. Fractures of the Ankle. In Medina LS, Applegate KE, Blackmore CC (eds): *Evidence-Based Imaging in Pediatrics: Optimizing Imaging in Pediatric Patient Care.* New York: Springer Science+Business Media, 2010.)

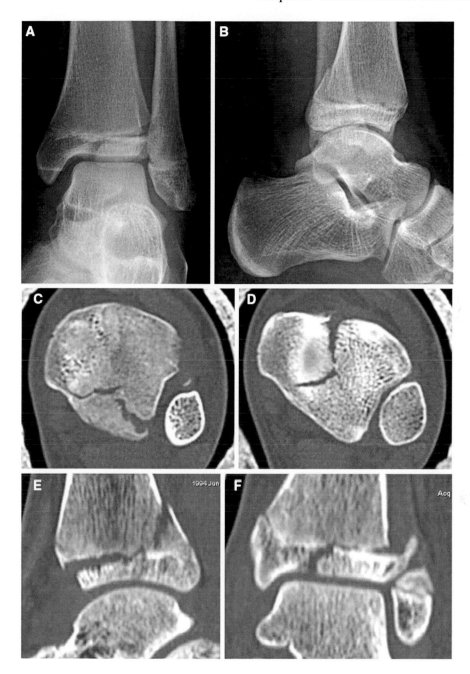

Figure 19.2. Triplane fracture in a 14-year-old boy. (**A, B**) Frontal and lateral X-rays. The metaphyseal component of the fracture in the coronal plane (**C**) is more clearly seen on the CT scan as is the epiphyseal component in the sagittal plane (**D**) as well as the degree of separation of the fragments. The extension through the growth plate in the axial plane is best seen on the sagittal (**E**) and coronal (**F**) reconstructions. These also show that a triplane fracture can be thought of as a combination of a Salter Type II fracture (**E**) and a Salter Type III fracture (**F**). (Reprinted with kind permission of Springer Science+Business Media from Reed MH, Black GB. Fractures of the Ankle. In Medina LS, Applegate KE, Blackmore CC (eds): *Evidence-Based Imaging in Pediatrics: Optimizing Imaging in Pediatric Patient Care.* New York: Springer Science+Business Media, 2010.)

Future Research

- To understand the barriers to implementation of the Ottawa Ankle Rule in the clinical setting (both Emergency Department and outpatient).
- To prospectively validate the decision rule developed by Boutis et al. (17).
- To determine the role of MRI in the management of acute ankle injuries in children.
- To assess the potential role of ultrasound in the diagnosis of ankle injuries in children.

References

1. MacNealy GA, Rogers LF, Hernandez R, Poznanski AK. AJR Am J Roentgenol 1982;138:683–689.
2. Horn BD, Crisci K, Krug M, Pizatillo PD et al. J Pediatr Orthop 2001;21:162–164.
3. Brown SD, Kasser JR, Zurakowski D, Jaramillo D. AJR Am J Roentgenol 2004;183:1489–1495.
4. Letts M, Davidson D, McCaffrey M. J Pediatr Orthop 2001;21:20–26.
5. Ogden JA, Lee J. J Pediatr Orthop 1990;10:306–316.
6. Lyons RA, Delahunty AM, Kraus D, Heaven M et al. Inj Prev 1999;5:129–132.
7. Cooper C, Dennison EM, Leufkens HG, Bishop N et al. J Bone Miner Res 2004;19:1976–1981.
8. Anis AH, Stiell IG, Stewart DG, Laupacis A. Ann Emerg Med 1995;26:422–428.
9. Stiell IG, Greenberg GH, McKnight RD et al. Ann Emerg Med 1992;4:384–390.
10. Stiell I, Wells G, Laupacis A, Brison R et al. BMJ 1995;311:594–597.
11. Auleley GR, Kerboull L, Durieux P, Cosquer M et al. Ann Emerg Med 1998;32:14–18.
12. Auleley GR, Ravaud P, Giraudeau B, Kerboull L et al. JAMA 1997;25:1935–1939.
13. Chande VT. Arch Pediatr Adolesc Med 1995;149:255–258.
14. Clark KD, Tanner S. Pediatr Emerg Care 2003;19:73–78.
15. Plint AC, Bulloch B, Osmond MH, Stiell I et al. Acad Emerg Med 1999;6:1005–1009.
16. Libetta C, Burke D, Brennan P, Yassa J. J Accid Emerg Med 1999;16:342–344.
17. Boutis K, Komar L, Jaramillo D, Babyn P et al. Lancet 2001;358:2118–2121.
18. Cutler L, Molloy A, Dhukuram V, Bass A. J Bone Joint Surg Br 2004;86:239–243.
19. Lohman M, Kivisaari A, Kallio P, Puntila J et al. Skeletal Radiol 2001;30:504–511.
20. Seifert J, Matthes G, Hinz P, Paris S et al. J Pediatr Orthop 2003;23:727–732.
21. Ecklund K, Jaramillo D. AJR Am J Roentgenol 2002;178:967–972.
22. Sailhan F, Chotel F, Guibal AL, Gollogly S et al. Eur Radiol 2004;14:1600–1608.
23. Simanovsky N, Hiller N, Leibner E, Simanovsky N. Pediatr Radiol 2005;35:1062–1065.
24. Singh AK, Malpass S, Walker G. Arch Emerg Med 1990;7:90–94.
25. Wang CL, Shieh JY, Wang TG, Hsieh FJ. J Clin Ultrasound 1999;27:421–425.

20

Imaging of Adults with Low Back Pain in the Primary Care Setting

Marla B. K. Sammer and Jeffrey G. Jarvik

Issues

I. What is the role of imaging in patients suspected of having a herniated disk?
   A. Plain radiography
   B. Computed tomography
   C. Magnetic resonance
II. What is the role of imaging in patients with low back pain suspected of having metastatic disease?
   A. Plain radiographs
   B. Computed tomography
   C. Magnetic resonance
   D. Bone scanning and single photon emission computed tomography
   E. Cost-effectiveness analysis
III. What is the role of imaging in patients with back pain suspected of having infection?
   A. Plain radiographs
   B. Computed tomography
   C. Magnetic resonance
   D. Bone scanning and single photon emission computed tomography
IV. What is the role of imaging in patients with low back pain suspected of having compression fractures?
   A. Plain radiographs
   B. Computed tomography
   C. Magnetic resonance
   D. Bone scanning and single photon emission computed tomography

J.G. Jarvik (✉)
Department of Radiology, University of Washington, Seattle, WA 98195, USA
e-mail: jarvikij@u.washington.edu

L.S. Medina et al. (eds.), *Evidence-Based Imaging: Improving the Quality of Imaging in Patient Care, Revised Edition*,
DOI 10.1007/978-1-4419-7777-9_20, © Springer Science+Business Media, LLC 2011

V. What is the role of imaging in patients with back pain suspected of having ankylosing spondylitis?
   A. Plain radiographs
   B. Computed tomography
   C. Magnetic resonance
   D. Bone scanning and single photon emission computed tomography
VI. What is the role of imaging in patients with back pain suspected of having spinal stenosis?
   A. Plain radiographs
   B. Computed tomography
   C. Magnetic resonance
   D. Bone scanning and single photon emission computed tomography
VII. What are patients' perceptions of the role of imaging in low back pain?
VIII. What is the role of vertebroplasty for patients with painful osteoporotic compression fractures?

Key Points

- The natural history of low back pain (LBP) is typically benign; in the absence of "red flags," imaging can safely be limited to a minority of patients with LBP in the primary care setting (strong evidence).
- LBP imaging is often performed to rule out a serious etiology, especially metastases. While the first-line study is plain radiographs, magnetic resonance (MR) is more sensitive. However, initial imaging with MR has not yet proven to be cost-effective (moderate evidence).
- Many incidental findings are discovered when imaging the lumbar spine, including disk desiccation, annular tears, bulging disks, and herniated disks. Their eventual correlation with back pain is not known. However, while disk bulges and protrusions are common in asymptomatic individuals, extrusions are not (strong evidence).
- Imaging can diagnose surgically treatable causes of radiculopathy (herniated disks and spinal stenosis). However, these are typically not the causes of LBP and are often incidental findings in asymptomatic individuals; furthermore, the long-term efficacy of corrective surgery for these conditions has not been established (moderate evidence).
- Vertebroplasty is not better than local anesthetic injection for the treatment of painful osteoporotic compression fractures and should not be routinely performed (strong evidence).

Definition and Pathophysiology

Low back pain (LBP) is a pervasive problem that affects two-thirds of adults at some time in their lives. Fortunately, the natural history of LBP is usually benign, and diagnostic imaging can be restricted to a small percentage of LBP sufferers. This chapter reviews the evidence regarding both the diagnostic accuracy of common imaging modalities for several common conditions, and the utility of imaging in patients with LBP in the primary care setting. The most common spine imaging tests are plain X-rays, computed tomography (CT), MR, and bone scanning. We do not review other modalities (conventional myelography, diskography, and positron emission tomography), which are usually ordered by specialists prior to surgical intervention. This work is based partly on an article we previously published in the *Annals of Internal Medicine* (1).

Epidemiology and Differential Diagnosis of LBP in Primary Care

Low back pain ranks among the most common reasons for physician visits and is the most common reason for work disability in the USA (2–4). Among those with uncomplicated back pain, it is often impossible to distinguish a precise anatomic cause, and early treatments are generally aimed at symptomatic relief, so a precise anatomic diagnosis is usually both unnecessary and impossible. In fact, a definitive diagnosis is not reached in as many as 85% of patients with LBP (5), and when the etiology cannot be determined it is frequently assumed to result from muscle sprains or strains, ligamentous injuries, and spinal degenerative changes.

Further complicating matters, there are numerous imaging findings in the spines of asymptomatic patients. These include spinal stenosis, mild scoliosis, transitional vertebra, spondylolysis, Schmorl's nodes, spina bifida, and degenerative changes (6). For example, spinal stenosis is present in up to 20% of asymptomatic adults over the age of 60. The relationship of these findings to back pain is questionable because they are equally prevalent among persons with and without pain (7). Steinberg and colleagues (6) studied the radiographs of a large group of male army recruits with and without LBP. While they attempted to find a correlation between numerous variables and LBP (including right and left scoliosis, lordosis, degree of lordosis, vertebral rotation, spina bifida at multiple levels, transitional vertebra, wedge vertebra, degenerative changes, Schmorl's nodes, unilateral spondylolysis, bilateral spondylolysis, spondylolisthesis, spinal canal anteroposterior diameter, interpedicular distance, and intra-apophyso-laminar space), they found an association with only six of the variables. The most statistically significant difference was the presence of right-sided scoliosis (16.8 vs. 5.6% in the control group, $p < 0.0001$). The study also found that lumbarization of S1, wedge vertebra, bilateral spondylolysis, and

spondylolisthesis had weaker associations with LBP, with p values up to 0.04. Since the authors did not have a priori hypotheses, their study suffers from the problem of multiple comparisons, limiting the conclusions that can be drawn. Except for right-sided scoliosis, all the other associations must be viewed as exploratory and require independent confirmation.

Still, researchers continue to explore the relationship between possibly incidental findings, especially of intervertebral disk herniation, and the symptoms of back pain. Herniated disks are clearly not the culprit in the vast majority of patients with LBP. Only 2% of persons with LBP actually undergo surgery for a disk herniation (8, 9). Moreover, imaging tests identify herniated disks among a large fraction of people without LBP (from 20 to 80%, depending on age, selection, and definition of disk herniation) (Fig. 20.1) (10–12). These asymptomatic herniations appear to be clinically unimportant. In a prospective study, our group found that the prevalence of most disk abnormalities, including desiccation, loss of disk height, bulge, annular tear, and protrusion, were not significantly different between asymptomatic subjects with and without a history of prior LBP (12). Boos and colleagues (13) followed asymptomatic individuals with a high rate of disk herniations (73%) for 5 years. They concluded that while the presence of disk abnormalities did not predict future LBP, psychosocial factors, mostly related to occupation, did. Certain imaging findings are likely quite important clinically. Disk extrusions, a subtype of herniation, are much less prevalent than disk protrusions in patients without LBP and are typically considered a clinically important imaging finding (10–12, 14).

Imaging is indicated when infection or malignancy is being considered, as well as when patients present with cauda equina syndrome, a true surgical emergency. These serious conditions occur less than 5% of the time in the primary care setting, with only 0.7% of LBP patients having metastatic cancer (with breast, lung, and prostate being the most common primary tumors), 0.01% having spinal infections, and 0.0004% having cauda equina syndrome (15). In their recent retrospective chart review of 2007 lumbar film reports, van den Bosch et al. (16) reported the overall likelihood of finding a serious condition, such as infection or possible tumor at <1%, with no tumors found in patients younger than 55.

Overall Cost to Society

In 1998, health care costs for LBP (inpatient care, office visits, prescription drugs, and emergency room visits) totaled $90.7 billion. This was 2.5% of the national health care expenditure, and did not include physical therapy, chiropractic care, or nursing home care. The data to calculate these figures came from a national database, and included only patients with back disorders, disk disorders, and back injuries, as per International Classification of Diseases (ICD-9) codes. Consequently, a substantial proportion of LBP patients, such as those with malignancy, infection, or osteoporotic compression fractures as the primary etiology of pain, were likely excluded from these estimates. Finally, this estimate does not include non-health care expenditures such as workers' compensation, sick leave, and disability, an important consideration since LBP is the largest cause of disability and workers' compensation claims in the USA (17, 18).

Goals

There are two major goals in imaging primary care patients with LBP: (1) to exclude serious disease (tumor, infection, or neural tissue compromise requiring decompression), and (2) to find a treatable explanation for the patient's pain.

Methodology

We performed three Medline searches using PubMed. The first covered the period 1966 to September 2001 and the second, to update the literature search from the original article on which this chapter is based, covered September 2001 through August 2004. The third was also performed to update the chapter, and covered 1996 through December 2009, searching specifically for randomized controlled trials related to vertebroplasty. For the first two searches we used the following search terms: (1) *back pain*, (2) *intervertebral disk displacement*, (3) *sciatica*, (4) *spinal stenosis*, and (5) *diagnostic imaging*. We applied the subheadings *diagnosis*, *radiography*, or *radionuclide imaging* to the first statement.

We excluded animal experiments and articles on pediatric patients. We also excluded case reports, review articles, editorials, and non-English-language articles. We included only articles describing plain X-rays, CT, MR (including MR myelography), and bone scanning. In the first search, the total number of citations retrieved was 1,468. Two reviewers (J.G.J. and Richard A. Deyo) reviewed all the titles and subsequently the abstracts of 568 articles that appeared pertinent; the full text of 150 articles was then reviewed. At each step, the articles' authors and institutions were masked. Disagreements regarding inclusion of particular articles, which occurred in approximately 15%, were settled by consensus. In the second search, the total number of citations retrieved was 558. Two reviewers (M.B.K.S. and J.G.J.) reviewed all the titles and subsequently the abstracts of 168 articles that appeared pertinent. Finally, we reviewed the full text of 75 articles. Disagreements regarding inclusion of particular articles, which occurred in 12%, were settled by consensus. Only those articles meeting our inclusion criteria were cited for this review.

Because most studies had several potential biases, our estimates of sensitivity and specificity must be considered imprecise. The most common biases were failure to apply a single reference test to all cases; test review bias (study test was reviewed with knowledge of the final diagnosis); diagnosis review bias (determination of final diagnosis was affected by the study test); and spectrum bias (only severe cases of disease were included).

I. What Is the Role of Imaging in Patients Suspected of Having a Herniated Disk?

Summary of Evidence: Radiculopathy is a common and well-accepted indication for imaging; however, it is not an urgent indication, and with 4–8 weeks of conservative care, most patients improve. Urgent MR and consultation are needed if the patient has signs or symptoms of possible cauda equina syndrome (bilateral radiculopathy, saddle anesthesia, or urinary retention). Current literature suggests that MR is slightly more sensitive than CT in its ability to detect a herniated disk. Plain radiography has no role in diagnosing herniated disks, though it does, like the other modalities, show degenerative changes that are sometimes associated with herniated disks. Finally, all three methods commonly reveal findings in asymptomatic subjects.

Supporting Evidence

A. Plain Radiography

Because radiographs cannot directly visualize disks or nerve roots, their usefulness is limited. Plain film signs of disk degeneration include disk space narrowing, osteophytes, and endplate sclerosis. Indirect signs of possible nerve root compromise include facet degeneration as manifested by sclerosis and hypertrophy.

In their recent prospective study examining patients with chronic LBP, Peterson and colleagues (19) considered whether a relationship existed between radiographic lumbar spine degenerative changes, and disability or pain severity. They found no link between the severity of lumbar facet degeneration and self-reported pain or disability levels. While they did find a weak link between the number of degenerative disk levels and the severity of degenerative changes at these levels with pain in the week immediately preceding the exam, they found no correlation to pain or disability over the patients' entire pain episode (which in some cases had lasted greater than 5 years) (moderate evidence). Furthermore, in greater than a quarter of the patients, all of whom were considered chronic LBP sufferers, no degenerative changes were evident on their radiographs. Even in those patients with degenerative findings, the severity of degeneration was rated as mild in approximately 50%. Lundin et al. (20) studied athletes for 12–13 years and found only a borderline correlation between loss of disk height at baseline and back pain ($p = 0.06$). However, they found a highly significant correlation between a decrease in disk height over the intervening 12–13 years and the development of LBP ($p = 0.005$) (strong evidence).

B. Computed Tomography

In an often-cited study by Thornbury and colleagues (21), CT had a sensitivity of 88–94% for herniated disks and a specificity of 57–64%,

similar to that for MR (Fig. 20.2) (moderate evidence). The area under a receiver operating characteristic (ROC) curve for CT was 0.85–0.86. Diagnosis review bias likely inflated these estimates of accuracy. Interestingly, a study by Jackson et al. (22) arrived at similar estimates of sensitivity and specificity (86 and 60%, respectively) despite the selective use of a surgical reference standard (moderate evidence). Not taken into account in these studies is that herniated disks are commonly present in asymptomatic persons. While likely representing real anatomic abnormalities, these findings are irrelevant for clinical decision making, and thus reduce test specificity (Table 20.1.). Finally, while these studies suggest CT is comparable to MR for diagnosing disk disease, an important drawback of CT compared with MR is that with only axial image acquisition, it is more difficult to subcategorize disk herniations into protrusions vs. extrusions (see section below on MR). However, multidetector CTs, with thin-section acquisition allows high-quality sagittal reformations to potentially overcome this limitation.

We did not find any data regarding the accuracy of CT for nerve root impingement. However, because surrounding fat provides natural contrast, CT, as opposed to plain radiography, can accurately depict the foraminal and extraforaminal nerve roots, directly visualizing nerve root displacement or compression. But CT is less effective in evaluating the intrathecal nerve roots (limited evidence) (32).

C. Magnetic Resonance

MR has good sensitivity and variable specificity for disk herniations. Thornbury et al. (21) (moderate evidence) demonstrated a sensitivity for herniated disks of 89–100%, but a specificity of only 43–57%. The area under the ROC curve was 0.81–0.84. In a cohort of 180 patients, Janssen et al. (33) found a sensitivity and specificity of 96 and 97%, respectively. Although this study avoided test review bias, diagnosis review bias was likely present, with selective application of the surgical reference standard (moderate evidence).

While data regarding sensitivity and specificity of MR for nerve root compromise is lacking, MR has several advantages over CT, including superior soft tissue contrast, multiplanar imaging, and the ability to characterize intrathecal nerve roots (12, 34–36). Still unclear is how best to evaluate nerve root compromise. In a prospective evaluation of 96 consecutive lumbar spine MRs, Gorbachova and Terk (37) found no correlation between nerve root sleeve diameter and disk pathology, concluding that measuring the nerve diameter is not a clinically useful (strong evidence). Pfirrmann and colleagues (38) devised a reliable grading system for nerve root compromise: (1) normal; (2) nerve root contacted; (3) nerve root displaced; and (4) nerve root compressed. They retrospectively evaluated 500 nerve roots in 250 symptomatic patients, and then compared their MR grading system to a similar surgical scale in the 94 nerve roots that were evaluated operatively. They found that their system correlated well with surgical findings, and that intra- and interobserver reliability for the grading scale was high with kappas of 0.72–0.77 for intraobserver, and 0.62–0.67 for interobserver (moderate evidence).

Despite the high prevalence of herniated disks (from 20 to 80%, depending on age, selection, and definition of disk herniation) (Table 20.1.) (10–12), and evidence of disk degeneration among asymptomatic individuals (on MR 46–93%), several studies have attempted to correlate disk disease with disability and pain. In a prospective study of 394 patients, Porchet et al. (39) found that leg pain (but not back pain), disability, and bodily pain (all $p < 0.005$) were significantly associated with MR disk disease severity. Beattie and colleagues (34) also studied MR abnormalities and their correlation to pain, finding relationships between distal leg pain and both disk extrusions and severe nerve compression ($p < 0.008$ and <0.005, respectively). Interestingly, however, in the majority of the participants, they found no MR abnormality that corresponded to the distribution of the patient's pain.

Brant-Zawadzki et al. argued that the distinction between protrusions and extrusions is important because extrusions are rare in asymptomatic subjects (1%), but bulges (52%) and protrusions (27%) are common. In a prospective trial, our group found that extrusions, but not bulges or protrusions, were significantly associated with a history of LBP ($p < 0.01$) (14). Ahn and colleagues (40), though they did not use the terms *protrusion or extrusion*, agreed that distinguishing the type of herniation is important. Comparing transligamentous herniations

(extrusions or migrated extrusions) to protrusions and bulges, they found that patients with transligamentous herniations had slightly better outcomes. In 2001, the North American Spine Society, the American Society of Neuroradiology, and the American Society of Spine Radiology jointly published recommendations regarding the use of a consensus nomenclature for describing disk abnormalities that incorporated these terms (protrusions and extrusions) (41).

In a series of 125 subjects, Brant-Zawadzki et al. (42) looked at the inter- and intraobserver agreement for four categories of disk morphologies (normal, bulge, protrusion, and extrusion). The authors defined a bulge as a circumferential and symmetrical extension of disk material beyond the interspace, while a herniation was a focal or asymmetrical extension of disk material. Protrusions and extrusions are subcategories of herniations. Protrusions are broad based, while extrusions have a "neck" that makes the base against the parent disk narrower than the extruded material itself (Fig. 20.3). Using these definitions for disk morphologies, the interreader kappa was 0.59, indicating moderate agreement. Intraobserver agreement was slightly higher, ranging from 0.69 to 0.72, indicating substantial agreement. Others have obtained comparable degrees of interreader agreement ($\kappa=0.59$) in cohorts of 34 and 45 patients, respectively (43, 44). In a study of the reliability of chiropractors' interpretations, Cooley and colleagues (45) found interexaminer reliability comparable to that of radiologists ($\kappa=0.60$).

Magnetic resonance myelography (MRM) is a relatively new method that uses heavily T2-weighted three-dimensional (3D) images to provide high contrast between cerebrospinal fluid (CSF) and the cord and nerve roots. Because of the high contrast of CSF, MRM has been used for diagnosing suspected spinal stenosis. However, its role in disk imaging has not been well established. In one prospective evaluation of preoperative candidates with prior diagnoses of disk herniation, Pui and Husen (46) found no difference between the sensitivity and specificity of MRM and conventional MR for diagnosis of disk herniation (strong evidence). Spectrum bias was likely present, since the reference standard, which was applied to all patients, was surgical confirmation. Also, MRM may be useful in the diagnosis of dorsal root pathology. In their prospective study of 83 patients with MR-verified lumbar disk herniation and sciatica, Aoto et al. (47) found that swelling in the dorsal root ganglia at clinically involved lumbar nerve segments was clearly seen on MRM, and the degree of root swelling correlated with pain severity.

The evidence for the use of gadolinium to detect nerve root enhancement, and thereby increase specificity, is conflicting (48–50) (moderate evidence). Autio and colleagues (51) prospectively studied 63 patients with unilateral sciatica to determine the relevance of enhancement patterns. They found a negative correlation between the duration of symptoms and the extent of enhancement. While they failed to find a correlation between enhancement and multiple clinical symptoms, they did find a significant correlation between percent rim enhancement (greater than 75%) and the presence of an abnormal Achilles reflex, with a sensitivity and specificity of 76 and 82%, respectively (moderate evidence). Currently, gadolinium is usually reserved for the evaluation of postoperative patients. But even in postoperative imaging, its role has recently been challenged. In a prospective study of postdiskectomy patients, Mullin et al. (52) found no significant difference between pre- and postcontrast sensitivity (92–93%) and specificity (97%) for recurrent disk herniation (strong evidence).

Aprill and Bogduk (53) proposed the term *high-intensity zone* (HIZ) to describe the presence of focal high signal in the posterior annulus fibrosus on T2-weighted images (Fig. 20.4). However, over a decade after publication of their manuscript, the clinical importance of annular tears remains uncertain. While some investigators have not found a strong relationship between the presence of an annular tear and either positive diskography (30) (moderate evidence) or clinical symptoms (54) (moderate evidence), others have found a correlation (53, 55) (limited evidence and moderate evidence). In a retrospective twin cohort study, Videman and colleagues (56) found that annular tears were present in 15% of their patients and were statistically significantly associated with many of the LBP parameters they studied. The most significant association existed between annular tears and pain intensity in the past year [odds ratio (OR) 2.2, 95% confidence interval (CI) 1.3–3.9] (moderate evidence). Similar associations existed between annular tears and any LBP in the past year, disability from LBP in the

past year, and LBP at the time of the study. But as with other imaging findings, the high prevalence of annular tears in subjects without LBP calls its clinical value into question (14, 30).

II. What Is the Role of Imaging in Patients with Low Back Pain Suspected of Having Metastatic Disease?

Summary of Evidence: Both radionuclide studies and MR are sensitive and specific studies for detecting metastases. We did not identify studies supporting the use of CT for detecting bony spinal metastases; however, CT does depict cortical bone well. Plain films are the least sensitive imaging modality for detecting metastases. Nevertheless, current recommendations still advocate using plain films as the initial imaging in selected patients.

Supporting Evidence

A. Plain Radiographs

Radiographs are a specific, but relatively insensitive test for detecting metastatic disease. A primary limitation is that 50% of trabecular bone must be lost before a lytic lesion is visible (limited evidence) (57, 58). If only lytic or blastic lesions are counted as a positive study, radiographs are 60% sensitive and 99.5% specific for metastatic disease [limited evidence (57, 58); strong evidence (59)]. If one includes compression fractures as indicating a positive examination, then sensitivity is improved to 70% but specificity is decreased to 95%.

B. Computed Tomography

We found no adequate data on the accuracy of CT for metastases.

C. Magnetic Resonance

While the sensitivity of MR for metastases is likely high, the variable quality of the available literature makes arrival at a summary estimate difficult. In five studies of patients with metastatic cancer or other infiltrative marrow processes, MR appeared more sensitive than bone scintigraphy. The sensitivity of MR ranged from 83 to 100% and specificity was estimated at 92%. These studies used a combination of biopsy and follow-up imaging as the reference standard. Several biases (selection, sampling, nonuniform application of reference standard, and diagnosis review) likely inflated apparent performance (60–64) (Albra, moderate evidence; Avrahami, moderate evidence; Carroll, moderate evidence; Carmody, limited evidence; and Kosuda, moderate evidence).

D. Bone Scanning and Single Photon Emission Computed Tomography

In seven studies, the sensitivity of radionuclide bone scans for tumor ranged from 74 to 98% (all moderate evidence except for McNeil, which was limited evidence) (65–72). Spectrum bias, incorporation bias, test review bias, and diagnosis review bias were all present and likely inflated the accuracy estimates.

E. Cost-Effectiveness Analysis

Despite advances in imaging over the past decade, there is no compelling evidence to justify substantial deviation from the diagnostic strategy published by the Agency for Health Care Research and Quality (AHRQ) in 1994 (73). These guidelines reflect the growing evidence-based consensus that plain radiography is unnecessary for every patient with back pain because of the low yield of useful findings, potentially misleading results, high dose of gonadal radiation, and interpretation disagreements. However, in patients in whom the pretest probability of a serious underlying condition is elevated (e.g., patients older than the age of 50, patients with a history of a primary cancer, etc.), the combination of radiographs and laboratory tests such as an erythrocyte sedimentation rate (ESR) or CBC is likely the appropriate first step.

MR is clearly a more accurate diagnostic test for detecting tumor than are radiographs; nevertheless, it is not a cost-effective initial option. This is nicely illustrated in the recent paper by Joines et al. (74). Building a decision analytic model to compare strategies for detecting cancer in primary care patients with LBP, they combined information from the history, ESR, and radiographs, and compared this strategy to one that used MR on all patients. They found that to detect a case of cancer, the MR strategy costs approximately ten times as much as the radiograph strategy ($50,000 vs. $5,300). Even more impressive was that the incremental cost of performing MR on all patients was $625,000 per additional case found. The authors did not attempt to convert cost per case detected into cost per life year saved or cost per quality-adjusted life year (QALY). However, since metastatic cancer presenting with back pain is usually incurable, the life year costs would likely be much greater. Hollingworth and colleagues (75) attempted to further elaborate on Joines et al.'s conclusions by limiting the MR imaging to rapid MR. In a decision model created for a hypothetical cohort of primary care patients referred to exclude cancer as the etiology of their back pain, they also found that there was not enough evidence to advocate routine rapid MR for this purpose. While there was a small increase in quality-adjusted survival (0.00043 QALYs), the incremental cost was large ($296,176). Using rapid MR rather than radiographs, fewer than one new case of cancer was detected per 1,000 patients imaged.

III. What Is the Role of Imaging in Patients with Back Pain Suspected of Having Infection?

Summary of Evidence: When infection is suspected, MR is the imaging modality of choice. Its sensitivity and specificity are superior to the alternatives, and the images obtained provide the anatomic information needed for surgical planning.

Supporting Evidence

A. Plain Radiographs

In contrast to metastatic disease, radiographic changes in infection are generally nonspecific. Furthermore, radiographic changes occur relatively late in the disease course. Findings of infection after several weeks include poor cortical definition of the involved end plate with subsequent bony lysis and decreased disk height. A paraspinous soft tissue mass may also be present. In one study, the overall sensitivity of radiographs for osteomyelitis was 82%, and the specificity was 57% (strong evidence) (76).

B. Computed Tomography

We found no adequate data on the accuracy of CT for infection in the lumbar spine.

C. Magnetic Resonance

In the single best-designed study, the sensitivity of MR for infection was 96% and the specificity was 92%, making MR more accurate than radiographs or bone scans (76) (strong evidence). Perhaps more importantly, MR delineates the extent of infection better than other modalities, which is critical to surgical planning.

The characteristic MR appearance of pyogenic spondylitis is diffuse low marrow signal on T1-weighted images and high signal on T2-weighted images (Fig. 20.5). These changes reflect increased extracellular fluid. Although classically two vertebral bodies are involved along with their intervening disk, the early imaging is more variable, occasionally with only one vertebral body being involved (77). The disk itself is high in signal and may herniate through a softened end plate. Gadolinium may increase the specificity of MR, with enhancement of an infected disk and end plates, although rigorous evidence is lacking (78).

We found no studies quantifying the accuracy of MR for epidural abscesses, but because of greater soft tissue contrast, MR should be better able to characterize the extent of an epidural process than CT.

D. Bone Scanning and Single Photon Emission Computed Tomography

In one study investigating bone scanning and infection, the sensitivity was moderately high

at 82%, but specificity poor; only 23% (79) (moderate evidence). In the same study, gallium-67 SPECT had a 91% sensitivity and 92% specificity.

IV. What Is the Role of Imaging in Patients with Low Back Pain Suspected of Having Compression Fractures?

Summary of Evidence: There are no good estimates on which imaging modality is best for compression fracture imaging. When differentiation between metastatic and osteoporotic collapse is sought, MR is currently the method of choice.

Supporting Evidence

A. Plain Radiographs

Various biases (diagnosis review bias, test review bias, and selective use of reference standards) make it difficult to provide a summary estimate of the radiographic sensitivity and specificity for acute compression fractures. While radiographs are likely reasonably sensitive, they probably cannot distinguish between acute and chronic compression fractures. Clues that a fracture is old include the presence of osteophytes or vertebral body fusion. Because MR identifies marrow edema or an associated hematoma, and because bone scan evaluates metabolic activity, they provide more useful information regarding fracture acuity (limited evidence) (80).

B. Computed Tomography

We found no adequate data on the accuracy of CT for compression fractures.

C. Magnetic Resonance

We were unable to identify accurate sensitivity and specificity estimates for MR imaging in compression fractures. While there is an abundance of literature on MR and compression fractures, the overwhelming majority of articles focus on differentiating malignant from osteo-porotic etiologies.

D. Bone Scanning and Single Photon Emission Computed Tomography

Bone scans are widely used for differentiating acute from older (subacute or chronic) com-pression fractures. Old fractures should be metabolically inactive, while recent fractures should have high radiotracer uptake (61). We did not identify articles that allowed us to cal-culate sensitivity and specificity for this condition.

V. What Is the Role of Imaging in Patients with Back Pain Suspected of Having Ankylosing Spondylitis?

Summary of Evidence: There are only a few studies that attempt to determine which imag-ing modality is best for diagnosing ankylosing spondylitis (AS). Plain radiographs and bone scans with SPECT both have relatively high specificity; specificity on CT and MR is cur-rently not available. Plain radiographs appear to be adequate for initial imaging in a patient suspected of having AS.

Supporting Evidence

A. Plain Radiographs

The characteristic imaging findings in AS are osteitis, syndesmophytes, erosions, and sacroil-iac joint erosions, with joint erosions occurring relatively early and being readily detectable by radiography. While the sensitivity of radio-graphs is poor (45%), the specificity appears high (100%), although in the single study exam-ining this issue, spectrum bias likely inflated both estimates (moderate evidence) (81).

B. Computed Tomography

We found no adequate data on the accuracy of CT for AS.

C. Magnetic Resonance

In a small study by Marc et al. (81), MR showed abnormalities in 17 of 31 subjects with spondy-loarthropathies yielding a sensitivity of 55%. Specificity could not be determined (81) (mod-erate evidence).

D. Bone Scanning and Single Photon Emission Computed Tomography

In two studies, bone scan sensitivity ranged from 25 to 85%, with the higher sensitivity achieved by using SPECT (81, 82) (both studies moderate evidence). Specificity ranged from 90 to 100%. These studies suffered from a lack of high-quality reference standards and indepen-dent interpretations.

VI. What Is the Role of Imaging in Patients with Back Pain Suspected of Having Spinal Stenosis?

Summary of Evidence: Both CT and MR can be used to diagnosis central stenosis. On MR, the radiologists' general impression, rather than a millimeter measurement, is valid.

Supporting Evidence

A. Plain Radiographs

No studies provided good estimates of radio-graphic accuracy in detecting central stenosis. Since radiographs can only estimate bony canal compromise, the sensitivity for central stenosis is undoubtedly poorer than that of CT or MR, which depict soft tissue structures.

B. Computed Tomography

A meta-analysis by Kent et al. (83) reported CT sensitivity for central stenosis of 70–100% and specificity of 80–96% (limited evidence). Methodologic quality was variable but gener-ally poor, making pooling of the data impracti-cal. Central stenosis is also common in asymptomatic persons, with a prevalence of 4–28% (limited evidence) (84), and thus the specificity of CT for central stenosis, as it is for disk herniations, is likely less than the reported estimates.

C. Magnetic Resonance

In the 1992 meta-analysis by Kent et al. (83) the sensitivity of MR for stenosis was 81–97% while specificity ranged from 72 to 100% (limited evidence). Using stricter criteria for false positives, specificity was 93–100%.

Of note, two recent studies suggest that the readers' general impression of central stenosis is valid. In a retrospective study comparing electromyogram (EMG) findings to radiologists' MR interpretations, Haig et al. (85) found that the radiologists' subjective sense of central stenosis (normal, mild, moderate, or severe) was statistically significantly correlated with the EMG ($r = 0.4$, $p < 0.017$) (moderate evidence). Speciale et al. (86) assessed the intra- and interobserver reliability of physicians for classifying the degree of lumbar stenosis. Two neurosurgeons, two orthopedic spine surgeons, and three radiologists reviewed MRs from patients with a clinical and radiologic diagnosis of lumbar spinal stenosis. While the interobserver reliability was fair among all specialties ($\kappa < 0.26$), it was highest among radiologists (moderate with $\kappa = 0.40$), and considerably lower among the surgeons ($\kappa = 0.21$ for neurosurgeons and $\kappa = 0.15$ for orthopedic surgeons). In concordance with Haig's work, they found that the readers' subjective evaluation of stenosis significantly correlated with the calculated cross-sectional area ($p < 0.001$).

D. Bone Scanning and Single Photon Emission Computed Tomography

Bone scanning has no role in central stenosis imaging.

VII. What Are Patients' Perceptions of the Role of Imaging in Low Back Pain?

Summary of Evidence: The majority of patients with LBP think imaging is an important part of their care. However, in patients who are imaged, results of satisfaction with care are conflicting and overall not significantly higher than in those who were not imaged. Additionally, when plain radiographs are obtained, outcome is not significantly altered (and in some cases, is worse). But when MR or CT is used early in the workup of LBP, there is a very slight improvement in patient outcome.

Supporting Evidence: While the majority of studies attempt to validate a modality by its diagnostic accuracy, possibly more important is whether the test actually alters patient outcomes. In their recent randomized controlled trial, Kerry et al. (87) studied 659 patients with LBP, randomizing 153 patients to either lumbar spine radiographs or care without imaging, while also studying 506 patients in an observational arm (strong evidence). At 6 weeks and at 1 year, there was no difference between the groups in physical functioning, disability, pain, social functioning, general health, or need for further referrals. However, in the treatment arm at both 6 weeks and 1 year, there was a small improvement in self-reported overall mental health (Table 20.2). In a similar randomized controlled trial of 421 patients, Kendrick and colleagues (88) actually found a slight increase in pain duration, and a decrease in overall functioning in the radiograph group at 3 months, though at 9 months there was no difference between the groups (strong evidence).

A few studies have attempted to demonstrate how CT and MR relate to outcome. In a large randomized study, Gilbert et al. (90) studied 782 patients, randomizing them to early imaging with CT or MR, or imaging only if a clear indication developed (strong evidence). They found that treatment was not influenced by early imaging. However, while both groups improved from baseline, there was slightly more improvement in the early imaging arm at both 8 ($p = 0.005$) and 24 ($p = 0.002$) months. In a subgroup of these patients, Gillan et al. (91) found that while there was an increase in diagnostic confidence in the early imaging group (Table 20.2), imaging did not change diagnostic or therapeutic impact (strong evidence). Our group also performed a randomized controlled trial assigning primary care patients with LBP to receive either lumbar spine radiographs or a rapid lumbar spine MR (92) (strong evidence). We found nearly identical outcomes in the two groups. Vroomen and colleagues (93), however, did find in patients with leg pain, utilizing early MR helped predict the patient's prognosis (strong evidence).

Patient satisfaction and expectations must also be accounted for when developing an imaging strategy. Many patients with LBP believe imaging is important or necessary to their care (94–96). However, there are conflicting results regarding improved satisfaction of care when imaging is actually performed. In their randomized trial using plain radiographs, Kendrick and colleagues (88) discovered that if participants had been given the choice, 80% would have elected to be imaged (strong evidence). They also found that while satisfaction was similar at 3 months in both the imaging and nonimaging groups (Table 20.3), by 9 months, the intervention group was slightly more satisfied with their care. In the same cohort, Miller et al. (96) reported that the imaging group had a higher overall satisfaction score at 9 months. In a comparable study, Kerry and colleagues (87) found no difference in early patient satisfaction (strong evidence). They did not provide data for long-term satisfaction. Finally, in our comparison of rapid MR to radiographs, there was no difference in overall patient satisfaction between the two groups, but patients who received an MR were more reassured (92) (strong evidence).

VIII. What Is the Role of Vertebroplasty for Patients with Painful Osteoporotic Compression Fractures?

Summary of Evidence: Percutaneous vertebroplasty, first described by Galibert et al. (97) in 1987, is the injection of polymethylmethacrylate (PMMA) into a painful vertebra, with the intention of stabilizing it, relieving pain, and restoring function. Rarely, serious complications from bone cement leaks can occur. What is unknown is whether vertebroplasty increases the rate of adjacent vertebral fractures (98). Uncontrolled studies indicated that vertebroplasty was a promising therapy for patients with painful osteoporotic compression fractures, but two blinded, randomized controlled trials failed to confirm that promise (99, 100).

Supporting Evidence: Osteoporotic vertebral compression fractures occur annually in about 700,000 Americans, including 25% of postmenopausal women (101, 102) and often produces psychologically and physically devastating pain, as well as an increased risk of death. Although the pain of an acute fracture is usually relieved within several weeks by conservative treatment (bed rest, antiinflammatory and analgesic medications, calcitonin, or external bracing), it occasionally requires narcotics, and even then may persist (103–105).

To date, there have been only two randomized controlled trials of vertebroplasty, both published in 2009 (99, 100). These two studies shared common outcome metrics and had similar methods. They recruited only patients with osteoporotic fractures and randomly allocated them to have either a true vertebroplasty or a control intervention consisting of a simulated vertebroplasty using only lidocaine without PMMA. Both studies used pain and functional disability as measures of outcome. The primary outcome time point was slightly different between studies, being 1 month in the Kallmes trial and 3 months in the Buchbinder trial. Both studies arrived at the same conclusion – although both the vertebroplasty and control groups improved from baseline to follow-up, there was no difference in the degree of improvement in the primary outcomes between the vertebroplasty and control groups. These results were in contrast to the case series, uncontrolled prospective studies and controlled but not randomized cohort studies that had been published previously (106–120). In light of these two blinded, randomized controlled trials both showing no advantage of vertebroplasty compared with local anesthetic injection for osteoporotic fractures, vertebroplasty should not be routinely performed for this indication.

Overall Modality Accuracy Summary

Table 20.4 summarizes the diagnostic accuracy parameters for each of the four modalities described. The likelihood ratio (LR) summarizes the sensitivity and specificity information in a single number, comparing the probability of having a positive test result in patients with the disease with the probability of a positive test in patients without the disease, or LR+ = [Probability (+test | disease)]/ [Probability (+test | no disease)]. This is equivalent to [sensitivity/(1 − specificity)]. Similarly, the LR for a negative test is [(1 − sensitivity)/ specificity]. The larger the LR, the better the test is for ruling in a diagnosis; conversely, the smaller the LR, the better it is for excluding a diagnosis. LRs greater than 10 or less than 0.1 are generally thought to be clinically useful. A LR equal to 1 provides no clinically useful information.

Suggested Imaging Protocols

Plain Radiographs

Lateral and anteroposterior (AP) radiographs should be obtained for initial imaging in primary care patients with LBP; recent evidence supports lateral radiographs alone.

Supporting Evidence: The 1994 AHRQ evidence-based guidelines for the diagnosis and treatment of patients with acute LBP (73) recommend only two views of the lumbar spine be obtained routinely (121, 122). More recently, a prospective study by Khoo et al. (123) suggests that a single lateral radiograph may be as effective as the standard two view examination. In 1,030 lumbar spine radiographs, the AP film significantly altered the diagnosis in only 1.3% of cases (all cases of possible sacroiliitis or pars defects). More importantly, infection and malignancy were not missed on the lateral film alone. In certain circumstances, other views are important. When compared with AP views alone, oblique films better demonstrate the pars interarticularis in profile to assess for spondylolysis. Flexion-extension films are used to assess instability, and angled views of the sacrum are used to assess sacroiliac joints for AS. Limiting the number of views is particularly important to younger females, because the gonadal dose of two views alone are equal to the gonadal radiation of daily chest X-rays for several years (124–126).

Computed Tomography

For routine lumbar spine imaging in the University of Washington health system, we use a multidetector CT with 2.5-mm detector collimation and 2.5-mm intervals at 140 kVp and 200–220 mA. If the radiologist determines prior to the study that sagittal and coronal reformats are needed, we scan at 1.25 mm with 1.25-mm intervals.

Supporting Evidence: We found no studies to support specific CT imaging protocols.

Magnetic Resonance

The MR sequences we use for routine lumbar spine imaging in the University of Washington system are as follows:

1. Sagittal T1-weighted 2D spin echo, TR 400/TE minimum, 192 × 256 matrix, 26-cm field of view (FOV), 4-mm slice thickness, and 1-mm skip.
2. Sagittal T2-weighted fast recovery (frFSE) fast spin echo 2D spin echo, TR 4000/TE 110, echo train length (ETL) 25, 224 × 320 matrix, 26-cm FOV, 4-mm slice thickness, and 1-mm skip.
3. Axial T1-weighted 2D spin echo, TR 500/ TE minimum, 192 × 256 matrix, 20-cm FOV, 4-mm slice thickness, and 1-mm skip.
4. Axial T2-weighted FSE-XL, TR 4000/TE 102, ETL 12, 192 × 256 matrix, 20-cm FOV, 4-mm slice thickness, and 1-mm skip.

Supporting Evidence: We found no studies to support specific MR imaging protocols.

Take Home Tables and Figures

Tables 20.1–20.4 and Figs. 20.1–20.5 serve to highlight key recommendations and supporting evidence.

Table 20.1. Studies of lumbar spine imaging in asymptomatic adults

Modality (references)	Age group description	Prevalence of anatomic conditions				
		Herniated disk	Bulging disk	Degenerated disk	Stenosis	Annular tear
Plain X-rays (23)	14–25 years, high performance athletes (n = 143)			20%		
Plain X-rays (6)	Army recruits, 18 years old ± 2 months			4% (vs. 5% of sx pts.)		
Myelography (24)	Mean age = 51, referred for posterior-fossa acoustic neuroma (n = 300)	31%				
CT (25)	Mean age = 40					
	<40 years (n = 24)	20%			0%	
	>40 years (n = 27)	27%			3%	
MR (26)	Women mean age = 28 (n = 86)	9%	44%			
MR (10)	Under age 60 (n = 53)	22%	54%	46%	1%	
	≥Age 60 (n = 14)	36%	79%	93%	21%	
MR (11)	Mean age = 42 (n = 98)	28%[a]	52%		7%	14%
MR (12)	Mean age = 36, matched age + occupation exposure to pts. having diskectomy (n = 46)	76%[b]	51% of disks	85%		
MR (27)	Mean age = 28 (n = 41)					
MR (28)	Median age = 42 referred for head or neck imaging (n = 36)	33%[c]	81%	56%		56%
MR (29)	Mean age = 35 (n = 60)	56–60%	20–28%	72%		19–20%
MR (30)	Mean age = 40 (n = 54)					24%
MR (14)	Mean = 54 (n = 148)	38%[d]	64%	91%	10%	38%
MR (13, 31)	20–50, unrelated trauma	73% (7% with extrusion)		49%	29%	
MR (14)	Mean age = 54, VA patients	38%	64%	91%	10%	38%
MR (30)	Mean age = 40.1; cohort of prior cervical diskectomy					39%

Source: Adapted with permission from Jarvik and Deyo (1).
sx symptomatic.
[a]Sixty-four percent had disk bulge, protrusion, or extension; only 1% had extrusions.
[b]Nerve root compression in 4%; contact or displacement of nerve root in 22%.
[c]Zero percent had extrusions.
[d]Six percent had extrusions, 3% had nerve root compromise.

Table 20.2. Patient outcome

Imaging type	Comparison	Difference (95% CI, p)
Plain radiographs		
Kerry et al. (87)	Radiograph vs. no radiograph	Mental health
	6 weeks	−8 (−14 to −1, $p < 0.05$)
	1 year	−8 (−15 to −2, $p < 0.05$)
Kendrick et al. (88, 89)	Radiograph vs. no radiograph	
	Pain at 3 months	1.26 (1.0–1.6, $p < 0.04$)
	Disability at 3 months	−1.90 (CI not provided, $p < 0.05$)
CT/MR		
Gilbert et al. (90)	Early CT or MR vs. selective delayed	Acute LBP score
	8 months	−3.05 (−5.16 to −0.95, $p < 0.005$)
	2 years	−3.62 (−5.92 to −1.32, $p < 0.002$)
Gillan et al. (91)	Early CT or MR vs. selective delayed	
	Treatment altered	$p = 0.733$
	Median change in diagnostic confidence	$p = 0.001$
Jarvik et al. (92)	Early MR vs. plain radiograph	
	Mean back-related disability (Roland) at 12 months	−0.59 (−1.69 to 0.87, $p = 0.53$)
Vroomen et al. (93)	Prognostic value of MR for sciatic	
	Favorable prognosis, anular rupture	$p = 0.02$
	Favorable prognosis, nerve root compression	$p = 0.03$
	Poor prognosis, disk herniation into foramen	$p = 0.004$

Table 20.3. Patient satisfaction

Study	Comparison	Difference (95% CI, p when provided)
Kendrick et al. (88, 89) and Miller et al. (96)	Radiograph vs. no radiograph	
	Satisfaction at 3 months	−1.50 (CI not provided, $p = 0.13$)
	Satisfaction at 9 months	−2.69 (CI not provided, $p < 0.01$)
Kerry et al. (87)	Radiograph vs. no radiograph	
	Satisfaction with initial consultation/6 weeks	
	Very satisfied	1.0/1.0
	Satisfied	0.87 (0.40–1.9)/0.89 (0.37–2.1)
	Indifferent or dissatisfied	0.41 (0.12–1.3)/0.54 (0.19–1.5)
Jarvik et al. (92)	Rapid MR vs. radiograph	
	Overall satisfaction at 12 months	0.30 (−0.42 to 0.99)
	Correlation of satisfaction with reassurance at 1, 3, and 12 months	Pearson correlation coefficients $p < 0.001$ for all

Table 20.4. Accuracy of imaging for lumbar spine conditions[a]

	Sensitivity	Specificity	Likelihood ratio +	Likelihood ratio −
X-ray				
Cancer	0.6	0.95–0.995	12–120	0.40–0.42
Infection	0.82	0.57	1.9	0.32
Ankylosing spondylitis	0.26–0.45	1	Not defined	0.55–0.74
CT				
Herniated disk	0.62–0.9	0.7–0.87	2.1–6.9	0.11–0.54
Stenosis	0.9	0.8–0.96	4.5–22	0.10–0.12
MR				
Cancer	0.83–0.93	0.90–0.97	8.3–31	0.07–0.19
Infection	0.96	0.92	12	0.04
Ankylosing spondylitis	0.56			
Herniated disk	0.6–1.0	0.43–0.97	1.1–33	0–0.93
Stenosis	0.9	0.72–1.0	3.2–Not defined	0.10–0.14
Radionuclide				
Cancer				
Planar	0.74–0.98	0.64–0.81	3.9	0.32
SPECT	0.87–0.93	0.91–0.93	9.7	0.14
Infection	0.90	0.78	4.1	0.13
Ankylosing spondylitis	0.26	1.0	Not defined	0.74

Source: Reprinted with permission from Jarvik and Deyo (1).
[a]Estimated ranges derived from multiple studies. See specific test sections in text for references.

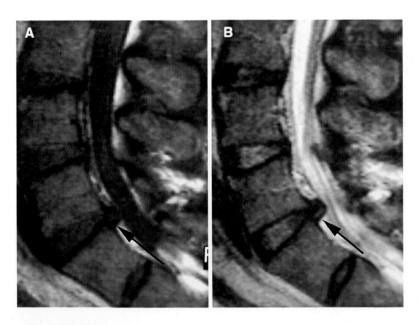

Figure 20.1. Magnetic resonance (MR) of the lumbar spine in a patient without low back pain (LBP) (rigorously determined for entry into a longitudinal study of people without LBP). T1-weighted (**A**) and T2-weighted (**B**) sagittal images demonstrate a moderate sized disk extrusion (*arrow*) at L5/S1. This is one example of many incidental findings. (Reprinted with kind permission of Springer Science+Business Media from Sammer MBK, Jarvik JG. Imaging of Adults with Low Back Pain in the Primary Care Setting. In Medina LS, Blackmore CC (eds): *Evidence-Based Imaging: Optimizing Imaging in Patient Care.* New York: Springer Science+Business Media, 2006.)

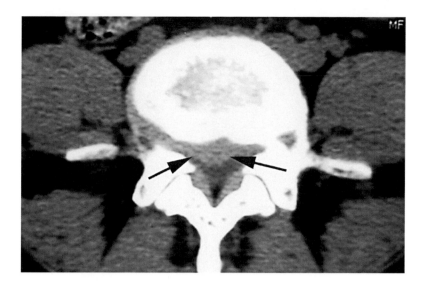

Figure 20.2. Axial computed tomography (CT) image demonstrates a relatively hyperdense focal disk herniation (*arrows*) outlined by lower density cerebrospinal fluid (CSF) within the spinal canal. This example shows CT's ability to depict disk herniations. (Reprinted with kind permission of Springer Science+Business Media from Sammer MBK, Jarvik JG. Imaging of Adults with Low Back Pain in the Primary Care Setting. In Medina LS, Blackmore CC (eds): *Evidence-Based Imaging: Optimizing Imaging in Patient Care*. New York: Springer Science+Business Media, 2006.)

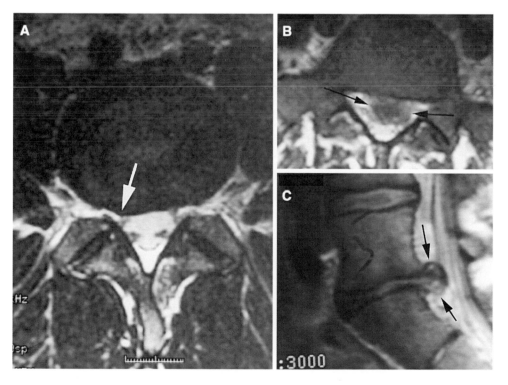

Figure 20.3. T2-weighted MR images in two different patients showing a disk protrusion (*arrow*) (**A**) vs. disk extrusion (*arrows*) (**B** and **C**). See text for definition. Protrusions are common in asymptomatic individuals and may clinically act as false positives. (Reprinted with kind permission of Springer Science+Business Media from Sammer MBK, Jarvik JG. Imaging of Adults with Low Back Pain in the Primary Care Setting. In Medina LS, Blackmore CC (eds): *Evidence-Based Imaging: Optimizing Imaging in Patient Care*. New York: Springer Science+Business Media, 2006.)

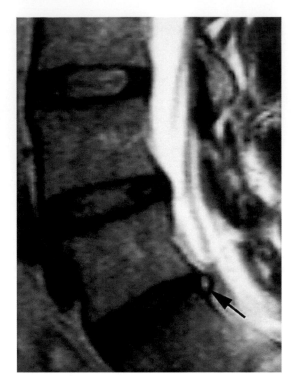

Figure 20.4. Sagittal T2-weighted MR demonstrating high-intensity zone (HIZ) (*arrow*) in an asymptomatic subject. (Reprinted with kind permission of Springer Science+Business Media from Sammer MBK, Jarvik JG. Imaging of Adults with Low Back Pain in the Primary Care Setting. In Medina LS, Blackmore CC (eds): *Evidence-Based Imaging: Optimizing Imaging in Patient Care*. New York: Springer Science+Business Media, 2006.)

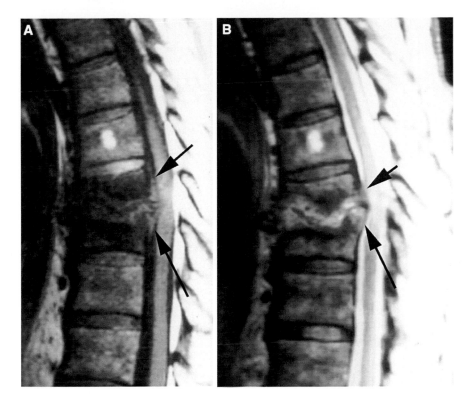

Figure 20.5. Sagittal MR of the thoracic spine demonstrating characteristic findings of diskitis and osteomyelitis, with virtual obliteration of the intervertebral disk, low signal on T1-weighted (**A**) and high signal on T2-weighted (**B**) images adjacent to the destroyed disk. Note the posterior extension of the process into the spinal canal and epidural space, causing compression of the cord (*arrows*). (Reprinted with kind permission of Springer Science+Business Media from Sammer MBK, Jarvik JG. Imaging of Adults with Low Back Pain in the Primary Care Setting. In Medina LS, Blackmore CC (eds): *Evidence-Based Imaging: Optimizing Imaging in Patient Care*. New York: Springer Science+Business Media, 2006.)

Future Research

- It is uncertain which imaging findings are the best predictors of surgical benefit in patients undergoing fusion for degenerative disease. Prospective cohort studies and randomized treatment trials could help to determine which imaging variables are key determinants of outcome.
- While compression fractures are readily identified on imaging, their natural history, including identifying which fractures will lead to chronic pain and what their best management is, has not yet been described.
- Both MR and bone scans are highly effective in identifying metastases. Because MR is more costly than bone scans, future studies may compare the cost-effectiveness of each option and may focus on whether patient outcome is changed from use of either method.
- With infection, molecular imaging techniques may eventually be developed that can identify specific organisms based on imaging properties.
- Data on the best imaging technique to diagnose AS are sparse. Future studies may determine the role and cost-effectiveness of MR in early diagnosis.
- In patients with spinal stenosis and symptomatic herniated disks, definitive studies to document patient outcomes from surgical intervention are needed.

Acknowledgment: This work is supported in part by grant 1 P60 AR48093 from the National Institute for Arthritis, Musculoskeletal, and Skin Diseases.

References

1. Jarvik JG, Deyo RA. Ann Intern Med 2002;137(7):586–597.
2. Frymoyer JW. N Engl J Med 1988;318:291–300.
3. Barondess JA. Ann Intern Med 1993;119(2): 153–160.
4. Salkever DS. DHHS Publication 1985;1–13. PHS Report #86–3343.
5. White AAD, Gordon SL. Spine 1982;7(2):141–149.
6. Steinberg EL et al. Clin Radiol 2003;58(12): 985–989.
7. van Tulder MW et al. Spine 1997;22(4):427–434.
8. Deyo R, Tsui-Wu Y. Spine 1987;12:264–268.
9. Currey HL et al. Rheumatol Rehabil 1979;18(2): 94–104.
10. Boden SD et al. J Bone Joint Surg Am 1990;72(3): 403–408.
11. Jensen MC et al. N Engl J Med 1994;331(2): 69–73.
12. Boos N et al. Spine 1995;20(24):2613–2625.
13. Boos N et al. Spine 2000;25(12):1484–1492.
14. Jarvik JJ et al. Spine 2001;26(10):1158–1166.
15. Deyo RA, Rainville J, Kent DL. JAMA 1992; 268(6):760–765.
16. van den Bosch MA et al. Clin Radiol 2004; 59(1):69–76.
17. Luo X et al. Spine 2004;29(1):79–86.
18. Klein BP, Jensen RC, Sanderson LM. J Occup Med 1984;26:443.
19. Peterson CK, Bolton JE, Wood AR. Spine 2000;25(2):218–223.
20. Lundin O et al. Scand J Med Sci Sports 2001; 11(2):103–109.
21. Thornbury JR et al. Radiology 1993;186(3): 731–738.
22. Jackson RP et al. Spine 1989;14(12):1362–1367.
23. Hellstrom M et al. Acta Radiol 1990;31(2): 127–132.
24. Hitselberger WE, Witten RM. J Neurosurg 1968;28(3):204–206.
25. Wiesel S et al. Spine 1984;9:549–551.
26. Weinreb JC et al. Radiology 1989;170(1 pt 1): 125–128.
27. Burns JW et al. Aviat Space Environ Med 1996; 67(9):849–853.
28. Stadnik TW et al. Radiology 1998;206(1):49–55.
29. Weishaupt D et al. Radiology 1998;209(3): 661–666.
30. Carragee EJ, Paragioudakis SJ, Khurana S. Spine 2000;25(23):2987–2992.
31. Elfering A et al. Spine 2002;27(2):125–134.
32. Wilmink JT. AJNR Am J Neuroradiol 1989; 10(2):233–248.
33. Janssen ME et al. Orthopedics 1994;17(2): 121–127.
34. Beattie PF et al. Spine 2000;25(7):819–828.
35. Vroomen PC, de Krom MC, Wilmink JT. J Neurosurg 2000;92(suppl 2):135–141.
36. Rankine JJ et al. Spine 1998;23(15):1668–1676.
37. Gorbachova TA, Terk MR. Skeletal Radiol 2002;31(9):511–515.
38. Pfirrmann CW et al. Radiology 2004;230(2): 583–588.
39. Porchet F et al. Neurosurgery 2002;50(6):1253–1259; discussion 1259–1260.
40. Ahn SH, Ahn MW, Byun WM. Spine 2000;25(4): 475–480.
41. Fardon DF, Milette PC. Spine 2001;26(5): E93–E113.
42. Brant-Zawadzki MN et al. Spine 1995;20(11): 1257–1263; discussion 1264.
43. Milette PC et al. Spine 1999;24(1):44–53.
44. Jarvik J et al. Acad Radiol 1996;528–531.
45. Cooley JR et al. J Manipulative Physiol Ther 2001;24(5):317–326.
46. Pui MH, Husen YA. Australas Radiol 2000;44(3): 281–284.
47. Aota Y et al. Spine 2001;26(19):2125–2132.
48. Kikkawa I et al. J Orthop Sci 2001;6(2):101–109.
49. Lane JI, Koeller KK, Atkinson JL. AJNR Am J Neuroradiol 1994;15(7):1317–1325.
50. Crisi G, Carpeggiani P, Trevisan C. AJNR Am J Neuroradiol 1993;14(6):1379–1392.
51. Autio RA et al. Spine 2002;27(13):1433–1437.
52. Mullin WJ et al. Spine 2000;25(12):1493–1499.
53. Aprill C, Bogduk N. Br J Radiol 1992;65(773): 361–369.
54. Rankine JJ et al. Spine 1999;24(18):1913–1919; discussion 1920.
55. Lam KS, Carlin D, Mulholland RC. Eur Spine J 2000;9(1):36–41.
56. Videman T et al. Spine 2003;28(6):582–588.
57. Sartoris DJ et al. Radiology 1986;160(3): 707–712.
58. Sartoris DJ et al. Radiology 1986;160(2): 479–483.
59. Deyo RA, Diehl AK. J Gen Intern Med 1988;3: 230–238.
60. Algra PR et al. Radiographics 1991;11:219–232.
61. Avrahami E et al. J Comput Assist Tomogr 1989;13(4):598–602.
62. Carroll KW, Feller JF, Tirman PF. J Magn Reson Imaging 1997;7(2):394–398.
63. Carmody RF et al. Radiology 1989;173:225.
64. Kosuda S et al. J Nucl Med 1996;37(6):975–978.
65. McDougall IR, Kriss JP. JAMA 1975;231(1): 46–50.
66. Corcoran RJ et al. Radiology 1976;121(3 pt 1): 663–667.
67. Savelli G et al. Anticancer Res 2000;20(2B): 1115–1120.

68. Petren-Mallmin M. Acta Radiol Suppl 1994;391:1–23.
69. McNeil BJ. Semin Nucl Med 1978;8(4):336–345.
70. Jacobson AF. Arch Intern Med 1997;157(1):105–109.
71. Even-Sapir E et al. Radiology 1993;187(1):193–198.
72. Han LJ et al. Eur J Nucl Med 1998;25(6):635–638.
73. Bigos S et al. Acute Low Back Problems in Adults. Clinical Practice Guideline No. 14. Rockville, MD: Agency for Health Care Policy and Research, Public Health Service, U.S. Department of Health and Human Services, 1994.
74. Joines JD et al. J Gen Intern Med 2001;16:14–23.
75. Hollingworth W et al. J Gen Intern Med 2003;18(4):303–312.
76. Modic M et al. Radiology 1985;157:157–166.
77. Gillams AR, Chaddha B, Carter AP. AJR Am J Roentgenol 1996;166(4):903–907.
78. Breslau J et al. AJNR Am J Neuroradiol 1999;20(4):670–675.
79. Love C et al. Clin Nucl Med 2000;25(12):963–977.
80. Yamato M et al. Radiat Med 1998;16(5):329–334.
81. Marc V et al. Rev Rhum Engl Ed 1997;64(7–9):465–473.
82. Hanly JG et al. J Rheumatol 1993;20(12):2062–2068.
83. Kent D et al. AJR Am J Roentgenol 1992;158:1135–1144.
84. Porter RW, Bewley B. Spine 1994;19(2):173–175.
85. Haig AJ et al. Spine 2002;27(17):1918–25; discussion 1924–1925.
86. Speciale AC et al. Spine 2002;27(10):1082–1086.
87. Kerry S et al. Br J Gen Pract 2002;52(479):469–474.
88. Kendrick D et al. BMJ 2001;322(7283):400–405.
89. Kendrick D et al. Health Technol Assess 2001;5(30):1–69.
90. Gilbert FJ et al. Radiology 2004;231(2):343–351.
91. Gillan MG et al. Radiology 2001;220(2):393–399.
92. Jarvik JG et al. JAMA 2003;289(21):2810–2818.
93. Vroomen PC, Wilmink JT, de Krom MC. Neuroradiology 2002;44(1):59–63.
94. Espeland A et al. Spine 2001;26(12):1356–1363.
95. Kerry S et al. Health Technol Assess 2000;4(20):i–iv, 1–119.
96. Miller P et al. Spine 2002;27(20):2291–2297.
97. Galibert P et al. Neurochirurgie 1987;33(2):166–168.
98. Kim SH et al. Acta Radiol 2004;45(4):440–445.
99. Buchbinder R et al. N Engl J Med 2009;361(6):557–568.
100. Kallmes DF et al. N Engl J Med 2009;361(6):569–579.
101. Melton LJ 3rd. Spine 1997;22(suppl 24):2S–11S.
102. Riggs BL, Melton LJ 3rd. Bone 1995;17(suppl 5):505S–511S.
103. Gold DT. Bone 1996;18(suppl 3):185S–189S.
104. Kado DM et al. Arch Intern Med 1999;159(11):1215–1220.
105. Silverman SL. Bone 1992;13(suppl 2):S27–S31.
106. Diamond TH et al. Med J Aust 2006;184(3):113–117.
107. Alvarez L et al. Spine 2006;31(10):1113–1118.
108. McKiernan F, Faciszewski T, Jensen R. J Bone Joint Surg Am 2004;86-A(12):2600–2606.
109. Legroux-Gerot I et al. Clin Rheumatol 2004;23(4):310–317.
110. Perez-Higueras A et al. Neuroradiology 2002;44(11):950–954.
111. Dudeney S, Lieberman I. J Rheumatol 2000;27(10):2526.
112. Jensen ME, Dion JE. Neuroimaging Clin N Am 2000;10(3):547–568.
113. Heini PF, Walchli B, Berlemann U. Eur Spine J 2000;9(5):445–450.
114. Martin JB et al. Bone 1999;25(suppl 2):11S–15S.
115. Wenger M, Markwalder TM. Acta Neurochir (Wien) 1999;141(6):625–631.
116. Cortet B et al. J Rheumatol 1999;26(10):2222–2228.
117. Jensen ME et al. AJNR Am J Neuroradiol 1997;18(10):1897–1904.
118. Cotten A et al. Radiology 1996;200(2):525–530.
119. Weill A et al. Radiology 1996;199(1):241–247.
120. Gangi A, Kastler BA, Dietemann JL. AJNR Am J Neuroradiol 1994;15(1):83–86.
121. Robbins SE, Morse MH. Clin Radiol 1996;51(9):637–638.
122. Scavone JG, Latshaw RF, Weidner WA. AJR Am J Roentgenol 1981;136(4):715–717.
123. Khoo LA et al. Clin Radiol 2003;58(8):606–609.
124. Hall FM. Radiology 1976;120:443–448.
125. Webster E, Merrill O. N Engl J Med 1957;257:811–819.
126. Antoku S, Russell W. Radiology 1957;101:669–678.

21

Imaging of the Spine in Victims of Trauma

C. Craig Blackmore and Gregory David Avey

Imaging of the Cervical Spine

I. Who should undergo cervical spine imaging?
   A. NEXUS prediction rule
   B. Canadian cervical spine prediction rule
   C. Applicability to children
II. What cervical spine imaging is appropriate in high-risk patients?
   A. Cost-effectiveness analysis
III. Special case: defining patients at high fracture risk
   A. Applicability to children
IV. Special case: the unconscious patient

Imaging of the Thoracolumbar Spine

V. Who should undergo thoracolumbar spine imaging?
   A. Applicability to children
VI. Which thoracolumbar imaging is appropriate in blunt trauma patients?

- Cervical spine imaging is not necessary in subjects with all five of the following: (1) absence of posterior midline tenderness, (2) absence of focal neurologic deficit, (3) normal level of alertness, (4) no evidence of intoxication, and (5) absence of painful distracting injury (strong evidence).

C.C. Blackmore (✉)
Department of Radiology, Center for Healthcare Solutions, Virginia Mason Medical Center, Seattle, WA 98111, USA
e-mail: craig.blackmore@vmmc.org

L.S. Medina et al. (eds.), *Evidence-Based Imaging: Improving the Quality of Imaging in Patient Care, Revised Edition*, 357
DOI 10.1007/978-1-4419-7777-9_21, © Springer Science+Business Media, LLC 2011

- Computed tomography (CT) scan of the cervical spine is cost-effective as the initial imaging strategy in patients at high probability of fracture (neurologic deficit, head injury, high energy mechanism) who are already to undergo head CT (moderate evidence).
- No adequate data exist on the appropriate cervical spine evaluation in subjects who cannot be examined due to a head injury (insufficient evidence).
- Imaging of the thoracolumbar spine is not necessary in blunt trauma patients with all five of the following: (1) absence of thoracolumbar back pain, (2) absence of thoracolumbar spine tenderness on midline palpation, (3) normal level of alertness, (4) absence of distracting injury, and (5) no evidence of intoxication (moderate evidence).

Definition and Pathophysiology

The majority of spine fractures occur from high-energy trauma such as high-speed motor vehicle accidents and falls from heights (1, 2). However, an important minority occur from relatively low-energy mechanisms such as falls from a standing height or low-velocity automobile accidents (3, 4).

Epidemiology

Cervical spine fractures occur in approximately 10,000 individuals per year in the USA, most the result of blunt trauma (5, 6). Among patients with a fracture, approximately one third will sustain severe neurologic injury (6, 7). Unfortunately, fractures of the cervical spine may not be clinically obvious. Patients may be neurologically intact initially, but if not treated appropriately and promptly, progress to severe neurologic compromise (8). Delayed onset of paralysis occurs in up to 15% of missed fractures, and death due to unidentified cervical spine fracture is possible (9, 10). Furthermore, the mechanism of injury is also not always useful for excluding cervical spine fracture.

Thoracolumbar spine injury has been estimated to occur in between 2 and 4% of all blunt trauma patients (11, 12). These injuries were judged to require treatment in approximately three fourths of those identified (13). Much like cervical spine fractures, a resulting neurologic deficit is noted in approximately one third of those with thoracolumbar injury

(14, 15). Given the potentially serious consequences of these injuries, it is unsettling to find that studies have noted a significant delay in diagnosis in 11–22% of patients with spine fractures (9, 16, 17).

Overall Cost to Society

There is enormous variability in the practice of cervical spine imaging (18, 19), but in most centers, imaging is used liberally. As a result, the yield from cervical spine imaging is low, with only 0.9–2.8% of such imaging studies demonstrating injury (20, 21). Overall, the total cost of the imaging, evaluation, and care of patients with cervical spine trauma in the USA is an estimated $3.4 billion per year (22). The yield of thoracolumbar imaging is somewhat higher than cervical spine imaging, with positive studies accounting for 7.6–9% of blunt trauma thoracolumbar exams (23). The total societal cost of thoracolumbar spine injury has been estimated at $1 billion per year (24).

Goals

The overall goal of initial spine imaging is to detect potentially unstable fractures to enable immobilization or stabilization and prevent development or progression of neurologic injury. Additional imaging studies may be performed to inform prognosis and guide surgical intervention for unstable injuries.

Methodology

A Medline search was performed using PubMed (National Library of Medicine, Bethesda, Maryland) for original research publications discussing the diagnostic performance and effectiveness of imaging strategies in the cervical and thoracolumbar spine. Clinical predictors of cervical and thoracolumbar spine fracture were also included in the literature search. The search for cervical spine-related publications covered the period 1966 to March 2002. The search strategy employed different combinations of the following terms: (1) *cervical spine*, (2) *radiography* or *imaging* or *computed tomography*, and (3) *fracture* or *injury*. The search for thoracolumbar spine-related publications covered the period 1980 to March 2004. The search strategy included the MESH headings (1) *spine* and *diagnosis* and (2) *imaging* and *trauma*. Additional articles were identified by reviewing the reference lists of relevant papers. This review was limited to human studies and the English-language literature. The authors performed an initial review of the titles and abstracts of the identified articles followed by review of the full text in articles that were relevant.

I. Who Should Undergo Cervical Spine Imaging?

Summary of Evidence: Determination of which blunt trauma subjects should undergo cervical spine imaging, and which should not undergo imaging, is a question that has been studied in detail in literally tens of thousands of subjects. The two major level I (strong evidence) studies, the NEXUS trial (Table 21.1), and the Canadian C-spine rule (Table 21.2) were comprehensive multicenter investigations of this topic. The NEXUS rule (Table 21.1) has undergone extensive validation and demonstrates high sensitivity for detection of fractures. The Canadian C-spine rule (Table 21.2) also has high sensitivity, and potentially higher specificity than the NEXUS. However, neither of these rules has been tested in an implementation trial to determine their impact outside the research setting.

Supporting Evidence: The low yield of cervical imaging has prompted a number of investigators to attempt to identify clinical factors that

can be used to predict cervical spine fracture. Early studies of this question were largely level III (limited evidence) investigations consisting of unselected case series. For example, in 1988, Roberge and colleagues (25) studied 467 consecutive subjects who underwent cervical spine radiography and found that subjects with cervical discomfort or tenderness were more likely to have a fracture than those without such symptoms or signs. Additional investigators identified associations between cervical spine fracture and mechanism of injury (26, 27), level of consciousness (20, 21, 27), and intoxication (20, 28). However, all of these investigations involved small numbers of subjects with fracture and a single or small number of centers.

A. NEXUS Prediction Rule

The first major cohort investigation of clinical indicators for cervical spine imaging was the National Emergency X-Radiography Utilization Study (NEXUS) (5, 29). This was a large Level I study performed at 23 different emergency departments across the USA. The goal of the NEXUS study was to assess the validity of four predetermined clinical criteria for cervical spine injury (Table 21.1). These criteria were (1) altered neurologic function, (2) intoxication, (3) midline posterior bony cervical spine tenderness, and (4) distracting injury. The NEXUS investigators prospectively enrolled over 34,000 patients who underwent radiography of the cervical spine following blunt trauma. Of these, 818 (2.4%) had cervical spine injury. These authors found that the clinical predictors had a sensitivity of 99.6% for clinically significant injury (Table 21.3) (5, 29). The authors also reported high interobserver agreement ($\kappa = 0.73$) for the prediction rule (30), and reported that use of the rule would have decreased the overall ordering of cervical radiography by an estimated 12.6% (29).

B. Canadian Cervical Spine Prediction Rule

A second level I clinical prediction rule, the Canadian C-spine rule for radiography (25) was published subsequent to the NEXUS trial, but with a similar objective: to derive a clinical decision rule that is highly sensitive for detecting acute cervical spine injury. The Canadian

C-spine rule was a prospective cohort study of 8,924 subjects from ten community and university hospitals in Canada. Excluded were patients who had neurologic impairment, decreased mental status, or penetrating trauma. Like the NEXUS study, the Canadian C-Spine Study was an observational study performed without informed patient consent. However, patients who were eligible for the study but did not undergo radiography were followed up with a structured telephone interview 14 days following their discharge from the emergency department (ED). Thus, any patients who had not undergone radiography, and who had missed fracture would potentially be discovered during the investigation. The Canadian study investigated the predictive ability of 20 factors, and based on the reliability and predictive properties of these factors, developed a prediction rule consisting of three questions. According to the Canadian C-spine rule (Table 21.2), the probability of cervical spine injury is extremely low, and imaging is not indicated if the following three determinations are made: (1) absence of high-risk factor (age >65 years, dangerous mechanism, paresthesias in extremities); (2) presence of a low-risk factor (simple rear-end motor vehicle collision, sitting position in ED, ambulatory at any time since injury, delayed onset of neck pain, or absence of midline cervical C-spine tenderness); or (3) patient is able to actively rotate neck 45° to left and right. The Canadian study group reported sensitivity of 100% and specificity of 42.5% for this clinical prediction rule and also reported that the rate of ordering radiography would be 58.2% of the current rate (Table 21.3) (31).

The Canadian C-spine rule was validated using a prospective cohort study of 8,283 patients presenting at the same ten Canadian community and academic hospitals as the original study (32). The results of this verification trial noted a sensitivity of 99.4% and a specificity of 45.1%, very similar to the results of the derivation study. It was noted during the course of this study that physicians failed to evaluate neck range of motion, as required by the Canadian C-spine rule, in 10.2% of patients. While virtually all of this group of incompletely evaluated patients underwent cervical spine imaging (98.8%), this group was found to have a lower rate of injury (0.8%) than the cohort as a whole (2.0%).

The data supporting the adoption of one cervical spine prediction rule over the other is limited. Two studies, the validation study for the Canadian C-spine rule and a retrospective analysis of the Canadian C-spine derivation cohort have attempted to compare the NEXUS and Canadian rules (32, 33). However, both cohorts excluded those with altered levels of consciousness, effectively eliminating one of the NEXUS criteria. In addition, others have voiced concerns regarding physician familiarity with the various rules, side-by-side comparison, and the definitions of the NEXUS criteria used in these trials (34, 35). The choice of clinical prediction rule in a broader clinical context is also unclear, as no trial has examined the impact of implementing these prediction rules outside of the research setting.

C. Applicability to Children

Evidence for who should undergo imaging is less complete in children than in adults. Determination of clinical predictors of injury in pediatric patients is complicated by the decreased incidence of injury in children, requiring a larger sample size for adequate study (36, 37). In addition, children may sustain serious cervical cord injuries that are not radiographically apparent (37, 38). Among the level I studies, the Canadian clinical prediction rule development study excluded children (31). The NEXUS trial included children, but there were only 30 injuries in patients under age 18, and only four in patients under age 9 (36). Although no pediatric injuries were missed in the NEXUS study, sample size was too small to adequately assess the sensitivity of the prediction rule in this group. Therefore, no adequate evidence exists regarding appropriate criteria for imaging in children.

II. What Cervical Spine Imaging Is Appropriate in High-Risk Patients?

Summary of Evidence: Cervical spine CT is more sensitive than radiography, and more specific in patients at high risk of fracture. But CT has higher direct costs than radiography. However, cost-effectiveness analysis demonstrates that CT is cost-effective, and may actually be cost-saving from the societal perspective in patients at high probability of fracture. Cost savings with CT are from a decreased number of second imaging examinations resulting from inadequate radiograph studies, and to the high cost in dollars and health for the rare fracture missed from radiography that leads to severe neurologic deficit. Radiography remains the most cost-effective imaging option in patients at low probability of injury (Fig. 21.1).

Supporting Evidence: There are multiple investigations of radiography accuracy, although most are retrospective, level III (limited evidence) studies (39, 40). Further, sensitivity of radiography is dependent on the selected reference standard. Studies incorporating CT as the reference standard suggest that radiography misses 23–57% of fractures (41, 42). However, the clinical relevance of these missed fractures is uncertain. Studies using fractures that become apparent clinically as the reference standard are probably more relevant for clinical practice. No formal meta-analyses of radiograph accuracy exist. However, weighted pooling of the larger studies using a clinical gold standard suggests that radiography is relatively accurate, with a sensitivity of approximately 94% and a specificity of approximately 95% when all trauma patients are considered (Table 21.3) (4).

Cervical radiography has substantial limitations in patients at the highest probability of fracture. Patients involved in high-energy trauma are commonly on backboards, have other injuries, and may be uncooperative. Cervical radiography in this group has been found to be more difficult to perform adequately, resulting in lower specificity, and requiring longer time, more repeat radiographs, and higher costs (43, 44). Radiograph specificity ranges from approximately 96% in patients with only minor noncervical injuries, to 89% in patients with head injury, to 78% in patients with head injury and a high-energy mechanism such as motorcycle crash (44). Radiographs are relatively inexpensive, with direct, short-term resource ranging from $34 to $60 (43).

More recently, CT has been proposed as an initial cervical spine evaluation modality in patients who are victims of major trauma. Nuñez and colleagues studied the use of CT in the initial evaluation of trauma patients and demonstrated high sensitivity for fracture (99%) in a large, level II prospective series (moderate evidence) (42). This has been subsequently confirmed by other studies (45, 46). Also, CT

demonstrated high specificity (93%), even in patients at high-risk of fracture (Table 21.3) (45).

Direct, short-term resource costs of cervical spine CT likely exceed those of radiography, but no comprehensive cost analyses of CT have been published. Assessment of cost of cervical spine CT is difficult as many institutions obtain economies of scale by performing CT of the cervical spine in the same setting as CT of the head (4, 46). However, CT may be faster than radiography, and Nuñez and colleagues (42) have suggested that use of CT may decrease patient time in the emergency department. Therefore, CT has higher sensitivity and specificity for cervical spine fracture in high-risk patients, but at potentially higher cost.

The appropriateness of CT as initial cervical spine imaging strategy in patients who are also undergoing head CT has been examined with cost-effectiveness analysis (4). This analysis, taken from the societal perspective, was based on a decision-analysis model, and compared the cost effectiveness of radiography and CT for patients at different probabilities of cervical spine fracture. The cervical spine cost-effectiveness model, taken from the societal perspective, was dependent on radiograph sensitivity, radiograph specificity, CT sensitivity, CT specificity, probability of fracture, and the probability of paralysis or the likelihood that a patient will become paralyzed if a fracture was missed by cervical imaging. In addition, the cost-effectiveness model was dependent on the short-term resource cost of radiography and CT, as well as the cost of the imaging that was induced by the initial strategy, and the cost of any neurologic deficit (paralysis) that developed from missed fracture. Costs were estimated from Medicare reimbursement data, and literature estimates, and the analysis was limited to adults (4).

A. Cost-Effectiveness Analysis

Cost-effectiveness analysis revealed that in patients at high risk (>10%) of cervical spine fracture, CT was actually a dominant strategy, both saving money and improving health through the prevention of paralysis. The cost savings associated with the use of CT was due to fewer inadequate exams, and to the very high medical and financial cost of the rare case of paralysis. The probability of a patient developing paralysis from missed fracture was actually extremely low, as fractures were uncommon, and the sensitivity of imaging was very high. However, the lifetime medical costs of a patient who became paralyzed were high, with estimates ranging from $525,000 to $950,000 (1995 dollars), and not including societal costs such as lost wages. In addition to the cost, there were obvious health consequences of paralysis. The dominance of CT over radiography in these high-probability patients was robust to sensitivity analysis testing of the uncertainty in the estimates. In patients at moderate probability of fracture (4–10%), CT cost more overall than radiography, but with a cost-effectiveness ratio on the order of $25,000 per quality-adjusted life year. In patients at low probability of cervical spine fracture (<4%) CT was clearly not cost-effective, and radiography was the preferred strategy (4).

III. Special Case: Defining Patients at High Fracture Risk

Summary of Evidence: Selection of patients for cost-effective use of cervical spine CT is dependent on probability of fracture. The Harborview high-risk cervical spine criteria have been developed and validated by a single institution level II (moderate evidence) study. Using these criteria, patients can be identified with injury probabilities ranging from 0.2 to 12.8%.

Supporting Evidence: Patients at risk for cervical spine fracture are a heterogeneous group. Some patients have sustained major trauma and will be at high probability of injury, while others will have sustained only minor trauma and will be at low probability of having sustained cervical spine fracture. Given that cost-effectiveness of imaging is dependent on the probability of cervical spine fracture, optimization of imaging in the cervical spine requires stratification of patients into different levels of probability of fracture. This stratification must be based on clinical findings that are apparent when patients are first evaluated in the ED, prior to any imaging.

To identify patients at high probability of fracture, Blackmore and colleagues (47) developed and validated a clinical prediction rule. This level II study employed a case–control study design, in which 160 patients were evaluated at Harborview Medical Center in the years 1994–1995 who had cervical spine fracture. Controls were 304 randomly selected adult blunt trauma

patients from the same institution. The authors used logistic regression and recursive partitioning to develop a clinical prediction rule, which was then validated internally using the bootstrap technique. Using likelihood ratios from the clinical prediction rule and the known base prevalence of cervical spine fracture in the institution's population, the authors developed a series of fracture probability estimates for patients of different clinical circumstances (47). Although derived retrospectively, this prediction rule was subsequently prospectively validated on a separate patient group at the same institution (Table 21.4) (48). To date, this prediction rule has not been validated at other institutions. A clinical prediction rule has also been developed (but not validated) to evaluate predictors of cervical spine fracture in the elderly. The elderly prediction rule was identical to that in all adults, except that a higher proportion of injured patients were missed by the prediction rule criteria (49).

A. Applicability to Children

Comparison of CT versus radiography has not been well explored in children. The cost-effectiveness analysis of Blackmore and colleagues (4) excluded children, as did the studies of the Harborview high-risk cervical spine criteria (47, 48). Further, the lower frequency of injury in children (36, 37) and the increased radiosensitivity of pediatric patients (50) suggest that cost-effectiveness results from adults may not be relevant.

IV. Special Case: The Unconscious Patient

Summary of Evidence: The theoretical risk of radiographically occult unstable ligamentous injury in patients who are unexaminable due to head injury has led to a variety of imaging approaches. There is insufficient evidence to support any particular approach.

Supporting Evidence: Standard radiologic and CT examinations of the cervical spine allow assessment of bony alignment. However, anecdotal reports exist in the literature describing unstable ligamentous injuries without malalignment on imaging (51, 52). Accordingly, organizations including the Eastern Association for the Surgery of Trauma recommend additional imaging of the neck soft tissues to exclude unstable ligamentous injury. Proposed imaging approaches include magnetic resonance imaging (MRI), flexion and extension radiography, and fluoroscopy.

To date, there have been no reported level I or level II studies of the accuracy or clinical utility of any of the proposed imaging algorithms. Case-series data suggest that approximately 2% of obtunded patients may have unstable cervical spine injuries not detectable on initial CT or radiography (51, 53, 54). The clinical significance of these injuries has not been established.

V. Who Should Undergo Thoracolumbar Spine Imaging?

Summary of Evidence: Clinical prediction rules to determine which patients should undergo thoracolumbar spine imaging have been developed but not validated. Although these prediction rules have high sensitivities for detecting thoracolumbar fractures, their low specificities and low positive predictive values would require imaging a large number of patients without thoracolumbar injuries. This drawback limits the clinical utility of these prediction rules (moderate evidence).

Supporting Evidence: Given the relative lack of clarity regarding which blunt trauma patients require thoracolumbar imaging, several level III (limited evidence) studies have examined potential risks for thoracolumbar fracture. These limited studies have identified associations among the risk of thoracolumbar injury and high-speed motor vehicle accident (52, 53), fall from a significant height (13, 55, 56), complaint of back pain (12–14, 55, 57), elevated injury score (13, 55), decreased level of consciousness (14, 55–57), and abnormal neurologic exam (14, 56).

Two separate clinical predication rules to guide thoracolumbar spine imaging decisions have been validated. The smaller study, conducted by Hsu et al. (58), examined the effect of six clinical criteria on two retrospective groups (58). The first group consisted of a cohort of 100 patients with known thoracolumbar fracture, while the second group consisted of 100 randomly selected multitrauma patients. The criteria evaluated were (1) back pain/midline tenderness, (2) local signs of injury, (3) neurologic deficit, (4) cervical spine fracture, (5) distracting injury, and

(6) intoxication. The results of this small-scale, retrospective trial found that 100% of the patients in the known thoracolumbar fracture group would have been imaged appropriately using the proposed criteria. This proposed pathway was then tested retrospectively in the group of randomly selected blunt trauma patients, and was found to have a sensitivity of 100%, a specificity of 11.3%, and a negative predictive value of 100%. Implementing these criteria would still require imaging the thoracolumbar spine in 92% of the selected multitrauma patients.

A much larger prospective, single center study by Holmes et al. (11) evaluated similar criteria in 2,404 consecutive blunt trauma patients who underwent thoracolumbar imaging (moderate evidence). These clinical criteria were (1) complaints of thoracolumbar spine pain, (2) thoracolumbar spine pain on midline palpation, (3) decreased level of consciousness, (4) abnormal peripheral nerve examination, (5) distracting injury, and (6) intoxication (Table 21.5). This prediction rule was successful in achieving 100% sensitivity for detecting thoracolumbar fracture; however, the specificity was only 3.9%. Due to this low specificity, implementing this prediction rule in this patient population would have decreased the rate of thoracolumbar imaging by merely 4%.

A. Applicability to Children

It is unknown if these clinical prediction rules may be applied to children. The largest study by Holmes et al. (11) did allow the enrollment of children; however, they do not report the actual number of children enrolled. The youngest patient enrolled in the small trial by Hsu et al. (58) was 14 years.

VI. Which Thoracolumbar Imaging Is Appropriate in Blunt Trauma Patients?

Summary of Evidence: Multiple studies have shown that some CT protocols used for imaging the chest and abdominal visceral organs are more sensitive and specific for detecting thoracolumbar spine fracture than conventional radiography. In patients undergoing such scans, conventional radiography may be eliminated (limited evidence). The effect of primary screening with CT scan on cost and radiation exposure has not been thoroughly studied for the thoracolumbar spine.

Supporting Evidence: Multiple level III (limited evidence) studies examine the possibility of eliminating conventional radiography in those patients who are candidates for both conventional thoracolumbar radiographs and CT evaluation of the chest or abdominal viscera; however, many of these trials are hampered by small sample sizes or verification bias (59–63). Studies that combine the results of both CT and conventional radiography as the reference standard suggest that CT has a sensitivity of 78.1–97%, while conventional radiographs have a sensitivity of 32.0–74% for detecting thoracolumbar fracture (60–62). The clinical importance of thoracolumbar fractures not found with conventional radiography is unknown, as no studies with clinically based outcome measures were located.

A single level III (limited evidence) trial examined the use of CT as an initial evaluation in patients for whom a CT scan is not indicated for other reasons (61). This prospective, single center trial examined 222 trauma patients with both CT and conventional radiographs as initial screening exams. The reported sensitivity was 97% for CT examination and 58% for conventional radiographs. The results of this trial are limited in that only 36 patients were diagnosed with thoracolumbar fracture during the course of the trial.

Take Home Tables and Figures

Tables 21.1–21.5 and Fig. 21.1–21.2 serve to highlight key recommendations and supporting evidence.

Table 21.1. NEXUS criteria: imaging of the cervical spine is not necessary if all five of the NEXUS criteria are met

1. Absence of posterior midline tenderness
2. Absence of focal neurologic deficit
3. Normal level of alertness
4. No evidence of intoxication
5. Absence of painful distracting injury

Source: Adapted from Hoffman et al. (29).

Table 21.2. The Canadian C-spine rule

If the following three determinations are made, then imaging is not indicated
1. No high-risk factor, including:
Age >64 years
Dangerous mechanism, including:
Fall from >3 m/5 stairs
Axial load to head (diving)
High-speed motor vehicle accident (60 mph, rollover, ejection)
Bicycle collision
Motorized recreational vehicle
Paresthesias in extremities
2. Low-risk factor is present
Simple rear-end vehicular crash, excluding:
Pushed into oncoming traffic
Hit by bus/large truck
Rollover
Hit by high-speed vehicle
Sitting position in emergency department
Ambulatory at any time
Delayed onset of neck pain
Absence of midline cervical tenderness
3. Able to actively rotate neck (45° left and right)

Source: Adapted from Dickinson et al. (33).

Table 21.3. Diagnostic performance

Test (reference)	Sensitivity	Specificity	Potential decrease in radiography
C-spine prediction rules			
NEXUS (29)	99.6	12.9	12.6
Canadian C-spine rule (31)	100	42.5	41.8
TL-spine prediction rules			
Holmes et al. (11)	100	3.9	3.7
C-spine imaging			
Radiography (4, 44)			
Overall	93.9	95.3	N/A
Low risk		96.4	N/A
High risk		78.1–89.3	N/A
CT (39, 41, 42, 45)[a]			
Overall	99.0	93.1	N/A
TL-spine imaging			
Radiography (59, 63)[a]	63.0	94.6	N/A
CT (59–63)	97.8	99.6	N/A

N/A not applicable.

Reprinted with kind permission of Springer Science+Business Media from Blackmore CC, Avey GD. Imaging of the Spine in Victims of Trauma. In Medina LS, Blackmore CC (eds): *Evidence-Based Imaging: Optimizing Imaging in Patient Care.* New York: Springer Science+Business Media, 2006.
[a]Pooled from these references.

Table 21.4. Harborview high-risk cervical spine criteria

Presence of any of the following criteria indicates a patient at sufficiently high-risk to warrant initial use of CT to evaluate the cervical spine
1. High-energy injury mechanism High-speed (>35 mph) motor vehicle or motorcycle accident Motor vehicle accident with death at scene Fall from height greater than 10 ft
2. High-risk clinical parameter Significant head injury, including intracranial hemorrhage or unconscious in emergency department Neurologic signs or symptoms referable to the cervical spine Pelvic or multiple extremity fractures

Source: Adapted from Hanson et al. (48).

Table 21.5. Thoracolumbar spine imaging criteria

1. Thoracolumbar spine pain
2. Thoracolumbar spine tenderness on midline palpation
3. Decreased level of consciousness
4. Abnormal peripheral nerve examination
5. Distracting injury
6. Intoxication

Reprinted with kind permission of Springer Science+Business Media from Blackmore CC, Avey GD. Imaging of the Spine in Victims of Trauma. In Medina LS, Blackmore CC (eds): *Evidence-Based Imaging: Optimizing Imaging in Patient Care.* New York: Springer Science+Business Media, 2006.

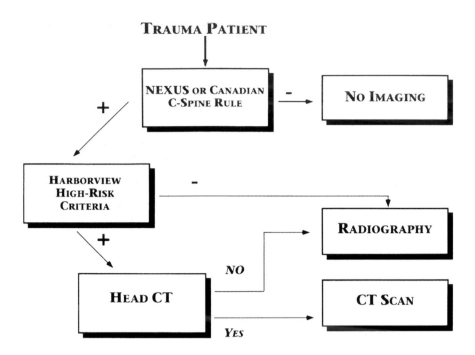

TRAUMA PATIENT

NEXUS OR CANADIAN C-SPINE RULE → − → NO IMAGING

+ → HARBORVIEW HIGH-RISK CRITERIA

− → RADIOGRAPHY

+ → HEAD CT

NO → RADIOGRAPHY

YES → CT SCAN

Figure 21.1. Evidence-based decision tree for imaging of the cervical spine in victims of trauma. The NEXUS or Canadian prediction rules are used to select patients for imaging. If imaging is appropriate, the Harborview prediction rule is used to select patients for CT rather than radiography. However, cervical spine CT is only used as the initial imaging strategy in patients who are to undergo head CT. Patients who are not to undergo head CT are imaged with radiography. (Reprinted with kind permission of Springer Science+Business Media from Blackmore CC, Avey GD. Imaging of the Spine in Victims of Trauma. In Medina LS, Blackmore CC (eds): *Evidence-Based Imaging: Optimizing Imaging in Patient Care.* New York: Springer Science+Business Media, 2006.)

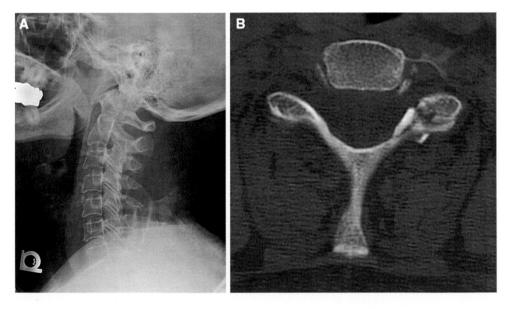

Figure 21.2. Imaging case study. Victim of a motor vehicle accident who met criteria for initial cervical spine imaging with CT scan. A potentially unstable C6–C7 facet and pars interarticularis fracture is apparent on CT (**A**), but may be missed on contemporaneous radiography (**B**). CT has higher sensitivity for fracture than radiography. (Reprinted with kind permission of Springer Science+Business Media from Blackmore CC, Avey GD. Imaging of the Spine in Victims of Trauma. In Medina LS, Blackmore CC (eds): *Evidence-Based Imaging: Optimizing Imaging in Patient Care.* New York: Springer Science+Business Media, 2006.)

Future Research

- Studies in both cervical spine and thoracolumbar spine imaging indicate that CT is more sensitive than traditional radiography in detecting fractures. However, the clinical relevance of these fractures is uncertain.
- The applicability of spine injury clinical prediction rules in pediatric patients is unknown. In addition, the sensitivity, specificity, and cost-effectiveness of the various imaging exams in the pediatric population are not well established.
- Clinical prediction rules for imaging of the thoracolumbar spine have been developed, but further research is necessary to validate such approaches. The effect of implementing these rules on cost, cost-effectiveness, and radiation exposure has not been determined.
- Appropriate imaging to detect unstable ligamentous injury, particularly in clinically unexaminable patients remains unresolved.

Suggested Imaging Protocols

- Cervical spine radiography: anteroposterior, open mouth, lateral, swimmer's lateral (optional: 45° oblique views with 10° cephalad tube angulation).
- Cervical spine CT (multidetector): C0 to T4, detector collimation 1.25 mm. Sagittal reformations: 3-mm intervals, right neuroforamen to left neuroforamen. Coronal reformations: 3-mm intervals, front of vertebral body through spinal canal, C0–C5 only.
- Thoracolumbar spine radiography: anteroposterior and interval. Swimmer's lateral of cervicothoracic junction if no CT cervical spine.
- Thoracolumbar spine CT (reconstructions from trauma abdomen pelvis CT). Axial images at 2.5-mm slice interval and sagittal reformations at 2.5-mm intervals.

References

1. DeVivo MJ, Rutt RD, Black KJ, Go BK, Stover SL. Arch Phys Med Rehabil 1992;73:424–430 [published erratum appears in Arch Phys Med Rehabil 1992;73(12):1146].
2. Kalsbeek WD, McLaurin RL, Harris BS III, Miller JD. J Neurosurg 1980;31:S19–S31.
3. Lomoschitz F, Blackmore C, Mirza S, Mann F. AJR Am J Roentgenol 2002;178:573–577.
4. Blackmore CC, Ramsey SD, Mann FA, Deyo RA. Radiology 1999;212:117–125.
5. Hoffman J, Wolfson A, Todd K, Mower W. Ann Emerg Med 1998;32:461–469.
6. Bracken MB, Freeman DH, Hellenbrand K. Am J Epidemiol 1981;113:615–622.
7. Fine PR, Kuhlemeier KV, DeVivo MJ, Stover SL. Paraplegia 1979;17:237–250.
8. Rogers WA. J Bone Joint Surg 1957;39-A:341–376.
9. Reid DC, Henderson R, Saboe L, Miller JD. J Trauma 1987;27:980–986.
10. Gerrelts BD, Petersen EU, Mabry J, Petersen SR. J Trauma 1991;31:1622–1626.
11. Holmes JF, Panacek EA, Miller PQ, Lapidis AD, Mower WR. J Emerg Med 2003;24:1–7.
12. Samuels LE, Kerstein MD. J Trauma 1993;34:85–89.
13. Durham RM, Luchtefeld WB, Wibbenmeyer L, Maxwell P, Shapiro MJ, Mazuski JE. Am J Surg 1995;170:681–684.
14. Meldon SW, Moettus LN. J Trauma 1995;39:1110–1114.
15. Saboe LA, Reid DC, Davis LA, Warren SA, Grace MG. J Trauma 1991;31:43–48.
16. van Beek E, Been H, Ponse K, Mass M. Injury 2000;31:219–223.
17. Dai LY, Yao WF, Cui YM, Zhou Q. J Trauma 2004;56:348–355.
18. Blackmore CC, Mann FA, Nuñez DB. Emerg Radiol 2000;7:142–148.
19. Mirvis SE, Diaconis JN, Chirico PA, Reiner BI, Joslyn JN, Militello P. Radiology 1989;170:831–834.
20. Hoffman JR, Schriger DL, Mower W, Luo JS, Zucker M. Ann Emerg Med 1992;21:1454–1460.
21. Kreipke DL, Gillespie KR, McCarthy MC, Mail JT, Lappas JC, Broadie TA. J Trauma 1989;29:1438–1439.
22. Berkowitz M. J Emerg Med 1993;1:63–67.
23. Terregino C, Ross S, Lipinski M, Foreman J, Hughes R. Ann Emerg Med 1995;26:126–129.
24. DeVivo MJ, Fine PR, Maetz HM, Stover SL. Arch Neurol 1980;37:707–708.
25. Roberge RJ, Wears RC, Kelly M et al. J Trauma 1988;28:784–788.
26. Jacobs LM, Schwartz R. Ann Emerg Med 1986;15:44–49.

27. Cadoux CG, White JD, Hedberg MC. Ann Emerg Med 1987;16:738–742.
28. Bachulis BL, Long WB, Hynes GD, Johnson MC. Am J Surg 1987;153:473–478.
29. Hoffman J, Mower W, Wolfson A, Todd K, Zucker M. N Engl J Med 2000;343:94–99.
30. Mahadevan S, Mower W, Hoffman J, Peeples N, Goldberg W, Sonner R. Ann Emerg Med 1998;31: 197–201.
31. Stiell I, Wells G, Vandemheen K et al. JAMA 2001;286:1841–1848.
32. Stiell IG, Clement CM, McKnight RD et al. N Engl J Med 2003;349:2510–2518.
33. Dickinson G, Stiell IG, Schull M, Brison R, Clement C, Vandemheen K. Ann Emerg Med 2004;43:507–514.
34. Yealy DM, Auble TE. N Engl J Med 2003;349: 2553–2555.
35. Mower WR, Wolfson AB, Hoffman JR, Todd KH. N Engl J Med 2004;350:1467–1468.
36. Viccellio P, Simon H, Pressman B, Shah M, Mower W, Hoffman J. Pediatrics 2001;108:E20.
37. Kokoska E, Keller M, Rallo M, Weber T. J Pediatr Surg 2001;36:100–105.
38. Finch G, Barnes M. J Pediatr Orthop 1998;18: 811–814.
39. Acheson MB, Livingston RR, Richardson ML, Stimac GK. AJR Am J Roentgenol 1987;148:1179–1185.
40. Clark CR, Igram CM, el Khoury GY, Ehara S. Spine 1988;13:742–747.
41. Woodring JH, Lee C. J Trauma 1993;34:32–39.
42. Nuñez DB, Ahmad AA, Coin CG et al. Emerg Radiol 1994;1:273–278.
43. Blackmore CC, Zelman WN, Glick ND. Radiology 2001;220:581–587.
44. Blackmore CC, Deyo RA. Emerg Radiol 1997;4:283–286.
45. Hanson JA, Blackmore CC, Mann FA, Wilson AJ. Emerg Radiol 2000;7:31–35.
46. Nuñez DB, Quencer RM. AJR Am J Roentgenol 1998;171:951–957.
47. Blackmore CC, Emerson SS, Mann FA, Koepsell TD. Radiology 1999;211:759–765.
48. Hanson JA, Blackmore CC, Mann FA, Wilson AJ. AJR Am J Roentgenol 2000;174:713–718.
49. Bub L, Blackmore C, Mann F, Lomoschitz F. Radiology 2005;234:143–149.
50. National Research Council. Health Effects of Exposure to Low Levels of Ionizing Radiation: BEIR V. Washington, DC: National Academy Press, 1990.
51. Ajani A, Cooper D, Scheinkestel C et al. Anaesth Intensive Care 1998;26:487–491.
52. Beirne J, Butler P, Brady F. Int J Oral Maxillofac Surg 1995;24:26–29.
53. Davis JW, Parks SN, Detlefs CL, Williams GG, Williams JL, Smith RW. J Trauma 1995;39: 435–438.
54. Sees D, Rodriguez C, Flaherty S et al. J Trauma 1998;45:768–771.
55. Cooper C, Dunham CM, Rodriguez A. J Trauma 1995;38:692–696.
56. Frankel HL, Rozycki GS, Ochsner MG, Harviel JD, Champion HR. J Trauma 1994;37:673–676.
57. Stanislas MJ, Latham JM, Porter KM, Alpar EK, Stirling AJ. Injury 1998;29:15–18.
58. Hsu JM, Joseph T, Ellis AM. Injury 2003;34: 426–433.
59. Gestring ML, Gracias VH, Feliciano MA et al. J Trauma 2002;53:9–14.
60. Wintermark M, Mouhsine E, Theumann N et al. Radiology 2003;227:681–689.
61. Hauser CJ, Visvikis G, Hinrichs C et al. J Trauma 2003;55:228–234; discussion 234–225.
62. Sheridan R, Perlata R, Rhea J, Ptak T, Novelline R. J Trauma 2003;55:665–669.
63. Rhee PM, Bridgeman A, Acosta JA et al. J Trauma 2002;53:663–667; discussion 667.

22

Imaging of Spine Disorders in Children: Dysraphism and Scoliosis

L. Santiago Medina, Diego Jaramillo,
Esperanza Pacheco-Jacome, Martha C. Ballesteros,
Tina Young Poussaint, and Brian E. Grottkau

Issues

Spinal Dysraphism

I. How accurate is imaging in occult spinal dysraphism?
II. What are the clinical predictors of OSD?
III. What are the natural history and role of surgical intervention in Occult Spinal Dysraphism?
IV. What is the cost-effectiveness of imaging in children with Occult Spinal Dysraphism?

Scoliosis

V. How should the radiographic evaluation of scoliosis be performed?
VI. What radiation-induced complications result from radiographic monitoring of scoliosis?
VII. What is the role of magnetic resonance imaging in idiopathic scoliosis?

Key Points

Spinal

Dysraphism

- The prevalence of occult spinal dysraphism (OSD) ranges from as low as 0.34% in children with intergluteal dimples to as high as 46% in newborns with cloacal malformation (moderate evidence).
- *Radiographs are relatively insensitive and nonspecific for this diagnosis.* MRI and ultrasound have high overall diagnostic performances (i.e., sensitivity and specificity) in children with suspected OSD (moderate evidence).

L.S. Medina (✉)
Division of Neuroradiology and Brain Imaging, Department of Radiology, Miami Children's Hospital,
Miami, FL 33155, USA
e-mail: smedina@post.harvard.edu

L.S. Medina et al. (eds.), *Evidence-Based Imaging: Improving the Quality of Imaging in Patient Care, Revised Edition*,
DOI 10.1007/978-1-4419-7777-9_22, © Springer Science+Business Media, LLC 2011

- Early detection and prompt neurosurgical correction of OSD may prevent upper urinary tract deterioration, infection of dorsal dermal sinuses, or permanent neurologic damage (moderate and limited evidence).
- Cost-effectiveness analysis suggests that, in newborns with suspected OSD, appropriate selection of patients and diagnostic strategy may increase quality-adjusted life expectancy and decrease cost of medical workup (moderate evidence).

Scoliosis

- Radiographic measurements of scoliosis are reproducible, particularly when the levels of the end plates measured are kept constant (moderate evidence). Unexpected findings on radiographs are unusual (limited evidence).
- Radiographic monitoring of scoliosis results in a clear increase in the radiation-induced cancer risk, particularly to the female breast (moderate evidence). It also results in a high dose of radiation to the ovaries and worsens reproductive outcome in females (moderate evidence). Therefore, it is very important to reduce the radiation exposure. Posteroanterior projection greatly reduces exposure. Some digital systems also decrease radiation.
- Significant controversy exists on the use of MRI in "idiopathic" scoliosis. MRI is recommended for children at higher risk of CNS lesions (1) patients with idiopathic scoliosis and an abnormal neurological exam; (2) children under the age of 11 years; and (3) patients with levoconvex or atypical curves (limited to moderate evidence). However, exceptions to these rules have been reported in the literature (limited to moderate evidence). Therefore, patients with scoliosis considered for surgical intervention should have preoperative MRI to avoid the potential irreversible neurological complications that could occur if any underlying CNS lesion was undetected or misdiagnosed.

Definition and Pathophysiology

Spinal Dysraphism

Spinal dysraphism is a wide spectrum of congenital anomalies that results from abnormal development of one or more of the midline mesenchymal, bony, and neural elements of the spine (1). This entity can be divided into open and closed spina bifida. Open spina bifida is characterized by a dorsal herniation of all or part of the spinal content without full skin coverage. Open spina bifida entities include meningocele and myelomeningocele. Closed or occult spinal dysraphism (OSD) is characterized by a spinal anomaly covered with skin and hence with no exposed neural tissue (2, 3). OSD spectrum includes dorsal dermal sinus, thickened filum terminale, diastematomyelia, caudal regression syndrome, intradural lipoma, lipomyelocele, lipomyelomeningocele, anterior

spinal meningocele, and other forms of myelodysplasia (Figs. 22.3 and 22.4).

Scoliosis

Scoliosis is defined as an abnormal spinal curvature most apparent in the coronal plane (4). Scoliosis can be classified as idiopathic, congenital, neuromuscular, or degenerative. Most pediatric cases are idiopathic in nature. Idiopathic scoliosis is further subdivided according to the age at which the disease presents: infantile (birth to 3 years), juvenile (4–9 years), and most commonly adolescent (10 years and beyond) (5). Congenital scoliosis is caused by vertebral anomalies of embryologic etiology (e.g., hemivertebra, butterfly, or block vertebra) (6). Neuromuscular scoliosis is typically seen in cerebral palsy and muscular dystrophy. Scoliosis can also be seen in disorders such as neurofibromatosis (Figs. 22.5 and 22.6) and Marfan syndrome (4). Degenerative scoliosis is primarily a disease of adults.

Conus Medullaris Position

Controversy has existed about the normal position of the conus medullaris. The normal level of the conus medullaris was thought to vary with the age of the child (7–9). Cross-sectional imaging studies, however, indicate that the normal conus medullaris position can vary from the middle of T11 to the bottom of L2 by the age of 2 months (7, 9) and probably at birth (7, 10). More recent study by Soleiman et al. (11) studied 635 adult patients with no spinal deformity and demonstrated the mean position of the tip of the conus medullaris at the level of the middle third of L1. The range extended from the lower third of T11 to the upper third of L3 (11). Although a spinal cord terminating at these normal levels can be tethered (8), the conus that terminates caudal to the L2–L3 disc space is at much higher risk of being tethered (7, 9, 12). Neuroimaging can define the anatomical location of the conus medullaris, but the concept and word of "tethered" is a neurophysiological concept which requires clinical input (13). Small fibrolipomas in the filum terminale may be seen in untethered as well as tethered cords. Five to six percent of normal individuals can have variable amounts of fat in the filum terminale (14, 15).

Epidemiology

Spinal Dysraphism

Three percent of neonates have major central nervous system or systemic malformations (16). Furthermore, 5–15% of pediatric neurology hospital admissions are related to cerebrospinal anomalies (17). The incidence of neural tube defects in the USA is 1.2–1.7 per 1,000 births (18, 19). Almost half of neural tube defects are caused by anencephaly (0.6–0.8 per 1,000 births), and the majority of the remaining are caused by spinal dysraphism (0.5–0.8 per 1,000 births) (18, 19). OSD is the most prevalent spinal axis malformation (20) and the most common indication for spinal imaging in children (21).

Occult spinal dysraphic lesions are commonly associated with urinary tract anomalies (22). One well-recognized risk factor for this disorder is folate deficiency in the mother.

The clinical spectrum of occult dysraphism is broad, ranging from skin stigmata such as a dimple, sinus tract, hairy patch, or hemangioma to motor, bladder, or bowel dysfunction (23–25). About 50–80% of occult spinal dysraphic cases exhibit a dermal lesion (15–28). However, 3–5% of all normal children have skin dimples (29, 30).

Scoliosis

Adolescent idiopathic scoliosis, by far the most common form, has a prevalence between 0.5 (31) and 3% (31, 32) and occurs more often in females. In a UK study of 15,799 children and young adolescents, Stirling et al. (31) found that the prevalence ratio of girls to boys was 5.2 [95% confidence interval (CI), 2.9–9.5]. In a study of 26,947 students, Rogala et al. (33) found that for curves ranging from 6 to 10°, the girl-to-boy ratio was 1:1, whereas the ratio was 5.4:1 for curves greater than 20°. The more severe the curve, the greater the predominance of girls over boys. Infantile scoliosis constitutes approximately 8% of idiopathic scoliosis, whereas juvenile scoliosis represents 18% (34). Male predominance is seen in infantile scoliosis. Congenital scoliosis is caused by failure of segmentation and normal formation of spinal elements (4). In a series of 60 cases of congenital scoliosis, Shahcheraghi and Hobbi (6) found that the most common type of anomaly was a hemivertebra (failure of formation), and that the most severe deformity was associated with a unilateral unsegmented bar (failure of segmentation) with a contralateral hemivertebra.

The etiology of adolescent scoliosis remains a mystery; however, some principles are generally agreed upon (34):

1. The progression of scoliosis is related to severity and skeletal maturity. The younger the onset and the greater the severity of the curve, the faster the progression. Although previously it was believed that scoliosis remained stable after skeletal maturity was attained, Weinstein and Ponseti (35) demonstrated that 68% of curves worsened after bone maturity.

2. The typical scoliosis curve is not associated with pain or neurologic signs and symptoms. Painful curves, especially if rapidly progressive or if associated with an atypical curve pattern, are frequently caused by underlying diseases (36).
3. Less than 10% of the curves require treatment (37).

Goals

Spinal Dysraphism

In patients with spinal dysraphism, the goal of imaging is to detect early neurosurgical correctable occult dysraphic lesions in order to prevent neurologic damage, upper urinary tract deterioration, and potential infection of the dorsal dermal sinuses.

Scoliosis

In patients with scoliosis, the goal of imaging is to detect and characterize the type of curve and its severity, to track disease progression and monitor changes related to treatment, and to identify those cases in which occult etiologies exist (4).

Methodology

The authors performed a MEDLINE search using Ovid (Wolters Kluwer US Corporation, NY City) and PubMed (National Library of Medicine, Bethesda, MD) for data relevant to the diagnostic performance and accuracy of both clinical and radiographic examination of patients with OSD or scoliosis during the years 1966 to January 2008. Animal studies and non-English articles were excluded. The titles, abstracts, and full text of the relevant articles were reviewed at each step.

I. How Accurate Is Imaging in Occult Spinal Dysraphism?

Summary of Evidence: Several studies have shown that MRI and ultrasound have better overall diagnostic performances (i.e., sensitivity and specificity) than do plain radiographs (moderate evidence) for detection of OSD (21, 26, 38, 39). The sensitivity of spinal MRI and ultrasound has been estimated at 95.6 and 86.5%, respectively (31, 39). The specificity of spinal MRI and ultrasound has been estimated at 90.9 and 92.9%, respectively (21, 39). Conversely, the sensitivity and the specificity of plain radiographs have been estimated at 80 and 18%, respectively (26, 38).

Supporting Evidence: The diagnostic performance of the imaging tests available is shown in detail in Table 22.1.

II. What Are the Clinical Predictors of OSD?

Summary of Evidence: The prevalence of OSD ranges from as low as 0.34% in children with intergluteal dimples to as high as 46% in newborns with cloacal malformation (moderate evidence). Table 22.2 summarizes the spectrum of OSD into low-, intermediate-, and high-risk groups.

Supporting Evidence: Children in the low-risk group included those with simple skin dimples as the sole manifestation or newborns of diabetic mothers. Intergluteal dimples over the sacrococcygeal area rarely extend into the spinal canal (40–42). Caudal regression syndrome occurs at higher rates in children born to diabetic mothers (43). The prevalence (pretest probability) of a dysraphic lesion among low-risk patients has been estimated at 0.3–3.8% (Table 22.2). In the low range (0.3%) are children with low intergluteal dimples, while in the upper range (3.8%) are children with higher lumbosacral dimples (19, 26, 31) (moderate and limited evidence).

Children in the intermediate-risk group included those with complex skin stigmata (hairy patch, hemangiomas, lipomas, and well-defined dorsal dermal sinus tracks) or low and intermediate anorectal malformations. The prevalence (pretest probability) of a dysraphic lesion among intermediate-risk patients has been estimated at 27–36% (Table 22.2) (moderate evidence). Children in the high-risk group included those with high anorectal malformations, cloacal malformation, and cloacal exstrophy. The prevalence (pretest probability) of a dysraphic lesion among high-risk patients has been estimated at 44–100% (Table 22.2) (moderate evidence).

III. What Are the Natural History and Role of Surgical Intervention in Occult Spinal Dysraphism?

Summary of Evidence: Early detection and prompt neurosurgical correction of OSD may prevent upper urinary tract deterioration, infection of dorsal dermal sinuses, or permanent neurologic damage (44–48) (moderate and limited evidence). Several studies have demonstrated that motor function, urologic symptoms, and urodynamic patterns may be improved, stabilized, or prevented by early surgical intervention in patients with OSD (49, 50) (moderate and limited evidence). The surgical outcome may be better if intervention occurs before the age of 3 years (49–51) (moderate and limited evidence). Spinal neuroimaging, therefore, has the important role in determining the presence or the absence of an occult spinal dysraphic lesion so that appropriate surgical treatment can be instituted in a timely manner.

At our institution, occult dysraphic lesions diagnosed in the newborn period are usually operated at the age of 2–3 months. Therefore, if ultrasound is indicated, it is performed in the early newborn and infancy period to avoid a limited sonographic window from posterior element mineralization (52, 53). If MRI is required, it is usually performed a few days before surgery.

Supporting Evidence: In the newborn period, most children with OSD are neurologically asymptomatic (29). Symptoms from OSD are often not apparent until the child becomes older and is ambulating (29) (moderate evidence). The most common clinical presentations for occult dysraphic patients later in life include delay in walking, delay in the development of sphincter control, asymmetry of the legs or abnormalities of the feet (i.e., pes cavus and pes equinovarus), and pain in the lower extremities or back (44, 45, 49, 54–57).

Several studies have demonstrated improvement of the multiple symptoms associated with occult dysraphism if surgical intervention is performed (49–51) (moderate and limited evidence). However, there are differences in outcome depending on the timing of surgery (51). Using surgical outcome data from the study by Satar et al. (51), in the children diagnosed and surgically treated before the age of 3 years, 60% became asymptomatic, 30% were unchanged, and 10% worsened. Conversely, the same study data for the children diagnosed and surgically treated after the age of 3 years demonstrated that 27% became asymptomatic, 27% improved, 27% were unchanged, and 19% worsened (51).

Dysraphic patients with a central nervous system communicating dorsal dermal sinus (i.e., 10% of all dysraphic patients) are at risk for infection (26). The most dreaded infection is meningitis. Meningitis in the patient with a communicating dorsal dermal sinus may be caused by gram-negative or anaerobic bacteria (58, 59). The meningitis mortality rate in patients with communicating dorsal dermal sinus ranges between 1 and 12% (57–61) (limited evidence).

Severely symptomatic patients with dysraphism are at high risk of upper urinary tract deterioration (30, 62). In this population, up to 15% may have upper urinary tract deterioration (30, 62) and of those with progressive renal damage, 7.5% may develop end-stage renal disease over a 10-year period if undiagnosed (30, 62) (limited evidence).

IV. What Is the Cost-Effectiveness of Imaging in Children with Occult Spinal Dysraphism?

Summary of Evidence: Cost-effectiveness analysis (CEA) suggests that, in newborns with suspected OSD, appropriate selection of patients and diagnostic strategy may increase quality-adjusted life expectancy and decrease cost of medical workup (30).

Supporting Evidence: A CEA in children with OSD has been published in *Pediatrics* (30). This study assessed the clinical and economic consequences of four diagnostic strategies, MRI, ultrasound, plain radiographs, and no imaging with close clinical follow-up, in the evaluation of newborns with suspected OSD (30).

A decision-analytic Markov model and CEA was performed incorporating (1) pretest or prior probability of disease in three different risk groups, (2) sensitivity and specificity of diagnostic tests, and (3) morbidity and mortality rates of early versus late diagnosis and treatment of dysraphism. Outcomes were based on quality-adjusted life year (QALY) gained and incremental cost per QALY gained.

Medina et al. (30) found that in low-risk children with intergluteal dimple or newborns of diabetic mothers (pretest probability = 0.3–0.34%), ultrasound was the most effective strategy with an incremental cost-effectiveness ratio of $55,100 per QALY gained. The cost for QALY is less than $100,000 and hence considered a reasonable cost-effective strategy. For children with lumbosacral dimples who have a higher pretest probability of 3.8%, ultrasound was less costly and more effective than MRI, plain radiographs, or no imaging with close clinical follow-up.

In intermediate-risk newborns with low anorectal malformation (pretest probability 27%), ultrasound was more effective and less costly than radiographs and no imaging. However, MRI was more effective than ultrasound at an incremental cost-effectiveness ratio of $1,000 per QALY gained. Therefore, this diagnostic strategy has a very low cost per QALY gained. In the high-risk group that included high anorectal malformation, cloacal malformation, and exstrophy (pretest probability 44–46%), MRI was actually cost saving when compared with the other diagnostic strategies.

For the intermediate-risk group, the CEA was sensitive to the costs and diagnostic performances (sensitivity and specificity) of MRI and ultrasound. Lower MRI cost or greater MRI diagnostic performance improved the cost-effectiveness of the MRI strategy, while lower ultrasound cost or greater ultrasound diagnostic performance worsened the cost-effectiveness of the MRI strategy. Therefore, individual or institutional expertise with a specific diagnostic modality (MRI versus ultrasound) may influence the optimal diagnostic strategy.

V. How Should the Radiographic Evaluation of Scoliosis Be Performed?

Summary of Evidence: Radiographic measurements of scoliosis are reproducible, particularly when the levels of the vertebral body end

plates measured are kept constant at each radiographic study over time (moderate evidence). Unexpected findings on radiographs are unusual (limited evidence) (4).

Supporting Evidence: Many articles have addressed the variability in measurement of the Cobb angle in adolescent idiopathic scoliosis. In a 1990 study by Morrisy et al. (67), four orthopedic surgeons performed six measurements on 50 frontal radiographs. The 95% CIs were 4.9°, and the variation was greatest when the end-plate vertebrae were not preselected (moderate evidence). Similar variability was noted in the sagittal and coronal planes. Carman et al. (68) had five observers perform two measurements on 28 radiographs showing kyphosis or scoliosis and found 95% CIs of 8° for scoliosis and 7° for kyphosis (moderate evidence). A more recent study (69) comparing manual versus computer-assisted radiographic measurements (24 radiographs, six observers) found a statistically significant difference between the 95% CIs of manual measurements (3.3°) and computer-generated measurements (2.6°).

Variability is greater for congenital scoliosis versus idiopathic scoliosis. Using six observers and 54 radiographs, Loder et al. (70) found 95% CIs of 11.8° (moderate evidence).

The contribution of radiologists' reports of scoliosis radiographs to clinical management was studied by Crockett et al. (71). These investigators retrospectively reviewed 161 charts and analyzed them for the presence or the absence of information about certain key parameters. There was no mention of how the review was done or whether there was any attempt to correct for bias. Radiologists added information in 1.9% of the cases that, although not specified, was not deemed clinically significant (limited evidence) (71).

VI. What Radiation-Induced Complications Result from Radiographic Monitoring of Scoliosis?

Summary of Evidence: Patients with severe scoliosis are monitored with the use of serial radiographs that expose the body to radiation. Radiographic monitoring of scoliosis results in a clear increase in the radiation-induced cancer risk, particularly to the breast (4) (moderate evidence). It also results in a high dose of radiation to the ovaries and worsens reproductive outcome in females (4) (moderate evidence). Therefore, it is very important to reduce the radiation exposure. Posteroanterior projection greatly reduces exposure, and some digital systems also decrease radiation (72).

Supporting Evidence: In 2000, Morin Doody et al. (73) published a retrospective cohort study of 5,573 female patients with scoliosis diagnosed before the age of 20 years. The average length of follow-up was 40.1 years, with complete follow-up in 89%. The average number of radiographs per patient was 24.7 (range, 0–618), and the mean estimated cumulative radiation dose to the breast was 10.8 cGy (range, 0–170). This dose is equivalent to 54 two-view mammograms (average breast dose of 2 mGy) (0.2 cGy). Seventy-seven breast cancer deaths were observed compared with 45.6 expected deaths on the basis of US mortality rates. Women with scoliosis had a 1.7-fold risk of dying of breast cancer (95% CI, 1.3–2.1) when compared with the general population. The data suggested that radiation was the causative factor, with risk increasing significantly with the number of radiographic exposures and the cumulative radiation dose (moderate evidence). Potential confounding was noted because the severity of disease was related to radiation exposure and reproductive history; patients with more severe disease were less likely to become pregnant and had a greater risk of breast cancer.

In a large retrospective cohort study of 2,039 patients, Levy et al. (74) found an excess lifetime cancer risk of 1–2% (12–25 cases per 1,000) among women (moderate evidence). The same group suggested that supplanting the anteroposterior (AP) view with the posteroanterior (PA) view would result in a three- to sevenfold reduction in cumulative doses to the thyroid gland and the female breast, three- to fourfold reductions in the life-time risk of breast cancer, and a halving of the lifetime risk of thyroid cancer (75). The same cohort of women was evaluated for adverse reproductive outcomes (76). Of the initial group of 1,793 young women evaluated for scoliosis between 1960 and 1979, 1,292 women returned questionnaires in 1990. This cohort was compared with a reference group of 1,134 women selected randomly from the general population. The adolescent idiopathic scoliosis cohort had a higher risk of spontaneous abortions [odds ratio (OR), 1.35; 95% CI, 1.06–1.73] (moderate evidence). The odds of unsuccessful attempts at pregnancy (OR, 1.33; 95% CI, 0.84–2.13) and of congenital malformations in their offspring (OR, 1.2; 95% CI, 0.78–1.84) were also higher, but not statistically significant (moderate evidence).

Digital radiography seems to reduce radiation exposure. The results are varied (77–79), and the technology is evolving (limited evidence). Recent studies report an 18-fold reduction with some systems (72) versus an almost twofold increase with others (80).

VII. What Is the Role of Magnetic Resonance Imaging in Idiopathic Scoliosis?

Summary of Evidence: Significant controversy exists on the use of MR in idiopathic scoliosis. (1) Patients with idiopathic scoliosis and an abnormal neurological exam; (2) children under the age of 11 years; and (3) patients with levo-convex or atypical curves are at higher risk of CNS lesions and hence MRI is recommended (limited to moderate evidence). However, significant exceptions to these rules have been reported in the literature (limited to moderate evidence). Therefore, patients with scoliosis considered for surgical intervention should have preoperative MRI to avoid the potential irreversible neurological complications that could occur if any underlying CNS lesion was undetected or misdiagnosed.

Supporting Evidence: Cheng et al. (81) studied 36 healthy control subjects, 135 patients with moderately severe adolescent idiopathic scoliosis (Cobb angle less than 45°), and 29 similar patients with Cobb angles greater than 45°. All of the patients were evaluated prospectively with MR imaging looking specifically for tonsillar ectopia and with somatosensory-evoked potentials. Tonsillar herniation was found in none of the controls versus 4 of 135 (3%) and 8 of 29 (27.6%) of the two scoliotic groups ($P<0.001$) (moderate evidence). Similarly, the percentages of patients with abnormal somatosensory-evoked potentials were 0, 11.9, and 27.6%, respectively. There was a significant association between tonsillar ectopia and abnormal somatosensory function ($P < 0.0011$; correlation coefficient, 0.672) (moderate evidence). Tonsillar ectopia was defined as any inferior displacement of the tonsils, and none of the patients had a displacement greater than 5 mm, which is considered the usual threshold for the diagnosis (82–84).

Several studies have addressed the prevalence of MR abnormalities in patients with severe idiopathic scoliosis who are otherwise asymptomatic. Do et al. (85) studied a consecutive series of 327 patients with idiopathic scoliosis requiring surgical intervention (average preoperative curve of 57°) but without neurologic findings. The patients, aged 10–19 years, were evaluated from the base of the skull to the sacrum. Seven patients had abnormal MR images, including two with syrinx, four with Chiari malformation type I, and one with a fatty vertebral body. None of them required specific treatment for these findings (moderate evidence). In four other cases, equivocal MR findings necessitated additional workup. In a similar prospective double-blinded study of 140 patients evaluated preoperatively, Winter et al. (86) found four patients with abnormalities, three with Chiari I malformations, and one with a small syrinx, none of whom required treatment. In another study of MR examinations performed preoperatively, Maiocco et al. (87) found 2 of 45 patients with syrinx, one requiring decompression (moderate evidence).

To study whether the severity of the curve increased the risk of associated abnormalities, O'Brien et al. (88) performed MR evaluation on 33 consecutive patients with adolescent idiopathic scoliosis and Cobb angles greater than 70°. No neural axis abnormalities were found (limited evidence).

In a recent prospective study by Maenza (89) of 56 patients with juvenile and adolescent scoliosis, 11 patients (19.6%) had spinal axis lesions (Chiari I, $n = 5$; Chiari I and syringomyelia, $n = 4$; diastematomyelia and tethered cord, $n = 1$; and tethered cord, $n = 1$) (moderate evidence). In this group, the right and left thoracic curve patterns were seen in the same number of patients (4 of 11 each) (89) (moderate evidence). Thirty-six percent of the patients in this group were under the age of 11 years. Four patients (7.1%) had intracranial lesions (Dandy Walker syndrome,

$n = 1$; hydrocephalus, $n = 2$; and cerebellar angioma, $n = 1$). Four of the 15 patients (26.7%) with CNS abnormalities (spinal axis or intracranial lesions) had a normal neurological exam. Aria et al. found in 1,059 patients with scoliosis screened with MRI a total of 43 patients with syringomyelia and 38 of them associated with a Chiari I malformation (90) (moderate evidence). Charry et al. found in 25 patients with scoliosis and syringomyelia, 10 patients with a levothoracic and 9 patients with a dextrothoracic curve pattern (limited evidence) (91).

Several studies have shown that, with scoliosis types that are different from the typical adolescent idiopathic form, there is a high prevalence of neural abnormalities (4). Of 30 consecutive children with congenital scoliosis studied by Prahinski et al. (92), nine had syringomyelia. Of these children, one required release of the tethered cord and one correction of a diastematomyelia (limited evidence). Two studies of prepubertal children suggest a high incidence of neural abnormalities in juvenile and infantile scoliosis. In a study of 26 consecutive children aged less than 11 years, Lewonowski et al. 93) found five (19.2%) with abnormalities of the cord. Three required surgical intervention, two with hydromyelia, and one with a mass (93) (limited evidence). Gupta et al. (94) found that 6 of 34 patients under 10 years of age studied prospectively had neural axis abnormalities, including two patients with syrinx requiring syringopleural shunting (one with a Chiari I malformation). Other abnormalities included dural ectasia, tethered cord, and a brainstem astrocytoma (limited evidence).

In a retrospective review of 95 patients with idiopathic scoliosis who had been studied for various indications, Schwend et al. (95) found that 12 had a syrinx, one a cord astrocytoma, and one dural ectasia (limited evidence). Left thoracic scoliosis was the most important predictor of abnormality (10 abnormalities in 43 patients). Mejia et al. (96) then performed a prospective study (level 2) of 29 consecutive patients with idiopathic left thoracic scoliosis, finding only two with syrinx and no other abnormalities (limited evidence). Barnes et al. (36) retrospectively analyzed 30 patients with atypical idiopathic scoliosis and found 17 abnormalities in 11 patients, including seven cases of syringohydromyelia and five Chiari I malformations (limited evidence).

Take Home Figures and Tables

How Should Physicians Evaluate Newborns with Suspected Occult Spinal Dysraphism?

The decision tree in Fig. 22.1 reinforces the primary importance of a careful acquisition of a medical history and performance of a thorough examination in newborns with suspected spinal dysraphism (30). For those patients in the high-risk group, imaging of the spine with MRI is recommended. For those patients in the intermediate-risk group, imaging of the spine with MRI or ultrasound is suggested, while in the low-risk group, the strategies of ultrasound or no imaging may be indicated. Selection between these two strategies per risk group may be based on individual and institutional diagnostic performance and cost per test. In newborns with suspected occult dysraphism, appropriate selection of patients for imaging based on these risk groups may maximize health outcomes for patients and improve health-care resource allocation.

Tables 22.1 and 22.2 discuss the diagnostic performance of imaging tests in children with OSD and the risk groups for OSD, respectively.

How Should Scoliosis Be Evaluated?

Figure 22.2 summarizes the decision tree for patients with suspected scoliosis.

Imaging Case Studies

Case 1: Spinal Dysraphism

Imaging case study illustrates a child with skin stigmata (Fig. 22.3) who has an occult dysraphic lesion of the intradural lipoma type (Fig. 22.4).

Case 2: Scoliosis

Imaging case study illustrates a child with atypical levoconvex thoracic scoliosis (Fig. 22.5) who has neurofibromatosis type 1 with underlying plexiform neurofibromas (Fig. 22.6).

Suggested Imaging Protocols

Spinal Dysraphism

Spinal Ultrasound
Should be performed before the age of 3 months to avoid limited acoustic window from mineralization of posterior elements. An experienced operator should perform the study using a high-frequency 5–15 MHz linear array transducer (52).

Entire Spine MRI
A retrospective case–control study including 101 patients (moderate evidence) suspected of having occult lumbosacral dysraphism demonstrated that conventional three-plane, T1-weighted lumbosacral MR imaging in children and young adults provided better diagnostic information than did a fast-screening, two-plane, T1-weighted MRI because of its higher specificity and interobserver agreement (21). T2-weighted images in the axial and sagittal plane are often added to the protocol to assess intrinsic cord abnormalities. Intravenous paramagnetic contrast is not routinely used unless the patient has a communicating dorsal dermal sinus tract or clinical concerns of underlying infection.

Scoliosis

Scoliosis Radiographs
Should be performed only when clinically indicated. Using the posteroanterior projection greatly reduces exposure, and some digital systems also decrease radiation (4, 72). Use of gonads and breast lead shields further decreases the radiation exposure.

Entire Spine MRI
Patients with scoliosis may represent an imaging challenge. In patients with scoliosis being evaluated with MRI, the entire spine should be covered. Three-plane, T1- and T2-weighted images should be obtained with different obliquities to optimize imaging information. Another approach is to obtain three-dimensional FSE volumetric imaging. Weinberger et al. (97) recommend using a TR of 500 ms, TE_{eff} of 21 ms, echo train length (ETL) of 8, 20–38 cm

field of view, 256×256 in-plane matrix, 1 mm sagittal partition thickness, one excitation, and 16 kHz of receive bandwidth. Intravenous paramagnetic contrast is important in the evaluation of intramedullary and extramedullary neoplasm.

Table 22.1. Diagnostic performance of imaging tests in children with occult spinal dysraphism

Variable	Baseline value (%)	95% Confidence interval[a] (%)	References
Ultrasound			
Sensitivity	86.5	75–98	(30, 39)
Specificity	92.0	84–100	(30, 39)
MRI			
Sensitivity	95.6	89.8–99.7	(20, 30)
Specificity	90.9	75.7–98.1	(20, 30)
Plain radiographs			
Sensitivity	80	80–100	(26, 30, 38)
Specificity	18	11–25	(30, 38)

Modified with kind permission of Springer Science+Business Media from Medina LS, Jaramillo D, Pacheco-Jacome E, Ballesteros MC, Grottkau BE. In Medina LS, Blackmore CC (eds): *Evidence-Based Imaging: Optimizing Imaging in Patient Care*. New York: Springer Science+Business Media, 2006.
[a]95% Confidence intervals were estimated from the available literature.

Table 22.2. Risk groups for occult spinal dysraphism

Variable	Baseline risk (%)	References
Low-risk group		
Offsprings of diabetic mothers	0.3	(30, 63–65)
Intergluteal dimples	0.34	(15, 30)
Lumbosacral dimple	3.8	(29)
Intermediate-risk groups		
Low anorectal malformation	27	(66)
Intermediate anorectal malformation	33	(66)
Complex skin stigmata[a]	36	(29)
High-risk group		
High anorectal malformation	44	(66)
Cloacal malformation	46	(22)
Cloacal exstrophy	100	(22)

Modified with kind permission of Springer Science+Business Media from Medina LS, Jaramillo D, Pacheco-Jacome E, Ballesteros MC, Grottkau BE. In Medina LS, Blackmore CC (eds): *Evidence-Based Imaging: Optimizing Imaging in Patient Care*. New York: Springer Science+Business Media, 2006.
[a]Hemangiomas, hairy patches, and subcutaneous masses.

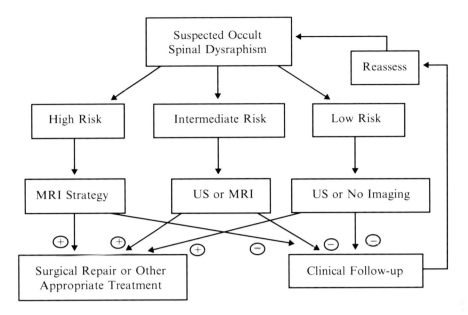

Figure 22.1. Suggested decision tree for use in newborns with suspected occult spinal dysraphism. For those patients in the high-risk group, MRI is recommended. For patients in the intermediate-risk group, ultrasound (US) or MRI is the strategy of choice, while for the low-risk group, ultrasound or no imaging is recommended. For patients with negative imaging studies, close clinical follow-up with periodic reassessment is recommended. (Reproduced with permission from Medina et al. (30). Copyright© 2001 by the AAP.)

Figure 22.2. Suggested decision tree for use in patients with suspected scoliosis. Decision tree emphasizes the importance of clinical history, physical exam, and radiographs in determining the need for MRI. (Modified with kind permission of Springer Science+Business Media from Medina LS, Jaramillo D, Pacheco-Jacome E, Ballesteros MC, Grottkau BE. In Medina LS, Blackmore CC (eds): *Evidence-Based Imaging: Optimizing Imaging in Patient Care.* New York: Springer Science+Business Media, 2006.)

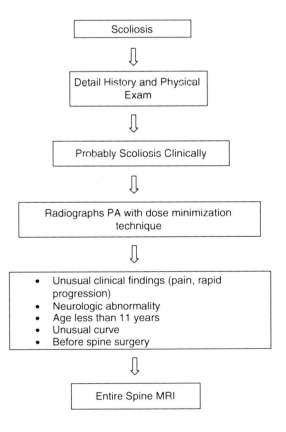

380

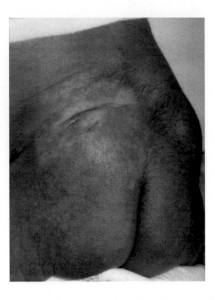

Figure 22.3. Photograph of the lower back reveals skin discoloration, hairy patch, and dorsal lipoma. (Reprinted with kind permission of Springer Science+Business Media from Medina LS, Jaramillo D, Pacheco-Jacome E, Ballesteros MC, Grottkau BE. In Medina LS, Blackmore CC (eds): *Evidence-Based Imaging: Optimizing Imaging in Patient Care*. New York: Springer Science+Business Media, 2006.)

Figure 22.4. Sagittal T1-weighted imaging shows a dorsal lipoma extending into the spinal canal with an associate low-lying conus medullaris. (Reprinted with kind permission of Springer Science+Business Media from Medina LS, Jaramillo D, Pacheco-Jacome E, Ballesteros MC, Grottkau BE. In Medina LS, Blackmore CC (eds): *Evidence-Based Imaging: Optimizing Imaging in Patient Care*. New York: Springer Science+Business Media, 2006.)

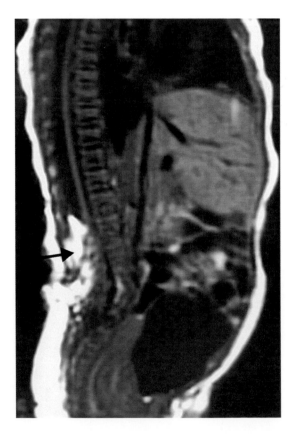

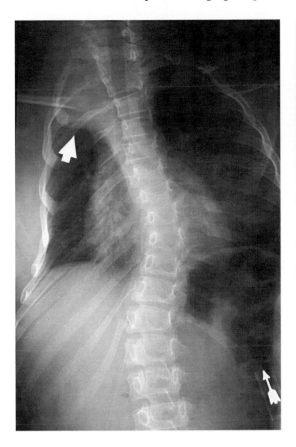

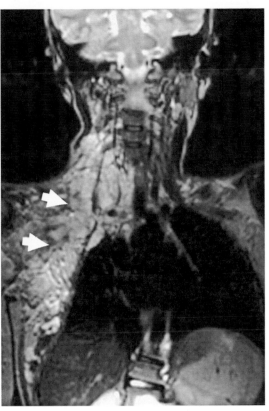

Figure 22.5. Frontal radiograph of the spine reveals atypical levoconvex thoracic scoliosis and right thoracic apical mass. (Reprinted with kind permission of Springer Science+Business Media from Medina LS, Jaramillo D, Pacheco-Jacome E, Ballesteros MC, Grottkau BE. In Medina LS, Blackmore CC (eds): *Evidence- Based Imaging: Optimizing Imaging in Patient Care*. New York: Springer Science+Business Media, 2006.)

Figure 22.6. Coronal T2-weighted image shows a large right neck and chest plexiform neurofibroma. (Reprinted with kind permission of Springer Science+Business Media from Medina LS, Jaramillo D, Pacheco-Jacome E, Ballesteros MC, Grottkau BE. In Medina LS, Blackmore CC (eds): *Evidence-Based Imaging: Optimizing Imaging in Patient Care*. New York: Springer Science+Business Media, 2006.).

Future Research

- Formal CEA of imaging in children with scoliosis.
- Further development of low- or no-radiation imaging techniques for patients with scoliosis.
- Large series studying the role of MRI in scoliosis.

References

1. Pacheco-Jacome E, Ballesteros MC, Jayakar P, Morrison G, Ragheb J et al. Neuroimaging Clin N Am 2003;13:327–334.
2. Soonawala N, Overweg-Plandsoen WCG, Brouwer OF. Clin Neurol Neurosurg 1999;101: 11–14.
3. Tortori-Donati P, Cama A, Rosa ML, Andreussi L, Taccone A. Neuroradiology 1990;31:512–522.
4. Jaramillo D, Poussaint TY, Grottkau BE. Neuroimaging Clin N Am 2003;13:335–341.
5. Oestreich AE, Young LW, Young Poussaint T. Skeletal Radiol 1998;27(11):591–605.
6. Shahcheraghi GH, Hobbi MH. J Pediatr Orthop 1999;19(6):766–775.
7. DiPietro MA. Radiology 1993;188:149–153.
8. Rowland Hill CA, Gibson PJ. AJNR Am J Neuroradiol 1995;16:469–472.
9. Wilson DA, Prince JR. AJNR Am J Neuroradiol 1989;10:259–262.
10. Beek FJ, de Vries LS, Gerards LJ, Mali WP. Neuroradiology 1996;38(suppl 1):S174–S177.
11. Soleiman J, Demaerel P, Rocher S et al. Spine 2005;30(16):1875–1880.
12. Barson AJ. J Anat 1970;106:489–497.
13. Warder DE, Oakes WJ. Neurosurgery 1993;33: 374–378.
14. Haworth JC, Zachary RB. Lancet 1955;2:10–14.
15. Milhorat TH, Miller JI. In Avery GB, Fletcher MA, Mhairi GM (eds.): Neonatology, 4th ed. Philadelphia: J.B. Lippincott, 1994;1155–1163.
16. Kalter H, Warkany J. N Engl J Med 1983;308: 424–431.
17. Bird TD, Hall JG. Neurology 1977;27:1057–1060.
18. Vintzileos AM, Ananth CV, Fisher AJ, Smulian JC, Day-Salvatore D, Beazoglou T et al. Am J Obstet Gynecol 1999;180(5):1110–1114.
19. Knight GJ, Palomaki GF. In Elias S, Simpson JL (eds.): Maternal Serum Screening for Fetal Genetic Disorders. New York: Churchill Livingstone, 1992;41–58.
20. Egelhoff JC, Prenger EC, Coley BD. In Ball W, Jr (ed.): Pediatric Neuroradiology. Philadelphia: Lippincott-Raven Publishers, 1997;717–778.
21. Medina LS, Al-Orfali M, Zurakowski D, Poussaint TY, DiCanzio J et al. Radiology 1999;211:767–771.
22. Appignani BA, Jaramillo D, Barnes PD, Poussaint TY. AJR Am J Roentgenol 1994;163:1199–1203.
23. Raghavan N, Barkovich AJ, Edwards M, Norman D. AJR Am J Roentgenol 1989;152:843–852.
24. Brophy JD, Sutton LN, Zimmerman RA, Bury E, Schut L. Neurosurgery 1989;25:336–340.
25. Moufarrij NE, Palmer JM, Hahn JF, Weinstein MA. Neurosurgery 1989;25:341–346.
26. Volpe JJ. Neurology of the Newborn, 4th ed. Philadelphia: W.B. Saunders, 2001.
27. Hoffman HJ, Hendrick EB, Humphreys RP. Childs Brain 1976;2:145–155.
28. Hoffman HJ, Taecholarn C, Hendrick EB, Humphreys RP. J Neurosurg 1985;62:1–8.
29. Kriss VM, Desai NS. AJR Am J Roentgenol 1998;171:1687–1692.
30. Medina LS, Crone K, Kuntz KM. Pediatrics 2001; 108:E101.
31. Stirling AJ, Howel D, Millner PA, Sadiq S, Sharples D et al. J Bone Joint Surg Am 1996;78(9): 1330–1336.
32. Newton PO, Wenger DR. In Morrissy RT, Weinstein SL (eds.): Lovell & Winter's Pediatric Orthopaedics, 5th ed. Philadelphia: Lippincott Williams & Wilkins, 2000;677–740.
33. Rogala EJ, Drummond DS, Gurr J. J Bone Joint Surg Am 1978;60(2):173–176.
34. Al-Arjani AM, Al-Sebai MW, Al-Khawashki HM, Saadeddin MF. Saudi Med J 2000;21(6):554–557.
35. Weinstein SL, Ponseti IV. J Bone Joint Surg Am 1983;65(4):447–455.
36. Barnes PD, Brody JD, Jaramillo D, Akbar JU, Emans JB. Radiology 1993;186(1):247–253.
37. Weinstein SL. Spine 1999;24(24):2592–2600.
38. Horton D, Barnes P, Pendleton BD, Polly M. J Okla State Med Assoc 1989;82:15–19.
39. Rohrschneider WK, Forsting M, Darge K, Tröger J. Radiology 1996;200:383–388.
40. Powell KR, Cherry JD, Hougen TJB, Blinderman EE, Dunn MC. J Pediatr 1975;87:744–750.
41. Byrd SE, Darling CF, McLone DG. Radiol Clin North Am 1991;29:711–752.
42. Herman TE, Oser RF, Shackelford GD. Clin Pediatr 1993;32:627–628.
43. Estin MD, Cohen AR. Neurosurg Clin N Am 1995;6:377–391.
44. Kaplan JO, Quencer RM. Radiology 1980;137: 387–391.
45. McLone DG, Naidich TP. In McLaurin RL, Schut L, Venes JL, Epstein F (eds.): Surgery of the Developing Nervous System. Philadelphia: W.B. Saunders, 1989;71–96.
46. Yamada S, Iacono RP, Andrade T, Mandybur G, Yamada BS. Neurosurg Clin N Am 1995;6: 311–323.
47. Davis PC, Hoffman JC, Ball TI, Wyly JB, Braun IF, Fry SM et al. Radiology 1988;166:679–685.

48. Scatliff JH, Kendall BE, Kingsley DPE, Britton J, Grant DN et al. AJNR Am J Neuroradiol 1989;10:269–277.

49. Pang D, Wilberger JE. J Neurosurg 1982;57:32–47.

50. Fone PD, Vapnek JM, Litwiller SE, Couillard DR, McDonald CM, Boggan JE et al. J Urol 1997;157:604–609.

51. Satar N, Bauer SB, Shefner J, Kelly MD, Darbey MM. J Urol 1995;154:754–758.

52. Coley BD, Siegel MJ. In Siegel MJ (ed.): Pediatric Sonography. Philadelphia: Lippincott Williams & Wilkins, 2002;671–698.

53. Rubin JM, Di Pietro MA, Chandler WF et al. Radiol Clin North Am 1988;26:1–27.

54. Page LK. In Wilkins RH, Rengachary SS (eds.): Neurosurgery. New York: McGraw Hill, 1992;2053–2058.

55. Westcott MA, Dynes MC, Remer EM, Donaldson JS, Dias LS. Radiographics 1992;12:1155–1173.

56. Atala A, Bauer SB, Dyro FM et al. J Urol 1992;148:592–594.

57. Reigel DH, Tchernoukha K, Bazmi B, Kortyna R, Rotenstein D. Pediatr Neurosurg 1994;20:30–42.

58. Law DA, Aronoff SC. Pediatr Infect Dis J 1992;11:968–971.

59. Rogg JM, Benzil DL, Haas RL, Knuckey NW. AJNR Am J Neuroradiol 1993;14:1393–1395.

60. DiTullio MV, Jr. Surg Neurol 1977;7:351–354.

61. Feigen RD, Cherry JD. Textbook of Pediatric Infectious Diseases, 2nd ed. Philadelphia: W.B. Saunders Co, 1987.

62. Capitanucci ML, Iacobelli BD, Silveri M, Mosiello G, De Gennaro M. Eur J Pediatr Surg 1996;6 (suppl 1):25–26.

63. Mills JL. Teratology 1982;25:385–394.

64. Rusnak SL, Discoll SG. Pediatrics 1965;35:989–995.

65. Becerra JE, Khoury MJ, Cordero JF, Ericson JD. Pediatrics 1990;85:1–9.

66. Long FR, Hunter JV, Mahboubi S, Kalmus A, Templeton JM. Radiology 1996;200:377–382.

67. Morrissy RT, Goldsmith GS, Hall EC, Kehl D, Cowie GH. J Bone Joint Surg Am 1990;72(3):320–327

68. Carman DL, Browne RH, Birch JG. J Bone Joint Surg Am 1990;72(3):328–333.

69. Shea KG, Stevens PM, Nelson M, Smith JT, Masters KS et al. Spine 1998;23(5):551–555.

70. Loder RT, Urquhart A, Steen H, Graziano G, Hensinger RN, Schlesinger A et al. J Bone Joint Surg Br 1995;77(5):768–770.

71. Crockett HC, Wright JM, Burke S, Boachie-Adjei O. Spine 1999;24(19):2007–2009; discussion 2010.

72. Kalifa G, Charpak Y, Maccia C, Fery-Lemonnier E, Bloch J, Boussard JM et al. Pediatr Radiol 1998;28(7):557–561.

73. Morin Doody M, Lonstein JE, Stovall M, Hacker DG, Luckyanov N et al. Spine 2000;25(16):2052–2063.

74. Levy AR, Goldberg MS, Hanley JA, Mayo NE, Poitras B. Health Phys 1994;66(6):621–633.

75. Levy AR, Goldberg MS, Mayo NE, Hanley JA, Poitras B. Spine 1996;21(13):1540–1547; discussion 1548.

76. Goldberg MS, Mayo NE, Levy AR, Scott SC, Poitras B. Epidemiology 1998;9(3):271–278.

77. Kalmar JA, Jones JP, Merritt CR. Spine 1994;19(7):818–823.

78. Kling TF, Jr, Cohen MJ, Lindseth RE, De Rosa GP. Spine 1990;15(9):880–885.

79. Stringer DA, Cairns RA, Poskitt KJ, Bray H, Milner R et al. Pediatr Radiol 1994;24(1):1–5.

80. Geijer H, Beckman K, Jonsson B, Andersson T, Persliden J. Radiology 2001;218(2):402–410.

81. Cheng JC, Guo X, Sher AH, Chan YL, Metreweli C. Spine 1999;24(16):1679–1684.

82. Barkovich AJ, Wippold FJ, Sherman JL, Citrin CM. AJNR Am J Neuroradiol 1986;7(5):795–799.

83. Elster AD, Chen MY. Radiology 1992;183(2):347–353.

84. Mikulis DJ, Diaz O, Egglin TK, Sanchez R. Radiology 1992;183(3):725–728.

85. Do T, Fras C, Burke S, Widmann RF, Rawlins B et al. J Bone Joint Surg Am 2001;83:577–579.

86. Winter RB, Lonstein JE, Heithoff KB, Kirkham JA. Spine 1997;22(8):855–858.

87. Maiocco B, Deeney VF, Coulon R, Parks PF, Jr. Spine 1997;22(21):2537–2541.

88. O'Brien MF, Lenke LG, Bridwell KH, Blanke K, Baldus C. Spine 1994;19(14):1606–1610.

89. Maenza RA. J Pediatr Orthop Sept 2003;12(5):295–302.

90. Arai S, Ohtsuka Y, Moriya H, Kitahara H, Minami S. Spine 1993;18:1591–1592.

91. Charry O, Koop S, Winter RB, Lonstein J, Denis F et al. J Pediatr Orthop 1994;14:309–317.

92. Prahinski JR, Polly DW, Jr, McHale KA, Ellenbogen RG. J Pediatr Orthop 2000;20(1):59–63.

93. Lewonowski K, King JD, Nelson MD. Spine 1992;17(suppl 6):S109–S116.

94. Gupta P, Lenke LG, Bridwell KH. Spine 1998;23(2):206–210.

95. Schwend RM, Hennrikus W, Hall JE, Emans JB. J Bone Joint Surg Am 1995;77(1):46–53.

96. Mejia EA, Hennrikus WL, Schwend RM, Emans JB. J Pediatr Orthop 1996;16(3):354–358.

97. Weinberger E, Murakami J, Shaw D, White K, Radvilas M et al. J Comput Assist Tomogr 1995;19:721–725.

Part V

Cardiovascular and Chest Imaging

23

Imaging of the Solitary Pulmonary Nodule

Anil Kumar Attili and Ella A. Kazerooni

Issues

I. Who should undergo imaging?
    A. Nodule stability in size
    B. Nodule morphology: calcification
    C. Nodule morphology: fat
    D. Nodule morphology: feeding artery and draining vein
    E. Nodule morphology: rounded atelectasis
    F. Applicability to children
II. Which imaging is appropriate?
    A. Computed tomography densitometry
    B. Thin-section computed tomography
    C. Computed tomography contrast enhancement
    D. Dual-energy computed tomography
    E. Positron emission tomography
    F. Single photon emission computed tomography
    G. Percutaneous needle biopsy
    H. Cost-effectiveness
III. Special case: estimating the probability of malignancy in solitary pulmonary nodules
IV. Special case: solitary pulmonary nodule in a patient with a known extrapulmonary malignancy

A.K. Attili (✉)
Department of Radiology, University of Kentucky, 800 Rose St, HX315B, Lexington, KY 40536, USA
e-mail: anil.attili@uky.edu

L.S. Medina et al. (eds.), *Evidence-Based Imaging: Improving the Quality of Imaging in Patient Care, Revised Edition*, DOI 10.1007/978-1-4419-7777-9_23, © Springer Science+Business Media, LLC 2011

- Further evaluation of a solitary pulmonary nodule (SPN) incidentally detected on chest radiography is not needed when either of the following two criteria (moderate evidence) is met: Nodule is stable in size for at least 2 years when compared to prior chest radiographs; there is a benign pattern of calcification demonstrated on chest radiography.
- Further evaluation of a pulmonary nodule showing a benign pattern of calcification, fat, or stability for 2 years or more on thin-section computed tomography (CT) is not needed (moderate evidence).
- In the absence of benign calcification, fat, or documented radiographic stability for at least 2 years, the choice of subsequent imaging strategy to differentiate between benign and malignant nodules is critically dependent on the pretest probability of malignancy.
- CT should be the initial test for most patients with radiographically indeterminate pulmonary nodules (moderate evidence).
- 18-Fluorodeoxyglucose positron emission tomography (^{18}FDG-PET) has a high sensitivity and specificity for malignancy (strong evidence), and is most cost-effective when used selectively in patients where the CT findings and pretest probability of malignancy are discordant.
- The use of multidetector CT (MDCT) scanners with improved spatial resolution for lung cancer screening has led to the increased detection of small (<1 cm) pulmonary nodules. Nodules are categorized on CT as (1) solid, (2) part-solid (mixed solid and ground-glass attenuation), or (3) nonsolid (pure ground-glass attenuation).
- The imaging strategy for the further evaluation of small solid pulmonary nodules in the absence of a known primary malignancy is based on nodule diameter (moderate evidence).
- For solid nodules 4–10 mm in diameter, a strategy of careful observation with serial thin-section CT scanning is recommended at 6, 12, and 24 months. In patients with a known primary neoplasm, initial reevaluation at 3 months is recommended.
- For solid nodules larger than 10 mm in diameter, further evaluation with ^{18}FDG-PET, percutaneous needle biopsy, or video-assisted thoracoscopic surgery (VATS) is recommended.
- Part-solid nodules (solid and ground-glass components) and nonsolid nodules (pure ground glass) detected at lung cancer screening have a higher likelihood of malignancy than solid nodules; therefore, tissue sampling (percutaneous CT-guided biopsy or VATS) is recommended (moderate evidence). For nodules less than 1 cm where this may not be possible, close serial CT evaluation at 3-month intervals in recommended.

Definition and Pathophysiology

Fleischner Society nomenclature defines nodule as "any pulmonary or pleural lesion represented in a radiograph by a sharply defined, discrete, nearly circular opacity 2–30 mm in diameter" and should always be qualified with respect to "size, location, border characteristics, number and opacity." A mass is defined as any similar lesion "that is greater than 30 mm in diameter (without regard to contour, border characteristics, or homogeneity), but explicitly shown or presumed to be extended in all three dimensions" (1). The differential diagnosis for an SPN is extensive, as listed in Table 23.1.

Epidemiology

An SPN may be found on 0.09–0.20% of all chest radiographs (2, 3). With the advent of CT scanning and screening for lung cancer, the discovery of SPNs has increased. From lung cancer screening studies, 23–51% of cigarette smokers over 50 years of age will have at least one SPN detected on screening CT (4, 5). The reported incidence of malignancy in SPNs varies from 5 to 69% (6–9). This wide range in part depends on the modality used for detection and the characteristics of the patient population studied. Compared to chest X-ray (CXR), low-dose helical CT detects three to four times more nodules, the majority of which are benign (5, 10). Large-scale screening studies with CXR report a 5–10% incidence of malignancy in SPNs, vs. less than 1% rate of malignancy in CT screening trials (5). In comparison, the incidence of malignancy in SPNs taken from series of surgically resected nodules is higher, due to selection bias and the high pretest probability of cancer in patients undergoing surgery (8, 9, 11). For nonselected adult populations, a new SPN on CXR has a 20–40% likelihood of being malignant (12–14). Infectious granulomas are responsible for approximately 80% of benign SPNs, and hamartomas approximately 10% (15, 16).

Overall Cost to Society

See Chap. 4 for the overall cost of lung cancer to society. A review of the literature reveals no information on the cost of evaluation of SPNs. In many ways, this subject is a moving target. As more nodules are detected with evolving MDCT scanners using thinner and thinner collimation, there are more and more nodules to evaluate. The majority of these nodules are too small to evaluate with PET scan or biopsy, leaving them to serial CT follow-up for at least 2 years to document stability as an indicator of benign biologic behavior. Needless to say, detecting and then following more nodules increases the total cost to society.

Goals

The goal for the imaging evaluation of an SPN is to accurately distinguish benign nodules from malignant nodules, enabling resection of malignant nodules without undue delay and avoiding exploratory thoracotomy, percutaneous biopsy, or additional testing such as CT or PET scanning, for patients with benign nodules.

Methodology

A Medline search was performed using PubMed (National Library of Medicine, Bethesda, Maryland) for original research publications discussing the diagnostic performance and effectiveness of imaging strategies in the evaluation of an SPN. The search covered the period 1966 to May 2004. The search terms were also entered into a Google search. The search strategy employed different combinations of the following subject headings and terms: (1) *coin lesion, pulmonary,* or *solitary pulmonary nodule;* (2) *lung neoplasms* or *lung cancer;* (3) *mass screening* or *lung cancer screening;* (4) *costs* and *cost analysis;* (5) *cost–benefit analysis,* (6) *socioeconomic factors,* (7) *incidence,* (8) *radiography* or *imaging* or *tomography,* X-ray computed or *tomography, emission-computed* or *tomography, emission-computed, single-photon* or *magnetic resonance imaging.* Additional articles were identified by reviewing the reference list of relevant papers. The review was limited to the English-language literature. The authors performed an initial review of the titles and abstracts of the identified articles followed by review of the full text in articles that were identified.

I. Who Should Undergo Imaging?

Summary of Evidence: Pulmonary nodules are commonly discovered incidentally on chest radiographs or CT examinations. There are four imaging findings that are highly predictive of benignity. If one or more of these four features is identified, no further diagnostic evaluation is required. If there is doubt on CXR about the presence of these findings, CT should be performed for better anatomic resolution:

1. Nodule calcification on CXR or CT that is either central, diffuse, popcorn, or laminar (concentric rings) (Fig. 23.1).
2. Fat within a nodule on CT is highly specific for hamartoma (Fig. 23.2).
3. A feeding artery and draining vein indicate an arteriovenous malformation.

4. A pleural-based opacity with incurving bronchovascular bundles associated with adjacent pleural thickening or effusion is a characteristic of rounded atelectasis (comet tail sign).

Stability on CXRs for 2 years or more has been considered an indicator of benignity. This is based on retrospective case series in which surgical resection was performed. A recent reevaluation of the original data shows that the 2-year stability criterion on CXR has a predictive value of only 65% for benignity, limiting the use of this criterion; 10–20% of small or subtle lesions interpreted as possible SPNs on CXRs do not actually represent SPNs, but rather lesions in the ribs, pleura, or chest wall or artifacts. When there is doubt about the presence of a nodule on CXR, further imaging is required.

Supporting Evidence

A. Nodule Stability in Size

An imperative step in determining the significance of an SPN is determining how long the nodule has been present. The widely accepted radiographic criterion for identifying nodules as benign is stability for 2 years or more. The evidence on which this is based was reanalyzed by Yankelevitz and Henschke (17), who traced the concept to articles by Good and Wilson (18). These include retrospective reviews of 1,355 patients who underwent surgical lung resection between 1940 and 1951. Using no growth on chest radiographs has only a 65% positive predictive value for benignity, with sensitivity of 40% and specificity of 72%. In view of these retrospective studies and bias only for nodules undergoing resection in the pre-CT era, this constitutes only limited evidence for 2 years or longer stability in size as a marker of benignity.

Fundamental to nodule stability is the concept of tumor doubling time. Collins et al. (19) advanced the theory of exponential tumor growth from a single cell, providing a methodology for predicting growth rates of human tumors that were previously evaluated only in animal models (20, 21). Nathan et al. (22), in a level II (moderate evidence) study, determined malignant growth rates of pulmonary nodules using Collins exponential equations; their predictions were verified in several subsequent using CXR studies (23–25). Malignant nodules

had a volume doubling time of 30–490 days. Lesions that doubled more rapidly were usually infection, and nodules with a slower doubling time are usually benign. Two-year stability implies a doubling time of well more than 730 days (26). Using the stability criterion assumes nodule diameter can be accurately measured on CXR; however, the limit of detectable change in size with CXR is 3–5 mm; smaller changes are better evaluated with thin-section CT, with a 0.3-mm lower limit of resolution. However, even using thin-section CT, human observers measuring small nodules (<5 mm) are prone to inter- and intraobserver variation (27).

Recently, calculating volumetric tumor growth rate from serial CT examinations has been investigated in a small number of retrospective level II (moderate evidence) studies (28, 29). Volumetric CT measurements are highly accurate for determining lung nodule volume, and useful to evaluate growth rate of small nodules by calculating nodule doubling time (30). Winer-Muram et al. (28) in a level II (moderate evidence) retrospective study evaluated CT volumetric growth of untreated stage I lung cancers in 50 patients. The median doubling time was 181 days (ranging from unchanged to 32 days). Of note, 11 lung cancers (22%) had a doubling time of 465 days or more. A wide variability in tumor doubling times was also demonstrated by Aoki et al. (31) in a retrospective level II (moderate evidence) CT study of peripheral lung adenocarcinomas. The group of nodules appearing as focal ground-glass opacity grew slowly (doubling time mean 2.4 years, range 42–1,486 days), while the group of solid nodules grew more quickly (doubling time mean 0.7 years, range 124–402 days).

Stability as an indicator of a benign process precluding further evaluation requires accurate measurement of growth using reproducible high-resolution imaging techniques. The CXR dictum of 2-year stability indicating a benign process should be used with caution. Every effort should be made to obtain prior comparison examinations, preferably from at least 2 years earlier. Stability of a nodule for 2 years on thin-section CT may be a more reasonable guideline for predicting benignity.

B. Nodule Morphology: Calcification

Several morphologic features can be used to indicate benignity with a high degree of specificity.

The first is identifying a benign pattern of calcification. In an early case series of 156 SPNs surgically resected between 1940 and 1951, Good et al. (32) found no calcification on chest radiographs in any of the malignant lesions. Subsequently, O'Keefe et al. (33), in a 1957 level II (moderate evidence) study, performed careful analysis of the specimen radiographs from 207 resected pulmonary nodules. Calcification was found histologically in 49.6% of the benign nodules and 13.9% of the malignant nodules. The patterns of diffuse, central, laminated, and popcorn calcification were only found in the benign pulmonary nodules. Eccentric calcifications were found both in malignant (Fig. 23.3) and benign nodules (34). Calcification in primary bronchogenic carcinomas is usually amorphous or stippled (35, 36). A later large case series demonstrated a popcorn pattern of calcification in one third of hamartomas.

Berger et al. (37) in a level II (moderate evidence) study evaluated the effectiveness of standard chest radiographs for detecting calcification in SPNs, using thin-section CT (1.5- to 3-mm slice thickness) as the reference standard. Chest radiographs were 50% sensitive and 87% specific for detecting any calcification, with a positive predictive value of 93%. The overall ability of CXR to detect calcification of any kind in SPNs is low. The superiority of CT for detecting calcification that is occult on CXR has been shown in several subsequent level II (moderate evidence) studies (8, 38, 39). These will be discussed further in the following section.

Without documentation of radiographic stability for a noncalcified pulmonary nodule detected on CXR, there should be a very low threshold for recommending further imaging with CT for these indeterminate pulmonary nodules.

C. Nodule Morphology: Fat

For nodules detected incidentally on CT, the additional finding of intranodular fat is a highly specific indicator of a hamartoma, a benign lung tumor. Fat may be found on CT in up to 50% of pulmonary hamartomas, and when present negates the need for further evaluation. In a prospective level II (moderate evidence) study of 47 hamartomas (31 pathology proven, 16 presumed by serial follow-up CT examinations) with thin-section CT, the correct diagnosis of hamartoma could be made based on the detection of fat alone in 18 nodules, and by the presence of fat and calcification in 12 nodules; together, this represented 69% of the hamartomas studied (40).

D. Nodule Morphology: Feeding Artery and Draining Vein

The third morphologic feature that indicates a benign nodule with a high degree of specificity is the presence of a feeding artery and a draining vein. While occasionally seen on chest radiographs, it is more easily seen on contrast-enhanced CT, and is a very reliable indicator of an arteriovenous malformation (41). No further noninvasive imaging to prove this diagnosis is required (strong evidence).

E. Nodule Morphology: Rounded Atelectasis

Rounded atelectasis is atelectasis of a peripheral part of the lung due to pleural adhesions and fibrosis, causing deformation of the lung and inward bending of adjacent bronchi and blood vessels, known as the "comet tail sign." It occurs in a variety of pleural abnormalities, but is typically associated with asbestos exposure and asbestos-related pleural plaques. In one series, 86% of cases were associated with asbestos exposure (12). To suggest the diagnosis of rounded atelectasis on thin-section CT, the opacity should be (1) round or oval in shape, (2) subpleural in location, (3) associated with curving of pulmonary vessels or bronchi into the edge of the lesion (comet tail sign), and (4) associated with ipsilateral pleural abnormality either effusion or pleural thickening.

Rounded atelectasis may show significant enhancement after the injection of intravenous contrast agents (43). If the criteria for rounded atelectasis listed above are met, a confident diagnosis can usually be made (42). No further invasive imaging is necessary (moderate evidence). However, if there is any question about the findings, follow-up serial CT examinations are recommended.

F. Applicability to Children

The evidence to determine who should undergo imaging is less complete in children than in adults. The vast majority of pulmonary nodules and masses in children are benign. Pneumonia may present as a spherical nodule or mass in children, referred to as round pneumonia. Clinical features and prompt response to antibiotic treatment serve to differentiate round pneumonia from malignancy (44). Most pediatric nodular disease is granulomatous in origin (45). Infections and congenital lesions in children together outnumber neoplastic lesions. Pulmonary metastases in children are most often secondary to Wilms' tumor, followed in frequency by sarcomas (45). Primary pulmonary malignancy is rare.

II. Which Imaging Is Appropriate?

Summary of Evidence: Management strategies for an SPN are highly dependent on the pretest probability of malignancy. The strategies include observation, resection, and biopsy. A CT should be the initial test in most patients with a new radiographically detected indeterminate SPN. Advances in technology have improved the ability to differentiate benign and malignant nodules using nodule perfusion and metabolic characteristics, as can be evaluated with intravenous contrast enhanced CT, [18]FDG-PET, and single photon emission computed tomography (SPECT); [18]FDG-PET should be selectively used when the pretest probability and CT probability of malignancy are discordant. If the pretest probability of malignancy after CT is high, [18]FDG-PET is not cost-effective. Recommendations for the use of CT, PET, watchful waiting, transthoracic needle biopsy, and surgery in the evaluation of an indeterminate SPN are shown in Table 23.2. The diagnostic algorithm for the SPN is detailed in Fig. 23.4.

Supporting Evidence: The limited ability of CXR to distinguish between benign and malignant SPNs has prompted development of CT-based techniques for noninvasive assessment. CT is more accurate than CXR in determining where an abnormality is located in the lungs, and if it is in the lung, CT optimally evaluates the morphologic characteristics of the nodule. Several different CT techniques for the evaluation of SPNs have been described including, thin-section CT, CT densitometry, dual-energy CT, and CT nodule enhancement studies.

A. Computed Tomography Densitometry

In the mid-1980s the use of a representative CT number and a reference phantom, known as CT densitometry, was applied to CT to improve its accuracy for the detection of calcification. A large multi-institutional level II (moderate evidence) study of 384 visibly noncalcified nodules on conventional thick-section nonhelical CT used CT nodule densitometry with 264 Hounsfield units (HU) or more to classify a nodule as benign (9). In the 118 confirmed benign nodules, calcification not present on thick-section CT was present in an additional 65 nodules, either visibly ($n = 28$) on CT or by CT densitometry alone ($n = 37$), yielding a sensitivity of 55% and specificity of 99% for identifying benign nodules. The sensitivity and specificity of this technique for benign disease depends on the cutoff point above which benign nodules are diagnosed and scanner calibration. The results of different studies using this technique are summarized in Table 23.3. The overall sensitivity (50–63%) and specificity (78–100%) of this technique for benign disease is variable, not optimal, and this technique has fallen out of favor. While a high specificity of 99–100% for benign disease has been reported using this technique in study samples with a high prevalence of malignancy (8, 9, 38), lower specificity, 78%, is reported when the prevalence of malignancy is lower (46).

B. Thin-Section Computed Tomography

Visual inspection of thin-section CT images is more accurate than CXR for identifying calcification in pulmonary nodules. Thin-section CT enables more accurate differentiation of benign from malignant nodules through a more detailed assessment of nodule morphology. However, the application of different criteria for identifying malignancy, as illustrated by the studies detailed in below and in Table 23.4, yields different sensitivity and specificity for identifying malignancy. For example, Takanashi et al. (47) studied thin-section CT for the evaluation of SPNs. This level II (moderate evidence) prospective study demonstrated 56% sensitivity and 93% specificity for identifying malignancy. Seemann et al. (48) in a level I (strong evidence) prospective study achieved a higher sensitivity of 91% at the sacrifice of a lower specificity of 57% by applying different criteria. In both studies the prevalence of malignancy was higher (53–78%) than a general population of indeterminate SPNs detected on radiography. In a comparative prospective level I (strong evidence) study of thin-section CT vs. helical CT at 8-mm collimation, malignant SPNs were identified with 88% sensitivity and 60.9% specificity on helical CT, vs. 91.4% sensitivity and 56.5% specificity on thin-section CT (49).

C. Computed Tomography Contrast Enhancement

Dynamic contrast-enhanced CT uses nodule vascularity to distinguish between benign and malignant nodules. Malignancies are thought to enhance more than benign nodules due to tumor neovascularity. In a multi-institutional level II (moderate evidence) prospective study, the absence of significant lung nodule enhancement (≤15 HU) on a CT enhancement study was strongly predictive of benignity (50). On nonenhanced, thin-section CT, the 356 solid, relatively spherical nodules studied measured 5–40 mm in diameter, and were homogeneously of soft tissue attenuation without visible calcification or fat on CT. The CT images at 3-mm collimation were obtained before and at 1, 2, 3, and 4 min after intravenous contrast administration. Of the 356 nodules, 171 (48%) were malignant. Malignant nodules enhanced a median of 38.1 HU (range 14.0–165.3 HU), while granulomas and benign neoplasms enhanced a median of 10 HU (range −20 to 96 HU; $p < 0.001$). Using 15 HU or more of enhancement from baseline as the threshold, the technique was 98% sensitive and 58% specific for identifying malignancy, with a negative predictive value of 96%. The results of this prospective study corroborate earlier, smaller case series, as summarized in Table 23.5 (50–52).

Several potential practical limitations exist to the widespread clinical application of the CT nodule enhancement technique. Nodules less than 5 mm do not fulfill the selection criteria used for the published studies. They are too small to reliably place a region of interest to measure attenuation and are difficult to consistently use due to differences in depth of a patient respiration. However, advances in MDCT technology with submillimeter collimation and isotropic resolution in the z-axis may

lower this size threshold in the future. The imaging protocol and nodule selected for evaluation, as described above, should be carefully followed to obtain similar results. The technique should be performed only on nodules that are relatively homogeneous in attenuation and without evidence of fat, calcification, cavitation, or necrosis on thin-section CT images. Patients considered for this technique must be able to perform repeated, reproducible breath holds. Finally, while the absence of significant enhancement is strongly predictive of benignity (high negative predictive value for malignancy), a significant number of benign nodules enhance above threshold. These nodules remain suspicious for malignancy after a CT enhancement study, and require further radiologic evaluation or tissue diagnosis.

D. Dual-Energy Computed Tomography

This technique is based on increased photon absorption by calcium as the beam energy is decreased, resulting in an increase in the CT attenuation number of calcified nodules imaged at 80 kVp compared to 140 kVp. Despite initial reports in level III studies (53, 54), a multicenter prospective level II (moderate evidence) study demonstrated the technique to be unreliable for distinguishing between benign and malignant nodules (3-mm-collimation CT at 140 and 80 kVp; 157 noncalcified, relatively spherical, solid, 5- to 40-mm-diameter nodules without visible calcification or fat) (55). The median increase in nodule mean CT number from 140 to 80 kVp was 2 HU for benign nodules and 3 HU for malignant nodules, not significantly different.

E. Positron Emission Tomography

The uptake of [18]FDG is used to measure glucose metabolism on PET. Pulmonary malignancies demonstrate higher [18]FDG uptake than normal lung parenchyma and benign nodules, due to their increased metabolic activity (Fig. 23.5). In a multicenter prospective level I (strong evidence) investigation of [18]FDG-PET of 89 lung nodules, 92% sensitivity and 90% specificity for malignancy was reported, using a standardized uptake value (SUV) of ≥2.5 as the criterion for malignancy (56). All patients in this study had newly identified indeterminate SPNs on chest radiographs or CT, with pathology (either by surgical resection or biopsy) as the reference test. Several other studies confirm the high sensitivity and moderately high specificity of ^{18}FDG-PET for identifying malignancy in pulmonary nodules (56–68). A summary of several investigations is presented (Table 23.6). In a meta-analysis of 13 studies using ^{18}FDG-PET for the evaluation of CT indeterminate SPNs, Gould et al. reported mean 93.9% sensitivity (98% median) and 85.5% specificity (83.3% median) for identifying malignancy (56, 58–69). A summary receiver operating characteristic (ROC) curve based on the meta-analysis is shown in Fig. 23.6.

Limited spatial resolution for nodules less than 8–10 mm in diameter may result in false-negative results for malignancy (56). False-negative results may also occur with carcinoid tumors and bronchoalveolar carcinoma (70, 71). False-positive results may occur with inflammatory and infectious lesions, such as tuberculous and fungal granulomas (56).

F. Single Photon Emission Computed Tomography

Pulmonary nodules can be evaluated using SPECT, and ^{18}FDG, ^{201}thallium, or the somatostatin analog ^{99}technetium depreotide; SPECT imaging is considerably less expensive and more widely available than PET. A prospective level I (strong evidence) study of ^{18}FDG-SPECT to evaluate indeterminate lung nodules reported 100% sensitivity and 90% specificity for malignancy for nodules 2 cm or larger in diameter, but only 50% sensitivity and 94% specificity for nodules 1–2 cm diameter (72). Similar to PET, the sensitivity for SPECT is dependent on nodule size; however, the lower limit of nodule size that can reliably be evaluated with SPECT is larger than PET. A retrospective level II (moderate evidence) study by Higashi et al. (73) compared ^{18}FDG-PET and ^{201}thallium SPECT in the evaluation of 33 patients with histologically proven lung cancer; ^{18}FDG-PET was significantly more sensitive than ^{201}thallium SPECT for the detection of malignancy in nodules less than 2 cm in diameter (85.7 vs. 14.3%). The sensitivity in nodules greater than 2 cm was not significantly different. In addition, ^{18}FDG-PET detected mediastinal lymph node metastases not detected on ^{201}thallium SPECT (three of four lymph nodes on PET vs. one of four on SPECT).

Depreotide is a somatostatin analog that can be complexed to ^{99m}technetium (^{99m}Tc depreotide) for optimal imaging properties. Blum and colleagues (74) demonstrated 99.6% sensitivity and 73% specificity for identifying malignancy in SPNs using ^{99m}Tc depreotide in a multicenter level I (strong evidence) prospective series. The study subjects were 114 patients with indeterminate pulmonary nodules (no benign pattern of calcification; no demonstrable radiologic stability for the prior 2 years), 30 years of age or more with nodules ranging from 0.8 to 6.0 cm in diameter (mean 2.8 ± 1.6 cm); 88 patients had malignant nodules. ^{99m}Technetium depreotide scintigraphy correctly identified 85 of 88 of the malignancies (sensitivity 96.6%). The three false-negative results were adenocarcinomas (one colon cancer metastasis and two primary lung cancers), ranging in diameter from 1.1 to 2.0 cm. There were seven false-positive results, including six granulomas and one hamartoma (specificity 73.1%). The sensitivity and diagnostic accuracy of ^{99m}Tc depreotide compare favorably with that of ^{18}FDG-PET for differentiating between benign and malignant nodules, with a lower projected cost for ^{99m}Tc depreotide than ^{18}FDG-PET, and therefore a more favorable cost–benefit analysis (75).

G. Percutaneous Needle Biopsy

There have been numerous investigations of CT-guided percutaneous transthoracic needle biopsy of pulmonary nodules (61, 76–83). A prospective randomized level I (strong evidence) study of immediate cytologic evaluation vs. offsite cytology demonstrated significantly greater diagnostic accuracy using immediate cytologic evaluation without a significant increase in complication rates (79). Adequate samples were obtained in 100% of procedures when the cytologist evaluated the adequacy of the sample immediately, compared to 88% in the group without immediate cytologic assessment. If the onsite cytologist determined the sample was inadequate, additional aspiration was performed without requiring an additional procedure at a later date. With immediate cytologic evaluation, 99% sensitivity and 100%

specificity for malignancy was obtained, vs. 90 and 96%, respectively, without it.

CT-guided percutaneous fine-needle aspiration biopsy of small pulmonary lesions less than or equal to 1 cm has been reported with diagnostic accuracy rates approaching that of larger nodules (84). In a retrospective level II (moderate evidence) study of 61 patients with pulmonary nodules 1 cm or smaller, adequate samples were obtained in 77% of patients. Overall 82% sensitivity and 100% specificity were reported for malignancy in 57 patients; four patients were not included in the analysis due to lack of follow-up. Results for 0.8- to 1.0-cm lesions were significantly better than for 0.5- to 0.7-cm lesions (sensitivity 88 vs. 50%; $p = 0.013$). The percentage of nondiagnostic percutaneous lung biopsies ranges from 4 to 40% in various series. This wide variation reflects no differences in technique, study population, and prevalence of malignancy. The most important complication of imaging-guided percutaneous lung biopsy is pneumothorax, with a 20–30% incidence, and a chest tube rate of 5% or less. In a small retrospective level II (moderate evidence) study comparing [18]FDG-PET with percutaneous needle aspiration biopsy for the evaluation of pulmonary nodules, [18]FDG-PET was more sensitive for malignancy (100 vs. 81%), while transthoracic needle aspiration was more specific (100 vs. 78%) (61).

H. Cost-Effectiveness

The cost-effectiveness of management strategies for SPNs was evaluated by Gould et al. (85) in an analysis taken from a societal perspective. The decision-analysis model compared the cost-effectiveness of 40 clinically plausible combinations of five diagnostic interventions (CT, [18]FDG-PET, percutaneous needle biopsy, surgery, and watchful waiting) for the evaluation of a newly identified 2-cm noncalcified pulmonary nodules on a CXR in adults with no known extrathoracic malignancy who were hypothetically 62 years of age. Strategies that did and did not include [18]FDG-PET were specifically compared. The CT sensitivity and specificity for malignancy used were 96.5 and 55.8%, respectively, and for [18]FDG-PET the values were 94.2 and 83.3%, respectively. A logistic regression model using three clinical characteristics (age, cigarette smoking, and history of

cancer) and three radiologic characteristics (diameter, spiculation, and upper lobe location) was used to stratify patients into three categories of pretest probability of malignancy. A separate analysis was performed for patients with low (10–50%), intermediate (51–76%), and high (77–90%) pretest probabilities of malignancy. A final diagnosis was established at surgery or after 24 months of observation with serial CXRs. In the watchful waiting strategy, serial CXRs were obtained at 1, 2, 4, and 6 months from baseline and every 3 months thereafter; a nodule that had no growth after 24 months was considered benign. The accuracy and complications of diagnostic tests were estimated from meta-analysis and a literature review. Cost estimates were derived from Medicare reimbursements. The effectiveness and cost-effectiveness of management strategies depended critically on the pretest probability of malignancy, and to a lesser extent on the patients risk for experiencing surgical complications, as listed in Table 23.2. An algorithm for clinical management of patients with a new noncalcified SPN and average risk of surgical complications based on the analysis by Gould et al. (85) is shown in Fig. 23.4. The selective use of [18]FDG-PET was the most cost-effective when the pretest probability of malignancy and CT findings were discordant, or in patients with an intermediate pretest probability of malignancy who were at high risk for surgical complications. In most other circumstances, CT-based strategies resulted in similar quality-adjusted life years and lower cost. The only circumstance in which CT was not the first test of choice was when the pretest probability of malignancy was extremely high, defined as greater than 90%. In summary, CT should be the initial test in the management of most SPNs. It is relatively inexpensive, noninvasive, and highly specific for identifying some benign nodules.

- In patients with a low pretest probability of malignancy (10–50%), [18]FDG-PET should be used selectively when the CT results are indeterminate for malignancy:

  - For an indeterminate SPN on CT coupled with a positive [18]FDG-PET result, surgery is highly cost-effective, and slightly more effective than performing percutaneous needle biopsy before surgery.

- For an indeterminate SPN on CT coupled with a negative ^{18}FDG-PET result, percutaneous needle biopsy is more effective than observation alone due to the possibility of a false-negative ^{18}FDG-PET result that may potentially lead to a delayed diagnosis of malignancy and missed opportunity for curative surgery.
- When CT results are benign, observation or needle biopsy were recommended; however, the definition of a benign nodule on CT is stated to be "negative for malignancy" and the imaging characteristics attributed to a benign nodule on CT were not further specified.

• In patients with an intermediate pretest probability of malignancy (51–76%):

- Surgery or percutaneous needle biopsy was recommended when CT results are possibly malignant.
- Needle biopsy or observation was recommended when CT results are benign.
- More aggressive use of surgery and needle biopsy resulted in slightly better health outcomes and slightly higher costs. The choice between more or less aggressive approaches should depend on factors such as the risk for surgical complications, expected yield of needle biopsy, and patient preference.
- Percutaneous needle biopsy is warranted in patients with a contraindication to surgical resection, such as severe lung or cardiovascular disease, or in the setting of a known extrapulmonary malignancy.

• In patients with high pretest probability of malignancy (77–90%):

- Surgery was recommended when CT results are possibly malignant, and there are no surgical contradictions.
- ^{18}FDG-PET was recommended when CT results are benign; if ^{18}FDG-PET is positive, surgery is recommended. When ^{18}FDG-PET results are negative,

percutaneous needle biopsy was marginally more effective than watchful waiting.

The results of this study support and extend the findings of others. In a decision analysis Cummings et al. (86) also found that the choice of evaluation strategy depended on the pretest probability of malignancy. Watchful waiting was preferred over biopsy when the pretest probability of cancer was less than 3%. Surgery was preferred over biopsy when the probability of cancer was greater than 68%. This study did not evaluate PET or cost-effectiveness. To examine the potential role of contrast-enhanced dynamic CT, Gould et al. (85) evaluated six additional strategies for dynamic CT when noncontrast CT indicated a possible malignancy. The use of contrast-enhanced dynamic CT was most cost-effective when used selectively in patients with a low-to-intermediate pretest probability of malignancy with a possibly malignant result on noncontrast CT.

III. Special Case: Estimating the Probability of Malignancy in Solitary Pulmonary Nodules

Summary of Evidence: The effectiveness and cost-effectiveness of management strategies for evaluation of SPNs is highly dependent on the pretest probability of malignancy. Bayesian analysis and multivariate logistic regression models can be used to predict the likelihood of malignancy for a given nodule, and perform equal to or better than expert human readers of imaging tests. Using Bayesian analysis, ^{18}FDG-PET as a single test is a better predictor of malignancy in SPNs than standard CT criteria.

Supporting Evidence: Given that the cost-effectiveness of imaging a SPN is dependent on the pretest probability of malignancy, optimum use of imaging requires stratification of subjects by their probability of malignancy. Bayesian analysis uses likelihood ratios (LRs) for radiologic findings and clinical features to estimate the probability of cancer (pCa) (13, 87). The LR for a given characteristic is derived as follows:

$$LR = \frac{\text{Number of malignant nodules with feature}}{\text{Number of benign nodules with feature}}.$$

An LR of 1 indicates a 50% chance of malignancy. An LR of less than 1 favors a benign lesion, whereas an LR greater than 1 favors malignancy. LRs for various clinical and radiologic features of SPNs derived from the literature are presented in Table 23.7 (87). The odds of malignancy are calculated as below. The LR prior is the likelihood of malignancy in all nodules based on the local prevalence of malignancy.

$$\frac{Odds\ of}{malignancy} = LR\ prior \times LR\ size \times LR\ edge \times LR, etc.$$

The probability of malignancy is calculated as follows below.

$$\frac{Probability}{of\ malignancy} = \frac{Odds\ of\ malignancy}{(1 + Odds\ of\ malignancy)}.$$

The probability of malignancy for a nodule can be calculated using Bayesian analysis at http://www.chestx-ray.com. Gurney et al. (13) in a level II (moderate evidence) study showed that readers using Bayesian analysis performed significantly better at identifying malignancy than expert readers alone, classifying fewer malignant nodules as benign when presented with the same clinical and radiological data.

Swensen's group (88) initially developed and then internally validated a clinical prediction model to estimate the probability of malignancy in SPNs. This level II (moderate evidence) retrospective study used a cohort of 629 patients with 4- to 30-mm indeterminate SPNs newly discovered on chest radiographs. Using multivariate logistic regression analysis a clinical prediction model was developed from a random sample of two thirds of the patients, then tested on the remaining third. Three clinical features (age, cigarette-smoking status, and history of cancer diagnosed more than 5 years ago) and three radiologic characteristics (diameter, spiculation, and upper lobe location) were identified as independent predictors of malignancy. A further level II (moderate evidence) study by the same investigators comparing the performance of the clinical prediction model to physician estimates of malignancy demonstrated no statistically significant differences (2).

Dewan et al. (65) compared Bayesian analysis to the results of ^{18}FDG-PET scans in a level II (moderate evidence) retrospective study. Fifty-two patients with noncalcified, solid nodules less than 3 cm in size were studied. The probability of malignancy was calculated using standard criteria (patient age, history of prior malignancy, smoking history, and nodule size and border), and compared to the probability of malignancy based on the ^{18}FDG-PET scan, with histology as the reference test. The LR for malignancy in a SPN was 7.11 with an abnormal ^{18}FDG-PET scan compared to 0.06 with a normal ^{18}FDG-PET scan. The LRs for malignancy were higher with an abnormal ^{18}FDG-PET scan compared to most LRs for age, size, history of previous malignancy, smoking history, and nodule edge in the literature. ROC curves were drawn to compare the standard criteria using Bayesian analysis, standard criteria plus ^{18}FDG-PET, and ^{18}FDG-PET alone. Analysis of the ROC curves revealed that ^{18}FDG-PET alone had the highest sensitivity and specificity at different levels of probability of cancer, the standard criteria the least, and the standard criteria plus ^{18}FDG-PET was intermediate; ^{18}FDG-PET as a single test had the highest percentage of nodules correctly classified as malignant or benign and was a better predictor of malignancy in SPNs than Bayesian analysis.

IV. Special Case: Solitary Pulmonary Nodule in a Patient with a Known Extrapulmonary Malignancy

An SPN in a patient with an existing extrapulmonary malignancy warrants special consideration, as it is often detected on staging, follow-up chest radiographs, or CT. The etiology of these nodules is important in determining the appropriate therapy and in differentiating a new lung cancer from a pulmonary metastasis or nodule of another etiology, such as infection.

In a level II (moderate evidence) retrospective study, Quint et al. (89) demonstrated that the likelihood of primary lung malignancy in such nodules depends on the histologic characteristics of the extrapulmonary neoplasm and the patient's cigarette smoking history. The medical records of 149 patients with an extrapulmonary malignancy and a SPN at chest CT were reviewed. The histologic characteristics of the nodule were correlated with the extrapulmonary malignancy, patient age, and cigarette smoking history. Patients with carcinomas of the head and neck, bladder, breast, cervix, bile ducts, esophagus, ovary, prostate, or stomach were more likely to have primary bronchogenic carcinoma than lung metastasis (ratio 8.3:1 for patients with head and neck cancers; 3.2:1 for all other malignancies combined). Patients with carcinomas of the salivary glands, adrenal gland, colon, parotid gland, kidney, thyroid gland, thymus, or uterus had fairly even odds of having bronchogenic carcinoma or pulmonary metastasis (ratio 1:1.2). Patients with melanoma, sarcoma, or testicular carcinoma were more likely to have a solitary metastasis than bronchogenic carcinoma (ratio 2.5:1). The results of this study were similar to an earlier study performed by Cahan et al. (90) in the

pre-CT era. The authors analyzed thoracotomy results obtained for 35 years in over 800 patients with a history of cancer, and obtained similar odds ratios for bronchogenic carcinoma vs. solitary pulmonary metastases in different primary malignancies, based on conventional radiographic detection of the SPN.

Take Home Tables and Figures

Tables 23.1–23.7 and Figs. 23.1–23.6 serve to highlight key recommendations and supporting evidence.

Table 23.1. Differential diagnosis of a solitary pulmonary nodule

Neoplastic	*Malignant*	Primary bronchogenic carcinoma Pulmonary lymphoma Carcinoid tumor Metastasis Chondrosarcoma Pulmonary blastoma Hemangiopericytoma Epithelioid hemangioendothelioma
	Benign	Hamartoma Chondroma Teratoma Hemangioma Lipoma Leiomyoma Endometriosis Neurofibroma and neurilemmoma Benign clear cell tumor Chemodectoma
Infectious		Granuloma (tuberculosis and histoplasmosis) Parasites (hydatid) Round pneumonia Lung abscess
Inflammatory		Rheumatoid arthritis Wegener's granulomatosis Sarcoidosis Intrapulmonary lymph node Inflammatory pseudotumor (synonym: plasma cell granuloma)
Vascular		Arteriovenous malformation Hematoma Pulmonary infarct
Developmental		Bronchial atresia Bronchogenic cyst Sequestration

Reprinted with kind permission of Springer Science+Business Media from Attili AK, Kazerooni EA. Imaging of the Solitary Pulmonary Nodule. In Medina LS, Blackmore CC (eds): *Evidence-Based Imaging: Optimizing Imaging in Patient Care.* New York: Springer Science+Business Media, 2006.

Table 23.2. Recommendations for the use of computed tomography, positron emission tomography, watchful waiting, transthoracic needle biopsy, and surgery in the evaluation of an indeterminate solitary pulmonary nodule

Intervention	Indications
CT	When pretest probability is <90%
^{18}FDG-PET	• When pretest probability is low (10–50%) and CT results are indeterminate (possibly malignant) • When pretest probability is high (77–89%) and CT results are benign • When surgical risk is high, pretest probability is low to intermediate (65%), and CT results are possibly malignant • When CT results suggest a benign cause and the probability of nondiagnostic biopsy is high, or the patient is uncomfortable with a strategy of watchful waiting
Watchful waiting	• In patients with very small, radiographically indeterminate nodules (<10 mm in diameter) • When the pretest probability is very low (<2%) or when pretest probability is low (<15%) and ^{18}FDG-PET results are negative • When pretest probability is low (<35%) and CT results are benign • When needle biopsy is nondiagnostic in patients who have benign findings on CT or negative findings on ^{18}FDG-PET
Percutaneous transthoracic needle aspiration/biopsy	• When ^{18}FDG-PET results are positive and surgical risk or aversion to the risk of surgery is high • When pretest probability is low (20–45%) and ^{18}FDG-PET results are negative • When pretest probability is intermediate (30–70%) and CT results are benign
Surgery	• When pretest probability is high and CT results are indeterminate (possibly malignant) • When ^{18}FDG-PET results are positive • As the initial intervention when pretest probability is very high (>90%)

Source: Adapted from (85), with permission.

Table 23.3. Investigations of computed tomography densitometry for the evaluation of solitary pulmonary nodules

Study, year (reference)	No. of subjects	No. of nodules or masses	Lesion diameter (cm)	Prevalence of malignancy (%)	Reference test	Definition of a positive test	Sensitivity for benign disease (%)	Specificity for benign disease (%)
Zerhouni et al., 1986 (9)	384	295	<6.0	60	Tissue diagnosis 207; observation >18–30 months in 195	Greater than reference phantom	55	99
Siegelman et al., 1986 (8)	720	634	Any size (564 nodules >3.0)	56	Tissue diagnosis 367; observation >2 years in 195; NS in 72	>164 HU; <2.5 cm with smooth edge	63	100
Proto et al., 1985 (38)	218	177	0.6–4.5	54	Observation 15–24 months 14; tissue diagnosis 111; observation >22 months 52; calcification on chest radiographs in 14	>200 HU	54	99
Khan et al., 1991 (46)	75	62	Any size (59 nodules <2.0)	15	Tissue diagnosis in 20; observation >2 years in 42	NS	58	78

NS not specified.
Reprinted with kind permission of Springer Science+Business Media from Attili AK, Kazerooni EA. Imaging of the Solitary Pulmonary Nodule. In Medina LS, Blackmore CC (eds): *Evidence-Based Imaging: Optimizing Imaging in Patient Care*. New York: Springer Science+Business Media, 2006.

Table 23.4. Investigations of thin-section CT for the evaluation of solitary pulmonary nodules

Study, year (reference)	No. of subjects	No. of lung nodules	Prevalence of malignancy	Reference test	Definition of a positive result (malignancy)	Sensitivity for malignancy (%)	Specificity for malignancy (%)
Takanashi et al., 1995 (47)	60	60	53	Bronchoscopy or surgery	Three or more of the following: irregular margin, spiculation, convergence, air bronchogram, >3 vessels involved	56 (18/32)	93 (26/28)
Seemann et al., 1999 (91)	104	104	78	Surgical resection	Any one of the following: pleural retraction or thickening, bronchus sign, vessel sign, ground glass, spiculation with or with extension to visceral pleura	91 (74/81)	57 (13/23)

Reprinted with kind permission of Springer Science+Business Media from Attili AK, Kazerooni EA. Imaging of the Solitary Pulmonary Nodule. In Medina LS, Blackmore CC (eds): *Evidence-Based Imaging: Optimizing Imaging in Patient Care*. New York: Springer Science+Business Media, 2006.

Table 23.5. Studies of dynamic computed tomography lung nodule enhancement

Study, year (reference)	No. of nodules or masses	Prevalence of malignancy (%)	Reference test	Definition of a positive test (malignancy)	Sensitivity for malignancy (%)	Specificity for malignancy (%)
Swensen et al., 2000 (50)	356	48	Tissue diagnosis 237 Observation 119	Enhancement ≥15 HU	98	58
Yamashita et al., 1995 (92)	32	56	Surgical resection or biopsy	Enhancement ≥20 HU	100	93
Potente et al., 1997 (93)	40	25	68	Thoracotomy 18 Needle biopsy 6	100	75

Reprinted with kind permission of Springer Science+Business Media from Attili AK, Kazerooni EA. Imaging of the Solitary Pulmonary Nodule. In Medina LS, Blackmore CC (eds): *Evidence-Based Imaging: Optimizing Imaging in Patient Care.* New York: Springer Science+Business Media, 2006.

Table 23.6. Selected investigations of ¹⁸FDG-PET for the evaluation of solitary pulmonary nodules

Study, year (reference)	No. of nodules or masses	Lesion diameter (cm)	Prevalence of malignancy (%)	Reference test	Sensitivity for malignancy (%)	Specificity for malignancy (%)
Lowe et al., 1998 (56)	89	0.7–4.0	66	Needle biopsy or open lung biopsy	92	90
Prauer et al., 1998 (68)	54	0.3–3.0	57	Surgery	90	83
Gupta et al., 1998 (66)	19	1.0–3.5	63	Needle biopsy 10 Thoracotomy 8 Bronchoscopy 1	100	100
Dewan et al., 1997 (65)	52	<3	65	Thoracotomy 36 Needle biopsy 9 Bronchoscopy 3 Mediastinoscopy 3 Observation 1	95	87

Table 23.7. Likelihood ratios (LRs) for malignancy in solitary pulmonary nodules (87)

Feature or characteristic	LR
>70 years of age	4.16
30–39 years of age	0.24
Current cigarette smoker	2.27
Never smoked	0.19
Growth rate 7–465 days	3.40
Growth rate <7 days	0
Growth rate >465 days	0.01
Spiculated margin	5.54
Smooth margin	0.30
Upper/middle lobe location	1.22
Lower lobe location	0.66
Size >3 cm	5.23
Size <1 cm	0.52
Previous malignancy	4.95

Reprinted with kind permission of Springer Science+Business Media from Attili AK, Kazerooni EA. Imaging of the Solitary Pulmonary Nodule. In Medina LS, Blackmore CC (eds): *Evidence-Based Imaging: Optimizing Imaging in Patient Care.* New York: Springer Science+Business Media, 2006.

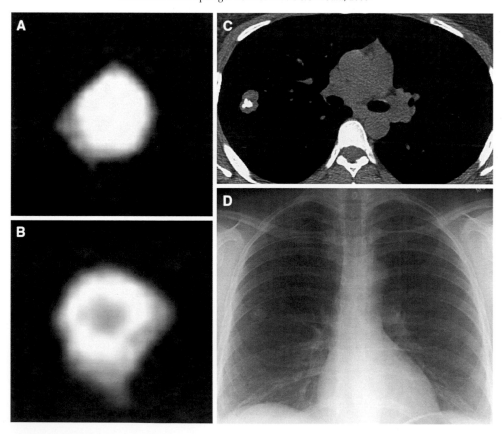

Figure 23.1. Benign patterns of calcification in solitary pulmonary nodules. (**A**) Central calcification on CT. (**B**) Target or concentric calcification on CT. (**C**) Popcorn pattern in a hamartoma on CT. (**D**) Chest X-ray. (Reprinted with kind permission of Springer Science+Business Media from Attili AK, Kazerooni EA. Imaging of the Solitary Pulmonary Nodule. In Medina LS, Blackmore CC (eds): *Evidence-Based Imaging: Optimizing Imaging in Patient Care.* New York: Springer Science+Business Media, 2006.)

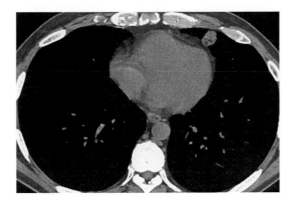

Figure 23.2. Hamartoma with both calcification and fat on CT. (Reprinted with kind permission of Springer Science+Business Media from Attili AK, Kazerooni EA. Imaging of the Solitary Pulmonary Nodule. In Medina LS, Blackmore CC (eds): *Evidence-Based Imaging: Optimizing Imaging in Patient Care.* New York: Springer Science+Business Media, 2006.)

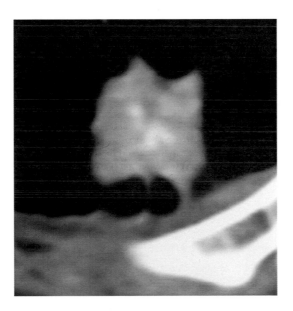

Figure 23.3. Indeterminate pattern of calcification for malignancy in a solitary pulmonary nodule in a histologically proven carcinoid tumor. (Reprinted with kind permission of Springer Science+Business Media from Attili AK, Kazerooni EA. Imaging of the Solitary Pulmonary Nodule. In Medina LS, Blackmore CC (eds): *Evidence-Based Imaging: Optimizing Imaging in Patient Care.* New York: Springer Science+Business Media, 2006.)

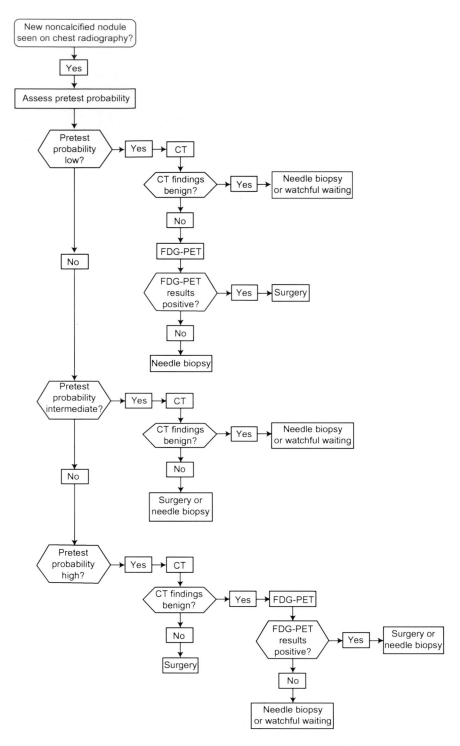

Figure 23.4. Suggested algorithm for clinical management of patients with SPNs and average risk of surgical complications. (*Source*: (85), with permission.)

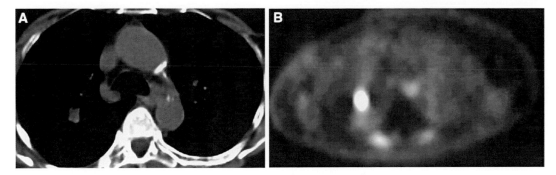

Figure 23.5. Concordant CT and PET scans for bronchogenic cancer in a 60-year-old woman. At resection this was a squamous cell carcinoma. (**A**) A 1.6-cm indeterminate noncalcified right upper lobe nodule on CT. (**B**) Corresponding [18]FDG-PET image shows increased radiotracer uptake corresponding to the nodule. (Reprinted with kind permission of Springer Science+Business Media from Attili AK, Kazerooni EA. Imaging of the Solitary Pulmonary Nodule. In Medina LS, Blackmore CC (eds): *Evidence-Based Imaging: Optimizing Imaging in Patient Care*. New York: Springer Science+Business Media, 2006.)

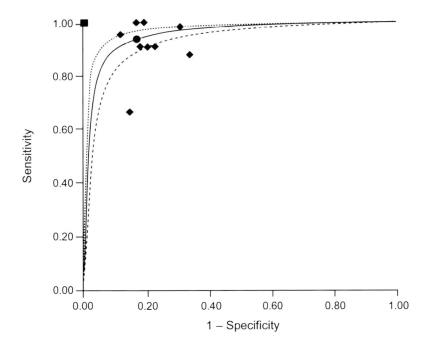

Figure 23.6. Summary receiver operating characteristic (ROC) curve for [18]FDG-PET. The ROC curves illustrate the trade-off between sensitivity and specificity as the threshold that defines a positive test result varies from most stringent to less stringent. The ROC curve for [18]FDG-PET is shown with 95% confidence intervals (*dotted lines*). *Black diamonds* represent individual study estimates of sensitivity and specificity. Four studies reported perfect sensitivity and specificity (*black square*). The point on the summary ROC curve that corresponds to the median specificity reported in 13 studies of [18]FDG-PET for pulmonary nodule diagnosis is shown (*black circle*). At this point, sensitivity and specificity were 94.2 and 83.3%, respectively. (*Source*: (85), with permission.)

Future Research

- Computer-aided diagnosis (CAD) both to assist with nodule detection on CXR and CT and to distinguish benign from malignant SPNs is under development, with some programs currently available for use. Their role in practice and effectiveness in clinical practice are currently unknown. While preliminary results are promising, further studies are necessary prior to the use of CAD schemes in actual clinical situations.
- Imaging techniques combined with patient biomarker evaluation from blood, sputum, or urine samples may help guide which patients need more aggressive, serial follow-up examinations and which patients do not.

References

1. Tuddenham WJ. AJR Am J Roentgenol 1984;143:509–517.
2. Earnest F, Ryu JH, Miller GM et al. Radiology 1999;211:137.
3. Holin SM, Dwork RE, Glaser S, Rikli AE, Stocklen JB. Am Rev Tuberc 1959;79:427–439.
4. Swensen SJ, Jett JR, Sloan JA et al. Am J Respir Crit Care Med 2002;165:508–513.
5. Henschke CI, McCauley DI, Yankelevitz DF et al. Lancet 1999;354:99–105.
6. Comstock GW, Vaughan RH, Montgomery G. N Engl J Med 1956;254:1018–1022.
7. Stelle JD. J Thorac Cardiovasc Surg 1963;46: 21–39.
8. Siegelman SS, Khouri NF, Leo FP, Fishman EK, Braverman RM, Zerhouni EA. Radiology 1986; 160:307–312.
9. Zerhouni EA, Stitik FP, Siegelman SS et al. Radiology 1986;160:319–327.
10. Kaneko M, Eguchi K, Ohmatsu H et al. Radiology 1996;201:798–802.
11. Steele JD. J Thorac Cardiovasc Surg 1963;46: 21–39.
12. Yankelevitz DF. Semin Ultrasound CT MR 2000;21:95–96.
13. Gurney JW, Lyddon DM, McKay JA. Radiology 1993;186:415–422.
14. Bateson EM. Clin Radiol 1965;16:51–65.
15. Ray JFD, Lawton BR, Magnin GE et al. Chest 1976;70:332–336.
16. Higgins GA, Shields TW, Keehn RJ. Arch Surg 1975;110:570–575.
17. Yankelevitz DF, Henschke CI. Am J Roentgenol 1997;168:325–328.
18. Good CA, Wilson TW. The solitary circumscribed pulmonary nodule; study of seven hundred five cases encountered roentgenologically in a period of three and one-half years. J Am Med Assoc 1958;166(3):210–215.
19. Collins VP, Loeffler RK, Tivey H. Am J Roentgenol 1956;76:988–1000.
20. Brues AM WA, Andervant HB. Proc Soc Exp Biol Med 1939;43:375–377.
21. Mottram J. J Pathol 1935;40:407–414.
22. Nathan MH, Collins VP, Adams RA. Radiology 1962;79:221–232.
23. Steele JD, Buell P. J Thorac Cardiovasc Surg 1973; 65:140–151.
24. Geddes DM. Br J Dis Chest 1979;73:1–17.
25. Weiss W. Am Rev Respir Dis 1971;103:198–208.
26. Lillington GA. Dis Mon 1991;37:271–318.
27. Wormanns D, Diederich S, Lentschig MG, Winter F, Heindel W. Eur Radiol 2000;10:710–713.
28. Winer-Muram HT, Jennings SG, Tarver RD et al. Radiology 2002;223:798–805.
29. Henschke CI, Yankelevitz D, Westcott J et al. ACR appropriateness criteria. Radiology 2000;215S: 607–609.
30. Yankelevitz DF, Reeves AP, Kostis WJ, Zhao B, Henschke CI. Radiology 2000;217:251–256.
31. Aoki T, Nakata H, Watanabe H et al. Am J Roentgenol 2000;174:763–768.
32. Good CA, Hood RT Jr, Mc D Jr. Am J Roentgenol 1953;70:543–554.
33. O'Keefe ME, Good CA, McDonald JR. Am J Roentgenol 1957;77:1023–1033.
34. Bateson EM, Abbott EK. Clin Radiol 1960;11: 232–247.
35. Stewart JG, MacMahon H, Vyborny CJ, Pollak ER. Am J Roentgenol 1987;148:29–30.
36. Mahoney MC, Shipley RT, Corcoran HL, Dickson BA. Am J Roentgenol 1990;154:255–258.
37. Berger WG, Erly WK, Krupinski EA, Standen JR, Stern RG. Am J Roentgenol 2001;176:201–204.
38. Proto AV, Thomas SR. Radiology 1985;156: 149–153.
39. Zerhouni EA, Boukadoum M, Siddiky MA et al. Radiology 1983;149:767–773.
40. Siegelman SS, Khouri NF, Scott WW Jr et al. Radiology 1986;160:313–317.
41. Remy J, Remy-Jardin M, Wattinne L, Deffontaines C. Radiology 1992;182:809–816.
42. Hillerdal G. Chest 1989;95(4):313–317.
43. Westcott JH, Volpe JP. Radiology 1991;181(P):182.
44. Rose RW, Ward BH. Radiology 1973;106: 179–182.
45. Eggli KD. Radiol Clin North Am 1993;31: 651–666.

46. Khan A, Herman PG, Vorwerk P, Stevens P, Rojas KA, Graver M. Radiology 1991;179:477–481.

47. Takanashi N, Nobe Y, Asoh H, Yano T, Ichinose Y. Lung Cancer 1995;13:105–112.

48. Seemann MD, Staebler A, Beinert T et al. Eur Radiol 1999;9:409–417.

49. Seemann MD, Seemann O, Luboldt W et al. Lung Cancer 2000;29:105–124.

50. Swensen SJ, Viggiano RW, Midthun DE et al. Radiology 2000;214:73–80.

51. Potente G, Iacari V, Caimi M. Comput Med Imaging Graph 1997;21:39–46.

52. Yamashita K, Matsunobe S, Takahashi R et al. Radiology 1995;196:401–408.

53. Bhalla M, Shepard JA, Nakamura K, Kazerooni EA. J Comput Assist Tomogr 1995;19:44–47.

54. Higashi Y, Nakamura H, Matsumoto T, Nakanishi T. J Thorac Imaging 1994;9:31–34.

55. Swensen SJ, Yamashita K, McCollough CH et al. Radiology 2000;214:81–85.

56. Lowe VJ, Fletcher JW, Gobar L et al. J Clin Oncol 1998;16:1075–1084.

57. Abe Y, Matsuzawa T, Fujiwara T et al. Int J Radiat Oncol Biol Phys 1990;19:1005–1010.

58. Gupta NC, Frank AR, Dewan NA et al. Radiology 1992;184:441–444.

59. Dewan NA, Gupta NC, Redepenning LS, Phalen JJ, Frick MP. Chest 1993;104:997–1002.

60. Patz EF Jr, Lowe VJ, Hoffman JM et al. Radiology 1993;188:487–490.

61. Dewan NA, Reeb SD, Gupta NC, Gobar LS, Scott WJ. Chest 1995;108:441–446.

62. Duhaylongsod FG, Lowe VJ, Patz EF Jr, Vaughn AL, Coleman RE, Wolfe WG. J Thorac Cardiovasc Surg 1995;110:130–139; discussion 139–140.

63. Duhaylongsod FG, Lowe VJ, Patz EF Jr, Vaughn AL, Coleman RE, Wolfe WG. Ann Thorac Surg 1995;60:1348–1352.

64. Gupta NC, Maloof J, Gunel E. J Nucl Med 1996; 37:943–948.

65. Dewan NA, Shehan CJ, Reeb SD, Gobar LS, Scott WJ, Ryschon K. Chest 1997;112:416–422.

66. Gupta N, Gill H, Graeber G, Bishop H, Hurst J, Stephens T. Chest 1998;114:1105–1111.

67. Orino K, Kawamura M, Hatazawa J, Suzuki I, Sazawa Y. Jpn J Thorac Cardiovasc Surg 1998;46: 1267–1274.

68. Prauer HW, Weber WA, Romer W, Treumann T, Ziegler SI, Schwaiger M. Br J Surg 1998;85: 1506–1511.

69. Kubota K, Matsuzawa T, Fujiwara T et al. J Nucl Med 1990;31:1927–1932.

70. Erasmus JJ, McAdams HP, Patz EF Jr, Coleman RE, Ahuja V, Goodman PC. Am J Roentgenol 1998;170:1369–1373.

71. Higashi K, Ueda Y, Seki H et al. J Nucl Med 1998;39:1016–1020.

72. Mastin ST, Drane WE, Harman EM, Fenton JJ, Quesenberry L. Chest 1999;115:1012–1017.

73. Higashi K, Nishikawa T, Seki H et al. J Nucl Med 1998;39:9–15.

74. Blum J, Handmaker H, Lister-James J, Rinne N. Chest 2000;117:1232–1238.

75. Gambhir SS, Handmaker H. J Nucl Med 1999;41(S):57P.

76. van Sonnenberg E, Casola G, Ho M et al. Radiology 1988;167:457–461.

77. Garcia Rio F, Diaz Lobato S, Pino JM et al. Acta Radiol 1994;35:478–480.

78. Li H, Boiselle PM, Shepard JO, Trotman-Dickenson B, McLoud TC. Am J Roentgenol 1996;167:105–109.

79. Santambrogio L, Nosotti M, Bellaviti N, Pavoni G, Radice F, Caputo V. Chest 1997;112: 423–425.

80. Westcott JL, Rao N, Colley DP. Radiology 1997;202:97–103.

81. Yankelevitz DF, Henschke CI, Koizumi JH, Altorki NK, Libby D. Clin Imaging 1997;21: 107–110.

82. Hayashi N, Sakai T, Kitagawa M et al. Am J Roentgenol 1998;170:329–331.

83. Laurent F, Latrabe V, Vergier B, Montaudon M, Vernejoux JM, Dubrez J. Clin Radiol 2000;55: 281–287.

84. Wallace MJ, Krishnamurthy S, Broemeling LD et al. Radiology 2002;225:823–828.

85. Gould MK, Sanders GD, Barnett PG et al. Ann Intern Med 2003;138:724–735.

86. Cummings SR, Lillington GA, Richard RJ. Am Rev Respir Dis 1986;134:453–460.

87. Gurney JW. Radiology 1993;186:405–413.

88. Hartman TE, Tazelaar HD, Swensen SJ, Muller NL. Radiographics 1997;17:377–390.

89. Quint LE, Park CH, Iannettoni MD. Radiology 2000;217:257–261.

90. Cahan WG, Shah JP, Castro EB. Ann Surg 1978;187:241–244.

91. Seemann MD, Beinert T, Dienemann H et al. Eur J Med Res 1996;1:371–376.

92. Yamashita K, Matsunobe S, Tsuda T et al. Radiology 1995;194:399–405.

93. Potente G, Guerrisi R, Iacari V et al. Radiol Med 1997;94:182–188.

24

Cardiac Evaluation: The Current Status of Outcomes-Based Imaging

Andrew J. Bierhals and Pamela K. Woodard

Issues

   I. Does coronary artery calcification scoring predict outcome?
  II. Special case: high-risk patients
 III. Which patients should undergo coronary angiography?
 IV. Which patients should undergo noninvasive imaging of the heart?
  V. What is the appropriate use of coronary artery computed tomography and magnetic resonance?

Key Points

- A strong recommendation can be made for initial coronary angiography among high-risk patients and those who are post myocardial infarction (MI) that was transmural or with ischemic symptoms (strong evidence).
- A strong recommendation can be made for performing a noninvasive imaging examination [e.g., single photon emission computed tomography (SPECT) or stress echo] prior to coronary angiography in low-risk patients and those who have had a non-Q-wave MI (strong evidence).
- Aside from coronary angiography, the appropriate usage of cardiac imaging studies remains unclear, and more research is required to evaluate the outcomes, as well as the cost-effectiveness of the aforementioned modalities (insufficient evidence).
- Coronary artery calcium scoring has been shown in asymptomatic patients to be predictive of coronary artery disease (CAD); however, there have been no data to support the position of added predictive value over and above the clinical Framingham model (insufficient evidence).

A.J. Bierhals (✉)
Mallinckrodt Institute of Radiology, Washington University School of Medicine, St. Louis, MO 63110, USA
e-mail: bierhalsa@mir.wustl.edu

L.S. Medina et al. (eds.), *Evidence-Based Imaging: Improving the Quality of Imaging in Patient Care, Revised Edition*, DOI 10.1007/978-1-4419-7777-9_24, © Springer Science+Business Media, LLC 2011

Definition and Pathophysiology

The etiology of CAD is multifactorial involving both interaction of lifestyle and genetic predispositions. While some factors are not modifiable, those risks that may be altered are often neglected until there evidence of disease. As a result, a multitude of tests and clinical assessment tools have been developed to risk stratify patients in order to direct short- and long-term treatments. The modifiable risk factors (e.g., hypertension, hyperlipidemia, and diabetes) have been on the rise over the past decade (1, 2); therefore, a greater urgency has arisen to identify patients with CAD.

Coronary artery disease begins as fatty streaks in the coronary arteries that may begin as early as 3 years of age. The fatty streaks are composed of large cells with intracellular lipids (foam cells) that are located in the subendothelial region. As patients age, the fatty streaks develop into fibrous plaques that narrow the vessel lumen, reducing blood flow. The fibrous plaques over time may calcify, reducing vessel compliance and increasing fragility. This further reduces blood flow and increases the chance of the plaque rupturing, resulting in an acute coronary artery occlusion.

Epidemiology

Coronary artery disease is a nationwide epidemic involving 6.4% of the entire population (3, 4) and is the largest cause of mortality, accounting for one in every five deaths (4). This translates into a death rate of 177.8 per 100,000 (based on 2001 estimates) (4). In the USA, over 1.5 million people will have a MI, and the majority of the patients will initially present with symptoms in their 50s and 60s.

A large volume of literature has been generated investigating these modalities, but little has focused on the impact the modalities have on the patient outcomes even though there has been a steady increase in the use of costly diagnostic testing and treatment (5). This chapter reviews the literature on the outcomes research of cardiac imaging, and makes recommendations concerning the utilization of the techniques in patient management.

Overall Cost to Society

In the USA, the estimated 2004 cost of heart disease to society is $238 billion, with over half secondary to CAD ($133 billion) (4, 6). The cost of heart disease is substantial in comparison to other disease processes, such as cancers ($189 billion) and AIDS ($29 billion) (4, 6). The costs of CAD include direct health care of $66 billion, and $67 billion in indirect costs (e.g., loss of productivity secondary to morbidity and mortality) (4, 6).

The expenditures for health care are consistently increasing, because of new technologies and the current medicolegal environment. An ever-declining budget results in a need for clinicians to incorporate cost-effective strategies in patient evaluations. However, cost-effective does not mean withholding evaluations or always ordering the seemingly least expensive test, but rather understanding what is most efficient with respect to a specific clinical situation, based on current research. The purpose of this approach is to direct a finite amount of resources and limit costs to society without affecting the quality of health care. This chapter reviews the cost-effectiveness and outcomes of various imaging modalities of heart disease, and makes recommendations concerning these techniques in patient care. Specifically, coronary artery calcification scoring, myocardial SPECT, angiography, stress echocardiography, and cardiac magnetic resonance (MR) and computed tomography (CT) will be evaluated in their potential roles in the evaluation of heart disease.

Goals

The goals of imaging related to CAD are based on the a priori risk to the patient. In a low-risk population, the goals of imaging are to identify those with early disease. Subsequently, interventions directed toward risk factors and lifestyle may be initiated in order to reverse disease or halt progression before any long-term effects result. However, risk stratification becomes the goal of cardiac imaging among those patients who are considered high risk. The imaging in the aforementioned population is to determine if any coronary artery intervention (i.e., endovascular or bypass graft) is required over and above medical management.

Methodology

The outcomes and cost-effectiveness literature was evaluated by performing a literature review on Medline from 1999 to 2004 using a keyword search including the terms *calcium scoring and outcomes* and *calcium scoring and cost-effectiveness*. Of the over 2,000 reports identified in the literature review, fewer than 50 addressed any issues concerning patient outcomes and not one evaluated cost-effectiveness.

A similar literature review was performed for coronary angiography using Medline. The keyword search from 1999 to 2004 included *coronary angiography and outcomes* and *coronary angiography and cost-effectiveness*. Over 5,000 reports were identified, with approximately 100 addressing patient outcomes and 10 evaluating cost-effectiveness.

Lastly, a literature review was performed on Medline from 1999 to 2004 for noninvasive techniques including SPECT, positron emission tomography (PET), echocardiogram, and coronary CT and MR using the same method, as described above. The review yielded over 100 articles addressing patient outcomes and five evaluating cost-effectiveness; however, there were no reports that evaluated either topic for MR or CT angiography.

I. Does Coronary Artery Calcification Scoring Predict Outcome?

Summary of Evidence: Coronary artery calcium scoring has been shown in asymptomatic patients to be predictive of CAD; however, there have been no data to support the position of added predictive value over and above the clinical Framingham model. Therefore, coronary artery calcification scoring cannot be recommended as a screening tool at this time. The lack of cost-effectiveness data necessitates further investigations before a final position can be determined on the utility of calcium scoring (insufficient evidence).

Supporting Evidence: Coronary artery calcium scoring performed by CT has been utilized in asymptomatic patients to assess their risk of an acute coronary event (7). However, the literature has debated the utility of calcium scoring. Some researchers support its use (8, 9), while others are less enthusiastic concerning the utilization in patient care (10).

Computed tomography calcium scoring, despite conflicting reports, has been shown to be associated with a fourfold increased risk in MI and coronary death in a meta-analysis by O'Malley et al. (11) in 2000. The study included nine reports that had a diverse asymptomatic population that was evaluated for coronary artery calcification by electron beam CT. The authors also reported a ninefold increased risk of coronary events (i.e., nonfatal MI, sudden death, or revascularization) among those with a coronary artery calcium score above the median. There is moderate evidence to suggest that coronary artery calcification score is predictive of coronary events.

More recent reports have echoed these results regarding the predictive value of CT calcium scoring. A 2003 study by Shaw et al. (8) developed a multivariate model on a sample of greater than 10,000 asymptomatic individuals incorporating calcium score with typical clinical risk factors (i.e., hypertension, hypercholesterolemia, diabetes, age, and sex) to predict all-cause mortality. The results of the study indicated that calcium score predicted all-cause mortality ($p < 0.001$) over and above the effects of other risk factors. The study also found that there was a trend with the coronary artery calcium score such that as the calcium burden increased there was a greater risk of all-cause mortality. The relative risk in patients with elevated calcium scores ranged from 1.6 to 4.0 above individuals with the lowest calcium burden; as the calcium burden increased, the risk increased (Fig. 24.1). Based on the results, the authors concluded that calcium scoring of the coronary arteries provides additional information in the prediction of all-cause mortality (8); however, morbidity and mortality secondary to CAD was not specifically addressed. In addition, the authors did not investigate if the added explanation would have any clinical impact and thus provide information that would have proved clinically important.

Other authors have found similar results in the prediction of mortality from calcium scoring. For example, Arad et al. (12) demonstrated that moderate calcium scores were associated with a ten times increase in cardiac death or MI. In addition, a small study of 676 subjects demonstrated that coronary artery calcification scores incrementally predicted cardiac events (13). These studies, as with the aforementioned larger sample, were able to show that coronary artery calcification on CT predicted health outcomes (e.g., MI and mortality). But of all the studies that have been evaluated, none has shown any extra value in risk stratification and patient management.

Aside from the earlier described reports, there has been a multitude of similar studies with varying patient population that have reached the same conclusion concerning the ability of coronary artery calcium scoring to predict heart disease and mortality (14–19). Other investigators utilized calcium scoring in conjunction with laboratory tests, such as C-reactive protein to model the mortality of heart disease (20), but no interactive effects were noted, although each independently predicted coronary events and mortality. However, a review of the literature to date has failed to identify any direct data suggesting that calcium scoring has any clinical benefit over the current Framingham risk model (21).

Currently, coronary artery calcium scoring on CT is utilized as a risk stratification tool for CAD. The major proportion of the data to date has shown that calcium scoring can predict CAD as well as mortality related to heart disease among asymptomatic patients. A literature review did not uncover any data that show that calcium scoring adds any additional information over current clinical predictive models in the asymptomatic patient. In addition, there have been no studies specifically evaluating the cost-effectiveness of coronary calcium scoring as a screening tool. As a result, calcium scoring, while predictive of CAD and mortality, has yet to be shown to add any additional information over and above current clinical models. Therefore, at this time there is insufficient data to recommend calcium scoring as a screening or risk stratification tool in the asymptomatic population. However, the dearth of cost-effectiveness data precludes stating that calcium scoring should not be performed as a screening test. Subsequently, additional cost-effectiveness studies should be instituted to evaluate the role of calcium scoring in the screening for CAD.

II. Special Case: High-Risk Patients

Summary of Evidence: Among high-risk symptomatic populations coronary artery calcium scoring on CT has failed to show any predictive value for a coronary event or mortality. Thus, among high-risk populations calcium scoring cannot be recommended for screening or risk stratification (insufficient evidence).

Supporting Evidence: The data in the asymptomatic populations consistently indicated that coronary artery calcium scoring can predict cardiac events and may be helpful in risk stratifying patients. However, the results in populations with a known risk are not as straightforward. Qu et al. (22) evaluated calcium scoring in a diabetic population. The data showed that when adjusting for other risk factors in a diabetic sample, calcium scores did not predict coronary events, but calcium scoring was predictive among nondiabetics (Fig. 24.2). Although the results have not been as clear among an elderly population that coronary artery calcification is associated with the degree of CAD, some researchers have found that the calcium score has variability among an elderly population, and thus may have the potential to discriminate risk within this group (9). However, other authors have concluded that there is limited utility of using calcium scoring among elderly patients (23, 24) because of comorbidities limiting the effect of interventions. Lastly, Detrano et al. (10) concluded that neither clinical risk assessment nor calcium scoring is an accurate predictor of cardiac events in a high-risk population, based on the Framingham model. Currently, there is insufficient evidence to recommend coronary artery calcium scoring in a high-risk population as a means of risk predicting coronary events (insufficient evidence).

III. Which Patients Should Undergo Coronary Angiography?

Summary of Evidence: Coronary angiography has been studied with a greater degree of rigor than the other modalities, with several studies investigating the cost-effectiveness. Based on the large amount of extant data, a strong recommendation can be made for initial coronary angiography among high-risk patients and those who are post-MI that was transmural or with ischemic symptoms. Also, a strong recommendation can be made for performing a noninvasive imaging examination (i.e., SPECT or stress echo) prior to coronary angiography in low-risk patients and those who have had a non-Q-wave MI (Fig. 24.3) (strong evidence).

Supporting Evidence: Over the past 20 years, coronary angiography has been the mainstay in the diagnosis of acute occlusion of the coronary arteries as well as in the quantification of CAD to direct management, whether surgical, medical, or endovascular. Throughout this period, angiography has become the gold standard for the diagnosis of CAD, but unlike other imaging studies of the heart there is greater risk associated with the procedure. Subsequently, the risk and technical factors preclude all patients from undergoing an angiogram.

Several cost-effectiveness models have been proposed to evaluate the role of coronary angiography in the diagnosis of CAD (25–27). Patterson et al. (26) utilized decision analysis to evaluate angiography versus other noninvasive modalities [i.e., SPECT, PET, exercise electrocardiogram (ECG)]. This model incorporated both direct and indirect costs as well as quality-adjusted life years (QALYs) to evaluate the different diagnostic modalities. The diagnostic evaluations included noninvasive testing followed by angiography (among those with an initial abnormal test) or angiography alone. The results of the study indicate that cost-effectiveness of the diagnostic modality is based on the initial pretest likelihood of disease. The authors found angiography was the most cost-effective modality in those with a high pretest probability ($p > 0.70$). However, populations with low risk ($p < 0.70$) noninvasive testing was the most cost-effective with PET > SPECT > exercise ECG. In addition, the authors found that there was little impact on the cost-effectiveness from the differing treatment modalities (i.e., surgical, medical, or endovascular). Similar results have been described by Garber and Solomon (27). Their decision analysis demonstrated that while stress echocardiography was the least costly per QALY saved, immediate angiography was an acceptable cost-effective alternative to SPECT and stress echocardiography among patients who are at high risk of cardiac disease. In their model, the relative cost-effectiveness for the modalities remained the same regardless of the patient's age or gender (Fig. 24.4). There is

strong evidence to recommend that among low-risk populations a noninvasive cardiac imaging study should be performed prior to coronary angiography (strong evidence).

Coronary angiography seemingly has a specific role in the diagnosis and risk stratification of patients with heart disease and has been shown to be cost-effective in given populations (25–27); however, the data in post-MI populations is not as clear. In a decision analysis by Kuntz et al. (28), the decision analytic model incorporated clinical history and symptoms in the post-MI patient to evaluate the cost-effectiveness of angiography versus medical care. While the authors incorporated clinical elements into the analyses, there was a failure to account for type of MI to address the issue of noninvasive evaluation of cardiac perfusion (e.g., SPECT or stress echo). Based on the model outcomes, angiography was found to be cost-effective in almost all patients in the post-MI setting, and among those at highest risk the cost-effectiveness ratios were less than $50,000 for each QALY saved. Only in those women at low to moderate risk for coronary disease was angiography found not to be cost-effective. Similar results on the patient survival and outcomes have been found in other studies that have included all post-MI patients (29, 30), and the largest effects were among the patients with transmural infarctions. There is strong evidence to support the use of angiography in the transmural infarction while those with a nontransmural infarction should undergo a noninvasive study prior to angiography (strong evidence).

Several authors have evaluated low to moderate risk (probability of CAD < 0.7) subpopulations in the post-MI state to determine the cost-effectiveness and outcomes among those treated with noninvasive image guidance versus immediate angiography. Barnett et al. (31) utilized a randomized controlled trial to evaluate the cost-effectiveness of angiography versus selective angiography (i.e., performing angiography in patients with an abnormal finding on a noninvasive study) in a population with a non-Q-wave MI. The results indicate a conservative management program is more cost-effective than immediate angiography in patients with a non-Q-wave MI. In the acute setting, image-directed angiography resulted in a cost of $14,700 versus $19,200 for immediate angiography and persisted after 2 years of follow-up, at which time there was an approximate $2,100 difference in cost. In addition, the conservative group had a better survival (1.86 years) over a 2-year follow-up relative to immediate angiography (1.76 years). Thus, conservative management (i.e., noninvasive image-directed angiography) is the dominant strategy over angiography in the non-Q-wave post-MI patient with resulting lower cost and improved outcome. There is strong evidence to show that noninvasive testing prior to angiography is more cost-effective than angiography alone in patients who have had a nontransmural infarction (strong evidence).

An earlier report by Boden et al. (32) came to a supporting conclusion regarding patient outcome in the post-MI setting. They evaluated the impact of post-MI angiography in a population with non-Q-wave MIs. Through 2 years of follow-up among the aforementioned patient population (Fig. 24.5), a noninvasive image-directed approach to patient management was found to have a significantly lower mortality and reinfarction rates than those patients who had undergone an initial angiogram in the acute MI state. The findings have been supported by the recommendations of other groups and researchers (33, 34).

Coronary angiography has a specific role in the evaluation of heart disease that is based on the patient's clinical history and symptoms. The data support the position that in an asymptomatic population with a low clinical suspicion of heart disease, noninvasive testing should be performed prior to angiography (25–27, 35), whereas in situations where there is a high clinical suspicion of CAD, angiography should be the initial test of choice. A similar picture develops in post-MI patients. For instance, individuals who have had a transmural MI or who have clinical signs of ischemia should undergo a coronary angiogram, but those with a non-Q-wave MI without clinical ischemia would best be evaluated by noninvasive imaging (28–34). Therefore, the utilization of coronary angiography is based on the clinical situation and the initial use may not always be the most prudent or cost-effective method to manage patients who are suspected of CAD or recently in the post-MI state.

IV. Which Patients Should Undergo Noninvasive Imaging of the Heart?

Summary of Evidence: There is a moderate amount of support to suggest that stress echo should be recommended prior to coronary angiography in the low-risk patients. However, several authors have suggested that stress echo is highly operator dependent and at times SPECT may be a viable alternative. Both modalities have an acceptable cost-effectiveness profile; as a result, there is insufficient evidence to recommend SPECT over stress echo. More comprehensive cost-effectiveness reports are needed to completely evaluate these modalities (insufficient evidence).

Supporting Evidence: A few cost-effectiveness evaluations have been performed incorporating the aforementioned noninvasive studies that have had some conflicting results. A decision analysis was performed by Kuntz et al. (35) that modeled immediate angiography versus a stepwise approach to angiography. In this situation angiography would be performed only if the initial noninvasive test were positive. The analysis incorporated SPECT, stress echocardiography, and stress electrocardiography. The results indicated that stress echocardiography was more cost-effective than SPECT in the low-risk population with an incremental cost effectiveness ratio of $26,800/QALY versus $27,600/QALY, respectively. Although the model does assume an idealized performance of echocardiography, slight changes in sensitivity of either SPECT or echo affect the results of the model. Thus, decisions concerning the performance of a specific test should be based on the test characteristics at a given institution (35). The model also supported the results of other angiographic studies in which immediate angiography is more cost-effective in the high-risk patient.

Another decision analysis performed by Garber and Solomon (27) included PET in their analyses along with angiography, stress echo, planar thallium, exercise electrocardiography, and SPECT. The results indicated that the initial use of stress echo was the most cost-effective followed by SPECT and angiography (Fig. 24.4). PET was not cost-effective in the diagnosis, resulting in higher cost without improved outcomes. The study also brings to the forefront the idea that there is variability in cost and performance of SPECT and stress echo; subsequently, SPECT may be the initial modality of choice in some regions (27).

However, a single study evaluating the cost-effectiveness of SPECT versus exercise electrocardiography was performed to evaluate any additional prognostic value of SPECT (36).

The authors found that SPECT provided additional information, which translated into $5,500 per level of risk reclassification.

Other researchers have also included PET in decision analysis along with SPECT and angiography (25). The findings of this study contradicted the prior model, such that PET was found to be the most cost-effective modality in diagnosing CAD among low-risk patients (27). Aside from the two prior studies, no other reports were found in the literature review to evaluate the cost-effectiveness of PET in the diagnosis of CAD. Subsequently, there is insufficient evidence to recommend PET in the evaluation of CAD (insufficient evidence).

Similarly, only the previously described studies could be found to evaluate the cost-effectiveness of stress echocardiography (27, 35, 37). However, several other studies evaluating the cost-effectiveness of SPECT were identified in the literature review. In a small patient sample ($n = 29$), SPECT was found to increase the diagnostic ability in cardiologist who were treating emergency room patients with acute chest pain (38). The study also found a decrease in hospitalizations and a savings of $800 per patient (38), although this study had a small sample size and did not rigorously evaluate cost and outcomes. Lastly, Udelson et al. (39) assessed the effect of SPECT in the evaluation of acute chest pain in the emergency department. There was a lower hospitalization rate among patients without coronary ischemia who had undergone a SPECT in the emergency department (42%) versus usual care (52%). The results suggest that SPECT may have an effect on decision making and possibly lower the costs by reducing hospitalization; however, to date there is insufficient evidence to recommend SPECT in the emergency setting.

In conclusion, multiple decision analyses and randomized studies agree that in a low-risk patient a noninvasive study should be preformed prior to an angiogram. Also, the models seem to support stress echocardiography as the most cost-effective, but also have suggested that SPECT may be as cost-effective depending on the institutional performance. Subsequently, there is little definitive data to use one of these studies over the other. The use of SPECT or echo should be based on the institutional efficacy. Although there is an early suggestion that SPECT may be useful in the emergent chest pain setting for patient triage, there is not enough data at this time to support this position.

Lastly, there is conflicting evidence concerning the cost-effectiveness of PET in the diagnosis of CAD and ischemia; more studies are needed to determine the role of PET in the cardiac evaluation (insufficient evidence).

In symptomatic post-MI patients or those at high risk for CAD, coronary angiography is the most cost-effective method to evaluate, diagnose, and plan treatments. However, among those without symptoms, noninvasive modalities (i.e., PET, SPECT, and stress echocardiography) are the more cost-effective means to evaluate heart disease. But the research to date is somewhat unclear as to the utilization of the aforementioned modalities. The current literature is somewhat limited in the cost-effective evaluations of noninvasive studies.

V. What Is the Appropriate Use of Coronary Artery Computed Tomography and Magnetic Resonance?

Summary of Evidence: The newer noninvasive modalities of cardiac MR and CT have a paucity of cost-effectiveness research and outcomes data available at this time and cannot be recommended for the evaluation of ischemic cardiac disease (insufficient evidence).

Supporting Evidence: In the past decade there have been advances in CT and MR in the evaluation of many aspects of the heart and heart disease. The current literature has limited data on the performance of MR and CT with respect to evaluation of the coronary arteries or for assessment of atherosclerosis aside from calcium scoring. However, our literature review found no reports evaluating the cost-effectiveness of either modality.

Huniak et al. (40) performed a decision analysis and developed a model incorporating current initial diagnostic modalities (i.e., SPECT and stress echo) prior to coronary angiography. In addition, coronary MR and CT were also included to determine those cost and performance characteristics necessary for the new modalities to possess in order to be cost-effective. For a new diagnostic study to be more cost-effective than stress echo, a cost of less than $1,000 and a sensitivity and specificity greater than 89 and 88%, respectively, should be obtained.

The results were similar for replacing SPECT, such that the new imaging study must have a sensitivity and specificity greater than 85 and 80%, respectively. Lastly, as would be expected, a new testing modality required a sensitivity and specificity of 99% to replace angiography (40). While the prior study is a good start in the evaluation of the cost-effectiveness of coronary MR and CT, dedicated studies are required to fully evaluate these aspects of the imaging modalities, in order to have a complete understanding of their role in patient care.

In addition, as opposed to the traditional modalities, cardiac MRI can assess simultaneously a multitude of aspects of the heart and cardiac function. Thus, a modality with such versatility may have higher costs that are offset by evaluating several cardiac dimensions at once, resulting in a greater cost-effective modality. Therefore, studies need to be designed to address cardiac MR's role in a complete heart evaluation encompassing ejection fraction, wall motion, coronary arteries, perfusion, and valvular disease. All of these aspects of cardiac MR have been addressed, but no single study has encompassed all aspects to evaluate cost-effectiveness.

Studies have shown that cardiac perfusion abnormalities can be detected with similar sensitivity and specificity with MR, SPECT, and PET (41–43). Cardiac MRI has been found to comparable to stress echo in the evaluation of wall motion (43, 44). In addition, it is better than SPECT in the assessment of myocardial viability as it is of higher resolution and able to differentiate between subendocardial and transmural infarct. Cardiac MR has also been utilized to evaluate the coronary arteries for aberrant vessel course and bypass graft complications, all with a relatively high degree of sensitivity of about 90% (43). Cardiac MR has been found to correlate with Doppler ultrasound findings in the estimation of valvular area size (45, 46). Aside from the potential utilization for heart disease, cardiac MR has been shown to have applications for patients with congenital heart disease (47) that assist with surgical planning and medical management. The current cardiac MR data are extremely promising but remain limited and require further investigation regarding a future role in patient care.

Cardiac CT also suffers from a paucity of data evaluating the cost-effectiveness in patient management; as a result, its role in patient care remains unclear. Cardiac CT has made great strides over the past 5 years with the introduction of multidetector scanners, which has improved resolution and speed, allowing for improved performance of multiphase and arterial phase studies. These characteristics do provide some advantage over MR in terms of speed and in the evaluation of stents and patients with pacemakers. But due to the novelty of the modality, the literature remains more limited than that for cardiac MR. Therefore, even before cost-effectiveness studies can be performed, data must be generated on the performance of cardiac CT. Preliminary studies have shown that cardiac CT can evaluate coronary artery stents (48), and others have used cardiac CT to evaluate congenital heart disease (49). Also, preliminary data have been generated in the use of cardiac CT for coronary angiography (50); however, the sample sizes are not substantial enough to generate any accurate assessment of performance.

Recommended Imaging Protocols Based on the Evidence

Cardiac Catheterization

- Selective injection of left coronary artery with at least the projections anteroposterior (AP), left anterior oblique (LAO) cranial, and right anterior oblique (RAO) caudal is the minimum needed to cover the course of the left main anterior descending and circumflex arteries.
- Selective injection of the right coronary artery with at least the projections lateral, RAO, LAO, and LAO cranial are required to evaluate the right coronary artery.

Stress Echo

In a nonpharmacologic stress echocardiogram, the target for an adequate study is similar to that of SPECT or a treadmill test. Failure to meet the stress limits the sensitivity of the examination. The heart rate should reach at least 85% of predicted. However, the study should be terminated if cardiac symptoms arise or there are ECG changes.

Cardiac SPECT

- In the nonpharmacologic stress SPECT, 85% of the maximum heart rate needs to be achieved to prevent limitations in sensitivity.
- Dipyridamole is infused at a rate of 0.6 mg/kg over 4 min. Then imaging with thallium 201 begins 10 min after infusion. No caffeinated products or xanthines should be taken prior to the study as they will eliminate the effects of dipyridamole. This should not be given to asthmatics as it may precipitate bronchospasm.
- Adenosine is infused intravenously at 140 µg/kg/min over 4–6 min. The thallium 201 is injected 3 min after infusion. Adenosine is contraindicated in individuals with heart block and bronchospasm.

Take Home Figures

Figs. 20.1–20.5 serve to highlight key recommendations and supporting evidence.

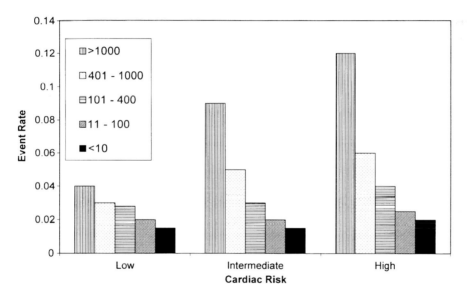

Figure 24.1. Graph shows risk stratification for each category of Framingham risk (from low to high) according to baseline calcium score. Event rate is predicted mortality at 5 years (8). Low risk <0.30 (no risk factors), intermediate risk <0.70 (one to two risk factors), and high risk <0.9 (three or more risk factors) probability of cardiac disease. [*Source*: Shaw et al. (8), with permission from the Radiological Society of North America.]

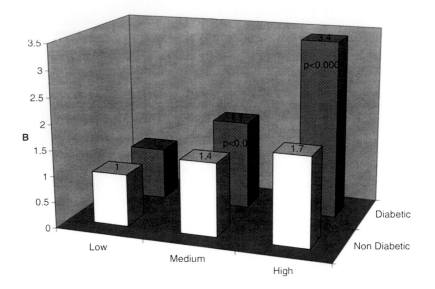

Figure 24.2. (**A**) Relative risks (RRs), stratified by diabetes status, of nonfatal myocardial infarction (MI), or coronary death associated with calcium score risk groups (low, <2.8; medium, 2.8–117.8; high, >117.8). (**B**) RRs, stratified by diabetes status, of nonfatal MI, coronary death, percutaneous transluminal coronary angioplasty (PTCA), coronary artery bypass graft (CABG), or stroke associated with calcium score risk groups (low, <2.8; medium, 2.8–117.8; high, >117.8). [*Source*: Qu et al. (22).]

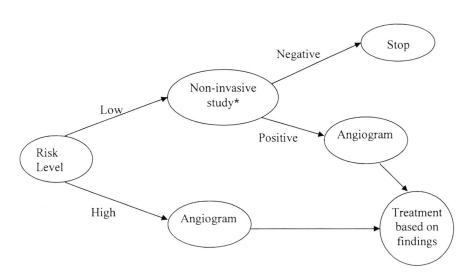

Figure 24.3. The recommended decision tree for the evaluation of CAD based on the patients' initial clinical status. *Noninvasive study can represent SPECT or stress echo depending on the institutional performance characteristics of the imaging study. (Reprinted with kind permission of Springer Science+Business Media from Bierhals AJ, Woodard PK. Cardiac Evaluation: The Current Status of Outcomes-Based Imaging. In Medina LS, Blackmore CC (eds): *Evidence-Based Imaging: Optimizing Imaging in Patient Care*. New York: Springer Science+Business Media, 2006.)

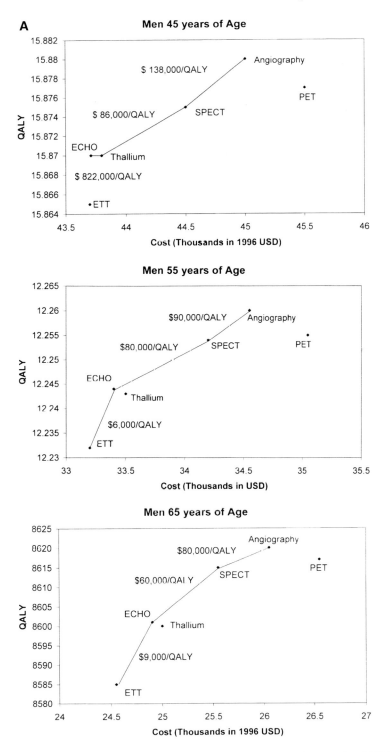

Figure 24.4. (**A**) Cost-effectiveness of tests for coronary artery disease, in thousands of 1996 US dollars per quality-adjusted life year (QALY), for men at 50% pretest risk for disease. (**B**) Cost-effectiveness of tests for coronary artery disease, in thousands of 1996 US dollars per QALY, for women at 50% pretest risk for disease. ECHO, stress echocardiography; ETT, exercise electrocardiography; PET, positron emission tomography; SPECT, single photon emission computed tomography. [*Source*: Garber and Solomon (27).]

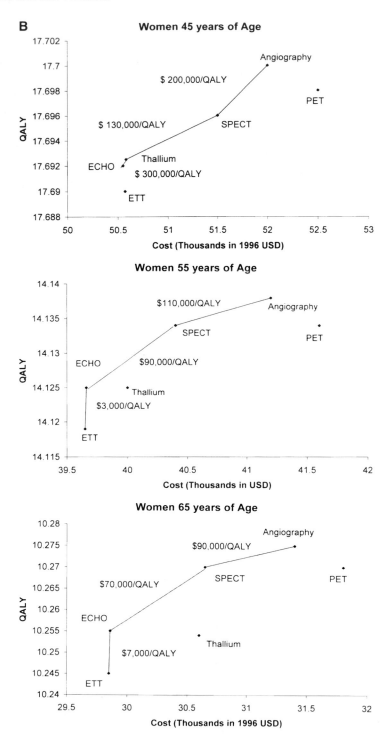

Figure 24.4. *Continued*

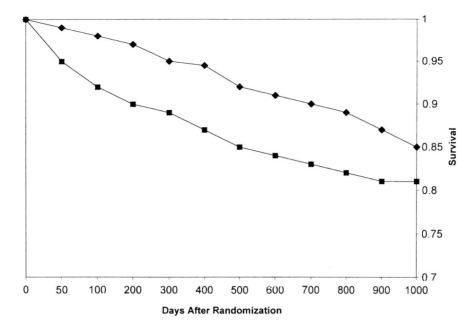

Figure 24.5. Kaplan–Meier analysis of the probability of survival according to strategy group during 12–44 months of follow-up. Death from any cause was included in this analysis. The Cox proportional-hazards ratio for the conservative as compared with the invasive strategy was 0.72 (95% confidence interval, 0.51–1.01). [*Source*: Boden et al. (32).]

Future Research

- In the future, cost-effectiveness research should focus on incorporating calcium scoring and clinical risk stratification in the screening for early heart disease. Coronary artery calcification scoring has been shown in the asymptomatic patient to predict a coronary event, but cost-effectiveness has not been adequately evaluated. By evaluating calcium scoring in this manner, a determination can be made concerning the modalities' additional benefits as well as the cost that may be incurred.
- Future research should focus on the potential utilization and outcomes of novel coronary artery imaging modalities, such as CT and MRI. These modalities are promising for the evaluation of coronary arteries in multiple clinical circumstances (51). Prior to any cost-effectiveness studies, an understanding of modality performance characteristics (e.g., sensitivity and specificity) is needed, along with evaluation of the impact on patient management and outcome.

References

1. Hurst W. The Heart, Arteries, and Veins, 10th ed. New York: McGraw-Hill, 2002.
2. CDC/NCHS. National Health and Nutrition Examination Survey III (NHANES III), 1988–1994.
3. American Heart Association. Annual Report. 1996.
4. American Heart Association. Heart Disease and Stroke Statistics – 2004 update.
5. Health Resources Utilization Branch, CDC/NCHS. National Hospital Discharge Survey.
6. National Health Expenditures, Amounts, and Average Annual Percent Change, by Type of Expenditure: Selected Calendar Years 1980–2012. http://cms.hhs.gov.
7. O'Rourke RA, Brundage BH, Froelicher VF et al., American College of Cardiology. Circulation 2000;102:126–140.
8. Shaw LJ, Raggi P, Schisterman E, Daniel S, Berman DS, Callister TQ. Radiology 2003;228: 826–833.
9. Newman AB, Naydeck BL, Sutton-Tyrrell K, Feldman A, Edmundowicz D, Kuller LH. Circulation 2001;104:2679–2684.
10. Detrano RC, Wong ND, Doherty TM et al. Circulation 1999;99:2633–2638.
11. O'Malley PG, Taylor AJ, Jackson J et al. Am J Cardiol 2000;85:945–948.
12. Arad Y, Spadaro LA, Goodman K, Newstein D, Guerci AD. J Am Coll Cardiol 2000;36:1253–1260.

13. Raggi P, Cooil B, Callister TQ. Am Heart J 2001; 141:375–382.
14. Detrano RC, Doherty TM, Davies MJ, Stary HC. Curr Probl Cardiol 2000;25:374–402.
15. Raggi P. Herz 2001;26:252–259.
16. Raggi P, Callister TQ, Cooil B et al. Circulation 2000;101:850–855.
17. Shaw LJ, O'Rourke RA. J Am Coll Cardiol 2000;36:1261–1264.
18. Detrano R, Hsiai T, Wang S et al. J Am Coll Cardiol 1996;27:285–290.
19. Arad Y, Spadaro LA, Goodman K et al. Circulation 1996;93:1951–1953.
20. Park R, Detrano R, Xiang M et al. Circulation 2002;106:2073–2077.
21. Lipid Research Clinics Program. JAMA 1984;251:365–374.
22. Qu W, Le TT, Azen ST et al. Diab Care 2003;26:905–910.
23. Sangiorgi G, Rumberger JA, Severson A et al. J Am Coll Cardiol 1998;31:126–133.
24. Janowitz WR, Agatston AS, Kaplan G et al. Am J Cardiol 1993;72:247–254.
25. Patterson RE, Eisner RL, Horowitz SF. Circulation 1995;91:54–65.
26. Patterson RE, Eng C, Horowitz SF, Gorlin R, Goldstein SR. J Am Coll Cardiol 1984;4:278–289.
27. Garber AM, Solomon NA. Ann Intern Med 1999;130:719–728.
28. Kuntz K, Tsevat J, Goldman L, Weinstein MC. Circulation 1996;94:957–965.
29. FRagmin and Fast Revascularisation during InStability in Coronary artery disease (FRISC II) Investigators. Lancet 1999;354:708–715.
30. Cannon CP, Weintraub WS, Demopoulos LA et al. N Engl J Med 2001;344:1879–1887.
31. Barnett PG, Chen S, Boden WE et al. Circulation 2002;105:680–684.
32. Boden W, O'rourke R, Crawford M et al. N Engl J Med 1998;338:1785–1792.
33. Pepine CJ, Allen HD, Bashore TM et al. J Am Coll Cardiol 1991;18:1149–1182.
34. Ryan TJ, Anderson JL, Antman EM et al. J Am Coll Cardiol 1996;28:1328–1428.
35. Kuntz K, Fleischmann KE, Hunick MGM, Douglas PS. Ann Intern Med 1999;130: 709–718.
36. Hachamovich R, Berman DS, Kiat H et al. Circulation 2002;105:823–829.
37. Fleischmann KE, Hunink MG, Kuntz KM, Douglas PS. JAMA 1998;280:913–920.
38. Weissman IA, Dickinson CZ, Dworkin HJ, Oneil WW, Juni JE. Radiology 1996;199:353–357.
39. Udelson JE, Beshansky JR, Ballin DS et al. JAMA 2002;288:2693–2700.
40. Hunink MGM, Kuntz K, Fleischmann KE, Brady TJ. Ann Intern Med 1999;131:673–680.
41. Hartnell G, Cerel A, Kamalesh M et al. AJR Am J Roentgenol 1994;163:1061–1067.
42. Muzik O, Duvernoy C, Beanlands RS et al. J Am Coll Cardiol 1998;31:534–540.
43. Wagner A, Mahrholdt H, Sechtem U, Kim R, Judd R. Magn Reson Imaging Clin N Am 2003;11:49–66.
44. Baer FM, Voth E, Larosee K et al. Am J Cardiol 1996;78:415–419.
45. Nishimura T, Yamada N, Itoh A et al. AJR Am J Roentgenol 1989;153:721–724.
46. Aurigemma G, Reichek N, Schiebler M et al. Am J Cardiol 1990;66:621–625.
47. Boxt LM, Rozenshtein A. Magn Reson Imaging Clin N Am 2003;11:27–48.
48. Fidler JL, Cheatham JP, Fletcher L et al. AJR Am J Roentgenol 2000;174:355–359.
49. Choi BW, Park YH, Choi JY et al. AJR Am J Roentgenol 2001;177:1045–1049.
50. Herzog C, Dogan S, Diebold T et al. Radiology 2003;229:200–208.
51. Schoepf UJ, Becker CR, Ohnesorge BM, Yucel EK. Radiology 2004;232:18–37.

25

Imaging in the Evaluation of Pulmonary Embolism

Krishna Juluru and John Eng

I. What is the performance of various imaging modalities in the evaluation of pulmonary embolism?
   A. Modality 1: angiography
   B. Modality 2: nuclear ventilation-perfusion imaging
   C. Modality 3: computed tomography pulmonary angiography (scanners with fewer than four detectors)
   D. Modality 4: multidetector computed tomography
   E. Modality 5: electron beam computed tomography
   F. Modality 6: magnetic resonance angiography
   G. Modality 7: ultrasound of lung and pleura
   H. Method 8: echocardiography
   I. Modality 9: chest radiography
II. How can imaging modalities be combined in the diagnosis of pulmonary embolism?

Issues

- When using a clinical outcome reference standards, angiography, VQ scan, non-multidetector computed tomography (MDCT) pulmonary angiography, MDCT pulmonary angiography, and electron beam computed tomography (EBCT), are all associated with negative predictive values of 94% or greater for diagnosing pulmonary embolism (PE).
- Differences in negative predictive values of non-MDCT in diagnosis of PE between studies using an imaging reference standard and studies using clinical outcome reference standard may be due to clinically insignificant pulmonary emboli at the subsegmental level.
- The performance of magnetic resonance angiography (MRA) in evaluation of PE has not been adequately studied.

Key Points

K. Juluru (✉)
Department of Radiology, Weill Cornell Medical College, 525 E. 68th Street, New York, NY 10065, USA
e-mail: kjuluru@med.cornell.edu

L.S. Medina et al. (eds.), *Evidence-Based Imaging: Improving the Quality of Imaging in Patient Care, Revised Edition*,
DOI 10.1007/978-1-4419-7777-9_25, © Springer Science+Business Media, LLC 2011

- The performances of ultrasound of the lung and pleura, echocardiography, and plain radiographs are insufficient to justify the use of these modalities in the primary evaluation of PE.
- Several pathways in the diagnosis of PE have been described using combinations of imaging modalities, clinical exam, and laboratory data. These pathways are equally effective with respect to clinical outcome, but differ in imaging utilization and may differ in safety.

Definition and Pathophysiology

Pulmonary emboli originate from blood clots in the venous system, blood clots in the right side of the heart, neoplasms invading the venous system, and other substances such as air, bone marrow fat, and amniotic fluid. Over 90% of pulmonary emboli originate from clots in the deep veins of the lower extremities. Major risk factors include advanced age, recent surgery, immobilization, malignancy, obesity, cigarette smoking, congestive heart failure, and history of deep venous thrombosis (DVT) (1).

Epidemiology

The incidence of PE has been estimated to be 0.2–0.6 per 1,000 per year (2, 3) with an estimated mortality rate of 11–15% (1).

Overall Cost to Society

Estimating the economic impact of PE is difficult since the overall incidence of this disease is hard to ascertain. However, in one well-defined group of patients at risk for developing DVT, patients who have undergone total hip replacement surgery, the average discounted lifetime cost of long-term DVT complications has been estimated to be $3,069 per patient, of which $333 is attributed to PE (4).

Goals

The goal of imaging is to identify evidence of clot in the pulmonary arterial system. Identification of any clot generally results in treatment with anticoagulant therapy.

Methodology

The medical literature was searched using PubMed (National Library of Medicine, Bethesda, Maryland) for original research publications that address the use of various imaging modalities in the evaluation of PE. The search parameters were *pulmonary embolism AND (CT OR ultrasound OR sonography OR echo OR nuclear OR ventilation perfusion OR MRI OR angiography OR imaging OR radiography) AND (evaluation OR diagnosis OR diagnostic)*. The search covered the period 1990 to April 2004 and was limited to human studies in the English language. Relevant articles from the search were entered into a database and classified into the following categories: (1) article type (systematic review vs. primary literature), (2) subject of evaluation (diagnostic imaging vs. diagnostic pathway), (3) imaging modality (if applicable), and (4) diagnostic reference standard (imaging vs. clinical outcome). The authors then rated the articles based on the quality of evidence.

Comment

It is important to recognize the limitations of studies reporting clinical outcomes in patients who receive diagnostic testing for pulmonary embolism. These studies can only report negative predictive values and rates of false negative results. The number of false negatives is the number of patients initially diagnosed as not having PE but who later return within a specified period of time with PE symptoms and imaging findings. This value is also known as the recurrence rate. Studies using clinical outcome as a reference standard did not follow patients initially diagnosed with PE, as these patients were treated. Therefore, positive predictive values and rates of false-positive results could not be determined.

I. What Is the Performance of Various Imaging Modalities in the Evaluation of Pulmonary Embolism?

A. Modality 1: Angiography

Summary of Evidence: Pulmonary angiography has traditionally been considered the gold standard diagnostic test in the evaluation of PE. Consequently, the major articles that evaluated the accuracy of pulmonary angiography itself have used clinical outcome as a reference standard. The risk of recurrent PE following negative pulmonary angiography is low, even though interobserver agreement is relatively low for subsegmental pulmonary arteries (5).

Supporting Evidence: One major level I (strong evidence) systematic review and three major level II (moderate evidence) primary studies were identified in our search that evaluated pulmonary angiography against a clinical outcome reference standard. Van Beek et al. (6) performed a systematic review of the literature from 1965 to 1999 for prospective studies of untreated patients with suspected PE and negative pulmonary angiograms who were followed-up for a minimum of 3 months. Eight articles were selected on the strength of the study design, comprising a total study population of 1,050 patients with negative pulmonary angiograms. Of these, 51 patients were lost to follow-up, 15 patients had nonfatal PE during the follow-up period, and three patients had fatal pulmonary embolism. In the worst-case scenario, if all patients who were lost to follow-up died from fatal PE, the recurrence rate of PE would have been 6.3% [95% confidence interval (CI), 4–7%]. In the best-case scenario, if all patients who were lost to follow-up did not have PE in the follow-up period, the recurrence rate of PE would have been 1.6% (95% CI, 1.0–2.6%). The study's authors note that the three oldest studies in the review, performed between 1978 and 1988, accounted for the majority of cases of recurrent PE as well the majority of cases that were lost to follow-up, and they argue that the lower recurrence rate in the more recent studies may be due to improvements in imaging technology. Excluding the three oldest studies from the analysis, the overall recurrence rate of PE drops to 5.4% in the worst-case scenario.

Of the three major primary articles identified in our search (5, 7, 8) (all level II), one article by Nilsson et al. (5) was not included in the van Beek analysis. In this study, 269 consecutive patients with clinical suspicion for PE were evaluated. Ninety-nine patients (37%) were excluded because of disease other than PE, refusal to participate, being too ill to participate, unavailability of diagnostic catheterization, contraindication to pulmonary angiography, or inadequate completion of protocol. The remaining 170 patients all underwent pulmonary angiography regardless of scintigraphic findings, and all had 6-month follow-up. Three of 119 patients (2.5%) with negative angiograms were later determined to have PE.

Our search identified no major studies that evaluated conventional angiography against an imaging reference standard.

B. Modality 2: Nuclear Ventilation-Perfusion Imaging

Summary of Evidence: Using imaging reference standards, the sensitivity of normal VQ scan is 98% and the specificity of a high-probability VQ scan is 97%. By both imaging and clinical outcome reference standards, negative predictive values of a normal scan range between 96 and 100%, while positive predictive values of high-probability scans range between 86 and 88%. A VQ scan with a normal result can be used to safely withhold anticoagulation in a patient suspected of PE, and a high probability scan can be used to justify treatment. A high percentage of patients have indeterminate probability, so nondiagnostic scans limit the usefulness of this modality.

Supporting Evidence: One major level II (moderate evidence) study used an imaging reference, though applied nonuniformly, to evaluate the performance of VQ scanning. The 1990 Prospective Investigation of Pulmonary Embolism Diagnosis (PIOPED) study (9) established the convention of reporting VQ scans as normal, low probability, indeterminate, or high probability; 931 patients with a PE prevalence of 27% were studied prospectively, with 731 obtaining both a VQ scan and diagnostic pulmonary angiogram. Based on patients who obtained a pulmonary angiogram, this study established the sensitivity and negative predictive values of a normal VQ scan as 98 and 96%, respectively. The specificity and positive predictive values of a high-probability scan were 97 and 87%, respectively. Of note, 150 patients who had low-probability or normal VQ scans either did not obtain an angiogram or had angiograms with uncertain interpretations. These patients were followed clinically for 1 year, with none experiencing recurrent symptoms of PE. A frequently cited deficit of the PIOPED reporting criteria is that 39% of patients fell into an intermediate probability category, of whom 30% were positive for PE.

Level II (moderate evidence) studies by Hull et al. (10) and van Beek et al. (11) both addressed the risk of withholding anticoagulation in patients with normal perfusion scans in a total of 628 patients who were followed for a minimum of 3 months. Only one of these patients (0.2%) developed symptomatic PE, establishing a negative predictive value of nearly 100%. A level III (limited evidence) study by Rajendran and Jacobson (12) found the 6-month mortality of low-probability lung scans due to PE to be 0%. However, it is not clear whether anticoagulation was withheld in patients with low-probability scans in this study.

One systematic review by van Beek et al. (13) reported negative and positive predictive values of 99.7 and 88%, respectively.

C. Modality 3: Computed Tomography Pulmonary Angiography (Scanners with Fewer than Four Detectors)

Summary of Evidence: Computed tomography pulmonary angiography (CTPA) is increasingly being used for the diagnosis of PE. Level I (strong evidence) studies using a clinical outcome reference standard find rates of PE recurrence to be 0–6%, with negative predictive values of 94–100%. Studies using a conventional pulmonary angiography reference standard find broad variations in sensitivities, specificities, and positive and negative predictive values, likely due to variations in detection of subsegmental emboli. Despite these variations, there is strong evidence to show that it is safe to withhold anticoagulation in patients with negative CTPA.

Supporting Evidence: A systematic review of all published literature from 1966 to 2003

(38) identified eight primary prospective levels I to II (strong to moderate evidence) studies in which all subjects underwent both CTPA and conventional angiography, the latter being considered the reference standard. Among the eight primary studies, the sensitivities ranged from 45 to 100%, and specificities ranged from 78 to 100%.

Nine major studies were found in our search that evaluated the negative predictive value of CTPA using clinical outcomes. One prospective level I (strong evidence) study with a total PE prevalence of 25% followed 378 patients with negative CTPA for 3 months (14). No patients were lost to follow-up, none were anticoagulated during the follow-up period, and no patients were excluded for other reasons. Four out of 378 patients developed PE (recurrence rate = 1%, negative predictive value = 99%). In all studies, recurrence rates ranged from 0 to 6%, and negative predictive values ranged from 94 to 100%. The study with the highest recurrence rate and lowest negative predictive value (level II) followed 81 hospitalized patients from cardiology and pulmonary wards with a PE prevalence of 38%, a majority of whom (82%) had underlying cardiorespiratory disease (15).

D. Modality 4: Multidetector Computed Tomography

Summary of Evidence: Multidetector computed tomography, with higher image acquisition rates than non-MDCT scanners, reduces the rate of respiratory and motion artifacts, particularly in sections obtained during the end of the scan when patients may not be able to maintain apnea, and improves overall spatial resolution. Limited evidence in clinical outcome studies demonstrates that the recurrence rate in patients with MDCT findings negative for PE is 1%, with a negative predictive value of 99%. Although definitive evidence is still forthcoming, it is reasonable to assume the performance of MDCT is at least as good as that of non-MDCT. It is safe, therefore, to withhold anticoagulation in patients with negative MDCT findings.

Supporting Evidence: There have been no major direct comparisons of conventional CTPA with MDCT. While we expect MDCT to be more sensitive for clots, negative predictive values cannot be much improved beyond the 94–100% achievable by conventional CTPA with clinical outcome as a reference standard. It is possible that subsegmental clots missed by conventional CTPA may have no clinical significance. The benefit of MDCT over non-MDCT appears to be the reduction in the number of patients with inconclusive scan results.

Two prospective level III (limited evidence) studies were identified in our search evaluating MDCT against a clinical outcome reference standard (16, 17). The studies evaluated a total of 236 patients, with PE prevalence of 18–19%. Patients were referred for MDCT scanning by clinicians who also had the option to choose other imaging modalities (e.g., nuclear imaging), thus introducing potential selection bias. Both studies reported a PE recurrence rate of 1% and negative predictive value of 99%. In comparison to non-MDCT scan, MDCT scans had fewer respiratory and cardiac motion artifacts, higher rates of interpretation down to subsegmental arterial levels, and fewer inconclusive results (17).

In our search, there were no major systematic reviews of MDCT or articles that evaluated MDCT against an imaging reference standard. A multicenter clinical trial, the PIOPED II sponsored by the National Heart, Lung, and Blood Institute, is currently obtaining data to assess the efficacy of multidetector CT (among other tests) in patients suspected of having acute PE (18).

E. Modality 5: Electron Beam Computed Tomography

Summary of Evidence: Electron beam computed tomography has undergone limited evaluation in the detection of PE, probably because this technology is not widely available. One major level I (strong evidence) study using clinical outcome as a reference standard has shown that it is safe to withhold anticoagulation in patients with negative EBCT findings. When using conventional pulmonary angiography as a reference standard, EBCT has sensitivities and specificities similar to those of CTPA.

Supporting Evidence: A level I (strong evidence) study by Swensen et al. (19) evaluated 993 patients with a PE prevalence of 34% who had negative EBCT findings and were not anticoagulated. At 3-month follow-up, seven patients developed PE or died from PE. No history was available in 19 patients who were known to have lived by the 3-month follow-up period. Recurrence of PE therefore ranged from 0.7% (7/993) to 2.6% [(7 + 19)/993].

One major level III (limited evidence) study evaluated EBCT against a pulmonary angiography reference standard (20). Sixty consecutive patients who had already been referred for conventional pulmonary angiography were imaged with EBCT. In this population with a PE prevalence of 38%, the sensitivity, specificity, and positive predictive and negative predictive values were 65, 97, 93, and 82%, respectively.

There have been no major systematic reviews evaluating EBCT.

F. Modality 6: Magnetic Resonance Angiography

Summary of Evidence: Magnetic resonance angiography has undergone limited evaluation, predominantly in populations referred for conventional pulmonary angiography. There is incomplete evidence to suggest that MRA can be used as the primary imaging modality in the evaluation of PE.

Supporting Evidence: In four level III (limited evidence) studies, patients were selected from a population referred for conventional pulmonary angiography. The oldest study in 1994 (21), with a PE prevalence of 52%, reported problems with identification of pulmonary emboli at the segmental levels. Sensitivity and specificity of MRA in this study were 83 and 100%, respectively. In the remaining three studies performed between 1997 and 2002 (22–24) with PE prevalences ranging from 25 to 36%, problems with identification of PE occurred mostly at the subsegmental levels. Sensitivities and specificities ranged from 77 to 100% and 95 to 98%, respectively. All three studies had at least two readers with interobserver agreement ranging from 57 to 91%, with lower values again noted mostly at subsegmental levels.

In our search, there were no major systematic reviews of MRA, and there were no major studies that evaluated MRA against a clinical outcome reference standard.

G. Modality 7: Ultrasound of Lung and Pleura

Summary of Evidence: Evidence on the use of transthoracic ultrasound imaging of the lung and pleura to diagnose PE is limited. The available data show that this method does not have adequate sensitivity or specificity for the detection of PE.

Supporting Evidence: One major level II (moderate evidence) study was identified in our search that used ultrasound imaging of the lung and pleura for evaluation of suspected PE against an imaging reference standard (25). Ultrasound diagnosis of PE was made by the identification of (1) wedge-shaped hypoechoic homogeneous pleural-based lesions or (2) sharply outlined pleural-based lesions with central hyperechoic reflection. Final diagnosis was established by a combination of nuclear lung imaging, clinical probability, CT, lower extremity Doppler ultrasound, and conventional angiography. In this study with a PE prevalence of 42%, the sensitivity, specificity, positive predictive, and negative predictive values were 71, 77, 69, and 79%, respectively.

There were no major systematic reviews of ultrasound in our search, and there were no major studies that evaluated ultrasound against a clinical outcome reference.

H. Method 8: Echocardiography

Summary of Evidence: Studies on the use of transthoracic echocardiography (TTE) have employed various criteria in the evaluation of pulmonary embolism. These include tricuspid regurgitation, right ventricular dilatation, right ventricular dyskinesis, right-sided cardiac thrombus, and flattening of the interventricular septum. Combinations of these criteria have yielded inadequate sensitivities and variable specificities.

Data on the effectiveness of transesophageal echocardiography (TEE) for direct pulmonary thrombus visualization is limited, and this modality also suffers from poor sensitivity and specificity. The limited data on both TTE and TEE show that both modalities are inadequate as a primary imaging modality in the evaluation of PE.

Supporting Evidence: Two level II studies (moderate evidence) and one level III (limited evidence) study were identified in our search that utilized TTE for the diagnosis of PE against an imaging reference standard (26–28). Miniati et al. (28) studied a group of 110 patients with a PE prevalence of 39%. All patients had TTE followed by VQ scan. Conventional angiography was performed when the VQ scan was not normal. Echocardiographic criteria for diagnosis of PE included enlarged right ventricle, tricuspid regurgitation, or right ventricular hypokinesis. Sensitivity, specificity, and positive and negative predictive values were 56, 90, 77, and 76%, respectively. Sensitivities in the other studies ranged from 19 to 52%, and specificities from 87 to 100%.

A level III (limited evidence) study by Steiner et al. (29) utilized TEE and TTE for diagnosis of PE in 35 patients with a PE prevalence of 63%, using helical CT as a reference standard. Pulmonary embolism was diagnosed by visualization of thrombus in the main pulmonary artery, dilatation of the right ventricle or pulmonary artery, tricuspid regurgitation, or abnormal motion of the interventricular septum. Sensitivity, specificity, and positive and negative predictive values were 59, 77, 81, and 53%, respectively.

There were no major systematic reviews of echocardiography in our search, and there were no major studies that evaluated echocardiography against a clinical outcome reference standard.

I. Modality 9: Chest Radiography

Summary of Evidence: There is limited evidence on the use of chest radiography in the evaluation of PE. Various chest radiographic findings are associated with poor sensitivity and only modest specificity. Chest radiography should not be the primary modality in PE evaluation.

Supporting Evidence: In one major level II (moderate evidence) study by Worsley et al. (30), 1,063 patients from the PIOPED group who underwent both diagnostic angiography and chest radiography were retrospectively evaluated. Radiographic signs evaluated included prominent central artery (Fleischner sign), enlarged hilum, enlarged mediastinum, pulmonary edema, chronic obstructive pulmonary disease (COPD), oligemia (Westermark's sign), vascular redistribution, pleural-based areas of increased opacity (Hampton hump), pleural effusion, and elevated diaphragm. The highest sensitivity obtained was 36% for pleural effusion, and the highest specificity obtained was 96% for COPD. Combinations of the signs were not assessed.

There were no major systematic reviews of chest radiography in our search, and there were no major studies that evaluated chest radiography against a clinical outcome reference standard.

II. How Can Imaging Modalities Be Combined in the Diagnosis of Pulmonary Embolism?

Summary of Evidence: Various proposed strategies have employed combinations of clinical exams, serum D-dimer measurement, lower extremity ultrasound, CTPA, VQ imaging, venography, impedance plethysmography, and conventional pulmonary angiography in the diagnosis of PE. Despite the heterogeneity in test utilization, recurrence rates for venous thromboembolism (VTE) in patients determined to be negative for PE were less than 2% in all major strategies identified. Safety, cost-effectiveness, and availability of resources may help to further differentiate these algorithms, and these issues require further investigation.

Supporting Evidence: Nearly all of the pathway articles identified in our search employed clinical pretest probability in the diagnostic algorithm. We excluded those articles in which clinical pretest probability was not explicitly defined. All six of the major studies identified included a 3-month follow-up on patients who were determined to be negative for PE by the algorithm (31–36), and all had recurrence rates of VTE of less that 2%, although in one study (33), the high percentage of patients who were lost to follow-up may make the reported recurrence rate unreliable. One algorithm by Kruip et al. (34) employed only clinical exam, D-dimer, and lower extremity ultrasound, but with a notably high conventional angiography rate of 63%. Another study by Hull et al. (36) published in 1994 is also less than ideal because it relied on impedance plethysmography, a diagnostic modality that is no longer widely available.

A level I (strong evidence) study by Wells et al. (31) deserves special mention because it most effectively limited the number of patients receiving intravenous contrast, thereby reducing the overall risk of contrast-induced renal insufficiency. The study included 1,252 patients with a PE prevalence of 15% who presented with symptoms of PE, had no contraindications to contrast media, and had an expected survival of greater than 3 months. Following clinical assessment, all patients received VQ scans, followed by single or serial lower extremity ultrasound exams (Fig. 25.1). Lower extremity venography or conventional pulmonary angiography was performed in only 2% of patients. Although this algorithm limited the number of contrast examinations, it did so at the expense of a high number of lower extremity ultrasound examinations. An estimated 3,093 lower extremity ultrasounds were performed on 1,252 patients in this study (2.5 ultrasounds per patient). At most 19 patients (including 13 who were lost to follow-up) out of 1,070 who were not anticoagulated by the algorithm developed VTE, equal to a recurrence rate of 1.8%.

A more recent level I (strong evidence) study by Perrier et al. (32) placed greater emphasis on D-dimer measurement and CTPA (D-dimer measurements were not performed in the Wells algorithm). This study involved 965 patients (PE prevalence of 24%) with suspected PE who had no contraindications to CT and who could be followed for 3 months. Following clinical probability assessment (Table 25.1), serum D-dimer was obtained in all patients, and a value less than 500 µg/L excluded PE. None of these patients had recurrent VTE on 3-month follow-up. The remaining patients received combinations of venous ultrasound, CTPA, and conventional angiography. Sixty-two percent of patients obtained a contrast study (compared to 2% in the Wells algorithm), and complications from contrast administration were not discussed. However, ultrasound examinations were performed in only 71% of patients (compared to 2.5 ultrasounds per patient in the Wells algorithm). At most 10 patients (including three who were lost to follow-up) out of 685 who were not anticoagulated developed VTE, equivalent to a recurrence rate of 1.5%.

Take Home Tables and Figures

The findings of this review are summarized in Table 25.2. Note that the sensitivities, specificities, and positive and negative predictive values shown in the table are derived from studies that range from level I (strong evidence) to level III (limited evidence). Therefore, comparison of these values between imaging modalities must be done with caution because of the heterogeneity in evidence strength.

All of the diagnostic algorithms for suspected PE were associated with similar performances. The algorithm developed by Wells et al. (31) (Fig. 25.1) most effectively limited the use of intravenous contrast. However, the high number of ultrasound examinations and the use of serial compression ultrasound up to 2 weeks following initial presentation challenge the practicality of this approach. Furthermore, although the algorithm may be effective in diagnosing pulmonary embolism, alternative etiologies of the presenting symptoms are more often discovered with CT.

In Fig. 25.2, we suggest an algorithm that is a modification of that proposed by Perrier et al. (32). The Perrier et al. algorithm makes use of enzyme-linked immunosorbent assay (ELISA) D-dimer as an initial screen, followed by lower extremity venous ultrasound in all patients with positive D-dimer values. Studies have shown that DVT is unlikely in the absence of the clinical features noted in Table 25.3 (37). In our algorithm, we propose that only patients with clinical features of DVT undergo venous ultrasound, followed by CTPA when venous ultrasound is negative. In the absence of clinical features of DVT, we propose that patients immediately undergo CTPA. The remainder of the investigation matches the Perrier et al. algorithm. We feel this approach provides rapid diagnosis of PE and offers the opportunity to identify alternative etiologies for the patients' symptoms through use of chest CT. Overall cost-effectiveness and safety need further study.

Table 25.1. Criteria for evaluating the clinical probability of pulmonary embolism (PE) according to Perrier et al. (32)

Variable	Score
Previous PE or deep vein thrombosis	+2
Heart rate >100 beats per minute	+1
Recent surgery	+3
Age (years)	
60–79	+1
≥80	+2
$PaCO_2$	
<4.8 kPa (36 mmHg)	+2
4.8–5.19 kPa (36–38.9 mmHg)	+1
PaO_2	
<6.5 kPa (48.7 mmHg)	+4
6.5–7.99 kPa (48.7–59.9 mmHg)	+3
8–9.49 kPa (60–71.2 mmHg)	+2
9.5–10.99 kPa (71.3–82.4 mmHg)	+1
Chest radiograph	
Platelike atelectasis	+1
Elevated hemidiaphragm	+1

Clinical probability according to total score: low, 0–4 points; intermediate, 5–8 points; high, nine or more points.

Reprinted with kind permission of Springer Science+Business Media from Juluru K, Eng J. Imaging in the Evaluation of Pulmonary Embolism. In Medina LS, Blackmore CC (eds): *Evidence-Based Imaging: Optimizing Imaging in Patient Care*. New York: Springer Science+Business Media, 2006.

Table 25.2. Summary of representative performance of various imaging modalities in detection of pulmonary embolism

| Modality | Imaging reference studies | | | | Clinical outcome reference studies |
	Sn (%)	Sp (%)	PPV (%)	NPV (%)	NPV (%)
Angiography	–	–	–	–	95[a]
Nuclear ventilation-perfusion imaging	98[b]	97[c]	86–88[c]	96–100[b]	99.8
Non-multidetector CT pulmonary angiogram	45–100	78–100	60–100	60–100	94–100
Multidetector CT pulmonary angiogram	–	–	–	–	99
Electron beam CT	–	–	–	–	97
MR angiography	–	–	–	–	–
Ultrasound of lung and pleura	71	77	69	79	–
Echocardiography	56	90	77	76	–
Plain film	36[d]	92[e]	38[f]	76[g]	–

Sn sensitivity; *Sp* specificity; *PPV* positive predictive value; *NPV* negative predictive value. Reprinted with kind permission of Springer Science+Business Media from Juluru K, Eng J. Imaging in the Evaluation of Pulmonary Embolism. In Medina LS, Blackmore CC (eds): *Evidence-Based Imaging: Optimizing Imaging in Patient Care*. New York: Springer Science+Business Media, 2006.
[a]Excludes three of the oldest studies, performed between 1978 and 1988.
[b]For a normal scan.
[c]For high-probability scan.
[d]Highest sensitivity obtained using pleural effusion.
[e]Highest specificity obtained using oligemia.
[f]Highest positive predictive value obtained, using oligemia.
[g]Highest negative predictive value obtained, using oligemia, pleural-based areas of increased opacity, pleural effusion, or elevated diaphragm.

Table 25.3. Clinical features of DVT according to Wells et al. (37)

Active cancer (treatment ongoing or within previous 6 months or palliative)
Paralysis, paresis, or recent plaster immobilization of the lower extremities
Recently bedridden for more than 3 days or major surgery within 4 weeks
Localized tenderness along the distribution of the deep venous system
Entire leg swollen
Calf swelling by more than 3 cm when compared with the asymptomatic leg (measured 10 cm below tibial tuberosity)
Pitting edema (greater in the symptomatic leg)
Collateral superficial veins (nonvaricose)

Reprinted with kind permission of Springer Science+Business Media from Juluru K, Eng J. Imaging in the Evaluation of Pulmonary Embolism. In Medina LS, Blackmore CC (eds): *Evidence-Based Imaging: Optimizing Imaging in Patient Care*. New York: Springer Science+Business Media, 2006.

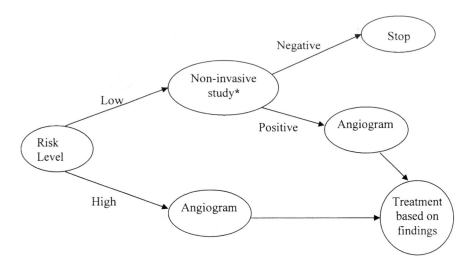

Figure 25.1. Clinical pathway proposed by Wells et al. (*Source:* Wells et al. (31), with permission from the *Annals of Internal Medicine.*)

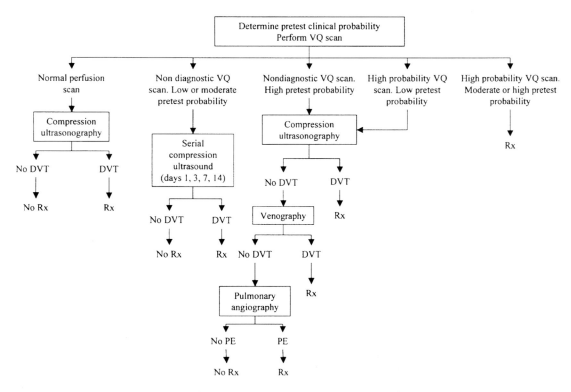

Figure 25.2. Suggested algorithm for evaluation of pulmonary embolism. Refer to Table 25.1 for method of determining clinical probability and Table 25.3 for clinical features of DVT. (Reprinted with kind permission of Springer Science+Business Media from Juluru K, Eng J. Imaging in the Evaluation of Pulmonary Embolism. In Medina LS, Blackmore CC (eds): *Evidence-Based Imaging: Optimizing Imaging in Patient Care.* New York: Springer Science+Business Media, 2006.)

Imaging Case Studies

These cases highlight the advantages and limitations of the different imaging modalities.

Case 1

History

A 20-year-old woman with sickle cell trait was diagnosed with right popliteal vein thrombosis. She presents with shortness of breath, fever, and bilateral leg pain.

Imaging

Multiple planar perfusion images demonstrate decreased perfusion to the left lung (Fig. 25.3A).

Ventilation images demonstrate normal ventilation to both lungs (Fig. 25.3B). These findings suggest central left-sided pulmonary emboli or a mass compressing the left main pulmonary artery. The CTPA demonstrates bilateral pulmonary emboli (Fig. 25.3C).

Discussion

This case demonstrates an instance in which both nuclear ventilation-perfusion imaging and CTPA detected evidence of pulmonary emboli necessitating treatment. However, it is notable that CTPA detected emboli in the right lung, where perfusion imaging was interpreted as normal.

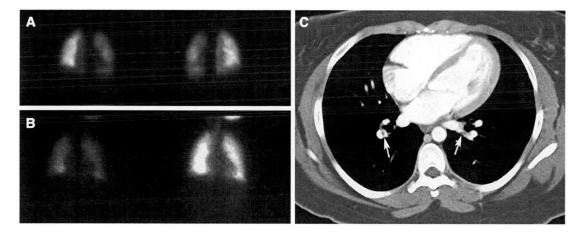

Figure 25.3. (**A**) Anterior and posterior technetium 99m (Tc-99m) macroaggregated albumin (MAA) planar perfusion images demonstrate decreased perfusion to the left lung. (**B**) Anterior single-breath and equilibrium-phase ^{133}Xe ventilation images in same patient demonstrate normal ventilation to both lungs. In combination with perfusion imaging, these findings led to an interpretation of high probability for pulmonary embolism. (**C**) The CTPA demonstrates filling defects in right and left pulmonary arteries (*arrows*) consistent with pulmonary emboli. (Reprinted with kind permission of Springer Science+Business Media from Juluru K, Eng J. Imaging in the Evaluation of Pulmonary Embolism. In Medina LS, Blackmore CC (eds): *Evidence-Based Imaging: Optimizing Imaging in Patient Care.* New York: Springer Science+Business Media, 2006.)

Case 2

History

A 41-year-old woman has an extensive vascular history and DVT in both lower extremities. She presents with pleuritic chest pain and shortness of breath.

Imaging

Multiple planar perfusion images demonstrate heterogeneous activity throughout both lungs with large perfusion defects in the basal segments of both lower lobes (Fig. 25.4A). Additional small perfusion defects are seen in the right and left apices. The perfusion defects in the lower lobes do not correspond to any defects in ventilation imaging (not shown). These findings led to an interpretation of a high probability for pulmonary embolism. Findings on perfusion imaging also include abnormal activity in the liver, raising the suspicion for collateral circulation and vascular shunting. The CTPA demonstrates occlusion of the superior vena cava (Fig. 25.4B) and multiple collateral vessels around the liver (Fig. 25.4C). No pulmonary emboli were identified on CTPA.

Discussion

This case demonstrates an instance in which nuclear ventilation-perfusion imaging findings and CTPA findings are discordant. The CTPA detected occlusion of the superior vena cava with collateral vessels around the liver that were suggested by VQ scanning. The patient received anticoagulation therapy based on VQ findings without further imaging.

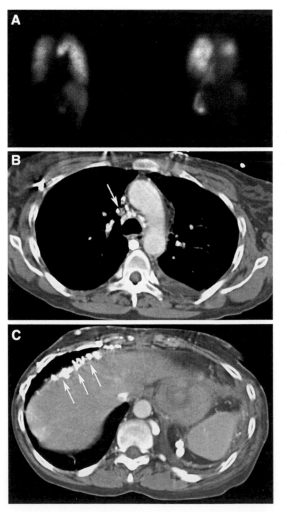

Figure 25.4. (**A**) Right and left posterior oblique Tc-99m MAA planar perfusion images demonstrate heterogeneous activity in both lungs with large perfusion defects in the basal segments of both lower lobes. Additional perfusion defects are seen in the apices. Ventilation imaging (not shown) demonstrated no corresponding defects, which led to an interpretation of high probability for pulmonary embolism. There is abnormal activity in the liver, suggesting collateral circulation and vascular shunting. (**B**) The CTPA in the same patient demonstrates occlusion of the superior vena cava (*arrow*). In discordance with the VQ scan findings, no evidence of PE was identified on CTPA. (**C**) CTPA in the same patient demonstrates multiple perihepatic collateral vessels (*arrows*), explaining the abnormal liver activity present in the perfusion scan. (Reprinted with kind permission of Springer Science+Business Media from Juluru K, Eng J. Imaging in the Evaluation of Pulmonary Embolism. In Medina LS, Blackmore CC (eds): *Evidence-Based Imaging: Optimizing Imaging in Patient Care*. New York: Springer Science+Business Media, 2006.)

Protocols Based on the Evidence

The following protocols are employed at Johns Hopkins Hospital based on a literature review and clinical experience.

A. Ventilation/Perfusion Imaging

Ventilation imaging is performed prior to perfusion. After the patient takes one or two normal breaths through a mask, 10–30 mCi (370–1,110 MBq) of ^{133}Xe gas is introduced into the mask at end expiration. Images are obtained in anterior and posterior projections on a 128×128 matrix using a parallel-hole collimator centered at 80 keV. A single breath image is first obtained for 100,000 counts. Equilibrium images are obtained for 300,000 counts after the patient breathes normally in the closed system for 3 min. After obtaining three 5-s pre-washout images, the system is placed in washout phase, and twelve 5-s washout images are obtained, followed by four 1-min delayed washout images.

Perfusion imaging is performed after intravenous injection of 4 mCi (111 MBq) of technetium 99m (Tc-99m) macroaggregated albumin (MAA). Images are obtained in the posterior, right and left posterior oblique, right and left lateral, right and left anterior oblique, and anterior projections. All images are obtained for a minimum of 600,000 counts on a 256×256 matrix using a parallel hole collimator centered at 140 keV.

B. Computed Tomography Pulmonary Angiography

Computed tomography pulmonary angiography is performed with an intravenous injection of 100–120 cc nonionic iodinated contrast agent at a rate of 3–4 cc/s. The scan is performed from the lung apices to bases after a 23- to 28-s delay at 120 kV, 0.5-s rotation time, and 1- to 2-mm slice thickness. The mAs varies according to scanner manufacturer.

Future Research

- Assess the clinical significance of subsegmental emboli.
- Determine the performance of CTPA in the detection of PE, with attention to the benefits of MDCT over non-MDCT and safety. The PIOPED II study will address some of these important questions.
- Determine the performance and role of MRA in detection of PE.
- Further develop diagnostic algorithms that can adequately exclude PE while being safe and cost-effective.
- Clarify the role of imaging relative to other types of diagnostic tests.

Acknowledgments: The authors would like to specially thank Marge Sturgill and Christine Simmons for their help in obtaining many references used in writing this chapter.

References

1. Goldhaber SZ. Semin Vasc Med 2001;1:139–146.
2. Anderson FA, Wheeler HB, Goldberg RJ et al. Arch Intern Med 1991;151:933–938.
3. Oger E. Thromb Haemost 2000;83:657–660.
4. Caprini JA, Botteman MF, Stephens JM et al. Value Health 2003;6:59–74.
5. Nilsson T, Turen J, Billstrom A, Mare K, Carlsson A, Nyman U. Eur Radiol 1999;9(2):276–280.
6. van Beek EJ, Brouwerst EM, Song B, Stein PD, Oudkerk M. Clin Radiol 2001;56(10):838–842.
7. van Beek EJ, Reekers JA, Batchelor DA, Brandjes DP, Buller HR. Eur Radiol 1996;6(4):415–419.
8. van Rooij WJ, den Heeten GJ, Sluzewski M. Radiology 1995;195(3):793–797.
9. The PIOPED Investigators. JAMA 1990;263(20):2753–2759.
10. Hull RD, Raskob GE, Coates G, Panju AA. Chest 1990;97(1):23–26.
11. van Beek EJ, Kuyer PM, Schenk BE, Brandjes DP, ten Cate JW, Buller HR. Chest 1995;108(1):170–173.
12. Rajendran JG, Jacobson AF. Arch Intern Med 1999;159(4):349–352.
13. van Beek EJ, Brouwers EM, Song B, Bongaerts AH, Oudkerk M. Clin Appl Thromb Hemost 2001;7(2):87–92.
14. van Strijen MJ, de Monye W, Schiereck J et al. Ann Intern Med 2003;138(4):307–314.
15. Bourriot K, Couffinhal T, Bernard V, Montaudon M, Bonnet J, Laurent F. Chest 2003;123(2):359–365.
16. Kavanagh EC, O'Hare A, Hargaden G, Murray JG. AJR Am J Roentgenol 2004;182(2):499–504.
17. Remy-Jardin M, Tillie-Leblond I, Szapiro D et al. Eur Radiol 2002;12(8):1971–1978.

18. Gottschalk A, Stein PD, Goodman LR, Sostman HD. Semin Nucl Med 2002;32:173–182.
19. Swensen SJ, Sheedy PF II, Ryu JH et al. Mayo Clin Proc 2002;77(2):130–138.
20. Teigen CL, Maus TP, Sheedy PF II et al. Radiology 1995;194(2):313–319.
21. Loubeyre P, Revel D, Douek P et al. AJR Am J Roentgenol 1994;162(5):1035–1039.
22. Meaney JF, Weg JG, Chenevert TL, Stafford-Johnson D, Hamilton BH, Prince MR. N Engl J Med 1997;336(20):1422–1427.
23. Gupta A, Frazer CK, Ferguson JM et al. Radiology 1999;210(2):353–359.
24. Oudkerk M, van Beek EJ, Wielopolski P et al. Lancet 2002;359(9318):1643–1647.
25. Mohn K, Quiot JJ, Nonent M et al. J Ultrasound Med 2003;22(7):673–678; quiz 680–681.
26. Bova C, Greco F, Misuraca G et al. Am J Emerg Med 2003;21(3):180–183.
27. Kurzyna M, Torbicki A, Pruszczyk P et al. Am J Cardiol 2002;90(5):507–511.
28. Miniati M, Monti S, Pratali L et al. Am J Med 2001;110(7):528–535.
29. Steiner P, Lund GK, Debatin JF et al. AJR Am J Roentgenol 1996;167(4):931–936.
30. Worsley DF, Alavi A, Aronchick JM, Chen JT, Greenspan RH, Ravin CE. Radiology 1993;189(1):133–136.
31. Wells PS, Ginsberg JS, Anderson DR et al. Ann Intern Med 1998;129(12):997–1005.
32. Perrier A, Roy PM, Aujesky D et al. Am J Med 2004;116(5):291–299.
33. Lorut C, Ghossains M, Horellou MH, Achkar A, Fretault J, Laaban JP. Am J Respir Crit Care Med 2000;162(4 pt 1):1413–1418.
34. Kruip MJ, Slob MJ, Schijen JH, van der Heul C, Buller HR. Arch Intern Med 2002;162(14):1631–1635.
35. Leclercq MG, Lutisan JG, van Marwijk Kooy M et al. Thromb Haemost 2003;89(1):97–103.
36. Hull RD, Raskob GE, Ginsberg JS et al. Arch Intern Med 1994;154(3):289–297.
37. Wells PS, Anderson DR, Bormanis J et al. Lancet 1997;350(9094):1795–1798.
38. Eng J, et al. AJR 2004;183(6):1819–1827.

26

Aorta and Peripheral Vascular Disease

Max P. Rosen

I. Aorta: what are the appropriate imaging studies for suspected acute aortic dissection or traumatic rupture?

II. Aorta: what is the impact and cost-effectiveness of screening for abdominal aortic aneurysms on mortality from abdominal aortic aneurysms rupture?

III. Aorta: endovascular versus surgical treatment of abdominal aortic aneurysms: which is the best choice?

IV. Peripheral vascular disease: what are the appropriate noninvasive imaging studies for patients with suspected peripheral vascular disease?
   A. Magnetic resonance angiography
   B. Computed tomography angiography

V. Special case: evaluation of abdominal aortic aneurysms graft endoleak

VI. Special case: evaluation of the renal donor

VII. Special case: evaluation of renal artery stenosis

Issues

Key Points

- Due to the need for rapid diagnosis of patients with suspected acute aortic rupture or dissection, computed tomographic angiography (CTA) is preferable to magnetic resonance angiography (MRA) (limited evidence).
- Screening with ultrasound for abdominal aortic aneurysms (AAA) among men between the ages of 60 and 74 has been shown to be cost-effective with a mean cost-effectiveness ratio of £28,400 per life year gained (strong evidence).

M.P. Rosen (✉)
Department of Radiology, Beth Israel Deaconess Medical Center, Boston, MA 02215, USA
e-mail: mrosen2@bidmc.harvard.edu

L.S. Medina et al. (eds.), *Evidence-Based Imaging: Improving the Quality of Imaging in Patient Care, Revised Edition*, DOI 10.1007/978-1-4419-7777-9_26, © Springer Science+Business Media, LLC 2011

■ Endovascular repair of AAA has been shown to significantly reduce 30-day mortality from repair of AAA rupture. However, the procedural cost of endovascular repair is greater than that for open surgical repair (strong evidence).

■ CTA is preferred to catheter angiography for detection of aortic stent-graft endoleak (moderate evidence).

■ Computed tomographic angiography is comparable to MRA for evaluation of peripheral vascular disease (PVD) and for the preoperative evaluation of renal artery stenosis (moderate evidence).

■ The most cost-effective imaging strategy for the evaluation of the living renal donor varies and is dependent on the perspective of the analysis (renal donor or recipient), as well as the specificity of digital subtraction angiography (DSA) (moderate evidence).

Definition, Pathophysiology, and Epidemiology

Imaging of the aorta and PVD poses a unique set of challenges and benefits in medical imaging. For almost all clinical settings, the gold standard is catheter-based angiography. While advances in catheter design and imaging equipment over the past decade have greatly enhanced the field of diagnostic angiography, the basic tenets of the field have changed little in the past 20 years. Thus, there is an extensive body of literature based on catheter-based imaging. With the advent of multidetector CT scans and concurrent advances in MRA, CTA and MRA have become viable alternatives to catheter-based diagnostic angiography. However, unlike any other diagnostic modality, a catheter-based diagnostic study may rapidly be converted to an interventional procedure. Thus, any new modality for imaging the aorta or PVD must be compared to the gold standard of angiography, both for its diagnostic accuracy and for its cost-effectiveness in the context of immediately converting a catheter-based diagnostic study to a therapeutic intervention.

Aortic rupture is usually caused by blunt or penetrating trauma. Aortic dissection can be precipitated by traumatic or nontraumatic causes such as hypertension and aortitis; the latter may be infectious or inflammatory in nature. Aortic aneurysms are caused by a weakening in the aortic wall resulting in either saccular or fusiform dilatation.

While most AAAs are the result of atherosclerosis, they may also have traumatic, infectious, and inflammatory etiologies. In men over 65 years of age, ruptured AAAs are responsible for 2.1% of all deaths in England and Wales (1). Approximately 50% of these deaths occur before the patient reaches the hospital. Operative mortality for the 50% of patients with ruptured AAAs who reach the hospital alive is between 30 and 70%.

Peripheral vascular disease is most often caused by hypertension, diabetes, hypercholesterolemia, or cigarette smoking and can be classified as either acute or chronic. Acute limb ischemia (ALI) is defined as a sudden decrease in limb perfusion that may result in threatened viability of the extremity. Chronic manifestations of peripheral arterial disease (PAD) are divided clinically into (1) intermittent claudication and (2) chronic critical limb ischemia.

Overall Cost to Society

Data on the societal cost of imaging for these indications is not available, except for the cost-effectiveness of screening for AAA with ultrasound among men 65–74 years of age (see section "II. Aorta", below).

Goals

The goals and method of imaging of the aorta and peripheral vascular branches depend on the clinical setting. In the case of suspected traumatic injury or aortic dissection, the goal of imaging is twofold. The most immediate goal is to identify as quickly as possible the patients in need of immediate surgical repair. The secondary goal in this acute setting is to help the surgeon identify the extent of vascular injury and plan the appropriate repair.

The goal of screening asymptomatic patients for AAA is to identify patients with AAA and provide immediate intervention if the size of the AAA at the time of screening warrants repair. For those patients with AAA, the size of which does not warrant immediate repair, the goal of screening is to identify any change in the size of the AAA over time, and to initiate therapy when the rate of expansion of the AAA reaches a threshold that justifies repair.

When vascular insufficiency or ischemia is suspected, the goal of imaging is to identify the level and extent of the stenosis or occlusion. The optimal imaging strategy is somewhat dependent on the most likely method for intervention. If a catheter-based intervention is likely, then a catheter-based imaging study is often warranted as the initial imaging study. On the other hand, if a surgical intervention is likely, then a less invasive initial imaging study such as CTA or MRA may be optimal.

Methodology

PubMed searches for the following index terms were performed from January 2000 to August 2004: *computed tomography (CT) angiography, magnetic resonance (MR), vascular studies, arteries, stenosis* or *occlusion, angiography, comparative studies, aneurysms, aortic, cost-effectiveness,* and *abdominal aortic aneurysms.* Relevant articles in English were obtained and read for appropriateness. The search was limited to articles published in January 2000 or later to ensure that only studies employing current noninvasive technologies would be included. Selected articles published before 2000 and after August 2004 (2) were also included at the time of manuscript review by the book's editors.

I. Aorta: What Are the Appropriate Imaging Studies for Suspected Acute Aortic Dissection or Traumatic Rupture?

Summary of Evidence: Due to the need for rapid diagnosis of patients with suspected acute aortic rupture or dissection (Fig. 26.1), CTA is preferable to MRA. Most modern emergency departments are equipped with helical CT scanners, and unlike MRA, CTA of the entire aorta can be performed in a less than 60s.

Supporting Evidence: Yoshida et al. (3) assessed the sensitivity, specificity, and accuracy of CTA among 57 patients with surgically proven type A dissection who underwent helical CT, and reported 100% sensitivity of helical CT to detect aortic dissection in the thoracic aorta. Sensitivity for detection of arch branch vessel involvement was 95 and 83% for detection of pericardial effusion. (The authors explain that the lower sensitivity for detection of pericardial effusion may be due to the delay between CTA and surgery, with the pericardial effusion developing during the delay.) Due to the lack of reported follow-up of the 64 patients in whom the CTA did not show dissection, this study represents limited (level III) evidence. Several other studies support the use of CTA to exclude aortic injury (4, 5), but are based on older single detector technology. Although not commonly available in emergency situations, Pereles et al. (6) reported excellent 100% sensitivity for diagnosis of thoracic aortic dissection using true fast imaging with steady-state precision (FISP).

Cost-Effectiveness Analysis: An older paper by Hunink and Bos (7) published in 1995 evaluated the cost-effectiveness of CT compared with plain film chest radiography and immediate angiography in deciding when angiography should be performed in hemodynamically stable patients with suspected aortic injury after blunt chest trauma. This study was performed before the widespread use of multidetector CT, and investigated the use of CT as a triage tool rather than as a definitive diagnostic study. The authors conclude that selecting patients for triage to angiography based on the CT findings yielded higher effectiveness at a lower cost-effectiveness ratio than doing so based on chest radiographs, and that the incremental cost-effectiveness ratio was $242,000 per life saved for the strategy of CT followed by angiography for positive cases.

II. Aorta: What Is the Impact and Cost-Effectiveness of Screening for Abdominal Aortic Aneurysms on Mortality from Abdominal Aortic Aneurysms Rupture?

Summary of Evidence: The Multicenter Aneurysm Screening Study (MASS) (1) investigated the impact of ultrasound screening for AAA in a population of 67,800 men between the ages of

65 and 74 years. The study was a randomized controlled study conducted at four centers in the United Kingdom and provides strong evidence that screening for AAA with ultrasound significantly reduced AAA related deaths.

Supporting Evidence: The MASS group (1) investigated the effect of AAA screening on mortality in men using a randomized controlled trial design of 67,800 men aged 65–74 years. Men in whom AAA (>3 cm in diameter) were detected were followed with repeat ultrasound for a mean of 4.1 years. Surgery was considered if the diameter of the AAA was >5.5 cm or if the AAA expanded >1 cm/year, or if symptoms related to the AAA developed. Health-related quality of life was measured using the standardized medical Outcomes Study short-form 36-item survey (SF-36) (8) and the EuroQol EQ-5D (9). The primary outcome measure was mortality related to AAA.

There were 65 (0.19%) AAA-related deaths in the screened group, and 113 (0.33%) in the control group ($p = 0.0002$) with a 53% risk reduction [95% confidence interval (CI), 30–64%] among those who underwent screening. Thirty-day mortality following elective surgery was 6% versus 37% following emergency surgery.

Cost-Effectiveness Analysis: Data from the MASS study (1) were used to estimate the cost-effectiveness of AAA screening using ultrasound over a 4-year period and they provide strong evidence. Costs included in the analysis were costs associated with the initial screening program: clinic staff and study administration, office space, equipment, and costs associated with any follow-up scans. Costs associated with surgery were calculated from the actual costs incurred by the cohort of patients who underwent surgery and any hospital admission during the 12 months after surgery. No costs related to patient death from aneurysm rupture were included if the patient had not been admitted to the hospital for attempted emergency surgery. Cost-effectiveness was measured as survival free from mortality related to AAA for each patient for up to 4 years and was expressed as incremental cost per additional life year gained.

Over 4 years, the mean estimated cost-effectiveness ratio for screening was $51,000 per life year gained, equivalent to $64,600 per quality-adjusted life year (QALY) gained.

III. Aorta: Endovascular Versus Surgical Treatment of Abdominal Aortic Aneurysms: Which Is the Best Choice?

Summary of Evidence: Endovascular treatment of AAA is associated with a significant reduction in 30-day mortality and hospital length of stay, compared to surgical repair. However, the cost of endovascular repair is greater than that of surgical repair, due to the cost of the endograft (strong evidence).

Supporting Evidence: Several recent papers have addressed the clinical effectiveness of endovascular aneurysm repair (EVAR) (10) and calculated the cost-effectiveness of EVAR compared to standard therapy. The short-term (30-day) outcome of patients treated with EVAR has been reported from a prospective registry in which 611 patients were enrolled at 31 centers in the UK (11). The aneurysm was successfully excluded in 465/611 (76%) of patients. Additional endovascular procedures were required in 71/611 (12%) and additional surgical procedures were required in 30/611 (5%). An additional 32/611 (5%) patients required conversion to open repair. Thirty-day complication rates were as follows: technical, 6%; wound complications, 8%; renal failure, 4%; and other medical complications, 13%. Thirty-day mortality for all patients was 6.6%. For patients considered fit, 30-day mortality was 4%, but increased to 18% for unfit patients. Complications of persistent endoleaks and 30-day mortality were significantly greater for AAAs > 6 cm than for AAAs ≤ 6 cm.

Zeebregts et al. (12) compared the outcome of AAA repair with EVAR ($n = 93$) versus open surgical repair ($n = 195$) in a nonrandomized prospective trial. All consecutive patients undergoing AAA repair at one institution during a 10-year period were included in the study. Detailed patient characteristics of the two groups were not provided, but the authors state, "The study confirmed that patients were mainly selected on anatomic grounds to undergo either open repair or EVAR." Compared to open surgical repair, patients undergoing EVAR had significantly ($p < 0.05$) shorter stays in the intensive care unit (ICU); shorter hospital stays; fewer bleeding complications, pulmonary complications, and episodes of multiple organ failure; and lesser 30-day morality.

A randomized controlled trial (EVAR 1 trial) (13), comparing EVAR with open repair, has recently been reported in which 1,082 elective patients (age >60 with AAA diameter >5.5 cm) were randomized to receive either EVAR ($n = 543$) or open repair ($n = 39$) at 41 British hospitals. Thirty-day mortality by intention to treat was the outcome reported and was significantly less in the EVAR group, 1.7% (9/531), compared to 4.7% (24/516) in the open group (odds ratio 0.35; 95% CI, 0.16–0.77; $p = 0.009$).

A second, multicenter trial, the Dutch Randomized Endovascular Aneurysm Management (DREAM) trial (14) is also being conducted with 345 patients enrolled. Initial results from 153 patients at 1 year demonstrated cumulative survival of 95% in the EVAR group compared to 89% in the operative group, ($p = 0.21$). The cumulative event-free survival at 12 months was 76% in the EVAR group and 72% in the operative group. Data from all 345 patients analyzed from the point of view of 30-day mortality found that endovascular repair was associated with a lower 30-day mortality, 1.2% (95% CI, 0.1–4.2%), compared to 4.6% (95% CI, 2.0–8.9%) for open repair, resulting in a risk ratio of 3.9 (95% CI, 0.9–32.9) (15). The DREAM trial has also reported quality of life (QoL) using the SF-36 and EuroQol(-)5D questionnaires at regular intervals during the first year (16). From 6 months onward the operative group reported a significantly higher score on the EuroQol EQ-5D than the EVAR group ($p = 0.045$).

The cost of EVAR has been compared to open repair using data from a retrospective analysis of 131 patients undergoing AAA repair and 49 patients undergoing open repair as part of a US Food and Drug Administration phase II prospective multicenter study (17). Total inpatient hospital costs of EVAR were significantly higher than that of open repair ($19,985 ± $7,396 vs. $12,546 ± $5,944, $p = 0.0001$). The cost of the Endograft ($10,400) accounted for 52% of the total cost of EVAR.

Cost-Effectiveness Analysis: While the expected robust cost-effectiveness data from the EVAR 1 and EVAR 2 trials has not yet been published, moderate data calculating the cost per hospital day saved of EVAR versus open repair from a single institution in which seven patients

underwent EVAR and 31 patients underwent open repair have been reported (18). The mean total cost for EVAR ($14,967) was significantly greater than that for open repair ($4,823) ($p = 0.004$), even though the mean length of stay for the EVAR group (2.09 days) was significantly less than the mean length of stay for the open repair group (4.45 days) ($p = 0.009$). The cost of the Endograft accounted for 57% of the total cost of EVAR. The cost of reducing the hospital stay by 1 day by performing EVAR was $1,604.

IV. Peripheral Vascular Disease: What Are the Appropriate Noninvasive Imaging Studies for Patients with Suspected Peripheral Vascular Disease?

MRA and CT angiography are the most commonly used noninvasive imaging studies in PVD.

A. Magnetic Resonance Angiography

Summary of Evidence: Numerous studies compare various MRA techniques with catheter angiography for evaluation of patients with suspected PVD. However, almost all of these studies provide only limited evidence in support of MRA. Many studies are retrospective and suffer from selection bias. Further complicating the analysis is a lack of standardization in the reporting of arterial segments.

Supporting Evidence: Several studies compare the sensitivity and specificity of MRA with DSA. However, synthesizing these studies into a comprehensive summary is difficult, due to heterogeneous patient populations, disparate reporting methods, and variations in MRA technique. For example, among patients with known or suspected PVD, Loewe et al. (19) reported positive and negative predictive values for overall stenosis detection of 91.2 and 97.3%, respectively. However, when nondiagnostic segments were included, the positive and negative predictive values decreased to 89.9 and 95.9%, respectively. Binkert et al. (20) compared the diagnostic accuracy of dedicated calf MRA versus standard bolus-chase MRA with catheter angiography and found that dedicated calf studies were superior to standard bolus-chase MRA, 81.5 versus 67.8% (reader 1) and 79.1 versus 63.4% (reader 2). Among patients with symptoms and signs of aortoiliac occlusion, MRA has been shown to yield sensitivity of 87.5% and specificity of 100% for diagnosing aortic occlusion, compared to catheter angiography (21). In a retrospective study of 45 patients with lower-limb ischemia at high risk for catheter angiography, none of 28 who subsequently underwent above-knee surgical reconstruction required complementary catheter angiography. However, in seven of ten patients who underwent below-knee surgical reconstruction, pre- or intraoperative catheter angiography was required (22). Khilnani et al. (23) retrospectively compared the concordance of three readers' selection of inflow and outflow segments for preoperative treatment planning with MRA and catheter angiography and found that the mean percentage of agreement between MRA and catheter angiography ranged from 91 to 97%.

B. Computed Tomography Angiography

Summary of Evidence: There is limited evidence supporting the diagnostic accuracy of CTA for the evaluation of patients with suspected PVD. Compared to MRA, there is less variability in CTA protocols and techniques, which reduces some of the variability in study design. The current literature reports diagnostic performance of four-row multidetector CT (MDCT), which is currently being replaced by up to 32- to 64-row MDCT.

Supporting Evidence: An initial study of the technical feasibility of MDCT for the evaluation of lower extremity arterial inflow and runoff was published in 2001 (24). The study evaluated patients with symptomatic lower extremity arterial occlusive ($n = 19$) or aneurysmal disease ($n = 5$). Indications for CTA among the 19 patients with suspected occlusive disease included calf or thigh claudication, nonhealing foot ulcers, or gangrene. Eighteen of the 24 patients underwent conventional angiography within 3 months of the CTA. The authors reported the degree of arterial enhancement and the number of arterial segments analyzable

with CTA. As the scope of this study was limited to technical issues, sensitivity and specificity were not reported.

A more clinically relevant paper was published in 2004 by Romano et al. (25) in which they compared the diagnostic accuracy of four-row multidetector CTA (MDCTA) with DSA in patients with peripheral occlusive disease. Forty-two patients underwent MDCTA and DSA within 5 days. Images were blindly interpreted by two radiologists. The overall sensitivity and specificity of MDCTA, compared to DSA, was 93 and 95%, respectively. Positive and negative predictive values were 90 and 97%, respectively. The accuracy of MDCT for each anatomic segment is provided in Table 26.1.

Normal arterial segments and 100% occluded segments were correctly identified in all cases by MDCT. Almost all cases in which the degree of arterial segment stenosis was misinterpreted were in the calf; 58% of misinterpreted stenotic segments were false positive and 42% were false negative. Interobserver agreement (κ) for DSA and MDCT were 0.817 and 0.802, respectively, and for MDCT versus DSA were 0.835 and 0.857 for reader 1 and reader 2, respectively.

Cost-Effectiveness Analysis: None available.

V. Special Case: Evaluation of Abdominal Aortic Aneurysms Graft Endoleak

Summary of Evidence: Immediate complications of endoluminal stent-graft placement for treatment of AAA include perigraft leaks (Fig. 26.2), occlusion of aortic branches, stent-graft collapse, incomplete stent-graft deployment, and graft thrombosis. Of these complications, perigraft leak is the most common. Endoleaks are classified according to their origin: type I, incomplete attachment; type II, retrograde filling; type III, device degeneration or junctional dehiscence; type IV, transient graft porosity; and type V, continued expansion of the aneurysm without detectable endoleak (endotension) (26). Type I, II, and III endoleaks are often amenable to treatment with a secondary endovascular procedure, whereas type V endoleaks must be corrected with surgical repair. Compared with catheter angiography, CTA has much greater sensitivity and specificity in detecting endoleaks and is the preferred method for imaging a patient with suspected endoleak. However, if an endoleak is detected during CTA, and the etiology of the endoleak is not demonstrated; in a 2004 case report of two patients (15), MR angiography identified the cause of an endoleak that was not detectable by CTA (limited evidence). The data provided from this single study provides moderate evidence in support of CTA as the modality of choice for evaluating patients with suspected endograft leak.

Supporting Evidence: Amerding et al. (27) conducted a retrospective, blinded study comparing the sensitivity and specificity of CTA and catheter angiography in detecting immediate complications of endoluminal stent-graft placement for treatment of AAA. The most common complication, perigraft leak, was observed in 20/46 (43%) of patients. All patients underwent both CTA and conventional angiography and each modality was reviewed by three independent reviewers. The reference standard interpretation was developed by consensus of a CT radiologist and the primary angiographer. Mean sensitivity and specificity for detecting perigraft leaks were 63% (range, 60–70%) and 77% (range, 58–100%) for catheter angiography and 92% (range, 80–100%) and 90% (range, 85–92%) for CTA. The mean k value for interpretation of catheter angiography was 0.41 (range, 0.27–0.63) and 0.81 (range, 0.73–0.91) for CTA. Wicky et al. (26) reported two cases in which the cause of an endoleak was not detected on CTA, but was detected on MRA.

Cost-Effectiveness Analysis: Not available.

VI. Special Case: Evaluation of the Renal Donor

Summary of Evidence: Several studies reported the sensitivity and specificity of CTA and MRA in identifying anatomic variations and arterial stenosis or occlusion, which are needed prior to selecting a donor kidney from a living donor. However, these studies only provide limited evidence, as most studies lack a gold standard (i.e., surgical confirmation of the anatomy of

the kidney that was not chosen as the donor). The majority of these studies simply report the interobserver agreement between two preoperative imaging modalities. However, using existing data from the literature, Liem et al. (28) evaluated the cost-effectiveness of several imaging strategies for the preoperative evaluation of living renal donors.

Supporting Evidence: Halpern et al. (29) compared CTA and MRA in the preoperative evaluation of living renal donors in which 35 donors underwent preoperative assessment with both CTA and gadolinium-enhanced MRA. Both CTA and MRA studies were evaluated by two independent reviewers and the following data were recorded: number and size of renal arteries found on each side, presence of arterial stenosis or a proximal arterial branch, and the anatomy of renal veins and ureters. Forty-one patients initially enrolled in the study, but only six underwent CTA. Surgical correlation with the transplanted kidney was available for 18 kidneys. The k-value for interobserver agreement for MRA was 0.74 and for CTA was 0.73, and for agreement between MRA and CTA was 0.74. Among the 18 kidneys for which surgical correlation was available, one proximal arterial branch to a left kidney was missed at both CTA and MRA, and two very small (<1 mm) accessory arteries suggested at CTA were not found at nephrectomy.

Rankin et al. (30) reported the correlation between CTA or gadolinium-enhanced MRA with findings at nephrectomy for living related kidney donors. Unlike the study of Halpern et al. (29), patients underwent either CTA or MRA. Both CTA and MRA were 100% sensitive in identifying the main renal arteries and renal veins; CTA visualized 37/40 arteries identified at surgery for a detection rate of 93%, and MRA visualized 18/20 arteries identified at surgery, for a detection rate of 90%.

Cost-Effectiveness Analysis: Liem et al. (28) reported a decision- and cost-effectiveness for the evaluation of living renal donors. Their conclusion depends on the perspective (donor versus recipient) and on the specificity of DSA. For the donor, MRA dominated all other strategies (DSA, CTA, DSA with MRA, MRA with CTA, no testing and transplantation always performed, and no testing and no transplantation performed). For the recipient, DSA and

DSA with MRA, both performed the same day, dominated all other strategies. For both donor and recipient (combined results) DSA dominated all other strategies. If the specificity of DSA was less than 99% for detection of renal disease, MRA with CTA performed the same day was superior. The authors point out the limitations of their study, which include that their model was based on multiple data sources, some of which may be subject to publication bias. Imaging protocols for each of the techniques varied among transplant centers. In addition, all cost data utilized in the analysis was obtained from their own center.

VII. Special Case: Evaluation of Renal Artery Stenosis

Summary of Evidence: There is no statistical difference between three-dimensional (3D) MRA and multidetector row CTA in the detection of hemodynamically significant renal artery stenosis identified in the current literature.

Supporting Evidence: Willmann et al. (31) reported the diagnostic performance of MRA compared with DSA in the detection of hemodynamically renal artery stenosis in 46 patients. Two independent readers participated in the study. The sensitivity for readers one and two were 86% (95% CI, 64–100%) and 100% (95% CI, 99–100%), respectively, and the specificity was 100% (95% CI, 99–100%) and 100% (95% CI, 95–100%), respectively. Stueckle et al. (32) reported the performance of CTA compared to DSA for identification of renal artery aneurysms, low- and high-grade renal artery stenosis, and renal artery occlusion. Data were reported for axial, 3D volume reconstruction and multiplanar imaging (MPI) CTA techniques. Compared to DSA, MPI achieved the greatest sensitivity (100%) and specificity (100%) for detection of low- and high-grade renal artery stenosis, as well as arterial occlusion.

Cost-Effectiveness Analysis: None available.

Take Home Tables and Figures

Tables 26.1–26.2 and Fig. 26.1–26.2 serve to highlight key recommendations and supporting evidence.

Table 26.1. Accuracy of multidetector computed tomography (MDCT), compared to digital subtraction angiography (DSA), according to anatomic segment (25)

	Sensitivity	Specificity	PPV	NPV	Diagnostic accuracy
Aortoiliac	95	99	99	97	98
Femoropopliteal	94	97	96	97	97
Infrapopliteal	85	92	74	96	89

PPV positive predictive value, *NPV* negative predictive value.
Reprinted with kind permission of Springer Science+Business Media from Rosen MP. Aorta and Peripheral Vascular Disease. In Medina LS, Blackmore CC (eds): *Evidence-Based Imaging: Optimizing Imaging in Patient Care.* New York: Springer Science+Business Media, 2006.

Table 26.2. Take-home table: questions and answers

Question	Answer	Level of evidence
What is the appropriate imaging study for suspected aortic injury?	CT angiography	Limited
Is screening for AAA with ultrasound cost-effective?	The MASS (1) study has shown a significant reduction in mortality from AAA among patients who underwent ultrasound screening The mean cost-effectiveness ratio for screening was £28,400 per life-year gained	Strong
Endovascular versus surgical repair of AAA – what is the best choice?	Endovascular repair of AAA has been shown to be associated with a significant reduction in mortality when compared with open surgical repair. However, the cost of endovascular repair is greater than that of open repair, mainly due to the cost of the stent-graft	Strong
What is the appropriate noninvasive imaging study for suspected peripheral vascular disease (PVD)?	Studies of CTA and MRA for PVD are limited to reporting the sensitivity and specificity of CTA and MRA compared to catheter angiography	Limited
What is the best way to evaluate the patient with suspected AAA endograft leak?	CTA is preferred to catheter angiography, with MRA reserved for cases in which the cause of the endoleak is not evident on CTA	Moderate
What is the best noninvasive imaging study for evaluation of the renal donor?	The most cost-effective imaging strategy varies and is dependent on the perspective of the analysis (renal donor or recipient), as well as the specificity of digital subtraction angiography (DSA)	Moderate
What is best noninvasive imaging study for evaluation of renal artery stenosis?	CTA and MRA are comparable MRA is preferred for the patients with impaired renal function	Moderate

Reprinted with kind permission of Springer Science+Business Media from Rosen MP. Aorta and Peripheral Vascular Disease. In Medina LS, Blackmore CC (eds): *Evidence-Based Imaging: Optimizing Imaging in Patient Care*. New York: Springer Science+Business Media, 2006.

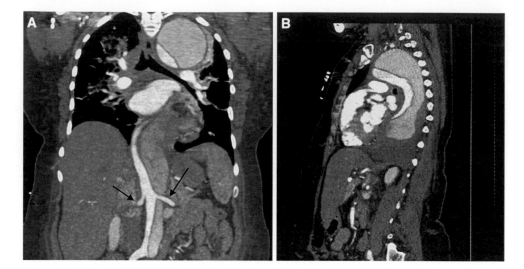

Figure 26.1. Coronal (**A**) and sagittal (**B**) computed tomographic angiography (CTA) demonstrating type B aortic dissection. Both renal arteries are supplied from the true lumen (*arrows*). (Reprinted with kind permission of Springer Science+Business Media from Rosen MP. Aorta and Peripheral Vascular Disease. In Medina LS, Blackmore CC (eds): *Evidence-Based Imaging: Optimizing Imaging in Patient Care.* New York: Springer Science+Business Media, 2006.)

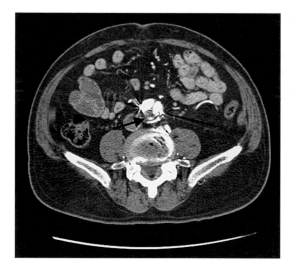

Figure 26.2. Axial CT scan cephalad to the aortic bifurcation. High density within the posterior aspect of the aorta represents an endoleak (*arrow*). (Reprinted with kind permission of Springer Science+Business Media from Rosen MP. Aorta and Peripheral Vascular Disease. In Medina LS, Blackmore CC (eds): *Evidence-Based Imaging: Optimizing Imaging in Patient Care.* New York: Springer Science+Business Media, 2006.)

Future Research

The following studies are needed to further define the cost-effectiveness of imaging of the aorta and PVD:

- Impact of CTA and MRA on treatment planning for patients with suspected PVD.
- Impact of CTA and MRA on outcome for patients evaluated for suspected renal artery stenosis.
- Standardization of CTA and MRA techniques to allow for more direct comparison of studies performed at different institutions.

Acknowledgment Dr. Bertrand Janne contributed to the definition and pathophysiology of peripheral vascular disease.

References

1. Multicenter Aneurysm Screening Study Group. Lancet 2002;360:1531–1539.
2. Olin JW, Kaufman JA, Bluemke DA et al. Circulation 2004;109:2626–2633.
3. Yoshida S, Akiba H, Tamakawa M et al. Radiology 2003;228:430–435.
4. Dyer DS, Moore EE, Mestek MF et al. Radiology 1999;213:195–202.
5. Fabian TC, Davis KA, Gavant ML et al. Ann Surg 1998;227:666–676.
6. Pereles FS, McCarthy RM, Baskaran V et al. Radiology 2002;223:270–274.
7. Hunink MG, Bos JJ. AJR Am J Roentgenol 1995;165:27–36.
8. Ware Jr., JE, Sherbourne CD. Med Care 1992;30: 473–483.
9. Rabin R, de Charro F. Ann Med 2001;33:337–343.
10. Brown LC, Epstein D, Manca A, Beard JD, Powel JT, Greenhalgh RM. Eur J Vasc Endovasc Surg 2004;27:372–381.
11. Thomas SM, Gaines PA, Beard JD. Eur J Vasc Endovasc Surg 2001;21:57–64.
12. Zeebregts CJ, Geelkerken RH, van der Palen J, Huisman AAB, de Smit P, van Det RJ. Br J Surg 2004;91:563–568.
13. The EVAR Trial Participants. Lancet 2004;364: 843–848.
14. Prinssen M, Buskens E, Blankensteijn JD. J Cardiovasc Surg (Torino) 2002;43:379–384.
15. Prinssen M, Verhoeven ELG, Buth J et al. N Engl J Med 2004;351:1607–1618.
16. Prinssen M, Buskens E, Blankensteijn JD, on behalf of the DREAM Trial Participants. Eur J Vasc Endovasc Surg 2004;27:121–127.
17. Sternbergh WC, Money SR. J Vasc Surg 2000;31: 237–244.
18. Forbes TL, DeRose G, Kribs S, Harris KA. Can J Surg 2002;45:420–424.
19. Loewe C, Schoder M, Rand T et al. AJR Am J Roentgenol 2002;179:1013–1021.
20. Binkert CA, Baker PD, Petersen BD, Szumowski J, Kaufman JA. Radiology 2004;232:860–866.
21. Torreggiani WC, Varghese J, Haslam P, McGrath F, Munk PL, Lee MJ. Clin Radiol 2002;57:625–632.
22. Brillet PY, Vayssairat V, Tassart M et al. J Vasc Interv Radiol 2002;14:1139–1145.
23. Khilnani NM, Winchester PA, Prince MR et al. Radiology 2002;224:63–74.
24. Rubin GD, Schmidt AJ, Logan RT, Sofilos MC. Radiology 2001;221:146–158.
25. Romano M, Mainenti PP, Imbriaco M et al. Eur J Radiol 2004;50:303–308.
26. Wicky S, Fan CM, Geller SC, Greenfield A, Santilli J, Waltman AC. AJR Am J Roentgenol 2003;181:736–738.
27. Armerding MD, Rubin GD, Beaulieu CF et al. Radiology 2000;215:138–146.
28. Liem YS, Kock MCJM, Ijzermans JNM, Weimar W, Visser K, Hunink MGM. Radiology 2003;226: 53–62.
29. Halpern EJ, Mitchell DG, Wechsler RJ, Outwater EK, Moritz MJ, Wilson GA. Radiology 2000;216: 434–439.
30. Rankin SC, Jan W, Koffman CG. AJT Am J Roentgenol 2001;177:349–355.
31. Willmann JK, Wildermuth S, Pfamatter T et al. Radiology 2003;226:798–811.
32. Stueckle CA, Haegele KF, Jendreck M et al. Australas Radiol 2004;48:142–147.

27

Imaging of the Cervical Carotid Artery for Atherosclerotic Stenosis

Alex M. Barrocas and Colin P. Derdeyn

I. What is the imaging modality of choice in symptomatic carotid stenosis? A. Catheter angiography B. Magnetic resonance angiography C. Computer tomography angiography D. Doppler ultrasound II. What is the imaging modality of choice in asymptomatic carotid stenosis? A. Cost-effectiveness analysis III. What is the role of carotid angioplasty and stenting? IV. What is the role of physiologic imaging in carotid stenosis and occlusion? A. Methods of hemodynamic assessment B. Association with stroke risk C. Cost-effectiveness analysis	**Issues**

▪ At present, carotid imaging is performed to identify the presence and measure the degree of atherosclerotic stenosis, in order to select appropriate candidates for surgical endarterectomy (strong evidence). Several different imaging strategies may be employed in symptomatic patients: Catheter angiography (CA) may be used for this purpose (strong evidence).	**Key Points**

C.P. Derdeyn (✉)
Mallinckrodt Institute of Radiology, Washington University School of Medicine, 510 S. Kingshighway,
St. Louis, MO 63110, USA
e-mail: derdeync@wustl.edu

L.S. Medina et al. (eds.), *Evidence-Based Imaging: Improving the Quality of Imaging in Patient Care, Revised Edition,*   **451**
DOI 10.1007/978-1-4419-7777-9_27, © Springer Science+Business Media, LLC 2011

> Doppler ultrasound (DUS), magnetic resonance angiography (MRA), and computed tomography angiography(CTA), or some combination, if adequately validated, may be used to screen patients (those with less than 50% stenosis) prior to CA (moderate evidence).
>
> Doppler ultrasound, MRA, and CTA, or some combination, if adequately validated, may be used to identify patients with severe stenosis (greater than 80%) for surgical endarterectomy (moderate evidence).
>
> ■ Screening of asymptomatic patients with noninvasive methods and highly specific thresholds may be cost-effective in certain high-risk populations, such as patients with known atherosclerotic disease in other circulations or the presence of bruit over the carotid artery on physical examination (moderate evidence).
>
> ■ More information regarding the safety and efficacy of angioplasty and stenting relative to surgical endarterectomy is expected in the near future. As treatment may be incorporated into the diagnostic catheter angiographic procedure, these recommendations may be revised.
>
> ■ Physiologic imaging tools identify higher-risk subgroups in patients with atherosclerotic carotid stenosis and occlusion (strong evidence).
>
> ■ The use of these physiologic imaging tools to improve guide therapy and improve outcome is unproven (insufficient evidence). A randomized clinical trial is underway for surgical revascularization of carotid occlusion in patients selected by positron emission tomography (PET).

Definition and Pathophysiology

Extracranial carotid bifurcation atherosclerotic disease is associated with ischemic stroke. The bifurcation of the common carotid artery into internal and external carotid arteries is a preferred site for the development of atherosclerotic plaque. Several biomechanical and physiologic factors are involved in the formation of atheroma at this location (1). As the atherosclerotic plaque builds, it can lead to ischemic stroke via two interrelated mechanisms: embolism and hemodynamic impairment. Embolism of plaque debris or thrombus that develops in or on the plaque may break free and lodge in a distal artery of the brain. Embolism likely accounts for the majority of stroke that occurs in association with carotid atherosclerotic disease. The second mechanism is that of low flow (2). Depending on the adequacy of collateral flow, primarily determined by the status of the circle of Willis, severe stenosis may limit the flow of blood to the distal cerebral hemisphere. Significant hemodynamic impairment due to severe stenosis or occlusion at the carotid bifurcation is an independent predictor of stroke, likely due to synergistic effects with embolic events. Primary

hemodynamic or low-flow stroke may also occur, but is uncommon relative to primary embolic or synergistic embolic and hemodynamic mechanisms.

At present, only the degree of luminal diameter narrowing as measured by CA has been proven as a predictor of outcome in large-scale clinical trials of intervention vs. medical therapy (3, 4). Many other features of atherosclerotic plaque, including length of stenosis, cross-sectional area reduction, blood flow velocity, and plaque ulceration or irregularity have been associated with higher risks of stroke on medical treatment, but none has been proven in randomized clinical trials as predictors of stroke risk.

Epidemiology

First-ever or recurrent ischemic stroke affects approximately 750,000 people in North America annually (5). A larger number of patients present with transient ischemic attacks (TIA), rather than a completed stroke. Associated carotid bifurcation disease is involved in 20–30% of patients with these neurologic symptoms (6).

Clinical trials of surgical endarterectomy in symptomatic patients (TIA and stroke) with severe stenosis (measured by CA) have shown substantial benefit for secondary stroke prevention over medical therapy (7). The issue of carotid imaging is relevant both for this population, for the purpose of secondary stroke prevention, as well as for patients with asymptomatic carotid stenosis. Asymptomatic carotid stenosis is present in up to 20% of patients with prior myocardial infarction or peripheral vascular disease.

period 1966 to June 2004. Search terms included combinations of the following key words: *carotid, stenosis, imaging, ultrasound, angiography, magnetic resonance, computed tomography, stroke,* and *ischemia*. Additional articles were identified from the reference lists of these papers. The review was limited to human studies and English-language literature. Abstracts and titles of articles were reviewed for relevance to this topic. Relevant articles were reviewed in full.

Overall Cost to Society

In 1999 the American Heart Association (AHA) estimated the total economic burden for stroke to be $51 billion. The large majority of this cost is for acute and long-term care after stroke. Consequently, even expensive diagnostic evaluation and expensive treatments aimed at primary or secondary stroke prevention are often cost-effective. For example, a recent analysis found that screening patients with complete occlusion of the carotid artery with a PET study of cerebral blood flow (CBF) and oxygen use followed by selective extracranial to intracranial arterial bypass for those patients with severe hemodynamic impairment would be cost effective (8).

Goals

The overall goal of carotid imaging is identifying appropriate candidates for surgical or endovascular revascularization. Patients with insignificant degrees of stenosis are treated medically. Imaging must detect, localize, and accurately measure the degree of stenosis in order to accomplish this goal.

Methodology

PubMed (National Library of Medicine, Bethesda, MD) was used to search for original research publications investigating the diagnostic performance and effectiveness of imaging strategies for the extracranial carotid artery bifurcation. The search included the

I. What Is the Imaging Modality of Choice in Symptomatic Carotid Stenosis?

Summary of Evidence: At present, carotid imaging is performed to identify the presence and measure the degree of atherosclerotic stenosis, in order to select appropriate candidates for surgical endarterectomy (strong evidence). Several different imaging strategies may be employed in symptomatic patients:

- Catheter angiography can be used for this purpose (strong evidence).
- Doppler ultrasound, MRA, and CTA, or some combination, if adequately validated at the local institution with quality assurance data, may be used to screen patients for those with less than 50% stenosis prior to CA (moderate evidence).
- DUS or MRA, alone or in combination, if adequately validated locally, may be used to identify patients for surgical endarterectomy (limited evidence).
- DUS or MRA can be used both to screen for patients with less than 50% stenosis and reliably identify patients with severe, >80% stenosis. CA is used to investigate the degree of stenosis for the remaining patients (moderate evidence).

Supporting Evidence: Patients presenting with focal ischemic symptoms, either ocular or cerebral, or permanent or temporary, are considered symptomatic. High-grade carotid stenosis is common in patients with anterior circulation ischemic symptoms (6, 9). Carotid endarterectomy is highly effective in reducing stroke risk in patients with ≥70% stenosis. This has been established by two large multicenter randomized trials of endarterectomy vs. best medical therapy (level I, strong evidence) (3, 4). The decision for surgery for patients with 50–69% stenosis should consider other risk factors, as the benefit is not dramatic. Males, patients with recent symptoms, and cerebral rather than ocular ischemic symptoms have greater benefit with surgery.

Both the North American Symptomatic Carotid Endarterectomy Trial (NASCET) and the European Carotid Surgery Trial (ECST) used CA to select patients for surgery (3, 4). The degree of stenosis by deciles was correlated with surgical benefit in both studies. The use of CA, therefore, has been correlated to clinical outcome in a way that no other noninvasive imaging modality has been or will be validated (level I, strong evidence).

The use of noninvasive screening tools to reduce or eliminate the need for CA has been extensively investigated. These imaging tools have the advantage of reducing costs and risk to patients due to CA, but at the expense of both overestimating stenosis and subjecting patients to unnecessary operation and surgical risk, as well as underestimating stenosis and subjecting the patient to an increased risk of stroke from their underlying disease. Sound validation of these different modalities against CA with local quality assurance data is imperative (10).

DUS is the most widely employed and most heavily investigated of these methods. MRA is another commonly used technique. Newer MRA methods, such as contrast-enhanced first-pass methods may be better than time-of-flight techniques, but have fewer validation studies. CTA is also emerging, but very few validation studies have been done.

The noninvasive imaging strategies can be divided into three broad categories. First, patients with a very low likelihood of surgically significant disease can be screened out prior to angiography. This strategy has the strongest support behind it. Using a highly sensitive threshold, DUS can very reliably identify patients with less than 50% stenosis (level II, moderate evidence). MRA can also be used for this purpose (level II, moderate evidence). The data for CTA is emerging (level III, limited evidence).

The second strategy is to use noninvasive tools entirely. DUS or MRA alone or in some combination have all been advocated and are in common use. The data supporting this strategy are limited, given the wide margin for error between angiography and these methods for any given individual. Cost-effectiveness analyses of this and other strategies are discussed below.

The third strategy is to use noninvasive imaging to identify patients with less than 50% stenosis and those with very high-grade stenosis (level II, moderate evidence). CA is reserved for those patients with estimated stenoses between 50 and 80% stenosis. All modalities can reliably identify these patients with high-grade stenosis.

The results of cost-effectiveness analyses of these different strategies are variable (8, 11, 12). Critical and variable local data that have profound impact on these models are the local rate of stroke with angiography, the accuracy of local DUS or MRA studies, and surgical complication rates. Different imaging strategies may be the most cost-effective at different institutions, depending on these local factors.

Finally, the advent of carotid angioplasty and stenting adds a new wrinkle in that accurate imaging and intervention can be performed during the same procedure. One randomized trial supports the use of angioplasty and stenting over endarterectomy in patients at high risk for surgery (13). The benefit of angioplasty and stenting in patients who are good surgical candidates remains to be established. For these patients, screening with a noninvasive modality, followed by angiography, and treatment at that time, would be reasonable.

A. Catheter Angiography

Imaging of the cervical carotid artery in TIA or stroke victims (i.e., symptomatic) is entirely focused on determination of the degree of stenosis. This single parameter predicted outcome in two large, randomized, multicenter trials (14, 15). In the NASCET (3, 15), symptomatic patients included patients with TIA, amaurosis fugax, or stroke. Patients with ≥70% carotid stenosis, determined angiographically (Fig. 27.1), had a 2-year cumulative risk of ipsilateral stroke of 9% (including perioperative morbidity and mortality of 5.8%), compared to best medical treatment 2-year cumulative risk of 26%.

For fatal or severe stroke, again in patients with ≥70% carotid stenosis, the surgical arm had a 2-year cumulative risk of 2.5% (including perioperative morbidity and mortality of 2.1%), whereas the medical group had a 2-year cumulative risk of 13.1%. In patients who had 50–69% stenosis there was an absolute risk reduction of 6.5% over 5 years, but only if the 30-day postoperative morbidity and mortality does not exceed 2%. For those patients who had less than 50% stenosis, the risk of stroke was the same as in the medicine arm. There were no significant differences between the reanalyzed results of the ECST and the results of the NASCET (16).

B. Magnetic Resonance Angiography

The bulk of the validation literature has been for time-of-flight techniques (17). Fewer studies have evaluated the use of contrast-enhanced methods. Nederkoorn et al. (18) critically reviewed the recent literature (including both MRA techniques) from 1994 to 2003 and found a pooled sensitivity and specificity of time-of-flight MRA for the detection of greater than 70% stenosis of 95% [95% confidence interval (CI), 92–97] and 90% (95% CI, 86–93), respectively, and a sensitivity and specificity for the identification of complete occlusion of 98% (95% CI, 94–100) and 100% (95% CI, 99–100), respectively (Fig. 27.2).

Butz et al. (19) used the care-bolus technique combined with a nearly real-time two-dimensional (2D) FLASH (fast low-angle shot) sequence and a 3D FLASH with elliptical centric view order for the angiographic pulse time to report a sensitivity of 96% and a specificity of 90% for carotid stenosis of ≥70%. Randoux et al. (20) prospectively studied dynamic 3D gadolinium-enhanced MRA with digital subtraction angiography (DSA) and concluded that there was a tendency to overestimate the degree of ostial stenosis. Many authors report the use of multiple overlapping thin-slab acquisition (MOTSA) to directly measure stenosis of the carotid artery (12, 21–23). Development of first-pass contrast-enhanced MRA resulted in more rapid image acquisitions that are physiologically more similar to those of DSA with the advantage of being less prone to motion artifacts than standard time-of-flight MRA. Hathout et al. (24) presented their institution's 4-year retrospective study of all carotid arteries with stenosis from 10 to 90% diagnosed angiographically and compared to 3D gadolinium-enhanced MRA. They found a linear relationship between DSA and contrast-enhanced MRA, with a Spearman rank correlation coefficient of 0.82, $p < .001$, with increasing severity of stenosis correlating angiographically. However, MRA was less reliable at predicting the degree of stenosis in the individual patient. There were wide confidence intervals and the addition of ultrasound peak systolic velocity did not improve the predictive accuracy. They recommended use of MRA as a screening tool, where patients with 50% or less stenosis were treated medically, those with >80% were treated surgically, and those in between were evaluated with angiography. Older studies show the continuing improvement of sensitivity and specificity of this technique over time with modifications of technique and reduction of signal-to-noise ratios, but none has the validation of large numbers of patients and clinical correlation such as NASCET (25–33)

C. Computer Tomography Angiography

Koelemay et al. (34) reviewed data from 28 studies published between 1990 and 2003, using single-slice scanners. Eight of the 28 studies were considered to be methodologically sound, with blinded review of images and reduction of other sources of bias. The pooled sensitivity and specificity of CTA for the detection of 70% stenosis was 85% (95% CI, 79–89%) and 93% (95% CI, 89–96%), respectively. For detection of complete occlusion, the sensitivity and specificity was 97% (95% CI, 93–99%) and 99% (95% CI, 98–100%), respectively.

The advent of multirow detector machines has expanded the vascular imaging capabilities of CT scanners. There are very few reports with the newer hardware. Zhang et al. (35) have demonstrated that the interfering factors such as ulcerations, calcifications, and adjacent vessels can be circumvented by manually correcting the automated stenosis recognition software. This improved the correlation between CTA and DSA from 0.69 to 0.81. Prokop et al. (36) expand on the thinnest possible section collimation, multislice scanning, to image from the aortic arch through the intracranial vessels. They derive a pooled sensitivity of 95% and specificity of 98% for the detection of >70% stenoses (including single-slice techniques). The Carotide-Angiographic par Resonance Magnétigue-Echographic-Doppler-Angiosce (CARMEDAS) multicenter study (37) compared the concordance rates of contrast-enhanced MRA, DUS, and CTA prospectively in 150 patients for symptomatic stenoses ≥50% and ≥70% and for asymptomatic stenoses ≥60%, for occlusion. Using CTA alone resulted in the misclassification of the stenosis in 11 of 64 cases.

D. Doppler Ultrasound

The performance of DUS can be highly variable (Fig. 27.3) (38). In a pooled meta-analysis of studies published since 1994, Nederkoorn et al. (18) reported a sensitivity and specificity of DUS for the detection of greater than 70% stenosis of 86% (95% CI, 84–89) and 87% (95% CI, 84–90), respectively, and a sensitivity and specificity for the identification of complete occlusion of 96% (95% CI, 94–98) and 100% (95% CI, 99–100), respectively. These numbers may reflect several biases, including publication bias. A better, real-world estimate, of DUS may have been from the NASCET investigators (39). In this analysis, they reviewed the DUS and catheter angiographic findings in 1,011 symptomatic patients screened for inclusion in NASCET. As all patients were considered for inclusion, verification bias was minimal. The sensitivities and specificities of DUS for the identification of 70% stenosis ranged from 0.65 to 0.71. The risk of stroke at 18 months declined sharply as the degree of angiographically defined stenosis declined from 99 to 70%. No pattern of decline was apparent on the basis of the ultrasonographic data. The authors concluded that DUS could be used as a screening tool to exclude patients with no carotid artery disease from further testing.

Furthermore, different criteria are often better correlated with angiography in different laboratories. For example, in a study by Alexandrov et al. (40), peak systolic velocity was more accurate in one lab, while the use of ratios was more accurate in another. Because performance differs substantially among devices, validation of local vascular laboratories is required. With validation, ultrasound performance can be sufficient for the reliable identification of patients with no significant

stenosis and of those with severe stenosis (39). As with MRA, the wide confidence limits for degree of stenosis in individual patients limit the ability of this modality to accurately classify patients at the cut-points for clinical decision making (i.e., 70% stenosis). Without quality control, many ultrasound machines are not adequate to accurately predict the degree of carotid stenosis and should not be the only test to decide whether surgery is warranted.

II. What Is the Imaging Modality of Choice in Asymptomatic Carotid Stenosis?

Summary of Evidence: The benefit of surgery in patients with asymptomatic carotid stenosis is marginal. Two large randomized trials have found a 1% absolute annual risk reduction for surgery, compared to best medical therapy. Whether treatment should be pursued will depend on many factors, including patient age and gender (no definite benefit for women). In one of these two studies, restricted to highly selected, relatively healthy asymptomatic patients, 20% of the patients were dead at 5 years, many due to vascular disease.

Imaging of asymptomatic patients is necessarily a screening issue. The low risk of stroke in medically treated patients and the small risk reduction with surgery remove the harsh penalties for false-negative or false-positive noninvasive studies that are incurred in symptomatic patients. Well-validated DUS or MRA laboratories may be used for this purpose (level II, moderate evidence). The critical factors for screening are well-validated noninvasive methods and documented low surgical complication rates.

Supporting Evidence: Two randomized controlled trials show that patients with 60–99% ipsilateral carotid stenosis have slight risk reduction with surgery (1% annual absolute risk reduction with surgical complication rates less than 2%). Unlike symptomatic patients, no relationship between degree of stenosis and surgical benefit was found. The Asymptomatic Carotid Atherosclerosis Study (ACAS) (41) had 1,662 randomized patients with 60–99% diameter asymptomatic stenosis (NASCET measurements). The actuarial estimated 5-year risk of an ipsilateral stroke or operative stroke, or death was 5.1% in the surgery group vs. 11.0% in the nonsurgery group – a relative risk reduction of about 50% or an absolute risk reduction of 5.9%. If the other (i.e., contralateral) strokes are added in, the absolute risk reduction hardly changes at 5.1%, which is not surprising because one would not expect surgery to influence such strokes. The risk of surgical or angiographic stroke or death was 2.3%. Operating on 85 patients might prevent about one stroke per year, or, if the patients did not die of a cardiac death first, operating on about 17 patients might prevent one stroke in 5 years. However, because only half the strokes were disabling, their absolute risk reduction was 2.6%, which doubles the numbers of patients needed to treat to prevent one disabling stroke compared with any other stroke. Subgroup analyses show no benefit in women.

The Asymptomatic Carotid Surgery Trial (ACST) (42) yielded similar results. Surgical morbidity and mortality was 3.1%. The absolute risk reduction at 5 years was 5.4%. With good medical care, patients face only a 2% annual stroke rate, which falls below 1% after successful carotid endarterectomy. However, the benefits exceed the risks only if the 30-day postoperative morbidity and mortality remain low; otherwise there is no benefit.

A. Cost-Effectiveness Analysis

Screening of asymptomatic patients with noninvasive methods and highly specific thresholds may be cost-effective in certain high-risk populations, such as patients with known atherosclerotic disease in other circulations or the presence of bruit over the carotid artery on physical examination. Different studies addressing the cost-effectiveness of screening asymptomatic carotid stenosis resulted in divergent conclusions (43). The critical factor in whether intervention is effective is the surgical complication rates. A one-time screening program of a population with a high prevalence (20%) of ≥60% stenosis cost $35,130 per incremental quality-adjusted life year (QALY) gained. Decreased surgical benefit (less than 1% annual stroke risk reduction with surgery) or increased annual discount rate resulted in screening being detrimental, resulting in lost QALYs. Annual screening cost $457,773 per

incremental QALY gained. In a low-prevalence (4%) population, one-time screening cost $52,588 per QALY gained, while annual screening was detrimental (44).

III. What Is the Role of Carotid Angioplasty and Stenting?

Summary of Evidence: More information regarding the safety and efficacy of angioplasty and stenting relative to surgical endarterectomy is expected in the near future. As treatment may be incorporated into the diagnostic catheter angiographic procedure, these recommendations may be revised.

At present, angioplasty and stenting is accepted as a reasonable therapy for patients with severe stenosis and recent ischemic symptoms who are not good surgical candidates (level II, moderate evidence). Patients who are good surgical candidates should be treated surgically or within clinical trials of stenting vs. endarterectomy. Noninvasive screening of symptomatic but surgically ineligible patients for possible carotid stenosis should be done prior to angioplasty and stenting (level II, moderate evidence). The benefit of angioplasty and stenting for asymptomatic patients is unproven (level IV, insufficient evidence).

Supporting Evidence: One randomized controlled study of angioplasty vs. carotid endarterectomy in symptomatic patients has been published, the Carotid and Vertebral Artery Transluminal Angioplasty Study (CAVATAS) (45). All patients had recent ischemic symptoms and high-grade stenosis by CA. The 30-day major stroke and death rates were similar, as was the outcome at 1 year. Limitations of this study include a higher surgical complication rate than NASCET, long-term follow-up for only 3 years, and dated endovascular devices.

A second randomized study has been recently published (13). Enrollment was limited to patients considered to be at high risk for complications of surgery. Inclusion criteria included age greater than 80 years, congestive heart failure, chronic obstructive pulmonary disease, prior surgical endarterectomy, and local radiation therapy. Both symptomatic and asymptomatic patients were included. Subgroup analyses for presence or absence of ischemic symptoms did not achieve statistical significance. Thirty-day and 1-year outcomes were significantly better in the angioplasty group. A major issue raised by this study is whether these patients would have done better with medical therapy alone.

IV. What Is the Role of Physiologic Imaging in Carotid Stenosis and Occlusion?

Summary of Evidence: Physiologic imaging studies that identify compensatory hemodynamic mechanisms for low perfusion pressure have been shown to be powerful predictors of subsequent stroke in patients with symptomatic carotid stenosis or occlusion using some, but not all, physiologic imaging methods. The best evidence is for measurements of the oxygen extraction fraction (OEF) with PET and breath-holding transcranial Doppler (TCD) studies (level I, strong evidence). There is moderate evidence (level II) supporting the use of stable xenon CT and single photon emission computed tomography (SPECT) methods. At present, however, the use of this information to guide therapy has not been proven to change outcome (level III, limited evidence). The two patient populations in whom these tools are likely to become important are those with symptomatic complete carotid occlusion and those with asymptomatic carotid stenosis.

Supporting Evidence

A. Methods of Hemodynamic Assessment

A completely occluded carotid artery often has no effect on the pressure in the arteries of the brain beyond the occlusion. In some patients, the circle of Willis or pial collateral branches are sufficient to maintain normal arterial pressure and, consequently, normal CBF. In other patients, the pressure in the arteries of the brain beyond the occlusion will decrease. There are two compensatory mechanisms by which the brain can maintain normal oxygen metabolism, and thereby normal neurologic function, when arterial pressure falls. First, in autoregulation, blood flow can be maintained by reducing vascular

resistance. Second, as flow is reduced passively as a function of pressure and exceeded autoregulatory capacity, the brain can increase the amount of oxygen extracted from the blood.

Single measurements of CBF alone do not adequately assess cerebral hemodynamic status. First, normal values may be found when perfusion pressure is reduced, but CBF is maintained by autoregulatory vasodilation. Second, CBF may be low when perfusion pressure is normal. This can occur when the metabolic demands of the tissue are low. Reduced flow due to reduced metabolic demand may not cause confusion when low regional CBF is measured in areas of frank tissue infarction. However, blood flow can also be reduced in normal, uninfarcted tissue due to the destruction of normal afferent or efferent fibers by a remote lesion as well (46).

Three basic strategies have been developed to assess regional cerebral hemodynamic status noninvasively (2). The normal compensatory responses of the brain and its vasculature to reduced perfusion pressure, as outlined above, are assumed to be present. The first two strategies are used to indirectly identify the presence and degree of autoregulatory vasodilation. The third relies on direct measurements of the OEF.

The first strategy relies on paired blood flow measurements with the initial measurement obtained at rest and the second measurement obtained following a cerebral vasodilatory stimulus. Hypercapnia, acetazolamide, and physiologic tasks such as hand movement have been used as vasodilatory stimuli. Normally, each will result in a robust increase in CBF. If the CBF response is muted or absent, preexisting autoregulatory cerebral vasodilation due to reduced cerebral perfusion pressure is inferred. Quantitative or qualitative (relative) measurements of CBF can be made using a variety of methods, including xenon 133 by inhalation or intravenous injection, SPECT, stable xenon computed tomography (Xe-CT), PET, and magnetic resonance imaging (MRI). Changes in the velocity of blood in the middle cerebral artery (MCA) trunk or internal carotid artery (ICA) can be measured with TCD and MRI. The blood flow or blood velocity responses to these vasodilatory stimuli have been categorized into several grades of hemodynamic impairment: (1) reduced augmentation (relative to the contralateral hemisphere or normal controls);

(2) absent augmentation (same value as baseline); and (3) paradoxical reduction in regional blood flow compared to baseline measurement. This final category, also called the "steal" phenomenon, can only be identified with quantitative CBF techniques.

The second strategy uses the measurement of regional cerebral blood volume (CBV), alone or in combination with measurements of CBF, in the resting brain in order to detect the presence of autoregulatory vasodilation. The CBV/CBF ratio (or, inversely, the CBF/CBV ratio), mathematically equivalent to the vascular mean transit time, may be more sensitive than CBV alone for the identification of autoregulatory vasodilation. Quantitative regional measurements of CBV and CBF can be made with PET or SPECT. Magnetic resonance techniques for the quantitative measurement of CBV have been developed. Patients are identified as abnormal with these techniques based on comparison of absolute quantitative values or hemispheric ratios of quantitative values to the range observed in normal control subjects.

The third strategy relies on direct measurements of OEF to identify patients with increased oxygen extraction. At present, regional measurements of OEF can be made only with PET using O-15-labeled radiotracers. Both absolute values and side-to-side ratios of quantitative and relative OEF have been used for the determination of abnormal from normal.

B. Association with Stroke Risk

Complete occlusion of the carotid artery is found in up to 15% of patients with carotid territory TIAs or strokes (9). The risk of subsequent stroke in this population is high, approximately 5–7% per year (47). No preventive therapy has been proven effective. A randomized trial of extracranial to intracranial arterial bypass, the EC/IC bypass trial, found no benefit with bypass compared to medical therapy (48). One limitation of this study was that there was no method of hemodynamic assessment: a large percentage of the patients included in this study may have had normal flow due to circle of Willis and other sources of collateral flow and therefore nothing to gain from an extra-anatomic bypass (49). The presence of severe hemodynamic impairment has since been proven to be an independent and

powerful predictor of stroke in patients with carotid occlusion (2, 50).

As these methods are inferential and indirect, correlation with outcome is required (2). At present, the strongest evidence is for PET measurements of OEF and TCD measurements of cerebrovascular reserve (level I, strong evidence). The St. Louis Carotid Occlusion Study was a blinded, prospective study of 81 patients with symptomatic carotid occlusion that also specifically assessed the impact of other risk factors (50). The risk of all stroke and ipsilateral ischemic stroke in symptomatic subjects with increased OEF was significantly higher than in those with normal OEF (log rank $p = .005$ and $p = .004$, respectively). Univariate and multivariate analysis of 17 baseline stroke risk factors confirmed the independence of this relationship. The age-adjusted relative risk conferred by increased OEF was 6.0 (95% CI, 1.7–21.6) for all stroke and 7.3 (95% CI, 1.6–33.4) for ipsilateral ischemic stroke. Similar data were reported in a study by Yamauchi et al. (51). Based on these data, a randomized trial of extracranial to intracranial arterial bypass in patients with increased OEF has been funded and is under way.

Several investigators have studied the association of paired flow techniques with stroke risk. Six found an association with stroke risk and three found none. Two of the six positive studies used a TCD method (breath-holding) and provided level I (strong evidence) for patients with complete carotid occlusion and patients with asymptomatic carotid stenosis (52, 53). Vernieri et al. (54) enrolled 104 patients with complete carotid occlusion and followed them for a median period of 24 months. The blood velocity response to 30 s of breath-holding was measured by TCD on study entry. Baseline stroke risk factors were assessed. The threshold for an abnormal TCD was set prospectively. Eighteen patients suffered a stroke during the follow-up period. Age and abnormal TCD response were independent risk factors for subsequent stroke.

Kleiser and Widder (55) reported an association between abnormal blood velocity responses to hypercapnia (by TCD) and the risk of subsequent stroke in 85 patients with carotid occlusion. Both symptomatic and asymptomatic patients were included. The risk of contralateral stroke in the patients with a diminished or exhausted CO_2 reactivity was increased, which suggests that the groups were not matched for other stroke risk factors, which were not evaluated. A subsequent study by these same authors reported the outcome of 86 patients with carotid occlusion (56). A much lower risk of stroke was observed in this second study and the number of asymptomatic patients was not reported.

Yonas et al. (57) reported an association of the steal phenomena (reduced blood flow by Xe-CT) after acetazolamide and subsequent stroke. This study included patients with high-grade carotid stenosis and patients with carotid occlusion. The hemodynamic data of patients with subsequent stroke was analyzed retrospectively in order to establish threshold values for the categorization of high- and low-risk groups. These authors subsequently repeated the analysis with an additional 27 patients (58). The hemodynamic criteria used to establish high- and low-risk groups were different from the prior analysis. Three of the five new strokes that occurred did so in patients who would not have met criteria for the first study and the definition of clinical outcome included contralateral stroke. Only two of these five new strokes were in the hemodynamically compromised territory of the occluded vessel.

Three studies have failed to find an association of a paired flow technique and stroke risk (59–61). The largest and most methodologically sound study was reported by Yokota et al. (60). They prospectively evaluated 105 symptomatic patients with mixed lesions [unilateral occlusion or severe stenosis (>75% in diameter) of the ICA or proximal MCA] with a SPECT study of relative CBF using ^{123}I iodoamphetamine (IMP) and measurement of cerebrovascular reactivity using acetazolamide. Other stroke risk factors were prospectively assessed. Thirteen strokes occurred during a median follow-up of 2.7 years: 7 strokes occurred in 39 patients with abnormal hemodynamics and 6 in the 39 patients with normal hemodynamics. The investigators were not blind to the results of the hemodynamic study. A relatively large number of patients ($n = 16$) were censored from the study because of subsequent cerebrovascular surgery and a significant number of patients ($n = 11$) were lost to follow-up.

C. Cost-Effectiveness Analysis

Cost-effectiveness analysis suggests that the use of these physiologic tools, even expensive ones such as PET, would be cost-effective for patients with symptomatic carotid artery occlusion, provided there is a benefit with surgical bypass (8). The costs of acute and long-term care for stroke victims greatly exceed the costs of diagnostic workup and surgery.

In addition to patients with complete carotid occlusion, another promising application for hemodynamic assessment is in asymptomatic carotid stenosis. The prevalence of hemodynamic impairment in patients with asymptomatic carotid occlusive disease is very low (53, 62). This low prevalence may account in part for the low risk of stroke with medical treatment, and consequently, the marginal benefit with revascularization. The presence of hemodynamic impairment may be a powerful predictor of subsequent stroke in this population (53, 62). This is one area of research with enormous clinical implications: if a subgroup of asymptomatic patients at high risk due to hemodynamic factors could be identified, it would be possible to target surgical or endovascular treatment at those most likely to benefit.

Only one study has been performed in this population, to date. Silvestrini et al. (53) performed a prospective, blinded longitudinal study of 94 patients with asymptomatic carotid artery stenosis of at least 70% followed for a mean of 28.5 months. Breath-holding TCD was performed on entry, as well as the assessment of other stroke risk factors. An abnormal TCD study was shown to be a powerful and independent risk factor for subsequent stroke.

Take Home Tables (Tables 27.1–27.3)

Protocols Based on the Evidence

Carotid Angiography

The key is to obtain measurements of linear diameter reduction using selective carotid artery injections. For ICA lesions, the point of maximal stenosis is measured and expressed as a percentage of the normal distal ICA diameter (64). For eccentric stenoses, the maximal degree of stenosis in any projection is reported. If there is evidence of collapse of the ICA due to low flow, the denominator will be artifactually reduced. By convention this is termed "near occlusion," and the degree of stenosis is not reported. These procedures are optimally performed using a biplane digital subtraction unit. An arch injection is useful to evaluate for origin stenosis and arch morphology. Selective carotid injections are obtained in magnified anteroposterior (AP) and lateral projections with orthogonal oblique views, if necessary. If a complete occlusion is encountered, be certain to perform a long run in the neck run to look for string, as well as to assess external to internal collaterals. Subclavian or vertebral injections to assess for collateral flow are also useful.

Doppler Ultrasound

Five- or 7.5-MHz linear array transducers are generally used. The following measurements must be acquired: the highest angle-adjusted peak systolic velocity in the common, proximal, and distal ICAs, and at the point of maximal stenosis. Angle adjustment for Doppler measurements is based on flow direction by color Doppler. End-diastolic velocity measurements are also at these levels. Ratios of these velocities should be calculated. No one specific protocol or value can be recommended to use as a threshold for degree of stenosis. The optimal thresholds for different degrees of stenosis must be determined at each laboratory vs. angiography.

Contrast-Enhanced Magnetic Resonance Angiography

A 3D subtracted gradient-recalled echo sequence and turbo FLASH sequence (4/1.6, 25° flip angle, 120×256 matrix) is generally used. A total of 20 ml of MR contrast is injected by a power injector at approximately 3 cm^3/s. Some clinicians use a timing bolus followed by a saline flush to estimate the optimal time for the contrast-enhanced scan. Others generate up to three post-gadolinium runs and select the one with the best arterial visualization for subtraction.

Computed Tomographic Angiography

Helical CT acquisitions for coverage of the arch to the circle of Willis generally employ 3-mm helical beam collimation with a 3-mm/s table speed, 12-cm scan field of view from the origin of the great vessels through the circle of Willis, 140 kV, 240 mA, and 90 ml of nonionic contrast media injected at 3 ml/s by a power injector. A 25-s delay between injection and scan start is employed.

Table 27.1. Suggested algorithm for imaging symptomatic patients (39, 63)

Screening ultrasound, CTA, or MRA (after establishing accuracy of local laboratory vs. angiography) to exclude patients with less than 50% stenosis from further evaluation for carotid stenosis
Patients with less than 50% stenosis treated medically
Subsequent imaging decisions are based on the accuracy of local noninvasive tests for the presence of occlusion and for severe stenosis
If not reliable for severe stenosis or occlusion, all patients with suspected stenosis greater than 50% or occlusion should undergo angiography
If noninvasive tests are reliable for the identification of greater than 80% stenosis, then these patients go to surgery and patients with suspected 50–80% stenosis or occlusion go to angiography

Reprinted with kind permission of Springer Science+Business Media from Barrocas AM, Derdeyn CP. Imaging of the Cervical Carotid Artery for Arterosclerotic Stenosis. In Medina LS, Blackmore CC (eds): *Evidence-Based Imaging: Optimizing Imaging in Patient Care.* New York: Springer Science+Business Media, 2006.

Table 27.2. Suggested algorithm for imaging asymptomatic patients

If surgical complication rates (stroke and death) for asymptomatic patients are less than 2%, and the patient is a male in relatively good health with a life-expectancy of least 5 years, then a screening ultrasound, CTA, or MRA with highly specific threshold for greater than 60% stenosis, followed by surgery if positive may be reasonable.

Reprinted with kind permission of Springer Science+Business Media from Barrocas AM, Derdeyn CP. Imaging of the Cervical Carotid Artery for Arterosclerotic Stenosis. In Medina LS, Blackmore CC (eds): *Evidence-Based Imaging: Optimizing Imaging in Patient Care.* New York: Springer Science+Business Media, 2006.

Table 27.3. Suggested algorithm for imaging patients with carotid occlusion

If noninvasive screening tool is documented as accurate for complete occlusion, then no further imaging is necessary for asymptomatic patients. The risk for stroke with a missed high-grade asymptomatic stenosis is so low that the risk of angiography is not worth the benefit. There is no increased risk of stroke with higher degrees of stenosis in asymptomatic patients. If the patient is symptomatic, the diagnosis should be confirmed by angiography, as a missed high-grade stenosis has a very high chance of causing a future stroke.

Reprinted with kind permission of Springer Science+Business Media from Barrocas AM, Derdeyn CP. Imaging of the Cervical Carotid Artery for Arterosclerotic Stenosis. In Medina LS, Blackmore CC (eds): *Evidence-Based Imaging: Optimizing Imaging in Patient Care.* New York: Springer Science+Business Media, 2006.

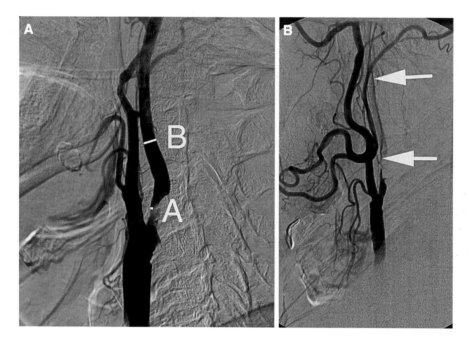

Figure 27.1. Selective arterial angiograms of carotid bifurcation showing 85% stenosis without near occlusion by the NASCET method of measurement (**A**) and near occlusion (severe stenosis with narrowing of the distal ICA) (**B**). To calculate the degree of stenosis, the lumen diameter at the point of maximum stenosis (point *A*) was measured as the numerator in NASCET. The lumen diameter of the distal ICA (point *B*) is used as the denominator. The percent stenosis is calculated as $(1 - A/B) \times 100$. In near occlusion (B), the denominator (*B* in A) is artifactually low. (Reprinted with kind permission from Springer Science+Business Media from Barrocas AM, Derdeyn CP. Imaging of the Cervical Carotid Artery for Artherosclerotic Stenosis. Medina LS, Blackmore CC (eds): *Evidence-Based Imaging: Optimizing Imaging in Patient Care.* New York: Springer Science+Business Media, 2006.)

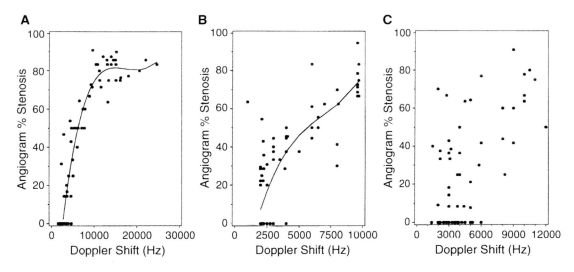

Figure 27.2. (**A**) Time-of-flight MRA in a patient with recent TIA shows a long segment of flow-gap, consistent with turbulent flow and suggesting high-grade stenosis. (**B**) The contrast-enhanced (CE) MRA depicts the lumen better than the time-of-flight method, but a segment of flow gap remains. (**C**) CA shows an 80% stenosis. This case illustrates the reliability of MRA, particularly CE-MRA to accurately identify severe stenosis. With less severe, but clinically relevant stenosis (50–70%), the wide error range for MRA makes it less reliable for individual patients. (Reprinted with kind permission from Springer Science+Business Media from Barrocas AM, Derdeyn CP. Imaging of the Cervical Carotid Artery for Artherosclerotic Stenosis. Medina LS, Blackmore CC (eds): *Evidence-Based Imaging: Optimizing Imaging in Patient Care.* New York: Springer Science+Business Media, 2006.)

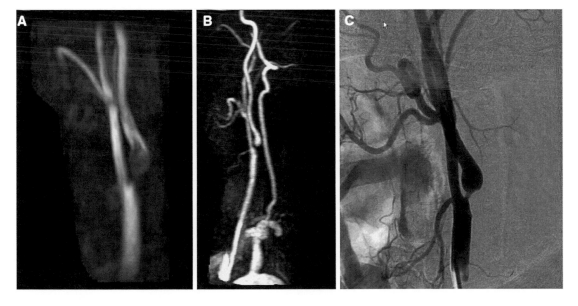

Figure 27.3. Relationship between Doppler frequency/velocity and percent stenosis by angiography for three specific devices: one with a device with a "strong" relationship (**A**), one with a "moderate" relationship (**B**), and one with a "poor" relationship (**C**) (38). This was a validation study performed as part of the Asymptomatic Carotid Surgery Study. (Reprinted with kind permission from Springer Science+Business Media from Barrocas AM, Derdeyn CP. Imaging of the Cervical Carotid Artery for Artherosclerotic Stenosis. Medina LS, Blackmore CC (eds): *Evidence-Based Imaging: Optimizing Imaging in Patient Care.* New York: Springer Science+Business Media, 2006.)

References

1. Malek AM, Alper SL, Izumo S. JAMA 1999;282(21):2035–2042.
2. Derdeyn CP, Grubb RL Jr, Powers WJ. Neurology 1999;53(2):251.
3. North American Symptomatic Carotid Endarterectomy Trial Collaborators. N Engl J Med 1991;325(7):445–453.
4. Rothwell PM, Gutnikov SA, Warlow CP. Stroke 2003;34(2):514–523.
5. Kissela B et al. Stroke 2001;32(6):1285–1290.
6. Bogousslavsky J et al. Arch Neurol 1986; 43(3):223–228.
7. Rothwell PM et al. Lancet 2003;361(9352): 107–116.
8. Derdeyn CP et al. J Nucl Med 2000;41(5):800–807.
9. Mead GE et al. Br J Surg 1997;84(7):990–992.
10. Howard G, Chambless LE, Baker WH. J Stroke Cerebrovasc Dis 1991;1:166–173.
11. Buskens E et al. Radiology 2004;233:101–112.
12. Kent KC et al. JAMA 1995;274(11):888–893.
13. Yadav JS et al. N Engl J Med 2004;351: 1493–1501.
14. Carotid Surgery Trialists' Collaborative Group. Lancet 1998;351(9113):1379–1387.
15. Barnett HJM et al. N Engl J Med 1998;339(20): 1415–1425.
16. Morgenstern L et al. Neurology 1997;48(4): 911–915.
17. Kallmes D et al. AJNR Am J Neuroradiol 1996;17(8):1501–1506.
18. Nederkoorn PJ, van der Graaf Y, Hunink MGM. Stroke 2003;34(5):1324–1331.
19. Butz B et al. Acta Radiol 2004;45(2):164–170.
20. Randoux B et al. Radiology 2003;229(3):697–702.
21. DeMarco JK, Huston J III, Bernstein MA. AJR Am J Roentgenol 2004;183(3):787–793.
22. Nederkoorn PJ et al. Stroke 2002;33(8): 2003–2008.
23. Huston J et al. AJNR Am J Neuroradiol 1998;19(2):309–315.
24. Hathout GM, Duh MJ, El-Saden SM. AJNR Am J Neuroradiol 2003;24(9):1747–1756.
25. Alvarez-Linera J et al. AJNR Am J Neuroradiol 2003;24(5):1012–1019.
26. Sundgren PC et al. Neuroradiology 2002; 44(7):592–599.
27. Remonda L et al. AJNR Am J Neuroradiol 2002;23(2):213–219.
28. Randoux B et al. Radiology 2001;220(1):179–185.
29. Serfaty JM et al. AJR Am J Roentgenol 2000; 175(2):455–463.
30. Sardanelli F et al. J Comput Assist Tomogr 1999;23(2):208–215.
31. Slosman F et al. AJR Am J Roentgenol 1998;170(2): 489–495.
32. Remonda L, Heid O, Schroth G. Radiology 1998;209(1):95–102.
33. Leclerc X et al. AJNR Am J Neuroradiol 1998; 19(8):1405–1413.
34. Koelemay MJW et al. Stroke 2004;35(10): 2306–2312.
35. Zhang Z et al. Eur Radiol 2004;14(4):665–672.
36. Prokop M, Waaijer A, Kreuzer S. JBR-BTR 2004; 87(1):23–29.
37. Nonent M et al. Stroke 2004;35(3):682–686.
38. Howard G et al. Stroke 1996;27(11):1951–1957.
39. Eliasziw M et al. Stroke 1995;26(10):1747–1752.
40. Alexandrov AV et al. Stroke 1997;28(2):339–342.
41. Executive Committee for the Asymptomatic Carotid Atherosclerosis Study. JAMA 1995; 273(18):1421–1428.
42. Halliday A et al. Lancet 2004;363(9420): 1491–1502.
43. Holloway RG et al. Stroke 1999;30(7):1340–1349.
44. Derdeyn CP, Powers WJ. Stroke 1996;27(11): 1944–1950.
45. CAVATAS Investigators. Lancet 2001;357(9270): 1729–1737.
46. Feeney DM, Baron JC. Stroke 1986;17:817–830.
47. Klijn CJM et al. Stroke 1997;28:2084–2093.
48. The EC/IC Bypass Study Group. N Engl J Med 1985;313:1191–2000.
49. Ausman Jr, Diaz FG. Surg Neurol 1986;26: 218–221.
50. Grubb RL Jr et al. JAMA 1998;280(12):1055–1060.
51. Yamauchi H et al. J Nucl Med 1999;40: 1992–1998.
52. Vernieri F et al. Stroke 1999;30:593–598.
53. Silvestrini M et al. JAMA 2000;283(16): 2122–2127.
54. Vernieri F et al. Stroke 2001;32:1552–1558.
55. Kleiser B, Widder N. Stroke 1992;23:171–174.
56. Widder B, Kleiser B, Krapf H. Stroke 1994; 25:1963–1967.
57. Yonas H et al. J Neurosurg 1993;79:483–489.
58. Webster MW et al. J Vasc Surg 1995;21:338–345.
59. Powers WJ, Tempel LW, Grubb RL Jr. Ann Neurol 1989;25:325–330.
60. Yokota C et al. Stroke 1998;29:1743–1744.
61. Hasegawa Y et al. Stroke 1997;28:242.
62. Powers WJ et al. Neurology 2000;54:878–882.
63. Derdeyn CP et al. Radiology 1995;197(3): 635–643.
64. Fox AJ. Radiology 1993;186(2):316–318.

28

Blunt Injuries to the Thorax and Abdomen

Frederick A. Mann

I. What imaging is appropriate for patients with blunt trauma to the chest?
   A. Chest wall
   B. Pleura and lung
   C. Diaphragm
II. What imaging is appropriate for patients with blunt trauma to the abdomen?
   A. Spleen and liver injuries
   B. Bowel and mesentery injuries
III. What is the optimal imaging approach in patients suspected of having retroperitoneal injury?

Issues

- Conventional radiography remains the appropriate initial screening evaluation of the chest in patients with major trauma. Computed tomography (CT) is appropriate for the definitive evaluation of abnormalities identified on initial radiography.
- Clinical evidence of hemodynamic instability or ongoing blood loss is the strongest indicator for operative intervention in the abdomen. Among patients with such indication of ongoing hemorrhage, trans-abdominal ultrasound and diagnostic peritoneal lavage (DPL) are diagnostically equivalent in identifying patients with intraperitoneal hemorrhage from solid organ injury.

Key Points

F.A. Mann (✉)
Department of Radiology/Medical Imaging, APC, Swedish Medical Centers,
1229 Madison, Suite 900, Seattle, WA 98104, USA
e-mail: fmann@searad.com

L.S. Medina et al. (eds.), *Evidence-Based Imaging: Improving the Quality of Imaging in Patient Care, Revised Edition*,
DOI 10.1007/978-1-4419-7777-9_28, © Springer Science+Business Media, LLC 2011

- CT has high sensitivity for surgically important injuries of the liver and spleen, but CT grading of injury shows poor correlation with outcome.
- In patients with clinical suspicion of retroperitoneal injury, CT is the diagnostic procedure of choice.
- CT is the preferred imaging modality for identification of hollow viscus injury, although DPL may have higher sensitivity at the expense of lower specificity.

Definition and Pathophysiology

Thoracic trauma is responsible for approximately 25% of trauma deaths in North America. Since death from thoracic trauma commonly occurs after presentation to the hospital, many of these deaths are presumed to be preventable with prompt and appropriate treatment. Important injuries leading to rapid death in trauma include aortic rupture, massive hemothorax, pericardial tamponade, and tension pneumothorax. Pulmonary contusion, myocardial contusion, tracheobronchial injury, and diaphragmatic rupture may also be fatal if not recognized and treated emergently. Fewer than 10% of chest injuries require thoracotomy for treatment (1).

In the abdomen, blunt trauma may result in compression or shear injury to the viscera, leading to hemorrhage and peritonitis. Among patients who undergo laparotomy for blunt trauma, the spleen, and liver are the most frequently injured organs. Because of the large potential space of the peritoneum, large volumes of hemorrhage can occur without tamponade, and exsanguination may occur rapidly from arterial and large venous injuries in the organ parenchyma.

Mechanisms of hollow viscus or mesenteric injury include direct blow to the abdomen (handlebars, kicks, or motor vehicle accident), and seatbelt injury, especially when associated with distraction-type spine injury. The spectrum of hollow viscus injuries (HVIs) includes wall contusions, serosal injuries ("deserosalization"), perforations and transection, and mesenteric rents and hematomas. When mural disruption occurs in the proximal gastrointestinal tract (stomach through proximal jejunum), leakage of alimentary tract contents into the peritoneum induce acute chemical peritonitis and related clinical findings. Distal small bowel and colon spillage tends to present later as peritoneal sepsis. Delays in diagnosis are associated with complicated clinical courses and increased mortality. Serial physical examination evaluation alone may be associated with delay in diagnosis in individuals who have concomitant distracting injuries, such as femur fractures.

Among retroperitoneal injuries, in adults, the duodenum and pancreas are rarely injured in isolation. However, children and adolescents may sustain isolated duodenal, or duodenal and pancreatic, injuries, especially from bicycle handlebar goring mechanisms. Pancreatic injuries range from contusions, lacerations, fractures, and duodenal–pancreatic disjunctions. In adults, injuries to the main pancreatic duct and combined pancreatoduodenal injuries necessitate intervention and are often associated with complicated treatment courses. In children, aggressive and early treatment remains controversial, and treatment directed at complications is more common.

Epidemiology

Injuries are the leading cause of death of individuals between the ages of 1 and 44 in the USA. In the 15–24 age group, injuries account for 78% of all deaths. Because trauma deaths tend to occur in younger individuals, there is a great burden on society in terms of years of life lost and lost lifetime earnings (2).

Motor vehicle accidents account for approximately half of unintentional injury deaths, followed by falls. Injury death rates are higher in the elderly population (over age 70), as well as in individuals in their early 20s. Males also have higher death rates than females (3).

Overall Cost to Society

Discounting lifetime earnings at 6%, the total lifetime cost of injuries that occurred in the year 1985 in the USA was estimated by Rice et al. (4)

to be $150 billion. This is more than the cost of cancer, heart disease, and stroke combined. Despite this, the US federal government spends only approximately a tenth as much money on injury research as on cancer research.

Goals

The goals of imaging in chest and abdominal trauma are twofold. Initial imaging must allow for rapid identification of life-threatening injuries to enable treatment of the injuries in the initial hour after presentation of the patient to the hospital. Secondary imaging provides a detailed evaluation of all injuries potentially leading to morbidity and mortality, including appropriate staging of these injuries.

Methodology

The literature review was based on combinations of the following terms: *imaging* and (*injury* or *wounds, nonpenetrating*) and *1990–2004* and (*chest wall, rib, pleura, scapulothoracic, hemothorax, pneumothorax, diaphragm, abdominal injuries, intestine-small, mesentery, spleen,* or *liver*) or (*lung* or *pulmonary* and *contusion* or *laceration*), and (*radiography* OR *tomography, X-ray computed*) and with this limit: *not case reports*. Studies that consisted of case series, case reports, and expert opinion after review were not included. Included were both English-language and non-English-language articles.

I. What Imaging Is Appropriate for Patients with Blunt Trauma to the Chest?

Summary of Evidence: Radiography remains the most appropriate initial imaging evaluation for blunt trauma to the chest. Radiography has high sensitivity for clinically important disease. Additional imaging, usually with CT or computed tomographic angiography (CTA) is often necessary to adequately evaluate abnormalities identified on conventional radiography (moderate evidence).

Supporting Evidence

A. Chest Wall

With the exception of medicolegal documentation purposes necessary for nonaccidental trauma, information necessary for recognition and treatment planning for important chest wall injuries may be achieved with conventional radiography. While bone scintigraphy is considerably more sensitive to the detection of rib fractures in the subacute setting, among polytrauma victims, it plays little or no role in treatment planning or an independent role in prognosis. While CT is an important adjunctive test in the evaluation of blunt chest trauma, it is less sensitive in the detection of rib fractures than conventional radiography. Where medicolegal documentation is necessary, such as in the evaluation of nonaccidental trauma, bone scintigraphy, ultrasound, and CT may provide additional evidence of characteristic injury to support the diagnosis (5–23).

When conventional radiography or clinical examination suggests the presence of scapulothoracic dissociation (closed forequarter amputation), angiography (CTA or catheter angiography) may be used to exclude the presence of the rare intrathoracic pseudoaneurysm of the subclavian or proximal axillary artery, whose intrapleural rupture may be catastrophic (24 29).

B. Pleura and Lung

Computed tomography is more sensitive in the detection of pneumothoraces than conventional radiography. However, the consequences of pneumothoraces that are occult to conventional radiography are generally benign, except when positive pressure ventilation is part of the management of the patient's pulmonary injury (including patients going emergently to the operating theater). CT is more sensitive in detecting lung hernias through muscular or osseous chest wall disruption, and better characterizes their need for surgical treatment (lung hernias with narrow necks are more likely to experience pulmonary infarctions than those with broad based necks). CT is also more accurate at assessing the size of hemothoraces. Hemothoraces exceeding 300–500 ml are more likely to be associated with delayed pulmonary complications, such as incarcerated lung and empyema (30–34).

In similar fashion, conventional radiography generally provides sufficient information for the diagnosis of pulmonary contusions and lacerations and their therapy. However, quantitative assessment of the volume of lung involved with pulmonary contusion may predict the likelihood of development of acute respiratory distress syndrome and delayed pneumonia (>20 and 30% of lung volume, respectively). CT is far more sensitive to the detection of pulmonary lacerations. However, there is no current evidence that earlier or more thorough detection of pulmonary laceration effects patient outcome. Certain CT findings, such as subpleural lucency associated with peripheral pulmonary opacity, facilitate confident diagnosis of contusion and distinguishing it from more common causes of pulmonary opacity in trauma (such aspiration and passive atelectasis). Disruption of the aerodigestive tract often leads to pneumomediastinum, and may be associated with mediastinal hematoma. Blunt injury to the esophagus usually occurs in the upper third of the esophagus and may be suggested by CT. However, esophagography and esophagoscopy remain the standard diagnostic modalities for detection and treatment planning. Tracheobronchial injuries may be suggested by massive pneumomediastinum and persistent air leak associated with pneumothorax, and may be directly imaged by CT. However, bronchoscopy remains the principal diagnostic tool in the acute and emergent setting (35–60).

Conventional radiography remains the primary survey for mediastinal abnormalities in blunt polytrauma of the chest. Where the cardiomediastinal silhouette is normal for a patient's age and sex, acute traumatic aortic injuries can be reliably excluded by conventional chest radiography. However, a large minority of patients who are subsequently shown to have normal aortic and great vessels do not show normal cardiomediastinal silhouettes by conventional radiography for various reasons, including low lung volumes, pulmonary or pleural opacities obscuring mediastinal margins, etc. In this setting, CT has largely supplanted catheter angiography in the evaluation of the aorta and its great vessels for acute traumatic injury, particularly when performed as CT angiography (61–63). Detailed discussion of aortic injury is included in Chap. 26.

C. Diaphragm

An high-index of suspicion for diaphragmatic ruptures is warranted in appropriate clinical circumstances (lateral impact crashes, especially when left-sided), because fewer than one third of cases present with classical findings (up to 40% of left-sided and less than 15% of right-sided ruptures) and 10–15% will have a false-negative DPL. Delayed diagnoses are not uncommon (10–15% greater than 24-h delay), especially if the commonly associated intrathoracic (~90%) and intraabdominal (~60%) injuries require endotracheal intubation and positive-pressure ventilation. Conventional radiography (chest radiographs with enteral tube placement; fluoroscopy) is abnormal in 60–90% of individuals with acute traumatic diaphragmatic rupture, but most findings are nonspecific (hemothorax, atelectasis, etc.). In unselected series, CT accuracy was equivalent, but not clearly superior to conventional radiographic techniques. At CT, the so-called dependent viscera sign (intraabdominal contents abutting the posterior thoracic wall where the scan level is in the upper third of the liver or spleen) and "collar" sign (narrowed waist of a herniated intraabdominal organ at the site of diaphragm rupture) are nearly 100% specific. Other findings, such as the discontinuous and thickened diaphragm signs, show intermediate sensitivity and specificity (40–75%). Among reported series in which magnetic resonance imaging (MRI) depicted no diaphragmatic disruptions, no delayed diagnoses have been reported (64–78).

II. What Imaging Is Appropriate for Patients with Blunt Trauma to the Abdomen?

Summary of Evidence: CT is the imaging modality of choice for evaluation of the abdomen in trauma patients (moderate evidence). However, clinical status is a more reliable predictor of requirement for operative intervention than imaging (moderate evidence). Ultrasonography is of insufficient sensitivity to allow exclusion of intraabdominal organ injury and hemoperitoneum (moderate evidence) (Fig. 28.1).

Supporting Evidence

A. Spleen and Liver Injuries

Hemodynamic status and evidence of ongoing blood loss are the strongest indicators of the need for intervention for injury to the spleen and liver, because the most common and life-threatening complication from abdominal trauma is surgically treatable hemorrhage. Among hemodynamically unstable patients that are not taken immediately to the operating suite, transabdominal ultrasound and DPL are diagnostically equivalent in selecting patients whose hemodynamic instability is due to intraperitoneal hemorrhage from solid organ (79–81).

Meta-analyses by Stengel et al. (82, 83) investigated the accuracy and positive and negative predictive values for the use of trauma ultrasound for the identification of hemoperitoneum. Ultrasound had relatively high specificity for intraperitoneal hemorrhage, indicating high reliability if hemoperitoneum was identified. However, the sensitivity of ultrasound for intraperitoneal fluid was relatively low, with a negative likelihood ratio of only 0.24. At the prevalence of injury encountered in major trauma centers, the posttest probability of disease following negative ultrasound was too high to exclude important injury. Subanalysis of pediatric patients revealed similar results. Accordingly, observation or CT following negative ultrasonography is warranted (strong evidence) (82–84).

Among hemodynamically stable patients, nonoperative management may be guided by information gleaned from adjunctive diagnostic tests and serial physical examination. CT shows a sensitivity in the middle to high 90s to the detection of surgically important injuries of the liver and spleen. However, CT grading of liver and spleen injuries shows generally poor correlation with the specific outcome of individual cases. Active hemorrhage detected by CT commonly leads to endovascular or surgical interventions in most patients where bleeding was focal [intraparenchymal: pseudoaneurysms vs. arteriovenous (AV) fistula], diffuse (intraperitoneal), or seen in multiple locations (most

common with pelvic ring fractures). Extravasated contrast presents as relatively discrete contrast collections that increase or "pool" on delayed imaging, and show measures within 10–20 Hounsfield units (HU) of contrast density of an adjacent major artery or aorta. At this time, contrast-enhanced CT does not reliably distinguish between pseudoaneurysms (>70% believed to progress to rupture) and AV fistulae (natural history is uncertain). Although not specifically studied, a clear trend is present in the literature for increasing proportions of blunt trauma patients to show extravasation when multidetector CT was used with higher injection rates (>2.5 cm^3/s) (85–92).

The likelihood of surgical intervention increases with the detection of multiple injuries (e.g., spleen and left kidney, left lobe of the liver and pancreas). In addition, liver lacerations that involve the hilum, particularly those associated with partial stripping of the gallbladder, may be benefit from repeat scanning or ultrasound, cholescintigraphy, or direct cholangiography to detect possible biliary complications. Liver lacerations involving the hepatic veins, especially when associated with large regions (>10 cm) of focal hypoperfusion, are thought to reflect retrohepatic vena caval injuries and are strongly predictive of surgically evident bleeding necessitating interventions (91–93).

Among patients who have otherwise uncomplicated postinjury courses (e.g., absent increasing abdominal pain, falling hematocrit, clinical features of intraabdominal sepsis, etc.), serial CT scans do not appear to be useful in altering therapy or determining the time for return to full activities, particularly in the pediatric population. Nonetheless, if serial follow-up imaging is believed indicated in specific cases, ultrasound is a more cost-effective alternative than CT (94–96).

B. Bowel and Mesentery Injuries

Controversy persist regarding the optimum and most cost-effective means of evaluating victims of blunt-force trauma perceived to be at risk for otherwise occult HVI. Diagnostic peritoneal lavage (DPL) may be a more sensitive test than CT for isolated HVI (sensitivity >97% vs. sensitivity 90–93%), albeit with lower specificity (~50–60% vs. 95%), even with intravenous contrast enhancement, thin sections, and multidetector technologies. Nonetheless, less than

5% of surgically important blunt-force HVIs occurring in adults are found in the absence of other, often more obvious and clinically immediate, intraabdominal injuries. Conventional radiography, ultrasound, and MRI have limited or no role in the routine diagnosis of bowel injuries (97–106).

Computed tomography, especially with appropriately timed data acquisition relative to intravenous contrast administration, is the currently preferred imaging modality, especially when performed with multidetector equipment at slice thickness of 5 mm or less. However, CT performed without oral or intravenous contrast enhancement may show intramural hematoma as focal, asymmetric hyperdensity within bowel thickened wall with adjacent mesenteric edema ("misty mesentery"). Although the role of oral contrast remains hotly contested, larger case series have failed to show a clinical advantage to its use, which may relate to failed opacification of the postduodenal small bowel in ~40% of patients 30 min following gastrointestinal contrast administration (107–109).

Numerous findings have been described: bowel wall thickening with or without dilation, bowel wall discontinuity, pathologic enhancement of bowel wall, mesenteric hematoma with adjacent bowel wall thickening, interloop (intramesenteric) fluid with abnormal adjacent bowel, extraluminal air or extravasation of alimentary positive contrast, acute abdominal wall hernias with bowel content, and active vascular extravasation from bowel. Bowel contusion may be suggested on intravenous contrast-enhanced CT by focal or multifocal bowel thickening and mural enhancement (sensitivity ~60%), and oral contrast (positive or negative) may help in appreciation of wall thickening. In contrast, diffuse bowel wall thickening and enhancement, especially associated with slit-like infrahepatic inferior vena cava and hypodense and contracted spleen, suggests underresuscitation and so-called hypoperfusion syndrome. While clear demonstration of spillage of positive alimentary contrast is essentially pathognomonic for bowel perforation, apparent bowel wall discontinuity has a sensitivity of ~60% and specificity of ~95% (110, 111). Almost all reports show that free intraabdominal gas is very strongly suggestive of bowel perforation or transaction (sensitivity ~40%; most reports provide a

specificity of ~100%). One unrepeated report found ~60% false-positive diagnoses based on CT-demonstrated pneumoperitoneum (112).

III. What Is the Optimal Imaging Approach in Patients Suspected of Having Retroperitoneal Injury?

Summary of Evidence: In general, retroperitoneal injuries must be suspected based on clinical history and physical examination findings, and laboratory tests (e.g., hematuria) (strong evidence). In adults, CT is currently the diagnostic procedure of choice, as neither trauma ultrasound nor DPL adequately assess the retroperitoneum (moderate evidence). In children, ultrasound may be useful to exclude surgically significant renal injury (color Doppler) (limited evidence). On occasion, conventional radiographic procedures (upper gastrointestinal positive-contrast fluoroscopy, intravenous or retrograde pyelography) may be helpful in secondary or follow-up evaluations of individuals known to have sustained injuries to the duodenum and upper urinary tracts, respectively.

Supporting Evidence: Compared to its performance at detecting acute injuries to intraperitoneal solid organ injury, CT is relatively insensitive to acute pancreatic injuries, even severe injuries completely disrupting the main pancreatic duct or pancreaticoduodenal junction (sensitivities <80%). Direct signs include a fracture plane traversing the neck, body, or tail of the pancreas, or separation of the duodenum from the head of the pancreas. Indirect findings on intravenous contrast-enhanced CT include heterogeneous enhancement of the pancreatic parenchyma, and fluid around the pancreas, especially when combined with fluid in the lesser sac. Fluid posterior to the pancreas, where it may separate the pancreas from the splenic vein, is nonspecific, especially when seen with diffuse anterior pararenal fluid collections, where it likely represents suffusions from aggressive resuscitation with crystalloid fluids. Definitive diagnosis and staging of main pancreatic duct injuries requires intraoperative, endoscopic, or magnetic resonance (MR) cholangiopancreatography. However, MR cholangiopancreatography may be less reliable in the acute than subacute setting (113–120).

Renal parenchymal injuries are more common, both as isolated retroperitoneal and as combined retro- and intraperitoneal injuries. Treatment choices are strongly guided by patients' hemodynamic status, and active arterial extravasation is commonly amenable to endovascular therapies. Interventions are more often required when the collecting systems or ureters are injured, especially when portions of the kidney appear devitalized and where renal injuries are combined with other intraabdominal injuries, such as liver, spleen, pancreas, or bowel lacerations.

Even where trauma ultrasound or DPL are negative, contrast-enhanced CT is indicated for the presence of posttraumatic gross hematuria (all age groups), and microscopic hematuria (>50 red blood cells per high-powered field, 3+ on urine dip) in children (regardless of their hemodynamic status) and in adults who have any documented systolic hypotension (<90 mmHg). Signs or symptoms (flank ecchymosis or pain) of retroperitoneal injury warrant imaging evaluation, even among victims of low-energy trauma, because up to 5–8% of surgically important renal injuries do not show any hematuria and preexisting renal abnormalities (e.g., congenital ureteropelvic junction (UPJ) stenosis, horseshoe kidney) have a much greater propensity for injury, and at least one third of such injured kidneys require intervention (121–123).

Dynamic, contrast-enhanced CT ideally evaluates vascular (vascular pedicle injuries including dissection, pseudoaneurysms, and AV fistulae), parenchymal (parenchymal lacerations), and pyelographic (lacerations involving the collecting system, and UPJ disruptions) physiologic phases. When low- or iso-osmolar intravenous contrast agents are employed, imaging during the late parenchymal phase and following an additional 5–10-min delay shows or strongly suggests the presence of essentially all important upper urinary tract injuries. However, the classic finding for renal infarct, the so-called cortical rim sign, may take 8 h or longer to develop following renal artery occlusion. Other findings, such as retrograde filling of the renal vein, suggest an acute arterial disruption as cause for nonopacification of the kidney. Indirect intravenous contrast-enhanced CT findings of upper urinary tract injury include perinephric stranding and hematoma, and heterogeneous parenchymal enhancement. Medial perinephric hematomas, especially when large and extending into the root of the mesentery, are associated with renovascular and UPJ injuries. Otherwise, the location of perinephric hematoma poorly correlates with the severity of parenchymal injury or the need to intervene. However, larger perinephric hematomas tend to be associated with more severe injuries. Direct intravenous contrast-enhanced CT findings of renal injury include parenchymal lacerations and extravasation, either vascular or urinary, and both of these extravasations may necessitate intervention or follow-up imaging. Although the frequency, timing, and optimum methods for follow-up examination remain subjects of debate, repeat contrast-enhanced CT or MR examinations 2–4 days following acute injury may guide selection of patients for early nonmedical interventions. In children, the initial assessment of severity of blunt renal injury (advancing grade) does not correlate with ultimate renal function or renal-related late complications (such as hypertension). However, advanced grades of renal injury do show morphologic changes on delayed follow-up. In adults, large subcapsular hematomas can be associated with subsequent renin-induced hypertension (Page kidney), and differential renal function is commonly associated with more advanced grades of renal injury (124–136).

Bladder ruptures may be intra- or extraperitoneal, or a combination of both. Almost all extraperitoneal bladder ruptures are associated with high-energy osseous disruptions of the pelvic ring. Although most intraperitoneal ruptures are also associated with high-energy osseous disruptions of the pelvis, the overdistended bladder (due to prostatism, etc.) rising out of the true pelvis may be subjected to direct blunt-force impact and rupture. Hematuria associated with pelvic ring fractures, especially if perivesical hematoma or bladder wall thickening is present, warrants positive-contrast cystography, which should not be considered adequate to exclude injury unless intravesical pressure is at least 40 cm H_2O (137).

With the advent of CT, adrenal injuries are now recognized as the most common retroperitoneal injury. The right is injured much more often than the left, and bilateral adrenal hemorrhage is relatively rare. An association exists between apparent right adrenal hemorrhage and liver lacerations involving the bare area. Despite their frequency (0.5–5%), adrenal hemorrhages very rarely require treatment: embolization for large, active extravasations associated with ongoing hemodynamic consequences, and adrenocortical replacement therapy for hypoadrenalism as a very infrequent sequel to bilateral adrenal hemorrhage. CT findings include irregular, globular enlargement of the gland, typically measuring 40–70 HU. However, definite distinction from extant nontraumatic adrenal pathology may require targeted follow-up CT, ultrasound, or MRI (138, 139).

Take Home Figures

Fig. 28.1–28.3 serve to highlight key recommendations and supporting evidence.

Imaging Case Studies

Case 1

A 56-year-old male passenger was ejected in an high-speed rollover motor vehicle accident (Fig. 28.2), sustaining left lower rib fractures (not shown) with associated pulmonary contusion, and left diaphragmatic rupture with gastric herniation.

Case 2

A 43-year-old woman sustained severe polytrauma (including adrenal, liver, gallbladder, and renal lacerations) in a 20-ft fall onto concrete (Fig. 28.3).

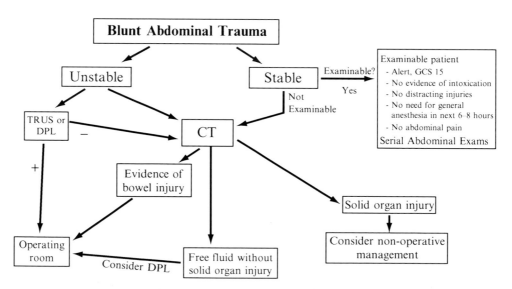

Figure 28.1. Flowchart of abdominal imaging protocol at Harborview Medical Center. The differentiation between hemodynamically stable and unstable is a continuum. With faster multidetector CT scanners and better trauma center design with on-site scanners mitigating the need for patient transport, less stable patients are now safe for CT. Nonoperative management of solid organ injury is preferred, but decision making is affected by hemodynamic stability and presence of arterial extravasation on CT. *DPL* diagnostic peritoneal lavage, *TUS* trauma ultrasound of the peritoneal space, *GCS* Glasgow Coma Scale. (Reprinted with kind permission of Springer Science+Business Media from Mann FA. Blunt Injuries to the Thorax and Abdomen. In Medina LS, Blackmore CC (eds): *Evidence-Based Imaging: Optimizing Imaging in Patient Care.* New York: Springer Science+Business Media, 2006.)

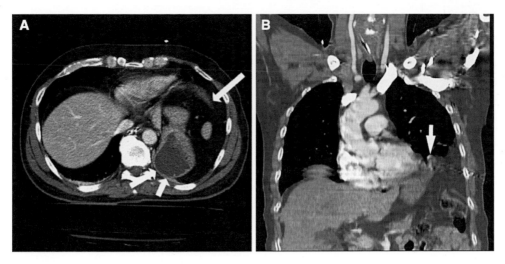

Figure 28.2. (**A**) Axial intravenous contrast-enhanced CT shows a discontinuous and thickened left hemidiaphragm at the 2 o'clock position (*arrow*), through which the stomach has herniated and abuts posterior chest wall ("dependent viscera" sign) (*double arrows*). (**B**) Coronal CT reformation shows the free edge of the lacerated diaphragm (*arrow*) with omentum and stomach herniated into the chest. (Reprinted with kind permission of Springer Science+Business Media from Mann FA. Blunt Injuries to the Thorax and Abdomen. In Medina LS, Blackmore CC (eds): *Evidence-Based Imaging: Optimizing Imaging in Patient Care.* New York: Springer Science+Business Media, 2006.)

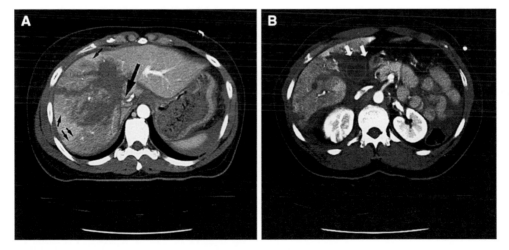

Figure 28.3. (**A**) Axial intravenous contrast-enhanced CT shows complex liver laceration extending to the inferior vena cava (IVC) through the course of the right hepatic vein (*large arrow*). Note geographic pattern of lesser enhancement involving most of the right lobe of liver (*small arrows*), which strong suggests disruption of the hepatic vein and may be associated with retrohepatic vena caval injury. (**B**) Axial intravenous contrast-enhanced CT shows complex liver laceration extending into gallbladder fossa, absent enhancement of the gallbladder wall (11–2 o'clock positions) suggestive of gallbladder rupture (*arrows*), and separation of gallbladder from liver, compatible with partial avulsion. (Reprinted with kind permission of Springer Science+Business Media from Mann FA. Blunt Injuries to the Thorax and Abdomen. In Medina LS, Blackmore CC (eds): *Evidence-Based Imaging: Optimizing Imaging in Patient Care.* New York: Springer Science+Business Media, 2006.)

Future Research

- Development of imaging modalities or imaging-based criteria that enable identification of subjects who require surgical rather than nonsurgical treatment for their injuries.
- Improvement in intravenous contrast agents to enable simultaneous imaging of arterial, venous, and organ parenchymal structures.
- Development of imaging equipment and procedures that enable rapid, accurate cross-sectional imaging of injured patients without transport or disruption of resuscitation efforts.
- Incorporation of imaging into injury-site triage to enable appropriate direction of patients within the trauma system.

Suggested Imaging Protocols

Trauma Computed Tomography of the Abdomen and Pelvis

Imaging protocols for CT of the abdomen and pelvis in trauma remain in flux as newer scanners are developed with higher numbers of detectors. In general, we scan from the dome of the diaphragm to the pelvic floor with a detector collimation of 2.5 mm. Images are reconstructed at 5-mm intervals for viewing on the workstation. Bone images may be reconstructed at 2.5-mm intervals for the bony pelvis and spine as indicated, with coronal and sagittal reformations. We use 150 cm³ of nonionic intravenous contrast and scan after a delay of 60 s. No oral contrast is used.

Trauma Ultrasound

Scanning is performed on a 3.5–5-MHz transducer depending on body habitus. Images are obtained prior to placement of the Foley catheter to preserve some fluid in the bladder. Otherwise, fluid may be inserted via the Foley. Transverse and sagittal images are obtained of the pelvis through the bladder window followed by transverse images of the bilateral upper quadrants and paracolic gutters. The pericardium is also visualized via a subxiphoid and/or left parasternal approach.

References

1. American College of Surgeons. Advanced Trauma Life Support Student Course Manual. Chicago: American College of Surgeons, 1997.
2. National Center for Health Statistics. Monthly Vital Statistics Report 1990;39:22–25.
3. Baker SP, O'Neill B, Ginsburg MJ, Li G. The Injury Fact Book. New York: Oxford University Press, 1992.
4. Rice DP, MacKenzie EJ et al. Cost of Injury in the United States: A Report to Congress. Baltimore, MD: Johns Hopkins University, 1989.
5. Kleinman PK, O'Connor B, Nimkin K et al. Pediatr Radiol 2002;32:896–901.
6. Kleinman PK, Nimkin K, Spevak MR et al. AJR Am J Roentgenol 1996;167:893–896.
7. Mandelstam SA, Cook D, Fitzgerald M, Ditchfield MR. Arch Dis Child 2003;88:387–390; discussion 387–390.
8. Carty H, Pierce A. Eur Radiol 2002;12: 2919–2925.
9. Fuhrman CR, Britton CA, Bender T et al. AJR Am J Roentgenol 2002;179:1551–1553.
10. Alkadhi H, Wildermuth S, Marincek B, Boehm T. J Comput Assist Tomogr 2004;28:378–385.
11. Ludwig K, Schulke C, Diederich S et al. Radiology 2003;227:163–168.
12. Herron JM, Bender TM, Campbell WL, Sumkin JH, Rockette HE, Gur D. Radiology 2000;215: 169–174.
13. Omert L, Yeaney WW, Protetch J. Am Surg 2001;67:660–664.
14. Park SH, Song HH, Han JH et al. Invest Radiol 1994;29:54–58.
15. Gupta A, Jamshidi M, Rubin JR. Cardiovasc Surg 1997;5:48–53.
16. Jelly LM, Evans DR, Easty MJ, Coats TJ, Chan O. Radiographics 2000;20(Spec. No.):S251–259; discussion S260–262.
17. Kara M, Dikmen E, Erdal HH, Simsir I, Kara SA. Eur J Cardiothorac Surg 2003;24:608–613.
18. Calculli L, Papa S, Spagnol A et al. Radiol Med (Torino) 1995;90:208–211.
19. Erhan Y, Solak I, Kocabas S, Sozbilen M, Kumanlioglu K, Moral AR. Ulus Travma Derg 2001;7:242–245.
20. LaBan MM, Siegel CB, Schutz LK, Taylor RS. Arch Phys Med Rehabil 1994;75:353–354.
21. Wippermann B, Schmidt U, Nerlich M. Unfallchirurg 1991;94:231–235.
22. Niitsu M, Takeda T. J Comput Assist Tomogr 2003;27:469–474.

23. Ciraulo DL, Elliott D, Mitchell KA, Rodriguez A. J Am Coll Surg 1994;178:466–470.

24. Lee L, Miller TT, Schultz E, Toledano B. Am J Orthop 1998;27:699–702.

25. Lange RH, Noel SH. J Orthop Trauma 1993;7:361–366.

26. Francois B, Desachy A, Cornu E, Ostyn E, Niquet L, Vignon P. J Trauma 1998;44:217–219.

27. Zelle BA, Pape HC, Gerich TG, Garapati R, Ceylan B, Krettek C. J Bone Joint Surg Am 2004;86-A:2–8.

28. Sampson LN, Britton JC, Eldrup-Jorgensen J, Clark DE, Rosenberg JM, Bredenberg CE. J Vasc Surg 1993;17:1083–1088; discussion 1088–1089.

29. Lahoda LU, Kreklau B, Gekle C, Muhr G. Unfallchirurg 1998;101:791–795.

30. Teh J, Firth M, Sharma A, Wilson A, Reznek R, Chan O. Clin Radiol 2003;58:482–486.

31. Abboud PA, Kendall J. J Emerg Med 2003;25:181–184.

32. Chen SC, Markmann JF, Kauder DR, Schwab CW. J Trauma 1997;42:86–89.

33. Sugimoto K, Asari Y, Hirata M, Imai H, Ohwada T. Injury 1998;29:380–382.

34. Shkrum MJ, Green RN, Shum DT. J Forensic Sci 1991;36:410–421.

35. Tyburski JG, Collinge JD, Wilson RF, Eachempati SR. J Trauma 1999;46:833–838.

36. Donnelly LF, Klosterman LA. Radiology 1997;204:385–387.

37. Liman ST, Kuzucu A, Tastepe AI, Ulasan GN, Topcu S. Eur J Cardiothorac Surg 2003;23:374–378.

38. Miller PR, Croce MA, Kilgo PD, Scott J, Fabian TC. Am Surg 2002;68:845–850; discussion 850–851.

39. Hoegerle S, Benzing A, Nitzsche EU et al. Nuklearmedizin 2001;40:44–50.

40. Hogerle S, Brautigam P, Benzing A et al. Nuklearmedizin 1997;36:137–141.

41. Holmes JF, Sokolove PE, Brant WE, Kuppermann N. Ann Emerg Med 2002;39:492–499.

42. Thaete FL, Fuhrman CR, Oliver JH et al. AJR Am J Roentgenol 1994;162:575–581.

43. Antonelli M, Moro ML, Capelli O et al. Chest 1994;105:224–228.

44. Kiev J, Kerstein MD. Surg Gynecol Obstet 1992;175:249–253.

45. Le Corre A, Genevois A, Hellot MF, Veber B, Dureuil B. Ann Fr Anesth Reanim 2001;20:23–27.

46. Miller PR, Croce MA, Bee TK et al. J Trauma 2001;51:223–228; discussion 229–230.

47. Putensen C, Waibel U, Koller W, Putensen-Himmer G, Beck E, Benzer H. Anaesthesist 1990;39:530–534.

48. Adegboye VO, Ladipo JK, Brimmo IA, Adebo AO. Afr J Med Med Sci 2002;31:315–320.

49. Bokhari F, Brakenridge S, Nagy K et al. J Trauma 2002;53:1135–1138.

50. Trupka A, Kierse R, Waydhas C et al. Unfallchirurg 1997;100:469–476.

51. Shiau YC, Liu FY, Tsai JJ, Wang JJ, Ho ST, Kao A. Ann Nucl Med 2003;17:435–438.

52. Gonzalez RP, Falimirski ME. Am Surg 1999;65:711–713; discussion 714.

53. Helm M, Hauke J, Esser M, Lampl L, Bock KH. Chirurg 1997;68:606–612.

54. Hyre CE, Cikrit DF, Lalka SG, Sawchuk AP, Dalsing MC. J Vasc Surg 1998;27:880–884; discussion 884–885.

55. Karaaslan T, Meuli R, Androux R, Duvoisin B, Hessler C, Schnyder P. J Trauma 1995;39:1081–1086.

56. Litmanovitz I, Dolfin T, Arnon S et al. J Perinat Med 2000;28:158–160.

57. Marts B, Durham R, Shapiro M et al. Am J Surg 1994;168:688–692.

58. Marzi I, Risse N, Wiercinski A, Rose S, Mutschler W. Langenbecks Arch Chir Suppl Kongressbd 1996;113:928–930.

59. von Oettingen G, Bergholt B, Ostergaard L, Jensen LC, Gyldensted C, Astrup J. Neuroradiology 2000;42:168–173.

60. Walz M, Muhr G. Unfallchirurg 1990;93:359–363.

61. Trupka AW, Trautwein K, Waydhas C, Nast-Kolb D, Pfeiffer KJ, Schweiberer L. Zentralbl Chir 1997;122:666–673.

62. Ho RT, Blackmore CC et al. Emerg Radiol 2002;9:183–187.

63. Hunink MGM, Bos JJ. AJR Am J Roentgenol 1995;165:27–36.

64. Boulanger BR, Milzman DP, Rosati C, Rodriguez A. J Trauma 1993;35:255–260.

65. Chen JC, Wilson SE. Am Surg 1991;57:810–815.

66. Gelman R, Mirvis SE, Gens D. AJR Am J Roentgenol 1991;156:51–57.

67. Guth AA, Pachter HL, Kim U. Am J Surg 1995;170:5–9.

68. Ilgenfritz FM, Stewart DE. Am Surg 1992;58:334–338; discussion 338–339.

69. Karnak I, Senocak ME, Tanyel FC, Buyukpamukcu N. Surg Today 2001;31:5–11.

70. Leung JC, Nance ML, Schwab CW, Miller WT Jr. J Thorac Imaging 1999;14:126–129.

71. Murray JG, Caoili E, Gruden JF, Evans SJ, Halvorsen RA Jr, Mackersie RC. AJR Am J Roentgenol 1996;166:1035–1039.

72. Nau T, Seitz H, Mousavi M, Vecsei V. Surg Endosc 2001;15:992–996.

73. Rodriguez-Morales G, Rodriguez A, Shatney CH. J Trauma 1986;26:438–444.

74. Scaglione M, Pinto F, Grassi R et al. Radiol Med (Torino) 2000;99:46–50.

75. Shanmuganathan K, Mirvis SE, White CS, Pomerantz SM. AJR Am J Roentgenol 1996;167:397–402.

76. Shapiro MJ, Heiberg E, Durham RM, Luchtefeld W, Mazuski JE. Clin Radiol 1996;51:27–30.

77. Voeller GR, Reisser JR, Fabian TC, Kudsk K, Mangiante EC. Am Surg 1990;56:28–31.
78. Worthy SA, Kang EY, Hartman TE, Kwong JS, Mayo JR, Muller NL. Radiology 1995;194:885–888.
79. Mehall JR, Ennis JS, Saltzman DA et al. J Am Coll Surg 2001;193:347–353.
80. Stylianos S. J Pediatr Surg 2002;37:453–456.
81. Leinwand MJ, Atkinson CC, Mooney DP. J Pediatr Surg 2004;39:487–490; discussion 487–490.
82. Stengel D, Bauwens K et al. Br J Surg 2001;88: 901–912.
83. Stengel D, Bauwens K et al. Zentralbl Chir 2003;128:1027–1037; German.
84. Sirlin CB, Brown MA, Andrade-Barreto OA et al. Radiology 2004;230:661–668.
85. Stengel D, Bauwens K, Sehouli J, Nantke J, Ekkernkamp A. J Trauma 2001;51:37–43.
86. Barquist ES, Pizano LR, Feuer W et al. J Trauma 2004;56:334–338.
87. Al-Shanafey S, Giacomantonio M, Jackson R. Pediatr Surg Int 2001;17:365–368.
88. Zabolotny B, Hancock BJ, Postuma R, Wiseman N. Can J Surg 2002;45:358–362.
89. Lutz N, Mahboubi S, Nance ML, Stafford PW. J Pediatr Surg 2004;39:491–494.
90. Catalano O, Lobianco R, Sandomenico F, Siani A. J Ultrasound Med 2003;22:467–477.
91. Willmann JK, Roos JE, Platz A et al. AJR Am J Roentgenol 2002;179:437–444.
92. Weishaupt D, Hetzer FH, Ruehm SG, Patak MA, Schmidt M, Debatin JF. Eur Radiol 2000;10: 1958–1964.
93. Pilleul F, Billaud Y, Gautier G et al. Gastrointest Endosc 2004;59:818–822.
94. Huebner S, Reed MH. Pediatr Radiol 2001;31: 852–855.
95. Lyass S, Sela T, Lebensart PD, Muggia-Sullam M. Isr Med Assoc J 2001;3:731–733.
96. Rovin JD, Alford BA, McIlhenny TJ, Burns RC, Rodgers BM, McGahren ED. Am Surg 2001;67:127–130.
97. Albanese CT, Meza MP, Gardner MJ, Smith SD, Rowe MI, Lynch JM. J Trauma 1996;40:417–421.
98. Kloppel R, Brock D, Kosling S, Bennek J, Hormann D. Aktuelle Radiol 1997;7:19–22.
99. Graham JS, Wong AL. J Pediatr Surg 1996;31: 754–756.
100. Hickey NA, Ryan MF, Hamilton PA, Bloom C, Murphy JP, Brenneman F. Can Assoc Radiol J 2002;53:153–159.
101. Jamieson DH, Babyn PS, Pearl R. Pediatr Radiol 1996;26:188–194.
102. Ruf C, Kohlberger E, Ruf G, Farthmann EH. Langenbecks Arch Chir Suppl Kongressbd 1997;114:1244–1246.
103. Sivit CJ, Eichelberger MR, Taylor GA. AJR Am J Roentgenol 1994;163:1195–1198.
104. Sivit CJ, Taylor GA, Bulas DI, Kushner DC, Potter BM, Eichelberger MR. Radiology 1992;182:723–726.
105. Sivit CJ, Taylor GA, Newman KD et al. AJR Am J Roentgenol 1991;157:111–114.
106. Butela ST, Federle MP et al. AJR Am J Roentgenol 2001;176:129–135.
107. Shankar KR, Lloyd DA, Kitteringham L, Carty HM. Br J Surg 1999;86:1073–1077.
108. Allen TL, Mueller MT, Bonk RT, Harker CP, Duffy OH, Stevens MH. J Trauma 2004;56: 314–322.
109. Federle MP, Yagan N, Peitzman AB, Krugh J. Radiology 1997;205:91–93.
110. Breen DJ, Janzen DL, Zwirewich CV, Nagy AG. J Comput Assist Tomogr 1997;21:706–712.
111. Brody JM, Leighton DB, Murphy BL et al. Radiographics 2000;20:1525–1536; discussion 1536–1537.
112. Kane NM, Francis IR, Burney RE, Wheatley MJ, Ellis JH, Korobkin M. Invest Radiol 1991;26: 574–578.
113. Jobst MA, Canty TG, Sr., Lynch FP. J Pediatr Surg 1999;34:818–823; discussion 823–824.
114. Soto JA, Alvarez O, Munera F, Yepes NL, Sepulveda ME, Perez JM. AJR Am J Roentgenol 2001;176:175–178.
115. Fulcher AS, Turner MA, Yelon JA et al. J Trauma 2000;48:1001–1007.
116. Bigattini D, Boverie JH, Dondelinger RF. Eur Radiol 1999;9:244–249.
117. Porter JM, Singh Y. Am J Emerg Med 1998;16: 225–227.
118. Coppola V, Vallone G, Verrengia D et al. Radiol Med (Torino) 1997;94:335–340.
119. Sivit CJ, Eichelberger MR. AJR Am J Roentgenol 1995;165:921–924.
120. Reaney SM, Parker MS, Mirvis SE, Bundschuh CV, Luebbert PD, Vingan HL. Clin Radiol 1995;50:834–838.
121. Bschleipfer T, Kallieris D, Hallscheidt P, Hauck EW, Weidner W, Pust RA. J Urol 2003;170: 2475–2479.
122. Mayor B, Gudinchet F, Wicky S, Reinberg O, Schnyder P. Pediatr Radiol 1995;25:214–218.
123. Brandes SB, McAninch JW. J Trauma 1999;47: 643–649; discussion 649–650.
124. Moudouni SM, Patard JJ, Manunta A, Guiraud P, Guille F, Lobel B. BJU Int 2001;87:290–294.
125. Rathaus V, Pomeranz A, Shapiro-Feinberg M, Zissin R. Emerg Radiol 2004;10:190–192.
126. Toutouzas KG, Karaiskakis M, Kaminski A, Velmahos GC. Am Surg 2002;68:1097–1103.
127. Perez-Brayfield MR, Gatti JM, Smith EA et al. J Urol 2002;167:2543–2546; discussion 2546–2547.
128. Nguyen MM, Das S. Urology 2002;59:762–766; discussion 766–767.
129. Pietrera P, Badachi Y, Liard A, Dacher JN. J Radiol 2001;82:833–838.

130. Ku JH, Jeon YS, Kim ME, Lee NK, Park YH. Int J Urol 2001;8:261–267.
131. Blankenship JC, Gavant ML, Cox CE, Chauhan RD, Gingrich JR. World J Surg 2001;25:1561–1564.
132. Sebastia MC, Rodriguez-Dobao M, Quiroga S, Pallisa E, Martinez-Rodriguez M, Alvarez-Castells A. Eur Radiol 1999;9:611–615.
133. McGahan JP, Richards JR, Jones CD, Gerscovich EO. J Ultrasound Med 1999;18:207–213; quiz 215–216.
134. Perry MJ, Porte ME, Urwin GH. J R Coll Surg Edinb 1997;42:420–422.
135. Mulligan JM, Cagiannos I, Collins JP, Millward SF. J Urol 1998;159:67–70.
136. Kawashima A, Sandler CM, Corriere JN Jr, Rodgers BM, Goldman SM. Radiology 1997;205:487–492.
137. Deck AJ, Shaves S, Talner L, Porter JR. World J Surg 2001;25:1592–1596.
138. Stawicki SP, Hoey BA, Grossman MD, Anderson HL 3rd, Reed JF 3rd. Curr Surg 2003;60: 431–436.
139. Schwarz M, Horev G, Freud E et al. Isr Med Assoc J 2000;2:132–134.

Part VI

Abdominal and Pelvic Imaging

29

Imaging of Appendicitis in Adult and Pediatric Patients

C. Craig Blackmore, Erin A. Cooke, and Gregory David Avey

Issues

I. What is the accuracy of imaging for diagnosing acute appendicitis in adults?
II. What is the accuracy of diagnostic imaging in pediatric patients?
III. Which subjects suspected of having appendicitis should undergo imaging?
IV. What is the effect of imaging on negative appendectomy rate?

Key Points

- In adult patients, CT demonstrates superior sensitivity and specificity for appendicitis compared to ultrasound, with less variability, and is the imaging modality of choice in nonpregnant patients (strong evidence).
- In pediatric patients, CT has higher sensitivity than ultrasound, but similar specificity, with the trade off of exposure to ionizing radiation (strong evidence).
- A protocol of initial use of ultrasound followed by CT for negative or equivocal cases may be warranted in (nonobese) pediatric patients in order to minimize the risks of ionizing radiation (moderate evidence). The presence of an elevated absolute neutrophil count, nausea, or maximal tenderness in the right lower quadrant shows high sensitivity, but poor specificity in identifying pediatric patients with appendicitis (moderate evidence). These patients may benefit from imaging.
- There is a moderate evidence of a decrease in the rate of negative appendectomy with use of preoperative imaging.
- MRI may be useful in pregnant women with suspected appendicitis, particularly beyond the first trimester (limited evidence). CT should be avoided in pregnant women.

C.C. Blackmore (✉)
Department of Radiology, Center for Healthcare Solutions, Virginia Mason Medical Center,
Seattle, WA 98111, USA
e-mail: craig.blackmore@vmmc.org

Definition and Pathophysiology

Appendicitis is defined as inflammation of the vermiform appendix, usually caused by obstruction of the appendiceal lumen (1, 2). Obstruction leads to bacterial overgrowth and an increase in intraluminal pressure, which in turn causes a decrease in mural perfusion. The resulting inflammation and decrease in vascular perfusion can lead to gangrene and perforation. Delayed diagnosis can result in serious complications, including gross perforation, abscess formation, peritonitis, wound infection, sepsis, infertility, adhesions, and bowel obstruction (1, 3).

Epidemiology

Acute appendicitis represents a relatively common condition, with an estimated lifetime incidence of 9% in males and 7% in females, and is most common (4) in those aged between 10 and 19 years (4, 5). Acute appendicitis is the most common reason for abdominal surgery in pediatric patients (3, 6, 7), with 70,000–90,000 pediatric cases each year, and is diagnosed in 1–8% of children presenting with abdominal pain to the emergency department (7, 8). The overall rate of perforation is 19–35.5%, with the risk proportionally greater in the pediatric and elderly populations (5, 9).

Overall Cost to Society

Comprehensive societal cost data for patients with suspected acute appendicitis is lacking. However, an analysis of the Nationwide Inpatient Sample of the Health Care Utilization Project estimated that there were 261,134 yearly hospitalizations due to suspected acute appendicitis. These admissions accrued an average hospital charge of $10,584, yielding an estimated national total of $2.76 billion dollars in hospital charges alone (10). In this same analysis, Flum and Koepsell estimated the national cost of negative appendectomy at $741.5 million dollars (10).

For pediatric patients, appendectomy is the most common surgical procedure performed in the hospital for nonneonatal or nonpregnancy related conditions (11). Nationwide, an average

of 238 pediatric appendectomies are performed daily. Annually, appendicitis accounts for approximately 87,000 pediatric hospital stays in the USA, representing 4.2% of all hospital stays for pediatric illness (11). Appendicitis is the second most common reason for hospitalization for children and adolescents 6–17 years old. The aggregate total charges related to care of pediatric patients with appendicitis nationwide sum to over $800,000,000 annually (11). At an institutional level, a retrospective chart review by Garcia Pena et al. showed that 308 pediatric patients who were observed for possible appendicitis collectively accumulated 487 inpatient observation days, with a per patient cost of $5,831 (12).

Goals

The goals of imaging in suspected acute appendicitis are to determine if the patient has appendicitis, enable earlier diagnosis, and identify complications, such as perforation or abscess, which may change surgical management.

Methodology

This report is based primarily on the meta-analyses of Terasawa and Doria and their colleagues. These studies were updated through a PubMed search of English-language articles through March 2010 using the MeSH terms *appendicitis* and *diagnostic imaging*. The bibliographies of relevant articles were searched for other potentially relevant articles. Studies were included if they were either prospective or retrospective evaluations of CT, graded compression ultrasound, or MRI with outcomes measured by surgical, pathological, or clinical follow-up.

I. What Is the Accuracy of Imaging for Diagnosing Acute Appendicitis in Adults?

Summary of Evidence: Computed tomography examination of adult patients has high sensitivity and specificity for acute appendicitis and is superior to graded compression ultrasound (moderate evidence).

Supporting Evidence: The meta-analysis by Terasawa et al. found 22 prospective trials of graded compression ultrasound or CT in adult and adolescent patients with suspected acute appendicitis. This meta-analysis identified 12 studies of CT in adult and adolescent patients, and demonstrated a combined sensitivity of 94% [95% confidence interval (CI), 91–95%], a combined specificity of 95% (95% CI, 93–96%), a combined positive likelihood ratio of 13.3 (95% CI, 9.9–17.9), and a combined negative likelihood ratio of 0.09 (95% CI, 0.07–0.12). When these test specifications are applied to a population with the mean prevalence of appendicitis found in the trials examined by Terasawa et al. (48%), the positive predictive value is 92% (range 67–98%), and the negative predictive value is 92% (range 76–99%) (Table 29.1) (13). The sensitivity and specificity of CT were homogeneous in these identified studies despite heterogeneous patient populations, differing prevalence of appendicitis, and varying contrast protocols.

There were 14 studies of graded compression ultrasound that met inclusion criteria in the Terasawa et al. study. There was significant heterogeneity in the outcome of the trials, requiring the use of a random effects model to combine study results. The summary sensitivity of ultrasound in adult and adolescent patients was 86% (95% CI, 78–84%), the summary specificity is 81% (95% CI, 78–84%), the summary positive likelihood ratio was 5.8 (95% CI, 9.4–22.2), and the summary negative likelihood ratio was 0.19 (95% CI, 0.13–0.27). The positive predictive value of graded compression ultrasound was 84% (range 46–95%) and the negative predictive value was 85% (range 60–97%) (Table 29.1) (13).

Several limitations were identified regarding imaging's efficacy in diagnosing adult and adolescent acute appendicitis. All studies reviewed by Terasawa et al. demonstrated differential reference standard bias, in that the imaging test results determined which subjects underwent appendectomy and which had clinical follow-up as the reference standard (13). Since the diagnostic test influenced the choice of reference standard, there is the possibility that the sensitivity and specificity for imaging were overestimated (14).

II. What Is the Accuracy of Diagnostic Imaging in Pediatric Patients?

Summary of Evidence:

- CT is more sensitive than ultrasound with similar specificity (moderate evidence) (Table 29.1).
- A protocol of US followed by CT in negative or equivocal subjects may achieve similar sensitivity and specificity to CT alone, with less radiation exposure (moderate evidence).
- A protocol of US followed by CT if negative may be cost-effective for the evaluation of pediatric patients suspected of having appendicitis (moderate evidence).
- There are no reliable data to support use of abdominal radiographs in the diagnosis of acute appendicitis (insufficient evidence).
- MRI appears to have moderately high diagnostic accuracy for appendicitis in pregnant patients (limited evidence).

Supporting Evidence: Abdominal radiography is generally considered to be both insensitive and nonspecific in the diagnosis of acute appendicitis, although there are limited data to support this (7). Some studies have indicated that abdominal radiographs are either normal or misleading in approximately 77% of children with appendicitis, and that they rarely affect management (8). Many of the findings that can be seen with appendicitis, such as localized ileus, bowel obstruction, and a right lower quadrant soft tissue mass, are very nonspecific. The purportedly most specific finding of that of a calcified appendicolith, is seen only in approximately 5–15% of patients with appendicitis, versus in less than 1–2% of children without appendicitis (2, 8).

Cross section imaging, therefore, is the mainstay of imaged guided diagnosis. The meta-analysis by Doria et al. (15) found 26 prospective and retrospective trials of graded compression US and/or CT in pediatric patients (mean age range of 7–12 years) with suspected acute appendicitis. Studies included results from ultrasound only, CT only, or combined ultrasound and CT in 6,850, 598, and 1,908 patients, respectively. The mean sample prevalence of appendicitis from these trials was 0.31 for both US and CT articles (range, 0.15–0.75). The weighted perforation rate in positive appendicitis cases was 26.5% (15).

This meta-analysis identified eight studies of CT in pediatric patients, which demonstrated a pooled sensitivity of 94% (95% CI, 92–97%), a combined specificity of 95% (95% CI, 94–97%), and a summary diagnostic odds ratio of 239 (95% CI, 118–487). For the extracted data, the positive and negative likelihood ratios were 18.8 and 0.06, respectively. When these test specifications were applied to a population with the mean prevalence of appendicitis found in the trials examined by Doria et al. (31%), the positive predictive value was 89% and the negative predictive value was 97% (Table 29.1) (15). A single small prospective trial of CT in pediatric patients with suspected acute appendicitis published since the Doria et al. paper yielded similar results (16).

There were 23 studies of graded compression ultrasound that met inclusion criteria in the Doria et al. study. With one outlier removed, the pooled sensitivity of ultrasound in pediatric populations was 88% (95% CI, 86–90%), the pooled specificity was 94% (95% CI, 92–95%), and the summary diagnostic odds ratio was 202 (95% CI, 159–258). The positive and negative likelihood ratios were 14.7 and 0.13, respectively (6). The positive predictive value of graded compression ultrasound was 87%, and the negative predictive value was 95% using the mean prevalence of 31% for calculations (Table 29.1) (15).

Thus, in patients with suspected acute appendicitis in whom further evaluation with imaging is desired, the Doria et al. article demonstrated that there is a significant difference in the weighted pooled sensitivities in favor of CT use, with no significant difference in specificity of CT compared to US. However, as the authors noted, pediatric patients in general demonstrate greater sensitivity to ionizing radiation, which is produced with CT scanning. This radiation risk of CT use must be weighed against the risk of additional false-negative cases with US.

Limitations in the pediatric appendicitis imaging literature included verification and selection bias, as in adults. Additional difficulties in analysis included lack of randomization of patients to imaging groups. Generalizability may also be an issue as CT was more commonly studied in North America whereas ultrasound was more prevalently used in Europe and Asia. In addition, relatively few children under the age of 5 years were included in many of the studies, so that the results may not hold true for infants and preschool age children.

Ideally, an imaging protocol would combine the sensitivity of CT with the lack of ionizing radiation afforded by US in order to maximize diagnostic accuracy, while minimizing patient risk. In our literature search, two prospective studies were identified which examined the combination of graded compression ultrasound as the initial imaging, followed by CT study if the appendix was not visualized by ultrasound or if the ultrasound was inconclusive for the diagnosis of appendicitis (17, 18). These trials enrolled a total of 585 patients with a prevalence of appendicitis ranging from 23 to 43% with a pooled prevalence of 39%. The sensitivity varied from 77 to 97% with a pooled sensitivity of 95% (95% CI, 83–100%). The range of specificity was 89–99%, with a pooled result of 93% (95% CI, 97–97%). As expected, these series demonstrated a greater sensitivity and lower specificity when the combined US followed by CT results were considered than when the US data were considered alone. Another randomized trial of 600 patients compared results of CT and ultrasound versus ultrasound alone in a pediatric population (19). This study demonstrated similar results to the two aforementioned series, with the combined CT and ultrasound protocol demonstrating a sensitivity of 99% and specificity of 89%, while ultrasound alone showed a sensitivity of 86% and specificity of 95%.

An additional consideration in deciding on the use of US versus CT is patient body habitus. An elevated body mass index (BMI) can limit visualization of the appendix with ultrasound, with nonvisualization of the appendix in 79% of overweight children compared to 33% in normal weight and 25% in underweight children (6). The majority of studies evaluating diagnostic imaging do not report weight or BMI, and thus it is difficult to define a cutoff as to which children of a given weight would benefit more from CT compared to US. A retrospective study by Grayson et al. found that increased intraperitoneal fat was correlated with a significantly increased likelihood of visualizing a normal appendix on CT of pediatric patients (20).

A recent formal cost-effectiveness analysis compared a protocol based on US followed by CT if negative to use of CT and US alone. The Markov decision analytic model indicated that the incremental cost effectiveness ratio (ICER) of the US followed by CT protocol was below $10,000 in both male and female pediatric patients (21). This falls well below the threshold for societal willingness to pay of $50,000. Thus, the protocol of US followed by CT was found to be a cost-effective imaging strategy (moderate evidence).

MRI has been promoted for the evaluation of possible appendicitis in pregnant patients, due to the lack of ionizing radiation. Gadolinium is not recommended. Data to date are limited, but small preliminary retrospective studies suggest that sensitivity of 90% and specificity 93% may be achievable (22, 23). No higher quality diagnostic accuracy studies are yet available.

III. Which Subjects Suspected of Having Appendicitis Should Undergo Imaging?

Summary of Evidence:

- No validated clinical prediction rules exist to determine which subjects should undergo imaging in appendicitis in adults.
- A pediatric clinical prediction rule that relies on signs and symptoms in conjunction with basic laboratory values may be useful in identifying subjects who do not need imaging (Table 29.2). This prediction rule has been validated at a single institution (moderate evidence).
- Limited data and modeling studies suggest that CT is most useful when the clinical probability of acute appendicitis is intermediate to high, as a confirmatory test in subjects for whom surgery is considered.

Supporting Evidence: Clinical exam and serum laboratory testing remains the standard initial method of determining which subjects may have appendicitis. However, given the historical rates of both missed diagnosis and unnecessary

laparotomy, a number of investigators have attempted to formalize the clinical exam into a valid scoring tool or decision rule for deciding which subjects are at risk of appendicitis. In 1986, Alvarado introduced a tool termed the MANTRELS criteria for scoring of appendicitis risk in adults (2). However, diagnostic accuracy in was low, with significant inter-provider variability in the successful use of these criteria (2). No useful adult clinical prediction rules for appendicitis imaging have been validated.

More recent efforts have focused on using clinical and laboratory examination as a triage tool in pediatric subjects to determine children who are at sufficiently low risk for appendicitis so that imaging could be avoided (24). Kharbanda et al. developed and validated a clinical prediction rule based on the presence of absolute neutrophil count $>6.75 \times 10^3/\mu L$, nausea, or maximal tenderness in the right lower quadrant to have a sensitivity of 98% and specificity of 32% in identifying patients with appendicitis (Table 29.2). Application of this rule could allow for a reduction in use of CT by 20% (24). Limitations in this study include the potential for interobserver variability and lack of validation in other locations.

Garcia Pena et al. also performed recursive partitioning analysis of a retrospective cohort of 958 children with equivocal acute appendicitis, who were risk stratified into three groups based on clinical signs and symptoms as well as laboratory values (25). Three different management guidelines with subsequent modeling of outcomes were developed. Outcomes included the number of negative appendectomies and missed or delayed diagnoses of appendicitis. The authors showed that management guidelines with more selective use of imaging could reduce the number of imaging exams ordered with minimal increase in the negative appendectomy rate and the number of missed diagnoses of appendicitis. However, these guidelines were not validated, so the effectiveness in clinical practice is uncertain.

There is only limited evidence on which subjects at risk for appendicitis should undergo imaging. Recent investigations by Nathan (26) and Kim et al. (27) suggest that imaging is more likely to be of value for clinical decision making when performed in subjects determined clinically to be high probability of acute appendicitis. In a study of community emergency physicians, Nathan found that when the emergency physicians determined that appendicitis was unlikely, the diagnostic yield from CT was extremely low. However, neither emergency physicians nor consulting surgeons were able to define when appendicitis was certain. Kim et al. found that CT would substantially decrease the rate of negative laparotomy in subjects with clinically evident appendicitis (26). In addition, modeling demonstrates the potential adverse effect of false-positive diagnoses if CT is used to screen a more low risk population (28). These results would suggest that the most appropriate use of CT is in subjects at intermediate risk as well as in subjects at high pretest probability for appendicitis. In effect, confirmatory CT should be performed in all subjects prior to being taken to the operating room for suspected appendicitis (26).

IV. What Is the Effect of Imaging on Negative Appendectomy Rate?

Summary of Evidence: There is moderate evidence that negative appendectomy rate decreases with increasing use of preoperative imaging, in particular CT.

Supporting Evidence: Historically, before the advent of routine CT and US use, history and physical exam were the key to the diagnosis of appendicitis and were associated with an approximately 20% negative appendectomy rate (29). In both adults and children, moderate evidence supports an association between imaging and a decrease in negative laparotomy rate.

In adults, the prospective Surgical Care and Outcomes Assessment Program (SCOAP) included 15 hospitals in Washington State, and reported a significantly lower negative appendectomy rate after imaging. The study included 3,450 patients who underwent urgent appendectomy, with a negative appendectomy rate of 9.8% in subjects without imaging, 8.1% in subjects who underwent ultrasound, and 4.5% in those who underwent CT (30). Smaller prospective trials, and retrospective studies are inconsistent, but generally support a similar effect (27, 31–34).

In children, the best available studies are retrospective. Rao et al. evaluated a consecutive group of 129 pediatric patients from 1992 to 1995, before introduction of appendiceal CT, and were compared to a group of 59 patients in 1997, after establishment of a standard appendiceal CT protocol (35). All of the patients in both groups underwent appendectomy. The NAR dropped with the advent of appendiceal CT availability, from 10 to 5% in boys and from 18 to 12% in girls. A second study, from Boston's Children Hospital by Garcia Pena et al., compared a retrospective cohort of consecutive patients admitted for suspected appendicitis before the use of a US–CT protocol, to a prospective cohort of patients who were evaluated during time the US–CT protocol was in use (36). The protocol involved obtaining US on all patients with equivocal appendicitis, followed by CT for equivocal or inconclusive US cases. The NAR dropped from 14.7% in the first group to 4.1% in the second group ($p < 0.001$). A third study, also from Children's Hospital Boston, found a decrease in the NAR from 11 to 5.5% ($p = 0.03$) with the use of selective CT or US imaging in the context of a clinical practice guideline compared to a control group of patients before the frequent utilization of imaging at their institution (37). However, this study evaluated the entire protocol and not the effects of imaging alone and thus other factors could have contributed to this result. One potential limitation of these three studies is the possible lack of generalizability as they were performed at urban academic institutions.

Take Home Tables and Figures

Tables 29.1–29.2 and Fig. 29.1–29.2 serve to highlight key recommendations and supporting evidence.

Imaging Case Studies

Case 1

Figure 29.1 presents the case of a 10-year-old girl in the emergency department complaining of less than 24 h of periumbilical abdominal pain as well as nausea and emesis.

Case 2

Figure 29.2 presents the case of a 54-year-old male presenting to the emergency department who complained of right lower quadrant abdominal pain and nausea for 2 days.

CT Protocols for Suspected Appendicitis

There is no consensus in the literature as to the ideal CT protocol with respect to use of intravenous contrast, oral contrast, rectal contrast, or noncontrast technique, with varying reports of the efficacy of these protocols (3, 38–43). There is also significant variability in terms of recommendations regarding focused imaging of the appendiceal region versus complete scan of the abdomen and pelvis, with tradeoffs between radiation dose and more complete exam (44, 45). In general, CT protocols are very institutional dependent, and the best technique for a given patient may vary depending on her ability to tolerate administration of oral or rectal contrast, and if there are any contraindications to intravenous contrast. Use of radiation dose reduction techniques is critical particularly given the relatively young age of most subjects (peak age 10–30 years) with clinically suspected appendicitis. There is, however a trend in the use of IV contrast alone without enteric contrast for emergency department patients to improve the throughput of patients (41).

Table 29.1. Sensitivity and specificity of imaging in patients with suspected acute appendicitis

	Sensitivity (%)	Specificity (%)	Positive predictive value[a] (%)	Negative predictive value[a] (%)
Adults[b]				
Ultrasound	86	81	81	86
CT	94	95	95	95
Pediatric[c]				
Ultrasound	88	94	87	95
CT	94	95	95	97
Ultrasound followed by CT[d]	95	93	86	98

Modified with kind permission of Springer Science+Business Media from Blackmore CC, Chang TA, Avey GD. In Medina LS, Blackmore CC (eds.): *Evidence-Based Imaging: Optimizing Imaging in Patient Care*. New York: Springer Science+Business Media, 2006.
[a]Calculated utilizing a prevalence of appendicitis of 48 and 31%, for the adult and pediatric trials respectively.
[b]From Terasawa et al. (13).
[c]From Doria et al. (15).
[d]Teo et al. (17), Garcia Pena et al. (18), and Kaiser et al. (19).

Table 29.2. Clinical decision rule for prediction of pediatric patients at elevated risk for acute appendicitis

Presence of any of the following three factors has a sensitivity of 98% and specificity of 32% in identifying pediatric patients with appendicitis
Absolute neutrophil count (ANC) > $6.75 \times 10^3/\mu L$
Nausea
Maximal tenderness in the right lower quadrant

Data from Kharbanda et al. (24).
Reprinted with kind permission of Springer Science+Business Media from Cooke EA, Blackmore CC. In Medina LS, Applegate KE, Blackmore CC (eds.): *Evidence-Based Imaging in Pediatrics: Optimizing Imaging in Pediatric Patient Care*. New York: Springer Science+Business Media, 2010.

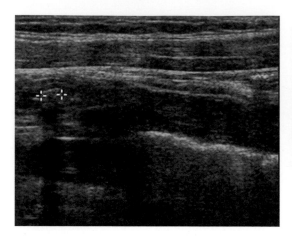

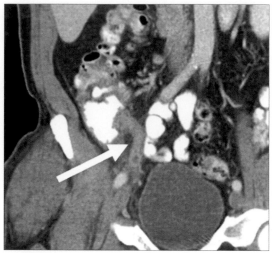

Figure 29.1. Ten-year-old female presented to the emergency department complaining of less than 24 h of periumbilical abdominal pain as well as nausea and emesis. On physical exam, she was afebrile and demonstrated right lower quadrant tenderness with guarding. Laboratory evaluation revealed an elevated white blood cell count of 16,700 cells/mm³. An ultrasound was obtained, demonstrating a blind-ending, noncompressible tubular structure in the right lower quadrant compatible with a dilated appendix measuring 13 mm in diameter and containing an echogenic, shadowing fecalith. On appendectomy, gross and histological findings established the presence of a nonperforated but friable, suppurative appendix. (Reprinted with kind permission of Springer Science+Business Media from Cooke EA, Blackmore CC. In Medina LS, Applegate KE, Blackmore CC (eds.): *Evidence-Based Imaging in Pediatrics: Optimizing Imaging in Pediatric Patient Care.* New York: Springer Science+Business Media, 2010.)

Figure 29.2. Fifty-four-year-old male presenting to the emergency department complained of right lower quadrant abdominal pain and nausea for 2 days. On physical exam, he was afebrile and demonstrated right lower quadrant tenderness with rebound pain. White blood cell count was mildly elevated at 10,800 cells/mm³. CT demonstrated a dilated, 11 mm appendix with mural thickening and inflammatory changes in the periappendiceal fat. Gross examination of the appendix after appendectomy revealed a necrotic dilated appendix containing purulent material.

Future Research

- Multicenter validation of proposed clinical decision rules aimed at determining when imaging is indicated patients with suspected appendicitis.
- Determination of the accuracy and role of MRI in pregnant women suspected of having appendicitis.
- Determination of the overall cost and cost-effectiveness of imaging in patients with suspected acute appendicitis.

References

1. Kumar V, Abbas AK, Fausto N, Aster J. Robbins and Cotran Pathological Basis of Disease, 8th ed. Philadelphia: WB Saunders, 2009.
2. Brennan CDG. Can J Emerg Med 2006;8: 425–432.
3. Sivit CJ, Applegate KE. Semin Ultrasound CT MR 2003;24:74–82.
4. Addiss DG, Shaffer N, Fowler BS, Tauxe RV. Am J Epidemiol 1990;132:910–925.
5. Al-Omran M, Mamdani M, McLeod RS. Can J Surg 2003;46:263–268.
6. Puig S, Staudenherz A, Feldr-Puig R, Paya K. Semin Roentgenol 2008;43:22–28.
7. Kwok MY, Kim MK, Gorelick MH. Pediatr Emerg Care 2004;20:690–698.
8. Rothrock SG, Pagane J. Ann Emerg Med 2000;36: 39–51.
9. Korner H, Sondenaa K, Soreide JA et al. World J Surg 1997;21:313–317.
10. Flum DR, Koepsell T. Arch Surg 2002;137: 799–804.
11. Agency for Healthcare Research and Quality (AHRQ). Care of Children and Adolescents in US Hospitals: HCUP Fact Book No. 4. Rockville, MD: AHRQ, 2003.
12. Garcia Pena BM, Taylor GA, Lund DP, Mandl KD. Pediatrics 1999;104:440–446.
13. Terasawa T, Blackmore C, Bent S, Kohlwes R. Ann Intern Med 2004;141:537–546.
14. Whiting P, Rutjes AW, Dinnes J, Reitsma J, Bossuyt PM, Kleijnen J. Health Technol Assess 2004;8:1–234.
15. Doria AS, Moineddin R, Kellenberger CJ et al. Radiology 2006;241:83–94.
16. Acosta R, Cain E, Goldman HS. Pediatr Radiol 2005;35:495–500.
17. Teo ELHJ, Tan KPAA, Lam SL, Ong CL, Wong CS. Singapore Med J 2000;41:387–392.
18. Garcia Pena BM, Mandl KD, Kraus SJ et al. JAMA 1999;282:1041–1046.
19. Kaiser S, Frenckner B, Jorulf HK. Radiology 2002;223:633–638.
20. Grayson DE, Wettlaufer JR, Dalrymple NC, Keesling CA. AJR Am J Roentgenol 2001;176: 497–500.
21. Wan MJ, Krahn M, Ungar WJ et al. Radiology 2009;250:378–386.
22. Oto A, Ernst RD, Ghulmiyyah LM. Abdom Imaging 2009;34:243–250.
23. Pedrosa I, Lafornara M, Pandharipande PV, Goldsmith JD, Rofsky NM. Radiology 2009;250:749–757.
24. Kharbanda AB, Taylor GA, Fishman SJ, Bachur RG. Pediatrics 2005;116:709–715.
25. Garcia Pena BM, Cook EF, Mandl KD. Pediatrics 2004;113:24–28.
26. Nathan RO. AJR Am J Roentgenol 2008;191: 1102–1106.
27. Kim K, Rhee JE, Lee CC et al. Emerg Med J 2008;25:477–481.
28. Blackmore CC, Terasawa T. J Am Coll Radiol 2006;3:115–121.
29. Bendeck SE, Nino-Murcia M, Berry GJ, Jeffrey RB. Radiology 2002;225:131–136.
30. Cuschieri J, Florence M, Flum DR et al. Ann Surg 2008;248:557–563.
31. Lee CC, Golub R, Singer AJ, Cantu R, Levinson H. Acad Emerg Med 2007;14:117–122.
32. Flum DR, Morris A, Koepsell TD, Dellinger P. JAMA 2001;286:1746–1753.
33. Morse C, Roettger RH, Kalbaugh MS, Blackhurst DW, Hines WB. Am Surg 2007;73:580–584.
34. Rao PM, Rhea JT, Novelline RA, Mostafavi AA, McCabe CJ. N Engl J Med 1998;338:141–146.
35. Rao PM, Rhea JT, Rattner DW. Ann Surg 1999;229:344–349.
36. Garcia Pena BM, Taylor GA, Fishman SJ, Mandl KD. Pediatrics 2002;110:1088–1093.
37. Smink DS, Finkelstein JA, Garcia Pena BM. J Pediatr Surg 2004;39:458–463.
38. Balthazar EJ, Birnbaum BA, Yee J, Megibow AJ, Roshkow J, Gray C. Radiology 1994;190:31–35.
39. Lowe LH, Penney MW, Stein SM et al. AJR Am J Roentgenol 2001;176:31–35.
40. Blackmore CC, Mann FA, Nunez DB. Emerg Radiol 2000;7:142–148.
41. Anderson SW, Soto JA, Lucey BC et al. AJR Am J Roentgenol 2009;193:1282–8.
42. Mun S, Ernst RD, Chen K, Oto A, Shah S, Mileski WJ. Emerg Radiol 2006;12:99–102.
43. Giuliano V, Giuliano C, Pinto F, Scaglione M. Emerg Radiol 2005;11:281–285.
44. Mullins ME, Kircher MF, Ryan DP. AJR Am J Roentgenol 2001;176:37–41.
45. Fefferman NR, Roche KJ, Pinkney LP. Radiology 2001;220:691–695.

Imaging in Non-appendiceal Acute Abdominal Pain

C. Craig Blackmore and Gregory David Avey

Given the broad range of diagnoses that may cause acute abdominal pain, several important diseases are examined in the other chapters of this book. Guidelines regarding the imaging of appendicitis, ureteral calculi, ectopic pregnancy, hepatobiliary disease, and vascular disease can be found in their respective chapters. Other frequent etiologies of acute abdominal pain are discussed in this chapter as individual entities.

Issues

   I. What is the accuracy of imaging for diagnosing small bowel obstruction?
  II. Diverticulitis:
II A. What is the accuracy of imaging for acute colonic diverticulitis?
II B. What is the accuracy of CT in predicting the success of conservative management in patients with suspected acute colonic diverticulitis?

Key Points

- CT has high sensitivity for detection of small bowel obstruction and is often able to identify the cause of obstruction (moderate evidence).
- CT has high negative predictive value for ischemic bowel in subjects with small bowel obstruction (moderate evidence).
- CT has high accuracy for detection of colonic diverticulitis (moderate evidence), but the effect on patient management and outcome has not been established (limited evidence).

C.C. Blackmore (✉)
Department of Radiology, Center for Healthcare Solutions, Virginia Mason Medical Center, 1100 Ninth Avenue, Seattle, WA 98111, USA
e-mail: craig.blackmore@vmmc.org

L.S. Medina et al. (eds.), *Evidence-Based Imaging: Improving the Quality of Imaging in Patient Care, Revised Edition*,
DOI 10.1007/978-1-4419-7777-9_30, © Springer Science+Business Media, LLC 2011

Definition and Pathophysiology

The term acute abdomen is defined as significant abdominal pain that develops over a course of hours (1, 2). The list of potential diagnoses is broad and encompasses potentially serious as well as relatively innocuous conditions (3). The initial presenting pain is often vague and diffuse reflecting the visceral innervation of the abdominal organs (4). These factors can make achieving an accurate clinical diagnosis difficult. For example, one series collected before the advent of graded compression ultrasound or helical CT demonstrated a change from the initial diagnosis to discharge diagnosis in 55% of patients admitted for abdominal pain (5).

The causes of *small bowel obstruction* are quite varied, with intra-abdominal adhesions, external and internal hernias, and neoplasms underlying the obstruction in the majority of patients (6). Other less common causes include volvulus, intussusception, inflammatory strictures, gallstones, feces, and bezoars. Mechanistically, the ischemic pathology of small bowel obstruction is thought to occur in a similar order as appendicitis; i.e., obstruction, bowel wall edema and interluminal fluid accumulation, followed by a decrease in vascular perfusion potentially causing ischemia and perforation (7). Progression to perforation does not occur in all patients presenting with small bowel obstruction, and the majority of patients with proximal, nonischemic obstruction due to adhesions will successfully resolve with non-operative management (6, 8, 9). Additionally, after each operation for small bowel obstruction due to adhesions there is an increasing risk of future episodes, with a recurrence rate of 81% after four such operations (10).

Three interdependent states have traditionally been defined in the study of *diverticular disease:* the prediverticular state, diverticulosis, and diverticulitis (11). The general term "diverticular disease," and diverticulosis refer to the presence of uninflamed diverticula, while the term diverticulitis describes the variety of inflammatory conditions associated with these lesions (12). Diverticulitis originates from both increased interluminal pressure and inherent weakness in the colonic wall near the areas of penetration of the vasa recta (12, 13). Epidemiologic studies suggest that a diet low in fiber presents an increased risk of formation of diverticuli in the sigmoid colon (14). Diverticulitis is thought to result from obstruction of diverticuli, resulting in inflammation and eventual microabscess formation (12). Severity of diverticulitis has been categorized by Hinchey et al. into four categories, with stage I being defined as those patients with microabscess formation. Patients with stage II disease have larger abscess collections, while stages III and IV are defined as peritonitis and fecal peritonitis respectively (15).

Epidemiology

Over seven million patients with *acute abdominal pain* present to an emergency department every year, making up 4–6% of all ED visits (16–18). Upon discharge, 25–41% will remain without a specific etiology for their abdominal pain (18, 19). These patients with undifferentiated abdominal pain typically have a benign course and a reassuring prognosis (20, 21). However, several life-threatening causes of abdominal pain have a high incidence of missed diagnosis, including ruptured aortic aneurysm, appendicitis, ectopic pregnancy, and myocardial infarction (22). For a more complete listing of the most prevalent diagnoses in patients with acute abdominal pain, see Table 30.1.

The Health Care Utilization Project, a weighted sample of hospital discharge data, estimated that there were 197,000 discharges with a primary diagnosis of *intestinal obstruction* in 2001 (23). Intra-abdominal adhesions are the most common cause of small bowel obstruction in the USA, accounting for 60% of the total incidence of obstruction (24). A previous abdominal operation was noted in 91% of those diagnosed with small bowel obstruction due to adhesions, with colorectal, gynecologic, and appendectomy accounting for the majority of the antecedent operations (9). Neoplasms, hernias, and Crohn's disease cause 20, 10, and 5% respectively of the small bowel obstructions in the industrialized world (24).

The presence of diverticuli increases with age in western societies, with a prevalence of 80% in patients over 85 years of age (12). However, only 10–35% of with diverticular disease develop diverticulitis, and of these (25), only 14–25% will require operative management (26–29).

Overall Cost to Society

Limited data is available to assess the societal cost of patients presenting *with acute abdominal pain*. One study has noted that the acute abdominal pain is the most prevalent diagnosis among those whose insurance claims are denied following an emergency department visit; a group whose average patient charge totaled $1,107 (30). When the previously noted seven million annual emergency department visits for acute abdominal pain are considered, it is clear that acute abdominal pain has a significant financial impact on the health care system.

The literature regarding small bowel obstruction and cost is largely limited to estimates of hospitalization costs. One study found that the cost of the average total charges for *small bowel obstruction* to be $23,900, with the mean patient requiring surgery acquiring charges of $37,000, and the mean nonoperative patient acquiring charges of $4,800 (31). The aggregate national charge estimated by the Health Care Utilization Project found that an estimated $4.6 billion in charges were accrued by patients discharged with a major diagnosis of bowel obstruction.

No epidemiologic studies explicitly examining the cost and incidence of *diverticulits* were identified in the literature, nor were any such data cited in the identified relevant articles. However, the significant and increasing incidence of diverticular disease with age and the estimated 20% rate of diverticulitis in those with diverticular disease suggest that diverticular disease is a considerable source of healthcare expenditure. Data from the Health Care Utilization Project, a weighted nationwide inpatient sample, estimated that 196,125 patients were discharged with a primary diagnosis of diverticulitis in 2002, with estimated hospital charges of 3.9 billion dollars (23).

Goals

The main goal of imaging in the setting of acute abdominal pain is to help identify the etiology of the pain, and to exclude the possibility of a life threatening condition. The secondary goal is to determine which subjects with acute abdominal pain require surgical intervention.

Methodology

Methodology A: Imaging in Small Bowel Obstruction

A literature search was performed of English language articles from 1996 to July 15, 2004, then updated on June 15, 2010 using the MEDLINE database. Search terms included the MeSH terms *diagnostic imaging* and *intestinal obstruction*, as well as the Mesh term *intestinal obstruction* or the plain text term *small bowel obstruction* paired with the terms *CT, computerized tomography, ultrasound, abdominal film, KUB, MRI,* and *Magnetic Resonance Imaging*. Inclusion criteria incorporated prospective studies of imaging in the setting of the evaluation of patients with suspected acute small bowel obstruction. To be eligible for inclusion, studies were required to use some combination of clinical, surgical, or pathologic follow-up to determine the presence of small bowel obstruction.

Methodology B: Imaging in Acute Diverticular Disease

A literature search was performed of English language articles from 1996 to July 15, 2004 then updated on June 15, 2010 using the MEDLINE database. Search terms included the MeSH terms *Diverticulitis, colonic* or the plain text term *diverticulitis* and the Mesh term *diagnostic imaging* or the plain text terms *CT, computerized tomography, ultrasound, sonography, radiography, MRI,* or *Magnetic Resonance Imaging*. Identified works were included if they were prospective studies of imaging in the setting of the evaluation of patients with suspected acute diverticulitis. To be eligible for inclusion studies, patients were required to use some combination of imaging, clinical, surgical, or pathologic follow-up in the determination of the presence of diverticulitis. Studies that only enrolled patients with positive imaging exams or that used imaging alone in the determination of the presence of diverticulitis were excluded.

I. What Is the Accuracy of Imaging for Diagnosing Small Bowel Obstruction?

Summary of Evidence: CT and ultrasound have higher sensitivity and specificity than conventional plain film abdominal imaging for diagnosing small bowel obstruction (moderate evidence).

Computerized tomography has a higher sensitivity in the detection of small bowel obstruction than ultrasound examination (limited evidence).

CT examination of patients with small bowel is highly sensitive and specific in detecting small bowel ischemia (moderate evidence).

Supporting Evidence: Four identified series, representing 199 patients, have prospectively examined the efficacy of *conventional abdominal imaging* in comparison to another imaging modality (31–34). No prospective trials examining conventional radiography outside of a comparison study were identified. The pooled sensitivity and specificity of conventional radiography were 65% (95% CI, 42–88%) and 75% (95% CI, 58–92%), respectively. If the prevalence of small bowel obstruction in those referred to imaging is similar to the pooled prevalence found in this review (68%), the positive predictive value of conventional radiography is 85%, and the negative predictive value is 50%. In direct comparison trials, conventional plain film examination was found to be less sensitive and specific in the diagnosis of small bowel obstruction than ultrasound (31, 32) or MRI (33). When directly compared to CT examination, conventional radiography was found to be both less specific and less sensitive in one study (32), and to have similar specificity, but lower sensitivity in another (34).

The reliability of *ultrasound* examination of patients with suspected small bowel obstruction has been examined in at least three prospective trials, representing 306 total exams (31, 32, 35, 36). The pooled sensitivity and specificity of ultrasound examination were 92% (95% CI, 87–96%) and 95% (95% CI, 87–100%), respectively. These test characteristics, evaluated with a prevalence of obstruction of 68%, yield a positive predictive value of 98%, and a negative predicative value of 84%.

A single, small ($n = 32$) prospective trial has compared ultrasound examination to computerized tomography for evaluation of this patient population, and found that ultrasound has lower sensitivity than CT exam in detecting bowel obstruction (32). This study did not find any difference in specificity between ultrasound and CT; however, this work was limited in that only two of 32 patients were not diagnosed with bowel obstruction.

The test characteristics of *CT* examination have the most prospective data in this area, with a total of seven studies representing 365 patients identified in the literature (32, 33, 37–41). The sensitivity of CT exam ranged from 71 to 100%, with a pooled sensitivity of 94% (95% CI, 86–100%). The specificity of CT exam was found to range from 57 to 100%, with a pooled result of 78% (95% CI, 63–93%). An additional small study has compared different methods of contrast enhancement at CT (oral, rectal, IV) without a demonstrable difference, though with small sample size. In a population referred for radiological imaging with a prevalence of small bowel obstruction of 68%, this would result in a positive predictive value of 90%, and a negative predictive value of 86%.

Two small investigatory studies have examined the possibility of utilizing specialized MRI protocols to detect small bowel obstruction (33, 41). These two trials, with a total sample size of 51 patients, suggest that MRI has a high sensitivity (range 93–95%), and a high specificity (100%). One study found that MRI had a higher sensitivity and specificity than CT exam; however, this trial was limited in that only 16 patients underwent both radiographic examinations (41).

All of the studies of imaging in patients with suspected small bowel obstruction demonstrate some common limitations. There is potential verification bias, as the imaging exams had a direct impact on the type of outcome verification that the patient was likely to receive. In addition, sample sizes were uniformly small in the eligible studies, with no study enrolling over 100 patients.

Detecting small bowel ischemia in patients with small bowel obstruction is important due to changes in the management of patients with suspected small bowel obstruction. While surgical tradition has dictated "never let the sun set or rise" on a small bowel obstruction, studies have suggested that up to 69% of patients may be safely observed and managed nonoperatively (42–44). The determination of bowel strangulation or ischemia is important in candidates for nonoperative management, as bowel ischemia is considered an indication for initial operative management. However, patient history, physical signs, and laboratory data are neither sufficiently sensitive nor specific to satisfactorily separate patients with and without small bowel ischemia (45, 46).

CT signs such as increased or decreased enhancement of the bowel wall, a *target* sign, closed loop bowel configuration, bowel wall thickening, increased mesenteric fluid, congestion of mesenteric veins, and a *serrated beak* sign have all been retrospectively described as indicating small bowel ischemia (47, 48).

Five studies, representing 399 *CT* exams, have prospectively examined the diagnostic accuracy of CT in detecting small bowel ischemia (37, 39, 49, 50). These studies have demonstrated a high sensitivity in detecting small bowel ischemia, ranging from 83 to 100%, with a pooled result of 95% sensitivity (95% CI, 88–100%). The demonstrated specificity at this high level of sensitivity ranged from 61–100%, with a pooled specificity of 90% (95% CI, 78–100%) When these results are evaluated at the pooled prevalence of small bowel ischemia found in these studies (24%), the positive predictive value of CT in predicting bowel ischemia due to small bowel obstruction was found to be 76%, and the negative predictive value 98%. Both MRI and CT enteroclysis have been promoted more recently for the evaluation of small bowel obstruction, but data to date is insufficient.

These results indicate that a patient with a negative CT exam is highly unlikely to be suffering from intestinal ischemia due to bowel obstruction. However, it should be acknowledged that the studies identified did not examine changes in overall patient outcome with CT exam. There is limited evidence that CT exam influences patient management. A single prospective study of 57 patients found that when surgeons were required to state management plans before and after CT examination, 23% of patients had a change in plan due to the CT findings (51).

All of the studies examining CT imaging of small bowel ischemia due to bowel obstruction are limited by verification bias and small individual study sample size. In addition, some trials were limited in that only patients with initial CT findings of small bowel obstruction were enrolled in these trials, possibly selecting for a patient population with increased probability for CT findings (49, 50). However, similar results were obtained in trials not limited to this patient population (37–39).

IIA. What Is the Accuracy of Imaging for Acute Colonic Diverticulitis?

Summary of Evidence: Computerized tomography demonstrates a higher sensitivity and specificity in detecting acute colonic diverticulitis than graded compression ultrasound (moderate evidence).

CT is considered more sensitive and specific than contrast enema for identification of diverticulitis, though data is limited.

Supporting Evidence: The radiographic imaging exam with the longest history of use in the diagnosis of acute colonic diverticulitis is a *contrast enema* in conjunction with conventional radiography (11). The accuracy of this exam has been examined by two small ($n = 86$ and $n = 38$) prospective trials as a comparison to CT exam (52, 53). Sensitivity of contrast enema in detection of acute diverticulitis ranged between 80 and 82%, while the specificity ranged between 80 and 100%. When these test characteristics are applied to a patient population with the prevalence of diverticulitis equivalent to the pooled prevalence in the eligible studies of imaging and diverticular disease (50%), the positive predictive value of contrast enema was found to be 84%, and the negative predictive value 82%. Both of these studies were performed to prospectively compare CT and contrast enema in patients with suspected acute diverticulitis. The older of these studies, by Stefannson et al. in 1990, found that CT had a lower sensitivity but higher specificity than contrast enema exam. However, another examination of this topic by Cho et al. determined that CT was more sensitive than contrast enema, but that no difference was found in the imaging modalities' specificities. Both studies were potentially limited due to small sample size and verification bias. In addition, the study by Cho et al. was limited by a failure to blind the image interpreters to the outcome of the other imaging result. No more recent studies of multidetector CT and contrast enema were identified. However, given recent increases in CT accuracy with multiplanar reformation and thinner collimation, CT is presumed to be superior to enema in both sensitivity and specificity (limited evidence). Two more recent studies looked at *CT* without direct comparison to radiography (54, 55). These four studies include 412 subjects, and indicate that CT is highly specific, with a pooled specificity of 99% (95% CI, 98–100%). The pooled sensitivity of CT was found to be 89% (95% CI, 78–100%), resulting in a positive predictive value of 99%, and a negative predictive value of 90%. No prospective studies comparing ultrasonography and CT examinations were identified.

Ultrasound examination has been proposed in cases of suspected acute diverticulitis due to its cross sectional capability, lack of ionizing radiation, and wide availability (12, 29). Four eligible prospective trials were identified, consisting of 571 imaging exams (56–59). The pooled sensitivity and specificity were found to be 91% (95% CI, 82–100%) and 92% (95% CI, 82–100%) respectively, resulting in a positive predictive and negative predictive value of 92 and 91% respectively. A recent meta-analysis reported superior sensitivity and specificity of CT over US, though without achieving statistical significance (60). No eligible studies performed a direct comparison between sonography and other imaging modalities. As with other investigations in this area, all the identified studies were limited by verification bias.

IIB. What Is the Accuracy of CT in Predicting the Success of Conservative Management in Patients with Suspected Acute Colonic Diverticulitis?

Summary of Evidence: Patients judged to have severe diverticular disease by computed tomography are more likely to require initial surgical management and to secondarily experience relapse, persistence, sigmoid stenosis, and fistula or abscess formation (limited evidence).

Supporting Evidence: A single study by Ambrosetti et al. (61) investigated the accuracy of *CT* in predicting patient management outcome during the initial episode of diverticulitis (medical versus surgical therapy) and likelihood of relapse of diverticulitis following initially successful medical therapy. This investigation of 542 patients with a positive imaging diagnosis of diverticulitis found that a significantly higher

proportion of those judged to have severe diverticulitis on CT examination (26%) went on to require surgical management during the initial hospitalization, compared to 4% of those judged to have mild diverticulitis. In addition, patients considered to have severe diverticulitis by CT exam were more likely to acquire a secondary complication (relapse, persistence, sigmoid stenosis, fistula formation, or abscess persistence) after the initial hospitalization, with secondary complication rates of 36 and 17% for the severe and moderate groups respectively. This study only enrolled those patients with positive imaging results, therefore it is unknown how accurately imaging predicts patient outcome in those with negative exams. This study was potentially limited by a lack of blinding and possible verification bias.

Take Home Tables (Tables 30.1–30.3)

Tables 30.1–30.3 and Fig. 30.1–30.2 serve to highlight key recommendations and supporting evidence.

Imaging Case Studies

Case 1

An abdominal and pelvic CT examination after intravenous contrast with axial (Fig. 30.1A) and coronal (Fig. 30.1B) reconstruction revealed multiple dilated loops of jejunum (arrowheads) with decompressed ileum distally. There was transition from dilated small bowel to normal caliber, but thick-walled ileum with surrounding inflammatory changes (arrow). Crohn's disease of the distal ileum with small bowel obstruction was diagnosed, and responded to conservative therapy.

Case 2

A 39-year-old woman presented to the emergency department with a 3-day history of left lower quadrant abdominal pain, fevers, chills, and vomiting, as well as leukocytosis. The studies cited in this chapter suggest that a clinical suspicion of diverticulitis, as in this case, is accurate approximately 50% of the time (Fig. 30.2).

CT revealed multiple diverticula and bowel wall thickening in the sigmoid colon, with fat stranding in the mesocolon, and an extraperitoneal abscess. Under CT guidance a percutaneous drainage catheter was placed into the abscess, with subsequent aspiration of 40 cc of purulent material. The patient recovered and was discharged 72 h after drainage catheter placement.

Suggested Protocols

Abdominal pain protocol
Patient Preparation: 1,000 ml oral contrast-drink over 90 min period
Give rectal contrast if patient is unable to tolerate oral contrast
IV Contrast: 125 cc IV contrast @ 3.0 cc/s
Imaging: Venous Phase (60 s scan delay) – dome of the diaphragm to ischial tuberosities, 2.5 mm detector collimation
Diverticulitis protocol (used for problem solving when the standard abdominal pain protocol is inadequate)

Patient Preparation: 1,000–1,500 ml rectal contrast instilled via soft rectal tube
IV Contrast: 125 cc IV contrast @ 3.0 cc/s
Imaging: Venous Phase (60 s scan delay) – dome of the diaphragm to ischial tuberosities, 2.5 mm detector collimation.

Future Inquiry

- While studies have demonstrated that CT has a high accuracy in the detection of ischemia in patients with suspected small bowel obstruction, no investigation has yet determined the impact of CT on overall patient outcome.
- The ability of imaging to differentiate medical from surgical causes of abdominal pain, and to influence patient management is not well established.
- Relatively little is known regarding the overall cost and cost-effectiveness of imaging for the set of conditions that make up the acute abdomen.

Table 30.1. Common diagnoses in patients presenting to the emergency department with acute abdominal pain

No.	Diagnosis	Percent (%)
1	Undiagnosed abdominal pain	25.1
2	Nausea/vomiting	9.8
3	Unspecified	9.0
4	Cystitis	6.7
5	Gastritis	5.3
6	Pancreatitis	3.9
7	Cholecystitis	3.6
8	Pelvic inflammatory disease	3.4
9	Constipation	3.3
10	Musculoskeletal	2.9
11	Ureteral calculus	2.8
12	Ovarian cyst	1.9
13	Dysmenorrhea	1.9
14	Bowel obstruction	1.6
15	GI ulcer	1.5
16	Cardiac	1.5
17	Hernia	1.4
18	Pyelonephritis	1.4
19	Appendicitis	1.4
20	Vaginitis/cervicitis	1.3

Source: Adapted with permission from Powers and Guertler (18).

Table 30.2. Sensitivity and specificity of imaging in patients with suspected small bowel obstruction

Modality	Sensitivity (%)	Specificity (%)	Positive predictive value[a] (%)	Negative predictive value[a] (%)
Detection of obstruction				
Plain film[b]	65	75	85	50
Ultrasound[c]	92	95	98	84
CT[d]	94	78	90	86
Detection of ischemia				
CT	95	90	76	98

Reprinted with kind permission of Springer Science+Business Media from Blackmore CC, Chang TA, Avey GD. Imaging in Acute Abdominal Pain. In Medina LS, Blackmore CC (eds): Evidence-Based Imaging: Optimizing Imaging in Patient Care. New York: Springer Science+Business Media, 2006.
[a]Calculated utilizing a prevalence of small bowel obstruction of 68% of those imaged and a prevalence of small bowel ischemia of 25%; these were the pooled prevalence found in the eligible studies.
[b]Adapted from (31, 32, 34).
[c]Adapted from (31, 32, 35).
[d]Adapted from (32, 33, 37–41).

Table 30.3. Sensitivity and specificity of imaging in patients with suspected acute colonic diverticulitis

Modality	Sensitivity (%)	Specificity (%)	Positive predictive value[a] (%)	Negative predictive value[a] (%)
Contrast enema[b]	81	85	84	82
Ultrasound[c]	91	92	92	91
CT[d]	89	99	99	90

Reprinted with kind permission of Springer Science+Business Media from Blackmore CC, Chang TA, Avey GD. Imaging in Acute Abdominal Pain. In Medina LS, Blackmore CC (eds.): *Evidence-Based Imaging: Optimizing Imaging in Patient Care.* New York: Springer Science+Business Media, 2006.
[a]Calculated utilizing a prevalence of diverticulitis of 50%, a prevalence equal to the pooled prevalence of the eligible studies.
[b]Adapted from (52, 53).
[c]Adapted from (56–59).
[d]Adapted from (52–55).

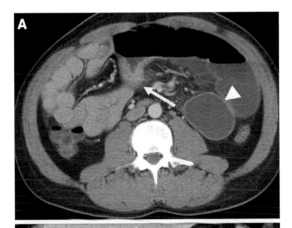

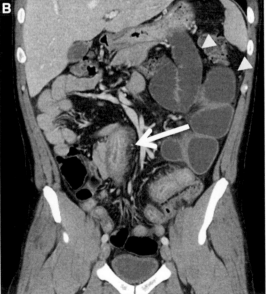

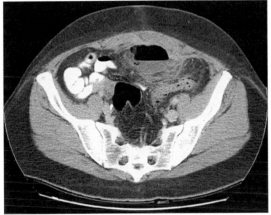

Figure 30.2. Diverticulitis with abscess formation. (Reprinted with kind permission of Springer Science+Business Media from Blackmore CC, Chang TA, Avey GD. Imaging in Acute Abdominal Pain. In Medina LS, Blackmore CC (eds): *Evidence-Based Imaging: Optimizing Imaging in Patient Care.* New York: Springer Science+Business Media, 2006.)

Figure 30.1. Small bowel obstruction. A 34-year-old male with a history of Crohn's disease presented to the emergency department with a 2-day history of crampy abdominal pain, nausea, and vomiting.

References

1. Tsushima Y et al. Clin Radiol 2002;57(6):507–513.
2. Urban BA, Fishman EK. Radiographics 2000; 20(3):725–749.
3. Ann Emerg Med 1994;23(4):906–922.
4. Martin RF, Rossi RL. Surg Clin North Am 1997; 77(6):1227–1243.
5. Adams ID et al. Br Med J (Clin Res Ed) 1986; 293(6550):800–804.
6. Townsend CM. Sabiston Textbook of Surgery, 16th ed. Elsevier, New York; 919–920.
7. Megibow AJ et al. Radiology 1991;180(2):313–318.
8. Shih SC et al. World J Gastroenterol 2003;9(3): 603–605.
9. Miller G et al. Br J Surg 2000;87(9):1240–1247.
10. Fevang BT et al. Ann Surg 2004;240(2):193–201.
11. Parks TG et al. Br Med J 1970;2(702):136–138.
12. Ferzoco LB, Raptopoulos V, Silen W. N Engl J Med 1998;338(21):1521–1526.
13. Diner WC, Barnhard HJ. Semin Roentgenol 1973;8(4):415–431.
14. Burkitt DP, Walker AR, Painter NS. JAMA 1974;229(8):1068–1074.
15. Hinchey EJ, Schaal PG, Richards JK. Adv Surg 1978;12:85–109.
16. McCaig LF, Nawar EW. Adv Data 2006;372:1–29.
17. Advanced data from Vital and Health Statistics. Hyattsville, MD: National Center for Health Statistics, 2004; 340.
18. Powers RD, Guertler AT. Am J Emerg Med 1995;13(3):301–303.
19. Brewer BJ et al. Am J Surg 1976;131(2):219–223.
20. Lukens TW, Emerman C, Effron D. Ann Emerg Med 1993;22(4):690–696.
21. Jess P et al. Am J Surg 1982;144(3):338–340.
22. Ann Emerg Med 2000;36(4):406–415.
23. Healthcare Cost and Utilization Project, AHRQ, 2003.
24. Tito SSM. Intestinal obstruction. In Zuidema GD (ed.): Surgery of the Alimentary Tract, 5th ed. New York: WB Saunders Company, 2001.
25. Pradel JA et al. Radiology 1997;205(2):503–512.
26. Kircher MF et al. AJR Am J Roentgenol 2002;178(6):1313–1318.
27. Rhea JT. Emerg Radiol 2000;7(4):237–244.
28. Brengman ML, Otchy DP. Dis Colon Rectum 1998;41(8):1023–1028.
29. Halligan S, Saunders B. Best Pract Res Clin Gastroenterol 2002;16(4):595–610.
30. Gresenz CR, Studdert DM. Ann Emerg Med 2004;43(2):155–162.
31. Ogata M, Mateer JR, Condon RE. Ann Surg 1996;223(3):237–241.
32. Suri S et al. Acta Radiol 1999;40:422–428.
33. Matsuoka H et al. Am J Surg 2002;183(6): 614–617.
34. Frager D et al. AJR Am J Roentgenol 1994;162: 37–41.
35. Czechowski J. Acta Radiol 1996;37:186–189.
36. Schmutz GR et al. Eur Radiol 1997;7(7): 1054–1058.
37. Frager D et al. AJR Am J Roentgenol 1996;166: 67–71.
38. Balthazar EJ, Liebeskind ME, Macari M. Radiology 1997;205:519–522.
39. Obuz F et al. Eur J Radiol 2003;48:299–304.
40. Peck JJ, Milleson T, Phelan J. Am J Surg 1999; 177:375–378.
41. Beall DP et al. Clin Radiol 2002;57(8):719–724.
42. Seror D et al. Am J Surg 1993;165(1):121–125; discussion 125–126.
43. Fevang BT et al. Eur J Surg 2002;168(8–9): 475–481.
44. Cox MR et al. Aust N Z J Surg 1993;63(11): 848–852.
45. Deutsch AA et al. Postgrad Med J 1989;65(765): 463–467.
46. Sarr MG, Bulkley GB, Zuidema GD. Am J Surg 1983;145(1):176–182.
47. Balthazar EJ. AJR Am J Roentgenol 1994;163(5): 1260–1261.
48. Ha HK et al. Radiology 1997;204(2):507–512.
49. Zalcman M et al. AJR Am J Roentgenol 2000;175: 1601–1607.
50. Donckier V et al. Br J Surg 1998;85:1071–1074.
51. Taourel PG et al. AJR Am J Roentgenol 1995;165: 1187–1192.
52. Cho KC et al. Radiology 1990;176(1):111–115.
53. Stefansson T et al. Acta Radiol 1997;38(2): 313–319.
54. Rao PM, Rhea JT. Radiology 1998;209(3):775–779.
55. Werner A et al. Eur Radiol 2003;13(12): 2596–2603.
56. Verbanck J et al. J Clin Ultrasound 1989;17(9): 661–666.
57. Zielke A et al. Br J Surg 1997;84(3):385–388.
58. Hollerweger A et al. AJR Am J Roentgenol 2000;175(4):1155–1160.
59. Schwerk WB, Schwarz S, Rothmund M. Dis Colon Rectum 1992;35(11):1077–1084.
60. Lameris W et al. Eur Radiol 2008;18:2498–2511.
61. Ambrosetti P, Becker C, Terrier TF. Eur Radiol 2002;12:1145–1149.

31

Intussusception in Children: Diagnostic Imaging and Treatment

Kimberly E. Applegate

I. What are the clinical predictors of intussusception? What are the clinical predictors of reducibility and bowel necrosis? Who should undergo imaging? II. Which imaging studies should be performed? III. How should therapeutic enema be performed? IV. What is appropriate management in recurrent cases? V. Special case: Intussusception limited to the small bowel VI. Special case: Intussusception with a known lead point mass	**Issues**

■ Children with clinically suspected intussusception should undergo enema reduction after surgical consultation. The only absolute contraindications to enema are signs of peritonitis on clinical exam or free air on abdominal radiographs. Air enema has better overall reduction rates than liquid enema, but the outcome depends on the experience of the radiologist (moderate evidence). ■ Ultrasound (US) should be the primary imaging modality in the initial diagnosis of intussusception because it is a noninvasive test with high sensitivity and specificity. US also plays a role in the evaluation of reducibility of intussusception, presence of a lead point mass, potential incomplete reduction after enema, and of intussusception limited to small bowel (limited evidence).	**Key Points**

K.E. Applegate (✉)
Department of Radiology, Emory University School of Medicine, 1364 Clifton Road NE,
Suite D112, Atlanta, GA 30322, USA
e-mail: keapple@emory.edu

L.S. Medina et al. (eds.), *Evidence-Based Imaging: Improving the Quality of Imaging in Patient Care, Revised Edition,*
DOI 10.1007/978-1-4419-7777-9_31, © Springer Science+Business Media, LLC 2011

- Barium should not be used due to the poorer outcomes compared with iodinated liquid contrast in those children who perforate (moderate evidence).
- Abdominal radiographs have poor sensitivity for the detection of intussusception, but may serve to screen for other diagnoses in the differential diagnosis, such as constipation, and for free peritoneal air. For evaluating children with a low probability for intussusception, sonography is the preferred screening test (limited evidence).
- The use of delayed repeat enema for the reduction of intussusception shows promise, but there are few data on the appropriate methods or time (limited evidence).
- For recurrence of intussusception, including multiple recurrences, enema is the preferred method for reduction (limited evidence).

Definition and Pathophysiology

Intussusception is an acquired invagination of the bowel into itself, usually involving both small and large bowel, within the peritoneal cavity. The more proximal bowel that herniates into more distal bowel is called the intussusceptum and bowel that contains it is called the intussuscipiens. It is an emergent condition where delay in diagnosis is not uncommon and leads to an increased risk of bowel perforation, obstruction, and necrosis. There may be an accompanying pathologic lead point (PLP) mass in approximately 5% of children (1). Intestinal intussusception may occur along the entire length of the bowel from the duodenum to prolapse of intussuscepted bowel through the rectum. It can also range from classic clinical presentations to asymptomatic transient intussusception seen increasingly on multichannel CT studies of the abdomen for other indications (2). Most cases are "idiopathic" in that the etiology of the intussusception is due to hypertrophied lymphoid tissue in the terminal ileum which results in ileocolic intussusception. Some reports have suggested a viral etiology, most commonly adenovirus but also enterovirus, echovirus, and human herpes virus 6 (3). The clinical signs and symptoms of intussusception are often nonspecific and overlap with those of gastroenteritis, malrotation with volvulus, and, in older children, Henoch–Schonlein Purpura (HSP). The large majority of clinically symptomatic cases occur in the infant and toddler, with a peak age of 5–9 months, although it has been reported on prenatal imaging and may occur in children who present without the typical clinical presentation of vomiting, bloody stools, palpable abdominal mass, and colicky abdominal pain (4). The classic triad of colicky abdominal pain, vomiting, and bloody stools is present in less than 25% of children (5–7).

Epidemiology

Intussusception is the most common cause of small bowel obstruction in children and occurs in at least 56 children per 100,000 per year in the USA (8). It is second only to pyloric stenosis as the most common cause of gastrointestinal tract obstruction in children. It occurs in boys more than girls at a ratio of 3:2. Some papers have reported associations with viruses, particularly adenovirus, although lack of seasonality suggests more than one pathogen (4, 8). Delay in diagnosis and treatment is not uncommon, making enema reduction less successful, bowel resection more likely, and death due to bowel ischemia possible (1, 4, 9, 10). There were 323 intussusception-associated deaths in American infants reported to the Centers for Disease Control (CDC) between 1979 and 1997. In a review of administrative discharge data of intussusception-associated hospitalizations and deaths in the USA, Parashar and colleagues (8) noted a peak age of 5–7 months, with two-thirds of patients under age 1 year, no consistent seasonality, hospitalization rates of approximately 56 per 100,000 children, and a general trend toward fewer hospitalizations over the past two decades. The mortality rates also decreased over this time period, from 6.4 per 1,000,000 to 2.3 per 1,000,000 live births.

They also reported an increased risk of intussusception-related deaths among infants whose mothers were <20 years old, unmarried, nonwhite, and had less than a grade 12 education. The authors concluded that these data suggest reduced access or delay in seeking care contributed to the risk of death. They did not investigate costs or rates of surgical versus enema reductions.

In another paper comparing worldwide data, Meier and colleagues noted that the most important difference between industrialized and developing countries' outcomes was the delay in presentation for treatment and consequent lower rates of enema reduction and higher rates of surgical mortality (18%) from bowel necrosis (10).

Rotavirus Vaccine

Shortly after the first and only rotavirus vaccine was introduced in the USA in 1998 for routine vaccination of infants at ages 2, 4, and 6 months, several reports to the CDC suggested an association between the vaccine and intussusception. This was noted particularly within 2 weeks after vaccination with the first dose. The vaccine was removed from the world market in 1999 (11). Although controversial, subsequent investigations have not found a higher rate of intussusception after rotavirus vaccination (12, 13). A new rotavirus vaccine is currently under development (14).

Overall Cost to Society

No data have been identified detailing the total cost to society of intussusception. Three recent surveys have documented practice patterns for the evaluation of intussusception (4, 15, 16). In centers without pediatric radiologists, the enema is the initial and often only imaging test performed for both diagnosis and treatment. In contrast, at the 2004 SPR annual meeting, a survey of pediatric radiologists showed that 57% now use sonography for initial diagnosis prior to enema (15). Overall, the total hospital cost for children with intussusception treated with surgery is approximately four times that of those treated with enema (17–19).

Goals

The goal of initial bowel imaging is early detection of intussusception to enable enema reduction of the intussusception. Additional imaging studies may be performed to further characterize indeterminate results. The ultimate goal that radiologists should strive for is nonoperative reduction for all children with idiopathic intussusception (approximately 95% cases), but delay in presentation and diagnosis makes this goal elusive.

Methodology

A MEDLINE search was performed using PubMed (National Library of Medicine, Bethesda, Maryland) for original research publications discussing the diagnostic performance and effectiveness of imaging strategies in intussusception. Clinical predictors of intussusception were also included in the literature search. The search covered the years 1966 to June 2008. The search strategy employed different combinations of the following terms: (1) *intussusception*, (2) *children, ages under 18 years*, (3) *diagnosis*, (4) *therapy* or *surgery* or *etiology*. Additional articles were identified by reviewing the reference lists of relevant papers, identifying appropriate authors, and use of citation indices for MeSH terms. This review was limited to human studies and the English language literature. The author performed an initial review of the titles and abstracts of the identified articles followed by review of the full text in articles that were relevant.

I. What Are the Clinical Predictors of Intussusception? What Are the Clinical Predictors of Reducibility and Bowel Necrosis? Who Should Undergo Imaging?

Summary of Evidence: At this point there are no reliable clinical prediction models that can accurately identify all patients with intussusception (limited evidence). Determination of children who should undergo imaging and who should not undergo imaging has not been studied in formal prospective trials.

Supporting Evidence

What Are the Clinical Predictors of Intussusception?

Ideally, children with intussusception should be diagnosed early to avoid bowel necrosis and surgery. However, one report found that only 50% of children were correctly diagnosed at initial presentation to a healthcare provider (20). The classic triad of colicky abdominal pain (58–100% cases), vomiting (up to 85% cases), and bloody stools is present in less than 25% of children (5, 21). Guaiac positive stool is present in 75% of children with intussusception (7, 22). Vomiting or diarrhea may lead to dehydration, which exaggerates lethargy. The mixture of stool, blood, and blood clots has been described as "current jelly stools" and is suggestive of intussusception.

Kupperman and colleagues published a cross-sectional study that evaluated the clinical factors that might predict intussusception in 115 children (23) (limited evidence). Using multivariate logistic regression and bootstrap sample analysis, they not only found that the presence of highly suggestive abdominal radiographs, rectal bleeding, and male sex were independent predictors of intussusception, but also noted that these factors were not specific. Harrington and colleagues investigated the positive and negative clinical predictors of intussusception in a prospective cohort study (5) (moderate evidence). They recorded signs and symptoms in 245 children and correlated them with sonographic and enema findings. Significant positive predictive factors for intussusception were the presence of right upper quadrant mass, gross blood in stool, guaiac positive stool, and the triad of colicky abdominal pain, vomiting, and right upper quadrant mass. They were unable to identify significant negative predictors. Klein and colleagues reviewed clinical history, physical exam, and radiographic findings to develop a prediction model of children with possible intussusception (24) (moderate evidence). Their univariate analysis identified several known factors associated with intussusception, including vomiting, abdominal pain, palpable abdominal mass, guaiac positive stool, and rectal bleeding. However, they concluded that they were "unable to develop a prediction model that would reliably identify all patients with the diagnosis of intussusception. Previously identified predictors of intussusception remain important in increasing suspicion of this important diagnosis. At this point there is no reliable prediction model that can accurately identify all patients with intussusception."

What Are the Clinical Predictors of Reducibility and Bowel Necrosis?

The most important factor that decreases the reduction rate of enema is a longer duration of symptoms. This finding is supported by multiple case series. A significant delay is typically 48 h, but some reports suggest 24 or 72 h as either one of several factors or the single factor predicting unsuccessful enema reduction (4, 25). Other factors associated with lower reduction rates include age less than 3 months, dehydration, small bowel obstruction, and intussusception encountered in the rectum (25% reduction rate) (4, 20, 21, 25, 26) (limited evidence).

II. Which Imaging Studies Should Be Performed?

Summary of Evidence: Ultrasound has higher accuracy in the diagnosis of intussusception than plain radiographs. Ultrasound also has higher diagnostic accuracy in identifying PLPs than plain radiographs or enema. The role of ultrasound findings in predicting success of reduction is not well known with available literature. Given current evidence, the diagnostic approach should include (a) abdominal radiographs if concern for other diagnoses or for perforation; (b) sonography for diagnosis or exclusion of intussusception; (c) if positive, a surgical consult should be obtained prior to the enema reduction attempt; and (d) air enema reduction (or if no experience with the air technique, liquid enema) (moderate evidence).

Supporting Evidence

What Is the Diagnostic Performance of Abdominal Radiographs?

The presence of a curvilinear mass within the course of the colon (the crescent sign), particularly in the transverse colon just beyond the hepatic flexure, is a nearly pathognomonic sign of intussusception. The absence of bowel gas in the ascending colon is one of the most specific sign of intussusception on radiographs (27). However, small bowel gas located in the right abdomen on radiographs may mimic ascending colon or cecal gas. Radiographs have low sensitivity and specificity, even when viewed by experienced pediatric radiologists (27, 28) (limited evidence). Sargent and colleagues (26) reported 45% sensitivity in 60 children when evaluated prospectively by pediatric radiologists, using the enema as the reference standard (Table 31.1). Others report similar poor sensitivity in the detection of intussusception (4). In a survey of the SPR 2004 attendees, Daneman found that 79% obtain radiographs, but this practice may not be under the control of radiologists (15). Only 10% of pediatric radiologists in this survey preferred radiographs for the diagnosis

What Is the Diagnostic Performance of Sonography?

Intussusception can be reliably diagnosed when a "donut," "target," or "pseudokidney" sign is seen using linear transducer sonography (29–32). The optimal US technique in this population is well described (30–34). There are no known contraindications or complications resulting from US for this purpose. US also plays a role in the evaluation of reducibility of the intussusception, the presence of a PLP mass, intussusception limited to small bowel, to diagnose or exclude residual intussusception after enema, and to identify alternative diagnoses (5, 31, 33, 34) (limited evidence). In a 2004 survey, 57% of North American pediatric radiologists reported the use of sonography to diagnose intussusception as compared to 93% of European pediatric radiologists in a 1999 survey (15, 35).

Sonography screening in children has been suggested to reduce cost, radiation exposure, and both patient and parental anxiety/discomfort with enema (34) (limited evidence). Published series from single institutions suggest high accuracy, approaching 100% in experienced hands, with sensitivity of 98–100% and specificity of 88–100% (5, 31, 36, 37) (limited evidence) (Table 31.1). Eshed and colleagues

found similar abilities in sonographic diagnosis of intussusception for staff radiologists as well as senior and junior radiology residents: sensitivity and specificity were 85 and 98% for staff radiologists, 75 and 96% for senior residents, and 83 and 97% for junior residents, respectively (38). Given that the theoretical cost-effectiveness of sonography is dependent on the prevalence of intussusception, optimization of imaging will require stratification of subjects into different levels of probability of intussusception (39). However, data are lacking for such stratification. Henrikson and colleagues noted a trend of decreased prevalence of intussusception (22%) in those children referred for enema and began sonographic screening (limited evidence). In their small series of 38 children, they were able to avoid 19 enemas in those with negative sonography, resulting in savings in both radiation exposure (an average of 8.2 mGy for negative enemas) and hospital charges (34). Future cost-effectiveness modeling research will be needed to define the population that should undergo sonography.

What Are the Sonographic Predictors of Reducibility and Bowel Necrosis?

Del-Pozo and colleagues performed sonography in 145 children with intussusception and found that fluid seen inside the intussusception represented trapped peritoneal fluid and was associated with significantly fewer reductions on enema and with bowel ischemia at surgery (40, 41) (limited evidence).

Some US reports have noted that thicker bowel wall was associated with fewer enema reductions (31, 42), but others did not find this association (41). Lack of color Doppler signal in the intussuscepted bowel wall suggested bowel ischemia in several small series (43–45). Free intraperitoneal fluid in small or moderate amounts is present in approximately half of children with intussusception and is not a contraindication for enema (32). There are conflicting reports that free peritoneal fluid is associated with fewer reductions (4, 21, 25, 33, 46). Some descriptive studies report that the presence of lymph nodes trapped in the intussusception is associated with fewer reductions (33, 47). For these US findings, due to the conflicting reports and/or small series, the evidence is inconclusive.

What Are the Pathologic Lead Points?

Approximately 5–6% of intussusceptions in children are caused by PLPs which are due to either focal masses or diffuse bowel wall abnormality. The most common focal PLPs are (in decreasing order of incidence) Meckel's diverticulum, duplication cyst, polyp, and lymphoma (1, 4, 48) (limited evidence). Diffuse PLPs are most commonly associated with cystic fibrosis or HSP. Although the common teaching remains that focal PLPs are more common in older children, this is somewhat misleading. The relative prevalence of PLP with intussusception is higher in children over the age of 3 years, particularly for lymphoma. However, the absolute number of PLP in infants versus older children is approximately equal (1).

The detection of lead points by imaging remains problematic (49), although US is the noninvasive standard of reference. Sixty-six percent of PLPs may be identified at US (50) and that of 40% of PLPs may be diagnosed on liquid enema (4). Air enema has a lower rate of detection of PLP of 11% (51), so that some researchers suggest that US be used afterward to search for PLP (4) (limited evidence).

III. How Should Therapeutic Enema Be Performed?

Summary of Evidence: The air enema is considered superior at reduction, cleaner (based on appearance of peritoneal cavity at surgery when perforation occurs), safer, and faster, with less radiation when compared to liquid enema (22, 52–56) (moderate evidence). The recurrence rates for air versus liquid enema reductions do not differ (both are approximately 10%). The "rule of threes" used to guide liquid enema technique is supported by limited evidence. Barium is no longer the liquid contrast medium of choice due to the risk of barium peritonitis, infection, and adhesions when perforation occurs during the enema (22, 46, 53, 57). Neither sedation nor medications increase the enema success rate (limited evidence). Direct comparison of reduction with fluoroscopy versus ultrasound has not been studied (insufficient evidence).

Supporting Evidence: There are multiple investigations of success rates for enema reduction,

although most are retrospective. Seventy-one published studies of this question were largely Level-3 (limited evidence) investigations consisting of unselected, but often consecutive case series. The average reduction rate for these 71 published studies was 74%. In 19 series with at least 150 children each, retrospective analysis demonstrated reduction rates averaging 80%, range 53–96% (25) (Table 31.2). The largest series from China, using air enema in 6,396 children, reported reduction rates of 95% (55) (limited evidence). However, while the air enema may be preferred in experienced hands, the liquid enema is also safe and effective. The air enema technique is well described in the literature (54, 56, 58). Briefly, the enema tip should be placed within the child's rectum and taped in place with abundant tape. The child is placed in a prone position to allow the radiologist or assistant to squeeze the buttocks closed and prevent air from leaking. Air is rapidly insufflated into the colon under fluoroscopic observation. Once the intussusception is encountered, its reduction is followed fluoroscopically until it is completely reduced. Air should flow freely from the cecum into the distal small bowel loops to signify complete reduction. One critical safety issue is to keep air pressure below a maximum limit of 120 mmHg to avoid the risk of perforation (22, 46, 56).

Air Versus Liquid Enema

Two randomized trials comparing outcomes with air versus liquid enema technique exist, yet their conclusions differ, with one stating there is no difference and the other showing the air enema superior to liquid enema (59, 60) (moderate evidence). In 1999, Hadidi and El Shah reported that air had a higher reduction rate than liquid enema ($p=0.01$). Children were randomized with less than 48 h of symptoms to saline reduction under sonographic guidance ($n=47$), air ($n=50$), or barium ($n=50$) under fluoroscopic guidance (59). In 1993, Meyer and colleagues randomized 101 children to air ($n=50$) or barium ($n=51$) enema and found success rates of 76% for air and 63% for liquid enema (60). The results were not statistically significant, but do support air as being more effective. In addition, the trial used sedation and had lower reduction rates than those not using sedation (25). The authors abandoned the use of sedation after this study. The use of sedation may reduce the intraabdominal pressure children create by the Valsalva maneuver and is reported to improve reducibility at enema (46, 56). More recent reports of air reduction show better results than liquid enema reduction (1). The superior air enema results may be due to the level of experience of those who use air reduction techniques as well as the presence of higher intraluminal pressure for air as compared to standard hydrostatic reduction (61, 62).

In a 1991 survey of American pediatric radiology chairs, Meyer found that only 24% were using air enema but 64% used barium and 12% water-soluble contrast (16) as compared to 35% of international pediatric radiologists who used air enema (63). More recently, in 2004, 65% of American pediatric radiologists reported using air enema, 33% used liquid enema (water-soluble contrast or barium), and 3% used liquid enema with sonographic guidance (15). Some pediatric radiologists will use air for children older than 3 months, but for younger infants, especially neonates, they prefer liquid contrast due to the greater differential diagnosis in this group (25).

All children should have surgical consultation prior to enema (a) to assess for peritoneal signs precluding enema, (b) to identify children who cannot be reduced with enema or who are found to have perforation, and (c) for post-reduction management. Prior to enema reduction, dehydration should be treated with intravenous fluid resuscitation. Children with evidence of peritonitis, shock, sepsis, or free air on abdominal radiographs are not candidates for enema. Radiologists should strive for enema reduction rates of 80%, but it will depend on their patient population (moderate evidence). Several reports estimate that the rate of spontaneous reduction based on sonographic and/or enema diagnosis prior to surgery is 10% (1, 21, 42, 51) (limited evidence).

Bratton and colleagues suggest that more experienced radiologists and caregivers at children's hospitals decrease the risk of surgical reduction, length of hospital stay, and cost of care (17) (moderate evidence). Surgical management is performed when the patient is too unstable (shock, dehydration, or sepsis) for enema reduction, when the enema is unsuccessful, or when PLP is diagnosed.

The Rule of Threes

A general guideline to the liquid enema technique, often taught to radiology residents, is the "rule of threes": three attempts of 3-min duration, with the liquid enema bag at 3 ft above the fluoroscopy table. There is little evidence to support this rule, particularly regarding the height of the enema bag (25, 64). Many experienced pediatric radiologists alter this general guide in response to the clinical status of the patient and the movement of the intussusceptum mass achieved with the initial enema (21, 64). For example, if the intussusception is partially reduced to where it most frequently hangs up, at the ileocecal valve, some radiologists will make further or longer attempts and/or raise the enema bag above 3 ft. The exam is tailored to the patient and performed in conjunction with the surgeon involved.

Radiation Dose

The dose deposited will depend on a number of factors, including the type of fluoroscopy equipment, the use of pulsed fluoroscopy, and the fluoroscopy time (1, 46). A 1993 study reported a very low mean effective dose of 0.055 mSv for enema reduction of an intussusception (65). Experienced pediatric radiologists using air enema averaged 95 s of fluoroscopy time to reduce an intussusception and 42 s to exclude one in a child without intussusception (56). Air enema radiation doses average one-third to one-half less the dose for liquid enema (46).

Alternative Enema Approaches

A number of different approaches have been described to try to improve intussusception reduction on enema that include sedation, anesthesia, use of glucagon, manual palpation, and delayed repeat enema. In the past, sedation and sometimes anesthesia were commonly used to improve reduction rates, but case series showed no improvement (16, 66, 67) (limited evidence). In a 1991 survey Meyer found that only 10% of respondents used sedation either always or almost always (16) as compared to 54% of international pediatric radiologists, and those using sedation reported lower reduction rates (59). Therefore, few pediatric radiologists currently use sedation in the USA. Glucagon was shown not to improve enema reduction rates in one study (68) and is no longer used (16). The use of manual palpation has been suggested to improve intussusception reduction at enema, but has not been systematically studied (46, 69). One study by Grasso et al. reported a reduction rate of 76% when manual palpation was used, less than the average of 80% in large series (69).

Fluoroscopy Versus Sonography

In the West (i.e., North America, parts of Europe, Australia), fluoroscopy is almost always used during enema reduction. There are other reports, primarily from Asia, on the use of sonography with either water (70–76) or air (77–79) that show reduction rates as high as or higher than those using fluoroscopy. However, the experience level required for these techniques has not been studied nor has the ability of sonography to detect perforations (limited evidence).

Delayed Repeat Enema

In the small percent of children who fail initial enema reduction, delayed repeat enema may avoid the need for surgical reduction. The use of delayed attempts at between 30 min and 19 h after initial attempt has shown promise in increasing the success of enema reductions (80–84) (limited evidence). These four small series showed further reduction rates of 50–82% by waiting at least 30 min prior to further attempts at enema reduction. Further research to understand optimal timing and technique for delayed repeat enemas is needed. Daneman and Navarro, with the largest reported experience to date, suggest a delay of 2–4 h until further research yields more rigorous guidelines (25). The child must remain clinically stable and be appropriately monitored during this time interval. Delayed enema should not be performed if the initial enema does not move the intussusception at all (25, 83).

Where Should Patients Be Treated?

Bratton and colleagues performed a retrospective cohort analysis of all children hospitalized with intussusception in the state of Washington from 1987 through 1996 (17) (moderate evidence). They investigated whether the rate of surgical management for these children varied by hospital pediatric caseload, measured by the annual number of pediatric hospital admissions. By reviewing the discharge data of all 507 children, they found an overall rate of surgical reduction of 53%, with 20% undergoing bowel resection. Rates of surgical reduction varied by pediatric caseload from 36% at hospitals with large pediatric caseloads to nearly double, 64%, at hospitals with low pediatric volumes. Children who underwent surgery versus enema reduction had similar gender and median age characteristics, but those who had bowel resection were more likely to have coexisting conditions. Median cost of hospital care for these children was $5,724 for surgical reduction and $1,184 for enema reduction.

What Are the Complications of Enema Therapy?

The most important potential complication of enema is bowel perforation. Sixty-six published studies of this question were largely Level-3 (limited evidence) investigations consisting of unselected, but often consecutive case series. The mean perforation rate was 0.8% (Table 31.2). In 18 case series with at least 150 children each, perforation rates averaged 0.6%, with a range of 0–1.6% (25). There were no statistically significant differences between air and liquid enema perforation rates (Table 31.3). When these averages were weighted to reflect the sample size of each published study, the perforation rates were even lower, at 0.3% for all 66 studies and 0.2% for the larger studies.

Ultimately, however, the risk of perforation depends on each radiologist's patient population and technique. Though determination of clinical predictors of perforation is complicated by lack of prospective studies, the one acknowledged key factor is symptom length greater than 48 h. Several reports in both pig models and children suggest that there may be preexisting focal perforation in the necrotic intussuscipiens or, less commonly, the intussusceptum that is rarely radiographically apparent as free air (20, 22, 25, 85–88) (moderate evidence). The most common site is at or just proximal to the intussusception in the transverse colon (88). Perforations with air tend to be smaller than those with liquid enema although the overall perforation rates are similar (22, 86).

In 1989, Campbell surveyed enema techniques and complications of North American pediatric radiologists (89). Respondents' combined experience was 14,000 intussusception enemas. Although they did not report enema reduction rates, the combined perforation rate was 0.39% (55/14,000), with only one death. This study remains the basis for the risk of perforation that is explained to parents for consent prior to enema reduction (one in 250 to one in 300) (limited evidence).

Barium is no longer the liquid contrast medium of choice for reduction of intussusception due to the risk of barium peritonitis, infection, and adhesions when perforation occurs during the enema (22, 46, 53, 57) (moderate evidence). While iodinated contrast is now preferred and is considered a safer agent than barium, one should be aware that it may produce fluid and electrolyte shifts if perforation occurs, since contrast is absorbed from the peritoneum.

One complication unique to air enema is the tension pneumoperitoneum. In an early report, two deaths occurred from this complication, leading the proponents of air enema to advise having an 18-gauge needle readily available in the fluoroscopy room for emergent decompression (25, 46, 53). Although theoretically possible, there have been no reports of air embolism.

What Are the Surgical Management and Complications?

Depending on the patient population, approximately 20–40% of children who undergo surgical reduction of their intussusception will require bowel resection [20% (17); 30–40% (1)]. If we estimate that 20% of children with intussusception will fail enema reduction and undergo surgical reduction, then only 4–8% of all children will require bowel resection. Ideally, only this population should need surgical intervention.

Short-term complications from laparotomy include infection and bowel perforation. The long-term risk of small bowel obstruction from adhesions is approximately 8% for neonates and 3–5% for those children older than 1 month (90).

Cost-Effectiveness Analysis

There are no known rigorous economic analyses on diagnosis and treatment strategies for intussusception, although one study evaluated the cost savings of more aggressive enema reduction compared to surgical reduction (19). Stein and colleagues analyzed single institution billing records of 703 children with intussusception to compare government DRG reimbursements of hospital care in Australia (limited evidence). In 1993 Australian dollars, the government paid, on average, $727 for enema reduction and $4,514 for surgical reduction in hospital care. With the broader indications for enema and the increased use of air, they noted decreased use of surgical reduction at their institution: in 1983, 65% children underwent surgical reduction decreasing to 25% in 1992 (19). Ironically, the authors noted that hospital profit, however, is greater for surgical reductions.

IV. What Is Appropriate Management in Recurrent Cases?

Summary of Evidence: Intussusception recurrence rates average 10% in large series, with a range of 5.4–15.4% (1, 91), regardless of air versus liquid enema technique (moderate evidence). The recurrence rates are =5% when surgical reduction is performed, presumably due to the development of adhesions (92). Repeat enema is both safe and effective in recurrent intussusception (1, 46, 92, 93) as long as the child remains clinically stable (limited evidence). There is insufficient evidence to support any particular approach beyond the performance of the enema and referral to a surgeon for shared decision-making with the patient.

Supporting Evidence: 50% of children who develop recurrent intussusception will present within 48 h, although recurrences have been reported up to 18 months later (53) (limited evidence). No clear risk factors are known for why some children have recurrences although some have focal PLP. In those with PLP, children with diffuse bowel abnormality such as cystic fibrosis, HSP, or celiac disease may be treated with enema reduction more aggressively than those with focal PLPs.

The risk of PLP in children with recurrent intussusception is low. In one large series of 763 children, it was 8% (5/69) (53), only slightly higher than the reported 5–6% incidence of PLP at first presentation of intussusception (1) (insufficient evidence). No predictive clinical factors have been identified for PLP in these children with recurrent intussusception. Reduction with air enema was possible in 95% of recurrences in the largest reported experience (1, 53) (limited evidence).

When there is concern for PLP, sonography may play an important role and may detect 60% of PLPs (1, 44, 92) (limited evidence). While US will not detect all PLPs, the risk of missing a PLP without other signs or symptoms to guide management is unlikely (48). Ein reviewed 1,200 intussusception cases covering 40 years' experience at one institution to analyze this risk. When the enema failed to detect lymphoma as a PLP, Ein noted the presence of clinical signs of illness of greater than 1 week, patient age greater than 3 years, weight loss, and palpable mass in all of these children (limited evidence).

In a randomized, double-blind trial comparing 144 children who received intramuscular corticosteroids versus 137 who received placebo before air enema reduction, Lin and colleagues reported significantly fewer intussusception recurrences at 6 months (3) (moderate evidence). In both groups, the initial reduction rate was 85%. There were no recurrences in the children who received dexamethasone, compared to 5% in the placebo group. They hypothesized that steroids decreased the volume of mesenteric adenopathy and lymphoid hyperplasia in the terminal ileum and thus the risk of recurrence. However, further investigation of the risks and benefits of this intervention is needed.

V. Special Case: Intussusception Limited to the Small Bowel

With the increasing use of multi-detector CT scanners, radiologists are reporting more frequent presence of small, asymptomatic small bowel–small bowel intussusception (2, 94) (limited evidence). These intussusceptions are typically transient and, since the children are asymptomatic, they are of no known clinical significance.

There is little evidence in the literature regarding the optimal diagnosis and treatment of symptomatic intussusception limited to the small bowel. Most authors agree, however, that the diagnosis is more difficult both clinically

and radiologically (1, 21, 26). Small bowel intussusceptions are unlikely to have associated abdominal mass or rectal bleeding. Treatment is virtually always surgical reduction. Special risk factors for small bowel intussusception include the early postoperative period after either intraperitoneal or retroperitoneal surgery, the presence of long enteric feeding tubes, diffuse PLP (cystic fibrosis or HSP), and small bowel polyps (1, 26, 95) (limited evidence).

VI. Special Case: Intussusception with a Known Lead Point Mass

The optimal imaging approach to children with intussusception and known PLP is unknown. However, Daneman surveyed the SPR members at their 2004 annual meeting and found that 76% of respondents attempt reduction in these patients (15). Some surgeons may request enema reduction in these children to partially reduce the intussusception and perhaps decrease the laparotomy incision size (82). There is insufficient evidence to support any particular approach beyond referral to a surgeon for shared decision-making with the patient and, if requested, the performance of an enema (25, 59, 93).

Take Home Tables

Table 31.1 summarizes the sensitivity and specificity of diagnostic imaging for intussusception. Table 31.2 summarizes the published intussusception enema reduction rates and perforation rates. Table 31.3 summarizes the comparison of air versus liquid contrast enema reduction and perforation rates.

Imaging Case Study

Case 1

Figures 31.1 and 31.2 present the case of a 9-month-old boy who comes to the emergency department with a 1-day history of irritability, vomiting, and intermittent crying.

Suggested Imaging Protocol for Intussusception in Children

Ultrasound for Clinically Suspected Intussusception

If there is a concern for alternative diagnoses such as constipation, 1–2 view abdominal radiographs (supine or prone and decubitus) (limited evidence). The abdomen is scanned with a 5 mHz or higher linear transducer using the graded compression technique and a bowel or high-contrast application package. All four quadrants of the abdomen must be scanned, typically in transverse planes, beginning with the right upper quadrant, to exclude an intussusception mass.

Air Enema for Reduction

Prior to performing the enema, consult the surgeon (moderate evidence). (If no experience with air or few cases seen per year, then perform liquid enema with water-soluble contrast using the guide of the "rule of threes" described previously.) The enema tip without a balloon should be placed within the child's rectum and taped in place with abundant tape. With the child prone, the radiologist squeezes the buttocks closed to prevent air leak. Air is rapidly insufflated into the colon under fluoroscopic observation until the intussusception is completely reduced, when air flows freely from the cecum into the distal small bowel loops. Air pressure must remain below a maximum limit of 120 mmHg to avoid the risk of perforation. Repeat enema for recurrences, including multiple recurrences (limited evidence).

Table 31.1. Summary of sensitivity and specificity of diagnostic imaging for intussusception

Test	Sensitivity (%)	Specificity (%)
Abdominal radiographs[a]	45	–
Ultrasound[b]	98–100	88–100
Enema[c]	100	100

Reprinted with the kind permission of Springer Science+Business Media from Applegate KE. Intussusception in Children: Diagnostic Imaging and Treatment. In Santiago LS, Blackmore CC (eds): *Evidence-Based Imaging: Optimizing Imaging in Patient Care.* New York: Springer Science+Business Media, 2006.
[a]Data from (4, 27).
[b]Data from (5, 31, 36, 37).
[c]Reference standard for ileocolic intussusception (does not include intussusception limited to small bowel); see (25).

Table 31.2. Summary of published intussusception enema reduction rates and perforation rates

Rates	All studies			Studies with cases>150		
	Number of studies	Mean (SD)	Wt mean (SD)	Number of studies	Mean (SD)	Wt mean (SD)
Reduction (%)	71	74.1 (16.8)	87.3 (12)	19	79.6 (12.5)	89.5 (9.3)
Perforation (%)	66	0.8 (1.4)	0.3 (0.7)	18	0.6 (0.8)	0.2 (0.4)

Summary data include a weighted average measure of reduction and perforation rates based on publications with at least 150 pediatric cases. The enema techniques varied and included air versus liquid media, with sonographic or fluoroscopic guidance.
Data from Daneman and Navarro (25).
Reprinted with the kind permission of Springer Science+Business Media from Applegate KE. Intussusception in Children: Diagnostic Imaging and Treatment. In Santiago LS, Blackmore CC (eds): *Evidence-Based Imaging: Optimizing Imaging in Patient Care.* New York: Springer Science+Business Media, 2006.
Wt mean weighted mean, *SD* standard deviation.

Table 31.3. Summary comparison of air versus liquid contrast enema reduction and perforation rates

		All studies			Studies with cases >150		
		Number of studies	Mean (SD)	Wt mean (SD)	Number of studies	Mean (SD)	Wt mean (SD)
Reduction (%)	Pneumatic	32	82.1 (11.9)	91.4 (5.2)	10	86.4 (6.3)	92.2 (3.3)
	Hydrostatic	39	67.5 (17.6)	69.1 (15.2)	9	72.1 (13.7)	70.0 (14.1)
	p-value		<0.001	<0.0001	0.009	<0.0001	
Perforation (%)	Pneumatic	31	1.0 (1.5)	0.3 (0.6)	11	0.8 (0.9)	0.2 (0.4)
	Hydrostatic	35	0.6 (1.4)	0.4 (1.0)	7	0.3 (0.6)	0.2 (0.4)
	p-value		0.30	0.53	0.28	0.99	

Note that while the liquid contrast media reduction rates are lower, a number of these studies are older than the newer air enema reports. There was no significant difference in perforation rates. *p*-values are based on the *t*-test.
Data from Daneman and Navarro (25).
Reprinted with the kind permission of Springer Science+Business Media from Applegate KE. Intussusception in Children: Diagnostic Imaging and Treatment. In Santiago LS, Blackmore CC (eds): *Evidence-Based Imaging: Optimizing Imaging in Patient Care.* New York: Springer Science+Business Media, 2006.

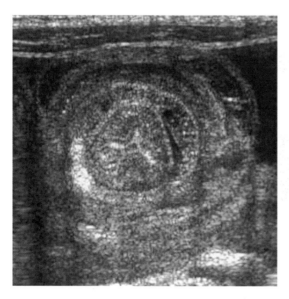

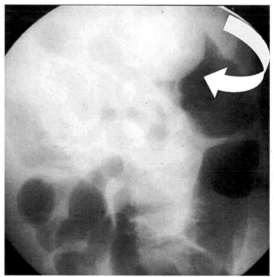

Figure 31.1. Linear sonography of the right mid-lower abdomen demonstrates the target sign of bowel intussusception. There is bowel within bowel and thickened walls of these loops due to edema. No primary lead point (PLP) is identified. (Reprinted with the kind permission of Springer Science+Business Media from Applegate KE. Intussusception in Children: Diagnostic Imaging and Treatment. In Santiago LS, Blackmore CC (eds): *Evidence-Based Imaging: Optimizing Imaging in Patient Care.* New York: Springer Science+Business Media, 2006.)

Figure 31.2. The appearance of the intussusception at air enema reduction. The intussusception is encountered at the hepatic flexure, with the baby in a prone position (*arrow*). Air is insufflated into the rectum to push the intussusception retrograde until it is no longer seen on fluoroscopy and there is air in multiple loops of small bowel. (Reprinted with the kind permission of Springer Science+Business Media from Applegate KE. Intussusception in Children: Diagnostic Imaging and Treatment. In Santiago LS, Blackmore CC (eds): *Evidence-Based Imaging: Optimizing Imaging in Patient Care.* New York: Springer Science+Business Media, 2006.)

Future Research Studies

- Investigate the optimal technique and timing of delayed, repeat enema reduction.
- Investigate the role of corticosteroids to decrease the rate of recurrence in a prospective controlled trial.
- Perform cost-effectiveness analyses of the role of US for the diagnosis of intussusception. This investigation would include the question: At what disease prevalence or individual case probability is US cost-effective prior to enema?

References

1. Navarro O, Daneman A. Pediatr Radiol 2004;34:305–312.
2. Strouse PJ, DiPietro MA, Saez F. Pediatr Radiol 2003;33(5):316–320. Epub 2003 Feb 26.
3. Lin SL, Kong MS, Houng DS. Eur J Pediatr 2000;159(7):551–552.
4. Daneman A, Navarro O. Pediatr Radiol 2003; 33:79–85.
5. Harrington L, Connolly B, Hu X, Wesson DE, Babyn P et al. J Pediatr 1998;132(5):836 839.
6. Lai AH, Phua KB, Teo EL, Jacobsen AS. Ann Acad Med Singapore 2002;31(1):81–85.
7. Losek JD, Fiete RL. Am J Emerg Med 1991; 9(1):1–3.
8. Parashar UD, Holman RC, Cummings KC, Staggs NW, Curns AT et al. Pediatrics 2000;106(6): 1413–1421.
9. Berlin L. Am J Roentgenol 1998;170:1161–1163.
10. Meier DE, Coln CD, Rescorla FJ, OlaOlorun A, Tarpley JL. World J Surg 1996;20(8):1035–1039; discussion 1040.
11. CDC and Prevention. MMWR Morb Mortal Wkly Rep 1999;48:1007.
12. Chang HG, Smith PF, Ackelsberg J, Morse DL, Glass RI. Pediatrics 2001;108(1):54–60.
13. Rennels MB, Parashar UD, Holman RC, Le CT, Chang HG et al. Pediatr Infect Dis J 1998;17(10): 924–925.
14. Dennehy PH, Bresee JS. Infect Dis Clin North Am 2001;15(1):189–207.
15. Daneman A. Personal communication, SPR meeting 2004 unpublished survey.
16. Meyer JS. Pediatr Radiol 1992;22:323–325.
17. Bratton SL, Haberkern CM, Waldhausen JH, Sawin RS, Allison JW. Pediatrics 2001;107(2): 299–303.
18. Leonidas JC. Am J Roentgenol 1985;145(4): 665–669.
19. Stein JE, Beasley SW, Phelan E. Aust N Z J Surg 1997;67(6):330–331.
20. Beasley S. Pediatr Radiol 2004;34:302–304.
21. Littlewood Teele R, Vogel SA. Pediatr Surg Int 1998;14(3):158–162; review.
22. Shiels WE II, Kirks DR, Keller GL, Ryckman FR, Daugherty CC et al. Am J Roentgenol 1993;160: 931–935.
23. Kuppermann N, O'Dea T, Pinckney L, Hoecker C. Arch Pediatr Adolesc Med 2000;154(3): 250–255.
24. Klein EJ, Kapoor D, Shugerman RP. Clin Pediatr (Phila) 2004;43(4):343–347.
25. Daneman A, Navarro O. Pediatr Radiol 2004;34: 97–108.
26. Sargent MA, Babyn P, Alton DJ. Pediatr Radiol 1994;24(1):17–20.
27. West KW, Stephens B, Vane DW, Grosfeld JL. Surgery 1987;102(4):704–710.
28. Eklof O, Hartelius H. Pediatr Radiol 1980;9(4): 199–206.
29. Bowerman RA, Silver TM, Jaffe MH. Radiology 1982;143:527–529.
30. Lee HC, Yeh HJ, Leu YJ. J Pediatr Gastroenterol Nutr 1989;8(3):343–347.
31. Pracros JP, Tran-Minh VA, Morin de Finfe CH, Deffrenne-Pracros P, Louis D et al. Ann Radiol (Paris) 1987;30(7):525–530.
32. Swischuk LE, Hayden CK, Boulden T. Pediatr Radiol 1985;15:388–391.
33. Del-Pozo G, Albillos JC, Tejedor D, Calero R, Rasero M et al. RadioGraphics 1999;19:299–319.
34. Henrikson S, Blane CE, Koujok K, Strouse PJ, DiPietro MA et al. Pediatr Radiol 2003;33: 190–193.
35. Schmit P, Rohrschneider WK, Christmann D. Pediatr Radiol 1999;29(10):752–761.
36. Shanbhogue RLK, Hussain SM, Meradji M, Robben SGF, Vernooij JEM et al. J Pediatr Surg 1994;29:324–328.
37. Verschelden P, Filiatrault D, Garel L, Grignon A, Perreault G et al. Radiology 1992;184:741–744.
38. Eshed I, Gorenstein A, Serour F, Witzling M. Pediatr Radiol 2004;34:134–137.
39. Bhisitkul DM, Listernick R, Shkolnik A et al. J Pediatr 1992;121(2):182–186.
40. Del-Pozo G, Gonzalez-Spinola J, Gomez-Anson B, Serrano C, Miralles M et al. Radiology 1996;201:379–383.
41. Britton I, Wilkinson AG. Pediatr Radiol 1999; 29(9):705–710.
42. Swischuk LE, John SD, Swischuk PN. Radiology 1994;192:269–271.
43. Lagalla R, Caruso G, Novara V, Derchi LE, Cardinale AE. J Ultrasound Med 1994;13(3): 171–174.

44. Lam AH, Firman K. Pediatr Radiol 1992;22(2): 112–114.
45. Lim HK, Bae SH, Lee KH, Seo GS, Yoon GS. Radiology 1994;191:781–785.
46. Kirks DR. Radiology 1994;191:622–623.
47. Koumanidou C, Vakaki M, Pitsoulakis G, Kakavakis K, Mirilas P. Am J Roentgenol 2002;178: 445–450.
48. Ein SH. J Pediatr Surg 1976;11(2):209–211.
49. Miller SF, Landes AB, Dautenhahn LW et al. Radiology 1995;197:493–496.
50. Navarro O, Dugougeat F, Kornecki A, Shuckett B, Alton DJ et al. Pediatr Radiol 2000;30(9):594–603.
51. Kornecki A, Daneman A, Navarro O, Connolly B, Manson D et al. Pediatr Radiol 2000;30:58–63.
52. Beasley SW, Glover J. J Pediatr Surg 1992;27(4): 474–475.
53. Daneman A, Alton DJ, Ein S, Wesson D, Superina R et al. Pediatr Radiol 1995;25:81–88.
54. Gu L, Alton D, Daneman A, Stringer DA, Liu P et al. Am J Roentgenol 1988;150:1345–1348.
55. Guo JZ, Ma XY, Zhou QH. J Pediatr Surg 1986;21:1201–1203.
56. Shiels WE II, Maves CK, Hedlund GL, Kirks DR. Radiology 1991;181:169–172.
57. Hernanz-Schulman M, Foster C, Maxa R, Battles G, Dutt P et al. Pediatr Radiol 2000;30(6): 369–378.
58. Stringer MD, Pablot M, J Brereton. J Surg 1992;79: 867–876.
59. Hadidi AT, El Shal N. J Pediatr Surg 1999;34: 304–307.
60. Meyer JS, Dangman BS, Buonomo C, Berlin JA. Radiology 1993;188:507–511.
61. Sargent MA, Wilson BP. Pediatr Radiol 1991;21(5):346–349.
62. Zambuto D, Bramson RT, Blickman JG. Radiology 1995;196:55–58.
63. Katz ME, Kolm P. Pediatr Radiol 1992;22:318–322.
64. McAlister WH. Radiology 1998;206(3):595–598; review.
65. Thomas RD, Fairhurst JJ, Roberts PJ. Clin Radiol 1993;48(3):189–191.
66. Suzuki M, Hayakawa K, Nishimura K, Koide M, Tateishi S et al. Radiat Med 1999;17(2):121–124.
67. Touloukian RJ, O'Connell JB, Markowitz RI, Rosenfield N, Seashore JH et al. Pediatrics 1987;79(3):432–434.
68. Franken EA, Smith WL, Chernish SM, Campbell JB, Fletcher BD et al. Radiology 1983;146: 687–689.
69. Grasso SN, Katz ME, Presberg HJ. Radiology 1994;191:777–779.
70. Gonzalez-Spinola J, Del Pozo G, Tejedor D, Blanco A. J Pediatr Surg 1999;34(6):1016–1020.
71. Khong PL, Peh WC, Lam CH, Chan KL, Cheng W et al. Radiographics 2000;20(5):E1.
72. Peh, WCG, Khong PL, Chan KL, Lam C, Cheng W et al. Am J Roentgenol 1996;167:1237–1241.
73. Riebel TW, Nasir R, Weber K. Radiology 1993; 188:513–516.
74. Rohrschneider WK, Troger J. Pediatr Radiol 1995;25:530–534.
75. Wang GD, Liu SJ. J Pediatr Surg 1988;23(9): 814–818.
76. Woo SK, Kim JS, Suh SJ, Paik TW, Choi SO. Radiology 1992;182:77–80.
77. Gu L, Zhu H, Wang S, Han Y, Wu X et al. Pediatr Radiol 2000;30(5):339–342.
78. Todani T, Sato Y, Watanabe Y, Toki A, Uemura S et al. Z Kinderchir 1990;45(4):222–226.
79. Yoon CH, Kim HJ, Goo HW. Radiology 2001;218:85–88.
80. Connolly B, Alton DJ, Ein SH, Daneman A. Pediatr Radiol 1995;25:104–107.
81. Gorenstein A, Raucher A, Serour F, Witzling M, Katz R. Radiology 1998;206:721–724.
82. Navarro OM, Daneman A, Chae A. Am J Roentgenol 2004;182(5):1169–1176.
83. Sandler AD, Ein SH, Connolly B, Daneman A, Filler RM. Pediatr Surg Int 1999;15(3–4): 214–216.
84. Saxton V, Katz M, Phelan E, Beasley SW. J Pediatr Surg 1994;29(5):588–589.
85. Armstrong EA, Dunbar JS, Graviss ER, Martin L, Rosenkrantz J. Radiology 1980;136:77–81.
86. Blane CE, DiPietro MA, White SJ, Klein ME, Coran AG et al. J Can Assoc Radiologists 1984;35: 113–115.
87. Daneman A, Alton DJ, Lobo E, Gravett J, Kim P et al. Pediatr Radiol 1998;28(12):913–919.
88. Mercer S, Carpenter B. Can J Surg 1982;25: 481–483.
89. Campbell JB. Pediatr Radiol 1989;19:293–296.
90. Janik JS, Ein SH, Filler RM, Shandling B, Simpson JS et al. J Pediatr Surg 1981;16:225–229.
91. Champoux AN, Del Beccaro MA, Nazar-Stewart V. Arch Pediatr Adolesc Med 1994;148:474–478.
92. Ein SH. J Pediatr Surg 1975;10:751–755.
93. Katz M, Phelan E, Carlin JB, Beasley SW. Am J Roentgenol 1993;160(2):363–366.
94. Cox TD, Winters WD, Weinberger E. Pediatr Radiol 1996;26:26–32.
95. Hughes UM, Connolly BL, Chait PG, Muraca S. Pediatr Radiol 2000;30(9):614–617.

32

Imaging of Infantile Hypertrophic Pyloric Stenosis

Marta Hernanz-Schulman, Barry R. Berch, and Wallace W. Neblett III

Issues

I.   What are the clinical findings that raise the suspicion for IHPS and direct further investigation?
II. What is the diagnostic performance of the clinical and imaging examinations in IHPS?
III. Is there a role for follow-up imaging in IHPS?
IV. What is the natural history of IHPS and patient outcome with medical therapy versus surgical therapy?

Key Points

- In advanced cases, the clinical presentation of IHPS is typical. However, in early cases, the presentation may overlap with other causes of vomiting, particularly gastroesophageal reflux.
- Clinical examination by palpation of the pyloric mass (olive) is specific, but less sensitive than imaging depending on the examiner and may be time consuming (moderate evidence).
- US is the preferred diagnostic imaging test in experienced hands (moderate to strong evidence).
- US is highly sensitive and specific to the diagnosis of IHPS, does not require radiation or additional gastric filling, and can be diagnostic within a few minutes. However, it requires operator and diagnostic expertise (moderate evidence).
- If US is negative, UGI series or nuclear medicine to evaluate for reflux may be necessary, depending on clinically assessed need to document presence and degree of reflux.
- UGI is effective in diagnosis of IHPS but may be time consuming, utilizes radiation which is of particular concern when fluoroscopic time is lengthy, and requires additional filling of the stomach, with the potential for aspiration.

M. Hernanz-Schulman (✉)
Department of Radiology, Monroe Carell Jr. Children's Hospital at Vanderbilt, Nashville, TN, 37232, USA
e-mail: marta.schulman@vanderbilt.edu

L.S. Medina et al. (eds.), *Evidence-Based Imaging: Improving the Quality of Imaging in Patient Care, Revised Edition*,
DOI 10.1007/978-1-4419-7777-9_32, © Springer Science+Business Media, LLC 2011

Definition, Clinical Presentation, and Pathophysiology

Infantile Hypertrophic Pyloric Stenosis (IHPS) is a condition that develops within the second to 12th week of postnatal life, in which there is abnormal thickening of the muscle and mucosa of the antropyloric portion of the stomach, leading to gastric outlet obstruction, protracted "projectile" vomiting, dehydration, electrolyte loss, and eventual emaciation (1, 2). The clinical presentation is dependent on the length of symptoms and initially can be confused with onset or exacerbation of reflux. Vomiting is at first intermittent, but increases to follow all feedings. As the frequency of vomiting increases, there is loss of fluid as well as hydrogen ion and chloride, with hypochloremic alkalosis, paradoxical aciduria as the kidney attempts to conserve sodium at the expense of hydrogen ion, and decreased urine output. The child is voraciously hungry, often gnawing his fists, and as weight loss and starvation supervene, the distended stomach and vigorous peristaltic waves may be visible through the emaciated body habitus.

The pathophysiology of IHPS remains elusive, despite the relatively high prevalence of this condition and the success of modern surgical management. Particular attention has been paid to the hypertrophied muscle, and multiple abnormalities have been identified. When compared to control specimens, the muscular layer has been found to have increased expression of insulin-like growth factor-I messenger RNA, increased platelet-derived, and insulin-like growth factors. Further, it is deficient in interstitial cells of Cajal, in the quantity of nerve terminals and markers for nerve-supporting cells, in peptide-containing fibers, and in messenger RNA production for nitric oxide synthase as well as in nitric oxide synthase activity (3–12). It is therefore hypothesized that, as a consequence of the abnormal innervation of the muscle, there is failure of muscle relaxation, increased synthesis of growth factors, and muscle hyperplasia, hypertrophy, and obstruction.

On the other hand, the hypergastrinemia hypothesis suggests that a genetically influenced congenital increase in parietal cells initiates a cycle of increased acid production, repeated pyloric contraction, and decreased gastric emptying, with histopathologic muscle abnormalities as secondary events.

Data supporting these contentions include induction of IHPS in puppies with pentagastrin infusion (13), the development of IHPS after inception of feeding (14), the thickening of the antropyloric mucosa and submucosal edema and cellular infiltrates (1, 2, 15), the development of IHPS with prokinetic agents such as erythromycin (15), and the resolution of the lesion and histopathologic abnormalities after obstruction is surgically relieved (16). However, further research is needed to extricate the etiology and pathophysiology of this intriguing condition from the multiplicity of associated findings and confounding variables.

Epidemiology

Ninety-five percent of cases of IHPS present between the third and 12th week of life, with a peak age at presentation of 4 weeks. The diagnosis is rare earlier than 10 days of life. The epidemiology of IHPS is variable, influenced by genetics and dependent on racial and geographic extraction. The genetic influence is likely to be polygenic, explaining the familial link. No single locus has been found to account for the greater than fivefold increase in incidence among first-degree relatives (17). Male and female children of affected mothers carry a 20 and 7% risk of developing IHPS, respectively, while male and female children of affected fathers carry a lower respective risk of 5 and 2.5%. Probandwise concordance in monozygotic and dizygotic twins is 0.25–0.44 and 0.05–0.10, respectively (18). The discordance in the incidence of pyloric stenosis among monozygotic twins suggests an environmental factor not yet identified. Among white populations of northern European extraction, the incidence of IHPS is approximately 2–5 per 1,000 live births, with a male:female ratio ranging from 2.5:1 to 5.5:1. This incidence falls by 20–30% among Caucasians in India and among Black (0.7 per 1,000 live births) and Asian populations.

An association has been described between pyloric stenosis and malrotation, esophageal atresia, and obstructive lesions of the urinary tract. Higher birth order, low birth weight, higher maternal age, and maternal educational status have also been described in association with pyloric stenosis (19).

Overall Cost to Society

The costs to society of caring for infants with IHPS vary with the decision tree for diagnosis, with the type of surgery performed, with the skill of the physicians involved, and with the rate of complications. In a retrospective study of 234 patients suspected of IHPS, White and colleagues (20) determined that the mean total charges for their patients with IHPS were $2,454, with a potential savings of $100 per patient in a model in which diagnostic imaging was applied after clinical evaluation by surgery, so long as the surgeon's sensitivity to palpate the olive was at least 38%. This model assumes that no further imaging will be performed if an olive is not palpated by the surgeon. A multi-institutional study by Campbell and colleagues (21) outlined minimum total hospital charges of $1,614 for patients with open pyloromyotomy and $5,075 for patients with laparoscopic pyloromyotomy. However, mean charges were $11,245 for open and $11,307 for laparoscopy surgery, largely secondary to complicating and comorbid events. In a retrospective study of 780 patients in North Carolina, Pranikoff et al. (22) found that mean hospital charges for patients treated for IHPS by general surgeons were $5,121, whereas the charges for those treated by pediatric surgeons were $4,496. This was compounded by the incidence of complications, which were significantly greater in the general surgeon group (2.9 versus 0.5%) and which raised the charges from $4,806 to $6,592. Safford et al. also showed that patients treated both by high-volume surgeons and at high-volume hospitals have improved outcomes at less cost (23).

Cost analyses have been performed that show (a) there is added cost without benefit if imaging is performed after positive palpation of the olive (20); (b) lower costs if patients are treated on a clinical pathway (24); and (c) UGI series as the initial test may be cost-effective when pyloric stenosis prevalence is low (25, 26) (limited evidence). However, to our knowledge, no studies have been published that assess the cost of surgical consult and surgeon's time in palpating the olive, versus performance of an imaging study, such as US, when the condition is initially suspected by the pediatrician or primary care physician or that have assessed the time delay in scheduling an outpatient surgical clinic appointment and its impact on patient care and its cost.

Goals

In patients with IHPS, the goal of imaging is to diagnose the condition as quickly and noninvasively as possible, so that treatment may be begun before electrolyte abnormalities, dehydration, and weight loss supervene.

Methodology

The authors performed a MEDLINE search using PubMed (National Library of Medicine, Bethesda, MD) for data relevant to the diagnostic performance and accuracy of both clinical and radiographic examinations of patients suspected of IHPS, as well as the surgical and medical therapy for this condition. The diagnostic performance of the clinical examination (history and physical exam) and surgical outcome was based on a systematic literature review performed in MEDLINE (National Library of Medicine, Bethesda, MD) during the years 1966 to June 2008. The search strategy used the following statements: (1) *pyloric stenosis*, (2) *US*, (3) *UGI*, (4) *clinical examination*, (5) *surgery*, (6) *laparoscopic surgery*, (7) *medical therapy*.

I. What Are the Clinical Findings that Raise the Suspicion for IHPS and Direct Further Investigation?

Summary of Evidence: The classic presentation of IHPS is that of nonbilious, often projectile vomiting in a young child 3–12 weeks of age. In severe cases, starvation may arise, with indirect hyperbilirubinemia and electrolyte abnormalities including hypochloremia, sodium and potassium imbalances, and alkalosis or acidosis. In emaciated children, the distended peristalsing stomach may be visible in the hypochondrium.

Supporting Evidence: The clinical presentation of IHPS is that of nonbilious vomiting in young infants. This scenario can be confusing, as reflux is common in this age group and is the major diagnostic differential. In patients with IHPS, forceful vomiting sometimes described as "projectile" develops acutely or as an exacerbation of preexistent reflux. The episodes of vomiting are initially intermittent, but progress to follow all or nearly all meals, and the infant may develop hematemesis with protracted vomiting, believed to be related to gastritis. Unlike patients with gastroenteritis, patients with IHPS are voraciously hungry. Starvation can exacerbate low glucuronyl transferase activity, and indirect hyperbilirubinemia may be present in 1–2% of patients. Electrolyte abnormalities (hypochloremic alkalosis and sodium and potassium deficits) are more specific findings which can be masked by dehydration. Renal mechanisms supervene to maintain intravascular volume by conservation of sodium at the expense of hydrogen ion, leading to aciduria in the face of systemic alkalosis; sodium may also be conserved at the expense of potassium, exacerbating potassium deficits. Emaciation in these infants is no longer common, but when it occurs, the distended stomach and active peristaltic activity may be visible in the hypochondrium.

In the vomiting infant, measurement of serum electrolyte levels can help differentiate the child with IHPS from the child with vomiting secondary to reflux. However, these findings are seen late in the course of the condition and are correlated with more severe dehydration. In a retrospective study of 65 infants with IHPS (27), investigators found that bicarbonate levels are normal in 29%, moderately elevated in 34%, and markedly elevated in 25%. Patients with elevated bicarbonate levels showed the most severe dehydration, the lowest chloride levels, the highest percentage of low urinary pH, and had the longest duration of symptoms. There was a decrease in bicarbonate levels in 12.3% of patients; these patients had otherwise normal electrolytes, the least dehydration, and the shortest duration of symptoms. The authors postulate that a slight metabolic acidosis from lack of nutrition occurs in IHPS, before the classic overlay of electrolyte disturbances supervenes secondary to gastric losses. In a subsequent study of 216 infants (28), the authors found that the alkalotic and hypochloremic infants had a significantly longer duration of illness, sodium, potassium, and chloride deficits. These sicker patients also had a higher percentage of palpable olives, and overrepresentation of female and black infants, likely because of a lower suspicion of IHPS in these populations.

Therefore, the patient with IHPS will present with new onset or exacerbation of postprandial nonbilious vomiting, with more advanced cases demonstrating dehydration, elevated serum bicarbonate, with chloride, sodium, and potassium deficits, and paradoxical aciduria. The evidence indicates that the typical electrolyte disturbances of IHPS occur later in the evolution of this condition, and that heightened clinical suspicion and further investigation before the full constellation of findings has appeared will aid in reaching the goal of early treatment.

II. What Is the Diagnostic Performance of the Clinical and Imaging Examinations in IHPS?

Summary of Evidence: Clinical examination has moderate sensitivity for pyloric stenosis of 72–74%, although this may be decreasing as reliance upon imaging increases and the diagnosis is made earlier. The specificity of abdominal palpation is high at 97–99%. Clinical examination is operator dependent, and may be time-consuming, requiring 10–29 min of palpation for high diagnostic sensitivity.

Ultrasound has high sensitivity and high specificity, approaching 100% in experienced hands. Ultrasound can be performed rapidly, without patient preparation. However, ultrasound is highly operator dependent.

UGI is considered to have high sensitivity and high specificity, although modern data are lacking. UGI has less operator dependency than ultrasound, but does require the use of ionizing radiation, which can be prolonged when there is poor gastric emptying.

In general, physical examination will be the first evaluation for suspected pyloric stenosis. When palpation for the olive is negative, US is the preferred initial imaging test. However, when there is little or no experience with using US for this diagnosis, UGI is the preferred imaging test (moderate evidence).

Supporting Evidence

Clinical Palpation

The clinical examination in IHPS refers to the ability to palpate the pyloric mass or olive.

The mainstay imaging examination for IHPS was the UGI or barium meal, standardized in 1932 by Meiweissen and Sloof (29); in 1977, US was first reported in the diagnosis of IHPS (30) and has now become the preferred diagnostic imaging modality for this condition. The sensitivity of each of these examinations varies with the skill of the examiner, particularly for clinical palpation and for US.

Success in palpating the enlarged pylorus is not easy in most circumstances and is possible only if the infant is calm. The use of a pacifier, decompression of the stomach via orogastric tube (which moves the pylorus more anteriorly), or a small feeding (5% dextrose in water) have been described as helpful. The examiner should be willing to commit 10–20 min of time in order to successfully palpate the pylorus, and repeat examinations may be required (31). The frequency of diagnosis by successful palpation of the pyloric mass has decreased over the past two decades; this is believed to be due in part to the time commitment needed for successful physical examination, the ease and reliability of the noninvasive US study, and the younger age at diagnosis today, addressed later in this section.

In a prospective investigation of 116 infants with vomiting, the physical examination was successful in 80% of 75 patients with proven IHPS. In this study, the physical examination had a sensitivity of 72%, specificity of 97%, positive predictive value of 98%, and negative predictive value of 61% (32).

In one retrospective study of 212 patients seen between 1974 and 1977 and of 187 patients seen between 1988 and 1991, Macdessi and Oates (33) found that the pyloric mass was successfully palpated by the surgeons in 99% of patients in the earlier group and in 79% of the patients in the second group; however, among the nonsurgeons to whom the patients initially presented, the pyloric mass was palpated in 47% of patients in the earlier group and in 33% of patients in the later group.

In another retrospective study of 234 patients, 150 of whom had pyloric stenosis, the pyloric mass was successfully palpated in 111 patients, with one false-positive examination, for a sensitivity of 74% and a specificity of 99%. However, the sensitivity ranged between 31 and 100% among the five surgeons in the group (20). Some authors suggest sedation in order to increase sensitivity of the manual examination, which increased from 70 to 100% after sedation in a reported series of ten patients with IHPS (34).

Abdominal Radiographs

Abdominal radiographs, if obtained, typically reveal a distended stomach with scarcity of bowel gas distal to the stomach. However, this is not a sensitive diagnostic test, and findings would need to be confirmed by palpation, US, or UGI. Therefore, if pyloric stenosis is suspected, this examination only adds delay and radiation exposure and is not recommended.

UGI Examination

The UGI examination is performed by introduction of a positive oral contrast agent, typically barium, into the stomach and observation of the abnormal antropyloric channel during passage of the contrast. The fluoroscopic examination can be lengthy, as diagnosis is dependent on passage of contrast through the abnormal channel, which can be markedly delayed. In addition, it necessitates further distension of the stomach with contrast, or passage of an orogastric tube to decompress the stomach, which allows improved visualization by eliminating dilution of the contrast by the gastric contents.

When performed by an experienced radiologist, the UGI is accurate in the diagnosis and exclusion of IHPS. There are few investigations today that specifically address the sensitivity and specificity of UGI in IHPS. In a study of 46 patients without a palpable olive published in 1967, UGI was diagnostic in 44 (96%) (35). These authors found the double track sign and string sign to be present in more than one-half of the patients, while beak, shoulder, and pyloric tit signs were present in slightly less than half; 7% of the patients had complete obstruction, with no passage of contrast from the stomach 30 min after completion of the fluoroscopic examination. There were no false positives in this series; however, without visualization of the muscle layer, overlap of IHPS and pylorospasm can lead to confusion between these two conditions. Continued fluoroscopy until the antropyloric channel opens can lead to protracted length of the examination and increased radiation exposure, even in infants without IHPS. In one patient reported by Hernanz-Schulman et al. (36) who did not have IHPS, findings in the UGI examination were diagnostic of the condition, although the US findings, which were not diagnostic of IHPS, resulted in surgery correctly not being performed. In that study, 45 UGIs were performed following US; the calculated UGI specificity was 98%. When there is little or no experience with the use of US for diagnosing pyloric stenosis, the UGI is the recommended initial imaging test.

Ultrasound Examination

The US examination, similar to abdominal palpation, requires a skilled and experienced examiner. Unlike the clinical examination, US is not time consuming, and diagnosis by an experienced examiner can be made very quickly, even in a hungry, crying infant, and without need to empty the stomach with an orogastric tube. Unlike the UGI examination, US diagnosis is not dependent upon gastric emptying, and both the lumen and the outer muscle are directly visualized. The child does not need to drink and there is no radiation exposure.

Uncertainty in the US diagnosis arises when absolute reliance is placed upon measurements of the antropyloric channel, with changing sensitivity and specificity based on the measurements used and the prevalence of the condition (37). The measurements most often used include muscle thickness, length of the hypertrophied pyloric channel typically termed pyloric length, and pyloric diameter. Analysis of the literature on this subject must be viewed with the understanding that the technique has evolved in unison with the equipment and our ability to visualize increasing details of the antropyloric junction.

The initial and seminal report of US for the diagnosis of IHPS, reported in the *New England Journal of Medicine* in 1977 (30), consisted of five patients examined with a static B-scanner and used the pyloric diameter, which ranged between 1.8 and 2.8 cm, with a mean of 2.3 cm. With the advent of real-time scanners soon thereafter, muscle thickness began to be reported as an important component of this diagnosis.

In a prospective study of 200 infants with vomiting (38) scanned with a mechanical sector transducer operating at 7.5 mHz, Stunden et al.

found a mean muscle thickness of 3.4 mm, with a range of 3–5 mm, a mean pyloric length of 22.3 mm with a range of 18–28 mm, and a pyloric diameter of 13.3 mm, with a range of 9–19 mm in positive cases. In their work, these investigators found the pyloric length the most discriminatory criterion, with a cutoff value at 18 mm. They additionally identified the importance of real-time evaluation, the lack of opening of the channel in patients with IHPS, and the variability in size of the normal channel secondary to normal muscular contractions. Using these criteria, these authors were able to discriminate between patients with and without IHPS with 100% success rate, without false-positive or false-negative results. In their patient population, a pyloric mass was palpated in two patients who had normal US examinations and subsequently were proven not to have IHPS.

In a subsequent study including 323 sonographic examinations scanned at 5.0 or 7.5 mHz, Blumhagen and colleagues (39) found an accuracy of 99.4% for US, despite classifying a positive case diagnosed as "suspicious" and a case diagnosed by sonography 4 days later, both scanned at 5.0 mHz, as false negatives. There were no false positives. In 8% of the normal patients, clinical examination had been false positive (specificity 91%). These authors found a mean muscle thickness of 4.8 with a range of 3.5–6.0 mm and a mean pyloric length of 17.8 with a range of 11–25 mm. They found some overlap in the pyloric length and identified muscle thickness as the criterion with the higher discriminatory value.

Graif et al. (40) examined a control group of 22 infants with gastrointestinal symptoms, and 22 patients suspected of IHPS, of whom 17 were shown to have IHPS. These investigators found a mean muscle thickness of 4.5, with a range of 3–6 mm, and pyloric length of 22.1 with a range of 16–26 mm. In the control group, mean muscle thickness was 2.3 with a range of 1.9–3.5 mm, and pyloric length was 12 with a range of 8–16 mm.

In a retrospective study of 145 consecutive infants with vomiting, O'Keefe et al. (41) determined that muscle thickness of 3 mm or greater is diagnostic of IHPS, while muscle thickness was <2 mm in 100% of normal patients and <1.5 mm in 98% of these normals. When appropriate referral for surgical therapy is taken as the endpoint of the examination, the sensitivity and specificity of US was 100 and 99%, respectively.

These results were validated in a study of 152 consecutive patients scanned with linear transducers at 7.5 mHz, with nonpalpable olive on initial physical examination. Hernanz-Schulman et al. (36) found that in the 66 patients with IHPS, a muscle thickness of 3 mm or greater was diagnostic of IHPS in their patient population, with no false-positive examinations. In the 77 normal patients, muscle thickness was evaluated only during the time when the antrum was relaxed and measured 1 mm or less in all the patients. There were no false-negative studies. These investigators identified seven patients in whom the muscle thickness ranged between 1.3 and 2.7 mm; these patients were observed and did not develop IHPS; although the muscle thickness in these patients did not reach 3 mm, the canal length overlapped with that of patients with IHPS. These authors also described thickening of the mucosa within the channel lumen, and protrusion into the gastric antrum, termed the antral nipple sign, variability in the thickness of the muscle of the unrelaxed normal antrum, as well as in the muscle thickness and pyloric length in patients with IHPS within the abnormal range.

III. Is There a Role for Follow-up Imaging in IHPS?

Summary of Evidence: Initially described as congenital hypertrophic pyloric stenosis, IHPS is now known to be a condition that develops after birth. The rate at which pyloric stenosis evolves is not known nor is it known whether pylorospasm is always a self-resolving condition, or whether it is one of the initial steps in the development of pyloric stenosis in some patients. Therefore, in the small minority of patients with equivocal findings, if symptoms do not resolve, a repeat examination is important to assess for the development of IHPS (limited evidence).

Supporting Evidence: In the retrospective evaluation of 145 consecutive patients, O'Keefe et al. (41) found six (4%) patients with equivocal findings and borderline muscle measurements >2 and <3 mm. In two of these patients, IHPS developed, with follow-up examination demonstrating a change in muscle thickness

from 2 to 4 mm 2 weeks later. Two patients had pylorospasm that resolved; one patient had milk allergy and one patient had eosinophilic gastroenteritis.

In a prospective Doppler study of vascularity of the pyloric muscle and mucosa, Hernanz-Schulman and colleagues (36) identified one child who was referred at 2 weeks for US evaluation of vomiting secondary to family history and heightened clinical suspicion. The initial examination found a muscle thickness of 2.8 mm with intermittent opening of the canal, which increased to 3.5 mm at 5 weeks of age without canal opening, at which time the diagnosis of IHPS was made and confirmed at surgery. In a manuscript addressing the accuracy of various muscle measurements, O'Keefe and colleagues illustrate the maturation of pyloric stenosis over a 2-week period, in an infant initially presenting at 5 weeks of age (41).

How long should one wait until a repeat sonogram is requested? The answer is not known; at this time, following the child's clinical status, requesting a follow-up examination is reasonable if initial findings lie in the borderline group as described previously, and the child's symptoms do not resolve, or exacerbate.

IV. What Is the Natural History of IHPS and Patient Outcome with Medical Therapy Versus Surgical Therapy?

Summary of Evidence: Although pyloromyotomy has been widely used and has been successful in the management of IHPS for the past century, experience with nonoperative management has been reported (42). However, the excellent outcomes achieved with the Ramstedt procedure have resulted in little enthusiasm for a nonoperative approach, particularly in North America. This procedure allows rapid return to oral feeding, with average length of stay in North America of less than 2 days.

Several recent publications from Japan have reported resurgent interest in medical therapy for this disorder (43–45). The theory that muscular spasm is a contributing factor to hypertrophy has led to trials of atropine (intravenous and oral) as the primary treatment. However, this approach has not been consistently successful, often requiring subsequent pyloromyotomy, and has the disadvantages of requirement for prolonged hospitalization, necessity of skilled nursing care, and careful follow-up while the patient is receiving this medication. Another approach has been endoscopic or image-guided balloon dilatation; however, these techniques are less reliable and do not convey significant advantage over standard operative surgical treatment but may have a limited application in rare patients in whom surgery may be contraindicated.

Supporting Evidence: In a prospective trial of 34 patients, Yamataka and colleagues (45) treated 14 patients with incremental doses of oral atropine, escalating to intravenous medication as needed, and 20 patients with pyloromyotomy. The stomach was decompressed via NG tube prior to each dose of atropine and trial feedings. Treatment was successful in 20/20 surgical cases and in 12/14 atropine patient cases (85%), with two patients requiring subsequent pyloromyotomy. Mean time to full feeds in the surgical group was 2.7 days with a range of 2–3 days and 5.3 days with a range of 1–10 days in the atropine group.

In a prospective trial of 85 patients with IHPS, Kawahara and colleagues (44) treated 52 patients medically with fixed doses of IV atropine, followed by oral atropine, and 33 patients with surgery. Medical therapy was successful in 87% of these, with the remaining needing pyloromyotomy with a mean hospital stay of 15 days and a range of 7–28 days. In the patients successfully treated, atropine was given for a mean of 51 days and a range of 29–137 days. Hospital stay was 13 days with a range of 6–36 days. Complications in this group consisted of urinary tract infection, upper respiratory tract infection, and transient increase in serum aspartate aminotransferase. Among the surgical group, mean hospital stay was 5 days, with a range of 4–29 days. Complications included wound infection in four patients requiring hospitalization in three, mucosal perforation in one patient, and postoperative hemorrhage resulting in hypoxic encephalopathy in one patient with hemophilia.

Balloon dilatation in infants with IHPS has been attempted unsuccessfully in a limited number of patients (46). However, it was reported to be successful in three infants with persistent vomiting after conventional pyloromyotomy (47).

The success of the muscle-splitting surgical correction of IHPS described by Ramstedt in 1912 (48) is unchallenged. However, the surgical approach to the pyloric mass has evolved from an upper midline laparotomy to an incision in the right hypochondrium and circumumbilical incision. In 1991, Alain reported laparoscopic pyloromyotomy in 20 infants, introducing a new approach to the Ramstedt procedure (49). Several retrospective and prospective studies have been performed comparing complications, postoperative recuperation, length of hospital stay, and expense between these operations. Mucosal perforation, a complication of both procedures, is more problematic with laparoscopy, as it may be unrecognized and require reoperation. On the other hand, wound infection appears to be slightly less with laparoscopy in some series. Although cosmetic results are superior with laparoscopy, the data to date suggest that once the learning curve for the laparoscopic approach is mastered, there is little difference in the overall outcome between these two procedures (21, 50–53).

Take Home Figures and Tables

Figure 32.1 is an algorithm for diagnosis of infants suspected of IHPS. Table 32.1 shows performance of diagnostic imaging in IHPS.

Imaging Case Studies

Case 1

Figure 32.2 presents a sonogram of an infant with IHPS.

Case 2

Figure 32.3 presents a UGI of an infant with IHPS.

Table 32.1. Performance characteristics of diagnostic examinations in IHPS

	Sensitivity (%)	Specificity (%)
Palpation by surgeon[a]	31–99 (mean 72.5) (20, 32–34, 37, 39)	85–99 (mean 93) (20, 32, 37, 39)
By nonsurgical clinician	26–47 (mean 37) (33, 37)	
Ultrasound (in experienced hands)	97–100 (mean 99) (20, 32, 36, 38–41)	99–100 (mean 99.8) (20, 32, 36, 38–41)
UGI	90–100 (mean 95) (20, 33, 35)	99 (20)

Reprinted with kind permission of Springer Science+Business Media from Hernanz-Schulman M, Berch BR, Neblett III WW. Imaging of Infantile Hypertropic Pyloric Stenosis (IHPS). In Medina LS, Applegate KE, Blackmore CC (eds): *Evidence-Based Imaging in Pediatrics: Optimizing Imaging in Pediatric Patient Care*. New York: Springer Science+Business Media, 2010.
[a]Reference (37). Assumption that palpation of olive pre-US examination was done by clinicians and post-US examination was done by surgeons, although actual examiner is not specified.

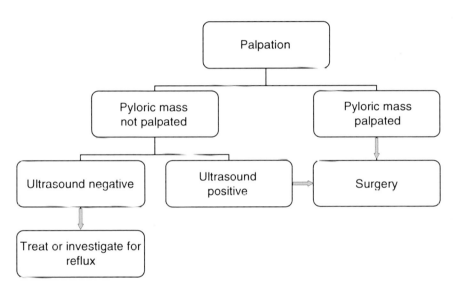

Figure 32.1. General algorithm for diagnosis of infants suspected of IHPS. (Reprinted with kind permission of Springer Science+Business Media from Hernanz-Schulman M, Berch BR, Neblett III WW. Imaging of Infantile Hypertropic Pyloric Stenosis (IHPS). In Medina LS, Applegate KE, Blackmore CC (eds): *Evidence-Based Imaging in Pediatrics: Optimizing Imaging in Pediatric Patient Care*. New York: Springer Science+Business Media, 2010.)

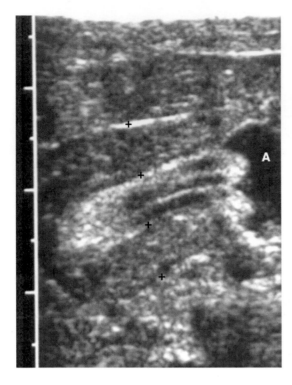

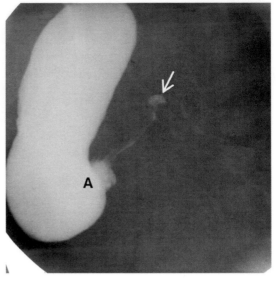

Figure 32.2. US of infant with IHPS. The length of the antropyloric channel with abnormally thickened muscle is 18 mm and the muscle (between cross-hairs) measures 4.5 mm in thickness. The thickened mucosa protrudes into the fluid-filled antrum (A). (Reprinted with kind permission of Springer Science+Business Media from Hernanz-Schulman M, Berch BR, Neblett III WW. Imaging of Infantile Hypertropic Pyloric Stenosis (IHPS). In Medina LS, Applegate KE, Blackmore CC (eds): *Evidence-Based Imaging in Pediatrics: Optimizing Imaging in Pediatric Patient Care*. New York: Springer Science+Business Media, 2010.)

Figure 32.3. UGI of infant with IHPS. The antropyloric portion of the stomach is narrowed by the thickened muscle, and contrast is seen coursing between the interstices of the thickened and compressed mucosa. *A* antrum; *arrow* points to the duodenal bulb. (Reprinted with kind permission of Springer Science+Business Media from Hernanz-Schulman M, Berch BR, Neblett III WW. Imaging of Infantile Hypertropic Pyloric Stenosis (IHPS). In Medina LS, Applegate KE, Blackmore CC (eds): *Evidence-Based Imaging in Pediatrics: Optimizing Imaging in Pediatric Patient Care*. New York: Springer Science+Business Media, 2010.)

Future Research

- Further research on the etiology of IHPS may prevent the condition or allow more effective and rapid medical management.
- Given the fact that pyloric ultrasound is the current standard of reference, further studies are required to determine learning curve and skills for general radiologists to be proficient with pyloric ultrasound.

References

1. Hernanz-Schulman M et al. J Ultrasound Med 1995;14(4):283–287.
2. Hernanz-Schulman M et al. AJR Am J Roentgenol 2001;177(4):843–848.
3. Kobayashi H, O'Briain D, Puri P. J Pediatr Surg 1994;29:651–654.
4. Kusafuka T, Puri P. Pediatr Surg Int 1997;12(8):576–579.
5. Langer JC, Berezin I, Daniel EE. J Pediatr Surg 1995;30(11):1535–1543.
6. Malmfors G, Sundler F. J Pediatr Surg 1986;21(4):303–306.
7. Ohshiro K, Puri P. J Pediatr Surg 1998;33(2): 378–381.
8. Ohshiro K, Puri P. Pediatr Surg Int 1998;13: 253–255.
9. Okazaki T et al. J Pediatr Surg 1994;29:655–658.
10. Vanderwinden J et al. N Engl J Med 1992; 327:511–515.

11. Vanderwinden JM et al. Gastroenterology 1996;111(2):279–288.
12. Wattchow D et al. Gastroenterology 1987;92:443–448.
13. Dodge JA, Karim AA. Gut 1976;17(4):280–284.
14. Rollins MD et al. Arch Dis Child 1989;64(1):138–139.
15. Callahan MJ et al. Pediatr Radiol 1999;29(10):748–751 [MEDLINE record in process].
16. Vanderwinden JM et al. J Pediatr Surg 1996;31(11):1530–1534.
17. Schechter R, Torfs CP, Bateson TF. Paediatr Perinat Epidemiol 1997;11(4):407–427.
18. Carter CO. Br Med Bull 1976;32(1):21–26.
19. Applegate MS, Druschel CM. Arch Pediatr Adolesc Med 1995;149(10):1123–1129.
20. White MC et al. J Pediatr Surg 1998;33(6):913–917.
21. Campbell BT et al. J Pediatr Surg 2007;42(12):2026–2029.
22. Pranikoff T et al. J Pediatr Surg 2002;37(3):352–356.
23. Safford SD et al. J Pediatr Surg 2005;40(6):967–972; discussion 972–973.
24. Michalsky MP et al. J Pediatr Surg 2002;37(7):1072–1075; discussion 1072–1075.
25. Hulka F et al. J Pediatr Surg 1997;32(11):1604–1608.
26. Olson AD, Hernandez R, Hirschl RB. J Pediatr Surg 1998;33(5):676–681.
27. Touloukian RJ, Higgins E. J Pediatr Surg 1983;18(4):394–397.
28. Breaux CW Jr, Hood JS, Georgeson KE. J Pediatr Surg 1989;24(12):1250–1252.
29. Meuwissen T, Slooff J. Maandschr Kindergeneeskd 1933;2:557–569.
30. Teele RL, Smith EH. N Engl J Med 1977;296(20):1149–1150.
31. Grosfeld JL, Coran AG, Fonkalsrud EW (eds). Pediatric Surgery, 6th ed. Philadelphia: Mosby, 2006.
32. Godbole P et al. Arch Dis Child 1996;75(4):335–337.
33. Macdessi J, Oates R. BMJ 1993;306:553–555.
34. Freund H et al. Lancet 1976;1(7982):473.
35. Shuman FI, Darling DB, Fisher JH. J Pediatr 1967;71(1):70–74.
36. Hernanz-Schulman M et al. Radiology 1994;193(3):771–776.
37. Yip WC, Tay JS, Wong HB. J Clin Ultrasound 1985;13(5):329–332.
38. Stunden RJ, LeQuesne GW, Little KE. Pediatr Radiol 1986;16(3):200–205.
39. Blumhagen JD et al. AJR Am J Roentgenol 1988;150(6):1367–1370.
40. Graif M et al. Pediatr Radiol 1984;14(1):14–17.
41. O'Keeffe FN et al. Radiology 1991;178(3):827–830.
42. Hernanz-Schulman M. Radiology 2003;227(2):319–331.
43. Kawahara H et al. Arch Dis Child 2002;87(1):71–74.
44. Kawahara H et al. J Pediatr Surg 2005;40(12):1848–1851.
45. Yamataka A et al. J Pediatr Surg 2000;35(2):338–341; discussion 342.
46. Hayashi AH et al. J Pediatr Surg 1990;25(11):1119–1121.
47. Khoshoo V et al. J Pediatr Gastroenterol Nutr 1996;23(4):447–451.
48. Ramstedt C. Med Klin 1912;8:1702–1705.
49. Alain JL, Grousseau D, Terrier G. Surg Endosc 1991;5(4):174–175.
50. Fujimoto T et al. J Pediatr Surg 1999;34(2):370–372.
51. Hall NJ et al. Ann Surg 2004;240(5):774–778.
52. Leclair MD et al. J Pediatr Surg 2007;42(4):692–698.
53. St Peter SD et al. Ann Surg 2006;244(3):363–370.

Imaging of Biliary Disorders: Cholecystitis, Bile Duct Obstruction, Stones, and Stricture

Jose C. Varghese, Brian C. Lucey, and Jorge A. Soto

Issues

I. What is the best imaging strategy for the diagnosis of acute calculous cholecystitis?
   A. Ultrasonography
   B. Cholescintigraphy
   C. Computed tomography
   D. Magnetic resonance imaging
   E. Imaging strategy

II. What is the best imaging strategy for the diagnosis of acute acalculous cholecystitis?
   A. Ultrasonography
   B. Cholescintigraphy
   C. Computed tomography
   D. Imaging strategy

III. What is the best imaging strategy for the diagnosis of chronic calculous cholecystitis?
   A. Ultrasonography
   B. Cholescintigraphy
   C. Imaging strategy

IV. What is the best imaging strategy for the diagnosis of chronic acalculous cholecystitis?
   A. Ultrasonography
   B. Cholescintigraphy
   C. Endoscopic retrograde cholangiopancreatography
   D. Imaging strategy

V. What is the best imaging strategy for the evaluation of bile duct obstruction?
   A. Ultrasonography
   B. Computed tomography
   C. Magnetic resonance cholangiopancreatography
   D. Endoscopic ultrasonography

J.C. Varghese (✉)
Department of Radiology, Boston University School of Medicine, Boston Medical Center and Quincy Medical Center, Boston, MA 02118, USA
e-mail: jvarghese@quincymc.org

L.S. Medina et al. (eds.), *Evidence-Based Imaging: Improving the Quality of Imaging in Patient Care, Revised Edition,*
DOI 10.1007/978-1-4419-7777-9_33, © Springer Science+Business Media, LLC 2011

VI. What is the best imaging strategy for the diagnosis of choledocholithiasis?
  A. Ultrasonography
  B. Computed tomography
  C. Endoscopic retrograde cholangiopancreatography
  D. Magnetic resonance cholangiopancreatography
  E. Endoscopic ultrasonography
  F. Imaging strategy
VII. What is the best imaging strategy for the evaluation of bile duct stricture?
  A. Ultrasonography
  B. Computed tomography
  C. Endoscopic retrograde cholangiopancreatography
  D. Magnetic resonance cholangiopancreatography
  E. Endoscopic ultrasonography
  F. Special case: Klatskin tumor
  G. Imaging strategy

Key Points

- Cholescintigraphy is significantly more accurate than ultrasonography in the diagnosis of acute calculous cholecystitis (ACC) (strong evidence).
- There is no one highly accurate test for the diagnosis of acute acalculous cholecystitis (AAC) (moderate evidence).
- Cholecystokinin stimulated cholescintigraphy is very helpful in the diagnosis of chronic acalculous cholecystitis (CAC) and is predictive of symptom relief after cholecystectomy (strong evidence).
- Magnetic resonance cholangiopancreatography (MRCP) and endoscopic ultrasonography (EUS) are superior to ultrasonography in visualizing the whole of the bile duct, and establishing the level of bile duct obstruction (strong evidence).
- Patients with a high likelihood of choledocholithiasis based on clinical, laboratory, and ultrasonography findings should proceed directly to therapeutic endoscopic retrograde cholangiopancreatography (ERCP) without further cholangiographic studies (strong evidence).
- Magnetic resonance cholangiopancreatography is useful in the diagnosis of bile duct obstruction and in directing further patient management (moderate evidence).
- Endoscopic ultrasound and MRCP have a complementary role in the comprehensive evaluation of patients with bile duct stricture (moderate evidence).

Definition and Pathophysiology

Acute cholecystitis is caused by chemical or bacterial inflammation of the gallbladder leading to mucosal ulceration, wall edema, and fibrinosuppurative serositis. In up to 90% of patients, gallstones are associated and lead to ACC. In the remaining 10% of patients, gallbladder inflammation occurs in the absence of stones and results in AAC. Repeated episodes of subacute gallbladder inflammation lead to chronic cholecystitis. Pathologically, the gallbladder is shrunken and fibrotic with a thickened wall. Gallbladder stones are associated in

95% of these patients leading to CCC. In the remaining minority of patients, chronic cholecystitis occurs in the absence of gallstones resulting in CAC.

Extrahepatic bile duct obstruction can result from intramural, mural, or extramural lesions of the biliary tract. The major causes of obstruction are stones, tumor, and benign strictures. Of these, choledocholithiasis is by far the commonest cause, accounting for up to 90% of bile duct obstruction. Bile duct strictures can be due to benign or malignant causes. Malignant lesions causing obstruction includes primary neoplasms of the bile ducts such as cholangiocarcinoma, and neoplasms extrinsic to the bile ducts. Most benign strictures of the bile duct are traumatic, infective, or inflammatory in origin.

Epidemiology

Approximately 25 million (10–20%) adults in the USA have gallstones. They occur far more commonly in women than men, with around 40% of women greater than 80 years of age having gallstones. Prevalence is high in fair-skinned people of northern European descent, but is highest in specific races such as the Pima Indians (up to 75%). It is least prevalent in African Americans, unless there is underlying genetic disorders such as sickle cell disease or thalassemia.

Acute cholecystitis typically occurs in women of reproductive age of 30–50 years. Chronic cholecystitis also occurs more frequently in women of the same age group. Although traditionally considered a disease of adults, cholecystitis is increasing in incidence in the pediatric population over the last 20 years with 1.3 pediatric cases occurring for every 1,000 adult cases. The prevalence is increased in children with chronic hemolysis such as hemolytic anemia. Up to 5% of all cholecystectomies are performed in the pediatric age group for this reason.

Acute acalculous cholecystitis occurs most commonly in hospitalized patients with severe underlying medical and surgical illness. There is no racial predilection. It occurs more commonly in males with a male-to-female ratio of 2–3:1, and occurs at an average age of over 50 years. It is more frequent in the pediatric population compared to adults. In the pediatric population,

prognosis is good due to earlier diagnosis and treatment with cholecystectomy.

The incidence of biliary obstruction in the USA is approximately 5 cases per 1,000 people, with gallstones being by far the commonest cause. However, the vast majority of patients with gallstones are asymptomatic, with only 20% presenting with related symptoms. Malignancy is the second commonest cause of biliary obstruction with cholangiocarcinoma (0.1–0.9%), and tumors of the surrounding organs (gallbladder, pancreas, and malignant nodes) being the commonest lesions. Benign strictures of the extrahepatic bile duct are the third commonest cause of bile duct obstruction with traumatic, infective, and inflammatory lesions being the leading causes.

Overall Cost to Society

Due to the high incidence of cholecystitis and the large number of cholecystectomies performed annually in the USA, a sizable portion of health care costs is devoted to treating this condition. In addition, 15% of 500,000 cholecystectomies performed in the USA each year require common bile duct exploration (75,000), further increasing the surgical costs. The advent of laparoscopic surgery has served to reduce some of these costs, although due to the large volume of cases the health economic burden still remains high.

There is very little information on the cost of managing patients with bile duct obstruction, particularly that due to malignancy. Only the minority of patients undergoes curative surgery. The majority is palliated with stent placement or chemoradiotherapy.

Goals

The goals of imaging in gallbladder disease are (1) to diagnose gallstones and (2) to identify underlying gallbladder disease (acute or chronic cholecystitis) that requires treatment. The goals of imaging in patients with suspected bile duct obstruction are (1) to confirm the presence of obstruction, (2) to determine the level of obstruction, and (3) to diagnose the cause of obstruction.

Methodology

A search of the Medline/PubMed (National Library of Medicine, Bethesda, MD) was performed using a single or combination of key words including *imaging, ultrasonography, computed tomography, magnetic resonance cholangiopancreatography, cholescintigraphy, endoscopic ultrasound, endoscopic retrograde cholangiopancreatography, acute cholecystitis, acalculous cholecystitis, chronic cholecystitis, sphincter of Oddi dysfunction, bile duct obstruction, choledocholithiasis, neoplasm,* and *stricture.* Reviewing the reference list of relevant papers identified additional articles. No time limits were applied for the searches, which were repeated up to several times up to April 16, 2004. Limits included English-language, abstracts, and human subjects. A search of the National Guideline Clearinghouse at http://www.guideline.gov was also performed.

I. What Is the Best Imaging Strategy for the Diagnosis of Acute Calculous Cholecystitis?

Summary of Evidence: Ultrasonography is useful primarily for the diagnosis of gallstones, and secondarily in the diagnosis of acute cholecystitis. Its accuracy for diagnosis of cholelithiasis is over 95%, but its accuracy for diagnosis of acute cholecystitis is reduced to around 80%. Cholescintigraphy is the most accurate test for the diagnosis of acute cholecystitis with an accuracy exceeding 90% (strong evidence). However, in the appropriate clinical setting, sonographic findings of gallstones and specific gallbladder changes are sufficient for management of most patients with suspected ACC. Cholescintigraphy should be performed where doubt exists.

Supporting Evidence: Patients with ACC usually present with the classical triad of right upper quadrant pain, fever, and leukocytosis. Unfortunately, clinical and laboratory findings alone are insufficient for accurate diagnosis (1, 2). Therefore, the diagnosis is often heavily dependent on imaging evaluation. Of all the imaging tests available, ultrasonography and cholescintigraphy have proven to be the two most useful tests for this task (3).

A. Ultrasonography

The accuracy for ultrasonography diagnosis of gallbladder stones exceeds 95% (4). However, its ability to diagnose acute cholecystitis is reduced. A meta-analysis by Shea et al. (5) showed ultrasonography to have an overall adjusted sensitivity of only 85%, and a specificity of 80% in the diagnosis of acute cholecystitis.

Despite this, some findings on ultrasonography have been more strongly associated with acute cholecystitis than others: a positive Murphy's sign is reported to have sensitivity as high as 88% (6); and an increased gallbladder wall thickness of >3.5 mm has been found to be a reliable and independent predictor of acute cholecystitis (7). In addition, combinations of ultrasonography findings have been found be very predictive of acute cholecystitis. In a study by Ralls et al. (8), a positive Murphy's sign and the presence of gallstones had a positive predictive value of 92%. In the same study, the findings of gallbladder wall thickening and gallstones had a positive predictive value of 95%. However, a single specific finding or several nonspecific findings alone were unreliable for diagnosis of acute cholecystitis (6). Thus, although ultrasonography is reduced in accuracy when broadly applied, in the right clinical setting and taken together with the above-mentioned specific imaging signs, ultrasonography alone is sufficient to direct patient management (9).

B. Cholescintigraphy

In the largest series published by Weissmann et al. (10), cholescintigraphy was found to have a sensitivity of 95% and a specificity of 99% in the diagnosis of acute cholecystitis. Across the board, investigators have consistently found a high sensitivity of over 90% in the diagnosis of acute cholecystitis. However, the specificity of cholescintigraphy has been less consistent and has varied from 73 to 99% (10–13).

When studies directly comparing cholescintigraphy with ultrasonography are evaluated, cholescintigraphy is consistently found to be superior in the diagnosis of ACC (Table 33.1). In a recent study by Alobaidi et al. (14), cholescintigraphy compared to ultrasonography had a sensitivity of 90.9 versus 62%. The results were even more striking in a study by Kalimi et al. (15), in which cholescintigraphy compared to ultrasonography had a sensitivity of 86 versus 48%. Cholescintigraphy is also found to be much more specific than ultrasonography (16). These findings have led some authors to suggest that cholescintigraphy should be the primary diagnostic modality used in patients with suspected acute cholecystitis, with ultrasonography used only for detection of gallbladder stones (5, 14, 15).

C. Computed Tomography

Computed tomography (CT) is not routinely used to diagnose ACC due to its poor sensitivity for detection of cholelithiasis (75%) and cholecystitis (17). However, a recent study by Bennett et al. (18) showed an extremely good overall sensitivity, specificity, and accuracy of 91.7, 99.1, and 94.3%, respectively, for the CT diagnosis of acute cholecystitis. In practice, CT is more commonly used for detection of complications of acute cholecystitis such as emphysematous cholecystitis, perforation, or abscess formation, rather than for primary diagnosis of acute cholecystitis (19–21).

D. Magnetic Resonance Imaging

Both conventional magnetic resonance imaging (MRI) (22–25) and magnetic resonance cholangiopancreatography (MRCP) (24, 26–29) have been evaluated in the diagnosis of ACC and its complications (30). When compared to ultrasonography, some have found MRI to be equivalent (31), some have found it to be superior (32), and others have found mixed results (33). As a primary tool, many workers have found MRI to be extremely accurate in the diagnosis of gallstones, which are seen as low signal intensity lesions surrounded by high signal bile (26, 28, 29). Similarly, the changes of acute cholecystitis have also been diagnosed with great accuracy (26, 28, 29). However, the lack of widespread availability of MRI and the relatively high cost prohibits its primary use for now.

E. Imaging Strategy

Based on literature evidence alone, there is no doubt that cholescintigraphy is the most accurate test for the diagnosis of acute cholecystitis.

However, due to a combination of reasons including availability, broad imaging capability, and clinician referral pattern, ultrasonography has emerged as the first-line imaging modality for the diagnosis ACC. Almost all patients presenting to the hospital with biliary symptoms undergo an initial ultrasonography examination. An evidence-based algorithm for evaluation of patients with suspected ACC based on clinical suspicion and sonographic findings is given in Fig. 33.1. Following such an algorithm should result in a diagnosis of ACC that is sufficiently accurate for clinical management, with the least time and cost burden to the patient.

II. What Is the Best Imaging Strategy for the Diagnosis of Acute Acalculous Cholecystitis?

Summary of Evidence: There is no ideal test for the diagnosis of AAC (moderate evidence). Ultrasonography, CT, and cholescintigraphy are all moderately accurate, with cholescintigraphy being the most accurate. Occasionally, an empirical trial of percutaneous cholecystostomy may be the only way to make the diagnosis.

Supporting Evidence: There are two well-documented reasons why it is important to promptly diagnose and treat patients with AAC: first, delay in treatment is associated with a high mortality ranging from 10 to 50% (34–37); and second, percutaneous cholecystostomy is effective in ameliorating sepsis (35–40).

A. Ultrasonography

Ultrasonography of the abdomen and pelvis is often the first test requested in the intensive care unit patient with sepsis of unknown etiology (39). Although easy to perform, evidence shows that ultrasonography is insensitive in the diagnosis of AAC (34, 40, 41), the reasons being that many of the usual indicators of acute cholecystitis are absent or difficult to elicit: gallstones are absent by definition, and the other helpful pointers such as sonographic Murphy's sign may not be elicited due to the patient's medical condition or heavy sedation (34). Thus, the diagnosis is dependent on the other findings such as gallbladder luminal distention (>5 cm transverse), presence of echogenic sludge, wall thickening (>4–5 mm), subserosal edema, and pericholecystic fluid (34). Unfortunately, these are all nonspecific findings that can also be found with other comorbidities that commonly afflict the intensive care unit patient.

In a study involving critically ill trauma patients, Puc et al. (41) found a sensitivity of only 30%, but a specificity of 93% in the sonographic diagnosis of AAC. They came to the conclusion that despite its convenience as a bedside procedure, ultrasonography was too insensitive to justify its use, and that a more sensitive diagnostic tool was required. However, others have found better sensitivities ranging from 60 to 70%. Apart from the poor sensitivities, reports also show a poor specificity for ultrasonography diagnosis of AAC (40). Overall, the reported accuracy for AAC is not sufficiently high to make ultrasonography definitive in the evaluation of patients with possible AAC.

B. Cholescintigraphy

Due to the above-mentioned reasons, cholescintigraphy has been advocated to increase diagnostic accuracy and avoid unnecessary percutaneous cholecystostomies. The reported sensitivities of cholescintigraphy in the diagnosis of AAC have ranged from 64 to 100%, with a mean of 79% and the specificities from 61 to 100%, with a mean of 87% (Table 33.2). In one direct comparative study, cholescintigraphy was found to be more sensitive than ultrasonography (100 versus 30%) in the diagnosis of AAC, although their specificities were similar (88 versus 93%) (41). Some studies have suggested that ultrasonography and cholescintigraphy are complementary, with each independently improving the overall diagnostic accuracy (42, 43).

C. Computed Tomography

Computed tomography of the abdomen and pelvis is sometimes the first test performed in the intensive care unit patient, particularly in the postoperative period when looking for an enteric leak, or when gastrointestinal symptoms predominate. When cholecystitis is present, CT can show features that can lead to this diagnosis (44, 45). The sensitivity and specificity of CT for the diagnosis of AAC can be as high as 90–95%. Thus, CT can be a very useful adjunct for diagnosis of AAC when ultrasonography is equivocal (45).

D. Imaging Strategy

There is as yet no ideal imaging test available for the diagnosis of AAC. Overall, cholescintigraphy has better test characteristics than ultrasonography. However, due to logistical and technical reasons, cholescintigraphy is not often performed or is equivocal in the intensive care unit patient. Although ultrasonography is more practicable, it too is poorly sensitive and specific (20). However, it is almost always performed because the finding of lesions such as gallstones, bile duct obstruction, or extrabiliary source of sepsis would alter patient management.

The management of patients with potential AAC remains difficult and controversial. The best strategy is for the interventional radiologist and the referring physician concerned to evaluate each patient based on the clinical, laboratory, and ultrasonography findings. Ideally, a CT or cholescintigraphy (Fig. 33.2) should be performed before percutaneous cholecystostomy. Sometimes when this is not possible or the imaging results are equivocal, there is no choice, but to proceed with a trial of percutaneous catheter drainage (36, 46).

III. What Is the Best Imaging Strategy for the Diagnosis of Chronic Calculous Cholecystitis?

Summary of Evidence: In the appropriate setting, ultrasonography is sufficient to make the diagnosis of CCC. Cholecystectomy is curative.

Supporting Evidence: CCC is the commonest manifestation of gallbladder disease. Patients present with biliary colic, nausea, and flatulent dyspepsia exacerbated by eating fatty foods.

A. Ultrasonography

Ultrasonography is the primary imaging test used in the diagnosis of CCC (47, 48), with a sensitivity of 86% and the specificity 90% (49). A contracted thick-walled gallbladder containing stones is the classical appearance (47). In some patients, the gallbladder may be so contracted that it is hard to visualize. Occasionally, associated findings of chronic cholecystitis such as cholesterolosis or adenomyomatosis may be evident.

B. Cholescintigraphy

This examination is performed with the patient fasting for 4–24 h. The diagnosis of chronic cholecystitis is suggested when there is delayed (1–4 h) filling of the gallbladder, either spontaneously or with the help of intravenous morphine (2 mg), given to induce spasm of the sphincter of Oddi. Once the gallbladder is filled, the ejection fraction is measured after intravenous administration of cholecystokinin (Sincalide) at a dose of 0.02 μg/kg weight. An ejection fraction of less than 35% after a slow infusion of cholecystokinin given over a period of 30–60 min is considered abnormal (50). Thus, the two findings of delayed gallbladder filling and a poor ejection fraction, in the appropriate clinical setting, are highly suggestive of chronic cholecystitis (51).

C. Imaging Strategy

In a patient with classic clinical and ultrasonography findings of CCC, the generally accepted practice is to perform cholecystectomy without necessarily pursuing further investigations. If there is doubt as to the diagnosis, cholescintigraphy should be performed. Also, if the patient's symptoms are more suggestive of pancreatic or gastrointestinal disease, other tests such as CT and endoscopy may be need before considering cholecystectomy.

IV. What Is the Best Imaging Strategy for the Diagnosis of Chronic Acalculous Cholecystitis?

Summary of Evidence: Cholecystokinin stimulated cholescintigraphy has a pivotal role in the diagnosis of patients with CAC who would benefit from cholecystectomy (strong evidence). The relative roles of quantitative cholescintigraphy versus ERCP with manometry in the diagnosis of sphincter of Oddi dysfunction have yet to be established.

Supporting Evidence: In less than 5% of patients, chronic cholecystitis occurs in the absence of gallbladder stones. The identification of these patients is not easy as a number of other biliary disorders can also give rise to similar symptoms. These include sphincter of Oddi dysfunction, ampullary stenosis, occult choledocholithiasis, and extrabiliary diseases such as peptic ulcer. The consequence of performing cholecystectomy in these patients includes the unnecessary risk of such an operation, and persistence of symptoms leading to the postcholecystectomy syndrome. The investigation of these patients includes ultrasonography, cholescintigraphy, MRCP, and ERCP with sphincter of Oddi manometry.

A. Ultrasonography

The gallbladder is usually normal in appearance without gallstones.

B. Cholescintigraphy

In patients with CAC, the gallbladder maintains its normal concentrating function but its contraction and emptying are reduced significantly. This may be due to intrinsic gallbladder disease, partial cystic duct obstruction, or a combination of both. Cholecystokinin cholescintigraphy with calculation of the gallbladder ejection fraction has been found to be a good predictor of pathology and symptom relief after cholecystectomy (51–60). The diagnostic findings are that of delayed (>4 h) filling of the gallbladder and an ejection fraction less than 35%. However, not all authors have found this test to be specific (61), or to correlate with histologic findings (62). Some have found reduced ejection fractions in control groups (61), and others have found spontaneous resolution of symptoms in patients with an abnormal study (63). However, the overall evidence remains strong that cholecystokinin-stimulated cholescintigraphy is highly predictive for CAC and relief of symptoms after cholecystectomy.

Shaffer et al. (64) demonstrated using quantitative cholescintigraphy, functional obstruction at the ampulla of Vater in a group of patients with the postcholecystectomy syndrome. These workers correctly identified patients with sphincter of Oddi dysfunction before papillotomy and showed functional improvement in the majority of patients following papillotomy. Furthermore, a recent direct comparison between cholescintigraphy and manometry found that cholescintigraphy was a better predictor of symptom relief after sphincterotomy than clinical symptoms or even manometry (65). However, others have found sensitivities ranging from only 69–83%, and specificities ranging from 60 to 88% in the cholangiographic diagnosis of sphincter of Oddi dysfunction (66–70). In a study by Pineau et al. (71), the specificity of cholescintigraphy was as low as 60%, making them question the value of this test in excluding the diagnosis of sphincter of Oddi dysfunction. For these reasons, quantitative cholescintigraphy is not widely used and its clinical utility yet remains to be determined.

C. Endoscopic Retrograde Cholangiopancreatography

Although technically challenging, ERCP with manometry is useful in the diagnosis of sphincter of Oddi dysfunction. At ERCP, pressures can be measured in the lower bile duct and sphincter zones by standard manometric techniques. A resting sphincter pressure of >40 mmHg is taken to be abnormal and predictive of patients likely to benefit from a therapeutic sphincterotomy (65, 72, 73).

D. Imaging Strategy

In patients without gallstones and persisting chronic biliary symptoms, cholescintigraphy should be used to select patients with CAC that may benefit from cholecystectomy. In the remaining patients, MRCP is indicated to exclude mechanical lesions of the bile duct. In patients with suspected functional disorders of the bile duct, the relative merits of quantitative cholescintigraphy versus ERCP with manometry have not been fully established. An evidence-based algorithm for imaging of

patients with chronic biliary symptoms is given in Fig. 33.3.

V. What Is the Best Imaging Strategy for the Evaluation of Bile Duct Obstruction?

Summary of Evidence: Ultrasonography is the initial test for detection of biliary obstruction by identifying intrahepatic or common bile duct dilatation. However, MRCP and EUS are superior to ultrasonography in visualizing the whole of the bile duct, and establishing the level of bile duct obstruction (strong evidence).

Supporting Evidence: The diagnosis of bile duct obstruction is based on a combination of clinical, laboratory, and imaging findings. The clinical findings of jaundice, pruritus, pale stools, and dark urine, in association with laboratory findings of elevated bilirubin, alkaline phosphatase, and transaminases, are highly suggestive of biliary tract obstruction (74, 75). The imaging modalities used for the evaluation of patients with suspected biliary tract obstruction include ultrasonography, CT, MRCP, ERCP, and EUS. The utility of these imaging modalities is based on a number of factors including their diagnostic accuracy, invasiveness, complication rate, availability, ease of use, local expertise, operator preference, and cost.

A. Ultrasonography

Transabdominal ultrasonography is universally accepted as the test of choice for distinguishing hepatocellular disease from mechanical bile duct obstruction, with a sensitivity of 70–95%, and a specificity of 80–100% (4, 76). Thus, together with the high sensitivity for diagnosis of bile duct obstruction, availability, ease-of-use, noninvasiveness, safety, and low cost, ultrasonography has established itself as the first-line imaging modality in the investigation of patients with suspected hepatobiliary disease (4).

Pitfalls in the ultrasonography diagnosis of bile duct obstruction include (1) nonobstructed but dilated common bile duct (CBD) in the elderly or postcholecystectomy patient, giving rise to a false-positive result; (2) bile duct dilatation lagging (as much as 1 week) behind the onset of mechanical obstruction, giving rise to a false-negative result; and (3) obstructive lesion not associated with significant bile duct dilation (as occurs in 10% to 25% of choledocholithiasis), resulting in a false-negative result (4, 77).

B. Computed Tomography

Computed tomography is superior to ultrasonography in the diagnosis of bile duct obstruction by revealing intrahepatic and extrahepatic bile duct dilatation (78). It is 96% accurate in determining the presence of biliary obstruction, 90% accurate in determining its level, and 70% accurate in determining its cause (78, 79). It is better able to visualize the middle to distal CBD compared to ultrasonography, particularly in the obese patient or those with overlying bowel gas (78).

C. Magnetic Resonance Cholangiopancreatography

With good-quality MRCP, the normal CBD is visualized in up to 98% of patients (80). A recent meta-analysis of 67 MRCP studies performed over a period of 16 years (from January 1987 to March 2003) evaluating a mixture of benign and malignant conditions found an overall sensitivity of 97% for the MRCP detection of the presence of obstruction, and a sensitivity of 98% for the MRCP determination of the level of obstruction (81).

D. Endoscopic Ultrasonography

Endoscopic ultrasonography is rapidly gaining momentum in the evaluation of the extrahepatic biliary system (78, 82–86) and other upper gastrointestinal disorders (87). It combines endoscopy with high-frequency (7.5–20 MHz) ultrasonography to visualize the whole of the bile duct in up to 96% of patients (78, 88). It is able to diagnose the presence of biliary obstruction with a diagnostic accuracy of 98%.

VI. What Is the Best Imaging Strategy for the Diagnosis of Choledocholithiasis?

Summary of Evidence: Ultrasonography is insensitive in the diagnosis of choledocholithiasis. ERCP is no longer indicated for the primary diagnosis of choledocholithiasis, but is reserved for its therapeutic role. Both MRCP and EUS are highly accurate alternatives in the diagnosis of choledocholithiasis. Patients with a high likelihood of choledocholithiasis based on clinical, laboratory, and ultrasonography findings should be referred directly for therapeutic ERCP, without further imaging (strong evidence).

Supporting Evidence

A. Ultrasonography

Most of the bile duct stones are found within the middle to distal portion of the CBD (89), a particularly difficult region of the biliary tract to visualize using ultrasonography (4, 77, 78). There is a further reduction in diagnostic information in patients who are obese. This results in a poor sensitivity for ultrasonography diagnosis of choledocholithiasis, ranging from 18 to 75% depending on the operator experience, the institution where performed, patient population studied, and quality of equipment used (78, 90–92). The specificity for diagnosis of choledocholithiasis can be as high as 95% (78), with false positives occurring due to pneumobilia, hematobilia, and overlying gas shadows from adjacent bowel (4, 77).

B. Computed Tomography

Bile duct stones are directly visualized or found by using the target or a crescent signs (79). The sensitivity for CT diagnosis of choledocholithiasis is only slightly higher than that for ultrasonography, ranging from 60 to 88%, with a specificity of 84–97% (78, 93, 94). This decreased detection rate is predominantly related to the varying density of gallbladder stones based on their cholesterol and calcium content (94). Up to 20–25% of stones are isodense with bile, making them almost impossible to detect.

Computed tomography cholangiography is a relatively new technique that is developed to overcome some of the limitations of CT in the diagnosis of bile duct disease. It provides cholangiographic images by opacification of the bile duct with contrast material administered through the oral or intravenous route. The low-density stones are now seen as filling defects within the contrast opacified bile duct. Improved stone detection rates with sensitivity and specificity of 92 and 92%, respectively, have been reported (93). However, this technique has not gained wide acceptance due to the small but finite incidence of contrast hypersensitivity reactions, poor bile duct opacification in patients with hepatocellular dysfunction/high-grade obstruction, and the availability of other more robust techniques such as MRCP and EUS.

C. Endoscopic Retrograde Cholangiopancreatography

Endoscopic retrograde cholangiopancreatography has a sensitivity of 89–90% and a specificity of 98–100% in the diagnosis of choledocholithiasis (95, 96). Although long considered the gold-standard test, its accuracy has been questioned (96). More recently, direct studies have shown EUS to be superior to ERCP in the diagnosis of choledocholithiasis (82, 96). It is highly likely that as the new technologies of MRCP and EUS mature, one of these will eventually emerge as the new standard of reference. They are already having a significant impact on the practice of ERCP with implications for future development and training (97, 98).

D. Magnetic Resonance Cholangiopancreatography

A recent meta-analysis has showed MRCP to have a sensitivity of 92% in the diagnosis of choledocholithiasis (81). The specificities have ranged from 84 to 100%, and the accuracy from 89 to 90% (89, 90, 93, 99, 100). In general, false-negative results occur due to small stones (<3 to <5 mm) found within nondilated bile ducts, particularly impacted at the ampulla (90, 101–103). False-positive results occur due to mistaking of stones for other low signal intensity lesions such as sludge, blood clots, air bubbles, tumor, and ampullary spasm (89, 90, 102).

E. Endoscopic Ultrasonography

The sensitivity, specificity, and accuracy for EUS in the diagnosis of choledocholithiasis have ranged from 93 to 98%, 97 to 100%, and 97%, respectively (78, 83, 86, 96, 104). A list of sensitivities and specificities for the EUS detection of choledocholithiasis is given in Table 33.3. In particular, EUS is sensitive in detecting small stones (<3 mm), even when situated at the distal bile duct or within a nondilated bile duct (78, 82, 105, 106). In patients with "idiopathic" pancreatitis, EUS was able to diagnose a cause in 77–92% patients where their symptoms were caused by small gallstones missed by conventional imaging (107, 108).

F. Imaging Strategy

To help direct therapy, classifications based on clinical, laboratory, and transabdominal ultrasonography findings have been developed to stratify patients according to their likelihood (low, intermediate, and high) of harboring CBD stones at presentation (89, 109–117). Calvo et al. (89) validated such a classification by finding bile duct stones at ERCP in 65.3, 33, and 0% of their patients with a high, intermediate, and low probability classification, respectively. Even better selection was achieved by Liu et al. (115), who found bile duct stones in over 90% of their patients classified as a high-probability group.

Many studies suggest that patients with a high probability for choledocholithiasis should directly undergo diagnostic ERCP with intent to treat (111–115). The needlessness of performing screening tests in such a high-probability group of patients was shown by Sahai et al. (111), who found that a screening MRCP would have prevented ERCP in only less than 4% of their patients. A recent cost-effectiveness study comparing MRCP-, EUS-, and ERCP-based strategies have also shown that outcomes were highly dependent on the pretest probability for choledocholithiasis and that at probabilities of >45%, ERCP alone was the most cost-effective option (112).

In patients with a low or intermediate probability for choledocholithiasis, the literature suggests that a relatively noninvasive screening test such as MRCP or EUS should be used first to select patients with common duct stone for therapeutic ERCP (89, 110, 118–120). In such a group of patients, Calvo et al. (89) showed that MRCP may replace ERCP without missing pronounced choledocholithiasis. A systematic review of 28 studies with economic evaluation has shown that the preliminary use of MRCP can also reduce cost and improve quality of life outcomes when compared to diagnostic ERCP (118).

The role of EUS has also been validated in a number of studies (119, 120). In a study of 55 patients with intermediate probability for choledocholithiasis by Kohut et al. (119), EUS selection for therapeutic ERCP only failed in one of five patients with CBD stones. Canto et al. (121) also found EUS to be a useful test in the low- to intermediate-probability group of patients. Evidence such as this has prompted the National Institutes of Health (NIH) state-of-the-science statement that in patients with a low likelihood of biliary stone disease, diagnostic ERCP should be avoided (120).

The question of whether to use MRCP or EUS as the primary screening tool has not yet been fully settled. They both consistently show diagnostic accuracies of greater than 90% in the diagnosis of choledocholithiasis (80, 88, 90, 110), resulting in the above-mentioned NIH statement declaring MRCP, EUS, and ERCP to be comparable in the diagnosis of choledocholithiasis (120). But MRCP has the advantages of being quick to perform, not requiring sedation, and being completely noninvasive. However, it is relatively expensive and is not yet widely available. EUS is less costly and facilitates interventions that are not possible with MRCP (86, 112, 122, 123). In practice, which of these two tests is used is dictated more by the availability of equipment, local expertise, and physician preference than by strict clinical or economic criteria.

Thus, it would appear that patients with a high pretest probability for choledocholithiasis should directly undergo ERCP for diagnosis and treatment of their probable stones. Performing screening tests such as MRCP or EUS would only serve to add a time and cost burden to the patient. However, in patients with a low or intermediate pretest probability for choledocholithiasis, a test such as MRCP or EUS should be performed to select patients for therapeutic ERCP. Doing so would result in considerable clinical benefit and cost savings by avoiding unnecessary diagnostic ERCP in the vast majority of these patients.

VII. What Is the Best Imaging Strategy for the Evaluation of Bile Duct Stricture?

Summary of Evidence: Ultrasonography is the initial test for diagnosis of biliary obstruction. MRCP is highly accurate in confirming the presence and level of obstruction, but is slightly inferior in diagnosing the cause of obstruction. However, it is able to provide a sufficiently accurate noninvasive cholangiographic image that is sufficient for directing further management (moderate evidence). Contrast-enhanced CT and MRI are helpful in diagnosis and staging most neoplastic lesions. In the hard-to-diagnose lesion, EUS with fine-needle aspiration is indicated. Thus, MRCP and EUS have complementary roles in the comprehensive evaluation of bile duct stricture (moderate evidence).

Supporting Evidence

A. Ultrasonography

Bile duct strictures can be due to benign or malignant lesions. Ultrasonography is highly accurate in detecting the presence of obstruction, but not accurate in diagnosing the level or cause of obstruction due to its inability to visualize the extrahepatic bile duct consistently (4, 124). It is able to diagnose some causes of obstruction such as liver metastasis, porta hepatis nodes, and pancreatic neoplasms (125). However, infiltrative lesions such as cholangiocarcinoma (77, 126) and small neoplasms of the pancreas/ampulla are difficult to diagnose (4). Once the presence of obstruction is established, further cholangiographic evaluation is often required, particularly if therapy is planned (125).

B. Computed Tomography

Oral and intravenous contrast-enhanced CT is moderately well suited to the diagnosis of biliary obstruction (79, 127, 128). Due to its tomographic capability, CT is able to clearly display neoplastic lesions and the surrounding anatomy, making the accurate diagnosis of cause and level of obstruction possible (77, 79, 129). The sensitivity, specificity, and accuracy of CT in the diagnosis of malignancy are 77, 63, and 83%, respectively (130, 131). CT can also be used to stage neoplasms; in a multimodality study using CT, EUS, and MRI to stage ampullary tumors, CT best predicted arterial vessel invasion, with an accuracy of 85% (131).

The limitations of CT include nonvisualization of very small neoplasms of the pancreas (132) and ampulla (77), and nonvisualization of infiltrative lesions of the bile duct such as cholangiocarcinoma (133). The sensitivity for CT diagnosis of benign strictures such as that arising from inflammatory (e.g., sclerosing cholangitis) and iatrogenic (e.g., surgical trauma) causes is also limited. Often cholangiographic techniques such as ERCP or MRCP are required for diagnosis and full delineation of biliary stricture, particularly if treatment options are being considered.

C. Endoscopic Retrograde Cholangiopancreatography

The role of ERCP in the management of biliary stricture is threefold: first, to distinguish benign from malignant stricture where doubt exists; second, to diagnose ampullary carcinoma as a cause of obstruction; and third, to relieve biliary obstruction using stent placement when indicated (120, 134–136). Due to its high spatial resolution and image quality, ERCP is able to distinguish benign from malignant strictures based on their radiographic appearance (77, 130, 137).

D. Magnetic Resonance Cholangiopancreatography

In patients with a stricture, MRCP is able to diagnose the presence of obstruction with an accuracy of 95–100%, and the level of obstruction with an accuracy of 97–100% (80, 89, 131, 138, 139). Unlike other cholangiographic methods such as ERCP or percutaneous transhepatic cholangiography (PTC), MRCP consistently and fully displays dilated biliary ducts proximal to a tight stricture. This is because MRCP does not require contrast opacification of the obstructed ducts for visualization, while ERCP and PTC can visualize only those ducts that are contrast filled. Thus, in patients with multiple segmentally obstructed intrahepatic biliary ducts, MRCP is often superior to ERCP or PTC in depicting the full extent of the obstruction

that is critical in the staging and management of their underlying disease (140, 141).

Despite the excellent MRCP accuracy for diagnosis of the presence and level of obstruction, its sensitivity in distinguishing malignant from benign stricture is only 88% (81). This reduced sensitivity is due to a combination of MR signal dropout within a stricture due to lack of fluid, and the lower spatial resolution of MR (142). However, at least in one study involving patients with pancreatic disease, MRCP has been found to be comparable with ERCP in differentiating malignant from benign disease (143). In this prospective controlled study of 111 patients with pancreatic lesions (54 malignant, 57 benign), MRCP compared to ERCP had a sensitivity of 84 versus 70% and a specificity of 97 versus 94%. Performing conventional MRI in the same setting as MRCP has been shown to increase the diagnostic accuracy for differentiating malignant from benign lesions by visualization of mural and extramural components of the disease process (127, 139, 144, 145).

The ability of MR to provide comprehensive staging of pancreaticobiliary neoplasms by adding conventional MRI (146–148) and MR angiography (149) to MRCP in the same setting is also very attractive (128, 131, 150–152). Thus, MR has the capacity to provide a one-stop imaging package for the compete staging of neoplasms that is suitable for directing therapy (99).

Diffuse stricturing conditions of the biliary tract such as primary sclerosing cholangitis (PSC) and ascending cholangitis can present with characteristic findings of multifocal strictures involving the intra- and extrahepatic biliary ducts with intervening areas of dilatation. In particular, PSC can be accurately diagnosed using MRCP in up to 90% of patients (137, 153). Furthermore, Talwalkar et al. (154) suggested that MRCP is comparable to ERCP in the diagnosis of PSC, and is cost-effective when MRCP is used as the primary test. However, in patients with a normal MRCP, ERCP may still be needed to diagnose the subtle ductal changes of early PSC, and in patients with advanced disease and dominant stricture ERCP will be required for therapeutic drainage (99).

E. Endoscopic Ultrasonography

Endoscopic ultrasonography is emerging as a powerful tool in the diagnosis, tissue characterization, and local staging of lesions causing biliary stricture (87, 135, 155–158). Compared to MRCP for the diagnosis of biliary stricture, at least one study (123) reported EUS to be more specific (100 versus 76%) and to have a much greater positive predictive value (100 versus 25%), although the two had equal sensitivity (67%). However, a second study (130) found the two tests to be comparable, with MRCP compared to EUS having a sensitivity of 85 versus 79%, and a specificity of 71 versus 62%.

Endoscopic ultrasonography is particularly useful in the diagnosis of small tumors causing distal bile duct obstruction; it is able to detect pancreatic carcinoma less than 3 cm in size causing obstruction undiagnosed by conventional imaging modalities (156, 159–161), and detect small ampullary tumors with a sensitivity of 100% (131). Due to the clear and detailed imaging provided by EUS, it is a very useful tool in the staging of distal bile duct neoplasms (135, 155). In a study of ampullary tumor staging by Cannon et al. (155) comparing EUS with CT and MRI, EUS was found to be significantly superior to the others in the assessment of T stage of tumor (78% versus 24% and 56%, respectively), while these methods were equally sensitive in the detection of lymph node spread (68% versus 59% and 77%, respectively).

In addition to diagnostic imaging, EUS facilitates tissue sampling through EUS-guided fine-needle aspiration (EUS-FNA) (157, 158, 162–164). The sensitivity of EUS-FNA for diagnosis of malignancy is reported to range from 75 to 90% (165–167), with an accuracy of 85–96% (168–171). The main cause of inaccuracies is false-negative findings in the presence of tumor. Performing EUS with EUS-FNA as the first endoscopic procedure in patients suspected of having obstructive jaundice can obviate the need for about 50% of ERCPs, help direct subsequent therapeutic ERCP, and substantially reduce costs (157, 162–164).

F. Special Case: Klatskin Tumor

Up to 50–60% of cholangiocarcinomas occur at the perihilar region (Klatskin tumor) and pose a particular challenge in diagnosis and treatment (128, 152). Accurate staging is important because treatment is based on the extent of bile duct involvement as defined by the Bismuth classification (172), and the extent of extrabiliary spread as diagnosed by CT or MRI (126, 128, 152). Medically fit patients undergo curative surgery

of varying severity based on their tumor staging (126, 133, 173). Patients unsuitable for surgery due to tumor spread or comorbidity, may be adequately palliated with biliary stenting performed using the endoscopic or percutaneous approach (133). The number of ducts and liver segments drained are also based on the cholangiographic findings (133, 140, 150, 174–176).

Although ERCP has traditionally been used for cholangiography, due to the risk of inducing cholangitis in patients with undrained obstructed bile ducts and the advent of noninvasive imaging its primary role for this application has been questioned. Once an obstructed system has been contaminated, it requires immediate drainage to prevent complications from sepsis (177–179). In patients with unresectable tumor requiring palliative stenting, immediate endoscopic stenting following diagnostic ERCP may be appropriate. However, in the remaining patients where surgery is a consideration, premature intervention may compromise the final clinical outcome (150, 175, 180, 181).

Magnetic resonance cholangiopancreatography provides cholangiographic images that are accurate in staging patients according to the Bismuth classification (131, 140, 141, 148–151) (Fig. 33.4). It is able to depict the length of extrahepatic bile duct involved with disease as well as accurately define its proximal extension, which is important for directing therapy (140, 141). If required, the local extent of the tumor can also be further evaluated using conventional MRI and MR angiography at the same sitting (126, 147–152). This allows for the prospective multidisciplinary planning of ideal treatment option for the patient (99, 101, 150), be it percutaneous (140, 182, 183), endoscopic (174, 183), or surgical (126, 128, 133, 173) in approach.

Endoscopic ultrasonography FNA has been used in the evaluation of patients with suspected cholangiocarcinoma (162, 163). In a study by Eloubeidi et al. (162), 67% of their patients had no mass identifiable by prior abdominal imaging studies but were found to have lesions measuring less than 2 cm in average size by EUS. They report that the use of EUS-FNA had a positive impact on patient management in 84% of their patients. Similarly, in a study by Fritscher-Ravens et al. (163) of 44 patients with indeterminate hilar strictures, the sensitivity, specificity, and accuracy for distinguishing malignant from benign lesions were 89, 100, and 91%, respectively. They found that EUS-FNA was useful for tissue diagnosis of hilar strictures that were indeterminate by other imaging modalities, resulting in a positive change in management in over half of their patients.

G. Imaging Strategy

Patients with suspected biliary stricture should initially undergo imaging using ultrasonography or CT to determine the presence and cause of biliary obstruction. CT is able to more consistently and comprehensively diagnose the cause of obstruction and define the extent of disease than ultrasonography (128, 133). In many patients, particularly in those with extensive metastatic disease, these may be the only imaging tests that are required to effect clinical management (133).

In patients requiring further delineation of disease, or when diagnostic doubt exists, a highly accurate noninvasive test such as MRCP or EUS should be used (128, 133). Although MRCP alone is limited at distinguishing malignant from benign stricture (81, 130), it is highly

accurate at defining the extent of the biliary duct involvement and accurately classifies patients according to the Bismuth classification (140, 152). EUS is highly accurate in diagnosing the cause of obstruction, particularly using its ability for FNA (88). Therefore, in patients with hard-to-diagnose stricture of the bile duct, there may be a complementary role for EUS, with MRCP used to define the extent of the stricture and EUS-FNA used to visualize the mass and obtain histologic diagnosis (97, 112

30). An evidence-based algorithm for investigation of patients with suspected bile duct obstruction is given in Fig. 33.5.

Take Home Tables (Tables 33.4 and 33.5)

Table 33.1-33.5 and Figs. 33.1–33.5 serve to highlight key recommendations and supporting evidence.

Table 33.1. Accuracy of ultrasonography compared with cholescintigraphy in the diagnosis of acute cholecystitis

Investigators	Cholescintigraphy Sensitivity/specificity (%)		Ultrasonography Sensitivity/specificity (%)	
Zeman et al. (184)	98	82	67	82
Worthen et al. (12)	95	100	67	100
Ralls et al. (185)	86	84	86	90
Freitas et al. (186)	98	90	60	81
Samuels et al. (187)	97	93	97	64
Chatziioannou et al. (188)	92	89	40	89

Reprinted with kind permission of Springer Science+Business Media from Varghese JC, Lucey BC, Soto JA. In Medina LS, Blackmore CC (eds.): *Evidence-Based Imaging: Optimizing Imaging in Patient Care.* New York: Springer Science+Business Media, 2006.

Table 33.2. Accuracy of cholescintigraphy in the diagnosis of acute acalculous cholecystitis

Investigators	Sensitivity (%) No. pts./total no. pts.	Specificity (%) No. pts./total no. pts.
Weissmann et al. (189)	14/15 (93)	
Shuman et al. (190)	14/19 (74)	
Ramanna et al. (191)	11/11 (100)	
Mirvis (44)	9/10 (90)	21/34 (62)
Swayne (192)	37/49 (76)	
Flancbaum and Choban (193)	12/16 (75)	29/29 (100)
Kalliafas et al. (194)	9/10 (90)	
Prevot et al. (42)	9/14 (64)	18/18 (100)
Mariat et al. (43)	8/12 (67)	16/16 (100)
Total	123/156 (79)	84/97 (87)

Reprinted with kind permission of Springer Science+Business Media from Varghese JC, Lucey BC, Soto JA. In Medina LS, Blackmore CC (eds.): *Evidence-Based Imaging: Optimizing Imaging in Patient Care*. New York: Springer Science+Business Media, 2006.

Table 33.3. Accuracy of endoscopic ultrasonography in the diagnosis of choledocholithiasis

Investigators	Sensitivity (%)	Specificity (%)	Accuracy (%)
Buscarini et al. (86)	98	99	97
Palazzo et al. (195)	95	98	96
Sugiyama and Atomi (78)	96	100	99
Kohut et al. (196)	93	93	94
Shim et al. (197)	89	100	97
Prat et al. (96)	93	97	95
Canto et al. (121)	84	95	94
Amouyal et al. (198)	97	100	98
Norton and Alderson (108)	88	96	92

Reprinted with kind permission of Springer Science+Business Media from Varghese JC, Lucey BC, Soto JA. In Medina LS, Blackmore CC (eds): *Evidence-Based Imaging: Optimizing Imaging in Patient Care*. New York: Springer Science+Business Media, 2006.

Table 33.4. Suggested parameters for performing computed tomography of the hepatobiliary system

Oral contrast material[a]	900 ml of 2.2% barium sulfate solution
Intravenous contrast material[a]	100–150 ml of Optiray 320 mg/ml at 2–5 ml/s
Slice thickness	2.5–5.0 mm
Reconstruction interval	1.0–3.0 mm
Pitch	1–6
kVp	120–140
mAs	200–300

Reprinted with kind permission of Springer Science+Business Media from Varghese JC, Lucey BC, Soto JA. In Medina LS, Blackmore CC (eds.): *Evidence-Based Imaging: Optimizing Imaging in Patient Care*. New York: Springer Science+Business Media, 2006.

[a]If CT is performed for the sole purpose of identifying bile duct stones, oral and intravenous contrast material is not administered.

Table 33.5. Suggested parameters for performing magnetic resonance cholangiopancreatography (for GE 1.5–T machine with torso phased array coil)

Sequence	Scout	FSE T2–W	Coronal SSFSE	Axial SSFSE	Thick slab SSFSE
Type	SSFSE	FRFSE-XL	SSFSE	SSFSE	SSFSE
TR	Infinite	2,200	Minimum	Minimum	Minimum
TE	96	84	60	60	600
FA			130	130	130
NEX	1	1	1	1	1
2D/3D	2D	2D	2D	2D	2D
ST (mm)	8	7	4	4	60
Gap (mm)	2	2	0	1	0
FOV (mm)	440	350	350	350	260
No. of partitions	20	22	20	20	5
Orientation	Coronal	Axial	Coronal	Axial oblique	Coronal
AT (s)	17	24	23	24	24
Phase × frequency steps	192 × 256	160 × 320	192 × 256	160 × 256	256 × 384
Fat suppression	No	Yes	No	No	Yes
ETL	192	15	n/a	n/a	n/a
BW (kHz)	62.5	31.25	62.5	62.5	62.5
Breath hold	Yes	Yes	Yes	Yes	Yes

Reprinted with kind permission of Springer Science+Business Media from Varghese JC, Lucey BC, Soto JA. In Medina LS, Blackmore CC (eds.): *Evidence-Based Imaging: Optimizing Imaging in Patient Care.* New York: Springer Science+Business Media, 2006.

SSFSE single shot fast spin echo, *FRFSE* fast recovery fast spin echo, *TR* time to repetition, *TE* time to echo, *FA* flip angle, *NEX* number of excitations, *ST* slice thickness, *FOV* field of view, *AT* acquisition time, *ETL* echo train length, and *BW* breath hold.

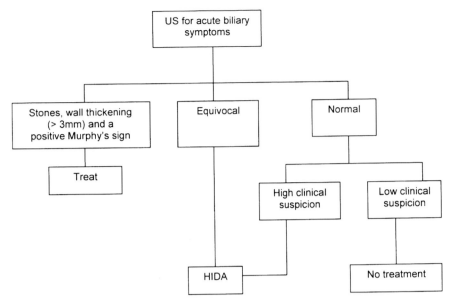

Figure 33.1.   An evidence-based algorithm for investigation of suspected acute cholecystitis. All patients with symptoms suggestive of acute cholecystitis should have ultrasonography performed in the first instance. If the three highly specific signs of acute calculous cholecystitis (ACC), that is, gallstones, wall thickening (>3.5 mm), and Murphy's sign, are all present, the patient has a high probability of ACC and should proceed directly to appropriate therapy without further investigations. If the ultrasonography findings are normal and the clinical suspicion is low, the patient should have no further imaging performed. If the ultrasonography findings are normal, but the clinical suspicion is strong, or the patient has equivocal ultrasonography findings, then the patient should proceed to cholescintigraphy. (Reprinted with kind permission of Springer Science+Business Media from Varghese JC, Lucey BC, Soto JA. In Medina LS, Blackmore CC (eds.): *Evidence-Based Imaging: Optimizing Imaging in Patient Care* New York: Springer Science+Business Media, 2006.)

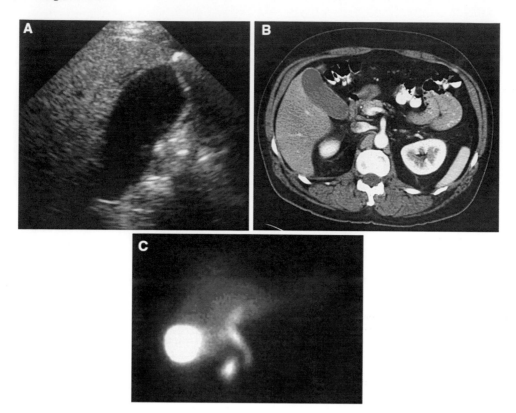

Figure 33.2. A 59-year-old man with a history of abdominal pain, leukocytosis, and abnormal liver function tests. (**A**) Ultrasonography shows a thin layer of fluid around the fundus of the gallbladder. Patient had an associated positive sonographic Murphy's sign. (**B**) Intravenous and oral contrast enhanced CT shows a normal gallbladder. (**C**) Technetium diisopropyl iminodiacetic acid (Tc-DISIDA) cholescintigraphy shows normal intense filling of the gallbladder, ruling out the diagnosis of acute cholecystitis. (Reprinted with kind permission of Springer Science+Business Media from Varghese JC, Lucey BC, Soto JA. In Medina LS, Blackmore CC (eds.): *Evidence-Based Imaging: Optimizing Imaging in Patient Care.* New York: Springer Science+Business Media, 2006.)

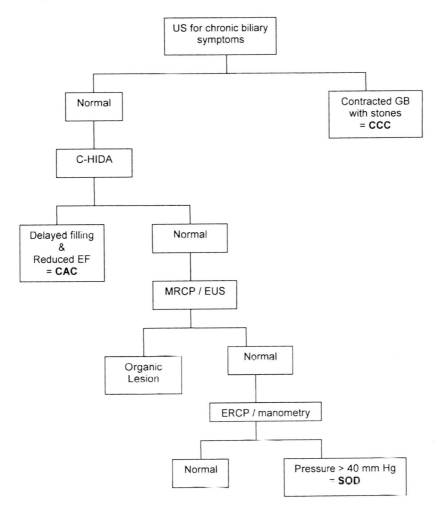

Figure 33.3. An evidence-based algorithm for investigation of suspected chronic biliary disease. *US* ultrasonography, *C-HIDA* cholecystokinin–hydroxy iminodiacetic acid, *SOD* sphincter of Oddi dysfunction, *CCC* chronic calculous cholecystitis, *CAC* chronic acalculous cholecystitis. All patients with symptoms suggestive of chronic biliary disease should have an initial ultrasonography performed. If a contracted gallbladder with stones is found, the patient should be treated for CCC. If the examination is negative, the patient should then proceed to a cholecystokinin cholescintigraphy. If there is delayed filling of a gallbladder, combined with a reduced ejection fraction, the patient should be treated for CAC. If the examination is negative, an MRCP of EUS should be performed to exclude occult choledocholithiasis or other mechanical cause of symptoms. If this test is negative, the patient should have an ERCP with manometry performed to assess sphincter pressure. If this is elevated, patient should be treated for sphincter of Oddi dysfunction. If the pressure is normal, other causes for patient cholestasis should be sought. (Reprinted with kind permission of Springer Science+Business Media from Varghese JC, Lucey BC, Soto JA. In Medina LS, Blackmore CC (eds.): *Evidence-Based Imaging: Optimizing Imaging in Patient Care.* New York: Springer Science+Business Media, 2006.)

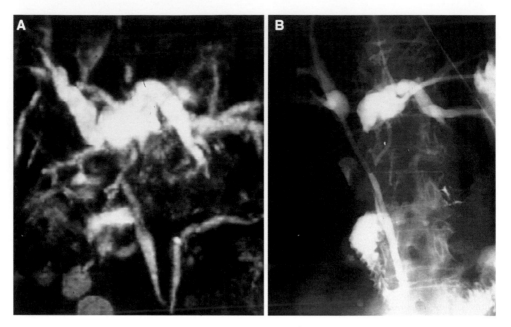

Figure 33.4. A 72-year-old man with a Klatskin tumor. **A**: Coronal maximum intensity projection MRCP showing Bismuth type 2 hilar obstruction. **B**: A percutaneous transhepatic cholangiogram confirms tumor involvement at the confluence with separation of the right and left hepatic ducts. (Reprinted with kind permission of Springer Science+Business Media from Varghese JC, Lucey BC, Soto JA. In Medina LS, Blackmore CC (eds.): *Evidence-Based Imaging: Optimizing Imaging in Patient Care.* New York: Springer Science+Business Media, 2006.)

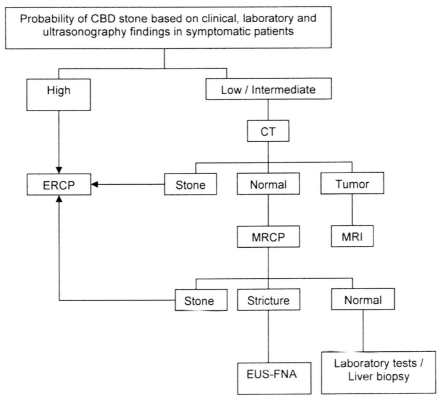

Figure 33.5. An evidence-based algorithm for investigation of suspected biliary obstruction. Patients with suspected bile duct obstruction should be stratified according to the likelihood of having choledocholithiasis based on clinical, laboratory, and ultrasonography findings. Those patients with a high probability of choledocholithiasis should be referred directly for therapeutic ERCP. Patients with a low to intermediate probability of CBD stones should have CT performed to rule out neoplasm or possibly stone. If choledocholithiasis is identified, the patient should be referred for therapeutic ERCP. If a tumor is identified, the investigation may be stopped if the neoplasm is sufficiently staged, or a contrast-enhanced MRI should be performed for complete staging. If CT is normal, an MRCP should be performed to diagnose occult choledocholithiasis or stricture. Patients with choledocholithiasis identified at MRCP should then undergo therapeutic ERCP. Those with a normal bile duct at MRCP should undergo further laboratory investigations to exclude hepatocellular disease as cause of their cholestasis. Patients with a stricture diagnosed at MRCP should undergo EUS-FNA for imaging and histologic diagnosis. (Reprinted with kind permission of Springer Science+Business Media from Varghese JC, Lucey BC, Soto JA. In Medina LS, Blackmore CC (eds.): *Evidence-Based Imaging: Optimizing Imaging in Patient Care*. New York: Springer Science+Business Media, 2006.)

Future Research

- Comparative studies of MRCP and EUS to determine the most cost-effective test for diagnosis of bile duct stricture.
- Further evaluation of quantitative cholescintigraphy in the diagnosis of biliary dyskinesia.
- Prospective evaluation of the utility of cholecystokinin stimulated cholescintigraphy in patients undergoing percutaneous cholecystostomy.

References

1. Trowbridge RL, Rutkowski NK, Shojania KG. JAMA 2003;289:80–86.
2. Singer AJ, McCracken G, Henry MC et al. Ann Emerg Med 1996;28:267–272.
3. Bree RL, Ralls PW, Balfe DM et al. Radiology 2000;215:153–157.
4. Laing FC. In Rumak CM, Wilson SR, Charboneau JW (eds.): Diagnostic Ultrasonography, 2nd ed. St. Louis: Mosby-Year Book, 1998;175–223.
5. Shea JA, Berlin JA, Escarce JJ et al. Arch Intern Med 1994;154:2573–2581.
6. Laing FC, Federle MP, Jeffery RB et al. Radiology 1981;140:449–455.
7. Imhoff M, Raunest J, Ohmann C et al. World J Surg 1992;16:1160–1165.
8. Ralls PW, Collette PM, Lapin SA et al. Radiology 1985;155:767–771.
9. Adam A, Roddie ME. Baillieres Clin Gastroenterol 1991;5:787–816.
10. Weissmann HS, Badia J, Sugarman LA et al. Radiology 1981;138:167–175.
11. Ziessman HA. Semin Nucl Med 2003;4:279–296.
12. Worthen NJ, Usler JM, Funamura JL. AJR Am J Roentgenol 1981;137:973–978.
13. Shuman WP, Mack LA, Rudd TG et al. AJR Am J Roentgenol 1982;139:61–64.
14. Alobaidi M, Gupta R, Jafri SZ et al. Emerg Radiol 2004;10:256–258.
15. Kalimi R, Gecelter GR, Capliin D et al. J Am Coll Surg 2001;193:609–613.
16. Lorberhoym M, Simon J, Horne T. J Nucl Med Technol 1999;27:294–297.
17. Paulson EK. Semin Ultrasound CT MR 2000;21:56–63.
18. Bennett GL, Rusinek H, Lisi V et al. AJR Am J Roentgenol 2002;178:275–281.
19. Fidler J, Paulson EK, Layfield L. AJR Am J Roentgenol 1996;166:1085–1088.
20. Bennett GL, Balthazar EJ. Radiol Clin North Am 2003;41:1203–1216.
21. Hanbidge AE, Buckler PM, O'Malley ME et al. Radiographics 2004;24:1117–1135.
22. Weissleder R, Stark DD, Compton CC et al. Magn Reson Imaging 1988;6:345–348.
23. Koenig T, Tamm EP, Kawashima A. Clin Radiol 2004;59:455–458.
24. Adusumilli S, Siegelman ES. Magn Reson Imaging Clin North Am 2002;10:165–184.
25. Loud PA, Semelka RC, Kettritz U et al. Magn Reson Imaging 1996;14:349–355.
26. Van Epps K, Regan F. Clin Radiol 1999;54:588–594.
27. Morikawa M, Fukuda T, Aso N et al. Nippon Rinsho 1998;56:2939–2945.
28. Regan F, Schaefer DC, Smith DP et al. J Comput Assist Tomogr 1998;22:638–642.
29. Ito K, Fujita N, Noda Y et al. Nippon Shokakibyo Gakkai Zasshi 2000;97:1472–1479.
30. Sood B, Jain M, Khandelwal N et al. Australas Radiol 2002;46:438–440.
31. Oh KY, Gilfeather M, Kennedy A et al. Abdom Imaging 2003;28:643–651.
32. Hakansson K, Leander P, Ekberg O et al. Acta Radiol 2000;41:322–328.
33. Park MS, Yu JS, Kim YH et al. Radiology 1998;209:781–785.
34. Cornwell EE, Rodriguez A, Mirvis SE et al. Ann Surg 1989;210:52–55.
35. Owen CC, Bilhartz LE. Semin Gastrointest Dis 2003;14:178–188.
36. Lee MJ, Saini S, Brink JA et al. AJR Am J Roentgenol 1991;156:1163–1166.
37. Babb RR. J Clin Gastroenterol 1992;15:238–241.
38. Akhan O, Akinci D, Ozmen MN. Eur J Radiol 2002;43:229–236.
39. Lameris JS, van Overhagen H. Baillieres Clin Gastroenterol 1995;9:21–36.
40. Berger H, Forst H, Nattermann U et al. Rofo 1989;150:694–698.
41. Puc MM, Tran HS, Wry PW et al. Am Surg 2002;68:65–69.
42. Prevot N, Mariat G, Mahul P et al. Eur J Nucl Med 1999;26:1317–1325.
43. Mariat G, Mahul P, Prevot N et al. Intensive Care Med 2000;26:1658–1663.
44. Mirvis SE. AJR Am J Roentgenol 1986;147:1171–1175.
45. Blankenberg F, Wirth R, Jeffery RB et al. Gastrointest Radiol 1991;196:149–153.
46. Menu Y, Vuillerme MP. Eur Radiol 2002;12:2397–2406.
47. Grossman SJ, Joyce JM. Emerg Med Clin North Am 1991;9:853–874.
48. Marton KI, Doubilet P. Ann Intern Med 1988;109:722–729.
49. Renfrew DL, Witte DL, Berbaum KS et al. Invest Radiol 1993;28:404–408.

50. Ziessman HA. Radiol Clin North Am 2001;39: 997–1006.
51. Khosla R, Singh A, Miedema BW et al. South Med J 1997;90:1087–1090.
52. Poynter MT, Saba AK, Evans RA et al. Am Surg 2002;68:382–384.
53. Chen PF, Nimeri A, Pham QH et al. Surgery 2001;130:578–581.
54. Goncalves RM, Harris JA, Rivera DE. Am Surg 1998;64:493–497.
55. Sorenson MK, Fancher S, Lang NP et al. Am J Surg 1993;166:672–674.
56. Reed DN Jr, Fernandez M, Hicks RD. Am Surg 1993;59:273–277.
57. Yap L, Wycherley AG, Morphett AD et al. Gastroenterology 1991;101:786–793.
58. Misra DC Jr, Blossom GB, Fink-Bennett D et al. Arch Surg 1991;126:957–960.
59. Zech ER, Simmons LB, Kendrick RR et al. Surg Gynecol Obstet 1991;172:21–24.
60. Kloiber R, Molnar CP, Shaffer FA. AJR Am J Roentgenol 1992;159:509–513.
61. Fink-Bennett D, DeRidder P, Kolozsi WZ et al. J Nucl Med 1991;32:1695–1699.
62. DeCamp JR, Tabatowski K, Schauwecker DS et al. Clin Nucl Med 1992;17:784–786.
63. Mishkind MT, Pruitt RF, Bambini DA et al. Am Surg 1997;63:769–774.
64. Shaffer EA, McOrmond P, Duggan H. Gastroenterology 1986;79:899–906.
65. Cicala M, Habib FI, Vavassori P et al. Gut 2002;50:665–668.
66. Oxford JL, Dibos PE, Soudry G. Clin Nucl Med 2000;25:670–675.
67. Thomas PD, Turner JG, Dobbs BE et al. Gut 2000;46:838–841.
68. Peng NJ, Lai KH, Tsay DG et al. Nucl Med Commun 1994;15:899–904.
69. Drane WE, Johnson DA. J Nucl Med 1990;9:1462–1468.
70. Fullerton GM, Allan A, Hilditch T et al. Gut 1988;1397–1401.
71. Pineau BC, Knapple WL, Spicer KM et al. Am J Gastroenterol 2001;96:3106–3109.
72. Choudhry U, Ruffolo T, Jamidar P et al. Gastrointest Endosc 1993;39:492–495.
73. Greene JE, Hogan WJ, Dodds WJ et al. N Engl J Med 1989;320:82–87.
74. Bilhartz MH, Horton JD. In Feldman M (ed.): Sleisenger and Fordtran's Gastrointestinal and Liver Disease, 6th ed. Philadelphia: WB Saunders, 1998;948–972.
75. Kaplan LM, Isselbacher KJ. In Fauci AS, Longo DL, Kasper DL et al. (eds.): Harrison's Principles of Internal Medicine, 14th ed. New York: McGraw-Hill, 1998;249–255.
76. Hulse PA, Nicholson DA. Br J Hosp Med 1994;52:103–107.
77. Baron RL, Tublin ME, Peterson MS. Radiol Clin North Am 2002;40:1325–1354.
78. Sugiyama M, Atomi Y. Gastrointest Endosc 1997;45:143–146.
79. Brant WE. In Webb WR, Brant WE, Helms CA (eds.): Fundamentals of Body CT, 2nd ed. Philadelphia: WB Saunders, 1998;213–222.
80. Soto JA, Barish MA, Yucel EK et al. Gastroenterology 1996;110:589–597.
81. Romangnuolo J, Bardou M, Rahme E et al. Ann Intern Med 2003;139:547–557.
82. Seifert H, Wehrmann T, Hilgers R et al. Gastrointest Endosc 2004;60:61–67.
83. Napoleon B, Dumortier J, Keriven-Souquet O et al. Endoscopy 2003;35:411–415.
84. Yusuf TE, Bhutani MS. J Gastroenterol Hepatol 2004;19:243–250.
85. Ainsworth AP, Rafaelsen SR, Wamberg PA et al. Scand J Gastroenterol 2004;39:579–583.
86. Buscarini E, Tansini P, Vallisa D et al. Gastrointest Endosc 2003;57:510–518.
87. Fickling WF, Wallace MB. J Clin Gastroenterol 2003;36:103–110.
88. Ahmad NA, Shah JN, Kochman ML. Radiol Clin North Am 2002;40:1377–1395.
89. Calvo MM, Bujanda L, Calderon A et al. Mayo Clin Proc 2002;77:422–428.
90. Varghese JC, Liddell RP, Farrell MA et al. Clin Radiol 2000;55:25–35.
91. Stott M, Farrands P, Guyer P et al. J Clin Ultrasound 1991;19:73–76.
92. Goodman A, Neoptolemos J, Carr-Locke D et al. Gut 1985;26:125–132.
93. Soto JA, Alvarez O, Munera F et al. AJR Am J Roentgenol 2000;175:1127–1134.
94. Neitlich JD, Topazian M, Smith RC et al. Radiology 1997;203:601–603.
95. Frey CF, Burbige EJ, Meinke WB et al. Am J Surg 1982;144:109–114.
96. Prat F, Amouyal G, Amouyal P et al. Lancet 1996;347:75–79.
97. Sahel J, Barthet M, Gasmi M. Eur J Gastroenterol Hepatol 2004;16:291–294.
98. Meenan J, Tibble J, Prasad P et al. Eur J Gastroenterol Hepatol 2004;16:299–303.
99. Fulcher AS, Turner MA. Radiol Clin North Am 2002;40:1363–1376.
100. Soto JA, Barish MA, Alvarez O et al. Radiology 2000;215:737–745.
101. Prasad SR, Sahani D, Saini S. J Clin Gastroenterol 2001;33:362–366.
102. David V, Reinhold C, Hochman M et al. AJR Am J Roentgenol 1998;170:1055–1059.
103. Zidi SH, Prat F, Le Guen O et al. Gut 1999;44:118–122.
104. Chak A, Hawes RH, Cooper GS et al. Gastrointest Endosc 1999;49:599–597.
105. Liu CL, Lo CM, Chan CK et al. Gastrointest Endosc 2000;51:28–32.
106. Dill JE. Endoscopy 1997;29:646–648.
107. Frossard J, Sosa-Valencia L, Amouyal G et al. Am J Med 2000;109:196–200.

108. Norton SA, Alderson D. Br J Surg 2000;87: 1650–1655.
109. Cotton PB. Am J Surg 1993;165:474–478.
110. Ainsworth AP, Rafaelsen SR, Wamberg PA et al. Endoscopy 2003;35:1029–1032.
111. Sahai AV, Devonshire D, Yeoh KG et al. Am J Gastroenterol 2001;96:2074–2080.
112. Arguedas MR, Dupont AW, Wilcox CM. Am J Gastroenterol 2001;96:2892–2899.
113. Nathan T, Kjeldsen J, Schaffalitzky De Muckadell OB. Endoscopy 2004;36:527–534.
114. Menenez N, Marson L, DeBeaux A et al. Br J Surg 2000;87:1176–1181.
115. Liu T, Consorti E, Kawashima A et al. Ann Surg 2001;234:33–40.
116. Barkun AN, Barkun JS, Fried GM et al. Ann Surg 1994;220:32–39.
117. Abboud PA, Malet PF, Berlin JA et al. Gastrointest Endosc 1996;44:450–459.
118. Kaltenthaler E, Vergel YB, Chilcott J et al. Health Technol Assess 2004;8:1–89.
119. Kohut M, Nowak A, Nowakowska-Dulawa E et al. World J Gastroenterol 2003;9:612–614.
120. Cohen S, Bacon BR, Berlin JA et al. Gastrointest Endosc 2002;56:808–809.
121. Canto MIF, Chak A, Stellato T et al. Gastrointest Endosc 1998;47:439–448.
122. De Ledingen V, Lecesne R, Raymond JM et al. Gastrointest Endosc 1999;49:26–31.
123. Scheiman JM, Carlos RC, Barnett JL et al. Am J Gastroenterol 2001;96:2900–2904.
124. Yoon JH, Gores GJ. Curr Treat Options Gastroenterol 2003;6:105–112.
125. Rubens DJ. Radiol Clin North Am 2004;42:257–278.
126. Khan SA, Davidson BR, Goldin R et al. Gut 2002;51:1–9.
127. Mortele KJ, Ji H, Ros PR. Gastrointest Endosc 2002;56:206–212.
128. Talamonti MS, Denham W. Radiol Clin North Am 2002;40:1397–1410.
129. Gulliver DJ, Baker ME, Cheng CA et al. AJR Am J Roentgenol 1992;159:503–507.
130. Rosch T, Meining A, Fruhmorgen S et al. Gastrointest Endosc 2002;55:870–876.
131. Schwartz LH, Coakley FV, Sun Y et al. AJR Am J Roentgenol 1998;170:1491–1495.
132. Saisho H, Yamaguchi T. Pancreas 2004;28:273–278.
133. Freeman ML, Sielaff TD. Rev Gastroenterol Disord 2003;3:187–201.
134. Flamm CR, Mark DH, Aronson N. Gastrointest Endosc 2002;56:218–225.
135. Skordilis P, Mouzas IA, Dimoulios PD et al. BMC Surg 2002;25:1.
136. Hawes RH. Gastrointest Endosc 2002;56: 201–205.
137. Fulcher AS, Turner MA, Franklin KJ et al. Radiology 2000;215:71–80.
138. Varghese JC, Farrell MA, Courtney G et al. Clin Radiol 1999;54:513–520.
139. Zhong L, Yao QY, Li L, Xu JR. World J Gastroenterol 2003;9:2824–2827.
140. Lopera JE, Soto JA, Munera F. Radiology 2001;220:90–96.
141. Fulcher AS, Turner MA. AJR Am J Roentgenol 1997;169:1501–1505.
142. Mehta SN, Reinhold C, Barkun AN. Gastrointest Endosc Clin North Am 1997;7:247–270.
143. Adamek HE, Albert J, Breer H et al. Lancet 2000;356:190–193.
144. Awaya H, Ito K, Honjo K et al. Clin Imaging 1998;22:180–187.
145. Lacomis JM, Baron RL, Oliver JH et al. Radiology 1997;203:98–104.
146. Kim MJ, Mitchell DG, Ito K et al. Radiology 2000;214:173–181.
147. Soto JA, Alvarez O, Lopera JE et al. Radiographics 2000;20:353–366.
148. Guthrie JA, Ward J, Robinson PJ. Radiology 1996;201:347–351.
149. Lee MG, Park KB, Shin YM et al. World J Surg 2003;27:278–283.
150. Zidi SH, Prat F, Le Guen O et al. Gut 2000;46:103–106.
151. Yeh TS, Jan YY, Tseng JH et al. Am J Gastroenterol 2000;95:432–440.
152. Manfredi R, Barbaro B, Masselli G et al. Semin Liver Dis 2004;24:155–164.
153. Textor HJ, Flacke S, Pauleit D et al. Endoscopy 2002;34:984–990.
154. Talwalkar JA, Angulo P, Johnson CD et al. Hepatology 2004;40:39–45.
155. Cannon ME, Carpenter SL, Elta GH et al. Gastrointest Endosc 1999;50:27–33.
156. Erickson RA, Garza AA. Am J Gastroenterol 2000;95:2248–2254.
157. Erickson RA, Garza AA. Gastrointest Endosc 2001;53:475–484.
158. Lee JH, Salem R, Aslanian H et al. Am J Gastroenterol 2004;99:1069–1073.
159. Muller MF, Myenberger C, Bertschinger P et al. Radiology 1994;190:745–751.
160. Nakaizumi A, Uehara H, Iishi H et al. Dig Dis Sci 1995;40:696–700.
161. Palazzo L, Roseau G, Gayet B et al. Endoscopy 1993;25:143–150.
162. Eloubeidi MA, Chen VK, Jhala NC et al. Clin Gastroenterol Hepatol 2004;2:209–213.
163. Fritscher-Ravens A, Broering DC, Knoefel WT et al. Am J Gastroenterol 2004;99:45–51.
164. Dewitt J, Ghorai S, Kahi C et al. Gastrointest Endosc 2003;58:542–548.
165. Binmoeller KF, Thul R, Rathod V et al. Gastrointest Endosc 1998;47:123–129.
166. Faigel DO, Ginsberg GG, Bentz JS et al. J Clin Oncol 1997;15:1439–1443.
167. Giovannini M, Seitz JF, Monges G et al. Endoscopy 1995;27:171–177.
168. Chang KJ, Nguyen P, Erickson RA et al. Gastrointest Endosc 1997;45:387–393.

169. Gress FG, Hawes RH, Savides TJ et al. Gastrointest Endosc 1997;45:243–250.
170. Suits J, Frazze R, Erickson RA et al. Arch Surg 1999;134:639–642.
171. Wiersema MJ, Vilmann P, Giovannini M et al. Gastroenterol 1997;112:1087–1095.
172. Bismuth H, Corlette MB. Surg Gynecol Obstet 1975;140:170–178.
173. Nordback IH, Coleman J, Venbrux AC et al. Surgery 1994;115:597–603.
174. Hintze RE, Abou-Rebyeh H, Adler A et al. Gastrointest Endosc 2001;53:40–46.
175. Chang WH, Kortan P, Harber GB. Gastrointest Endosc 1998;47:354–362.
176. De Palma GD, Galloro G, Siciliano S et al. Gastrointest Endosc 2001;53:547–553.
177. Nomura T, Shirai Y, Hatakeyama K. Dig Dis Sci 1999;44:542–546.
178. Freeman ML, Nelson DB, Sherman S et al. N Engl J Med 1996;335:909–918.
179. Deviere J, Motte S, Dumonceau JM et al. Endoscopy 1990;22:72–75.
180. Hochwald SN, Burke EC, Jarnagin WR et al. Arch Surg 1999;134:261–266.
181. Ducreux M, Liguory C, Lefebvre JF et al. Dig Dis Sci 1992;37:778–783.
182. Lammer J, Hausegger KA, Fluckiger F et al. Radiology 1996;201:167–172.
183. England RE, Martin DF. Cardiovasc Intervent Radiol 1996;19:381–387.
184. Zeman RK, Burell MI, Cahow CE et al. Am J Surg 1981;141:446–451.
185. Ralls PW, Colletti PM, Halls JM et al. Radiology 1982;144:369–371.
186. Freitas JE, Mirkes SH, Fink-Bennett DM et al. Clin Nucl Med 1982;8:363–367.
187. Samuels BI, Freitas JE, Bree RL et al. Radiology 1983;147:2017–2020.
188. Chatziioannou SN, Moore WH, Ford PV et al. Surgery 2000;127:6–9.
189. Weissmann HS, Berkowitz D, Fox MS et al. Radiology 1983;146:177–180.
190. Shuman WP, Rogers JV, Rudd TG et al. AJR Am J Roentgenol 1984;143:531–534.
191. Ramanna L, Brachman MB, Tanascescu DE et al. Am J Gastroenterol 1984;79:650–653.
192. Swayne LC. Radiology 1986;160:33–38.
193. Flancbaum L, Choban PS. Intensive Care Med 1995;21:120–124.
194. Kalliafas S, Ziegler DW, Flancbaum L et al. Am Surg 1998;64:471–475.
195. Palazzo L, Girollet PP, Salmeron M et al. Gastrointest Endosc 1995;42:225–231.
196. Kohut M, Nowakowska-Dulawa E, Marek T et al. Endoscopy 2002;34:299–303.
197. Shim CS, Joo JH, Park CW et al. Endoscopy 1995;27:428–432.
198. Amouyal P, Amouyal G, Levy P et al. Gastroenterology 1994;106:1062–1067.

34

Hepatic Disorders: Colorectal Cancer Metastases, Cirrhosis, and Hepatocellular Carcinoma

Brian C. Lucey, Jose C. Varghese, and Jorge A. Soto

Issues

I. How accurate is imaging in patients with suspected hepatic metastatic disease?
 A. Ultrasonography
 B. Computed tomography
 C. Magnetic resonance imaging
 D. Whole-body positron emission tomography
II. What is the accuracy of imaging in patients with cirrhosis for the detection of hepatocellular carcinoma?
 A. Ultrasonography
 B. Computed tomography
 C. Magnetic resonance imaging
 D. Whole-body positron emission tomography
III. What is the cost-effectiveness of imaging in patients with suspected hepatocellular carcinoma?

Key Points

- State-of-the-art magnetic resonance imaging (MRI) may be superior to state-of-the-art multidetector computed tomography (CT) for detection of liver metastases from colorectal cancer (insufficient and limited evidence).
- Fluorodeoxyglucose positron emission tomography (FDG-PET) is the most sensitive noninvasive test for detecting liver metastases (limited to moderate evidence).
- Periodic screening with imaging tests of patients with cirrhosis for early detection of hepatocellular carcinoma is beneficial (limited evidence).
- Magnetic resonance imaging may be superior to CT for detecting hepatocellular carcinoma (limited evidence).

B.C. Lucey (✉)
Department of Radiology, The Galway Clinic, Doughiski, County Galway, Ireland
e-mail: Brian.Lucey@galwayclinic.com

L.S. Medina et al. (eds.), *Evidence-Based Imaging: Improving the Quality of Imaging in Patient Care, Revised Edition,*
DOI 10.1007/978-1-4419-7777-9_34, © Springer Science+Business Media, LLC 2011

Definition and Pathophysiology

Liver Metastases

Hematogenous spread of tumor cells to the liver is a common problem in clinical practice. Although several explanations have been offered, this is likely the result of the dual blood supply through the hepatic artery and portal vein and the relatively common occurrence of primary malignancies of the gastrointestinal tract (such as colon, stomach, and pancreas), for which the liver serves as the first end-capillary bed and can therefore easily trap tumor cells or emboli that have escaped to the bloodstream. As metastases grow and reach a certain size threshold, they become detectable with imaging methods. Other tests that are commonly used to monitor patients with gastrointestinal malignancies and to identify patients who require further evaluation include measurement of serum carcinoembryonic antigen (CEA) and liver function tests. Unfortunately, the sensitivity of CEA assessments is low (50–60%) (1, 2) and its use in clinical practice is therefore limited. The decision regarding whether or not to perform an imaging test in a patient with possible liver metastases should also take into account the pretest probability of finding disease. An imaging test has the greatest impact when the pretest probability is intermediate (20–50%) (3). This means that patients with very low or very high likelihood of harboring metastases may not need any specific imaging test of the liver, if the indication is that of detecting possible lesions.

Cirrhosis and Hepatocellular Carcinoma

Cirrhosis is characterized by irreversible scarring of the liver that can lead to liver failure and death. Causes include excessive alcohol use, chronic viral hepatitis, including chronic hepatitis B (HBV) and hepatitis C (HCV), autoimmune disease, hemochromatosis, and drugs, among many others. These entities may result in inflammation of the liver, which may lead to fibrosis. Fibrosis results in the loss of liver parenchyma and impairs liver function. Cirrhosis is characterized by the formation of nodules within the liver. These nodules represent attempts by the liver to regenerate. These nodules may be large or small, resulting in macronodular or micronodular cirrhosis. These nodules may in turn undergo dysplasia and become dysplastic nodules that in turn may develop into hepatocellular carcinoma (HCC).

The pathophysiology of HCC is related to underlying liver dysfunction, and cirrhosis is a predisposing condition. In adults, infectious and autoimmune hepatitis, alcoholic cirrhosis, and hemochromatosis are strongly associated with HCC. Although children are less likely to have chronic liver disease, congenital liver disorders increase the chance of developing HCC. Hepatitis B carries a 100-fold increase in the risk for developing HCC. Hepatitis B is a DNA virus whose mechanism for tumor genesis involves integrating into the hosts DNA. The mechanism of tumor genesis with hepatitis C is less well defined, but is thought most likely to result from chronic inflammation. Although HCC is frequently indolent, it may undergo hemorrhage or necrosis. Vascular invasion, particularly of the portal veins, may occur. Invasion into the biliary system is less common. Occasionally, HCC may result in rupture and hemoperitoneum.

The annual risk of developing HCC among persons with cirrhosis is between 1 and 6%. Most patients with HCC die within 1 year after diagnosis. Survival is dependent on tumor size at the time of diagnosis and on associated diseases at the time of diagnosis. Patients with cirrhosis have a shorter survival. Surgical cure is possible in less than 5% of patients.

Despite the overall dismal prognosis of HCC, when diagnosed early it is a potentially curable cancer. Treatment is most likely to be successful when the number of foci of HCC in the cirrhotic liver and the size of the lesions is small. This implies that early detection is essential. Traditionally, either liver transplant or surgical resection has been the only treatment modality available to provide a cure for HCC. The results of surgery for HCC are poor and many patients with HCC and cirrhosis are not surgical candidates. More recently, with the advent of percutaneous treatment options including thermal therapy and alcohol injection, there is renewed interest in treating HCC in cirrhotic patients. These treatments show promise with success rates very much dependent on tumor size and number. With radiofrequency ablation (RFA), tumors less than 3 cm in size have an excellent chance of cure and tumors between 3 and 5 cm are often treated successfully. But RFA is less successful in attempting cure in tumors greater than 5 cm. The success rates are higher with smaller lesions and in patients with few lesions.

As a result of the close association between cirrhosis and HCC and the relative success of early treatment of HCC, enormous efforts are made to identify the early development of HCC in the cirrhosis population. Hematologic tests for HCC are limited to α-fetoprotein (AFP), a protein that may be elevated in patients with HCC. This is of limited value in the detection of HCC, with reported sensitivity for detection of HCC varying between 48 and 65% (4, 5). This leaves imaging as the test of choice for detecting the early development of HCC in patients with cirrhosis. As with the detection of hepatic metastatic disease, there are multiple imaging modalities available to detect HCC in the cirrhotic liver. These include sonography, CT, MRI, and PET. There is extensive literature available detailing the sensitivity and specificity of these imaging modalities for detecting HCC in cirrhotic patients. In evaluating these studies, direct comparison is often difficult given the wide differences in the study designs.

colorectal cancer. Several randomized studies have shown that aggressive therapy with wide resections of liver metastases from colorectal carcinoma leads to improved survival when compared to control groups receiving other forms of standard therapy. Not uncommonly, the liver is the only site of distant spread of the tumor in patients with colorectal carcinoma. Survival rates of up to 20–40% have been reported after wide resections of liver metastases from colorectal carcinoma (6–8). As imaging-guided interstitial therapies of liver tumors (including metastases), such as RFA, cryoablation, microwave ablation, and laser photocoagulation, increase in popularity, the need for accurate imaging of the liver will also increase. In a decision analysis study, Gazelle et al. (9) concluded that an aggressive approach with resection of six or sometimes more metastases from colorectal cancer has a positive impact in patient outcome, as measured by the dollar/quality-adjusted life year (QALY) index. Thus, in the patient with newly diagnosed colorectal carcinoma, a thorough evaluation of the liver to rule out metastases is mandatory prior to bowel resection with curative intent.

Epidemiology

Liver Metastases

In most cases, a liver metastasis is a poor prognostic sign and usually indicates incurable disease. One exception may be that of metastases from colorectal carcinoma. Colorectal cancer is the third most common cancer found in men and women in the USA. The American Cancer Society estimates that there were about 106,370 new cases of colon cancer and 40,570 new cases of rectal cancer in 2004 in the USA. Combined, they will cause about 56,730 deaths. The death rate from colorectal cancer has been going down for the past 15 years. One reason is that there are fewer cases. Also, they are being found earlier, and treatments have improved. The liver is a common site of metastatic spread of colorectal cancer, and therefore early detection of liver metastases is critical for guiding decisions regarding therapy.

Liver metastases develop in nearly 40% of patients who undergo "curative" resection for

Cirrhosis

Cirrhosis is the seventh leading cause of disease-related death in the USA. It is twice as common in men as in women. The disease kills approximately 25,000 people a year in the US and is the third most common cause of death in adults between the ages of 45 and 65.

HCC is relatively uncommon in the US. The reported prevalence is four cases per 100,000 population or 2% of all malignancies. Approximately 5,000–10,000 cases per year are seen. Worldwide, HCC is the fourth most common cancer. It is more common in Asia and Africa than in the US. The highest incidence of HCC is in Japan, and other high-incidence regions include sub-Saharan Africa. The incidence of HCC continues to rapidly increase in the US. These findings are consistent with a true increase in HCC and could be explained by consequences of HCV acquired earlier in life during the 1960s and 1970s. In the US, chronic hepatitis B and C account for about 30–40% of HCC.

Goals

In patients with colorectal cancer imaging studies are acquired periodically in order to detect development of recurrent disease and to assess tumor burden and response to therapy. In the cirrhotic patient, the main goal of imaging is detection of developing complications, the most important of which is HCC. Many imaging modalities currently available have been used for detecting liver metastases, with variable success. Regardless of the technique used, the ability to detect a focal space-occupying lesion in the liver depends on the size of the tumor, the spatial and contrast resolution of the imaging method, the difference in contrast and perfusion between the tumor and background liver parenchyma, and the adequacy of the method used for displaying the images after acquired (10). All these factors affect the performance parameters of the various imaging techniques. A test is useful if sensitivity remains high at an acceptable specificity level. In a meta-analysis that studied the detection rate of liver metastases from gastrointestinal malignancies with multiple modalities, Kinkel et al. (3) suggest that, in order to be useful in clinical practice, the minimum acceptable specificity of imaging methods in this context should be 85%. Lower specificities would lead to excessive and unnecessary interventions such as biopsies, excessive complementary imaging tests, and follow-up examinations. When assessing cost-effectiveness of the imaging methods, other factors need to be considered: availability, cost, risks (such as radiation and use of toxic contrast agents), and potential benefit of tumor detection (i.e., likelihood of achieving long-term remission or cure with appropriate therapy).

Overall Cost to Society

On an individual level, cirrhosis results in impaired quality of life and indirect costs involving decreased productivity and lost days from work. The Centers for Disease Control and Prevention conservatively estimates US expenditures in excess of $600 million annually on patients with HCC. In 2002, in the US, a total of 15,654 patients were discharged from hospitals with the diagnosis of HCC and 2,522 patients died in the hospital with HCC. The mean length of hospital stay was 7.2 days with a mean cost of $32,193. This resulted in a total cost of $501,998,078.

Methodology

We performed a search of the Medline/PubMed electronic database (National Library of Medicine, Bethesda, Maryland) using the following keywords: (1) *hepatic metastases*, (2) *colorectal cancer*, (3) *cirrhosis*, (4) *hepatocellular carcinoma*, (5) *CT, computed tomography*, (6) *MR, magnetic resonance*, (7) *US, ultrasonography*, and (8) *PET or PET/CT*. No time limits were applied for the searches, which were repeated several times up to September 23, 2004. Limits included English language, abstracts, and human subjects. A search of the National Guideline Clearinghouse at www.guideline.gov was also performed using the following keywords: *hepatic metastases, cirrhosis, hepatocellular carcinoma*, and *imaging*.

I. How Accurate Is Imaging in Patients with Suspected Hepatic Metastatic Disease?

Summary of Evidence: CT and MRI (MRI) are the most widely used techniques for evaluating the liver in the initial staging and follow-up of cancer patients. For detecting liver metastases, carefully performed CT and MRI studies with state-of-the-art equipment and interpretation by experienced radiologists afford similarly good results. Some studies showed a slight advantage for MRI (11, 12) (moderate evidence). Others, including a multi-institutional study of 365 patients (13) (moderate evidence), have not. CT is usually preferred because it is more widely available and because it is a well-established technique for surveying the extrahepatic abdominal organs and tissues (such as the peritoneum and lymph nodes). However, MRI has an advantage in the characterization of focal lesions. Thus, MRI is commonly used as a problem-solving tool or for initial staging of a tumor. It is also preferred for patients who cannot receive intravenous iodinated contrast material. Finally, concerns about the risk of radiation from repeated exposure to CT examinations make MRI a valuable alternative for children or young adults with malignancies. As mentioned previously, a comparison of the performance of CT vs. MRI for this and other indications needs to be reassessed periodically, considering the rapid evolution of both technologies and the increase in therapeutic options available.

Kinkel et al. (3) reviewed a total of 111 studies that included over 3,000 patients. At a specificity of at least 85%, the weighted sensitivities were ultrasonography (US) 55%, CT 72%, MRI 76%, and PET 90% (moderate evidence). These data, however, need to be validated in prospective trials before broad conclusions can be drawn. Intraoperative ultrasonography (IOUS) has higher sensitivity than transabdominal ultrasonography, CT, and MRI (14, 15). The role of FDG-PET and PET-CT will continue to expand, but cost constraints will limit their use to patients in whom the possible impact is greatest.

Supporting Evidence: The most widely used imaging techniques today include US, CT, MRI, and more recently, PET. There is extensive literature available regarding the relative merits and limitations of each of these modalities for detecting metastases of primary tumors from various organs. When analyzing the multiple studies published on this topic, several limitations are evident: insufficient definition of inclusion and exclusion criteria, incomplete reporting of methods used, and lack of a uniform standard of reference. Although the best standard of reference available is findings at laparotomy with bimanual palpation or IOUS, this was used as the gold standard in only a minority of studies (14, 16, 17). As indicated by van Erkel et al. (18), use of a suboptimal standard of reference results in underreporting of lesions and overestimation of detection rate. Another confounding factor is the varying method for reporting sensitivity numbers: per patient (detection of at least one lesion per patient) and per lesion (detection of all lesions per patient). Thus, it is important to continually scrutinize the results of all available current studies as evolving and improving technology can make results of prior studies redundant. Following is a review of the available data regarding the benefits and limitations of the various imaging techniques commonly used for evaluating the liver in patients with colorectal cancer and other gastrointestinal primary malignancies.

A. Ultrasonography

Ultrasonography has the advantage of being widely available throughout the world, inexpensive, and essentially risk-free. The reported sensitivity of US for detecting liver metastases varies between 60 and 90% (3). Unfortunately, many of the published studies were performed in the 1980s (19, 20) (limited evidence) and were largely limited to reporting sensitivity results on a per patient basis. More recently, the advent of US contrast agents has led several investigators to evaluate the use of US with current equipment. For detecting liver metastases, the sensitivity and specificity of US improve substantially with the addition of microbubble contrast agents. Microbubbles are essentially blood pool agents that augment the Doppler and harmonic US signal. In addition, some of these agents have a hepatosplenic specific late phase, which enables visualization of tumor foci in the liver that were otherwise undetectable (21). In a multicenter study, Albrecht et al. (22) found that the addition of a microbubble contrast agent increased the per patient sensitivity of US from 94 to 98% (not significant), while the per lesion sensitivity increased from 71 to 87% (highly significant, $p < .05$).

IOUS has higher sensitivity than transabdominal US, CT, and MRI (14, 15). Conlon et al. (14) compared MRI with IOUS in 80 patients with colorectal cancer metastases who underwent hepatic resection and found that IOUS findings added important information in 37 patients and changed the surgical approach in 14 patients. They concluded that IOUS provides valuable information prior to hepatic resection of colorectal cancer metastases.

B. Computed Tomography

Multiple factors pertaining to technique need to be considered when planning CT scans of patients with suspected metastatic disease and when examining reports that deal with this topic. The typical colorectal cancer metastasis is hypoattenuating and hypovascular relative to liver parenchyma. Thus, detectability is maximized by administering intravenous contrast material and by acquiring the CT images during the time of peak enhancement of the liver parenchyma. This typically occurs during the portal venous dominant phase, which occurs approximately 60–80 s after the initiation of contrast injection. Ideally, hepatic parenchyma attenuation should increase by at least 50 Hounsfield units after the administration of intravenous contrast material. The addition of images acquired prior to the administration of intravenous contrast material or in the arterial-dominant or delayed phases of contrast enhancement are not routinely necessary when the indication for the scan is suspected hypovascular metastases. These are necessary when evaluating the cirrhotic liver, when attempting to characterize a focal lesion, or when the primary tumor is one that is known to be associated with hypervascular metastases, such as neuroendocrine and carcinoid tumors, thyroid cancer, melanoma, breast cancer, or renal cell carcinoma (Fig. 34.1).

Although specific protocols vary among institutions, most use a total load of 37–50 g of iodine (23). Although as little as 30 g have been used, detection of hypovascular focal lesions may be limited with this approach (24). In the patient with colorectal cancer who is being scanned to decide among the several therapeutic options available, the risk of overlooking a potentially resectable small liver metastasis needs to be outweighed vs. the benefit of limiting the amount of contrast material injected.

In a carefully performed study, Valls et al. (25) used contrast-enhanced helical CT to detect liver metastases in 157 patients with colorectal carcinoma. Using intraoperative palpation and US as the standard of reference, helical CT correctly depicted 247 (85.2%) of 290 metastases and had a 96.1% positive predictive value (moderate evidence). Surgical resection of the liver metastases was attempted in 112 patients and the authors achieved a 4-year survival rate of 58.6%. In their study, all false-negative interpretations occurred in lesions less than 1.5 cm in diameter. Other studies that also used surgical findings and IOUS as the standard of reference found similar high sensitivity and specificity (16), for detecting lesions as small as 4 mm in diameter.

Although with the multirow detector helical CT (MDCT) scanners that are now available it is possible to acquire CT images in multiple phases after administration of intravenous contrast material, it has not been convincingly demonstrated that detection of hypovascular metastases such as those from colorectal carcinoma is improved significantly by scanning in any phase other than the peak portal venous phase (16, 26, 27). The advent of MDCT has also

brought about new paradigms related to CT technique. Although scanning with slice thickness of less than 1 mm and often with isotropic voxels is tempting, there is debate as to what is the limit in thickness that achieves the performance that is adequate for demonstrating small metastatic lesions in clinical practice. Some studies have shown that scanning with a slice thickness of less than 5 mm does not result in a significant improvement in sensitivity for detecting small lesions (28). Other investigators have obtained better results using thinner collimation (29). However, detection of even small lesions in the patient with cancer is important, since approximately 12% of lesions less than 1 cm in diameter will prove to be metastatic in nature (30). The possible added benefit of images acquired with isotropic voxels remains to be determined and will undoubtedly be the focus of multiple studies in the near future.

Another CT technique that continues to be used at some institutions is CT during arterial portography (CTAP). This is an invasive technique that requires catheterization of the superior mesenteric or splenic artery for direct injection of contrast into the territory drained by the portal vein. This direct delivery of contrast into the portomesenteric circulation achieves the greatest degree of hepatic parenchymal enhancement and maximizes lesion detection with CT, with a sensitivity that exceeds 90% (17, 31). The technique, however, is invasive and has a false-positive rate as high as 25% (17, 31). This has led to decreased enthusiasm for this technique and its replacement with noninvasive CT and MRI methods using state-of-the-art equipment (32, 33).

C. Magnetic Resonance Imaging

MRI of the liver for detecting metastases requires the acquisition of multiple sequences and administration of intravenous contrast material. Although the appearance of metastatic lesions on MRI is variable, the T1 and T2 relaxation times of metastases are prolonged relative to normal liver parenchyma. In general, this results in hypointensity on T1-weighted sequences and hyperintensity on T2-weighted images (Fig. 34.2). T2-weighted MRI is also useful for characterizing focal lesions and differentiating nonsolid benign lesions such as cysts and hemangiomas from metastases. In multiecho

T2-weighted scans, metastases become less intense when the echo time (TE) is increased from <120 to 160 ms or more. Conversely, cysts and hemangiomas typically remain hyperintense as the TE increases. For lesions with equivocal behavior, MRI can be used to measure the T2 value; the T2 of malignant tumors is approximately 90 ms, while that of hemangiomas and cysts exceeds 130 ms (34, 35). However, metastases with liquefactive necrosis or cystic neoplasms may remain hyperintense on heavily T2-weighted images. Metastases can have a perilesional halo of high signal, indicating viable tumor, or demonstrate a doughnut or target appearance (36, 37).

For detection of liver metastases, a three-phase technique after administration of gadolinium is recommended; these phases are the arterial-dominant phase, the portal venous phase, and the hepatic venous or interstitial phase. Similar to CT, the detection of colorectal cancer metastases using MRI is maximized during the portal venous phase. In this phase, the lesions typically appear hypointense relative to the enhanced liver parenchyma and may exhibit variable degrees of enhancement (Fig. 34.2). In addition to lesion detection, this protocol also allows characterization of coexisting nonmetastatic focal lesions. This is important for staging recently detected malignant tumors, and has implications in determining the type of therapy to be offered. The reported sensitivity of MRI using multiple combinations of the sequences available varies between 65 and 95% (3, 33, 38–41), with a mean of approximately 76% (3) (moderate evidence).

The administration of organ-specific contrast agents increases the lesion-to-liver contrast-to-noise ratio (CNR), thereby improving the conspicuity and detection rate of metastatic lesions. These include hepatobiliary agents such as mangafodipir trisodium (MnDPDP) (40) and gadobenate dimeglumine (Gd-BOPTA), and reticuloendothelial agents such as superparamagnetic iron oxide (SPIO) particles (41). The available data regarding the need for these liver-specific agents is controversial, with some studies showing improved results (17, 42) while others do not (3, 43, 44). In addition to a lack of consensus regarding the benefits associated with their use, these agents are generally considered costly and not widely available. Thus, a broad use of liver-specific contrast material for detecting liver metastases is not recommended at this time.

D. Whole-Body Positron Emission Tomography

Whole body PET performed with fluorine-18-fluorodeoxyglucose (18F-FDG) has also been used successfully for detecting extracolonic spread of colorectal carcinoma, including liver metastases. Although published studies have included small groups of patients, early results are encouraging, with sensitivity and specificity exceeding 80% (45, 46). Kinkel et al. (3) performed a meta-analysis study comparing the data available for detection of liver metastases from gastrointestinal tract neoplasms with non-invasive tests: US, CT, MRI, and PET. They reviewed a total of 111 studies that included over 3,000 patients. At a specificity of at least 85%, the weighted sensitivities were US 55%, CT 72%, MRI 76%, and PET 90%. The strength of these data is moderate and they need to be validated in randomized trials before broad conclusions can be drawn.

II. What Is the Accuracy of Imaging in Patients with Cirrhosis for the Detection of Hepatocellular Carcinoma?

Summary of Evidence: Screening for HCC in patients with cirrhosis is not easy. No one imaging modality dominates over the others. All imaging modalities have advantages and disadvantages with no one modality offering both high sensitivity and specificity. The results of these individual studies often depend on the date of the study. This is primarily because of the rapid change in technology available in all imaging modalities. A reasonable consensus for screening includes biannual measurement of the AFP level. Annual sonography is the imaging modality most commonly used, as it is cheap, portable, and most widely available. If the AFP value increases and the sonogram does not show evidence of an HCC, either CT or MRI should be performed.

Although MRI at present has marginally higher specificity than CT, the recent improvement in CT technology may change this soon (Fig. 34.3). Published sensitivities for MRI range from 48 to 87% (47–50). The CT sensitivities for these studies range from 47 to 71% without the use of computed tomography hepatic arteriography (CTHA) or CTAP. These reports conclude that MRI is certainly as sensitive and perhaps a little more so than CT. The use of SPIO has increased the sensitivity of MRI.

The sensitivity of sonography for detecting HCC has been reported between 59 and 90% (51–55), with lower sensitivity for smaller lesions (55). Ultrasound may also lead to a high percentage of false-positive studies. Overall, there is little evidence to support the use of PET imaging in the detection of HCC. The value of PET in this patient population lies in detecting distant metastases, and PET may be useful in monitoring the response to treatment.

Supporting Evidence

A. Ultrasonography

The 59–90% sensitivity of sonography cited above varies with lesion size, with the sensitivity for detecting lesions 2 cm or less approaching 60%, with larger lesions having higher sensitivity (55). The sensitivity for detecting HCC also depends on patient selection. Screening a population at risk for developing HCC (i.e., chronic hepatitis carriers) is often performed differently from screening a population with documented cirrhosis. As a result, lesions missed by sonography in cirrhotic patients may be picked up by CT or AFP measurement, thus masking the false-negative cases that may be attributable to sonography (52). One major difficulty with sonography in the detection of HCC is the high percentage of false-positive studies. This is particularly difficult in the cirrhotic patient population as the risk of developing HCC is higher and therefore any focal geographic area of heterogeneity is concerning for HCC. This may lead to frequent percutaneous biopsy to obtain a definitive diagnosis with the attendant morbidity and mortality. Despite the difficulties of sonography, given the widespread availability, portability, and safety of the modality, sonography remains the imaging modality of choice for screening for HCC in cirrhotic patients. The time interval between sonograms remains controversial. There is no consensus as to when to perform repeat imaging; however, authors have suggested that annual or biannual interval imaging with sonography is the most effective approach to detecting HCC.

There is great interest in the use of intravenous contrast agents for enhancing the value of sonography to detect and characterize liver lesions. There are many reports describing the value of these agents in patients with HCC (56–59). There is no doubt that these microbubbles demonstrate increased vascularity in HCC when used, increasing the color flow within HCC from 33 to 92% in one study (57); however, there is little published evidence to support the value of these agents in identifying HCC from degenerative nodules in patients with cirrhosis. Increased flow may be detected in other hepatic lesions also and not just in HCC after injection of the microbubbles. One potential use for the microbubbles is in the evaluation of patients following RFA. The results for contrast-enhanced sonography for detecting tumor recurrence post-RFA have been reported to be similar to those for CT (60).

B. Computed Tomography

Computed tomography has benefited even more than sonography from recent advances in technology. With the move from incremental CT to single-detector CT to multidetector CT, the ability to detect HCC in the cirrhotic liver has improved. This difference in technology is the most important consideration when attempting to compare the results of studies performed to evaluate CT in the detection of HCC. This improvement allows for thinner slice collimation and improved image quality. Another technical parameter to consider is the use of dual-phase imaging. The liver has a dual blood supply from both the hepatic artery and portal vein. In normal livers, approximately three quarters of the blood supply comes from the portal system. In contrast, HCC depends more on the hepatic artery for blood supply. Therefore, ideally, imaging to detect HCC should include images obtained in the hepatic arterial phase, usually commencing at 30 s after contrast administration. With the advent of multidetector CT, imaging in dual phase became possible and this improved detection of HCC.

When examining the reports available for detecting HCC in cirrhotic patients, it is important to differentiate between identifying patients with HCC and identifying lesions that represent HCC. This fact may change the sensitivity of an imaging modality greatly. The effect of this is clearly demonstrated in a study by Peterson et al. (61) evaluating patients pre-liver transplant for HCC, in which CT had a prospective sensitivity to detect patients with HCC of 59%. This fell to 37% when attempting to detect HCC on a lesion-by-lesion basis.

Reported sensitivity for detecting HCC by CT varies greatly. Most recent reports yield sensitivities between 68 and 88% (5, 62). These reports generally refer to the percentage of patients in whom an HCC is found. Figures for detecting individual lesions are much lower. The value of some of these reports is always in some doubt, however, given the previously described rapid change in CT technology today. In an effort to improve detection of HCC using CT, CTAP is occasionally used. This involves placing a catheter into the splenic or superior mesenteric artery and directly injecting contrast. CTHA has also been used, in which a catheter is placed directly into the hepatic artery. These techniques have yielded high sensitivities when used together. Makita et al. (63) found the sensitivity of CTAP alone to be 85.5%, CTHA alone to be 88.1%, and combined to be 95%. Specificity, however, suffers and the combined specificity reported by that group was only 54%. Similar findings have been reported by others (64, 65) with sensitivities ranging from 82 to 97%, although the high number of false-positive studies with these techniques leads most authors to conclude that they have minimal role in the evaluation for HCC in cirrhotic patients, particularly given the relatively invasive nature of the procedures.

C. Magnetic Resonance Imaging

The MRI sequences used in the evaluation of the cirrhotic liver are the same as those used for the detection of liver metastases. The use of intravenous gadolinium is required in all cases. As with CT, the difficulty with MRI lies in differentiating early HCC from dysplastic nodules. As nodules change from regenerative to dysplastic to malignant, the T1 signal characteristics become more hypointense and the T2 signal characteristics become more hyperintense. As one moves along this spectrum, the primary blood supply of the mass changes from predominantly portal to predominantly hepatic arterial. As a result, HCC generally

demonstrates early enhancement in the arterial phase following gadolinium injection. In the same manner as CT, MRI technology is advancing rapidly. Some of the difficulties with MRI include respiratory and peristalsis motion artifact. With newer, faster sequences, these are becoming less of a problem. This therefore leaves us to decide which imaging modality is best for detecting HCC in a cirrhotic liver.

There are many reports published using MRI to detect HCC and many of these compare directly with CT. The results of many of the studies performed in the 1990s are extremely variable. Sensitivity in these studies for MRI in detecting HCC lies between 44 and 75% (66–71). Although all these studies compared MRI with CT, the results of some support CT as the imaging modality of choice (66, 67), others support MRI as the imaging modality of choice (69, 71), and yet others suggest that the imaging modalities have equal capability in detecting HCC (68, 70), with one report stating that intraarterial CT is an improvement over both CT and MRI using intravenous contrast (68). The reasons for such discrepancy are multiple, but certainly the lack of consistency in study design contributes to the variability. The results also vary considerably depending on the size of the HCC identified.

The figures published comparing CT to MRI since 2000 make interesting reading. Although there is not yet a clear advantage of MRI over CT, more studies give MRI a slight edge over CT. Published sensitivities for MRI range from 48 to 87% (47–50). Sensitivities for CT in these studies range from 47 to 71% without the use of CTHA or CTAP. These reports conclude that MRI is certainly as sensitive and perhaps a little more so than CT. The use of SPIO has increased the sensitivity of MRI. Its use by Kwak et al. (50) when combined with gadolinium-enhanced imaging increased the sensitivity of MRI from 87 to 95%, which surpassed the sensitivity of CTHA and CTAP combined. Other authors have reported similar advantages of using SPIO (49, 72), including increased sensitivity compared to CT imaging.

D. Whole-Body Positron Emission Tomography

Although PET has been around as an imaging modality for many years, it is only recently that the modality has been used with any frequency in the clinical setting. The studies available for detecting HCC using PET are few in number and generally have few patients evaluated. Three studies looking directly at the value of PET imaging in HCC all had 20 or fewer patients (73–75). In these studies, the sensitivity of PET for detecting HCC was low, varying from 20 to 55%. Well-differentiated HCCs are not identified using PET imaging. Moderately differentiated or poorly differentiated HCC may be identified. Tumors greater than 5 cm and tumors associated with elevated AFP levels are also more likely to be identified using PET. One advantage to the use of PET imaging in patients with HCC is the ability to detect extrahepatic metastases. This is especially important in the workup of patients with cirrhosis for liver transplant. In a larger study evaluating PET in HCC with 91 patients (76), PET had a clinical impact on the management of 28% of patients. This included not only detecting unsuspected metastases but also monitoring the response to therapy. Several other studies have evaluated PET in detecting HCC in patients with hepatitis C and cirrhosis prior to transplant (77–79). These show poor sensitivity for PET ranging from 0 to 30%.

III. What Is the Cost-Effectiveness of Imaging in Patients with Suspected Hepatocellular Carcinoma?

Summary of Evidence: A study concluded that screening all patients with cirrhosis is of limited value given the high cost, and the benefit in terms of patient survival is poor. However, targeted screening in high-risk patients with HCC and imaging may yet be of value.

Supporting Evidence: There are a number of reports on the cost-effectiveness of screening for HCC. The results of some of these studies conclude that there is little value to be gained from screening (80–82). One such report by Bolondi et al. (80) evaluated 324 patients with cirrhosis for HCC using sonography and AFP every 6 months. In all, 1,800 sonographic examinations and AFP titrations were obtained at a cost of $219,600 per patient. The cost of

diagnosing each of the successfully treated HCC was $24,400. The authors concluded that screening all patients with cirrhosis is of limited value given the high cost, and the benefit in terms of patient survival is poor. Targeted screening may yet be of value according to this group. Two similar studies reach similar conclusions (81, 82). Sarasin et al. (81) compared screening patients with cirrhosis for HCC with imaging for HCC only when clinically suspected. The cost for each year of life gained ranged between $48,000 and $284,000 in the screening group. The cost of each year of life gained in the group with predicted cirrhosis-related survival rate above 80% at 5 years ranged between $26,000 and $55,000. This suggests that screening to identify asymptomatic tumors provides a negligible benefit in life expectancy, yet targeted screening may increase life expectancy by 3–9 months at a lower cost. A meta-analysis type study by Yuen and Lai (82) concluded that AFP with sonography remains the screening modality of choice given that they are convenient, accessible, and noninvasive. They also concluded that screening for HCC in countries with a low prevalence of HCC was not cost-effective, but targeted screening of high-risk patients in countries with a higher incidence of HCC makes screening for HCC more cost-effective.

As with the studies based purely on detection of HCC, there is little consensus on the most cost-effective imaging modality to use to detect HCC. While acknowledging that screening for HCC may not be cost-effective at all, if one is to perform imaging, which modality is most cost-effective is open to debate. In a retrospective study, Gambarin-Gelwan et al. (83) compared AFP with sonography and with CT. They found that sensitivity and specificity of sonography and CT were similar and that sonography was preferable given the lower cost. A similar study by Lin et al. (84) compared AFP and sonography annually, biannually, biannual AFP with annual sonography, and biannual AFP with annual CT. They found that biannual AFP with annual sonography gave the most QALY gain while still maintaining a cost-effectiveness ratio <$50,000 per QALY. In addition, they found the cost-effectiveness ratio of biannual AFP with annual CT to be $51,750 per QALY. This compares to the $33,083 per QALY for sonography. The authors suggest that CT screening may be becoming cost-effective. This is supported by other work that evaluated the cost-effectiveness of no screening, AFP alone, and imaging with sonography, CT, and MRI all performed in conjunction with AFP levels (85). This study was performed in a patient population with high risk for developing HCC as all patients had cirrhosis secondary to hepatitis C. The results found that compared to no screening, sonography had a cost of $26,689 per QALY; CT had a cost of $25,232 per QALY and MRI had a cost of $118,000 per QALY. These figures would certainly support the value of CT for screening; however, this study did involve the so-called targeted screening described by the previous authors.

Take Home Tables and Figure (Tables 34.1 and 34.2; Fig. 34.4)

Table 34.1-34.2 and Figs. 34.1–34.4 serve to highlight key recommendations and supporting evidence.

Table 34.1. Performance of various tests for diagnosis of liver metastases from colorectal cancer

Test	Sensitivity (%)	References	Strength of evidence
CT	71–91	(10, 16, 25, 27–29, 40, 86)	Moderate
MRI	72	(11, 12, 32, 38–40)	Moderate
MRI with organ-specific contrast	87–90	(17, 31, 33, 38, 40–44)	Moderate
US	54–77	(3, 19, 20)	Moderate
PET and PET/CT	88	(41, 45, 46)	Weak to moderate

Reprinted with kind permission of Springer Science+Business Media from Lucey BC, Varghese J, Soto JA. Hepatic disorders: colorectal cancer metastases, cirrhosis, and hepatocellular carcinoma. In Medina LS, Blackmore CC (eds.): *Evidence-Based Imaging: Optimizing Imaging in Patient Care.* New York: Springer Science+Business Media, 2006.

Table 34.2. Sensitivity of various imaging tests for detecting hepatocellular carcinoma

Imaging modality	Sensitivity (%)
US	59–90
US with intravenous contrast	92
CT	47–88
CTAP	85
CTHA	88
CTAP + CTHA	95
MRI	44–87
MRI + SPIO	95
PET	0–55
AFP	48–65

Reprinted with kind permission of Springer Science+Business Media from Lucey BC, Varghese J, Soto JA. Hepatic disorders: colorectal cancer metastases, cirrhosis, and hepatocellular carcinoma. In Medina LS, Blackmore CC (eds.): *Evidence-Based Imaging: Optimizing Imaging in Patient Care.* New York: Springer Science+Business Media, 2006.

AFP α-fetoprotein, *CTAP* CT during arterial portography, *CTHA* computed tomography hepatic arteriography, *SPIO* superparamagnetic iron oxide.

Table 34.3. Liver magnetic resonance imaging for detection of metastases or hepatocellular carcinoma (minimum sequences)

Sequence	TR	TE	Flip angle	Slice thickness (mm)	Matrix	Fat suppression	Breath hold
T1 gradient-echo axial in and out of phase	200	4.6/2.3	80	7	192 × 256	No	Yes
T2 dual echo, fast spin-echo	2,350	40/140	90	6	256 × 512	Yes	No, respiratory triggered
Precontrast T1 fat-suppressed gradient-echo	200	4.6	80	7	192 × 256	Yes	Yes
Dynamic gadolinium 20cc IV	3.5	1.7	10	2	192 × 256	Yes	Yes
Precontrast T1 fat-suppressed gradient-echo	200	4.6	80	7	192 × 256	Yes	Yes

Reprinted with kind permission of Springer Science+Business Media from Lucey BC, Varghese J, Soto JA. Hepatic disorders: colorectal cancer metastases, cirrhosis, and hepatocellular carcinoma. In Medina LS, Blackmore CC (eds.): *Evidence-Based Imaging: Optimizing Imaging in Patient Care.* New York: Springer Science+Business Media, 2006.

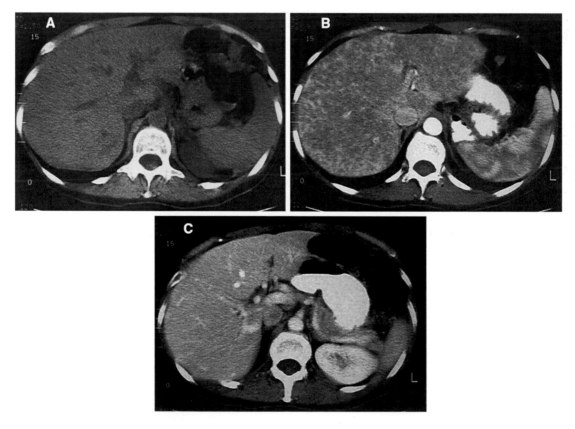

Figure 34.1. Importance of adequate technique for detecting computed tomography (CT) of metastatic disease to the liver. Noncontrast (**A**), arterial phase (**B**), and portal venous phase (**C**) CT images of a 57-year-old patient with breast cancer and abnormal results of liver function tests. There are multiple foci of hypervascular metastatic deposits seen exclusively in the arterial phase image (B). The appearance of the liver is near normal on the noncontrast (**A**) and portal venous phase (**C**) images. (Reprinted with kind permission of Springer Science+Business Media from Lucey BC, Varghese J, Soto JA. Hepatic disorders: colorectal cancer metastases, cirrhosis, and hepatocellular carcinoma. In Medina LS, Blackmore CC (eds.): *Evidence-Based Imaging: Optimizing Imaging in Patient Care.* New York: Springer Science+Business Media, 2006.)

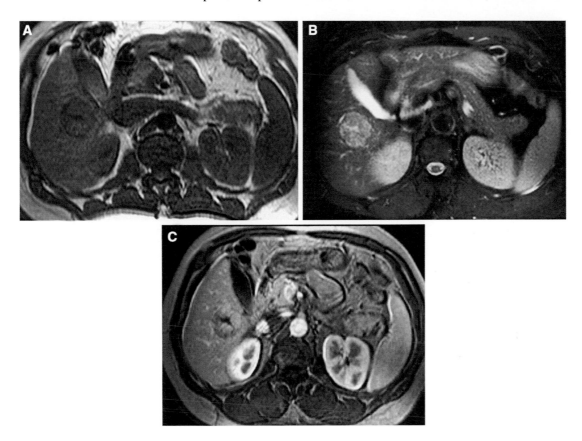

Figure 34.2. Typical appearance of hepatic metastasis on magnetic resonance imaging (MRI). T1-weighted (**A**), T2-weighted (**B**), and late arterial phase (**C**) MRI acquired in a patient with known colon cancer demonstrate a large metastatic deposit in the right hepatic lobe. The lesion is hypointense (relative to liver parenchyma) on the T1-weighted image, slightly hyperintense on the T2-weighted image, and demonstrates moderate enhancement after administration of gadolinium-DTPA. (Reprinted with kind permission of Springer Science+Business Media from Lucey BC, Varghese J, Soto JA. Hepatic disorders: colorectal cancer metastases, cirrhosis, and hepatocellular carcinoma. In Medina LS, Blackmore CC (eds.): *Evidence-Based Imaging: Optimizing Imaging in Patient Care.* New York: Springer Science+Business Media, 2006.)

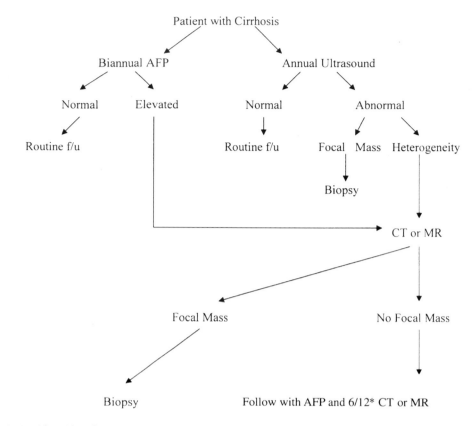

Figure 34.3. Algorithm for imaging to detect HCC in a patient with cirrhosis. *AFP* α-fetoprotein, *f/u* follow-up. *6/12 means 6 months. (Reprinted with kind permission of Springer Science+Business Media from Lucey BC, Varghese J, Soto JA. Hepatic disorders: colorectal cancer metastases, cirrhosis, and hepatocellular carcinoma. In Medina LS, Blackmore CC (eds.): *Evidence-Based Imaging: Optimizing Imaging in Patient Care.* New York: Springer Science+Business Media, 2006.)

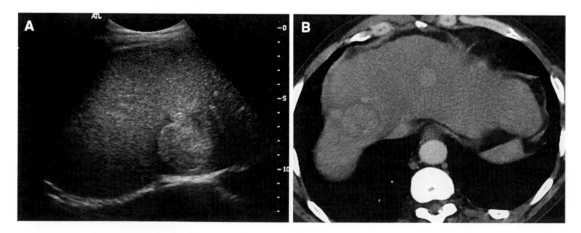

Figure 34.4. (**A**) Sonographic image showing large hyperechoic mass in the liver in a 67-year-old man with chronic hepatitis C. (**B**) CT image showing arterial enhancement of multiple masses, which proved to be hepatocellular carcinoma (HCC) following biopsy. (Reprinted with kind permission of Springer Science+Business Media from Lucey BC, Varghese J, Soto JA. Hepatic disorders: colorectal cancer metastases, cirrhosis, and hepatocellular carcinoma. In Medina LS, Blackmore CC (eds.): *Evidence-Based Imaging: Optimizing Imaging in Patient Care.* New York: Springer Science+Business Media, 2006.)

Imaging Technique Protocols

Abdominal Computed Tomography for Detection of Hepatocellular Carcinoma Using Multirow Detector Computed Tomography

Slice thickness: 2–3 mm

Scan parameters: 120–140 kVp; 180–220 mAs

Number of acquisitions: 3

Area of coverage first acquisition: top of diaphragm through the liver

Area of coverage second acquisition: top of diaphragm to inferior pubic ramus

Area of coverage third acquisition: top of diaphragm to inferior pubic ramus

Breath hold: full inspiration or full expiration

Reconstruction algorithm: standard

Oral contrast: 800 cc 2 h prior to imaging

Intravenous (IV) contrast: first acquisition performed without IV contrast; second acquisition 120–150 cc nonionic contrast injected at 3–4 cc/s; 30-s prescan delay; third acquisition obtained with a 60-s delay

Liver MRI for Detection of Metastases or Hepatocellular Carcinoma (Minimum Sequences)

See Table 34.3.

Future Research

1. A randomized, multicenter, trial comparing the performance of state-of-the-art CT, MRI and PET-CT for detecting colorectal cancer metastases is highly desirable at this time.
2. Need to develop an imaging modality that will differentiate dysplastic nodules from HCC.
3. Need to identify HCC earlier. Study design similar to the one shown for colorectal cancer metastases above is recommended – relates to 1 in this listing.

4. The role of PET and PET-CT in these populations of patients should continue to be explored.
5. Molecular imaging and tagging HCC cells will be the future of screening; CT and MRI are operating at the limits of their sensitivity and specificity.

References

1. Ohlsson B, Tranberg KG, Lundstedt C, Ekberg H, Helderestrom E. Eur J Surg 1993;159:275–281.
2. Moertel CG, Fleming TR, Macdonald JS, Haller DG, Laurie JA, Tangen C. JAMA 1993;270: 943–947.
3. Kinkel K, Lu Y, Both M, Warren RS, Thoeni RF. Radiology 2002;224:748–756.
4. Maringhini A, Cottone M, Sciarrino E et al. Dig Dis Sci 1988;33(1):47–51.
5. Chalasani N, Horlander JC Sr, Said A et al. Am J Gastroenterol 1999;94(10):2988–2993.
6. Scheele J, Stang R, Altendorf-Hofmann A, Paul M. World J Surg 1995;19:1959–1971.
7. Fong Y, Cohen AM, Fortner JG et al. J Clin Oncol 1997;15:938–946.
8. Fusai G, Davidson BR. Colorectal Dis 2003;5: 2–23.
9. Gazelle GS, Hunin MG, Kuntz KM et al. Ann Surg 2003;237:544–555.
10. Pijl MEJ, Wasser MNJM, Joekes EC, van de Velde CJH, Bloem JL. Radiology 2003;227:747–751.
11. Semelka RC, Shoenut JP, Asher SM et al. J Magn Reson Imaging 1994;4:319–323.
12. Semelka RC, Worawattanakul S, Kelekis NL et al. J Magn Reson Imaging 1997;7:1040–1047.
13. Zerhouni EA, Rutter C, Hamilton SR et al. Radiology 1996;200:443–451.
14. Conlon R, Jacobs M, Dasgupta D, Lodge JP. Eur J Ultrasound 2003;6:211–216.
15. Hartley JE, Kumar H, Drew PJ et al. Dis Colon Rectum 2000;43:320–324.
16. Soyer P, Poccard M, Boudiaf M et al. Radiology 2004;231:413–420.
17. Strotzer M, Gmeinwieser J, Schmidt J et al. Acta Radiol 1997;38:986–992.
18. van Erkel AR, Pijl MEJ, van den Berg-Husymans AA, Wasser MNJM, van de Velde CJH, Bloem JL. Radiology 2002;224:4040–4094.
19. Tempero MA, Williams CA, Anderson JC. J Clin Oncol 1986;4:1074–1078.
20. Grace RH, Hale M, Mackie G, Marks CG, Bloomberg TJ, Walker WJ. Br J Surg 1987;74:480–481.

21. Hohmann J, Albrecht T, Oldenburg A, Skrok J, Wolf KJ. Abdom Imaging 2004;29:669–681.
22. Albrecht T, Blomkey MJK, Burns PN et al. Radiology 2003;227:361–370.
23. Silverman PM, Kohan L, Ducic I. AJR Am J Roentgenol 1998;170:149–152.
24. Freeny PC, Gardner JC, von Ingersleben G, Heyano S, Nghiem HV, Winter TC. Radiology 1995;197:89–93.
25. Valls C, Andia E, Sanchez A et al. Radiology 2001;218:55–60.
26. Miller FH, Butler RS, Hoff FL, Fitzgerald SW, Nemcek AA, Gore RM. AJR Am J Roentgenol 1998;171:643–649.
27. Scott DJ, Guthrie JA, Arnold P et al. Clin Radiol 2001;56:235–242.
28. Haider MA, Amitai MM, Rappaport DC. Radiology 2002;225:137–142.
29. Weg N, Scheer MR, Gabor MP. Radiology 1998;209:417–426.
30. Schwartz LH, Gandras EJ, Colangelo SM, Ercolani MC, Panicek DM. Radiology 1999;210:71–74.
31. Soyer P, Levesque M, Caudron C, Elias D, Zeitoun G, Roche A. J Comput Assist Tomogr 1993;17:67–74.
32. Kondo H, Kanematsu M, Hoshi H et al. AJR Am J Roentgenol 2000;174:947–954.
33. Seneterre E, Taourel P, Bouvier Y et al. Radiology 1996;200:785–792.
34. McFarland EG, Mayo SW, Saini S, Hahn PF, Goldberg MA, Lee MJ. Radiology 1994;193:43–47.
35. Tello R, Fenlon HM, Gagliano T, de Carvalho VLS, Yucel EK. AJR Am J Roentgenol 2001;176:870–884.
36. Wittenberg J, Stark DD, Forman BH et al. AJR Am J Roentgenol 1988;151:79–84.
37. Outwater E, Tomaszewski JE, Daly JM, Kressel HY. Radiology 1991;180:327–332.
38. Yamashita Y, Tank Y, Namimoto T, Mitsuzaki K, Takahashi M. Radiology 1998;207:331–337.
39. Kanematsu M, Hoshi H, Murakami T et al. Radiology 1999;211:363–371.
40. Bartolozzi C, Donati F, Cioni D et al. Eur Radiol 2004;14:14–20.
41. Vogl TJ, Schwarz W, Blume S et al. Eur Radiol 2003;13:262–272.
42. Ward J, Naik KS, Guthrie JA, Wilson D, Robinson PJ. Radiology 1999;210:459–466.
43. Said B, McCart JA, Libutti SK, Choyke PL. Magn Reson Imaging 2000;18:305–309.
44. Matsuo M, Kanematsu M, Itoh K et al. AJR Am J Roentgenol 2001;177:637–643.
45. Kantorova I, Lipska L, Belohlavek O, Visokai V, Trubac M, Schneiderova M. J Nucl Med 2003;44:1784–1788.
46. Abdel-Nabi H, Doerr RJ, Lamonica DM et al. Radiology 1998;206:755–760.
47. Noguchi Y, Murakami T, Kim T et al. J Comput Assist Tomogr 2002;26(6):981–987.
48. Noguchi Y, Murakami T, Kim T et al. AJR Am J Roentgenol 2003;180(2):455–460.
49. Hori M, Murakami T, Kim T et al. J Comput Assist Tomogr 2002;26(5):701–710.
50. Kwak HS, Lee JM, Kim CS. Eur Radiol 2004;14(3):447–457.
51. Shinagawa T, Ohto M, Kimura K et al. Gastroenterology 1984;86(3):495–502.
52. Okazaki N, Yoshida T, Yoshino M, Matue H. Clin Oncol 1984;10(3):241–246.
53. Ikeda K, Saitoh S, Koida I et al. Hepatology 1994;20(1 pt 1):82–87.
54. Tanaka S, Kitamura T, Ohshima A et al. Cancer 1986;58(2):344–347.
55. Okano H, Shiraki K, Inoue H et al. Anticancer Res 2001;21(4B):2979–2982.
56. Angeli E, Carpanelli R, Crespi G, Zanello A, Sironi S, Del Maschio A. Radiol Med (Torino) 1994;87(5 suppl 1):24–31.
57. Maruyama H, Matsutani S, Sato G et al. Abdom Imaging 2000;25(2):164–171.
58. Khong PL, Chau MT, Fan ST, Leong LL. Australas Radiol 1999;43(2):156–159.
59. Choi BI, Kim AY, Lee JY et al. J Ultrasound Med 2002;21(1):77–84.
60. Shimizu M, Iijima H, Horibe T et al. Hepatol Res 2004;29(4):235–242.
61. Peterson MS, Baron RL, Marsh JW Jr, Oliver JH 3rd, Confer SR, Hunt LE. Radiology 2000;217(3):743–749.
62. Bhattacharjya S, Bhattacharjya T, Quaglia A et al. Dig Surg 2004;21(2):152–159.
63. Makita O, Yamashita Y, Arakawa A et al. Acta Radiol 2000;41(5):464–469.
64. Matsuo M, Kanematsu M, Inaba Y et al. Clin Radiol 2001;56(2):138–145.
65. Jang HJ, Lim JH, Lee SJ, Park CK, Park HS, Do YS. Radiology 2000;215(2):373–380.
66. Hori M, Murakami T, Oi H et al. Acta Radiol 1998;39(2):144–151.
67. Kanematsu M, Hoshi H, Murakami T et al. AJR Am J Roentgenol 1997;169(6):1507–1515.
68. Murakami T, Kim T, Oi H et al. Acta Radiol 1995;36(4):372–376.
69. Oi H, Murakami T, Kim T, Matsushita M, Kishimoto H, Nakamura H. AJR Am J Roentgenol 1996;166(2):369–374.
70. Kim T, Murakami T, Oi H et al. J Comput Assist Tomogr 1995;19(6):948–954.
71. Yamashita Y, Mitsuzaki K, Yi T et al. Radiology 1996;200(1):79–84.
72. Lee JM, Kim IH, Kwak HS, Youk JH, Han YM, Kim CS. Korean J Radiol 2003;4(1):1–8.
73. Trojan J, Schroeder O, Raedle J et al. Am J Gastroenterol 1999;94(11):3314–3319.
74. Khan MA, Combs CS, Brunt EM et al. J Hepatol 2000;32(5):792–797.

75. Verhoef C, Valkema R, de Man RA, Krenning EP, Yzermans JN. Liver 2002;22(1):51–56.

76. Wudel LJ Jr, Delbeke D, Morris D et al. Am Surg 2003;69(2):117–124.

77. Liangpunsakul S, Agarwal D, Horlander JC, Kieff B, Chalasani N. Transplant Proc 2003; 35(8):2995–2997.

78. Schroder O, Trojan J, Zeuzem S, Baum RP. Nuklearmedizin 1998;37(8):279–285.

79. Teefey SA, Hildeboldt CC, Dehdashti F et al. Radiology 2003;226(2):533–542.

80. Bolondi L, Gaiani S, Casali A, Serra C, Piscaglia F. Radiol Med (Torino) 1997;94(1–2):4–7.

81. Sarasin FP, Giostra E, Hadengue A. Am J Med 1996;101(4):422–434.

82. Yuen MF, Lai CL. Ann Oncol 2003;14(10): 1463–1467.

83. Gambarin-Gelwan M, Wolf DC, Shapiro R, Schwartz ME, Min AD. Am J Gastroenterol 2000;95(6):1535–1538.

84. Lin OS, Keeffe EB, Sanders GD, Owens DK. Aliment Pharmacol Ther 2004;19(11):1159–1172.

85. Arguedas MR, Chen VK, Eloubeidi MA, Fallon MB. Am J Gastroenterol 2003;98(3):679–690.

86. Lopez Hanninen E, Vogl TJ, Felfe R et al. Radiology 2000;216:403–409.

35

Imaging of Inflammatory Bowel Disease in Children

Sudha A. Anupindi, Rama Ayyala, Judith Kelsen, Petar Mamula, and Kimberly E. Applegate

Issues

I. What are the important clinical predictors of IBD?
II. What is the diagnostic performance of current endoscopic techniques in the evaluation of patients with IBD: Lower, upper endoscopies and WCE?
III. What Is the diagnostic performance of current imaging modalities in evaluating IBD of the small bowel (small bowel follow-through, CT, MR, US, enteroclysis)?
IV. Complications of IBD (intra abdominal abscess, intestinal fistulae, strictures and small bowel obstruction, primary sclerosing cholangitis): Which imaging should be performed and what is its diagnostic performance?
V. What Are the most important imaging features that lead to surgery in a child with crohn's disease and ulcerative colitis?
VI. What are the role and risk of repeat imaging in monitoring IBD response to treatment?
VII. Special situation: Which imaging modality provides the best performance for the evaluation of perianal/perirectal disease in Crohn's disease?

Key Points

- Children with clinically suspected IBD should have both upper and lower endoscopies as part of the initial workup (strong evidence). Fluoroscopic small bowel follow-through (SBFT) studies are typically performed as part of the initial diagnosis (limited evidence).
- Wireless capsule endoscopy (WCE) is a safe, moderately sensitive test for the detection of small bowel inflammatory changes and should be utilized in patients without small bowel obstruction and when other

S.A. Anupindi (✉)
Department of Radiology, The Children's Hospital of Philadelphia, University of Pennsylvania School of Medicine, 3rd Fl Main, 34th Str & Civic Center Blvd, Philadelphia, PA 19104, USA
e-mail: anupindi@email.chop.edu

L.S. Medina et al. (eds.), *Evidence-Based Imaging: Improving the Quality of Imaging in Patient Care, Revised Edition*, DOI 10.1007/978-1-4419-7777-9_35, © Springer Science+Business Media, LLC 2011

diagnostic small bowel exams are negative. However, the specificity and positive predictive value need to be further established (limited evidence).

■ MRI is superior to CT and is the preferred initial diagnostic and follow-up imaging exam of perirectal and perianal disease in Crohn's disease (CD) patients (moderate–strong evidence).

■ About 70–80% of CD patients and 30–40% of UC patients will require surgery for disease refractory to medical therapy, or severe disease with complications, or risk of malignancy (UC) (moderate evidence).

■ Repeat imaging with SBFT and CT results in significant ionizing radiation exposure and risk of later cancer induction so that alternative imaging methods, MRI and US, should be used (limited evidence).

Definition and Pathophysiology

Inflammatory bowel disease (IBD), comprised of the well-recognized CD and ulcerative colitis (UC), is one of the most serious, chronic gastrointestinal (GI) conditions affecting the growth, social well-being, and education in children worldwide. The pathogenesis is not completely understood; however, the general accepted hypothesis is that IBD occurs as the result of an inappropriate and exaggerated mucosal immune response to common environmental antigens including commensal microflora in a genetically susceptible host. Up to 25% of children with IBD will have a primary degree relative with this diagnosis. Generally both conditions result in suppurative inflammation of the bowel that results in abdominal pain, diarrhea (sometimes bloody), weight loss, and growth disturbance.

Ulcerative colitis is a diffuse chronic mucosal inflammation of the mucosa that is limited to the colon and invariably affects the rectum in an uninterrupted fashion, although 5% of UC patients have backwash ileitis. In contrast, CD features segmental transmural inflammation and fibrosis involving the entire GI tract. In 10% of cases a third entity termed "indeterminate colitis" (IC) is used when a firm diagnosis of CD or UC cannot be made. Although the etiology for IBD is not clear, some risk factors include first-degree relatives, smoking, NSAIDs, oral contraceptives. Several infectious agents that have been proposed as causative agents although with great controversy include *Listeria monocytogenes*, *Chlamydia trachomatis*, *Escherichia coli*, Cytomegalovirus, *Saccharomyces cerevisiae*, and *Mycobacterium avium paratuberculosis* (1, 2).

Epidemiology and Diagnosis

In the pediatric population, defined as ages 1–17, the incidence of IBD in North America is approximately 2/100,000 for UC and 4.5/100,000 for CD (1). The US prevalence of CD and UC combined is estimated to be 400 cases per 100,000 persons and these numbers are on the rise (2). Twenty-five percent of all IBD presents in the pediatric age group. The peak age of onset is in the adolescent years, with 4% of pediatric IBD cases occurring before the age of 5 years and 20% before the age of 10 years (3). While IBD incidence is equal in males and females, it occurs more commonly in the developed world and, in urban compared to rural areas, is higher in Caucasians, followed by African Americans and occurs less commonly in Asians and Hispanics.

One million Americans have IBD. There is a higher predisposition of IBD in northern latitudes than southern latitudes. Worldwide the incidence of IBD is increasing. There is minimal emerging data from Asia, Pacific regions, and South America; however, the incidence in these regions is not as great as that in North America or Europe. The current descriptive data are derived from European (Scotland and Sweden) and North American cohorts (4).

No single test can diagnose IBD. Patients presenting with signs and symptoms that suggest IBD, such as bloody or non-bloody diarrhea, or weight loss need to be evaluated with supportive laboratory testing, such as hemoglobin, albumin, inflammatory markers such as erythrocyte sedimentation rate (ESR) and C-reactive protein (CRP), stool cultures, radiographic studies, and endoscopy. Patients may appear ill on physical exam with some findings including pallor secondary to anemia, and pharyngeal aphthous lesions. The abdominal exam may be normal, nonspecific, or have "fullness" in right lower quadrant, indicating inflamed terminal ileum (TI) or thickened bowel. On perianal and rectal exam, the frequency of the findings of perianal/perirectal skin tags, fissures, and fistulae is 2–4.5% in newly diagnosed CD patients (1). Upper endoscopy, colonoscopy with biopsies, and radiologic studies are performed for confirmation of diagnosis. The differentiating features at biopsy are listed in Table 35.1.

Overall Cost to Society

A review of the current literature reveals that the overall cost burden of CD to society is quite high and a substantial portion of the direct costs is attributed to hospitalizations. There are several cost-effective analyses evaluating the overall cost to society regarding hospitalization and treatment (i.e., surgery), as well as loss of time from school and work. However, no cost-effectiveness data were found in the literature specifically incorporating imaging strategies in the evaluation and management of IBD. The total economic burden of CD in the United States is estimated to be between $10.9 and $15.5 billion (5). The estimated cost per patient with CD in the United States is close to $18,000–19,000 annually (5). The severity of the disease is directly proportional to the cost by as much as three- to ninefold, higher in children with severe disease than those with mild disease. Data from 1990 reported a total annual medical cost for patients with UC in the United States as approximately $0.4–0.6 billion (6). In keeping with annual inflation and rising medical costs this estimate is much higher today. Only a single study assessed the economic costs of different diagnostic exams including imaging studies but the focus was primarily on capsule endoscopy (7). Imaging costs are barely mentioned separately in the reviewed citations, but it is presumed that it is a significant portion of the costs, as imaging is widely used to help determine medical versus surgical treatment (2, 8, 9) (limited evidence).

Goals

The diagnosis of IBD encompasses use of clinical, tissue diagnosis, and imaging. The goals of imaging in IBD are to primarily determine the extent of small bowel involvement, assess complications, and help determine patients who are candidates for surgery. Using conventional endoscopic techniques (with the exception of emerging capsule endoscopy), the small bowel is difficult to assess and therefore imaging is relied upon. Imaging plays a key role in assessing complications such as abscesses, fistulae, strictures, and obstruction, which would require intervention. Patients with CD who present with acute exacerbations resulting in hospitalizations often require CT and MR imaging to evaluate the current status of disease and possible complications. These imaging techniques are used to help determine who might benefit from surgery.

Methodology

The authors performed a MEDLINE search using PubMed (National Library of Medicine, Bethesda, MD) for data relevant to the diagnostic performance and accuracy of both clinical and imaging examinations of patients with IBD. The cost analysis of diagnosis, treatment, and imaging strategies of IBD was searched on MEDLINE (National Library of Medicine, Bethesda, MD) using the following search criteria for the period 1990–2008: (1) *Inflammatory bowel disease*; (2) *diagnosis*; (3) *treatment*; (4) *health economics*; (5) *hospital costs*; (6) *imaging costs*. The diagnostic performance of the clinical examination (history and physical exam) and the surgical outcome were based on a systematic literature review performed in MEDLINE (National Library of Medicine, Bethesda, MD) during the years 1990–2008. The clinical examination search strategy used the following statements: (1) *Inflammatory bowel disease*; (2) *Crohn's disease*; (3) *ulcerative colitis*; (4) *pediatric*; (5) *children*;

(6) *epidemiology* or *physical examination* or *endoscopy* or *colonoscopy* or *capsule endoscopy*; (7) *treatment* or *surgery*. The review of the current diagnostic imaging literature was done with MEDLINE covering the years 1990 to September 2008. The search strategy used the following key statements and words: (1) *Inflammatory bowel disease*, (2) *Crohn's disease*, (3) *ulcerative colitis*, (4) *MRI* or *magnetic resonance imaging*, (5) *computed tomography* or *CT*, (6) *ultrasound*, (7) *PET imaging*, (8) *imaging*, as well as combinations of these searches. We excluded animal studies and non-English articles.

I. What Are the Important Clinical Predictors of IBD?

Summary of Evidence: The clinical signs and symptoms of IBD, although variable between UC and CD, most commonly include abdominal pain, diarrhea, weight loss, fever, hematochezia (in UC), and growth failure (10). These are the most common predictive signs and symptoms occurring in more than 90% of the cases (moderate evidence).

Routine blood and inflammatory markers including, but not limited to, cell blood count, ESR, and CRP are sensitive but not specific for IBD; however, serologic antibody studies such as perinuclear antineutrophil cytoplasm antibodies (pANCA) and anti-*S. cerevisiae* antibodies (ASCA-IgA and IgG) have a high degree of specificity (10, 11).The sensitivity and specificity of ASCA has been estimated as 37 and 97%, respectively, for the diagnosis of CD, whereas for the diagnosis of UC, the sensitivity and specificity of pANCA has been reported as 55 and 89% (10) (moderate evidence). When history, physical, and laboratory studies suggest ongoing symptoms not explained by infection, endoscopy is needed to diagnose (11) (strong evidence).

Supportive Evidence: IBD peak incidence is between 15 and 35 years. A delay in diagnosis is common and can be between 5 months and 2 years. Growth failure in children is identified in 10–40% of patients with IBD at presentation and is more common in CD. Atypical presentations occur in 10–20% of patients. Approximately 4% of IBD patients present with arthritis, usually pauciarticular and involving the large joints. Younger children are more likely to have atypical clinical presentations. In addition, 10% of patients with CD may initially present with perianal abscesses or fistulae or unusual dermatological manifestations such as erythema nodosum or pyoderma gangrenosum (12).

Laboratory Markers

There is also variability in the biological laboratory markers in children with IBD. There is usually an increased concentration of CRP, ESR, fecal calprotectin (FC) and a low albumin, anemia, and neutrophil leukocytosis (13). Certain autoantibodies such as pANCA and ASCA are abnormal in IBD, but the utility of these markers to diagnose IBD is limited by low sensitivity (10). The pANCA is detected in 50–80% of UC patients and 10–40% of CD patients while ASCA is detected in 46–70% of CD patients and only 6–12% of UC patients (11) (moderate evidence). These markers are useful to predict the risk of stricture or perforation and to distinguish Crohn's from UC patients since UC patients more often will have elevated levels of pANCA whereas Crohn's patients are more likely to have ASCA elevated (14). Canani and colleagues showed that if the values of FC, ANCA/pANCA, and bowel US were all negative, the probability of having IBD was 0.69%. If the laboratory exams described above were normal, this was a good negative predictive value for IBD (10, 11, 15, 16) (moderate evidence).

Children Under Age 5 Years

In a large analysis by Heyman et al. IBD specific symptoms were seen in 3% (37/1,370 patients) of children less than 1 year of age (17). The serologic markers were poor indicators of disease in younger children than in older children (18). Growth failure, as a presenting symptom, is more common in children with CD than UC or IC ($p = 0.004$). It has been estimated that 5% of fever of unknown origin in children is due to IBD (18). Chronic fever is associated with CD but not with UC and vomiting has been associated with CD but not with UC in children less than 5 years old (18) (strong evidence).

II. What Is the Diagnostic Performance of Current Endoscopic Techniques in the Evaluation of Patients with IBD: Lower, Upper Endoscopies and WCE?

Summary of Evidence: Lower and upper endoscopic techniques are the primary tests used to diagnose or exclude IBD (moderate to strong evidence). WCE, a newer technique, used to evaluate small bowel disease, has a high diagnostic yield compared to other modalities (limited evidence).

Colonoscopy with ileoscopy, defined as TI intubation, should be performed in the initial workup of IBD (strong evidence). This technique is the preferred way to both visualize mucosa and biopsy the colon and TI for diagnosis. Between 60 and 80% of the colonoscopies will have successful ileal intubation in children (19). Colonoscopy assesses disease severity, extent, evidence of disease complications (fistulae, ulceration), and allows surveillance of cancer, more common in UC. CT colonography (CTC) is not used for the evaluation of IBD; it is used to detect polyps (20).

Esophagogastroduodenoscopy (EGD) has an important place in the initial workup of IBD (21). Previously, EGD was not routinely performed unless a patient exhibited symptoms suggesting upper GI disease such as dysphagia, nausea, vomiting, or oral aphthous ulcers. It has become widely accepted only within the last decade with increasing recognition that UC, CD, and IC patients have upper GI tract inflammation (21, 22).

Supporting Evidence

Lower Endoscopy

Endoscopic biopsy data show up to 85% of patients with CD have terminal ileal disease. In a minority of adult patients (15–25%), CD is confined to the colon (23).

Ileal intubation (ileoscopy) is a vital part of the colonoscopy as the TI may be the only area of CD in up to 23% of pediatric Crohn's patients (24). Two or three biopsies are taken from each region of the bowel. Biopsy needs to be performed even if the colon and TI macroscopically

appear normal. Histologic diagnosis of CD is made when there is segmental involvement characterized by transmural inflammation, congested serosa, aphthous ulcers, granulomas and ulceration leading to nodularity. In distinction, UC does not show granulomas but has continuous bowel changes (Table 35.1) (25).

Colonoscopy with ileoscopy has been shown to be a safe, feasible, and accurate procedure. In a retrospective review of all colonoscopies performed in 164 children referred for suspicion of IBD, the percentage of successful ileoscopies increased from 20% in 1994 to 66% in 2000 (19). The rate of bowel perforation is estimated at 0.2%.

Upper Endoscopy

Overall upper GI tract inflammation is most common in the stomach, followed by esophagus and duodenum in children with IBD (22). Both CD and UC may have upper GI tract inflammation.

The incidence of an abnormal upper endoscopy in children with IBD is significant. A retrospective study of 115 patients with IBD (CD and UC) over a 7-year period revealed abnormal upper endoscopic findings in 64% of 82 subjects with CD and in 50% of the 34 subjects with UC. Findings included ulcers (20%), erythema (25%), and erosions (42%) in the esophagus, gastric mucosa, and duodenum. The most common finding, erosions, was more often seen in the stomach (22%) and duodenum (14%) (21). In a control blinded study evaluating endoscopic biopsies in IBD patients, Tobin et al. showed that esophagitis, gastritis, and duodenitis occurred more commonly in CD patients. Esophagitis occurred in 72% of CD, 50% of UC; gastritis in 92% of CD, 69% of UC; and duodenitis in 33% CD, 23% UC patients.

The histologic identification of granulomas is pathopneumonic for CD and can help distinguish it from UC. In a large series of 376 CD patients at a Children's Hospital, granulomas were found on endoscopic biopsies in 48% of all patients, the majority (61%) untreated. De Matos et al. found the presence of granulomas correlated with anti-*S. cerevisiae* antibodies, hypoalbuminemia, perianal disease, and gastritis at presentation ($p = 0.03$, $p = 0.008$, $p = 0.03$, and $p = 0.001$) (24).

As seen in the TI, microscopic mucosal disease can be present in the absence of symptoms. In a prospective study of 54 children with IBD upper GI inflammation was seen in 29/54 (22 CD, 7 UC) (22). However, nine (31%) of these patients were asymptomatic. Thus in all patients strongly suspected to have either CD or UC, EGD in conjunction with lower endoscopy is recommended at initial diagnosis (strong evidence).

Wireless Capsule Endoscopy

Summary of Evidence: WCE employs a small, ingestible capsule containing a videochip, transmitter, and battery. The capsule will pass through bowel and appear in the stool within 24–48 h. An average of 55,000 video images are transmitted to a portable device and downloaded to a computer for interpretation. WCE is used in patients with suspected small bowel pathology (Crohn's, polyps, unexplained hemorrhage) not seen in conventional studies. WCE is a safe and well-tolerated exam in adolescents and adults (26, 27) (limited evidence). In recent studies, WCE was also safe in infants and small children but the 25-mm-sized capsule must be placed in the stomach under endoscopic guidance (26, 28). The biggest risk with capsule endoscopy is capsule impaction above a small bowel stricture. To minimize this risk, small bowel lumen patency is initially evaluated by SBFT, patency capsule, or enterography (CT or MR).

While WCE is equivalent or superior to other modalities in the evaluation of known ileal CD, it is expensive and typically reserved for patients with unexplained GI bleeding or a hereditary polyposis syndrome (limited evidence).

Supporting Evidence: WCE has higher sensitivity than conventional small bowel exams (SBFT) or MDCT for the diagnosis of CD of the small bowel and for diagnosis of a cause of bowel hemorrhage when endoscopy is negative. Based on recent adult literature, capsule endoscopy has the highest diagnostic yield for identifying small bowel disease from any cause (including Crohn's) with a sensitivity of 87% versus only 13% for all other imaging modalities (29). The capsule appears to have greater sensitivity in identifying small bowel ulceration or stricture than conventional fluoroscopic barium

studies and enteroclysis. In an adult study of 17 patients suspected or known to have non-obstructive CD at the Mayo Clinic in Scottsdale, CD was detected by WCE in (12/17) 71%, by ileoscopy in (11/17) 65%, by CT enterography in (9/11) 53%, and by SBFT in only (4/17) 24% (27). It is advocated that WCE may be helpful in identifying non-obstructive CD when SBFT and ileoscopy are negative or inconclusive (27).

Currently WCE is not routinely used in the identification of CD in children. However, it has a role beyond IBD in diagnosing obscure small bowel lesions accurately in children over the age of 10 years. In a prospective study by Guilhon de Araujo et al., WCE correctly diagnosed or excluded a bleeding source, small-bowel polyps, or CD of the small bowel in 29 of 30 children (30).

There are limitations and pitfalls with WCE, which can lead to false positives or false negatives. Small children need the capsule placed by endoscopy and extra-intestinal abnormalities cannot be assessed. Limitations include submucosal lesions mimicking normal folds, poor localization of the pathology, capsule retention in patients with asymptomatic strictures, rapid transit resulting in decreased sensitivity, or slow transit which outlasts the capsule battery life (7–8 h). Also mucosal erosions can be seen in 14% of normal patients and in 28% of NSAID users (31, 32).

III. What Is the Diagnostic Performance of Current Imaging Modalities in Evaluating IBD of the Small Bowel (Small Bowel Follow-Through, CT, MR, US, Enteroclysis)?

Summary of Evidence: There are multidimensional considerations for which imaging test is the best to evaluate a child that include the patient's age and comfort, availability of the exam, radiation dose, and cost. Imaging studies are categorized as follows: conventional includes radiographs, SBFT, multidetector CT (MDCT); newer imaging comprised of enterography using CT/MR, and enteroclysis CT (CTE), or MR (MRE); and finally ultrasound (US). Despite the many new imaging tests, SBFT remains the most common initial exam performed (limited evidence).

Children with abdominal pain from IBD or its complications (particularly, abscess or bowel obstruction) may have conventional MDCT performed. However, it does not have a strong role in the diagnosis of IBD as it has a low sensitivity and specificity because of collapsed, underfilled bowel. CT enterography has improved sensitivity and specificity when compared with CT with positive enteral contrast. MR enterography has become increasingly desirable because of the lack of ionizing radiation and its high diagnostic accuracy.

The role of enteroclysis (CT or MRI) is to detect partial small bowel obstruction from either adhesions or stricture. CTE is more sensitive than fluoroscopic enteroclysis (FE) and has largely replaced it where CT is readily available. CT enteroclysis (CTE) should be reserved for complex cases of CD when a partial obstruction (from adhesion or stricture) is highly suspected but other imaging has been negative. MR enteroclysis has been shown to have high diagnostic performance in children but is not widely available and requires experienced personnel, nasal intubation, and sedation making it less practical. Like MRE, US may be used in the first assessment of a child with IBD and in monitoring disease but requires experienced and dedicated personnel.

Supporting Evidence

Abdominal Radiographs

Radiographs are used to evaluate for any patient with acute abdominal pain or in those with known IBD where complications are suspected such as bowel obstruction, free intraperitoneal air, and overall stool burden. Radiographs have no role in diagnosing IBD. The findings of "thumb-printing" (suggesting bowel wall edema or inflammation) and dilated bowel loops are nonspecific (33).

Small Bowel Follow-Through

The SBFT exam involves giving the patient oral barium taking immediate and delayed images of the upper GI tract and entire small bowel until the contrast reaches the cecum. Relative to ileoscopy, SBFT is not only less sensitive but also inexpensive, widely available, easy to perform,

and requires no sedation in diagnosing CD (19, 27) (moderate evidence). The diagnostic capability of SBFT in detecting CD in the small bowel has been conflicting in the literature. In a pediatric study of 84 subjects, the SBFT had a low sensitivity in detecting TI involvement, sensitivity of 45%, and a specificity of 96% (19). In an adult study by Hara et al. small bowel CD was detected in 4/17 patients (24%) (27). In an older pediatric study ($n = 46$), a sensitivity of 90% and specificity 96% in detection of CD in the small bowel was reported (34). The former two studies appear to reveal more realistic data as poor bowel opacification leads to equivocal exams, and substantial intra- and interobserver variations in interpretation are present (35). In a prospective blinded study of 30 adults with CD, the extent of CD and the presence of complications were imaged and compared by both SBFT and MR barium enterography (36). MRI has provided additional information in eight patients. SBFT revealed superficial mucosal lesions seen on MRI, but extra-intestinal pathology, colorectal disease, and potential to distinguish active from chronic disease were far better on MRI (36).

Multidetector CT

MDCT is performed using a low-dose technique with weight-based parameters, after the ingestion of a positive oral contrast agent and administration of IV contrast. CT adds information on extra-intestinal findings of UC and CD; from the earliest publications by Jabra et al. MDCT has had a high sensitivity but low specificity for bowel wall thickness (37, 38). Jabra et al. defined the role of CT as aiding in the management of children with known CD with changing clinical symptoms (limited evidence). CT is the most common examination used for assessing complications of CD such as abscesses, peritonitis, postoperative leaks, and anastomotic issues and has demonstrated a high sensitivity and specificity. These points and the diagnostic performance of CT are discussed in detail under Issue 4, a focus on complications of IBD.

Enterography

Enterography (CT or MR) differs from the conventional CT and MR studies in that a large volume (1,000 ml) of neutral oral contrast agent is given over 1 h followed by acquisition of a routine intravenously enhanced abdominopelvic CT or MR. The main advantage is that the particular enteric contrast agents used not only result in more bowel distension compared to the conventional enteric agents, but also provide low density on CT and low signal on MR imaging of the bowel lumen to allow improved depiction of the bowel wall.

A few CT enterography studies have included a small number of adolescents and the focus of these studies has been to describe data or correlate CT findings with biological markers of inflammation (limited evidence). In one retrospective adult study by Bodily et al. 96 patients underwent CT enterography with enteric water contrast and IV contrast and ileoscopy with or without biopsy. CT results were compared to endoscopic and histological data. CT enterography had a sensitivity of 90% for the detection of CD based on the quantitative mural enhancement which correlated with active CD on endoscopy and biopsy (39). In a large retrospective review of adult CT enterography studies by Paulsen et al. ($n = 700$), the sensitivity of CT enterography to detect IBD was >85% when the reference standard was FE or SBFT. However, when compared to endoscopy or surgery results, the sensitivity was between 77 and 92% (40).

The data on MR enterography versus the gold standard ileocolonoscopy are promising, but limited in children. The key advantage of MRE is its lack of radiation exposure. In a prospective study by Laghi et al. 75 children with IBD underwent ileocolonoscopy and MR enterography with a PEG solution. MRI had a sensitivity of 84% and specificity of 100% in detecting ileitis and differentiating it from other inflammatory conditions (41). Pilleul et al. examined 62 patients (median age 14 years) who had suspected or known CD and all underwent MR enterography with an oral preparation of mannitol solution. Imaging was compared to endoscopy and biopsy data. MRI had a sensitivity of 83% and a specificity of 100% in the diagnosis of CD and also identified complications in eight patients (42). There was also a positive correlation between bowel wall thickening and the Pediatric Crohn's Disease Activity Index ($p = 0.003$). Borthne et al. performed MR in 43 patients suspected of having CD using oral mannitol. MR compared with endoscopy had a sensitivity of 81%, specificity of 100%, and diagnostic accuracy of 90% (43). MR enterography is equally comparable to higher sensitivity compared to CT and US in detection of small bowel CD. Current limitations of MR are the artifacts from respiratory motion and bowel peristalsis and lack of patient cooperation leading to poor bowel distension (limited–moderate evidence).

Enteroclysis (MR or CT)

Enteroclysis is distinct from enterography in that it achieves maximal luminal distention by placement of a duodenal or jejunal tube for high volume, controlled contrast administration. This critical difference improves the detection of partial small bowel obstruction and polyps compared to routine CT or MR and enterography. CT enteroclysis (CTE) combines the advantages of MDCT and enteroclysis. CT enteroclysis has replaced the conventional fluoroscopic technique in many centers and consists of sedation and placement of a feeding tube into the duodenum. A variety of contrast media can be used (water, iodinated contrast, methylcellulose). Once the contrast reaches the cecum the patient is transferred from the fluoroscopic room to CT to undergo a routine abdominopelvic CT (35). CTE is more sensitive and superior to FE and may have a lower radiation dose as reported in an early study by Bender et al. (44, 45). In this adult study, CTE was performed to evaluate partial SBO and the sensitivity and specificity for localizing the site of obstruction were 82 and 88%, respectively (45). Brown et al. have recently published data evaluating the safety, feasibility, and outcomes of CTE in 175 children and comparing it with FE. CTE added additional diagnostic information over CT and FE and altered surgical management in 28% of the patients (44). The importance of a normal enteroclysis study in excluding an abnormality is an important clinical consideration. Barloon and colleagues followed 83 adults who had a normal enteroclysis for 3 years to assess its negative predictive value. Only six were found to have small bowel pathology, meaning that the enteroclysis had a 93% negative predictive value for ruling out any disease (46).

For many children and adults with IBD, repeat imaging is the norm rather than the exception. The main advantage of MR enteroclysis over CTE is the lack of ionizing radiation. The main disadvantage is the motion artifacts, as well as higher cost and possible delay in imaging patients that must be moved from fluoroscopy rooms to the MRI room. A recent evidence-based review of MR enteroclysis shows that this procedure has high diagnostic accuracy in children. Darbari et al. looked at 58 pediatric patients and found a positive predictive value of 96%, negative predictive value of 92%, and overall sensitivity and specificity of 96 and 92%, respectively, for the evaluation of IBD (47). However, MR enteroclysis is not universally available or practical. Currently there are no strong evidence-based studies comparing MR enteroclysis with capsule endoscopy or CT enteroclysis in children (limited evidence).

Ultrasound

Ultrasound of the bowel is performed using a high-frequency transducer with gray scale and color-Doppler compression technique. US oral contrast agents as well as intravenous contrast agents (SICUS) to evaluate the small bowel are not available in the USA, but are widely used in Europe. Their use increases the sensitivity and specificity of diagnosing CD over the conventional US techniques (48). Several studies using duplex and color Doppler show improved detection of inflammation of the bowel wall in IBD patients.

Alison and colleagues tabulated the diagnostic effectiveness of US for the few existing studies in children, which have small sample sizes ($n = 21$, $n = 26$). The overall sensitivity of US in detecting bowel IBD is 74–93%, specificity 78–93%; for terminal ileal bowel wall thickening and for stenosis the sensitivity is 85% (48). The variability of these numbers results from both the operator's experience and different cutoff values for abnormal bowel wall thickness.

Absence of bowel wall thickening, particularly when imaging the TI, has a good negative predictive value for CD. Increased bowel wall thickness in the colon proximal to the rectum and in the TI has a good positive predictive value for IBD, although it is not specific. In a double-blinded prospective study in 44 children who had endoscopy ($n = 33$) or SBFT ($n = 25$), US of ileal and colonic bowel wall was performed and compared to results of colonoscopy, biopsy, and barium studies (49). US showed significant difference in bowel wall thickness which correlated with active disease on endoscopy. Bowel wall thickness measurements >2.9 mm in the colon or >2.5 mm in the TI reliably indicated moderate or severe inflammation in children with IBD (49) (limited evidence). In experienced hands, US is an inexpensive imaging tool that avoids ionizing radiation exposure to both diagnose and assess treatment response of the TI.

IV. Complications of IBD (Intra-abdominal Abscess, Intestinal Fistulae, Strictures and Small Bowel Obstruction, Primary Sclerosing Cholangitis): Which Imaging Should Be Performed and What Is Its Diagnostic Performance?

Summary of Evidence: The most common complications of Crohn's disease include abscesses, strictures, fistulae, growth failure, decreased bone mineral density, and delayed puberty. On the other hand, patients with ulcerative colitis are at increased risk for toxic megacolon, peritonitis, and primary sclerosing cholangitis (PSC). Approximately 15–20% of adult patients with ulcerative colitis develop a fulminant colitis and 5% develop toxic megacolon (50). Toxic megacolon, perforation with peritonitis, and mucosal dysplasia are overall rare in children. Because the complications of CD are more frequent than those seen in UC, our discussion will focus primarily on the CD complications with a brief note on the importance of PSC in children.

When imaging complications, CT is preferred in emergent settings specifically for detecting small bowel obstruction, abscesses, peritonitis, postoperative leaks, anastomotic strictures, and perforation (37, 44). To minimize ionizing radiation exposure, US and MRI are recommended for repeat imaging at follow-up (limited to moderate evidence).

Supporting Evidence

Intra-abdominal Abscess

Intra-abdominal abscesses occur in approximately 10% of children with CD (51). It is rare in children with UC unless it is after colectomy. The most common location of an abscess is the right lower quadrant. However, they can also occur anywhere in the peritoneal cavity, abdominal wall, retroperitoneum, iliopsoas, and subphrenic regions. In nearly 50% of patients, the abscesses occur near an anastomosis following surgical resection. MDCT is the imaging test of choice for the detection of these abscesses unless they are limited to the abdominal wall when US may be sufficient.

Sensitivity and specificity of contrast-enhanced CT in detecting intra-abdominal abscesses in patients with severe CD was 87 and 95%, respectively (52). In experienced hands and using meticulous technique, the sensitivity and specificity of US in detecting abscesses in these same patients was 91 and 85%, respectively (52). CT showed higher specificity and positive predictive value [37]. There are both more false negatives (due to overlying bowel gas) and more false positives (fluid-filled bowel loops) with US and it requires more time and experience than CT.

In a small study, MR enterography had a sensitivity of 100%, in detecting abscesses compared to US (89%) (53). MR enteroclysis, although not performed in children for abscess evaluation, is also sensitive for the detection of abscesses, 100% sensitivity (54) (moderate evidence).

Intestinal Fistulae

The incidence of fistula is also approximately 10% in children, less than that of adults (30%). The gold standard for detection of fistulae is surgery. Using imaging, the gold standard to detect them is CT or MR (limited evidence).

Both CT and MR can detect small bowel fistulae in approximately 70% of patients although reports vary based on experience, technique, and patient populations. The sensitivity of US in the detection of fistulae varies from 31 to 87%. In a prospective study of 213 patients with CD, the US findings of fistulae were compared to surgical data and US showed a sensitivity of 87% and specificity of 90% (55). In patients with internal fistulae, CT showed a sensitivity and specificity of 68 and 91%, respectively, whereas MRI has an overall sensitivity of 87%. MDCT is more accurate for detecting enterovesical and enterocutaneous fistulae and sinus tracts from the bowel to the psoas muscle (50). For fistulae and abscesses extending into the perirectal and perianal regions, MRI is the test of choice with the highest sensitivity and specificity (56, 57) (limited evidence).

Strictures and Small Bowel Obstruction

Development of strictures is a big concern in children, primarily with CD. Symptomatic strictures can lead to partial or complete small bowel obstruction and often surgery. In the emergent setting, conventional CT is recommended for assessment of bowel obstruction. In children with subacute or chronic symptoms, CT or MR enteroclysis best detect partial small bowel obstructions. This topic is addressed in more detail in the issue of imaging features leading to surgery (see Issue V).

Primary Sclerosing Cholangitis

Any child who presents with PSC should have an evaluation for IBD. PSC is more commonly seen in patients with UC rather than CD. Equally, a child with IBD and elevated liver enzymes may need sonography to evaluate for dilated biliary ducts and if needed MRCP for the diagnosis. PSC is more prevalent in CD than originally thought. According to one adult series the incidence of PSC is 2–7% in UC rather than 0.7–3.4% in CD (58). Approximately 5% of patients with UC are found to have PSC, whereas 75% of patients with PSC are found to have UC. Although these numbers are primarily from data in adults, they are comparable to the limited reports in children. Feldstein et al. reported that in 52 children with PSC, 81% had IBD, and in 20% of these children PSC was diagnosed before IBD, thereby setting the impetus for an IBD workup in any child with PSC (58) (moderate evidence). MRCP is the diagnostic study of choice for the evaluation of PSC; when positive, a liver biopsy is not required (limited evidence).

V. What Are the Most Important Imaging Features that Lead to Surgery in a Child with Crohn's Disease and Ulcerative Colitis?

Summary of Evidence: Despite improvements in medical therapies, 70–80% of patients with CD will require an operation, whereas only 30–40% of UC patients will ultimately need surgery (59, 60). The main indications for surgery in a child with CD are (1) small bowel obstruction, SBO (complete or partial) that does not respond to medical therapy; (2) small bowel strictures with associated obstruction; and rarely (3) bowel perforation, appendicitis, or abscess formation (59). When these issues particularly impact the child's growth and development, surgery is warranted. In UC patients, surgery is warranted for the following reasons in the order of most common to least common: (1) disease refractory to medical management, (2) severe disease with complications, (3) risk of malignancy (60). Malignancy requires a colectomy and is a strong concern in adults but rare in children.

Supporting Evidence: The evidence in the pediatric surgical literature determining who needs surgery is limited to a few studies with small sample sizes. The existing large cohort studies evaluate only adults. In a large study by Hurst and colleagues including 513 adult patients, the indications for surgery were the following: failure of medical management in 220, obstruction in 94, intestinal fistula in 68, mass in 56, abscess in 33, peritonitis in 9, and bleeding in 7 (61). Unlike in adults, the impact on a child's growth and development is a vital part of surgical decision making. In one pediatric study, the decision for surgery in up to 50% of the patients was based on the presence of failure of medical therapy with significant growth retardation rather than a mechanical obstruction (62). In a small study of 26 patients, Dokucu et al. described chronic intestinal dysmotility and poor absorption with growth failure as an indication for surgery in 13 children, whereas the remaining 13 had surgery secondary to chronic mechanical intestinal obstruction (63) (limited evidence).

Role of Conventional Barium Fluoroscopy and Multidetector CT

Summary of Evidence: The imaging features of small bowel obstruction include dilated small bowel loops, a decompressed colon, and small bowel air–fluid levels. A symptomatic stricture requires surgery. The presence of a persistently narrowed, smooth walled, and non-thickened segment of bowel with proximal bowel dilatation represents a stricture. The imaging studies most commonly utilized until recently for evaluation of strictures and obstruction have been SBFT and MDCT. MDCT is the imaging test of choice for SBO with high sensitivity for a complete SBO in children but is less likely to detect a partial SBO (Table 35.2) (64) (limited evidence).

Supporting Evidence: Overall conventional fluoroscopic barium imaging is the least accurate in identifying strictures compared with surgical results. Otterson et al. retrospectively reviewed barium studies and surgical records of 118 patients having a total of 230 strictures. The data show that fluoroscopic exams incorrectly estimated the number of small bowel strictures in 43/118 (36%) patients (65). The original work by Jabra et al. has shown that MDCT is both sensitive and specific in diagnosing SBO in children, sensitivity 87%, specificity 86% (66). In this retrospective review MDCT correctly identified the level of obstruction in 12/14 scans, 86% of the cases, and etiology of obstruction in 14/30 scans, 47% of the cases (moderate evidence).

Role of Enteroclysis (CT/MR) and Enterography (CT/MR)

Summary of Evidence: In adults, enteroclysis has been shown to be the most accurate in diagnosing small bowel obstructions in CD (67–69). More recent publications in the pediatric imaging literature report that FE and CT enteroclysis (CTE) are more sensitive and specific in detecting small bowel strictures, partial bowel obstruction, and adhesions compared to conventional SBFT and MDCT, especially in children with IBD (44). MR enteroclysis (MREC) and MR enterography (MRE) have comparable high sensitivity for the detection of stenoses/ strictures (54, 69). In comparison, US has a moderate but lower sensitivity for the detection of ileal stenoses/strictures and post-operative reoccurrences (48). Both accessibility and experience often limit these specialized exams to tertiary care centers.

Supporting Evidence: In adults the sensitivity and specificity of CT enteroclysis (CTE) in accurately diagnosing a small bowel obstruction approaches 100% (Table 35.3) (67, 68). In a recent study by Brown et al. comparing FE and CTE with conventional imaging, FE and CTE added diagnostic information (identification of partial SBO and for CT, extra-intestinal abnormalities) over conventional exams such as SBFT. In particular, CTE definitively identified the etiology of small bowel obstruction, secondary to adhesion, internal hernia, or stricture and changed the surgical management in 28% of patients (44).

MR enteroclysis (MREC) has been shown to be equally sensitive to CTE. Masseli and colleagues found no difference in diagnostic ability of MR enteroclysis and MR enterography to detect stenoses (69). MREC like other enteroclysis procedures requires sedation, nasal–duodenal/ jejunal tube placement, and contrast administration. MR enterography is a practical alternative to CT enterography with equal overall sensitivity (limited evidence).

VI. What Are the Role and Risk of Repeat Imaging in Monitoring IBD Response to Treatment?

Summary of Evidence: Imaging is very important for assessing CD activity and complications, particularly to investigate the cause of abdominal pain, vomiting, weight loss, or fever; to select or change therapy; and to plan surgery. The imaging modalities most commonly used for follow-up include SBFT and CT because they are noninvasive, widely available, and reproducible. However, in experienced hands, US and MRI have comparable diagnostic accuracy and should be considered to avoid repeated exposure to ionizing radiation. Some children with UC or indeterminant IBD will also need repeat

imaging to assess their disease complications but to a lesser frequency than children with CD.

Supporting Evidence: The exact frequency of repeat imaging is not known, but based on current CT literature it is not insignificant. Repeat imaging is primarily performed in children with CD rather than UC and the radiation risk in this population is a big concern. A recent study by Gaca et al. (70) demonstrated that the effective dose (ED) from an abdominopelvic CT was approximately twice that of an average SBFT exam. One important point in this study is that the ED of SBFT studies was calculated based on institutional protocol and equipment, but with varying practices and varying number of images acquired elsewhere, this may potentially lead to ED values larger or equal to that of a CT. In this study of 176 children with CD, 78% of the patients had 0–1 SBFT and 74% patients had over 1.1 CT scans over a follow-up time frame of 3 years and 11 months. Only one patient had an excessive number of SBFT and CTs. The advantages of CT in monitoring these children are clear. CT is a fast, readily available, well-tolerated exam with high sensitivity for evaluation of complications in the emergency setting. Jabra et al. reported that CT should be the first line of imaging in a child with changing clinical symptoms (37). In a separate report of 18 patients with a diagnosis of IBD (including CD, UC, and IC), Jamieson et al. reported that the sensitivity of MDCT for identifying disease in the small bowel was equal to or greater than that of barium studies (71). When isolated TI or colonic disease is present or if CT has demonstrated an abscess, US with color Doppler can be used to follow these patients (48, 72). In the follow-up evaluation of the extent of bowel involvement or for abscesses and strictures, MRI can be very helpful. A prospective meta-analysis by Horsthuis et al. (73) comparing performance of US, MR, leukocyte-tagged scintigraphy, CT, and PET in the diagnosis of IBD revealed no significant differences in diagnostic accuracy among these techniques [19]. A total of 33 studies out of a search of 1,406 articles, in both the pediatric and adult literature, were evaluated in this meta-analysis and reviewed by two independent reviewers. A minimum of 15 patients were included in the reviewed studies and there were no age limits on the search. In this study sensitivity for the diagnosis of IBD by each modality per segment of diseased bowel was 73.5% (US), 70.4% (MR), 67.4% (CT), with specificity of 92.7% (US), 94% (MR), 90.2% (CT). CT proved to be significantly less sensitive and specific for intestinal and extra-intestinal pathologies. A limitation of these European studies included in this meta-analysis is that overall CT is much less frequently used in Europe and their experience is superior to North America in US and MRI imaging of bowel. The benefits of CT need to be carefully weighed against the potential long-term risks of radiation dose (74). When possible, based on indication, availability, experience, and cost, an alternative equally diagnostic test, US and MRI, should be obtained in patients requiring repeat imaging (limited–moderate evidence).

VII. Special Situation: Which Imaging Modality Provides the Best Performance for the Evaluation of Perianal/Perirectal Disease in Crohn's Disease?

Summary of Evidence: Pelvic MRI with gadolinium contrast enhancement is the imaging modality of choice for the evaluation of perianal disease, fistula, and adjacent abscesses (limited evidence). It is noninvasive and there is no concern for motion in the pelvis; therefore, high-resolution, high-contrast multiplanar images are feasible without sedation and little patient preparation. Exact differentiation of the sphincter muscles with high-resolution, contrast-enhanced sequences is a requirement for the detection of disorders of the anal canal and the perianal tissues (75). Perianal inflammation occurs overall in about 50% patients with CD. Lifetime risk of a patient with CD to develop a perianal fistula is approximately 20–40% (76) and the rate of recurrence is high. A recurrence rate of up to 48% has been reported in adults with tracts and abscesses inactive and healed after 1 year and up to 60% at 2 years of treatment (77, 78). Although fistulae are less common in children as compared to adults, the lack of ionizing radiation makes MRI ideal, especially when re-imaging children.

Supporting Evidence: A *pelvic* MRI for perianal disease is performed without any endorectal instrumentation or enteric contrast, only intravenous contrast. Perianal inflammation has several manifestations including (1) perirectal wall thickening and inflammation, (2) external cutaneous fistulae and tracts, (3) complex internal fistulae from the bowel to bowel, to bladder, or vagina with frank abscess formation.

Based on the current imaging literature, MR imaging is superior to anal endosonography (EUS/AES), CT, or surgical evaluation in showing disease extent but the optimal approach may be to combine two studies (57, 76). A prospective blinded study in 34 adult patients with CD compared the diagnostic accuracy of EUS, MRI, and rectal exam under anesthesia to identify and classify fistulae (76). The authors reported that the accuracy of identifying a fistula was the greatest, 100%, with any two tests combined rather than one exam alone. MR imaging is also superior to surgical evaluation for predicting clinical outcome (57, 77). In an evidence-based review in adult populations, Sahni et al. described the performance of MRI for the evaluation of perianal disease in CD patients. They concluded that MRI was able to distinguish between simple disease, limited to the perirectal region without fistula, and complex disease, defined as the presence of fistulae and abscesses. MRI overall has a 97% sensitivity and 96% specificity for detection of perianal fistulae (Table 35.4) (57). Essary and colleagues have shown that MRI in children can help differentiate perianal fistulae from other inflammatory conditions such as pilonidal sinus (56) (moderate evidence).

Take Home Tables and Figures

Table 35.1 shows endoscopic, histological, and bio-marker differences between CD and UC. Table 35.2 shows diagnostic performance of imaging in small bowel obstruction (adults). Table 35.3 shows MDCT small bowel obstruction diagnostic accuracy in children. Table 35.4 shows diagnostic performance of MRI for evaluation of perianal disease. Figures 35.1 and 35.2 are algorithms of imaging protocols for CD and US, respectively.

Table 35.1. Endoscopic, histological, and bio-marker differences between CD and UC

Modality	CD	UC
Endoscopy and visualization of oral and/ or perianal regions	Ulcers (aphthous, linear, or stellate)	Ulcers Erythema
	Cobblestoning	Loss of vascular pattern
	Skip lesions	Granularity
	Strictures	Friability
	Fistula	Spontaneous bleeding
	Abnormalities in oral and/or perianal regions	Pseudopolyps
	Segmental distribution	Continuous with variable proximal extension from rectum
Histology	Submucosal (biopsy with sufficient submucosal tissue) or transmural involvement (surgical specimen)	Mucosal involvement
	Crypt distortion	Crypt abscess
	Ulcers, crypt distortion	Gobler cell depletion
	Crypt abscess	Mucin granulomas (rare)
	Granulomas (non-caseating, non-mucin)	Continuous distribution
	Focal changes (within biopsy)	
	Patchy distribution (biopsies)	
Bio-markers		
pANCA detection in IBD	10–40% of CD patients	50–80% of UC patients
ASCA detection in IBD	46–70% of CD patients	6–12% of UC patients

Reprinted with kind permission of Springer Science+Business Media form Anupindi S, Ayyala R, Kelsen J, Mamula P, Applegate KE. Imaging of Inflammatory Bowel Disease in Children. In Medina LS, Applegate KE, Blackmore CC (eds): *Evidence-Based Imaging in Pediatrics: Optimizing Imaging in Pediatric Patient Care.* New York: Springer Science+Business Media, 2010.

Table 35.2. Diagnostic performance of imaging in small bowel obstruction (adults)

Modality	Sensitivity (%)	Specificity (%)	References
Radiographs ($n = 78$)	46–69	57	(79)
CT abdomen ($n = 78;55$)	57–64	63–79	(79–81)
High grade	81		(80)
Low grade	48		(80)
CT enteroclysis	100	100	(79)
CTE versus CT ($n = 15$)			

Reprinted with kind permission of Springer Science+Business Media from Anupindi S, Ayyala R, Kelsen J, Mamula P, Applegate KE. Imaging of Inflammatory Bowel Disease in Children. In Medina LS, Applegate KE, Blackmore CC (eds): *Evidence-Based Imaging in Pediatrics: Optimizing Imaging in Pediatric Patient Care.* New York: Springer Science+Business Media, 2010.

Table 35.3 MDCT small bowel obstruction diagnostic accuracy in children

Modality	Sensitivity (%)	Specificity (%)	Reference
MDCT abdomen ($n = 81$)	87	86	(64)

Reprinted with kind permission of Springer Science+Business Media from Anupindi S, Ayyala R, Kelsen J, Mamula P, Applegate KE. Imaging of Inflammatory Bowel Disease in Children. In Medina LS, Applegate KE, Blackmore CC (eds): *Evidence-Based Imaging in Pediatrics: Optimizing Imaging in Pediatric Patient Care.* New York: Springer Science+Business Media, 2010.

Table 35.4. Diagnostic performance of MRI for evaluation of perianal disease (*n* = 34)

Modality	Sensitivity (%)	Specificity (%)	Positive predictive value (%)	Negative predictive value (%)
MRI	97	96	97	96
AES (anal endosonography)	92	85	89	89
Clinical exam (under anesthesia)	75	64	73	67

Data from Schwartz et al. (76).

Reprinted with kind permission of Springer Science+Business Media from Anupindi S, Ayyala R, Kelsen J, Mamula P, Applegate KE. Imaging of Inflammatory Bowel Disease in Children. In Medina LS, Applegate KE, Blackmore CC (eds): *Evidence-Based Imaging in Pediatrics: Optimizing Imaging in Pediatric Patient Care*. New York: Springer Science+Business Media, 2010.

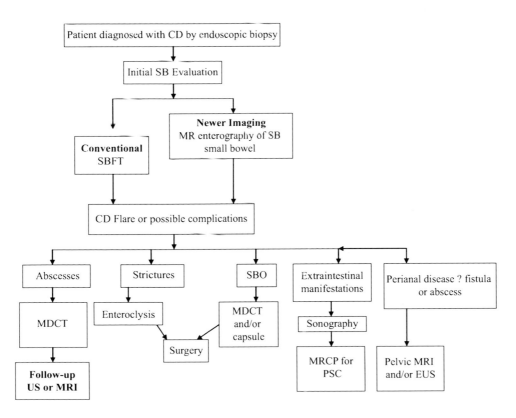

Figure 35.1. Clinical imaging pathways for CD. (Reprinted with kind permission of Springer Science+Business Media from Anupindi S, Ayyala R, Kelsen J, Mamula P, Applegate KE. Imaging of Inflammatory Bowel Disease in Children. In Medina LS, Applegate KE, Blackmore CC (eds): *Evidence-Based Imaging in Pediatrics: Optimizing Imaging in Pediatric Patient Care*. New York: Springer Science+Business Media, 2010.)

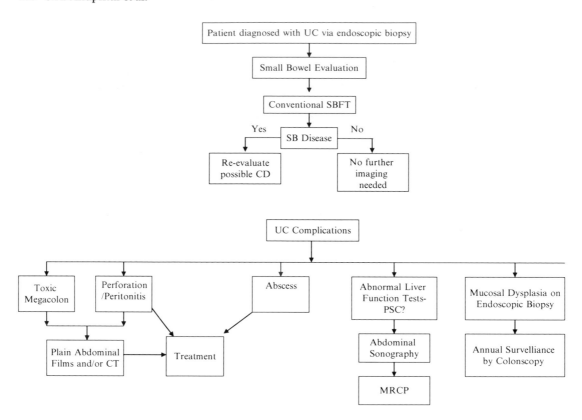

Figure 35.2. Clinical imaging pathways for UC. (Reprinted with kind permission of Springer Science+Business Media from Anupindi S, Ayyala R, Kelsen J, Mamula P, Applegate KE. Imaging of Inflammatory Bowel Disease in Children. In Medina LS, Applegate KE, Blackmore CC (eds): *Evidence-Based Imaging in Pediatrics: Optimizing Imaging in Pediatric Patient Care.* New York: Springer Science+Business Media, 2010.)

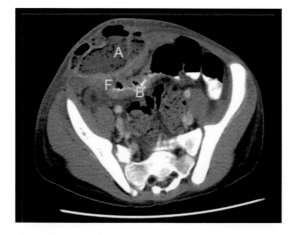

Figure 35.3. CT scan of Crohn's disease in a 14-year-old boy complicated by large fistula entering into an even larger abscess in the anterior abdominal wall. Axial contrast-enhanced CT image of the abdomen demonstrates an enterocutaneous fistula (F) arising from an abnormal loop of ileum (B) leading to a large abscess (A) in the anterior abdominal wall. (Reprinted with kind permission of Springer Science+Business Media from Anupindi S, Ayyala R, Kelsen J, Mamula P, Applegate KE. Imaging of Inflammatory Bowel Disease in Children. In Medina LS, Applegate KE, Blackmore CC (eds): *Evidence-Based Imaging in Pediatrics: Optimizing Imaging in Pediatric Patient Care.* New York: Springer Science+Business Media, 2010.)

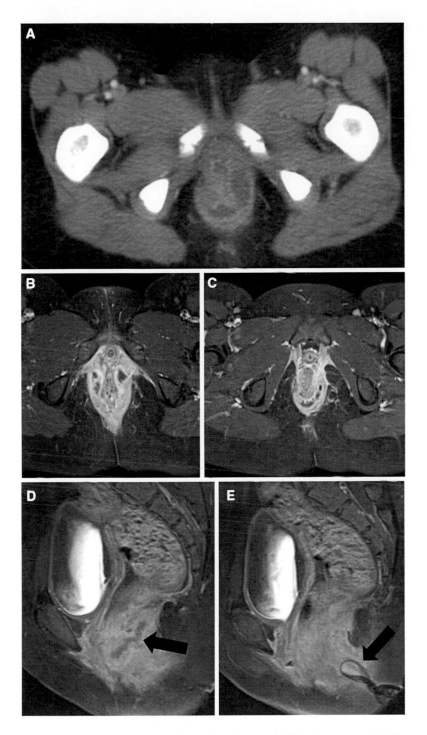

Figure 35.4. MRI of large perianal fistula with abscess in a 10-year-old girl who presented with acute abdominal pain and a new diagnosis of Crohn's disease. (**A**) is the initial axial MDCT image of the perianal inflammation and small abscesses around her anus. (**B**) and (**C**) demonstrate the superior image contrast of the findings on axial MRI with gadolinium and fat saturation technique. There are both exuberant inflammation (enhancement) and small abscesses that nearly circumscribe the anus. (**D**) demonstrates the perianal abscesses on sagittal view MRI (*black arrow*). (**E**) shows the superficial position of the drain (*black arrow*) relative to the more deep position of the perianal abscess. She had a large amount of stool in her colon and rectum. She required diverting colostomy to successfully treat her perianal disease. (Reprinted with kind permission of Springer Science+Business Media from Anupindi S, Ayyala R, Kelsen J, Mamula P, Applegate KE. Imaging of Inflammatory Bowel Disease in Children. In Medina LS, Applegate KE, Blackmore CC (eds): *Evidence-Based Imaging in Pediatrics: Optimizing Imaging in Pediatric Patient Care.* New York: Springer Science+Business Media, 2010.)

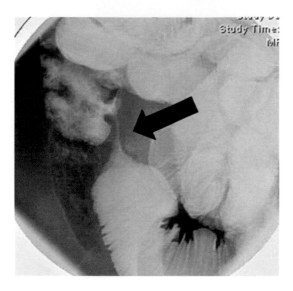

Figure 35.5. Crohn's disease in a 12-year-old girl with worsening abdominal pain. She underwent enteroclysis to evaluate for partial small bowel obstruction. The fluoroscopic enteroclysis image shows that the terminal ileum is strictured (*black arrow*). It produced dilation of the ileum proximal to it and required surgical resection. (Reprinted with kind permission of Springer Science+Business Media from Anupindi S, Ayyala R, Kelsen J, Mamula P, Applegate KE. Imaging of Inflammatory Bowel Disease in Children. In Medina LS, Applegate KE, Blackmore CC (eds): *Evidence-Based Imaging in Pediatrics: Optimizing Imaging in Pediatric Patient Care.* New York: Springer Science+Business Media, 2010.)

Imaging Case Studies

Case 1

Figure 35.3 presents a CT scan of Crohn's disease in a 14-year-old boy complicated by large fistula entering into an even larger abscess in the anterior abdominal wall.

Case 2

Figure 35.4 presents CT and MRI of large perianal fistula with abscess in a 10-year-old girl who presented with acute abdominal pain and a new diagnosis of Crohn's disease.

Case 3

Figure 35.5 presents a case of Crohn's disease in a 12-year-old girl with worsening abdominal pain.

Suggested Imaging Protocols for Inflammatory Bowel Disease in Children

Definition of Imaging Techniques

Upper Gastrointestinal Study with SBFT UGI/SBFT

A patient is given barium orally and immediate images of the esophagus, stomach, and proximal small bowel are acquired. Then delayed images every 30–45 min are obtained of the small bowel until the endpoint when the contrast reaches the cecum. The radiologist will compress the bowel intermittently to evaluate for abnormalities and to assess function of the small bowel loops. The most important anatomy to document on compression spot imaging is the TI, the most likely area of Crohn's disease.

Enterography (MDCT, MR)

The patient is given oral contrast (20 cc/kg) such as polyethylene glycol, or VoLumen, neutral contrast agents that provide more sustained bowel distention. The patient is given a large volume of contrast to drink over 1 h. A CT or MRI study is performed after the 1-h period using a standard institutional CT low-dose protocol with IV contrast.

Enteroclysis (CT, MR)

Three types of enteroclysis exist. All require nasal intubation with sedation for placement of a feeding tube into the duodenum or jejunum for high-volume contrast delivery. Unlike other imaging exams, enteroclysis can achieve the maximum luminal distension of the small bowel. Conventional FE requires contrast administration with a controlled flow rate and careful spot images taken under direct fluoroscopy. MR enteroclysis requires routine MR imaging of the entire abdomen and pelvis in the coronal and axial planes after contrast delivery, whereas CT enteroclysis requires a combination of fluoroscopy and CT. The enteric contrast is instilled under brief fluoroscopic guidance and then the patient undergoes a routine abdominopelvic CT.

Wireless Capsule Endoscopy

This procedure is comprised of a 2.5 cm, ingestible capsule containing a videochip, transmitter, and battery. The capsule will pass through the bowel and will evacuate through the stool within 24–48 h. An average of 55,000 video images are transmitted to a portable device and downloaded to a computer where images are reviewed.

General IBD Algorithm

In a patient suspected to have IBD, the initial workup includes a physical examination, laboratory testing, followed by upper and lower endoscopies for pathological diagnosis and imaging of the small bowel. There is no set rule that endoscopy precedes or follows imaging studies. Endoscopy with biopsy can determine if the patient has IBD and further classify the patient as CD, UC, or indeterminate. If the endoscopy results are normal, but there is continued concern for IBD, small bowel evaluation should be performed to exclude disease limited to the small bowel, including further laboratory tests or newer techniques such as capsule endoscopy. In some situations imaging of the small bowel by either SBFT or MDCT is performed before endoscopy and may yield information to direct the gastroenterologist especially if the disease process is something other than IBD, i.e., malrotation or malabsorption.

Clinical and Imaging Pathways for CD and UC

See algorithms presented in Figs. 35.1 and 35.2.

Future Research

- Determine the value of both current and as-yet unidentified serologies in the diagnosis and follow-up of IBD.
- Further understanding regarding the role of genetics in IBD.
- Cost-effective analyses on imaging strategies in the evaluation of inflammatory bowel disease activity both at diagnosis and in symptomatic children.
- Large pediatric cohort studies to optimize the techniques of MRI and US to avoid ionizing radiation.
- The role of double-balloon enteroscopy in children with IBD.
- The role of PET and PET–CT in the evaluation of IBD needs to be defined as it can provide both functional and anatomical information.

References

1. Kugathasan S, Judd RH, Hoffmann RG, Heikenen J, Telega G et al. J Pediatr 2003;143(4):525–531.
2. Loftus EV Jr. Gastroenterology 2004;126(6): 1504–1517.
3. Baldassano RN, Piccoli DA. Gastroenterol Clin North Am 1999;28(2):445–458.
4. Saeed S, Kugathasan S. In Mamula P, Markowitz JE, Baldassano RN (eds.): Pediatric Inflammatory Bowel Disease. New York, NY: Springer Science and Business Media, 2008;45–49.
5. Yu AP, Cabanilla LA, Wu EQ, Mulani PM, Chao J. Curr Med Res Opin 2008;24(2):319–328.
6. Hay AR, Hay JW. J Clin Gastroenterol 1992;14(4): 318–327.
7. Goldfarb NI, Pizzi LT, Fuhr JP Jr, Salvador C, Sikirica V et al. Dis Manag 2004;7(4):292–304.
8. Cohen RD, Thomas T. Gastroenterol Clin North Am 2006;35(4):867–882.
9. Bassi A, Dodd S, Williamson P, Bodger K. Gut 2004;53(10):1471–1478.
10. Hugot JP, Bellaiche M. Pediatr Radiol 2007;37(11): 1065–1070.
11. Gupta SK, Fitzgerald JF, Croffie JM, Pfefferkorn MD, Molleston JP et al. Inflamm Bowel Dis 2004;10(3):240–244.
12. Rabizadeh S, Oliva-Hemker M. In Mamula P, Markowitz JE, Baldassano RN (eds.): Pediatric

Inflammatory Bowel Disease. New York, NY: Springer Science and Business Media, 2008;94–95.

13. Solem CA, Loftus EV Jr, Tremaine WJ, Harmsen WS, Zinsmeister AR et al. Inflamm Bowel Dis 2005;11(8):707–712.

14. Papp M, Norman GL, Altorjay I, Lakatos PL. World J Gastroenterol 2007;13(14):2028–2036.

15. Dubinsky MC, Seidman EG. Curr Opin Gastroenterol 2000;16(4):337–342.

16. Canani RB, de Horatio LT, Terrin G, Romano MT, Miele E et al. J Pediatr Gastroenterol Nutr 2006;42(1):9–15.

17. Heyman MB, Kirschner BS, Gold BD, Ferry G, Baldassano R et al. J Pediatr 2005;146(1):35–40.

18. Mamula P, Telega GW, Markowitz JE, Brown KA, Russo PA et al. Am J Gastroenterol 2002;97(8): 2005–2010.

19. Batres LA, Maller ES, Ruchelli E, Mahboubi S, Baldassano RN. J Pediatr Gastroenterol Nutr 2002;35(3):320–323.

20. Anupindi S, Perumpillichira J, Jaramillo D, Zalis ME, Israel EJ. Pediatr Radiol 2005;35(5):518–524.

21. Abdullah BA, Gupta SK, Croffie JM, Pfefferkorn MD, Molleston JP et al. J Pediatr Gastroenterol Nutr 2002;35(5):636–640.

22. Castellaneta SP, Afzal NA, Greenberg M, Deere H, Davies S et al. J Pediatr Gastroenterol Nutr 2004;39(3):257–261.

23. Horsthuis K, Bipat S, Bennink RJ, Stoker J. Radiology 2008;247(1):64–79.

24. De Matos V, Russo PA, Cohen AB, Mamula P, Baldassano RN et al. J Pediatr Gastroenterol Nutr 2008;46(4):392–398.

25. Russo P. In Mamula P, Markowitz JE, Baldassano RN (eds.): Pediatric Inflammatory Bowel Disease. New York, NY: Springer Science and Business Media, 2008;245–248.

26. Deangelis GL, Fornaroli F, Deangelis N, Magiteri B, Bizzarri B. Am J Gastroenterol 2007;102(8):1749–1757; quiz 8, 58.

27. Hara AK, Leighton JA, Heigh RI, Sharma VK, Silva AC et al. Radiology 2006;238(1):128–134.

28. Arguelles-Arias F, Caunedo A, Romero J, Sanchez A, Rodriguez-Tellez M et al. Endoscopy 2004;36(10):869–873.

29. Maglinte DD, Sandrasegaran K, Chiorean M, Dewitt J, McHenry L et al. Am J Roentgenol 2007;189(2):306–312.

30. Guilhon de Araujo Sant'Anna AM, Dubois J, Miron MC, Seidman EG. Clin Gastroenterol Hepatol 2005;3(3):264–270.

31. Hara AK. Abdom Imaging 2005;30(2):179–183.

32. Maglinte DD. Radiology 2005;236(3):763–767.

33. Taylor GA, Nancarrow PA, Hernanz-Schulman M, Teele RL. Pediatr Radiol 1986;16(3): 206–209.

34. Lipson A, Bartram CI, Williams CB, Slavin G, Walker-Smith J. Clin Radiol 1990;41(1):5–8.

35. Applegate KE, Maglinte DD. Pediatr Radiol 2008;38(suppl 2):S272–S274.

36. Bernstein CN, Greenberg H, Boult I, Chubey S, Leblanc C et al. Am J Gastroenterol 2005;100(11): 2493–2502.

37. Jabra AA, Fishman EK, Taylor GA. Radiology 1991;179(2):495–498.

38. Jabra AA, Fishman EK, Taylor GA. Am J Roentgenol 1994;162(4):975–979.

39. Bodily KD, Fletcher JG, Solem CA, Johnson CD, Fidler JL et al. Radiology 2006;238(2):505–516.

40. Paulsen SR, Huprich JE, Fletcher JG, Booya F, Young BM et al. Radiographics 2006;26(3):641–657; discussion 57–62.

41. Laghi A, Borrelli O, Paolantonio P, Dito L, Buena de Mesquita M et al. Gut 2003;52(3):393–397.

42. Pilleul F, Godefroy C, Yzebe-Beziat D, Dugougeat-Pilleul F, Lachaux A et al. Gastroenterol Clin Biol 2005;29(8–9):803–808.

43. Borthne AS, Abdelnoor M, Rugtveit J, Perminow G, Reiseter T et al. Eur Radiol 2006;16(1): 207–214.

44. Brown S, Applegate KE, Sandrasegaran K, Jennings SG, Garrett J et al. Pediatr Radiol 2008;38(5):497–510.

45. Bender GN, Timmons JH, Williard WC, Carter J. Invest Radiol 1996;31(1):43–49.

46. Barloon TJ, Lu CC, Honda H, Berbaum KS. Abdom Imaging 1994;19(2):113–115.

47. Darbari A, Sena L, Argani P, Oliva-Hemker JM, Thompson R et al. Inflamm Bowel Dis 2004;10(2):67–72.

48. Alison M, Kheniche A, Azoulay R, Roche S, Sebag G et al. Pediatr Radiol 2007;37(11): 1071–1082.

49. Bremner AR, Griffiths M, Argent JD, Fairhurst JJ, Beattie RM. Pediatr Radiol 2006;36(9):947–953.

50. Carucci LR, Levine MS. Gastroenterol Clin North Am 2002;31(1):93–117; ix.

51. The Key Complications of Crohn's Disease. http://www.ccfa.org [last accessed November 2008].

52. Maconi G, Sampietro GM, Parente F, Pompili G, Russo A et al. Am J Gastroenterol 2003;98(7): 1545–1555.

53. Potthast S, Rieber A, Von Tirpitz C, Wruk D, Adler G et al. Eur Radiol 2002;12(6):1416–1422.

54. Ryan ER, Heaslip IS. Abdom Imaging 2008; 33(1):34–37.

55. Gasche C, Moser G, Turetschek K, Schober E, Moeschl P et al. Gut 1999;44(1):112–117.

56. Essary B, Kim J, Anupindi S, Katz JA, Nimkin K. Pediatr Radiol 2007;37(2):201–208.

57. Sahni VA, Ahmad R, Burling D. Abdom Imaging 2008;33(1):26–30.

58. Feldstein AE, Perrault J, El-Youssif M, Lindor KD, Freese DK et al. Hepatology 2003;38(1): 210–217.

59. Allmen D. In Mamula P, Markowitz JE, Baldassano RN (eds.). Pediatric Inflammatory Bowel Disease. New York, NY: Springer Science and Business Media, 2008;455–465.

60. Mattei P, Rombeau JL. In Mamula P, Markowitz JE, Baldassano RN (eds.): Pediatric Inflammatory Bowel Disease. New York, NY: Springer Science and Business Media, 2008;469–481.

61. Hurst RD, Molinari M, Chung TP, Rubin M, Michelassi F. Surgery 1997;122(4):661–667; discussion 7–8.

62. Patel HI, Leichtner AM, Colodny AH, Shamberger RC. J Pediatr Surg 1997;32(7):1063–1067; discussion 7–8.

63. Dokucu AI, Sarnacki S, Michel JL, Jan D, Goulet O et al. Eur J Pediatr Surg 2002;12(3):180–185.

64. Jabra AA, Fishman EK. Abdom Imaging 1997;22(5):466–470.

65. Otterson MF, Lundeen SJ, Spinelli KS, Sudakoff GS, Telford GL et al. Surgery 2004;136(4):854–860.

66. Jabra AA, Eng J, Zaleski CG, Abdenour GE Jr, Vuong HV et al. Am J Roentgenol 2001;177(2): 431–436.

67. Maglinte DD, Sandrasegaran K, Lappas JC. Radiol Clin North Am 2007;45(2):289–301.

68. Maglinte DD, Sandrasegaran K, Lappas JC, Chiorean M. Radiology 2007;245(3):661–671.

69. Masselli G, Brizi MG, Menchini L, Minordi L, Vecchioli Scaldazza A. Radiol Med (Torino) 2005;110(3):221–233.

70. Gaca AM, Jaffe TA, Delaney S, Yoshizumi T, Toncheva G et al. Pediatr Radiol 2008;38(3): 285–291.

71. Jamieson, DH et al. AJR Am J Roentgenol 2003;180(5):1211–1216.

72. Spalinger J, Patriquin H, Miron MC, Marx G, Herzog D et al. Radiology 2000;217(3):787–791.

73. Horsthuis K, Bipat S, Bennink RJ et al. Radiology 2008;247(1):64–79.

74. CT and Radiation Dose. http//:www.imagegently.com/CT [last accessed September 2008].

75. Schaefer O, Oeksuez MO, Lohrmann C, Langer M. J Comput Assist Tomogr 2004;28(2):174–179.

76. Schwartz DA, Wiersema MJ, Dudiak KM, Fletcher JG, Clain JE et al. Gastroenterology 2001;121(5):1064–1072.

77. Darge K, Anupindi SA, Jaramillo D. Magn Reson Imaging Clin N Am 2008;16(3):467–478; vi.

78. Makowiec F, Jehle EC, Starlinger M. Gut 1995;37(5):696–701.

79. Maglinte DD, Reyes BL, Harmon BH et al. AJR Am J Roentgenol 1996;167(6):1451–1455.

80. Maglinte DD, Gage SN, Harmon BH. Radiology 1993;188(1):61–64.

81. Walsh SE, Bender GN, Timmons JH. Emerg Radiol 1998;5:29–37.

36

Imaging of Nephrolithiasis and Its Complications in Adults and Children

Lynn Ansley Fordham, Julia R. Fielding, Richard W. Sutherland,
Debbie S. Gipson, and Kimberly E. Applegate

Issues

Imaging of Nephrolithiasis in Adults

   I. What is the appropriate test when there is clinical suspicion of obstructing ureteral stone in adults?
   II. How should stones be followed after treatment in adults?
   III. Special case: the pregnant patient

Imaging of Nephrolithiasis in Children

   IV. What are the clinical findings that raise the suspicion for stones in children?
   V. What is the diagnostic performance of the different imaging studies in nephrolithiasis and urinary tract calculi in the pediatric population?
   VI. What is the role of repeat imaging in children with known stone? In children with recurrent symptoms (suggesting obstructing stone)?

Imaging of Nephrolithiasis in Adults and Children

   VII. What is the natural history of nephrolithiasis and urinary tract calculi and what are the roles of medical therapy versus extracorporeal shock-wave lithotripsy or surgical management in both adults and children?
   VIII. Special Case: Will the stone pass on its own (adults and children)?

L.A. Fordham (✉)
Department of Radiology, University of North Carolina, North Carolina Children's Hospital,
3323 Old Clinic Building, Chapel Hill, NC 27599, USA
e-mail: fdh@med.unc.edu

L.S. Medina et al. (eds.), *Evidence-Based Imaging: Improving the Quality of Imaging in Patient Care, Revised Edition,*
DOI 10.1007/978-1-4419-7777-9_36, © Springer Science+Business Media, LLC 2011

Key Points

Nephrolithiasis in Adults

- Low radiation dose, noncontrast-enhanced computed tomography (MDCT) with 2.5-mm image reconstruction in at least one plane is the test of choice for the patient with a suspected obstructing ureteral stone. In the absence of an available MDCT scanner, intravenous urography (IVU) or a combination of plain radiograph (KUB) and ultrasonography (US) should be performed (moderate evidence).
- Plain radiograph may be used to follow the descent of stones along the ureter (moderate evidence).
- For the pregnant patient when US is not diagnostic, MRI avoids ionizing radiation and may be useful with suspected nephroureterolithiasis (insufficient evidence).

Nephrolithiasis in Children

- The clinical presentation of pediatric nephroureterolithiasis can be nonspecific (moderate evidence).
- A single abdominal radiograph (KUB) is recommended as the initial screening test (moderate evidence).
- The intravenous urogram (IVU) is no longer used for evaluating children for renal stones but has a limited role after complex ureteral surgery (moderate evidence).
- Ultrasound is the most frequently used imaging test for young children with suspected stones, but has a wide range of sensitivity and specificity because of limitations inherent in the modality and because it is user dependent (moderate evidence).
- MDCT is highly sensitive for the detection of nephrolithiasis and urinary tract calculi but incurs added cost and ionizing radiation (moderate evidence).
- In older and/or larger children, MDCT is the imaging modality of choice to evaluate for nephrolithiasis and urinary tract calculi. The ability to localize renal, ureteral, and bladder calculi and the inherent high spatial resolution allow exact anatomic detail that may be helpful for surgical planning (moderate evidence).
- MR is not currently recommended for evaluation of renal stones but shows promise for imaging in obstruction (limited evidence).

Definition and Pathophysiology

Urolithiasis is the presence of stones within the urinary tract. Some patients with stones in the kidney live out their lives without incident. Many patients suffer from hematuria as the stones grow and move within the renal pelvis and experience severe flank pain when the stone(s) become lodged in the ureter. The most common renal stones in the USA are calcium based and are formed at the tip of the papilla when excess calcium is excreted into the urine. Less common stone varieties include those made of uric acid, struvite (ammonium/magnesium/phosphate), cystine, and xanthine.

Epidemiology

Urolithiasis is the presence of stones anywhere in the collecting system within the urinary tract. Nephrolithiasis is defined as calculi within the collecting system in the kidney.

Nephrocalcinosis is defined as calcification within the renal parenchyma. Nephrocalcinosis can be further subdivided into cortical and medullary. Patients with nephrocalcinosis can also have nephrolithiasis or urolithiasis (1). Nephrolithiasis is a common problem of people living in temperate climates. It is estimated that at least 5% of female and 12% of the male population will have at least one episode of renal colic due to stone disease by the age of 70 years (2). In the USA, the majority of stone disease cases are seen in the southeastern part of the country where diet, genetic predisposition, and certain occupations all may predispose to stone formation. Nephrolithiasis is three times more common in males. The peak age for onset of renal stone disease is age 20–30 years, but stone formation is often a lifelong problem.

Urolithiasis is an increasingly common problem in the pediatric population (3). The increasing incidence of urinary system calculi in American children may be due to higher salt intake and inadequate oral hydration in children today. Stone disease can be an incidental finding in children imaged for other reasons or can present with acute symptoms. It accounts for between 1 in 1,000 and 1 in 7,600 pediatric inpatient admissions in North America (4). Most pediatric stones contain calcium, while uric acid stones are the most common cause of radiolucent kidney stones in children.

Medical therapy can be effective and includes encouraging the child in adequate oral hydration as well as therapy targeted to the type of stones formed (4, 5). Surgical intervention is utilized for large or symptomatic stones. With advances in miniaturization of instrument technology in the last two decades, pediatric stone management, similar to the management of adult stones, has changed from an open surgical approach to less invasive surgical procedures such as extracorporeal shock-wave lithotripsy (ESWL) and endoscopic techniques (5–9).

Overall Cost to Society

Because nephrolithiasis is such a common process, the cumulative expense of imaging and clinical evaluations is quite high. In 1995, Clark et al. (10) estimated the annual cost of nephrolithiasis in the USA to be $1.23 billion, with the cost of outpatient evaluation at $278 million. In the intervening years since their publication, the costs have most certainly increased due to higher salt intake, increasing obesity rates leading to more CT utilization and demand for imaging.

Goals

The goal of imaging in the case of nephrolithiasis is twofold: first, to determine the presence or absence of an obstructing ureteral stone; and second, to contribute to treatment planning. In a patient who chronically forms stones, imaging can also be used to follow renal stone burden.

Methodology

A Medline search was performed using PubMed (National Library of Medicine, Bethesda, MD) for original research publications relating the diagnostic performance and accuracy for imaging of nephrolithiasis and UTIs. Clinical indicators of urinary tract disease including hematuria and flank pain were also included. The search covered the period 1966 through May 2010. The search strategy employed different combinations of the following terms (1) *nephrolithiasis, nephrolithiasis, urolithiasis, renal* or *kidney, ureter* or *bladder, calcul(us)(i)* or *stone (?) radiography,* or *imaging,* or *computed tomography,* or *intravenous urography,* or *ultrasound* or *MRI,* (3) *infants and children,* (4) *treatment* or *surgery.* This search was limited to the English language and human studies. Using the limits feature of PubMed and the previously mentioned terms, the database was also searched specifically for clinical trials and meta-analyses. After review of the abstracts of the search results, we reviewed the entire text of relevant articles. In addition, additional pertinent publications were gleaned from a review of the reference lists.

I. What Is the Appropriate Test When There Is Clinical Suspicion of Obstructing Ureteral Stone in Adults?

Summary of Evidence: Patients with clinical signs and symptoms of renal obstruction should undergo unenhanced MDCT of the abdomen and pelvis. The accuracy of this test has been shown to be higher than that of IVU and a combination of US and plain radiograph in level II (moderate evidence) studies. In addition, MDCT is quick to perform and interpret and does not require the administration of intravenous contrast medium. Findings on the MDCT scan can be used by the referring physician to determine treatment. The drawbacks of the technique include cost and a relatively high dose of ionizing radiation, which can range up to 20–25 mSv using a nonoptimized abdominal protocol, and depending on the size of the patient. Careful patient positioning and use dose reduction software will yield radiation doses of 8–10 mSv. When MDCT is not available, either IVU or a combination of plain radiograph and sonography may be used.

Supporting Evidence: For many years, IVU served as the test of choice for identification of obstructing ureteral stones. Following administration of intravenous contrast medium, delayed renal enhancement and excretion and a filling defect within the ureter were diagnostic findings. Because this test dates to the beginning of modern radiology, no prospective studies were performed to determine its accuracy. It was one of the few imaging tests available. In recent years, level II and III (moderate and limited evidence) studies have revealed an accuracy between 85 and 90% (11, 12). Unfortunately, the IVU, while accurate, often requires several hours to perform, requires intravenous access, and is accompanied by contrast administration with its allergy and renal nephrotoxicity risks. In addition, the excretion of contrast into the dilated ureter tends to increase the patient's already severe pain.

An alternative imaging scenario used commonly in Europe and the Far East combines a plain radiograph with an ultrasound examination. In a level II (moderate evidence) study comparing IVU and US in the identification of ureteral stones, both modalities revealed 44 stones for a sensitivity of 64% (13). More recently, unenhanced, low dose MDCT has become the preeminent test for the diagnosis of renal colic in the USA. The low dose MDCT technique has similar sensitivity and specificity for renal and ureteral stone detection when compared to the standard dose technique (14). In one of the largest published series, 210 patients with a confirmed diagnosis for flank pain underwent helical CT (15); 100 stones were recovered and 30 patients were found to

have a source for pain beyond the urinary tract. There were three false negatives and four false positives for stone disease. These data yield a sensitivity of 97%, specificity of 96%, and accuracy of 97% for the diagnosis of obstructing ureteral stone. Of note, all stones are radiodense on CT with the exception of the urinary concretions formed by HIV patients taking protease inhibitors (16, 17). Similar level II (moderate evidence) clinical studies have been performed by multiple groups with reported diagnostic accuracies ranging from 0.90 to 0.97, high interobserver reliability, and accurate depiction of stone size (18–21). Level II (moderate evidence) and level III (limited evidence) studies have also shown that stone size, shape, and location can be used to determine whether the stone will pass spontaneously or is likely to require intervention (18, 20). Stones that are 5 mm or less in size, of regular shape, are located in the distal two-thirds of the ureter, and are present on one or two consecutive CT images 5 mm in thickness are most likely to pass spontaneously. These same studies also demonstrate an alternative source for flank pain in 15% of cases, including ovarian masses, appendicitis, and diverticulitis.

In a level II (moderate evidence) study comparing the combination of plain radiograph and sonography with unenhanced CT in 181 patients with flank pain, CT was found to have a greater sensitivity (92 vs. 77%), negative predictive value (87 vs. 68%), and overall accuracy (94 vs. 83%) for identification of flank pain (22). Sourtzis et al. (11) reported similar results in a level III (limited evidence) study. When CT was compared with both IVU and sonography in 64 patients with recovered ureteral stones, sensitivities were 94, 52, and 19%, respectively (12).

II. How Should Stones Be Followed After Treatment in Adults?

Summary of Evidence: Because plain radiograph has the highest spatial resolution of any imaging modality, has good contrast sensitivity, is inexpensive, and delivers minimal radiation dose, it is at present the best way to follow the passage of a stone down the ureter over time.

Supporting Evidence: Level II and III (moderate and limited evidence) studies report that 60% of ureteral stones are visible on plain radiography (23, 24). The low detection rate is likely due to overlying fecal material and the presence of some radiolucent stones, such as those composed of uric acid. Despite the relatively low detection rate, the use of repeat CT studies is likely not justified because of the cumulative radiation dose. An exception may be made when following the results of lithotripsy and the detection of small intrarenal stone fragments is of importance.

III. Special Case: The Pregnant Patient

Summary of Evidence: There is no compelling published evidence that IVU, plain radiograph, sonography or multidetector CT is the preferred test. Today, however, neither plain radiography nor IVU are performed in favor of cross-sectional imaging. MDCT is highly accurate, but exposes the fetus to ionizing radiation and the risk of later leukemia and solid cancer induction. Therefore, MDCT may still be used as a low dose protocol when MRI is not available. In dealing with the pregnant patient, fetal age and estimated radiation dose is of paramount importance. Pregnant patients routinely have right hydronephrosis as the enlarging uterus turns slightly to the right, compressing the ureter. Noncontrast single phase computed tomography, the most accurate test, delivers approximately 5–25 mSv effective dose to the fetus, depending on the gestational age and MDCT technique used. Two plain radiographs obtained prior to and after administration of intravenous contrast material deliver significantly less radiation, but can be more difficult to interpret because of the overlying bony fetal parts and lateral deviation of the ureters. Dilation of the left ureter is thought to be less common, and the presence of left hydronephrosis with flank pain or hematuria is often enough clinical evidence for clinicians to begin treatment for stone disease.

In order to avoid ionizing radiation exposure to the fetus, many institutions start with ultrasound to detect urinary tract obstruction and ureteral stone, especially in the first and early second trimester as well as to investigate other causes of abdominal pain such as appendicitis (insufficient evidence). When no diagnosis is made, an MRI is typically performed next. In the later second and in the third trimester, it may be more difficult to use ultrasound for determining the cause of abdominal pain so that MRI may be performed first rather than an ultrasound. There is growing but limited evidence that MRI may be useful in pregnant women with acute abdominal pain, including urological diagnoses (25–27).

IV. What Are the Clinical Findings that Raise the Suspicion for Stones in Children?

Summary of Evidence: Children with urolithiasis can present with a wide range of signs and symptoms. Presentations vary depending on whether there is a urinary tract infection or urinary tract obstruction. Children with urolithiasis can present with specific signs and symptoms of flank pain and hematuria or nonspecific symptoms such as irritability and nausea. Many children have an identifiable etiology to their stone disease. Therefore, every child with a urinary stone should have a metabolic evaluation (3, 5, 28). The younger child may present with nonspecific symptoms such as irritability, vomiting, fever, and hematuria. In the older, verbal child, symptoms include flank or abdominal pain and dysuria. Nephrocalcinosis is generally asymptomatic and identified incidentally on evaluation for some other abnormality or identified in the investigation of persistent microscopic hematuria.

Supporting Evidence: VanDervoort et al. (3) retrospectively identified 61 patients from 2003 to 2005 with urolithiasis as their primary diagnosis for their hospital/clinic visit. Patients presented with one or more of the following symptoms: abdominal pain (75%), dysuria (13%), gross hematuria (32%), and urinary tract infection (15%). In a recent study of 123 children who presented with urolithiasis between 1991 and 2003, 76% presented with pain, 15% hematuria, and 10% urinary tract infection (29). Nephrolithiasis can also be asymptomatic in both pediatric and adult populations (30).

Urolithiasis can be related to underlying structural urological abnormalities (11%) and neurogenic bladder (6%). Most commonly, they are related to metabolic abnormalities which include hypercalciuria in 12–50%, hyperoxaluria in 2–20%, hyperuricosuria in 2–10%, and cystinuria in 2–6% (4, 29, 31, 32). Metabolic causes are increasingly common etiologies of stone disease in children with neurogenic bladder due to improvements in management of urinary tract infection (33). Nephrolithiasis is relatively common in preterm infants, affecting 30% of children with chronic lung disease (34–36) and associated with short-term furosemide administration (37). Nephrolithiasis is seen in approximately 1–8% of children on ceftriaxone, and nearly all of these will resolve spontaneously (38, 39). Urolithiasis was reported in approximately 5% of the pediatric renal transplant recipients at a single center (40). Additives in infant formula such as silicate mild thickeners (41) and melamine (42, 43) have also been linked to the formation of renal calculi and renal failure.

V. What Is the Diagnostic Performance of the Different Imaging Studies in Nephrolithiasis and Urinary Tract Calculi in the Pediatric Population?

Summary of Evidence: Noncontrast MDCT is the imaging gold standard for diagnosing or excluding urinary tract calculi (44, 45) (moderate evidence). MDCT allows precise measurements, localization of stone(s), characterization of stone density, stone morphology, and body habitus that can predict the likelihood of successful stone passage or fragmentation with treatment (46–51) (moderate evidence). However, CT utilizes moderately high doses of ionizing radiation and can be expensive. A variety of approaches have been utilized to decrease the dose in MDCT. In addition, protocols using US (52) or a combination of US with CT in selected cases may yield relatively high sensitivity and specificity at lower radiation doses (moderate evidence) (22, 53). Plain radiographs play an important role as well.

Supporting Evidence

Abdominal Radiographs

Plain abdominal radiographs (KUB) are somewhat useful for the detection, localization, and measurement of radiopaque calculi (54–60) performing best for calcium-containing stones greater than 3 mm located over the kidneys or bladder. Scout images from the MDCT, also known as MDCT KUB or Scout KUB exams, are less sensitive and specific for stone detection than conventional KUB (23, 44, 56) (moderate evidence). In a study with stones ranging from 1 to 10 mm on CT, CT scout radiography detected 40% of the renal calculi compared with 52% seen on KUB (61).

Multidetector Computed Tomography

MDCT has very high sensitivity and specificity for detection of nephrolithiasis and urinary tract calculi. It is estimated to be 91–98% sensitive and 91–100% specific in children (58, 62–68) (moderate evidence). Limitations of MDCT include the cost, the occasional need for sedation, and the radiation dose.

MDCT can identify the stone directly, identify secondary findings of obstruction, or identify signs of renal stone passage including periureteral inflammatory changes, ureteral dilatation, and decreased renal attenuation (45, 69). Stone measurements are approximately 12% smaller by CT compared to measurements on KUB. Objects are magnified on plain radiographs and so CT measurements are more accurate (70). CT can evaluate stone density to predict the stone composition (45, 47, 49, 71–74) (moderate evidence) and treatment response including stone passage and fragmentation with lithotripsy (75, 76) (moderate evidence). In one recent study, CT was effective in identifying both dense and lucent residual stone, with 65% more stones detected at CT than antegrade pyelogram (77) (moderate evidence). CT can also be used to differentiate an obstructive stone from a nonobstructive stone (38). It correctly identifies obstructed from nonobstructed systems compared with diuretic renography (78) (moderate evidence). CT can also identify other causes of abdominal pain (79, 80) (moderate evidence).

Radiation dose is a significant issue particularly in the pediatric population, and decreasing the dose is a priority. CT dose is typically tenfold or more higher than a KUB though they can be equivalent (81) if using an ultra-low dose CT techniques (14, 81–88).

Different approaches to dose reduction have been studied (81–83, 85). Reduction in mA reduces radiation dose with an effective dose calculated at 1.4 mSv for males and 2.0 mSv for females in an adult group scanned at a pitch of 1.5 and 50 mA (85). In a recent study on adults using simulated added noise, 35 mA was effective at detecting renal calculi, but less so with ureteral calculi (88). Tube current modulation has also been effective in detecting stones while decreasing dose in the adult population (87). In an adult population, increasing the pitch to 2.5 or 3 decreases the dose with little diminution in image quality or accuracy (89) (limited evidence). CT in adults utilizing low-dose technique of 120 kV, 6.9 effective mA with a mean effective whole-body dose was 0.5 mSv in men and 0.7 mSv in women, and a sensitivity and specificity in detecting patients with calculi was 97 and 95% for CT compared with 67 and 90% for ultrasound in the same group (81) (moderate evidence).

Intravenous Urogram

Intravenous urogram is rarely utilized in the evaluation of the child with urolithiasis. It is occasionally used to evaluate the position of the ureters prior to or after complex urological surgery. CT is more effective than IVU both in stone detection (64, 89) and in identifying obstruction (12, 90). CT and IVU are equivalent in detecting obstruction (89). There is a moderate radiation dose with IVU calculated to be approximately 3.0–3.6 mSv in adults (89, 91, 92). The dose in children will depend on the age and size of the child, gender, and number of radiographs obtained. In a recent prospective randomized study of 200 patients presenting to the emergency room, CT was more sensitive and specific, but there was no difference in clinical outcomes between the IVU and the CT groups (92) (moderate evidence).

Ultrasound

Ultrasound has many advantages including low cost, no need for patient sedation, lack of ionizing radiation, and portability. Limitations of ultrasound include potential incomplete visualization of the entire urinary tract due to body habitus or overlying bowel gas (12, 59, 68, 93, 94) and variable skill levels among imagers as ultrasound is operator dependent. In general, children are easier to image than adults

due to their smaller body habitus. The range of reported sensitivities and specificities is broad. Improvements in technique, transducer design, and image processing continue to lead to improved image quality. Fluid ingestion has been shown to decrease visualization of the ureter in adults (95). In a prospective study of fasting adult patients with a full urinary bladder, urolithiasis was identified by US in 291 of 296 patients with urolithiasis. The five cases not identified by US were seen by CT ($n=3$), IVU ($n=1$), or by passing a stone ($n=1$) (52) (moderate evidence). US detection of hydronephrosis in the ER setting in adults with flank pain and hematuria has a reported 83% sensitivity and 92% specificity for the diagnosis of renal colic (96).

In one small retrospective study in children, all renal tract calculi seen on plain radiograph were also identified on sonography (53) (limited evidence). In a prospective study in 62 adults with proven ureterolithiasis, US was 93% sensitive and 95% specific compared with CT, which was 91 and 95%, respectively (94). In adults, ultrasound demonstrates 67–77% of renal calculi in the right kidney and 53–54% of the calculi in the left kidney compared with CT (67).

The renal artery resistive index has been shown to be useful in some studies for acute obstruction (97–100) but less so in others (101). The difference may be due to the timing or whether there is complete obstruction (102). Asymmetric ureteral jets can also help to identify obstruction (98, 100, 103–105) (moderate evidence). Three-dimensional reconstruction is another US technique which may prove helpful though the data are limited to date (106).

KUB Plus US

A combination of US and plain radiograph can improve the diagnostic performance of US while keeping the radiation dose relatively low (22, 53, 59, 93, 107, 108). In a prospective study of 66 adults, CT had a higher sensitivity and negative predictive value than the combination of KUB and ultrasound for the detection of urolithiasis. When stone visualization and signs of obstruction were combined the sensitivity and specificity of CT was 100% compared with 100% sensitivity and 90% specificity for KUB with US. All stones missed by the combination of KUB with US passed spontaneously (107) (moderate evidence). KUB with US using tissue harmonic imaging had a sensitivity of 96% and specificity of 91% compared with CT (108) (moderate evidence).

Ultrasound Followed by MDCT for Equivocal Cases

In a small retrospective study in 20 children, US was an effective screening tool with CT used as an adjunct in equivocal cases (109) (limited evidence). In a prospective study of 560 patients with unilateral flank pain, urolithiasis was identified by KUB and US in approximately 60% of the patients. CT was obtained in the remaining 40%; 60% of that group were found to have urolithiasis, 6% other diagnoses, and no etiology was identified for flank pain in the remainder (59) (moderate evidence).

Magnetic Resonance Imaging

MR has also been studied in adults. In a study of 51 adults, an MR urogram was used to select a level for targeted CT, which led to a fivefold decrease in radiation dose and was 98% specific compared with CT of the entire urinary tract (110) (moderate evidence). In another study in 64 adults, the combination of MR (HASTE sequence) and KUB was compared with noncontrasted CT. CT revealed more ureteral calculi than the combination of plain radiograph and MR while ureteral dilatation of perinephric stranding were more reliably detected with MR (111) (moderate evidence). MR urography compares favorably with conventional urography and noncontrast MDCT (112). MR is less sensitive than MDCT in the detection on obstructing renal calculi, but it is better than MDCT in identifying the noncalculus etiologies of urinary obstruction in patients with diminished renal function (113) (moderate evidence).

Special Case: Bladder Calculi

Bladder calculi are seen in children with dysfunctional bladder (e.g., neurogenic bladder), prior bladder surgery such as bladder augmentation (114–116), and from other infectious and metabolic causes (117, 118). These stones may be much larger and therefore easier to detect with a simple radiograph. Imaging strategies are similar to stone disease in the upper urinary tract (65).

VI. What Is the Role of Repeat Imaging in Children with Known Stone? In Children with Recurrent Symptoms (Suggesting Obstructing Stone)?

Summary of Evidence: After initial treatment, small residual stones may be asymptomatic and either remain in the kidney or pass on their own. Unfortunately, initial "clinically insignificant residual fragments" (CIRF) can become clinically symptomatic (119–121). Residual fragments can act as a nidus for new stone growth and subsequent symptoms (121). Secondary surgical procedures or medical treatment for residual stones requires accurate location of the remaining stones and the stone size and volume. Noncontrasted MDCT scan is the most sensitive radiologic procedure to identify residual stones. Repeat imaging is also utilized as a monitoring tool to assess the adequacy of preventive measures. Asymptomatic patients are monitored using ultrasound to avoid additional radiation exposure.

Supporting Evidence: During the era of open surgery for urolithiasis, the goal of treatment was to render the patient completely free of stones. With less morbid procedures that can be easily repeated, such as ESWL and endoscopy, success has been redefined as rendering the patient free of symptomatic stones but with small clinically insignificant residual stones (CIRF) (122). Future less invasive procedures can be performed if the fragments become symptomatic. Patients with small (<4 mm) residual stone fragments that are asymptomatic have a higher rate of future symptomatic stones presenting with fever, pain, obstruction, and infection as well as renal damage compared to patients who are rendered completely stone free: 6–15% versus 17–80% (119, 120, 123, 124). Stone position and the amount of residual stones will determine which technique will be most effective. Lower pole stones are poorly treated with ESWL and are best treated with ureteroscopy or PCNL (125). Upper pole, middle portion, and renal pelvis stones can be treated with subsequent ESWL, endoscopy, or PCNL. Abdominal radiography is effective in detecting dense calculi larger than 5 mm in size (50) (moderate evidence). MDCT is more sensitive for small fragments (126). Follow-up may not be required in patients who do not have residual fragments (127) (moderate evidence).

VII. What Is the Natural History of Nephrolithiasis and Urinary Tract Calculi and What Are the Roles of Medical Therapy Versus extracorporeal shock-wave lithotripsy or Surgical Management in Both Adults and Children?

Summary of Evidence: The natural history of urolithiasis is dependent on the chemical composition of the stone and on the stone size. Many stones of size <2–4 mm will pass on their own. Larger stones generally require either medical chemolysis or surgical intervention. Recurrent stones are common.

Supporting Evidence: In the USA, nephrolithiasis is identified in 1 in 1,000 to 1 in 7,600 hospital admissions. Stones are found most commonly in Caucasian patients and rarely in African-American children. The prevalence of urinary stones varies by region, being more common in the southeastern United States (128). Most children with urolithiasis (75–85%) will be found to have an underlying cause for stone formation, including metabolic abnormalities (52%), urinary tract infection (19%), and structural abnormality in the remainder (31, 128–131). The recurrence risk for stones is estimated to be approximately 5% per year in adults or 50% over a 10-year period (132). For children, conservative estimates are similar with an approximate 6% annual recurrence risk (133). Given this recurrence risk, targeted intervention to reduce or eliminate the underlying stone risk is coupled with routine monitoring for stone recurrence and adjustment of therapeutic interventions (134).

Medical chemolysis with oral potassium citrate is possible, particularly for uric acid stones. It may take several weeks and only 50% of the stones resolve completely (134–136). Medical therapy can also be utilized to facilitate stone passage (137). The other types of stones pass spontaneously if size permits. If they do not, they will require ESWL or surgical management. All symptomatic stones will require intervention for early resolution of symptoms. The initial treatment of the stones is dependent on the severity of the signs and symptoms. Infected stones associated with obstruction require immediate treatment with decompression of the infected system. Percutaneous nephrostomy tube placement or ureteral stenting is performed until the infection is cleared. Subsequent treatment can be accomplished electively.

Nonurgent surgical treatment of symptomatic stones can be performed utilizing ESWL, percutaneous nephrolithotripsy (PCNL), ureteroscopy with laser lithotripsy, or open surgical removal. ESWL has become the primary treatment for almost all renal stones regardless of size (6–8, 138–140). ESWL is less morbid than other surgical techniques with almost the same success rate. ESWL is less successful in mid-ureteral stones and distal ureteral stones secondary to bowel interference, cystine stones secondary to poor fragmentation, lower pole stones that are dependent in the kidney and do not fall down the ureter once fragmented, and staghorn calculus with a large stone burden (141). Treatment options for these include either PCNL, particularly for lower pole stones, or ureteroscopy with laser lithotripsy for ureteral stones (142, 143). Treatment with ESWL or PCNL has been shown to lead to an improvement in glomerular filtration rate (GFR) in children treated for stone disease (144).

VIII. Special Case: Will the Stone Pass on Its Own (Adults and Children)?

Summary of Evidence: Stone passage is difficult to predict accurately. Smaller stones are more likely to pass than larger stones as are more distal compared with more proximal ureteral stones (48, 145).

Supporting Evidence: The spontaneous passage rate for stones 1 mm in diameter was 87%; for stones 2–4 mm, 76%; for stones 5–7 mm, 60%; for stones 7–9 mm, 48%; and for stones larger than 9 mm, 25%. Spontaneous passage rate as a function of stone location was 48% for stones in the proximal ureter, 60% for mid-ureteral stones, 75% for distal stones, and 79% for ureterovesical junction stones (48). CT can be used in computer models which predict stone passage better than size criteria alone (146). The majority of stones 5 mm or less are likely to pass on their own (147).

Take Home Tables (Tables 36.1 and 36.2)

Table 36.1-36.2 and Figs. 36.1–36.4 serve to highlight key recommendations and supporting evidence.

Table 36.1. Diagnostic performance for CT, US, and IVU in detection of ureteral stones in adults

Lead author	Year of publication	N	Stones+	Test	Sensitivity	Specificity
Catalano	2002	181	82	CT	0.92	0.96
				US + plain radiography	0.77	0.96
Boulay	1999	51	49	CT	1.0	0.96
Sheley	1999	180	87	CT	0.86	0.91
Sourtzis	1999	36	36	CT	1.0	1.0
				IVU	0.66	1.0
Yilmaz	1998	97	64	CT	0.94	0.97
				US	0.19	0.97
				IVU	0.52	0.94
Smith	1996	210	100	CT	0.97	0.96

Reprinted with kind permission of Springer Science+Business Media from Fielding JR, Pruthi RS. In Medina LS, Blackmore CC (eds.): *Evidence-Based Imaging: Optimizing Imaging in Patient Care*. New York: Springer Science+Business Media, 2006.

Table 36.2. Performance characteristics of imaging studies of urolithiasis in children and adults

	Sensitivity (%)	Specificity (%)
Plain radiograph (55, 56, 58, 61, 108)	52–69	82
IVU (11, 12, 64, 89)	52–87	92–100
US (52, 53, 66, 68, 93, 94, 96, 98, 100, 108)	24–100	82–100
US with KUB (22, 93, 107)	77–100	90–100
CT (58, 62–64)	91–98	91–100
CT low dose[a] (81–88)	93–99	86–97
MRI (110–113)	69–93	95–100

Adapted with kind permission of Springer Science+Business Media from Fordham LA, Sutherland RW, Gipson DS. In Medina LS, Applegate KE, Blackmore CC (eds.): *Evidence-Based Imaging in Pediatrics: Optimizing Imaging in Pediatric Patient Care*. New York: Springer Science+Business Media, 2010.
[a] Low-dose MDCT defined as 50 mA technique.

Imaging Case Studies

Case 1: Pediatric

Figure 36.1 shows nephrocalcinosis in a 45-day-old preterm infant treated with repeated doses of Lasix.

Case 2: Pediatric

Figure 36.2 shows ureteral stones with ureteral dilatation identified by ultrasound.

Case 3: Adult

Figure 36.3 shows an adult CT study for nephrolithiasis. Figure 36.4 shows an adult CT study for urinary tract infection.

Suggested Adult Computed Tomography Imaging Protocols

Suspected obstructing ureteral stone: noncontrast-enhanced MDCT performed with 120 kV and the milliamperes (mA) approximately equal to the patient's weight in pounds (to minimize radiation dose). Volumetric data acquisition thickness and table speed vary with scanner type; reconstructed images should be ≤2.5 mm thickness in one plane. Viewing the images using cine mode facilitates stone detection.

Suggested Pediatric Imaging Protocols

Plain Radiograph

Collimated single abdominal radiograph to include the kidneys and the symphysis pubis.

Ultrasound

High-frequency probe (in younger children) 7–12 MHz with evaluation to include the

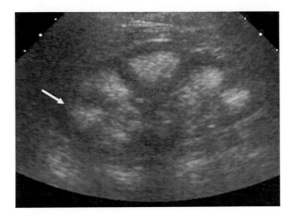

Figure 36.1. Nephrocalcinosis in a 45-day-old preterm infant treated with repeated doses of Lasix. The US image of the right kidney shows echogenic renal pyramids indicating nephrocalcinosis. (Reprinted with kind permission of Springer Science+Business Media from Fordham LA, Sutherland RW, Gipson DS. In Medina LS, Applegate KE, Blackmore CC (eds.): *Evidence-Based Imaging in Pediatrics: Optimizing Imaging in Pediatric Patient Care*. New York: Springer Science+Business Media, 2010.)

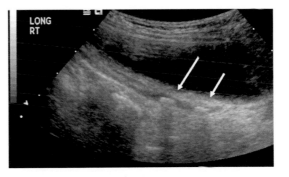

Figure 36.2. Two ureteral stones with ureteral dilatation visualized by sonography through a moderately full urinary bladder which were not identified on plain film. (Reprinted with kind permission of Springer Science+Business Media from Fordham LA, Sutherland RW, Gipson DS. In Medina LS, Applegate KE, Blackmore CC (eds.): *Evidence-Based Imaging in Pediatrics: Optimizing Imaging in Pediatric Patient Care*. New York: Springer Science+Business Media, 2010.)

kidneys, proximal and distal ureters, and urinary bladder. Color Doppler to assess for calcifications.

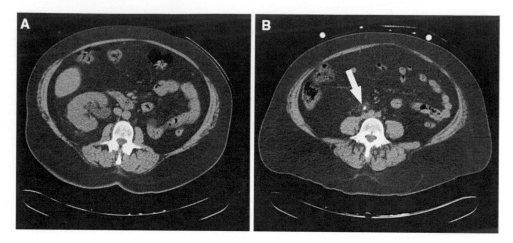

Figure 36.3. Imaging case study for nephrolithiasis. Woman with right flank pain underwent noncontrast-enhanced helical computed tomography (CT) that revealed a solitary right kidney with hydronephrosis (**A**) and an obstructing ureteral stone at the level of the mid-ureter (**B**). (Reprinted with kind permission of Springer Science+Business Media from Fielding JR, Pruthi RS. In Medina LS, Blackmore CC (eds.): *Evidence-Based Imaging: Optimizing Imaging in Patient Care.* New York: Springer Science+Business Media, 2006.)

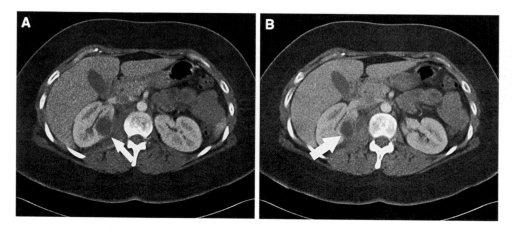

Figure 36.4. Imaging case study of urinary tract infection. Woman with UTI unresponsive to antibiotics for days and with interval development of flank pain and fever. An ovoid right renal mass is hypodense to the adjacent renal parencyma on a contrast-enhanced CT scan (**A**). There is rim enhancement of the developing renal abscess and stranding of the adjacent fat (**B**). (Reprinted with kind permission of Springer Science+Business Media from Fielding JR, Pruthi RS. In Medina LS, Blackmore CC (eds.): *Evidence-Based Imaging: Optimizing Imaging in Patient Care.* New York: Springer Science+Business Media, 2006.)

MDCT

Thin section (=2.5 mm) noncontrast MDCT. Low-dose technique. Recommend low-dose technique of 50 mA. The mA setting will depend on the size of the child; use of the auto mA option is recommended.

MRI

Axial and coronal T1-spin echo, axial and sagittal T2 FSE with fat saturation, coronal STIR or HASTE, axial and coronal T1 2D SPGR with fat saturation before and after intravenous gadolinium (in patients with acceptable renal function).

Alternative to imaging with MDCT. Not as sensitive for calcification, but can provide functional data.

Future Research

- Prospective trial of sonography for the diagnosis/management of obstruction in patients with recurrrent nephroureterolithiasis to potentially reduce both the cost of care and the ionizing radiation dose to this patient population.
- Can MRI replace MDCT in the evaluation of urolithiasis in children (to avoid ionizing radiation)?
- Can findings on imaging (KUB, CT, MR, and ultrasound) predict the likelihood of success of medical therapy alone and provide early triage to surgical therapy?

References

1. Cheidde L, Ajzen SA, Tamer Langen CH, Christophalo D, Heilberg IP. Nephron Clin Pract 2007;106(3):c119 c124.
2. Sierakowski R, Finlayson B, Landes RR et al. Invest Urol 1978;15:438–441.
3. VanDervoort K, Wiesen J, Frank R et al. J Urol 2007;177(6):2300–2305.
4. Bartosh SM. Urol Clin North Am 2004;31(3): 575–587, x–xi.
5. Dogan HS, Tekgul S. Curr Urol Rep 2007;8(2):163–173.
6. Delakas D, Daskalopoulos G, Metaxari M, Triantafyllou T, Cranidis A. J Endourol 2001;15(7):675–680.
7. Smaldone MC, Corcoran AT, Docimo SG, Ost MC. J Urol 2009;181(1):17–28. Epub 2008 Nov 13. Review.
8. D'Addessi A, Bongiovanni L, Sasso F, Gulino G, Falabella R et al. J Endourol 2008;22(1):1–12.
9. D'Addessi A, Bongiovanni L, Racioppi M, Sacco E, Bassi P. J Pediatr Surg 2008;43(4): 591–596.
10. Clark JY, Thompson IM, Optenber SA. J Urol 1995;154:2020–2024.
11. Sourtzis S, Thibeau JF, Damry N, Raslan A, Vandendris M, Bellemans M. AJR Am J Roentgenol 1999;172:1491–1494.
12. Yilmaz S, Sindel T, Arslan G et al. Eur Radiol 1998;8(2):212–217.
13. Sinclair D, Wilson S, Toi A, Greenspan L. Ann Emerg Med 1989;18(5):556–559.
14. Poletti PA, Platon A, Rutschmann OT, Schmidlin FR, Iselin CE et al. AJR Am J Roentgenol 2007; 188(4):927–933.
15. Smith RC, Verga M, McCarthy S, Rosenfield AT. AJR Am J Roentgenol 1996;166:97–101.
16. Blake SP, McNicholas MM, Raptopoulos V. AJR Am J Roentgenol 1998;171(3):717–720.
17. Schwartz BF, Schenkman N, Armenakas NA, Stoller ML. J Urol 1999;161(4):1085–1087.
18. Fielding JR, Silverman SG, Samuel S, Zou KH, Loughlin KR. AJR Am J Roentgenol 1998;171: 1051–1053.
19. Sheley RC, Semonsen KG, Quinn SF. Am J Emerg Med 1999;17(3):279–282.
20. Boulay I, Holtz P, Foley WD, White B, Begun FP. AJR Am J Roentgenol 1999;172:1485–1490.
21. Olcott EW, Sommer FG, Napel S. Radiology 1997;207:19–25.
22. Catalano O, Nunziata A, Altei F, Siani A. AJR Am J Roentgenol 2002;178:379–387.
23. Assi Z, Platt JF, Francis IR, Cohan RH, Korobkin M. AJR Am J Roentgenol 2000;175:333–337.
24. Levine JA, Neitlich J, Verga M, Dalrymple N, Smith RC. Radiology 1997;204(1):27–31.
25. Fielding JR, Chin BM. Magn Reson Imaging 2006;17(6):409–416.
26. Pedrosa I, Zeikus EA, Levine D, Rofsky NM. Radiographics. 2007;27(3):721–743
27. Oto A, Ernst RD, Ghulmiyyah LM, Nishino TK, Hughes D, Chaljub G, Saade G. Abdom Imaging 2009;34(2):243–250.
28. Srivastava T, Alon US. Adolesc Med Clin 2005;16(1):87–109.
29. Sternberg K, Greenfield SP, Williot P, Wan J. J Urol 2005;174(4 Pt 2):1711–1714; discussion 4.
30. Wimpissinger F, Turk C, Kheyfets O, Stackl W. J Urol 2007;178(4 Pt 1):1341–1344; discussion 4.
31. Coward RJ, Peters CJ, Duffy PG et al. Arch Dis Child 2003;88(11):962–965.
32. Acar B, Inci Arikan F, Emeksiz S, Dallar Y. World J Urol 2008;26(6):627–630.
33. Matlaga BR, Kim SC, Watkins SL, Kuo RL, Munch LC et al. J Urol 2006;175(5):1716–1719; discussion 9.
34. Cranefield DJ, Odd DE, Harding JE, Teele RL. Pediatr Radiol 2004;34(2):138–142.
35. Hein G, Richter D, Manz F, Weitzel D, Kalhoff H. Pediatr Nephrol 2004;19(6):616–620.
36. Hoppe B, Duran I, Martin A et al. Pediatr Nephrol 2002;17(4):264–268.
37. Ali SK. Congenit Heart Dis 2006;1(5):251–253.
38. Avci Z, Koktener A, Uras N et al. Arch Dis Child 2004;89(11):1069–1072.
39. Mohkam M, Karimi A, Gharib A et al. Pediatr Nephrol 2007;22(5):690–694.
40. Khositseth S, Gillingham KJ, Cook ME, Chavers BM. Transplantation 2004;78(9):1319–1323.

41. Ulinski T, Sabot JF, Bourlon I, Cochat P. Eur J Pediatr 2004;163(4–5):239–240.
42. Parry J. BMJ 2008;337:a1738.
43. Xin H, Stone R. Science 2008;322(5906): 1310–1311.
44. Chowdhury FU, Kotwal S, Raghunathan G, Wah TM, Joyce A et al. Clin Radiol 2007;62(10):970–977.
45. Akay H, Akpinar E, Ergun O, Ozmen CA, Haliloglu M. Diagn Interv Radiol 2006;12(3): 147–150.
46. Ege G, Akman H, Kuzucu K, Yildiz S. Clin Radiol 2003;58(12):990–994.
47. El-Nahas AR, El-Assmy AM, Mansour O, Sheir KZ. Eur Urol 2007;51(6):1688–1693; discussion 93–94.
48. Coll DM, Varanelli MJ, Smith RC. AJR Am J Roentgenol 2002;178(1):101–103.
49. Ketelslegers E, Van Beers BE. Eur Radiol 2006;16(1):161–165.
50. Olcott EW, Sommer FG, Napel S. Radiology 1997;204(1):19–25.
51. Zarse CA, Hameed TA, Jackson ME et al. Urol Res 2007;35(4):201–206.
52. Park SJ, Yi BH, Lee HK, Kim YH, Kim GJ et al. J Ultrasound Med 2008;27(10):1441–1450.
53. Smith SL, Somers JM, Broderick N, Halliday K. Clin Radiol 2000;55(9):708–710.
54. Tisdale BE, Siemens DR, Lysack J, Nolan RL, Wilson JW. Can J Urol 2007;14(2):3489–3492.
55. Katz D, McGahan JP, Gerscovich EO, Troxel SA, Low RK. J Endourol 2003;17(10):847–850.
56. Zagoria RJ, Khatod EG, Chen MY. AJR Am J Roentgenol 2001;176(5):1117–1122.
57. Jackman SV, Potter SR, Regan F, Jarrett TW. J Urol 2000;164(2):308–310.
58. Eray O, Cubuk MS, Oktay C, Yilmaz S, Cete Y et al. Am J Emerg Med 2003;21(2):152–154.
59. Kobayashi T, Nishizawa K, Watanabe J, Ogura K. J Urol 2003;170(3):799–802.
60. Narepalem N, Sundaram CP, Boridy IC, Yan Y, Heiken JP et al. J Urol 2002;167(3):1235–1238.
61. Ege G, Akman H, Kuzucu K, Yildiz S. Acta Radiol 2004;45(4):469–473.
62. Fielding JR, Steele G, Fox LA, Heller H, Loughlin KR. J Urol 1997;157(6):2071–2073.
63. Nachmann MM, Harkaway RC, Summerton SL et al. Am J Emerg Med 2000;18(6):649–652.
64. Miller OF, Rineer SK, Reichard SR et al. Urology 1998;52(6):982–987.
65. Myers MT, Elder JS, Sivit CJ, Applegate KE. Pediatr Radiol 2001;31(3):135–139.
66. Oner S, Oto A, Tekgul S et al. JBR-BTR 2004;87(5):219–223.
67. Ulusan S, Koc Z, Tokmak N. J Clin Ultrasound 2007;35(5):256–261.
68. Palmer JS, Donaher ER, O'Riordan MA, Dell KM. J Urol 2005;174(4 Pt 1):1413–1416.
69. Goldman SM, Faintuch S, Ajzen SA et al. AJR Am J Roentgenol 2004;182(5):1251–1254.

70. Dundee P, Bouchier-Hayes D, Haxhimolla H, Dowling R, Costello A. J Endourol 2006;20(12): 1005–1009.
71. Deveci S, Coskun M, Tekin MI, Peskircioglu L, Tarhan NC et al. Urology 2004;64(2):237–240.
72. Motley G, Dalrymple N, Keesling C, Fischer J, Harmon W. Urology 2001;58(2):170–173.
73. Perks AE, Schuler TD, Lee J et al. Urology 2008;72(4):765–769.
74. Stolzmann P, Scheffel H, Rentsch K et al. Urol Res 2008;36(3–4):133–138.
75. Kosar A, Sarica K, Aydos K, Kupeli S, Turkolmez K et al. Int J Urol 1999;6(3):125–129.
76. Osman Y, El-Tabey N, Refai H et al. J Urol 2008;179(1):198–200; discussion.
77. Halachmi S, Ghersin E, Ginesin Y, Meretyk S. J Endourol 2007;21(5):473–477.
78. Bird VG, Gomez-Marin O, Leveillee RJ, Sfakianakis GN, Rivas LA et al. J Urol 2002;167(4):1597–1603.
79. Eshed I, Kornecki A, Rabin A, Elias S, Katz R. Eur J Radiol 2002;41(1):60–64.
80. Hoppe H, Studer R, Kessler TM, Vock P, Studer UE et al. J Urol 2006;175(5):1725–1730; discussion 30.
81. Kluner C, Hein PA, Gralla O et al. J Comput Assist Tomogr 2006;30(1):44–50.
82. Heneghan JP, McGuire KA, Leder RA, DeLong DM, Yoshizumi T et al. Radiology 2003;229(2):575–580.
83. Kalra MK, Maher MM, D'Souza RV et al. Radiology 2005;235(2):523–529.
84. Karmazyn B, Frush D, Applegate KE, Maxfield C, Cohen M et al. AJR Am J Roentgenol 2009;192(1):143–149.
85. Kim BS, Hwang IK, Choi YW et al. Acta Radiol 2005;46(7):756–763.
86. Liu W, Esler SJ, Kenny BJ, Goh RH, Rainbow AJ et al. Radiology 2000;215(1):51–54.
87. Mulkens TH, Daineffe S, De Wijngaert R et al. AJR Am J Roentgenol 2007;188(2):553–562.
88. Paulson EK, Weaver C, Ho LM et al. AJR Am J Roentgenol 2008;190(1):151–157.
89. Niall O, Russell J, MacGregor R, Duncan H, Mullins J. J Urol 1999;161(2):534–537.
90. Wong SK, Ng LG, Tan BS et al. Ann Acad Med Singapore 2001;30(6):568–572.
91. Eikefjord EN, Thorsen F, Rorvik J. AJR Am J Roentgenol 2007;188(4):934–939.
92. Mendelson RM, Arnold-Reed DE, Kuan M et al. Australas Radiol 2003;47(1):22–28.
93. Ather MH, Jafri AH, Sulaiman MN. BMC Med Imaging 2004;4(1):2.
94. Patlas M, Farkas A, Fisher D, Zaghal I, Hadas-Halpern I. Br J Radiol 2001;74(886):901–904.
95. Ozden E, Gogus C, Turkolmez K, Yagci C. J Ultrasound Med 2005;24(12):1651–1657.
96. Gaspari RJ, Horst K. Acad Emerg Med 2005;12(12):1180–1184.

97. Onur MR, Cubuk M, Andic C, Kartal M, Arslan G. Urol Res 2007;35(6):307–312.

98. Pepe P, Motta L, Pennisi M, Aragona F. Eur J Radiol 2005;53(1):131–135.

99. Brkljacic B, Kuzmic AC, Dmitrovic R, Rados M, Vidjak V. Eur Radiol 2002;12(11):2747–2751.

100. Geavlete P, Georgescu D, Cauni V, Nita G. Eur Urol 2002;41(1):71–78.

101. Gurel S, Akata D, Gurel K, Ozmen MN, Akhan O. J Ultrasound Med 2006;25(9):1113–1120; quiz 21–23.

102. Coley BD, Arellano RS, Talner LB, Baker KG, Peterson T et al. Acad Radiol 1995;2(5): 373–378.

103. Burge HJ, Middleton WD, McClennan BL, Hildebolt CF. Radiology 1991;180(2): 437–442.

104. Cvitkovic Kuzmic A, Brkljacic B, Rados M, Galesic K. Eur J Radiol 2001;39(3):209–214.

105. Leung VY, Chu WC, Yeung CK, Metreweli C. Pediatr Radiol 2007;37(5):417–425.

106. Volkmer BG, Nesslauer T, Kuefer R, Engel O, Kraemer SC et al. Ultrasound Med Biol 2002; 28(2):143–147.

107. Ripolles T, Agramunt M, Errando J, Martinez MJ, Coronel B, Morales M. Eur Radiol 2004;14(1): 129–136.

108. Mitterberger M, Pinggera GM, Pallwein L et al. BJU Int 2007;100(4):887–890.

109. Eshed I, Witzling M. Pediatr Radiol 2002;32(3): 205–208.

110. Blandino A, Minutoli F, Scribano E et al. J Magn Reson Imaging 2004;20(2):264–271.

111. Regan F, Kuszyk B, Bohlman ME, Jackman S. Br J Radiol 2005;78(930):506–511.

112. Sudah M, Vanninen RL, Partanen K et al. Radiology 2002;223(1):98–105.

113. Shokeir AA, El-Diasty T, Eassa W et al. J Urol 2004;171(6 Pt 1):2303–2306.

114. DeFoor W, Minevich E, Reddy P et al. J Urol 2004;172(5 Pt 1):1964–1966.

115. Hernandez DJ, Purves T, Gearhart JP. J Pediatr Urol 2008;4(6):460–466.

116. Roberts WW, Gearhart JP, Mathews RI. J Urol 2004;172(4 Pt 2):1706–1708; discussion 9.

117. Salah MA, Holman E, Khan AM, Toth C. J Pediatr Surg 2005;40(10):1628–1631.

118. Sayasone S, Odermatt P, Khammanivong K et al. Southeast Asian J Trop Med Public Health 2004;35(suppl 2):50–52.

119. Candau C, Saussine C, Lang H, Roy C, Faure F et al. Eur Urol 2000;37(1):18–22.

120. Streem SB, Yost A, Mascha E. J Urol 1996; 155(4):1186–1190.

121. Zanetti G, Seveso M, Montanari E et al. J Urol 1997;158(2):352–355.

122. Miles SG, Kaude JV, Newman RC, Thomas WC, Williams CM. AJR Am J Roentgenol 1988;150(2): 307–309.

123. Afshar K, McLorie G, Papanikolaou F et al. J Urol 2004;172(4 Pt 2):1600–1603.

124. Osman MM, Alfano Y, Kamp S et al. Eur Urol 2005;47(6):860–864.

125. Cannon GM, Smaldone MC, Wu HY et al. J Endourol 2007;21(10):1179–1182.

126. Kupeli B, Gurocak S, Tunc L, Senocak C, Karaoglan U et al. Int Urol Nephrol 2005;37(2):225–230.

127. Karadag MA, Tefekli A, Altunrende F, Tepeler A, Baykal M et al. J Endourol 2008;22(2):261–266.

128. Gillespie RS, Stapleton FB. Pediatr Rev 2004;25(4):131–139.

129. Stapleton FB, McKay CP, Noe HN. Pediatr Ann 1987;16(12):980–981, 4–92.

130. Diamond DA. Br J Urol 1991;68(2):195–198.

131. Perrone HC, dos Santos DR, Santos MV et al. Pediatr Nephrol 1992;6(1):54–56.

132. Menon M, Resnick MI. In Walsh PC, Retik AB, Vaughan ED Jr et al. (eds.): Campbell's Urology, 8th ed. Philadelphia: WB Saunders, 2002;3276.

133. Diamond DA, Menon M, Lee PH, Rickwood AM, Johnston JH. J Urol 1989;142(2 Pt 2):606–608; discussion 19.

134. Dello Strologo L, Laurenzi C, Legato A, Pastore A. Pediatr Nephrol 2007;22(11):1869–1873.

135. Hoffman N, McGee SM, Hulbert JC. Urology 2003;61(5):1035.

136. Sarica K, Erturhan S, Yurtseven C, Yagci F. J Endourol 2006;20(11):875–879.

137. Hollingsworth JM, Rogers MA, Kaufman SR et al. Lancet 2006;368(9542):1171–1179.

138. Wadhwa P, Aron M, Seth A, Dogra PN, Hemal AK et al. J Endourol 2007;21(2):141–144.

139. Brinkmann OA, Griehl A, Kuwertz-Broking E, Bulla M, Hertle L. Eur Urol 2001;39(5):591–597.

140. Tanaka ST, Makari JH, Pope JC, Adams MC, Brock JW, 3rd, Thomas JC. J Urol 2008;180(5):2150–2153; discussion 3–4.

141. Tan MO, Kirac M, Onaran M, Karaoglan U, Deniz N et al. Urol Res 2006;34(3):215–221.

142. El-Assmy A, Hafez AT, Eraky I, El-Nahas AR, El-Kappany HA. J Endourol 2006;20(4):252–255.

143. Erturhan S, Yagci F, Sarica K. J Endourol 2007;21(4):397–400.

144. Wadhwa P, Aron M, Bal CS, Dhanpatty B, Gupta NP. J Endourol 2007;21(9):961–966.

145. Erdodru T, Aker O, Kaplancan T, Erodlu E. Int Braz J Urol 2002;28(6):516–521.

146. Parekattil SJ, Kumar U, Hegarty NJ et al. J Urol 2006;175(2):575–579.

147. Pietrow PK, Karellas ME. Am Fam Physician 2006;74(1):86–94.

37

Urinary Tract Infection in Infants and Children

Carol E. Barnewolt, Leonard P. Connolly, Carlos R. Estrada, and Kimberly E. Applegate

Issues

I. What is known about the natural history of urinary tract infections in infants and children?
II. What can imaging reveal in the setting of UTI?
III. What are reasonable imaging strategies when caring for a male infant or child with a history of a febrile urinary tract infection?
IV. What are reasonable imaging strategies when caring for a female infant or child with a history of a febrile urinary tract infection?
V. Special case: postnatal management of fetal hydronephrosis

Key Points

- The presence of fever, in the setting of an appropriately collected urine specimen and positive urine culture, reasonably distinguishes between cystitis (lower tract) and pyelonephritis (upper tract) infections (moderate evidence).
- Pyelonephritis, and hence renal scarring, can occur with or without the existence of vesicoureteric reflux (VUR) (strong evidence).
- Infants and children with their first febrile UTI should undergo imaging workup to detect congenital anomalies or high-grade VUR [with US and voiding cystourethrography (VCUG)] that increase the risk of renal scar and later dysfunction (limited evidence).
- Higher grades of upper urinary tract obstruction alone, without complicating factors such as stones or infection, may lead to progressive, focal renal damage, and progressive loss of renal function (moderate evidence).
- Unrelieved bladder outlet obstruction, caused by posterior urethral valves or neurogenic bladder, predisposes to infection and may result

C.E. Barnewolt (✉)
Department of Radiology, Children's Hospital Boston, 300 Longwood Avenue, Boston, MA 02115, USA
e-mail: carol.barnewolt@childrens.harvard.edu

L.S. Medina et al. (eds.), *Evidence-Based Imaging: Improving the Quality of Imaging in Patient Care, Revised Edition*,
DOI 10.1007/978-1-4419-7777-9_37, © Springer Science+Business Media, LLC 2011

in progressive voiding dysfunction, VUR, renal scarring, and dysplasia (strong evidence).

■ Low-grade VUR (grades I–III), in the absence of infection, is unlikely to result in progression of renal scarring (moderate evidence).

■ High-grade VUR (grades IV–V) is more likely than low-grade VUR to be associated with renal cortical scarring and with recurrent UTI (moderate evidence).

■ There is insufficient evidence that early detection of urinary tract obstruction, VUR, and/or renal scarring after UTI in infants and children, and instigation of therapy, either medical or surgical, minimizes or prevents further scarring (insufficient evidence).

■ There is insufficient evidence that instigation of low-dose prophylactic antibiotic therapy, after identification of urinary tract obstruction, lower grades of VUR, and/or renal scarring prevents development of recurrent infection and further scars (insufficient evidence). In addition, antibiotic prophylaxis leads to higher rates of resistant infections (limited to moderate evidence).

■ There is insufficient evidence that elimination of VUR with surgical reimplantation or endoscopic introduction of antireflux agents prevents development of recurrent infection and further scars (insufficient evidence).

Definitions and Pathophysiology

Cystitis is defined as inflammation or infection of the bladder and most commonly occurs from retrograde ascent of perineal bacteria up the urethra into the bladder. After infancy, girls, with much shorter urethras than boys, have an eightfold higher incidence.

The diagnosis of a febrile UTI is made when a urine culture produces growth of greater than 100,000 colony forming units per cubic centimeter of a single pathogen, from an adequately obtained urine specimen (a catheterized or suprapubic specimen in infants), in the setting of a fever of $\geq 38°C$. Fever is evidence for the presence of pyelonephritis (an upper tract infection), without the need for direct imaging evidence. The vast majority of infections in infants and children are caused by *Escherichia coli*. Non-*E. coli* infections tend to occur with greater frequency in boys and in association with underlying genitourinary abnormalities such as urinary tract obstruction or VUR. Infections with Enterobacteria and *Enterococci* also occur in young girls, *Staphylococcus aureus* in adolescent girls, and Proteus in young boys (1–3).

Pyelonephritis can result from blood-borne infection, particularly in the newborn period.

However, some infants and children with pyelonephritis acquire the renal infection by ascent of bacteria from the bladder (4–6), perhaps as a result of reflux of infected urine from the bladder. Some data indicate that higher grades of VUR, in combination with high fever and elevated C-reactive protein, have a tenfold increase in risk of persistent scars (7). Animal studies suggest that certain bacterial properties, such as those of the P-fimbriated *E. coli*, allow bacterial ascent without the presence of VUR (8, 9).

Finally, histologic examination of scarred kidneys that were surgically removed, in particular from young, refluxing males, shows focal renal dysplasia along side of segmental scarring. This raises the question that some observed renal abnormalities may be congenital in nature, rather than acquired from infection (10).

VUR is a congenital condition that most often resolves spontaneously in infancy or early childhood. In infants and children diagnosed with UTI, one-third will have VUR (11). VUR is more common in girls and has a peak age of detection before age 2 years. Family history and Caucasian race are risk factors for VUR. It is graded on a one to five scale: grade I is reflux from the bladder into the distal ureter, but not into the renal collecting system; grade II reflux extends into the renal collecting system; grade III reflux causes distention of the ureter and renal collecting system; grade IV reflux results in tortuosity of the dilated ureter; and grade V shows marked dilation and tortuosity of the ureter and renal collecting system with marked calyceal blunting.

Epidemiology

Urinary tract infection is one of the most common infections in children with approximately 19 episodes per 1,000 children annually. During the first 6 years of life, 8% of all girls and 2% of all boys will have a symptomatic UTI (12). In *febrile* infants and children, somewhere between 1 and 17% will prove to have a UTI (1, 12, 13). Results of DMSA scans performed soon after a first UTI in children 2 years of age and younger suggest that 75% of these children with coexisting fever and bacteriuria will prove to have pyelonephritis (14). Caucasian girls with fever are more likely to have a UTI than African American girls or boys of any ethnicity (15, 16). Uncircumcised male infants also have an increased risk of UTI in the first few months of life (17–20).

Even in children with no identifiable urinary tract abnormality, recurrent febrile UTIs cause significant morbidity. In a study of 850 children, 45% of girls and 14% of boys had recurrent UTI. In those with a negative-imaging workup (renal US and VCUG) after febrile UTI, 28% of girls and 4% of boys developed a recurrent febrile UTI (21). UTI recurrence rates were greater in young uncircumcised boys than in circumcised boys and in children older than 5 years with dysfunctional voiding patterns.

The incidence of VUR in healthy infants and children is estimated at 17–33% (22–27) and decreases with increasing age (Table 37.1) (1–6, 16, 28–39). During the first year of life, boys may have a higher rate and grade of VUR than girls (40–42). The overall incidence of VUR in siblings of infants and children with VUR was found to be about 37% in one study of 482 siblings, with decreasing incidence in older siblings as follows: 46% for siblings under 2 years, 33% for 2–6 years, and only 7% when older than 6 years of age (43). There is no known correlation between index patient reflux grade, sex, or cortical scars with the likelihood of sibling reflux (44).

Overall Cost to Society

In the USA, urinary tract infections account for more than one million outpatient visits among children younger than 18 years, and about 25,000 visits to urologists for evaluation and treatment of VUR annually (45). There were just under 0.1% children hospitalized annually in Australia for UTI (46).

Monetary costs of hospitalization, antibiotic therapy, loss of work for caregivers, imaging evaluation, and complications of infections and therapy have not been scientifically studied in the USA, though there has been some attempt to do so in other countries such as Britain, Australia, and Israel (46–48). It is clear that the approach to treatment and subsequent imaging, despite professional society guidelines, varies greatly from region to region throughout the USA (49–52). The reason for this discrepancy may reflect a lack of evidence to support current recommendations or a lack of awareness or consensus within the medical community (53–56). In fact, a recent review of the clinical effectiveness and cost-effectiveness of tests for the diagnosis and investigation of UTI in children stated that there were insufficient data to support an imaging workup after first UTI in children under 5 years (57).

Goals

There are two immediate goals of imaging in the setting of UTI: (1) to identify urinary tract obstruction and resultant urinary stasis that may warrant surgical intervention to lessen the risk of sepsis, recurrent infection, and preserve renal function; and (2) to prevent the formation and/or minimize the progression of renal scars by identifying patients at increased risk of progressive scar formation. The long-term goal is to prevent the complications of chronic renal scars, namely hypertension, chronic renal failure (CRF), and complications of pregnancy in women. Renal scars may form as a result of pyelonephritis both with and without accompanying VUR (10) (Table 37.1).

Methodology

A Medline search was performed by an experienced, trained medical librarian using PubMed (National Library of Medicine, Bethesda, MD) for original research and review articles, including clinical trials and meta-analyses, targeted at discussing the diagnosis, treatment, and imaging of UTI in infants and children. Both English language and non-English language searches were performed, though the non-English literature was only included if an English translation of the abstract was available and the content deemed vital and worthy of further investigation. Animal studies were included as well. The search covered the years 1966 through October 2008. After review of available abstracts, the entire text of relevant articles were obtained and read in detail by the first author.

I. What Is Known About the Natural History of Urinary Tract Infections in Infants and Children?

Summary of Evidence: It is clear that the approach to treatment and subsequent imaging, despite professional society guidelines, varies greatly from region to region throughout the USA (47–50). The reason for this discrepancy may reflect a perceived and real lack of evidence to support current recommendations (51–54).

Few studies provide us with the long-term outcomes of children with UTI (58), despite the large amount of literature since the earliest UTI study in children and young adults by Bright in the early nineteenth century (59). The modern study of UTIs began in earnest in the mid-twentieth century when children were evaluated with the evolving radiologic tools of VCUG and intravenous urography (IVU), a test only rarely used today (60).

Supporting Evidence: Table 37.1 summarizes the complex and at times conflicting literature that addresses the relationship between UTI, VUR, and renal cortical scarring in various cohorts, beginning in 1964. There is a lack of standardization of diagnostic criteria, imaging techniques, treatment regimes, or patient follow-up.

By following 389 patients with a first UTI, Oh et al. showed that higher grades of VUR (grades IV and V) are associated with the diagnosis of pyelonephritis on Tc-99m DMSA scans, but that later scars are independent of grade of VUR (61). More recent large studies suggest that prophylactic antibiotic therapy does not prevent recurrent UTI and therefore may not prevent progression of renal compromise. Further, surgical or endoscopic correction of VUR may not improve long-term outcome in these children. Wheeler et al. performed a meta-analysis of randomized controlled trials to evaluate the benefits and harms of treatments for VUR in children. They identified eight trials involving 859 evaluable children comparing long-term antibiotics with surgical correction of reflux (VUR) and antibiotics (seven trials), and antibiotics compared with no treatment (one trial). They concluded that there is no clear clinical benefit from identification and treatment of children with VUR. Further, they state "the additional benefit of surgery over antibiotics alone is small at best. Assuming a UTI rate of 20% for children with VUR on antibiotics for 5 years, nine reimplantations would be required to prevent one febrile UTI, with no reduction in the number of children developing any UTI or renal damage" (62).

The incidence of new cases of end-stage renal disease (ESRD) in Australia and New Zealand did not diminish with the use of prophylactic antibiotics and surgical treatment of VUR (63). Craig et al. concluded that "Treatment of children with VUR has not been accompanied by the hoped-for reduction in the incidence of ESRD attributable to reflux nephropathy."

Acute pyelonephritis is not always associated with VUR (2, 5, 6, 16, 28–35, 37–39); renal cortical scars occur in children with a history of UTI but no VUR (5, 6, 34, 35, 37, 38); and one can observe cortical defects, perhaps representing cortical dysplasia, without convincing evidence for antecedent UTI (64).

The prevalence of VUR markedly and spontaneously diminishes in the first few years of life. The likelihood of resolution of VUR increases with decreased grade and with unilateral VUR. Some data suggest that neither gender nor the presence or absence of renal cortical scars effect the rate of VUR resolution (36), while others suggest that resolution of VUR occurs more quickly in boys and in the absence of renal cortical scars (35, 65, 66). For asymptomatic children with low-grade VUR detected in a sibling-screening program, the likelihood of resolution did not vary with age at diagnosis, gender, and whether VUR was unilateral or bilateral (67).

An epidemiologic study from Sweden reports no case of nonobstructive pyelonephritis as a cause of CRF in a review of patients from a period of 1986–1994, perhaps reflecting the success of a screening program (68). On the other hand, a Chilean review of children with CRF reports that 17% of 227 patients resulted from reflux nephropathy (69). The very different economic and medical structures of each country make it impossible to know whether this apparent difference reflects a Chilean weakness in treatment of UTI or screening after UTI.

In 1812, Bell described the anatomy of the ureterovesical junction, explaining the configuration that prevents regurgitation of the urine into the ducts of the kidney, emphasizing the importance of the ureteral obliquity (70). Assuming that reflux of infected urine leads to a high incidence of pyelonephritis and resultant scars, prevention of such reflux should decrease the incidence of scarring, thus improving long-term outcomes. However, studies comparing outcomes of patients treated with prophylactic antibiotic (medical treatment) and antireflux procedures (surgical treatment) have not shown a distinct difference between the two groups (39, 62, 71–87). One paper suggests that males with higher grades of reflux have fewer UTIs with antibiotic prophylaxis therapy than without (88).

II. What Can Imaging Reveal in the Setting of UTI?

Summary of Evidence: Routine imaging during an acute episode of UTI is not necessary to make the diagnosis (moderate evidence). In nonroutine cases that require imaging, the gold standard imaging test to diagnose pyelonephritis is technetium-99m dimercaptosuccinic acid (Tc-99m DMSA) (moderate evidence), although ultrasound (particularly with the use of Doppler) (89), computed tomography (CT), and magnetic resonance imaging (MRI) are used with lower sensitivity and specificity.

After the first episode of UTI in infants and children, most will receive both a renal US and a VCUG in the USA. However, despite a common and recommended practice, a systematic review of the literature does not support imaging children under 5 years (90) (moderate evidence).

Table 37.2 provides information about the diagnostic performance of tests for UTI, pyelonephritis, VUR, and renal scarring. Currently, only the DMSA test can adequately predict the later development of renal scar (moderate evidence).

If the patient is not responding to usual medical therapy, a complication, such as abscess formation, may be suspected. Renal abscesses can be detected with cross-sectional imaging; the choice of US versus CT or MR depends on the size of the child and the availability and experience of the imager. The American College of Radiology has developed appropriateness criteria and provided the estimated radiation exposures for imaging subgroups of children after first UTI (91).

Supporting Evidence

Abdominal Radiographs

Plain radiographs have essentially no role in the evaluation of suspected UTI in infants and children, unless other diagnoses are under consideration. Radiographs can suggest the alternate diagnoses of the gastrointestinal tract, large abdominal masses, and abnormal abdominal/retroperitoneal calcifications.

Sonography

Ultrasound evaluation of the kidneys and bladder is a readily available, safe modality, but is insensitive for the diagnosis of acute pyelonephritis (moderate evidence) and even for the diagnosis of renal abscess. Acute pyelonephritis is suspected with focal swelling, loss of corticomedullary differentiation, and/or a decrease in relative vascularity. Doppler US only marginally improves sensitivity and specificity. It is a useful modality for the qualitative evaluation of urinary tract obstruction at the level of the ureteropelvic junction, ureterovesicular junction, and sometimes for bladder outlet obstruction with the observation of bladder wall thickening. Quantitative grading systems exist for the systematic description of hydronephrosis, though they are not universally adopted (92). Ultrasound provides no direct, quantifiable measure of renal function.

Ultrasound has poor sensitivity and specificity for the identification of VUR (93–101) (moderate evidence). Specifically, the observation of hydronephrosis does not indicate the presence of VUR, and the absence of hydronephrosis does not exclude the diagnosis of VUR. These limitations may be improved with documentation of changes in collecting system caliber (102).

Intravenous Pyelogram

Prior to the era of cross-sectional imaging, intravenous pyelogram was the mainstay of urologic imaging. It has the advantages of availability and assessment of renal function, obstruction, and overall anatomy. It has the disadvantages of venipuncture, risk of iodinated contrast reaction, and exposure to ionizing radiation. It is insensitive, when compared to Tc-99m DMSA, for detection of both acute infection and cortical scars. It has no role in the diagnosis or exclusion of VUR. Therefore, its role is limited to patients with complex ureteral anatomy or postoperative ureteral obstructions.

CT and MRI/MR Urography

Contrast-enhanced CT and MR do not play a role in routine UTI, although they may detect pyelonephritis during emergent imaging of a child with abdominal pain. CT and MR have lower sensitivity and specificity, on average, compared to DMSA for the detection of pyelonephritis and renal scar. Both provide moderate sensitivity and specificity for pyelonephritis, cortical scarring, abscess formation, urinary tract obstruction, and anatomic variants such as subtle duplex systems (103–107). In the case of CT and MR contrast agents, adverse reactions have been reported. Gadolinium administration with MRU is accompanied by risk of nephrogenic systemic fibrosis if the child has renal dysfunction (108).

Nuclear Medicine

Tc-99m DMSA is the gold standard for detection of both acute pyelonephritis, with the observation of flare-shaped regions of decreased radioactivity, and renal scars, as indicated by focal loss of cortical bulk (109). It is far more sensitive and specific in general than is ultrasound and CT/MR. It has the disadvantages of the need for venipuncture to administer the radiopharmaceutical and exposure to radiation.

Tc-99m MAG3 and Tc-99m DTPA each provide quantifiable data to diagnose and exclude urinary tract obstruction, often using intravenous furosemide challenge. Tc-99m MAG3 provides little other anatomic detail. Tc-99m DTPA can be used to assess physiologic parameters such as differential renal function, renal plasma flow, and glomerular filtration. Both also require venipuncture to administer the radiopharmaceutical and exposure to radiation.

Evaluation for Vesicoureteric Reflux

The only reliable way to diagnose or exclude VUR is with a voiding cystogram, either VCUG using iodinated contrast agents and fluoroscopy or radionuclide cystogram (RNC) using the radiotracer Tc-99m pertechnetate, instilled along with saline into the urinary bladder, with continuous observation with a gamma camera during the filling and voiding phases. Both require placement of a urethral catheter, which can be an uncomfortable procedure, particularly in inexperienced hands. While briefly uncomfortable, the examination is generally not associated with complications (110). Both tests use small amounts of ionizing radiation. Though the development of pulsed fluoroscopy equipment has lessened the discrepancy in dose between the two studies, RNC continues to have lower exposures than does VCUG (103–105, 111). However, RNC is less available in general and community hospitals and, therefore, fluoroscopic VCUG is more commonly performed. Contrast-enhanced ultrasound for VCUG is used in Europe to avoid ionizing radiation, but the contrast agents are not approved for use in the USA.

III. What Are Reasonable Imaging Strategies When Caring for a Male Infant or Child with a History of a Febrile Urinary Tract Infection?

Summary of Evidence: In boys, the incidence of infection, beyond the newborn period, is lower than in girls, and the grade of VUR tends to be higher in neonatal boys than in girls (42, 112). Some boys that present with first UTI will have posterior urethral valves, a correctable, mechanical obstruction to urinary flow. Therefore, most current guidelines state that renal US and fluoroscopic VCUG are recommended to identify upper urinary obstruction and/or posterior urethral valves (limited evidence). Renal US alone is inadequate for the evaluation of VUR and renal scar (96) (moderate evidence). These recommendations are emphasized in children under 5 years when detection of urinary system obstructive lesions, the presence of VUR, and the risk of renal scar are higher (limited evidence).

Figures 37.1A and 37.2A provide an imaging strategy for boys, depending on local confidence and use of antibiotic prophylaxis. Evidence is building that the use of antibiotic prophylaxis is not associated with improved outcomes, though data are lacking for higher grades of VUR. Additionally, surgical correction of higher grades of VUR may provide improved outcomes. This strategy, therefore, allows identification of obstruction and VUR, but incorporates evolving data, supporting a watch and wait approach to lower grades of VUR (113).

Supporting Evidence: Ultrasound is readily available, requires no sedation, does not use ionizing radiation, and can identify higher grades of obstruction, but does not identify VUR reliably (114). Widespread prenatal ultrasound has decreased the incidence of obstruction presenting as UTI, not all fetuses are screened, the quality of screening varies widely between geographic areas, and variation in maternal body habitus can effect the sensitivity of this tool (115, 116). Therefore, ultrasound is included as a first-line screen.

VCUG, rather than RNC, is employed to allow the diagnosis or exclusion of posterior urethral valves and to identify VUR. The incidence of PUV is 1 in 5,000–8,000 live male births (117). Modern equipment, and in particular pulsed fluoroscopic techniques, keeps radiation exposure low (118–120). The goal is to identify higher grades of VUR that warrant either antibiotic prophylaxis, periodic reassessment, or surgical reimplantation, depending on evolving data, local culture, and family preference. The goal of these tests and treatment is to prevent cortical scarring (Figs. 37.3 and 37.4). High-grade VUR, age of diagnosis of VUR greater than 5 years, and male gender were the most significant risk factors for renal scarring in a study of 98 infants and children (121).

Renal cortical scintigraphy with technetium-99m dimercaptosuccinic acid (Tc-99m DMSA) is more sensitive for scars than ultrasound, but is reserved for patients found to have high-grade reflux (89, 109, 122–125). The intention is to use the absence of scars, reliably identified, as a guide to clinical management (126). MRI is an appealing alternative because of its lack of use of ionizing radiation, but it tends to be less widely available and may require sedation of the infant or child (106, 107). Since only a minority of infants and children with proven pyelonephritis will develop scars, DMSA is not recommended for all cases (7, 14, 127, 128).

Finally, a quantitative assessment of obstruction is introduced if ultrasound reveals the presence of moderate to severe hydronephrosis. By definition, this includes kidneys shown to have gross calyceal dilatation, not just pelviectasis, in the absence of VUR. This can be performed with either Tc-99m mercaptoacetyltriglycine (Tc-99m MAG3), Tc-99m diethylenetriamine pentaacetic acid (Tc-99m DTPA), or magnetic resonance urography (MRU). MRU has the advantage of lack of use of ionizing radiation, but tends to be less widely available and may require sedation of the infant or child.

IV. What Are Reasonable Imaging Strategies When Caring for a Female Infant or Child with a History of a Febrile Urinary Tract Infection?

Summary of Evidence: Girls have a much higher incidence of UTI than boys. Similar to recommendations for boys, most current guidelines state that renal US and VCUG are recommended to identify upper urinary obstruction and VUR after first UTI (limited evidence). However, radionuclide cystography (RNC) may be used instead of fluoroscopic VCUG since the urethral anatomy is almost invariably normal. Renal US alone is inadequate for the evaluation of VUR and renal scar (moderate evidence). These recommendations are emphasized in children below 5 years of age when detection of urinary system obstructive lesions, the presence of VUR, and the risk of renal scar are higher (limited evidence).

The imaging strategy for female infants and children with UTI is provided in Figs. 37.1B and 37.2B, depending on local confidence and use of antibiotic prophylaxis.

Supporting Evidence: Ultrasound evaluation of both kidneys and the bladder is used to detect congenital anomalies and obstruction. The reasoning is similar to the situation for boys, with one additional motive: the possible identification of an obstructing ureterocele, usually as part of the upper moiety of a duplex collecting system. While ureteroceles can occur in boys, the incidence is far less in girls (129, 130) (Fig. 37.5). The approach in girls is modified to the use of RNC, a still lower radiation dose technique, rather than VCUG to evaluate for the possibility of VUR (131). If one subscribes to the belief that prophylactic antibiotic use may improve outcomes in the setting of high-grade VUR, the remainder of the scenario is the same for girls as for boys. The use of RNC may be limited to those radiology practices that are experienced and comfortable with children's imaging. Therefore, its use is less common than the fluoroscopic VCUG.

However, should the evidence for the use of prophylactic antibiotic be considered insufficient, the use of RNC is replaced with Tc-99m DMSA. Data suggest that this exam can be used as a surrogate for RNC as a way to eliminate the likelihood of lower grades of VUR, thus eliminating the need for urethral catheterization. This avoids the low, but potential risks and stress that catheterization can cause, even in expert hands (132). If scars are identified, RNC is warranted as a higher grade of VUR may be present, perhaps warranting surgical

reimplantation or periodic reassessment for evidence of progression of renal cortical scarring (Fig. 37.6).

V. Special Case: Postnatal Management of Fetal Hydronephrosis

Summary of Evidence: Fetal sonography detects hydronephrosis in 1–5% of all pregnancies (133). Currently, there has been limited standardization of fetal genitourinary system ultrasound technique and subsequent postnatal evaluation. The postnatal imaging with (a) resolution of hydronephrosis and (b) persistent hydronephrosis varies widely based on a lack of consensus. The most common current recommendation is to perform renal and bladder US in neonates that had moderate to severe prenatal hydronephrosis (insufficient evidence). Some centers also recommend VCUG (or RNC for girls).

Supporting Evidence: A meta-analysis was recently performed to determine whether the degree of antenatal hydronephrosis and related antenatal ultrasound findings are associated with postnatal outcome. Although the risk of VUR was similar for all degrees of fetal hydronephrosis, the risk of any postnatal pathology versus the degree of antenatal hydronephrosis was 12% for mild, 45% for moderate, and 88% for severe fetal hydronephrosis. Overall, children with any degree of antenatal hydronephrosis were at greater risk of postnatal pathology as compared with the normal population. Moderate and severe antenatal hydronephrosis has a significant risk of postnatal pathology, indicating that comprehensive postnatal diagnostic management should be performed. Mild antenatal hydronephrosis may carry a risk for postnatal pathology, but additional prospective studies are needed to determine the optimal management of these children (133).

Infants with a history of mild hydronephrosis may not require postnatal evaluation. Distinction between these two groups assumes that the fetal ultrasound examination attempts to characterize the degree of dilatation, does so correctly, and consistently and accurately conveys this information to the postnatal caregivers. This may not be the case (116).

A recent systematic study, evaluating a group of nearly 500 newborns with thorough prenatal and postnatal evaluation, found a VUR incidence of 9%. This study reports that approximately 75% of those with VUR have low-grade reflux that resolves rapidly (grades I–III), but about one-quarter have a high-grade reflux. In the group with high-grade VUR, spontaneous resolution by 2 years of age was rare. Encouragingly, persistent reflux was rarely associated with impaired renal function (134-136). A recent study of over 1,500 infants with persistent postnatal grade II hydronephrosis (Society for Fetal Urography grading system) showed that screening for VUR and treatment with prophylactic antibiotic decreased the risk of febrile UTI when compared with the group who were not screened (137). An increasingly popular approach to the postnatal evaluation of infants with fetal hydronephrosis is to use postnatal ultrasound as a tool to determine whether or not further imaging is recommended (134). If hydronephrosis, scarring, or renal dysplasia is discovered by careful postnatal ultrasound, further evaluation with a reflux study, either RNC or VCUG, is suggested. However, some infants with high-grade VUR will not be discovered by this technique. The challenge is to determine how much pelviectasis/hydronephrosis is required to warrant VCUG (Figs. 37.7 and 37.8).

It is important to realize that, throughout this analysis of imaging of UTI, we have been operating under the assumption that sterile VUR does not cause impairment in renal function. Some evidence shows that renal cortical defects are related to the presence of high-grade, sterile VUR (138–140).

Take Home Tables and Figures

Table 37.1 summarizes the literature on the role imaging of UTI in children. Table 37.2 provides information about the diagnostic performance of tests for UTI, pyelonephritis, VUR, and renal scarring.

Figures 37.1 and 37.2 show flowcharts that provide a strategy for the imaging evaluation of male and female infants and children; Fig. 37.1 assumes the use of prophylactic antibiotics, and Fig. 37.2 assumes that prophylactic antibiotics will not be used.

Imaging Case Studies

Case 1

Figure 37.3 shows the case of an adolescent boy who first presented at 14 years of age with a UTI and hematuria.

Case 2

Figure 37.4 shows the case of a boy who first presented at 4 years of age for evaluation after a sibling was found to have VUR.

Case 3

Figure 37.5 shows a case of a 2-month-old female infant who presented with a febrile UTI.

Case 4

Figure 37.6 shows a case of a 4-year-old little girl who presented with a febrile UTI and was found to have VUR.

Case 5

Figure 37.7 shows the case of a male fetus who was revealed to have bilateral hydronephrosis that was followed periodically throughout pregnancy and was last imaged prior to delivery at 35 weeks of gestation. Figure 37.8 shows postnatal ultrasound views of the kidney obtained at 2 weeks of age, after the fetal diagnosis of hydronephrosis.

Table 37.1. Summary data on the role of imaging in children with UTI*

First author	Specialty of first author	Prospective vs. retrospective	Year of publication	Number of patients	Number of kidneys	Population studied	Overall with reflux (%)	Overall with scars (%)	Scars in the population with VUR (%)	Scars in the population without VUR (%)	Period of follow-up
Kunin (1)	Preventive medicine	R	1964	107	NA	School age children with UTI	19%	13% (IVU)	NA	NA	NA
Smellie (16)	Pediatrics	R	1964	200	NA	3 days to 12 years	34%	17% (IVU)	NA	NA	NA
Rolleston (30)	Radiology	P	1970	175	350	3 days to 12 months UTI without obstruction	49%	NA	22% (IVU)	NA	5 years
Pylkkanon (31)	NA	P	1981	252	NA	Infants and children with UTI	8%	3% (IVU)	40%	0%	2 years
Bourchier (32)	NA	R	1984	100	NA	Infants with UTI	36%	10% (IVU)	NA	NA	NA
Jakobsson (34)	Pediatrics	P	1992	106	NA	0–15.9 years with symptomatic UTI	25%	52% (DMSA)	88%	40%	2 months
Ditchfield (33)	Radiology	P	1994	150	300	>5 years	33%	NA	NA	NA	NA
Benador (6)	Pediatrics	P	1997	107	NA	0–16 years	36%	60%	63%	63%	2+ months
Jakobsson (33)	Pediatrics	P	1997	185	NA	UTI in child <10 years	37%	36%	51%	27%	2 years
Wennerstrom (35)	Pediatrics	P	1998	688	NA	0–15 years with first symptomatic UTI	33%	11% (IVU)	26%	3%	NA
Gelfand (28)	Radiology	P	2000	919	NA	Birth to >10 years UTI, separated by age 0–1 year: 29%; ≥10 years: 46%; ≤10 years: 18%	—	NA	NA	NA	NA
Honkinen (2)	Pediatrics	R	2000	134	NA	UTI with bacteriuria (from birth to 15 years); 1 week to 3 months: 33%; 3–11 months: 41%; ≤12 months: 56%	—	NA	NA	NA	NA

Study	Specialty	Type	Year	No.	No.	Population				Follow-up
Smellie (36)	Pediatrics	P	2001	228 149	NA	Infants and children with UTI who were found to have reflux with follow-up at 5 and 10 years		43% 42% (DMSA)	NA NA	5 years 10 years
Ilyas (29)	Nephrology	R	2002	208	NA	>2 years 2–8 years >8 years	51% 47% 28%	NA	NA	NA
Moorthy (37)	Radiology	R	2005	108	216	<1 year with UTI	12% of kidneys	4% (DMSA) 16%	2%	NA
Gonzalez (38)	Pediatrics	P	2005	161	322	0–11.2 years with defects on DMSA during UTI	28%	32%	47% (varies with >60% reflux grade)	NA
Garin (39)	Pediatrics	P	2006	218	NA	3 months to 18 years with defects on DMSA during UTI (excludes reflux $ gr. IV)	52%	24%	NA	1 year

*Summary of investigations to identify the frequency with which urinary tract infections (UTI), vesicoureteric reflux (VUR), and renal cortical scars coexist. In the early years, the presence of scars tended to be evaluated with intravenous urography (IVU), the best available tool at the time. More recently, scars have been more sensitively identified with 99mTc-labeled dimercaptosuccinic acid (DMSA), enhanced further with the use of single photon emission computed tomography (SPECT). Each requires an intravenous puncture and ionizing radiation, but placement of a bladder catheter is rarely required.

Reprinted with kind permission of Springer Science+Business Media from Barnewolt CE, Connolly LP, Estrada CR, Applegate KE. Urinary Tract Infection in Infants and Children. In Medina LS, Applegate KE, Blackmore CC (eds): *Evidence-Based Imaging in Pediatrics: Optimizing Imaging in Pediatric Patient Care*. New York: Springer Science+Business Media, 2010.

R retrospective, *P* prospective, *IVU* intravenous urogram or pyelogram.

Table 37.2. Reference standard test and diagnostic test performance for the detection of UTI, pyelonephritis, renal scar, and VUR in infants and children

Test	Sensitivity (%)	Specificity (%)	Reference standard	References
UTI			Urine culture	
Cloudy appearing urine	90	72–82		
Urine dip stick[a]	96	99		
Urine culture (clean catch)	75–100	57–100		
Pyelonephritis			DMSA	
Fever >38.1°C	47	56		
Fever ≥39°C for 2 days (age <2 years)	95	31		
Ultrasound (with Power Doppler)	57	82		(107)
DMSA	50–91	–		(4)
CT or MRI	87–92	88–94		(107)
Renal or bladder congenital anomalies, obstruction			US	
VUR			VCUG	
RNC (radionuclide cystogram)	50–87	88		(141)
US	18	88		(142)
	50	77		(143)
Renal scarring			DMSA	
DMSA nuclear scintigraphy	94	100		(144)
Ultrasound				(145)
Diffuse scarring	47	92		
Focal scarring	5	98		
MRI[b]	77	87		(146)

Data from Whiting et al. (57) unless otherwise stated.

Reprinted with kind permission of Springer Science+Business Media from Barnewolt CE, Connolly LP, Estrada CR, Applegate KE. Urinary Tract Infection in Infants and Children. In Medina LS, Applegate KE, Blackmore CC (eds): *Evidence-Based Imaging in Pediatrics: Optimizing Imaging in Pediatric Patient Care*. New York: Springer Science+Business Media, 2010.

[a] Positive for protein, leukocyte esterase, and nitrate.

[b] MRI without gadolinium compared to DMSA as the gold standard (146).

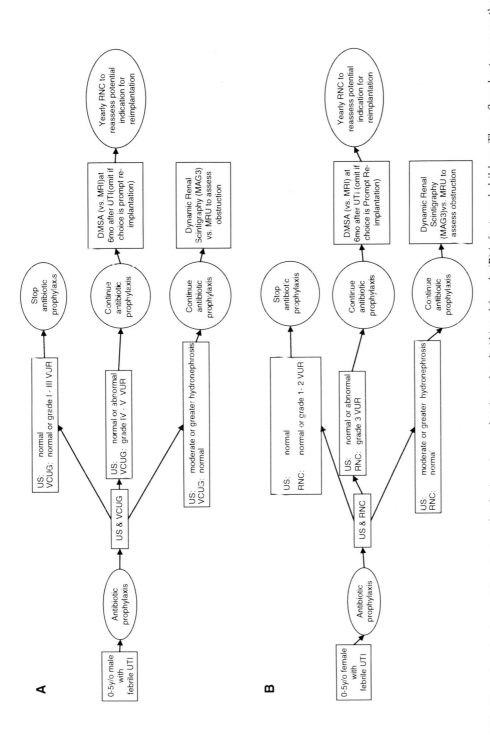

Figure 37.1. These flowcharts provide a strategy for the imaging evaluation of male (**A**) and female (**B**) infants and children. These flowcharts assume that the use of prophylactic antibiotic is of no demonstrable benefit in improving overall outcomes, but remains commonly used. (*US* ultrasound, *VCUG* voiding cystourethrogram, *DMSA* 99mTc-labeled dimercaptosuccinic acid, *MRI* magnetic resonance imaging, *MAG3* 99mTc-labeled mercaptoacetyltriglycine, *MRU* magnetic resonance urography, *RNC* radionuclide cystogram). (Reprinted with kind permission of Springer Science+Business Media from Barnewolt CE, Connolly LP, Estrada CR, Applegate KE. Urinary Tract Infection in: Infants and Children. In Medina LS, Applegate KE, Blackmore CC (eds): *Evidence-Based Imaging in Pediatrics: Optimizing Imaging in Pediatric Patient Care.* New York: Springer Science+Business Media, 2010.)

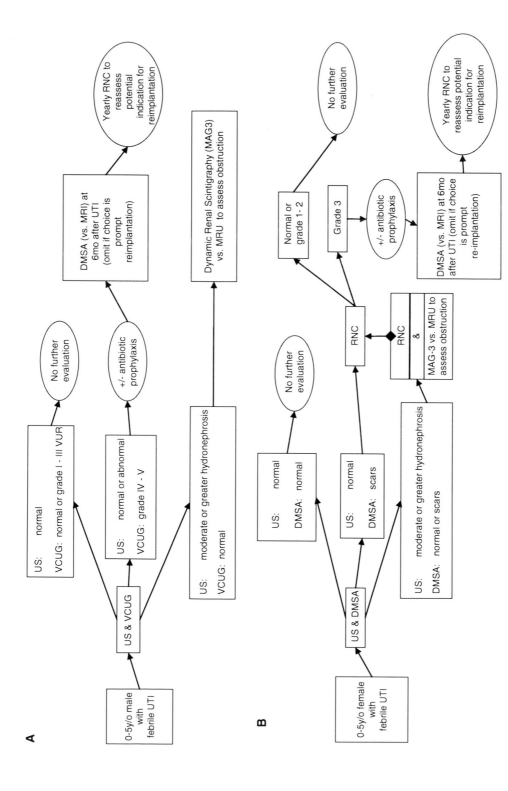

Figure 37.2. These flowcharts are a modified version of those in Fig. 37.1 and do not use prophylactic antibiotics. (*US* ultrasound, *VCUG* voiding cystoure-throgram, *DMSA* 99mTc-labeled dimercaptosuccinic acid, *MRI* magnetic resonance imaging, *RNC* radionuclide urography, *RNC* radionuclide cystography). (Reprinted with kind permission of Springer Science+Business Media from Barnewolt CE, Connolly LP, Estrada CR, Applegate KE. Urinary Tract Infection in Infants and Children. In Medina LS, Applegate KE, Blackmore CC (eds): *Evidence-Based Imaging in Pediatrics: Optimizing Imaging in Pediatric Patient Care.* New York: Springer Science+Business Media, 2010.)

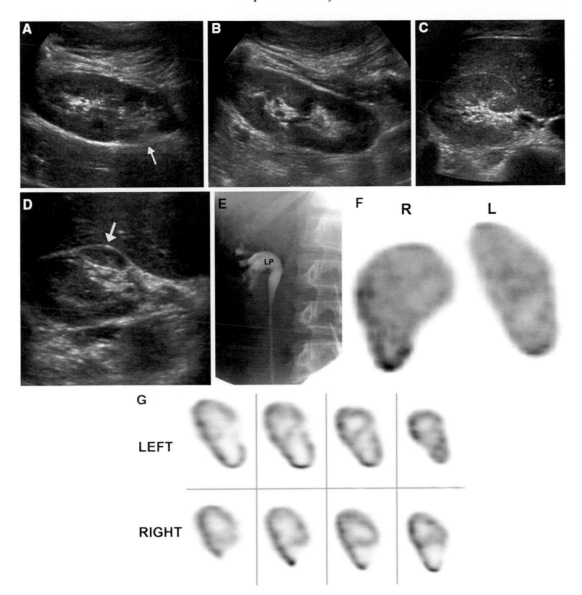

Figure 37.3. These series of images were performed over a period of 3 months for evaluation of an adolescent boy who first presented at 14 years of age with a UTI and hematuria. Evaluation began with ultrasound, where it was suspected that the right kidney contained a duplex collecting system and there was evidence for associated right lower pole scarring (**A**) prone sagittal view of the right kidney, *arrow* indicates site of focal cortical thinning; (**B**) prone sagittal view of normal appearing left kidney; (**C**) normal transverse view if the upper pole of the right kidney; (**D**) transverse view of the scarred right lower pole, *arrow* indicates site of anterior cortical thinning, raising the question of VUR into the lower moiety, which was subsequently proved by VCUG [(**E**) *LP* lower pole]. Tc-99m DMSA confirmed the suspicion of right lower pole scarring on reconstructed (**F**) and source SPECT views (**G**). (Reprinted with kind permission of Springer Science+Business Media from Barnewolt CE, Connolly LP, Estrada CR, Applegate KE. Urinary Tract Infection in Infants and Children. In Medina LS, Applegate KE, Blackmore CC (eds): *Evidence-Based Imaging in Pediatrics: Optimizing Imaging in Pediatric Patient Care*. New York: Springer Science+Business Media, 2010.)

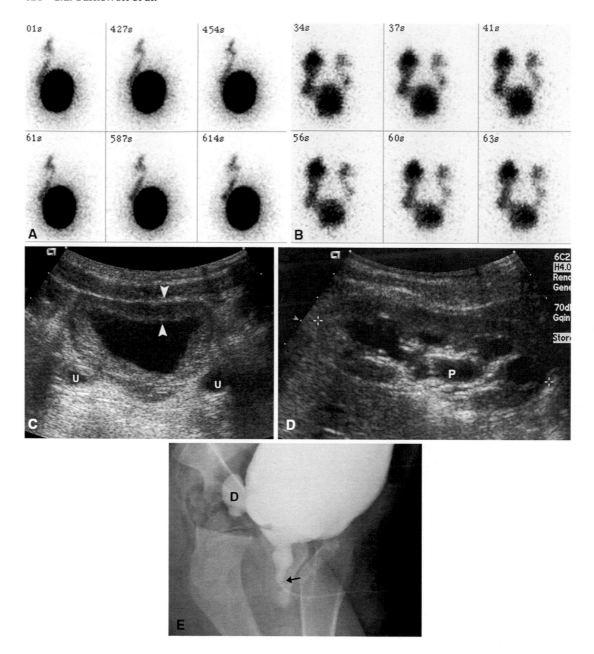

Figure 37.4. This example is a lesson in the importance of careful evaluation of urethral anatomy in boys. Interestingly, this little boy first presented at 4 years of age for evaluation after a sibling was found to have VUR. Radionuclide cystogram demonstrated left grade 2 VUR on prone views (**A**), which had become bilateral and increased in grade 1 year later (**B**). Subsequent reimplantation was performed and a postoperative ultrasound revealed bilateral, distal hydroureter, bladder wall thickening, and persistent hydronephrosis (**C**) transverse view of the urinary bladder, *u* distal hydroureter, *arrowheads* indicate a thickened bladder wall; (**D**) prone, sagittal view of the moderately hydronephrotic right kidney, *p* dilated renal pelvis. Subsequent VCUG (**E**) revealed the presence of previously unrecognized posterior urethral valves (*arrow*) and a moderate-sized bladder diverticulum (*D* diverticulum). Theoretically, progression of VUR and subsequent ureteral reimplantation may have been avoided had the presence of posterior urethral valves been recognized and addressed. (Reprinted with kind permission of Springer Science+Business Media from Barnewolt CE, Connolly LP, Estrada CR, Applegate KE. Urinary Tract Infection in Infants and Children. In Medina LS, Applegate KE, Blackmore CC (eds): *Evidence-Based Imaging in Pediatrics: Optimizing Imaging in Pediatric Patient Care.* New York: Springer Science+Business Media, 2010.)

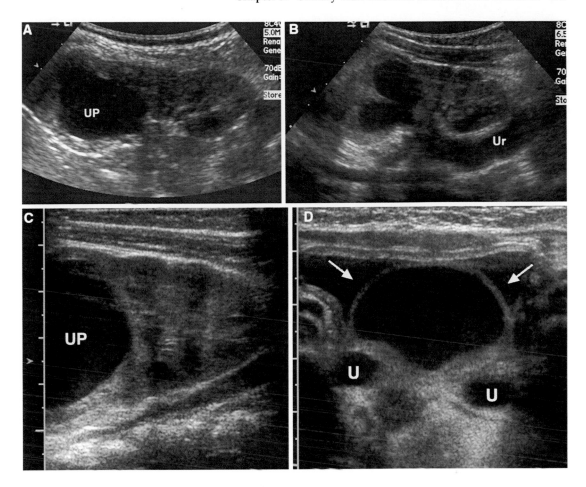

Figure 37.5. This 2-month-old female infant presented with a febrile UTI, where her initial ultrasound demonstrated the presence of a duplex left kidney, with upper pole hydroureteronephrosis [(**A–C**) sagittal views of the left kidney demonstrating a dilated upper pole pelvis (UP) and dilated upper pole ureter (Ur)], associated with a moderately large ureterocele and bilateral, distal hydroureter [(**D**) transverse view of the bladder demonstrating dilated distal ureters (u) and a ureterocele (*arrows*)]. VCUG performed on the same day reveals a filling defect within the urinary bladder on early-fill views of the bladder [(**E**), *arrowheads* outline left ureterocele] and on an oblique view of the right side [(**F**), *arrowhead* = left ureterocele, *arrow* = refluxing right ureter], with the additional observation of high-grade VUR on the right [(**G**), *B* bladder, *RU* dilated, refluxing right ureter]. With voiding, the ureterocele prolapsed into the urethra [(**H**), *arrowheads* = ureterocele prolapsing into the urethra]. Subsequent Tc-99m DMSA, both routine (**I**) and pinhole views (**J**), revealed a photopenic defect in the left upper pole. Without the ultrasound and VCUG findings, this may have been difficult to differentiate from a large focal scar. With the identification of a complex anatomic anomaly by ultrasound, it was important to redirect from RNC to VCUG to demonstrate the finer points of urinary tract anatomy that could not have been fully discerned by RNC. This is one of only a few situations where VCUG, rather than RNC, is preferable in girls and can be determined based on information provided by ultrasound. (Reprinted with kind permission of Springer Science+Business Media from Barnewolt CE, Connolly LP, Estrada CR, Applegate KE. Urinary Tract Infection in Infants and Children. In Medina LS, Applegate KE, Blackmore CC (eds): *Evidence-Based Imaging in Pediatrics: Optimizing Imaging in Pediatric Patient Care*. New York: Springer Science+Business Media, 2010.)

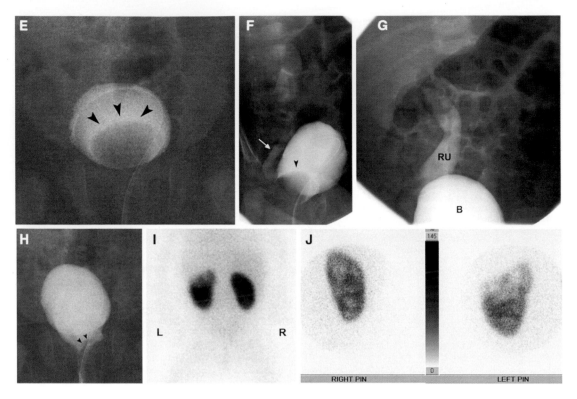

Figure 37.5. *Continued*

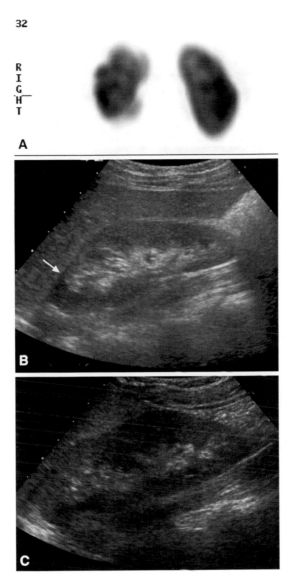

Figure 37.6. This 4-year-old little girl presented with a febrile UTI and was found to have VUR. Tc-99m DMSA revealed evidence of scarring of both the upper and lower poles of the right kidney, but no scars on the *left* (**A**). These scars were only faintly discernible on ultrasound, and perhaps only with knowledge of the Tc-99m DMSA findings (**B**), sagittal view of the right kidney, *arrow* = subtle, focal area of cortical thinning; [(**C**), sagittal view of the normal left kidney]. (Reprinted with kind permission of Springer Science+Business Media from Barnewolt CE, Connolly LP, Estrada CR, Applegate KE. Urinary Tract Infection in Infants and Children. In Medina LS, Applegate KE, Blackmore CC (eds): *Evidence-Based Imaging in Pediatrics: Optimizing Imaging in Pediatric Patient Care.* New York: Springer Science+Business Media, 2010.)

628   C.E. Barnewolt et al.

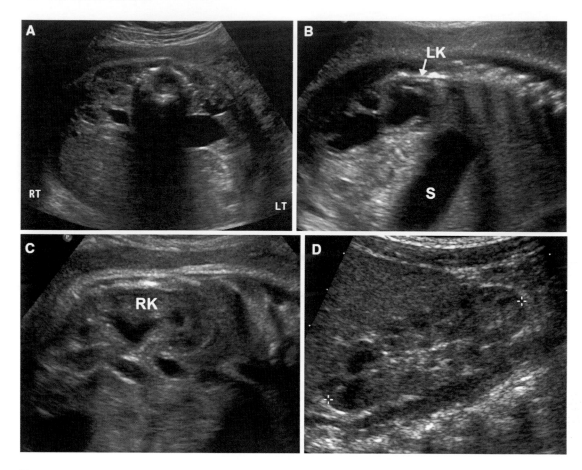

Figure 37.7. Routine prenatal ultrasound screening of this male fetus revealed bilateral hydronephrosis that was followed periodically throughout pregnancy and was last imaged prior to delivery at 35 weeks of gestation (**A**), transverse view showing mild right and moderate left hydronephrosis; (**B**), sagittal view of the moderately hydronephrotic left fetal kidney, *S* stomach, *LK* left kidney; [(**C**), sagittal view of the mildly hydronephrotic right fetal kidney, *RK* right kidney]. After delivery, at 3 weeks of life, postnatal renal ultrasound revealed a normal appearing right kidney and mild to moderate left hydronephrosis (**D**), supine view of normal right kidney; (**E**), supine view of moderately hydronephrotic left kidney; (**F**), prone view of normal right kidney; [(**G**), prone view of moderately hydronephrotic left kidney]. VCUG on the same day as the ultrasound revealed grade III VUR on the right (the side where the postnatal ultrasound had been normal) (**H**) and no VUR on the left (implying the presence of some degree of obstruction at the level of the left ureteropelvic junction). The urethra was normal (**I**). This example illustrates the great challenge in predicting or excluding the presence of VUR on ultrasound alone. (Reprinted with kind permission of Springer Science+Business Media from Barnewolt CE, Connolly LP, Estrada CR, Applegate KE. Urinary Tract Infection in Infants and Children. In Medina LS, Applegate KE, Blackmore CC (eds): *Evidence-Based Imaging in Pediatrics: Optimizing Imaging in Pediatric Patient Care.* New York: Springer Science+Business Media, 2010.)

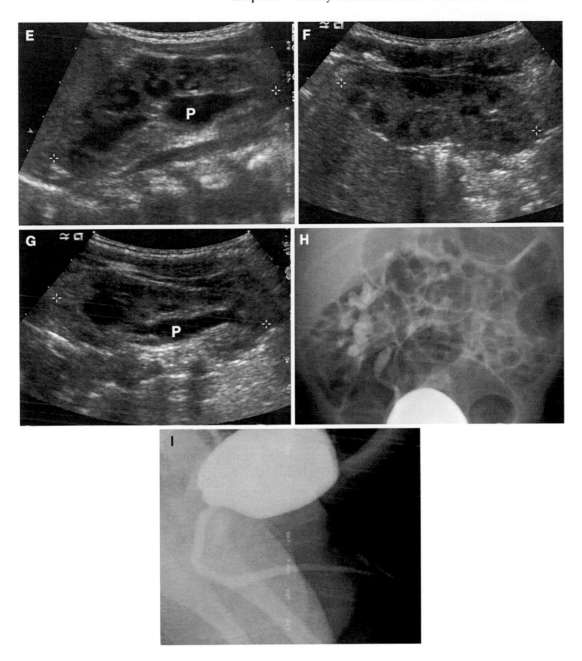

Figure 37.7. *Continued*

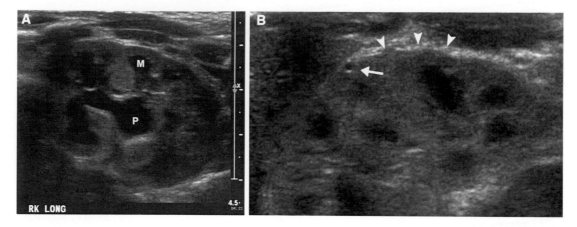

Figure 37.8. These postnatal ultrasound views of the kidney were obtained at 2 weeks of age, after the fetal diagnosis of hydronephrosis. At worst, one might describe this as mild to moderate hydronephrosis [(**A**), *p* renal pelvis, *m* medullary pyramid]. Nonetheless, high detail views reveal several very tiny cortical cysts along the renal cortical surface [(**B**), *arrow* = tiny cyst, *arrowheads* = cortical surface of kidney]. These subtle findings suggest the possibility of renal dysplasia and probably warrant formal evaluation for VUR, with VCUG in males, to exclude the possibility of posterior urethral valves, and RNC in girls, minimizing radiation exposure. (Reprinted with kind permission of Springer Science+Business Media from Barnewolt CE, Connolly LP, Estrada CR, Applegate KE. Urinary Tract Infection in Infants and Children. In Medina LS, Applegate KE, Blackmore CC (eds): *Evidence-Based Imaging in Pediatrics: Optimizing Imaging in Pediatric Patient Care.* New York: Springer Science+Business Media, 2010.)

Suggested Imaging Protocols for Urinary Tract Infections in Infants and Children

See Figs. 37.1 and 37.2.

Future Research

- Large, multi-center, prospective, controlled studies of infants and children with carefully diagnosed UTI, assessing the controversies of (a) prophylactic antibiotic use, and (b) whether surgical or endoscopic management of VUR provides improved renal function and decreased recurrent UTI.
- Development of nonimaging predictors of risk of UTI and/or progression of renal impairment after UTI.
- Standardization of prenatal evaluation of fetal and postnatal hydronephrosis, to predict outcome.
- Development of a standardized, automated protocol for MRU in infants and children.

References

1. Kunin CM, Deutscher R, Paquin A, Jr. Medicine 1964;43:91–130.
2. Honkinen O, Jahnukainen T, Mertsola J, Eskola J, Ruuskanen O. Pediatr Infect Dis J 2000;19: 630–634.
3. Marcus N, Ashkenazi S, Yaari A, Samra Z, Livni G. Pediatr Infect Dis J 2005;24:581–585.
4. Rushton HG, Majd M. J Urol 1992;148: 1726–1732.
5. Jakobsson B, Soderlundh S, Berg U. Arch Dis Child 1992;67:1338–1342.
6. Benador D, Benador N, Slosman D, Mermillod B, Girardin E. Lancet 1997;349:17–19.
7. Stokland E, Hellstrom M, Jacobsson B, Jodal U, Sixt R. J Pediatr 1996;129:815–820.
8. Roberts JA. J Urol 1983;129:1102–1106.
9. Roberts JA, Suarez GM, Kaack B, Kallenius G, Svenson SB. J Urol 1985;133:1068–1075.
10. Risdon RA, Yeung CK, Ransley PG. Clin Nephrol 1993;40:308–314.
11. http://kidney.niddk.nih.gov/Kudiseases/pubs/vesicoureteralreflux/.
12. Marild S, Jodal U. Acta Paediatr 1998;87: 549–552.
13. Hoberman A, Wald ER. Pediatr Infect Dis J 1997;16:11–17.
14. Hoberman A, Charron M, Hickey RW, Baskin M, Kearney DH et al. N Engl J Med 2003;348: 195–202.

15. Chen L, Baker MD. Pediatr Emerg Care 2006;22:485–487.
16. Smellie JM, Hodson CJ, Edwards D, Normand IC. Br Med J 1964;2:1222–1226.
17. Wiswell TE, Roscelli JD. Pediatrics 1986;78: 96–99.
18. Herzog LW. Am J Dis Child 1989;143:348–350.
19. Schoen EJ, Colby CJ, Ray GT. Pediatrics 2000;105:789–793.
20. Zorc JJ, Levine DA, Platt SL et al. Pediatrics 2005;116:644–648.
21. Mingin GC, Hinds A, Nguyen HT, Baskin LS. Urology 2004;63:562–565; discussion 565.
22. Sargent MA. Pediatr Radiol 2000;30:587–593.
23. Peters PC, Johnson DE, Jackson JH, Jr. J Urol 1967;97:259–260.
24. Iannaccone G, Panzironi PE. Acta Radiol 1955;44:451–456.
25. Gibson HM. J Urol 1949;62:40–43.
26. Forsythe WI, Whelan RF. Br J Urol 1958;30: 189–197.
27. Krepler P. Z Kinderheilkd 1968;104:103–114.
28. Gelfand MJ, Koch BL, Cordero GG, Salmanzadeh A, Gartside PS. Pediatr Radiol 2000;30:121–124.
29. Ilyas M, Mastin ST, Richard GA. Pediatr Nephrol 2002;17:30–34.
30. Rolleston GL, Shannon FT, Utley WL. Br Med J 1970;1:460–463.
31. Pylkkanen J, Vilska J, Koskimies O. Acta Paediatr Scand 1981;70:879–883.
32. Bourchier D, Abbott GD, Maling TM. Arch Dis Child 1984;59:620–624.
33. Ditchfield MR, De Campo JF, Cook DJ et al. Radiology 1994;190:413–415.
34. Jakobsson B, Svensson L. Acta Paediatr 1997;86:803–807.
35. Wennerstrom M, Hansson S, Jodal U, Stokland E. Arch Pediatr Adolesc Med 1998;152:879–883.
36. Smellie JM, Jodal U, Lax H, Mobius TT, Hirche H et al. J Pediatr 2001;139:656–663.
37. Moorthy I, Easty M, McHugh K, Ridout D, Biassoni L et al. Arch Dis Child 2005;90: 733–736.
38. Gonzalez E, Papazyan JP, Girardin E. J Urol 2005;173:571–574; discussion 574–575.
39. Garin EH, Olavarria F, Garcia Nieto V, Valenciano B, Campos A et al. Pediatrics 2006;117:626–632.
40. Chandra M, Maddix H, McVicar M. J Urol 1996;155:673–677.
41. Sillen U. Pediatr Nephrol 1999;13:355–361.
42. Silva JM, Oliveira EA, Diniz JS et al. Pediatr Nephrol 2006;21:510–516.
43. Connolly LP, Treves ST, Connolly SA et al. J Urol 1997;157:2287–2290.
44. Noe HN. J Urol 1992;148:1739–1742.
45. http://emedicine.medscape.com/article/439403 overview.
46. Craig JC, Irwig LM, Knight JF, Roy LP. J Paediatr Child Health 1997;33:434–438.
47. Stark H. Pediatr Nephrol 1997;11:174–177; discussion 180–181.
48. Cohen AL, Rivara FP, Davis R, Christakis DA. Pediatrics 2005;115:1474–1478.
49. American Academy of Pediatrics, Committee on Quality Improvement, Subcommittee on Urinary Tract Infection. Pediatrics 1999;103: 843–852.
50. Armstrong EP. Am J Manag Care 2001;7: 269–280.
51. Conway PH, Edwards S, Stucky ER, Chiang VW, Ottolini MC et al. Pediatrics 2006;118: 441–447.
52. Altemeier WA, III. Pediatr Ann 1999;28: 663–664.
53. Dick PT, Feldman W. J Pediatr 1996;128:15–22.
54. Newman TB. Pediatrics 2005;116:1613–1614.
55. Garin EH, Young L. Pediatrics 2007;120:249–250.
56. Greenfield SP, Chesney RW, Carpenter M et al. J Urol 2008;179:405–407.
57. Whiting P, Westwood M, Bojke L et al. Health Technol Assess 2006;10:iii–iv, xi–xiii, 1–154.
58. Verrier Jones K. Arch Dis Child 2005;90: 663–664.
59. Rosenheim ML. In The Richard Bright Memorial Lecture, delivered on the occasion of the Bright Centenary Celebrations at Guy's Hospital Medical School, 1958;403–423.
60. Bailey RR. Clin Nephrol 1973;1:132–141.
61. Oh MM, Jin MH, Bae JH, Park HS, Lee JG, Moon du G. J Urol 2008;180:2167–2170.
62. Wheeler D, Vimalachandra D, Hodson EM, Roy LP, Smith G et al. Arch Dis Child 2003;88:688–694.
63. Craig JC, Irwig LM, Knight JF, Roy LP. Pediatrics 2000;105:1236–1241.
64. Nguyen HT, Bauer SB, Peters CA et al. J Urol 2000;164:1674–1678; discussion 1678–1679.
65. Schwab CW, Jr., Wu HY, Selman H, Smith GH, Snyder HM, III et al. J Urol 2002;168:2594–2599.
66. Silva JM, Diniz JS, Lima EM, Vergara RM, Oliveira EA. BJU Int 2006;97:1063–1068.
67. Connolly LP, Treves ST, Zurakowski D, Bauer SB. J Urol 1996;156:1805–1807.
68. Esbjorner E, Berg U, Hansson S. Pediatr Nephrol 1997;11:438–442.
69. Lagomarsimo E, Valenzuela A, Cavagnaro F, Solar E. Pediatr Nephrol 1999;13:288–291.
70. Bell C. Med Chir Trans 1812;3:171.13–384.13.
71. Olbing H, Claesson I, Ebel KD et al. J Urol 1992;148(5 Pt 2):1653–1656.
72. Piepsz A, Tamminen-Mobius T, Reiners C, et al. Eur J Pediatr 1998;157:753–758.
73. Smellie JM, Barratt TM, Chantler C et al. Lancet 2001;357:1329–1333.
74. Jodal U, Smellie JM, Lax H, Hoyer PF. Pediatr Nephrol 2006;21:785–792.
75. Br Med J (Clin Res Ed) 1983;287:171–174.
76. Br Med J (Clin Res Ed) 1987;295:237–241.

77. Le Saux N, Pham B, Moher D. Can Med Assoc J 2000;163:523–529.

78. Thompson RH, Chen JJ, Pugach J, Naseer S, Steinhardt GF. Urology 2001;166:1465–1469.

79. Williams G, Lee A, Craig J. J Pediatr 2001;138:868–874.

80. Hellerstein S, Nickell E. Pediatr Nephrol 2002;17:506–510.

81. Wald ER. Pediatrics 2006;117:919–922.

82. Georgaki-Angelaki H, Kostaridou S, Daikos GL et al. Scand J Infect Dis 2005;37:842–845.

83. Faust WC, Pohl HG. Curr Opin Urol 2007;17: 252–256.

84. Conway PH, Cnaan A, Zaoutis T, Henry BV, Grundmeier RW et al. JAMA 2007;298:179–186.

85. Lee SJ, Shim YH, Cho SJ, Lee JW. Pediatr Nephrol 2007;22:1315–1320.

86. Larcombe J. Clin Evid 2005;13:444–457.

87. Al-Sayyad AJ, Pike JG, Leonard MP. J Urol 2005;174:1587–1589; discussion 1589.

88. Roussey-Kesler G, Gadjos V, Idres N et al. J Urol 2008;179:674–679; discussion 679.

89. Hitzel A, Liard A, Vera P, Manrique A, Menard JF et al. J Nucl Med 2002;43:27–32.

90. Westwood ME, Whiting PF, Cooper J, Watt IS, Kleijnen J. BMC Pediatr 2005;15:2

91. Podberesky DJ, Unsell BJ, Gunderman R et al. Urinary tract infection – child. [online publication]. Reston, VA: American College of Radiology (ACR) 7 p. [70 references]. In Imaging EPoP, ed., 2006.

92. Fernbach SK, Maizels M, Conway JJ. Pediatr Radiol 1993;23:478–480.

93. Blane CE, DiPietro MA, Zerin JM, Sedman AB, Bloom DA. J Urol 1993;150:752–755.

94. DiPietro MA, Blane CE, Zerin JM. Radiology 1997;205:821–822.

95. Davey MS, Zerin JM, Reilly C, Ambrosius WT. Pediatr Radiol 1997;27:908–911.

96. Rickwood AM, Carty HM, McKendrick T et al. Br Med J 1992;304:663–665.

97. Tibballs JM, De Bruyn R. Arch Dis Child 1996;75:444–447.

98. Yerkes EB, Adams MC, Pope JCT, Brock JW, III. J Urol 1999;162:1218–1220.

99. Jaswon MS, Dibble L, Puri S et al. Arch Dis Child Fetal Neonatal Ed 1999;80:F135–F138.

100. Brophy MM, Austin PF, Yan Y, Coplen DE. J Urol 2002;168:1716–1719; discussion 1719.

101. Phan V, Traubici J, Hershenfield B, Stephens D, Rosenblum ND et al. Pediatr Nephrol 2003;18: 1224–1228.

102. Anderson NG, Allan RB, Abbott GD. Pediatr Nephrol 2004;19:749–753.

103. Grattan-Smith JD. Pediatr Radiol 2008;38(suppl 2):S275–S280.

104. Jones RA, Schmotzer B, Little SB, Grattan-Smith JD. Pediatr Radiol 2008;38(suppl 1):S18–S27.

105. Kirsch AJ, Grattan-Smith JD, Molitierno JA, Jr. Curr Opin Urol 2006;16:283–290.

106. Lonergan GJ, Pennington DJ, Morrison JC, Haws RM, Grimley MS et al. Radiology 1998;207:377–384.

107. Majd M, Nussbaum Blask AR, Markle BM, et al. Radiology 2001;218:101–108.

108. Agarwal R, Brunelli SM, Williams K, Mitchell MD, Feldman HI et al. Nephrol Dial Transplant 2009;24:856–863.

109. Lavocat MP, Granjon D, Allard D, Gay C, Freycon MT et al. Pediatr Radiol 1997;27: 159–165.

110. Vates TS, Shull MJ, Underberg-Davis SJ, Fleisher MH. J Urol 1999;162:1221–1223.

111. Barnewolt CE, Paltiel HJ, Lebowitz RL, Kirks DR. In Kirks DR (ed.): Practical Pediatric Imaging – Diagnostic Radiology of Infants and Children, 3rd ed. Philadelphia: Lippincott Raven, 1998;1010–1019.

112. Goldraich NP, Goldraich IH. J Urol 1992;148: 1688–1692.

113. NICE Clinical Guideline 54. Urinary tract infection in children: diagnosis, treatment and long-term management. National Institute for Health and Clinical Excellence, developed by the National Collaborating Centre for Women's and Children's Health, August 2007 [online publication]. London, UK.

114. Smellie JM, Rigden SP, Prescod NP. Arch Dis Child 1995;72:247–250.

115. Gelfand MJ, Barr LL, Abunku O. Pediatr Radiol 2000;30:665–670.

116. Hohenfellner K, Seemayer S, Stolz G et al. Klin Padiatr 2000;212:320–325.

117. http://rad.usuhs.edu/medpix/medpix_home. html?mode=displayjactoid&recnun=2800.

118. Ward VL. Pediatr Radiol 2006;36:168–172.

119. Ward VL, Barnewolt CE, Strauss KJ et al. Radiology 2006;238:96–106.

120. Ward VL, Strauss KJ, Barnewolt CE et al. Radiology 2008;249:1002–1009.

121. Vachvanichsanong P, Dissaneewate P, Thongmak S, Lim A. Nephrology (Carlton) 2008;13:38–42.

122. Christian MT, McColl JH, MacKenzie JR, Beattie TJ. Arch Dis Child 2000;82:376–380.

123. Bjorgvinsson E, Majd M, Eggli KD. Am J Roentgenol 1991;157:539–543.

124. Benador D, Benador N, Slosman DO, Nussle D, Mermillod B et al. J Pediatr 1994;124:17–20.

125. Preda I, Jodal U, Sixt R, Stokland E, Hansson S. J Pediatr 2007;151:581–584, 584 e581.

126. Cascio S, Chertin B, Colhoun E, Puri P. J Urol 2002;168:1708–1710; discussion 1710.

127. Jakobsson B, Berg U, Svensson L. Arch Dis Child 1994;70:111–115.

128. Rushton HG, Majd M, Jantausch B, Wiedermann BL, Belman AB. J Urol 1992;147:1327–1332.

129. Friedland GW, Cunningham J. Am J Roentgenol Radium Ther Nucl Med 1972;116:792–811.

130. Husmann D. In Gonzalez E, Bauer S (eds.). Pediatric Urology Practice. Philadelphia: Lippincott Williams & Wilkins, 1999;295–311.

131. Treves ST, Gelfand MJ, Willi UV. In Treves ST (ed.). Pediatric Nuclear Medicine, 2nd ed. New York: Springer-Verlag, 1995;411–429.

132. Rachmiel M, Aladjem M, Starinsky R, Strauss S, Villa Y et al. Pediatr Nephrol 2005;20:1449–1452.

133. Lee RS, Cendron M, Kinnamon DD, Nguyen HT. Pediatrics 2006;118:586–593.

134. Ismaili K, Hall M, Piepsz A et al. J Pediatr 2006;148:222–227.

135. Coelho GM, Bouzada MC, Lemos GS, Pereira AK, Lima BP et al. J Urol 2008;179:284–289.

136. Walsh TJ, Hsieh S, Grady R, Mueller BA. Urology 2007;69:970–974.

137. Estrada CR, Peters CA, Retik AB, Nguyen HT. J Urol 2009;181:801–806; discussion 806–807.

138. Yeung CK, Godley ML, Dhillon HK, Gordon I, Duffy PG et al. Br J Urol 1997;80:319–327.

139. Stock JA, Wilson D, Hanna MK. J Urol 1998;160:1017–1018.

140. Hellerstein S. Curr Opin Pediatr 2000;12:125–128.

141. De Sadeleer C, De Boe V, Keuppens F, Desprechins B, Verboven M et al. Eur J Nucl Med 1994;21:223–227.

142. Zamir G, Sakran W, Horowitz Y, Koren A, Miron D. Arch Dis Child 2004;89:466–468.

143. Alshamsam L, Harbi AA, Fakeeh K, Al Banyan E. Ann Saudi Med 2009;29:46–49.

144. Shanon A, Feldman W, McDonald P, Martin DJ, Matzinger MA et al. J Pediatr 1992;120:399–403.

145. Moorthy I, Wheat D, Gordon I. Pediatr Nephrol 2004;19:153–156.

146. Kavanagh EC, Ryan S, Awan A, McCourbrey S, O'Connor R et al. Pediatr Radiol 2005;35:275–281.

38

Current Issues in Gynecology: Screening for Ovarian Cancer in the Average Risk Population and Diagnostic Evaluation of Postmenopausal Bleeding

Ruth C. Carlos

Issues

   I. Ovarian cancer screening: what is the role of biochemical markers such as CA 125?
  II. Ovarian cancer screening: what is the diagnostic performance (accuracy) of imaging?
 III. Ovarian cancer screening: what is the role of imaging?
     A. Screening with gray-scale ultrasound only
     B. Screening with ultrasound and color Doppler imaging
     C. Multimodality approach using CA 125 and ultrasound
  IV. Postmenopausal bleeding evaluation: when should a woman with PMB be referred for additional evaluation?
   V. Postmenopausal bleeding evaluation: what is the accuracy of imaging tests?
     A. Transvaginal ultrasonography
     B. Saline-infused hysterosonography
     C. Hysteroscopy
  VI. Postmenopausal bleeding evaluation: what is the role of imaging?
 VII. How should women on tamoxifen therapy be evaluated?

R.C. Carlos (✉)
Department of Radiology, University of Michigan Health System, 1500 E. Medical Center Drive,
UH B2 A209/5030, Ann Arbor, MI 48109, USA
e-mail: rcarlos@umich.edu

L.S. Medina et al. (eds.), *Evidence-Based Imaging: Improving the Quality of Imaging in Patient Care, Revised Edition*,
DOI 10.1007/978-1-4419-7777-9_38, © Springer Science+Business Media, LLC 2011

> ■ Current data do not support ovarian cancer screening in women who are at average risk, with any screening regimen (moderate evidence).
> ■ Transvaginal ultrasound (TVUS) is preferred as the initial test in evaluating women with postmenopausal bleeding (PMB) who are not on tamoxifen (moderate evidence).
> ■ Histologic sampling is necessary in women with PMB and a positive TVUS (moderate evidence).
> ■ Hysteroscopy and curettage is the preferred diagnostic test over Pipelle endometrial biopsy, to detect polyps and other benign lesions (limited evidence).
> ■ In women with PMB and tamoxifen use, hysteroscopy and curettage is preferred as the initial diagnostic test (limited evidence).

Key Points

Definition and Pathophysiology

Ovarian cancer is a heterogeneous group of malignancies that arises from the various cell types that comprise the organ (1). Epithelial tumors represent the most common histology (90%) of ovarian tumors. Other histologies include (1) low malignant or borderline ovarian tumors, (2) sex cord-stromal tumors, (3) germ cell tumors, (4) primary peritoneal carcinoma, and (5) metastatic tumors of the ovary. The etiology of ovarian cancer is poorly understood; however, its epidemiology and risk factors have been well described.

Endometrial cancer is also a heterogeneous disease with two apparent subtypes. The majority of women with endometrial cancer have a well-differentiated carcinoma with grade 1 or 2 endometrioid histology and well-defined risk factors. A minority of cases are diagnosed with poorly differentiated tumors (grade 3 endometrioid, clear cell, and papillary serous carcinoma), which occur spontaneously in postmenopausal women.

Epidemiology

Ovarian Cancer

Ovarian cancer is estimated to have caused over 25,000 new cancers in women in 2004 and is the most frequent cause of death from a gynecologic cancer (2). Ovarian cancers typically present few symptoms before having reached a large size or having disseminated. The vast majority of patients are diagnosed

with metastatic disease. Therefore, survival rates remain poor despite marked advances in surgery and chemotherapeutics. Women with metastatic disease have a less than 30% chance of surviving 5 years after diagnosis. In contrast, women diagnosed with stage I ovarian cancer (with cancer confined to the ovaries) have a greater than 90% chance of 5-year survival (3). Baseline lifetime risk for developing ovarian cancer is estimated at 1.4–1.8% (3, 4). The most significant risk factor for ovarian cancer is positive family history, increasing the baseline risk five- to sevenfold. Identification of *BRCA1* or *BRCA2* gene mutations increases the estimated risk to approximately 30–40% (5, 6). Approximately 90% of all familial ovarian cancers are attributable to these two mutations with the remaining 10% accounted for by mutations at other loci (7, 8).

Increasing parity has a protective effect against ovarian cancer. A review of 12 case-control studies demonstrated that having a single term pregnancy reduces the risk of ovarian cancer by half with progressive risk reduction with each additional pregnancy (9). The findings above were supported by additional findings from the Nurses Cohort study, where each pregnancy reduced the risk of ovarian cancer by approximately 15% (10). The linkage between infertility and increased risk of ovarian cancer is not as well established. After adjusting for confounding variables, a weak association [odds ratio (OR), 1.21; 95% confidence interval (CI), 0.83–1.77] between infertility and ovarian cancer was demonstrated in a large Australian population (11). Further, there appear to be subgroups of infertile women who are at higher risk for ovarian cancer, specifically nulliparous women and women with unexplained infertility (12). Although early menarche and late menopause have been implicated as risk factors for ovarian cancer, Whittemore et al. (9) and Hankinson et al. (10) independently demonstrated nonsignificant effects of early menarche and of late menopause on ovarian cancer risk. Oral contraceptive pill (OCP) use as a protective factor has been demonstrated in a United Kingdom-based study involving over 15,000 women, where OCP use for more than 8 years reduced the risk of ovarian cancer (OR, 0.4); these findings were confirmed in a large Australian case-control study.

In screening for ovarian cancer, as in all cancers, important time points to note are the lead time required to alter the natural history of the disease with intervention in order to increase survival, and the duration of marker-positive preclinical disease when disease can be detected using current tests at a stage sufficiently early to successfully intervene. Both of these time points have not been defined in the natural history of ovarian cancer.

Endometrial Cancer

The American Cancer Society estimated that cancer of the uterine corpus, of which endometrial cancer is the most common, caused greater than 40,000 new cancer cases and approximately 7,000 deaths in 2004 (2). The absolute risk of endometrial cancer in patients without hormone replacement therapy (HRT) who present with PMB ranges from 5.7 to 11.5% (13–15). Menopause, as defined by the World Health Organization, is the permanent cessation of menstruation resulting from the loss of ovarian follicular activity (16). In general, PMB represents an episode of bleeding occurring 12 months or more after the last period (17). Abnormal bleeding occurring during HRT can be difficult to define and depends on the type of HRT. Breakthrough bleeding or heavy/prolonged bleeding after the progestogen phase while on sequential HRT may be considered abnormal. Any bleeding occurring after the first 6 months of treatment or after amenorrhea has been established while on continuous combined HRT may be considered abnormal (18).

The primary genetic risk factor for endometrial cancer is hereditary nonpolyposis colorectal cancer, where endometrial cancer is the most commonly associated extracolonic cancer.

The lifetime risk for developing endometrial cancer in this population has been estimated at 42–60% (19, 20). In these women, endometrial cancer occurs prior to menopause, distinct from the sporadic type of endometrial cancer that occurs primarily in postmenopausal women (21).

The major reproductive risk factors increasing endometrial cancer risk are late menopause and early menarche, while increasing parity decreases risk with an approximately 30% reduction in risk with first birth compared to an approximately 15% reduction with each subsequent birth (22–26).

The use of OCP decreases the risk significantly. At premenopausal ages, the risk is reduced by approximately 10% per year of use (27, 28), but this declines with increasing age. Obesity greatly increases the risk (29). Unopposed estrogen therapy for menopausal symptoms increases the risk of endometrial cancer approximately 120% at doses commonly used in the USA when used for 5 years (29). The addition of progesterone markedly decreases the risk of endometrial cancer with continuous combined estrogen–progesterone therapy associated with essentially no increased risk. Women on tamoxifen are at a three to six times higher risk for endometrial cancer (30–33).

Overall Cost to Society

Ovarian Cancer

The average present value of the 15-year costs attributable to ovarian cancer is $21,285 for local-stage disease and $32,126 for distant-stage disease in 1990 dollars, using data derived from Medicare claims data linked with Surveillance, Epidemiology, and End Results (SEER) cancer registry data (34). Long-term costs attributable to ovarian cancer were $64,000 as measured in a health maintenance organization (35).

Endometrial Cancer

Unlike ovarian cancer, the symptom most associated with endometrial cancer, namely PMB, accounts for the majority of societal cost. It accounts for 5% of all office gynecologic visits, but indicates endometrial cancer only 10% of the time (36). Data do not exist on the total monetary cost of evaluation of PMB and subsequent staging and treatment of detected endometrial cancer.

Goals

Screening in Ovarian Cancer

The relationship between stage at diagnosis and survival has provided the rationale for screening. The focus of screening in ovarian cancer rests on the identification of disease at a stage early enough to allow intervention to change survival. However, the ability of current techniques, namely the cancer antigen 125 (CA 125) tumor marker and ultrasonography (US), for detecting ovarian cancer at this early stage has not been fully established.

Evaluation in Postmenopausal Bleeding

PMB is a common clinical complaint; however, the optimal algorithm for its evaluation has not been fully elucidated. One of the goals of this chapter is to review the evidence for diagnostic testing in PMB.

Methodology

A Medline search was performed using PubMed (National Library of Medicine, Bethesda, MD) for original research publications discussing the diagnostic performance and effectiveness of screening strategies in ovarian cancer screening. The search covered the years 1966–2003 and included the following search terms: (1) ovarian cancer screening, (2) CA 125, (3) ovarian cancer and ultrasound, and (4) ovarian cancer and imaging. Additional articles were identified by reviewing the reference lists of relevant papers. This review was limited to human studies and the English-language literature.

A separate Medline search was performed using PubMed for original research publications discussing the diagnostic performance and effectiveness of diagnostic strategies in PMB. The search covered the years 1966–2003 and included the following search terms:

(1) PMB, (2) endometrial cancer, (3) endometrial cancer and ultrasound, (4) endometrial cancer and hysteroscopy, and (5) endometrial biopsy. Additional articles were identified by reviewing the reference lists of relevant publications. This review was limited to human studies and the English-language literature.

I. Ovarian Cancer Screening: What Is the Role of Biochemical Markers Such as CA 125?

Summary of Evidence: CA 125 represents the most extensively studied biochemical marker used as a screening test for ovarian cancer. Elevated levels of CA 125 ($\geq$35 U/ml) have a high sensitivity for ovarian cancer at stage II or greater, with only low to moderate (approximately 50%) sensitivity in early-stage disease (moderate evidence). Longitudinal trends in CA 125 levels appear to be more predictive of developing ovarian cancer than a fixed upper limit, as increasing levels of CA 125 were associated with malignancy, whereas stable, though elevated levels of CA 125 were associated with benign disease (Limited evidence).

Supporting Evidence: Although other tumor markers have been recently developed, this review focuses on the use of CA 125, the most frequently used tumor marker. This tumor marker has been developed predominantly using samples from women with clinically detected disease, rather than from women with preclinical disease. Nevertheless, elevated CA 125 (>35U/ml) was demonstrated in 83% of women with epithelial ovarian cancer. As has been previously mentioned, reported sensitivity of elevated CA 125 for detecting ovarian cancer exceeds 90% in the women with greater than stage I disease, but drops to 50% in women with stage I disease (37, 38). A study of 59 serum samples obtained 5 years before the diagnosis of ovarian cancer found that 25% had elevated levels of CA 125, suggesting the potential use of CA 125 for screening for preclinical disease.

The use of trends in serial CA 125 values may be more predictive than a fixed cut-off. Skates et al. (39, 40) observed that CA 125 levels tended to rise in women with malignancy, but remained the same or decreased in women without malignancy. Incorporating trends in serial CA 125 levels increases the sensitivity of the screening regimen as women with normal, but rising CA 125 levels are identified at increased risk of malignancy; identifying women with elevated though stable CA 125 at lesser risk of malignancy increases the specificity (40).

II. Ovarian Cancer Screening: What Is the Diagnostic Performance (Accuracy) of Imaging?

Summary of Evidence: The diagnostic performance of gray-scale US imaging in screening for ovarian cancer in the general population has variable sensitivity ranging from 85 to 97% with lesser specificity of 56–97% (limited evidence). Color Doppler has more variability in its accuracy for detecting ovarian cancer with much weaker supporting evidence, such that there is insufficient evidence to warrant use of color Doppler alone as a screening tool.

Supporting Evidence: Real-time TVUS represents the current state of the art in imaging ovarian changes associated with ovarian cancer. Increased ovarian volume (greater than 10 ml in postmenopausal women) and alterations in normal ovarian morphology have been associated with malignancy (41). Specifically, complex ovarian cysts with multilocularity, wall or septal thickening, internal echogenicity, mural nodules, papillary projections, or solid components are have been used as imaging markers for ovarian cancer (42–45). Typically, repeat imaging at 4–6 weeks to verify stability of abnormal findings is recommended to decrease false positives. The sensitivity of morphologic analysis with US in predicting malignancy in ovarian tumors has been shown to be 85–97%, whereas its specificity ranges from 56 to 95% (44, 46–49).

Gray-scale imaging of the ovaries can be augmented with duplex and color Doppler imaging to detect low resistance flow induced by tumoral neovascularity. In general, lower mean pulsatility indices have been previously demonstrated to be associated with malignancy compared to benign lesions. Resistive indices less than 0.4–0.8 (50–56) and pulsatility indices less than 1.0 are generally considered to

be suspicious for malignancy (50, 51, 53–59). Despite these reports, the duplex Doppler parameters consistently differentiating ovarian malignancies from benign lesions have not been established. A comparison of different studies shows that no standard has been established concerning which Doppler index to use or what cutoff value is most appropriate. Doppler US has yielded variable results in distinguishing benign from malignant masses, with a sensitivity of 50–100% and a specificity of 46–100% (44, 45, 47, 48, 52, 57, 60, 61). Different results are partly due to varying threshold values and corresponding trade-offs between sensitivity and specificity.

Jeng et al. (62) demonstrated that in 740 benign masses, all tumors had a resistive index of greater than 0.4, with 354 having no intratumoral blood flow. In the same study, five of six cases of borderline ovarian malignancies had resistive indices of 0.5–0.6, with the sixth case without intratumoral flow, while 52 of the 55 malignancies had resistive indices less than 0.4. Jeng et al. and others have demonstrated that color Doppler improves performance characteristics of gray-scale US (52, 62, 63). However, there appears to be little support for the use of color duplex Doppler imaging alone as a screening tool for detecting malignant ovarian masses.

Use of prediction rules and neural networks incorporating US imaging characteristics has been reported. To improve the sensitivity and specificity of gray-scale imaging, Timmerman et al. (64) incorporated patient characteristics such as age, menopausal status, and CA 125 level with specific US characteristics of the ovarian mass to derive a risk of malignancy index. The characteristics most predictive of malignancy were postmenopausal status, CA 125 level, the presence of one or more papillary growths, and a color score indicating tumor vascularity and blood flow. The optimized prediction model had a sensitivity of 95.9% and a specificity of 87.1%. Others have also derived morphologic indices by weighting specific US characteristics. However, the application of these indices or prediction rules can be difficult, as there is no consensus on the number and type of characteristics to include in the model (42, 43, 45, 64–66). Furthermore, at least one investigator has demonstrated no significant difference in clinician estimate of probability of malignancy and estimate of malignancy made with a prediction model, using a standardized set of cases (66).

The use of magnetic resonance imaging or computed tomography has not been tested as a screening test (insufficient evidence).

III. Ovarian Cancer Screening: What Is the Role of Imaging?

Summary of Evidence: There is marked heterogeneity in the available evidence for screening in the asymptomatic population with limited to moderate evidence. The specificities from the above studies range from 91 to 98.9%, although the low incidence of ovarian cancer in the general population precluded sufficient assessment of sensitivity. Only one study reported survival, which was increased to 73 months in the screening group, compared to 42 months. Limited evidence supports the use of imaging alone as a screening tool. Even though the evidence is more robust for the use of initial CA 125 level followed by TVUS if CA 125 is elevated, current evidence does not support population-based screening for ovarian cancer in the general population regardless of screening algorithm (limited evidence).

Supporting Evidence: To present the best available evidence for ovarian cancer screening in the general population, only prospective studies with clear enrollment criteria are included in this review. If multiple publications using the same population were identified, only the most recent publication reporting the longest term follow-up was included.

A. Screening with Gray-Scale Ultrasound Only

Campbell et al. (67) evaluated 5,479 self-referred women without symptoms of ovarian cancer using serial transabdominal US conducted annually, with subsequent referral for laparoscopy, laparotomy, or both if positive. Participants without a family history of ovarian cancer were enrolled if they were 45 years and older. All participants with a family history of ovarian cancer (4%) were included regardless of age. A total of 326 women screened positive. Of the nine women who were eventually diagnosed

with ovarian cancer, five had stage I cancers. Despite a 97.7% specificity of the screening regimen, individual US characteristics were insufficient to differentiate benign from malignant lesions.

Tabor et al. (68) conducted a population-based randomized control trial of ovarian cancer screening using TVUS in women 45–65 years old. A total of 950 participants were randomized into either no screening (400 women) or one-time screening with TVUS (450 women). Women with abnormal ovarian morphology on TVUS were referred to laparotomy. A total of nine women were referred for operative evaluation, none of whom had ovarian cancer. Overall specificity for the screening arm was 98%.

van Nagell et al. (41) performed annual TVUS screening on a total of 14,469 women – 11,170 asymptomatic women 50 years and over without a family history of ovarian cancer and 3,299 asymptomatic women 25 years and older with a family history of ovarian cancer received a TVUS at enrollment. Women with a normal TVUS received a follow-up TVUS at 12 months after enrollment. Ultrasound was repeated in women with an abnormal initial TVUS at 4–6 weeks. If the TVUS was persistently abnormal, women received CA 125, color Doppler sonography, and referral for surgery. The TVUS was classified as abnormal if ovarian volume exceeded 10 cm^3 in postmenopausal women (20 cm^3 in premenopausal women) or a papillary or complex tissue projection was identified in a cystic ovarian mass. A total of 180 women with persistently abnormal TVUS received salpingo-oophorectomy with or without hysterectomy. Seventeen women eventually were diagnosed with ovarian cancer, 11 of which were stage I cancers. Specificity of the screening algorithm was 98.9%. But TVUS did not reliably distinguish between benign and malignant tumors.

B. Screening with Ultrasound and Color Doppler Imaging

Vuento et al. (69) enrolled 1,364 asymptomatic women of ages 56–61 years using gray-scale TVUS (96%) or transabdominal US (4%) and color Doppler imaging. Repeat imaging was performed 1–3 months later in women with an abnormal US, with referral to exploratory laparotomy in women with persistently abnormal

US. The US examination was classified as abnormal if ovarian volume equaled or exceeded 8 cm³, ovarian echogenicity was inhomogeneous, or pulsatility index of the ovarian artery or tumor vessel did not exceed 1.0. Women who had a normal screening US were followed using the Finnish Cancer Registry to identify women who subsequently developed ovarian cancer. Eighteen women had persistent sonographic abnormalities; only three women had an abnormal pulsatility index. Of these 18 women, only one ovarian cancer (stage I) was identified. Specificity of the screening algorithm was 98%.

C. Multimodality Approach Using CA 125 and Ultrasound

Einhorn et al. (70) evaluated 5,550 women 40 years and older randomly identified through the Stockholm Population registry. Elevated CA 125 was defined as greater than 35 U/ml in the first 3,455 women enrolled. The threshold for CA 125 was subsequently lowered to 30 U/ml for the latter 2,095. A total of 175 women with elevated CA 125 with age-matched controls were subjected to additional workup with serial CA 125 every 3 months and transabdominal US and pelvic examination every 6 months. Of the 175 women with elevated CA 125, six were found to have ovarian cancer, only two of which were stage I. Of the remainder of women with normal CA 125, three women with ovarian cancer were identified through the Swedish Cancer Registry, only one of which was stage I. In women 50 years and older, the specificity of CA 125 was 98.5% using 35 U/ml as a threshold, and 97% using 30 U/ml. In women under 50 years old, specificity for CA 125 using 35 and 30 U/ml were 94.5 and 91%, respectively.

Jacobs et al. (39) randomized 21,955 postmenopausal women 45 years and older who were asymptomatic to screening or follow-up without screening. The screening regimen consisted of CA 125 and ultrasound if CA 125 was 30 U/ml or greater. The screening regimen was performed annually for 3 years. Transabdominal US was used for the first screen and TVUS for the second and third screens. Women with elevated CA 125 and an abnormal US were referred for surgical evaluation. Follow-up for women who screened negative for ovarian cancer and women in the control group was performed through the National Health Service Central Register. A total of 29 patients were referred for surgical evaluation after detection of elevated CA 125 and abnormal ultrasounds, six of whom had an ovarian cancer. Through the Central Register, an additional ten women in the screening group and 20 women in the control group were identified with ovarian cancer. The median survival time of women with a diagnosed cancer in the screened group was 72.9 months compared to 41.8 months in the control group.

IV. Postmenopausal Bleeding Evaluation: When Should a Woman with PMB Be Referred for Additional Evaluation?

Summary of Evidence: Although there is limited evidence supporting mandatory evaluation of PMB, clinician or patient concern regarding the risk of endometrial cancer warrants additional testing.

Supporting Evidence: As will be discussed in section "VI. Postmenopausal Bleeding Evaluation: What Is the Role of Imaging?" below, the risk for endometrial cancer varies widely in different populations. Although PMB previously represented an absolute indication for further evaluation, given the variable risk of endometrial cancer, the following considerations guide the need for additional workup:

1. Increased prevalence of irregular bleeding in women with HRT: Other causes of abnormal bleeding in this population includes skipped doses, especially progestogens, poor gastrointestinal absorption for oral preparations, drug interactions, coagulation disorders, or other gynecologic abnormalities such as cervical polyps.
2. Paucity of evidence on the clinical significance of bleeding patterns, where a single episode of bleeding should be of equal concern as persistent bleeding or if the magnitude of bleeding should precipitate evaluation.
3. Patient preference for additional evaluation can guide referral.

There is no evidence supporting mandatory referral, but rather the above points may be considered prior to additional testing. Despite this lack of evidence, the risk of endometrial cancer in women not on HRT with PMB or women on HRT with abnormal bleeding is sufficient to warrant further testing (71).

V. Postmenopausal Bleeding Evaluation: What Is the Accuracy of Imaging Tests?

Summary of Evidence: In women with PMB, TVUS is the most sensitive test (moderate evidence), detecting more abnormalities than saline-infused hysterosonography (moderate evidence) or hysteroscopy (moderate evidence).

Supporting Evidence

A. Transvaginal Ultrasonography

The best evidence available for the test performance of TVUS in post-menopausal bleeding results from two recent meta-analysis studies. In symptomatic postmenopausal women not on tamoxifen therapy, Smith-Bindman et al. (72), using a double wall measurement of 5 mm as an upper threshold, demonstrated that the sensitivity for endometrial disease detection reached 92% and for endometrial cancer detection reached 96%. Transvaginal US performed equally well in identifying endometrial disease in women using HRT and women not on HRT. The TVUS false positive rate was 8% in women not on HRT and 23% in women on HRT. Decreasing the threshold for endometrial thickness increases sensitivity (98% using a 3-mm cutoff) with a false-positive rate of 38%. The meta-analysis conducted by Gupta et al. (73) identified 1,243 cases of endometrial carcinoma among 8,890 patients reported in the literature, giving a pretest probability of 14.0%. Using double wall thickness of 5 mm as a cutoff yielded a sensitivity of 97% with a specificity of 45%.

B. Saline-Infused Hysterosonography

De Kroon et al. (74) conducted a meta-analysis to evaluate the diagnostic accuracy of saline contrast hysterosonography in the evaluation of the uterine cavity abnormalities in pre- and postmenopausal women with symptoms of abnormal uterine bleeding.

The main outcome measure was the test performance in detection of any endometrial abnormality in the evaluation of the uterine cavity in cases of abnormal uterine bleeding. The authors did not segregate test results (i.e., they did not separate findings of endometrial cancer from benign etiologies of bleeding). The gold standard used was variable, but inclusion criteria maximized the gold standard by hysteroscopy or avoidance of verification bias in the selection of studies. Pooled sensitivity and specificity were 95 and 88%, respectively. Heterogeneity in sensitivity was not influenced by menopausal status, but specificity was. Baseline prevalence of any uterine abnormality was 56%, much higher than the generally accepted prevalence of endometrial cancer. Pooled likelihood ratio for a positive saline-infused hysterosonogram was 8.23 with an increase in posttest probability to 91%. For a negative test, the likelihood ratio was 0.06, with reduction in posttest probability to 7%.

C. Hysteroscopy

Meta-analysis of observational studies by Clark et al. (75) evaluated 65 primary studies including 26,346 women and assessed the diagnostic accuracy of hysteroscopy in detecting endometrial cancer and hyperplasia. The review included summarized studies including both premenopausal and postmenopausal women. The diagnostic reference standard was endometrial histologic findings. The authors presented pooled sensitivity and specificity across the population. In the detection of endometrial cancer, the variations in sensitivity were much greater than the variations in specificity. Weighted by the number of cases, the overall sensitivity was 86.4% and specificity was 99.2%. Diagnostic accuracy was lower for endometrial disease than for endometrial cancer, with weighted overall sensitivity of 78.0% and specificity of 95.8%. The authors noted that heterogeneity in test performance for detection of endometrial cancer was not explained by menopausal status; however, performance for detection of endometrial disease increased in postmenopausal women.

Other measures of the clinical impact of hysteroscopy, namely likelihood ratios and changes in posttest probability, were segregated by menopausal status. For endometrial cancer, pretest probability (prevalence in women with PMB) increased from 3.9 to 61% with a positive hysteroscopy (positive likelihood ratio 38.3) and decreased to 0.5% with a negative hysteroscopy (negative likelihood ratio 0.13). For endometrial disease, pretest probability (prevalence in women with PMB) increased from 10.6 to 71% with a positive hysteroscopy (positive likelihood ratio 20.4) and decreased to 1.6% with a negative hysteroscopy (negative likelihood ratio 0.14).

VI. Postmenopausal Bleeding Evaluation: What Is the Role of Imaging?

Summary of Evidence: Transvaginal US is recommended as the best initial test for PMB, as a negative test effectively excludes an underlying endometrial abnormality (moderate evidence). Hysteroscopy is recommended as a complementary test to a positive TVUS (moderate evidence). There is insufficient evidence for the routine use of saline-infused hysterosonography unless hysteroscopy is unavailable or more difficult to obtain due resource or expertise limitations.

Supporting Evidence: The high sensitivity of TVUS makes it an excellent noninvasive test for determining which women with vaginal bleeding do not require endometrial biopsy. The specificity is low, and thus US is not very accurate in predicting endometrial disease (72, 73). Therefore, an abnormal TVUS result in a woman with vaginal bleeding needs to be followed by a histologic biopsy.

Hysteroscopy is highly accurate and thereby clinically useful in diagnosing endometrial cancer in women with abnormal uterine bleeding. However, its high accuracy relates to diagnosing cancer rather than excluding it (74). Therefore, this test is more useful as a diagnostic tool complementary to a test such as TVUS, which has a high sensitivity and low specificity.

VII. How Should Women on Tamoxifen Therapy Be Evaluated?

Summary of Evidence: There is insufficient evidence for routine imaging in asymptomatic women on tamoxifen. Symptomatic women should be evaluated with hysteroscopy and biopsy (limited evidence) as the initial algorithm as tamoxifen causes increased false positives with TVUS (moderate evidence).

Supporting Evidence: Long-term use of tamoxifen increases risk of endometrial cancer, as previously mentioned. Furthermore, differentiating potential cancers from other tamoxifen-induced endometrial changes is challenging using any diagnostic test. The evidence does not support the use of investigating asymptomatic women on tamoxifen (76–82). Assigning an absolute upper limit in endometrial thickness detected by TVUS in the setting of tamoxifen administration is difficult as tamoxifen, even in the absence of pathology, causes endometrial thickening, thus increasing false positives using the standard upper limit of 5 mm employed in the postmenopausal woman (83, 84). At least one investigator has proposed increasing the limit to 9 mm, although further studies are required to support this limit. Clearly, the use of TVUS in patients with abnormal bleeding while on tamoxifen is less accurate. As physician and patient concern should be taken into account in the evaluation of abnormal bleeding, hysteroscopy combined with biopsy as the initial test may be more appropriate in this high-risk group (17).

Take Home Tables and Figures (Tables 38.1 and 38.2; Figs. 38.1–38.4)

Protocol: Transvaginal Ultrasound

Sonography should be performed using a 5- to 10-MHz transducer, and the patient's bladder should be empty for sufficient resolution of the endometrial cavity, uterine morphology, and adnexal morphology. Imaging of the uterus should be performed in short axis and long axis relative to the uterus. Sagittal and transverse imaging of the adnexa should be performed.

Table 38.1. Summary of screening regimens in ovarian cancer detection

Screening regimen	Study type	Subjects (cancers)	Specificity (%)
Gray-scale transvaginal ultrasound (TVUS)			
Campbell	Observational	5,479 (9)	98
Tabor	RCT	950 (0)	98
Van Nagell	Observational	14,469 (17)	99
Gray-scale and Doppler TVUS			
Vuento	Observational	1,364 (1)	98
CA 125 + gray-scale TVUS			
Einhorn	Observational	5,500 (7)	99
Jacobs	RCT	21,955 (36)	97

Note: Due to the extremely low prevalence of ovarian cancer in the screening population, none of the studies presented reliable information on sensitivity.

Reprinted with kind permission from Springer Science+Business Media from Carlos RC. Current Issues in Gynecology: Screening for Ovarian Cancer in the Average Risk Population and Diagnostic Evaluation of Postmenopausal Bleeding. In Medina LS, Blackmore CC (eds): *Evidence-Based Imaging: Optimizing Imaging in Patient Care*. New York: Springer Science+Business Media, 2006.

RCT randomized controlled trial.

Table 38.2. Summary of imaging techniques in the evaluation of postmenopausal bleeding

Imaging technique	HRT use	Endometrial disease detection			Endometrial cancer detection		
		Sensitivity (%)	Specificity (%)	PLR (NLR)	Sensitivity (%)	Specificity (%)	PLR (NLR)
Transvaginal ultrasound							
Smith-Bindman, 5-mm threshold	Yes	95	92	11.9 (0.12)			
	No	91	77	4.0 (0.5)			
	Pooled				96	61	nr
Gupta, 5-mm threshold	Pooled	nr	nr	nr	97	45	2.17 (0.15)
Saline-infused sonography							
de Kroon	Pooled	95	88	8.23 (0.06)			
Hysteroscopy							
Clark	Pooled	78	96	20.4 (0.14)	86	99	38.3 (0.13)

Reprinted with kind permission from Springer Science+Business Media from Carlos RC. Current Issues in Gynecology: Screening for Ovarian Cancer in the Average Risk Population and Diagnostic Evaluation of Postmenopausal Bleeding. In Medina LS, Blackmore CC (eds): *Evidence-Based Imaging: Optimizing Imaging in Patient Care*. New York: Springer Science+Business Media, 2006.

PLR positive likelihood ratio, *NLR* negative likelihood ratio, *nr* not reported.

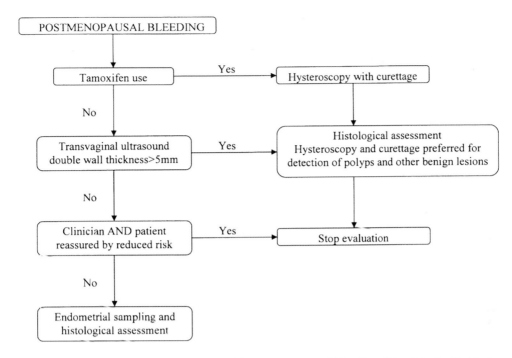

Figure 38.1. Algorithm for evaluating women with postmenopausal bleeding. (Reprinted with kind permission from Springer Science+Business Media from Carlos RC. Current Issues in Gynecology: Screening for Ovarian Cancer in the Average Risk Population and Diagnostic Evaluation of Postmenopausal Bleeding. In Medina LS, Blackmore CC (eds): *Evidence-Based Imaging: Optimizing Imaging in Patient Care.* New York: Springer Science+Business Media, 2006.)

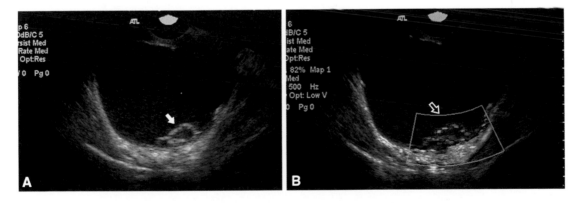

Figure 38.2. Ovarian cancer. (**A**) Large multiloculated cyst with internal echogenicity and a mural nodule (*solid arrow*) (**B**) with vascular flow demonstrated on power Doppler (*open arrow*). (Reprinted with kind permission from Springer Science+Business Media from Carlos RC. Current Issues in Gynecology: Screening for Ovarian Cancer in the Average Risk Population and Diagnostic Evaluation of Postmenopausal Bleeding. In Medina LS, Blackmore CC (eds): *Evidence-Based Imaging: Optimizing Imaging in Patient Care.* New York: Springer Science+Business Media, 2006.)

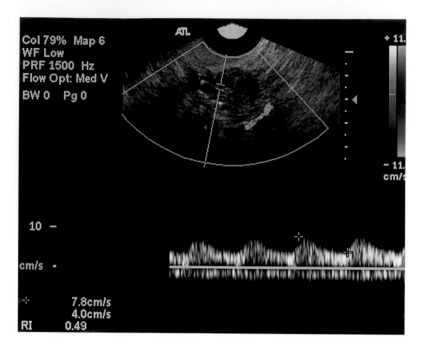

Figure 38.3. Benign ovarian mass. Complex adnexal mass with solid and cystic components. The solid component demonstrates vascular flow with a low resistive index (0.49). Mass was interpreted as an ovarian carcinoma, proved to be a fibroadenoma on resection. (Reprinted with kind permission from Springer Science+Business Media from Carlos RC. Current Issues in Gynecology: Screening for Ovarian Cancer in the Average Risk Population and Diagnostic Evaluation of Postmenopausal Bleeding. In Medina LS, Blackmore CC (eds): *Evidence-Based Imaging: Optimizing Imaging in Patient Care.* New York: Springer Science+Business Media, 2006.)

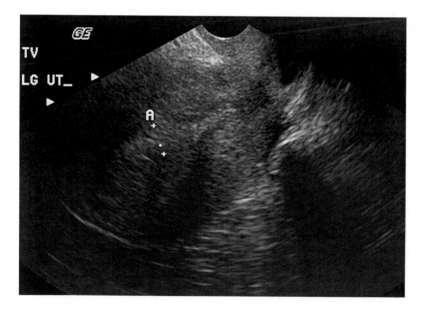

Figure 38.4. Proliferative endometrium. Thickening of the endometrium (10 mm) detected on transvaginal ultrasound in a postmenopausal woman on hormone replacement therapy. Repeat evaluation demonstrated similar thickening. Pathologic samples from intraoperative hysteroscopy and biopsy demonstrated proliferative endometrium, without evidence of endometrial cancer. (Reprinted with kind permission from Springer Science+Business Media from Carlos RC. Current Issues in Gynecology: Screening for Ovarian Cancer in the Average Risk Population and Diagnostic Evaluation of Postmenopausal Bleeding. In Medina LS, Blackmore CC (eds): *Evidence-Based Imaging: Optimizing Imaging in Patient Care.* New York: Springer Science+Business Media, 2006.)

Future Research

- Longitudinal analysis of population-based cohort for ovarian cancer screening.
- Randomized trial of different algorithms for ovarian cancer screening.
- High-quality cohort studies comparing saline-infused hysterosonography to a rigorous standard of reference.
- Analysis of a higher threshold for endometrial thickening in women on tamoxifen.

References

1. Chen VW, Ruiz B, Killeen JL, Cote TR, Wu XC, Correa CN. Cancer 2003;97(10 suppl):2631–2642.
2. Cancer Facts and Figures 2004. Available at http://www.cancer.org.
3. Holschneider CH, Berek JS. Semin Surg Oncol 2000;19(1):3–10.
4. Edmondson RJ, Monaghan JM. Int J Gynecol Cancer 2001;11(6):423–429.
5. Rubin SC, Blackwood MA, Bandera C et al. Am J Obstet Gynecol 1998;178(4):670–677.
6. Boyd J, Rubin SC. Gynecol Oncol 1997;64(2):196–206.
7. Boyd J. In Rubin S, Sutton G (eds.): Ovarian Cancer. Philadelphia: Lippincott Williams & Wilkins, 2001;3–17.
8. Marra G, Boland C. J Natl Cancer Inst 1995;87:1114–1125.
9. Whittemore AS, Harris R, Itnyre J et al. Am J Epidemiol 1992;136:1184–1203.
10. Hankinson SE, Colditz GA, Hunter DJ et al. Cancer 1995;76:284–290.
11. Purdie D, Green A, Bain C et al. Int J Cancer 1995;62:678–684.
12. Mosgaard BJ, Lidegaard O, Kjaer SK, Schou G, Andersen AN. Fertil Steril 1997;67:1005–1012.
13. Ferrazzi E, Torri V, Trio D, Zannoni E, Filiberto S, Dordoni D. Ultrasound Obstet Gynecol 1996;7:315–321.
14. Gredmark T, Kvint S, Havel G, Mattsson LA. Br J Obstet Gynaecol 1995;102:133–136.
15. Lidor A, Ismajovich B, Confino E, David MP. Acta Obstet Gynecol Scand 1986;65:41–43.
16. Research on the Menopause in the 1990s Report of a WHO Scientific Group. World Health Organization, WHO Technical Report Series No. 866, 1996.
17. Investigation of post-menopausal bleeding: a national clinical guideline. Scottish Intercollegiate Guidelines Network 2002. Available at http://www.guideline.gov/summary/summary.aspx?doc_id=3456.
18. Spencer CP, Cooper AJ, Whitehead MI. Br Med J 1997;315:37–42.
19. Dunlop MG, Farrington SM, Carothers AD et al. Hum Mol Genet 1997;6:105–110.
20. Aarnio M, Sankila R, Pukkala E et al. Int J Cancer 1999;81:214–218.
21. Vasen HF, Wijnen JT, Menko FH et al. Gastroenterology 1996;110:1020–1027.
22. Pettersson B, Adami HO, Bergstrom R, Johansson EDB. Acta Obstet Gynecol Scand 1986;65:247–255.
23. Kvale G, Heuch I, Ursin G. Cancer Res 1988;48:6217–6221.
24. Brinton LA, Berman ML, Mortel R et al. Am J Obstet Gynecol 1992;167:1317–1325.
25. Albrektsen G, Heuch I, Tretli S, Kvale G. Int J Cancer 1995;61:485–490.
26. Lambe M, Wuu J, Weiderpass E, Hsieh CC. Cancer Causes Control 1999;10:43–49.
27. Henderson BE, Casagrande JT, Pike MC, Mack T, Rosario I, Duke A. Br J Cancer 1983;47:749–756.
28. N Engl J Med 1987;316:650–655.
29. Pike MC, Peters RK, Cozen W et al. J Natl Cancer Inst 1997;89:1110–1116.
30. Rutqvist LE, Johansson H, Signomklao T, Johansson U, Fornander T, Wilking N. J Natl Cancer Inst 1995;87:645–651.
31. Fisher B, Costantino JP, Wickerham DL et al. J Natl Cancer Inst 1998;90:1371–1388.
32. Fornander T, Rutqvist LE, Cedermark B et al. Lancet 1989;1:117–120.
33. Curtis RE, Boice JD Jr., Shriner DA, Hankey BF, Fraumeni JF Jr. J Natl Cancer Inst 1996;88:832–834.
34. Etzioni R, Urban N, Baker M. J Clin Epidemiol 1996;49:95–103.
35. Fireman B, Quesenberry C, Somkin C et al. Health Care Financ Rev 1997;18:51–76.
36. Develioglu OH, Bilgin T, Yalcin OT, Ozalp S. Arch Gynecol Obstet 2003;268(3):175–180.
37. Fritsche HA, Bast RC. Clin Chem 1998;44:1379–1380.
38. Jacobs IJ, Menon U. Mol Cell Proteomics 2004;3(4):355–366.
39. Jacobs IJ, Skates SJ, Macdonald N et al. Lancet 1999;353:1207–1210.
40. Skates SJ, Pauler DK, Jacobs IJ. J Am Stat Assoc 2001;96:429–439.
41. van Nagell JR Jr., DePriest PD, Reedy MB et al. Gynecol Oncol 2000;77:350–356.
42. Sassone AM, Timor-Tritsch IE, Artner A, Westhoff C, Warren WB. Obstet Gynecol 1991;78:70–76.
43. Lerner JP, Timor-Tritsch IE, Federman A, Abramovich G. Am J Obstet Gynecol 1994;170:81–85.
44. Reles A, Wein U, Lichtenegger W. J Clin Ultrasound 1997;25:217–225.

45. Ferrazzi E, Zanetta G, Dordoni D, Berlanda N, Mezzopane R, Lissoni AA. Ultrasound Obstet Gynecol 1997;10:192–197.
46. Leibman AJ, Kruse B, McSweeney MB. AJR Am J Roentgenol 1988;151:89–92.
47. Hata K, Hata T, Manabe A, Sugimura K, Kitao M. Obstet Gynecol 1992;80:922–926.
48. Kurjak A, Predanic M. J Ultrasound Med 1992;11:631–638.
49. Franchi M, Beretta P, Ghezzi F, Zanaboni F, Goddi A, Salvatore S. Acta Obstet Gynecol Scand 1995;74:734–739.
50. Hamper UM, Sheth S, Abbas FM, Rosenshein NB, Aronson D, Kurman RJ. AJR Am J Roentgenol 1993;160:1225–1228.
51. Stein SM, Laifer-Narin S, Johnson MB et al. AJR Am J Roentgenol 1995;164:381–386.
52. Bromley B, Goodman H, Benacerraf BR. Obstet Gynecol 1994;83:434–437.
53. Brown DL, Frates MC, Laing FC et al. Radiology 1994;190:333–336.
54. Carter J, Saltzman A, Hartenbach E, Fowler J, Carson L, Twiggs LB. Obstet Gynecol 1994;83: 125–130.
55. Jain KA. Radiology 1994;191:63–67.
56. Levine D, Feldstein VA, Babcook CJ, Filly RA. AJR Am J Roentgenol 1994;162:1355–1359.
57. Salem S, White LM, Lai J. AJR Am J Roentgenol 1994;163:1147–1150.
58. Weiner Z, Thaler I, Levron J, Lewit N, Itskovitz-Eldor J. Fertil Steril 1993;59:743–749.
59. Rehn M, Lohmann K, Rempen A. Am J Obstet Gynecol 1996;175:97–104.
60. Timor-Tritsch LE, Lerner JP, Monteagudo A, Santos R. Am J Obstet Gynecol 1993;168: 909–913.
61. Schneider VL, Schneider A, Reed KL, Hatch KD. Obstet Gynecol 1993;81:983–988.
62. Jeng CJ, Lin SY, Wang KL, Yang YC, Wang KG. Ultrasound Med Biol 1994;20;180.
63. Fleischer AC, Cullinan JA, Kepple DM, Williams LL. J Ultrasound Med 1993;12:705–712.
64. Timmerman D, Bourne TH, Tailor A et al. Am J Obstet Gynecol 1999;181:57–65.
65. Ueland FR, DePriest PD, Pavlik EJ, Kryscio RJ, van Nagell JR Jr. Gynecol Oncol 2003;91:46–50.
66. Mol B, Boll D, DeKanter M et al. Gynecol Oncol 2001;80:162–167.
67. Campbell S, Bhan V, Royston P, Whitehead MI, Collins WP. Br Med J 1989;299:1363–1367.
68. Tabor A, Jensen FR, Bock JE, Hogdall CK. J Med Screen 1994;1:215–219.
69. Vuento MH, Pirhonen JP, Makinen JI, Laippala PJ, Gronroos M, Salmi TA. Cancer 1995;76: 1214–1218.
70. Einhorn N, Sjovall K, Knapp RC et al. Obstet Gynecol 1992;80:14–18.
71. Department of Health. Referral guidelines for suspected cancer. London: Department of Health, 2000. Available at url:http://www.doh.gov.uk/cancer/referral.htm.
72. Smith-Bindman R, Kerlikowske K, Feldstein VA et al. JAMA 1998;280:1510–1517.
73. Gupta JK, Chien PF, Voit D, Clark TJ, Khan KS. Acta Obstet Gynecol Scand 2002;81(9): 799–816.
74. de Kroon CD, de Bock GH, Dieben SW, Jansen FW. Br J Obstet Gynaecol 2003;110(10):938–947.
75. Clark TJ, Voit D, Gupta JK, Hyde C, Song F, Khan KS. JAMA 2002;288(13):1610–1621.
76. Timmerman D, Deprest J, Bourne T, Van den Berghe I, Collins WP, Vergote I. Am J Obstet Gynecol 1998;179:62–70.
77. Cecchini S, Ciatto S, Bonardi R et al. Tumori 1998;84:21–23.
78. Tepper R, Beyth Y, Altaras MM et al. Gynecol Oncol 1997;64:386–391.
79. Love CD, Muir BB, Scrimgeour JB, Leonard RC, Dillon P, Dixon JM. J Clin Oncol 1999;17: 2050–2054.
80. Berliere M, Charles A, Galant C, Donnez J. Obstet Gynecol 1998;91:40–44.
81. Gerber B, Krause A, Muller H et al. J Clin Oncol 2000;18:3464–3470.
82. Barakat RR, Gilewski TA, Almadrones L et al. J Clin Oncol 2000;18:3459–3463.
83. Bornstein J, Auslender R, Pascal B, Gutterman E, Isakov D, Abramovici H. J Reprod Med 1994;39:674–678.
84. Mourits MJ, Van der Zee AG, Willemse PH, Ten Hoor KA, Hollema H, De Vries EG. Gynecol Oncol 1999;73:21–26.

39

Imaging of Female Children and Adolescents with Abdominopelvic Pain Caused by Gynecological Pathologies

Stefan Puig

Issues

I. What is the diagnostic performance of the different imaging studies for the diagnosis or exclusion of ovarian torsion?
II. What is the best imaging technique for the diagnosis of PID?
III. What is the best imaging technique for the diagnosis of endometriosis?
IV. What is the best technique for the diagnosis of an ectopic pregnancy?

Key Points

- The clinical presentation of abdominopelvic pain and gonadal pathologies is often nonspecific and therefore difficult to diagnose (limited evidence).
- Surgical emergencies such as ovarian torsion should be considered when a girl presents with acute abdominopelvic pain (limited to moderate evidence).
- In menstruating girls and adolescents, pregnancy (orthotopic or ectopic) should be considered as a cause of abdominopelvic discomfort/pain (limited evidence).
- The initial imaging modality of choice for evaluating the uterus and adnexa is ultrasound (US) (limited to moderate evidence). If US is nondiagnostic and the clinical picture remains uncertain, MRI is the preferred next imaging test. CT may also be considered in patients with acute symptoms (limited evidence).
- Other gynecological causes of abdominopelvic pain such as endometriosis and PID have a significant impact on societal health care costs (limited to moderate evidence).
- Various complications associated with tumors may lead to acute abdominopelvic pain (limited evidence).

S. Puig (✉)
Paracelsus Medical University, Strubergasse 21, Salzburg 5020, Austria
e-mail: stefan.Puig@pmu.ac.at

L.S. Medina et al. (eds.), *Evidence-Based Imaging: Improving the Quality of Imaging in Patient Care, Revised Edition*, **649**
DOI 10.1007/978-1-4419-7777-9_39, © Springer Science+Business Media, LLC 2011

Definition

In general, acute pelvic or lower abdominal pain in girls (as in boys) is mainly associated with gastrointestinal disorders (1). However, it may be secondary to a wide range of gynecological disorders in girls and female adolescents (2). Therefore, a gynecological etiology should always be considered in young female patients with lower abdominal and/or pelvic discomfort or pain. In adolescents, a gynecological process is more commonly the cause for acute pain than appendicitis. Klein et al. found in 20% of girls older than 12 years of age a pelvic inflammation or gynecological process (including pregnancy) as a cause for pain, whereas appendicitis was only found in 4% (3). A gynecological problem (adnexitis or ovarian cysts) was identified in 12% of the populations studied by Puig et al., including children, adolescents, and young adults who received preoperative misdiagnosis of appendicitis and underwent a negative appendectomy (4). Specifically, in younger patients, it is difficult to localize the pain during physical examination, making it a diagnostic challenge.

The presentation and types of pain from gynecologic infectious and inflammatory conditions are variable. It may be intermittent and localized to one quadrant; severe, acute, and generalized; crampy; chronic and cyclical; chronic and noncyclical; or present as an acute abdomen. Nausea, vomiting, or bleeding may accompany the pain. In ovarian neoplasms, clinical presentation includes abdominal distension, a palpable abdominal mass, genitourinary symptoms, or constipation.

Gynecological conditions that should be considered and will be discussed in this chapter include congenital Müllerian anomalies, PID, ovarian tumors, ovarian cysts, ovarian torsion, trauma, and pregnancy (2, 5).

Pathology and Epidemiology

Congenital Anomalies

Congenital anomalies of the Müllerian system are estimated to occur in approximately 0.1–1.5% of women in the general population and approximately 90% of these anomalies involve the uterus (6, 7). Girls with uterovaginal anomalies may present with pain and occasionally with an abdominal/pelvic mass due to vaginal obstruction. Because of the complexity of the embryology, obstruction may occur at different levels and in various degrees, including imperforate hymen, complete vaginal membrane, or atresia of the vagina and/or uterus (2, 5, 6). These conditions are usually encountered either in the neonatal period or in adolescence at the time of menarche (2). Hydrometrocolpos, back-flow of uterine blood products into the fallopian tubes and adnexa, is associated with the development of endometriosis.

Endometriosis

Endometriosis is defined as the presence of endometrium-like tissue (endometrial glands) outside of the normal location in the uterus (8, 9). It is a relatively common disease affecting 0.5–15% of women, in general, and 25–80% of all women with pelvic pain and/or infertility (9–15). Endometriosis is the most common cause of pelvic pain, which may be noncyclical (15). The true prevalence of endometriosis remains unclear (16). Estimates of prevalence range up to 10% in the general population. Large-scale studies suggest a prevalence of 0.5–5% in fertile and 25–40% in infertile women (17, 18). For adolescents, a prevalence of 25–38% of patients with pelvic pain has been reported. If the pain is persistent, the prevalence increases to 70–79% (19–23) (limited evidence). Although endometriosis is generally accepted to be associated with infertility, its actual impact on fecundity and the mechanisms underlying this effect are less clear. Unfortunately, well-designed scientific studies are lacking on this issue (16, 24).

Pelvic Inflammatory Disease

Pelvic inflammatory disease is associated with *Chlamydia trachomatis* and *Neisseria gonorrhoeae* infections, and therefore the incidence increases with sexual activity (25–27). *Mycoplasma genitalium* and microorganisms of the vaginal flora including anaerobes, streptococci, staphylococci, *Escherichia coli*, and *Haemophilus influenzae* might also be implicated in the etiology of the disease. However, the importance of the different pathogens varies in different countries and regions (27). The infection spreads from the vagina to the fallopian tubes and leads to pelvic pain, vaginal discharge or dyspareunia, endometritis, salpingitis, parametritis, oophoritis, tubo-ovarian abscess, and/or pelvic peritonitis (27). In a large British screening study, the prevalence of Chlamydia was 6.2% (95% CI, 4.9–7.8%) in 16–24-year-old women and 5.3% (95% CI, 4.4–6.3%) in men (28). Factors associated with PID are related to sexual behavior (young age, multiple partners, recent new partners in the previous 3 months, and past history of sexually transmitted disease) and interruption of the cervical barrier (e.g., termination of pregnancy, insertion of an intrauterine device within the past 6 weeks, hysterosalpingography, in vitro fertilization, and intrauterine insemination) (27).

When present, clinical symptoms and signs in PID lack sensitivity. Compared to laparoscopic diagnosis, the positive predictive value of a clinical diagnosis of PID is 65–90% (27, 29–31). The clinical diagnosis includes a broad range of differential diagnoses: ectopic pregnancy, acute appendicitis, endometriosis, irritable bowel syndrome, complications of an ovarian cyst (e.g., rupture, torsion), or functional pain (pain of unknown physical origin) (27).

Adnexal Torsion

Adnexal torsion is defined as a complete or partial rotation of the ovary and/or fallopian tube including the vascular pedicle (32). While ovarian torsion is the twisting of an ovary on its ligamentous supports, which might result in a compromised blood supply, the term adnexal torsion describes a twisting of either the ovary or fallopian tube, or both. Concomitant torsion of an ovary and the ipsilateral fallopian tube occurs in up to 67% of patients with adnexal torsion (32–34). It is an important cause of abdominal pain, which may lead to initial compromise of the lymphatic and venous drainage, later to arterial occlusion and thrombosis, resulting in a hemorrhagic infarction (2, 25, 35). It may occur at any age, most commonly in the first two decades of life (2). Some authors reported a peak incidence after menarche (25) and others reported the highest prevalence in pregnant women with a peak of 17–20% (32, 36–39). Adnexal torsion is supposed to account for up to 2.7% of all cases with acute abdominal pain in children, and is the fifth most common

gynecologic emergency with a reported incidence of 3% in one series of acute gynecologic complaints (34, 40, 41). Despite the relatively uncommon nature of this condition, most reviews report three to five cases per year at large institutions (34, 42, 43). In any case, it is a medical/surgical emergency (25). Ovaries with any type of mass are predisposed to torsion (32, 33, 44). Torsion of normal ovaries is more common in adolescents. Postulated causes of normal adnexal torsion include mobile fallopian tubes or mesosalpinx, elongated pelvic ligaments, fallopian tube spasm, strenuous exercise, or abrupt changes in intra-abdominal pressure (32, 34, 43, 45). A limited number of studies have shown that the right ovary is more likely to twist, because the space in the lesser pelvis occupied by the sigmoid colon may protect the left ovary (32, 33, 46, 47). Adnexal torsion is often misdiagnosed as appendicitis. In a retrospective study, Pomeranz and Sabnis found 38% of children with adnexal torsion and abdominal pain, who had the preliminary diagnosis of appendicitis (48).

Abdominopelvic Mass

Functional cysts, ovarian torsion, and benign neoplasms are the most common ovarian masses among young adolescents. In pubescent girls and adult women, ovarian follicle size is up to 2.5 cm; cysts larger than 4 cm generally require a follow-up sonogram at 2 or 6 weeks to ensure resolution (during a different point in the girl's menstrual cycle).

In younger children, the ovaries are a solid and homogenous structure, which may contain primordial follicles. These follicles measure up to 9 mm in diameter in most children and usually regress spontaneously (25). Neonatal ovarian cysts develop under the influence of maternal, placental, and fetal hormones during the third trimester. The majority resolve spontaneously after birth. The prevalence of ovarian cysts in children is unclear. A small number of studies reported frequencies between 33 and 84% (49, 50) (limited evidence). Cohen et al. found macrocysts larger than 9 mm in diameter in 18% of children of up to 2 years of age (49). Uncomplicated cysts may present as palpable abdominopelvic mass lesions (25). Cysts may be complicated by torsion, hemorrhage, or rupture. Torsion is more common in cysts which have a diameter over 5 cm or a long pedicle.

Differential diagnosis of neonatal ovarian cysts includes hydronephrosis, hydrocolpos, enteric duplication cyst, choledochal cyst, urachal cyst, bowel atresia, or obstruction (25) (limited evidence). Older children and adolescents with ovarian cysts may present with acute abdominal pain due to hemorrhage or cyst rupture (25, 51).

Girls with an ovarian neoplasm may present with abdominal distension and a palpable abdominal mass. The tumors may be complicated by torsion and/or rupture (25). Ovarian dermoid/teratoma is the most common tumor of the ovaries, accounting for 50% of pediatric and 20% of adult ovarian tumors (52). Ovarian teratomas may be associated with various complications, leading to acute lower abdominal pain, such as adnexal torsion (16% of ovarian teratomas), rupture (1–4%), and infection (1%) (52–55). Epithelial tumors account for about 17% and sex cord-stromal tumors for about 13% of pediatric ovarian tumors (25).

Pregnancy

Pregnancy is not uncommon and should always be considered in adolescents who present with acute pelvic pain (2). The incidence of ectopic pregnancies is unclear. Zane et al. estimated a total number of 10,221–77,129 ectopic pregnancy cases per year in the USA (56). In the UK, nearly 32,000 ectopic pregnancies are diagnosed every year, resulting in an incidence of about 11 per 1,000 pregnancies (57). It is the second leading cause of maternal mortality and accounts for 80% of first trimester maternal deaths (25, 57). In younger women, ectopic pregnancy accounts for 0.5% of pregnancies (25). Menon et al. compared the incidence of ectopic pregnancies in symptomatic women, which was significantly lower in women under 20 years of age (9.7%) compared to those of 20 years of age and older (21.7%) (58) (limited evidence).

Overall Cost to Society

Pelvic Inflammatory Disease

There are numerous cost analyses on PID. Yeh et al. calculated the costs of major complications of PID based on a cohort of 100,000 women aged 20–24 years, in which 8,550 ectopic pregnancies, 16,800 cases of infertility, and 18,600 cases of chronic pelvic pain were projected to occur (59). They found an average per-person lifetime cost of US $2,150. Average lifetime costs for women who developed major complications were US $6,350 for chronic pelvic pain, US $6,840 for ectopic pregnancy, and US $1,270 for infertility. The majority of costs (79%) were due to upper genital tract infection (59) (moderate evidence).

Endometriosis

In 2006, Gao et al. published a systematic review on economic consequences of endometrioses and related symptoms (60). They included 13 relevant studies evaluating treatment costs, time lost from work, employment status, and other parameters. Only one of these 13 studies presented data of the entire hospitalization process (61), being based on data from the "Healthcare Cost and Utilization Project" (HCUP). The mean inpatient charges per admission for endometriosis were US $6,597 in 1991 and US $7,449 in 1992 (61). Based on the publication of Zhao et al., the HCUP data were reevaluated by Gao et al. for the year 2002, calculating an increase of 61% or a mean per-patient charge of US $12,644 (60). Simoens et al. published a systematic review of estimates and methodology of studies quantifying the costs of endometriosis (62). They found one study indicating that annual health care costs of endometriosis are substantial, amounting to direct costs of US $2,801 per patient in 2002 and annual indirect costs of US $1,023 per patient. The direct costs were broken down into hospitalization costs of US $2,518 (90%) and outpatient costs of US $283 (10%) (63). Delayed correct diagnosis of endometriosis is a major reason for costs in these patients. About 3–12 years may pass between symptom onset and definitive diagnosis (62, 64). In this period of time, unnecessary investigations and treatments are likely to be initiated.

For other specific diagnoses of pelvic pain, accurate cost analyses are not available. However, the economic and psychosocial impacts are important (65–68) and may be reduced due to earlier diagnosis (69, 70).

Goals

In cases of abdominopelvic pain, identification or exclusion of gonadal causes in girls and adolescents is mandatory, since it may be a surgical emergency. Clinical presentation is often nonspecific and may overlap with clinical presentation of other abdominal pathologies such as appendicitis.

In patients with chronic pelvic pain, early correct diagnosis of the underlying cause is desirable to avoid unnecessary treatments and costs as well as compromised quality of life.

Methodology

The diagnostic performance of the clinical examination (history and physical exam) and the accuracy of both clinical and radiographic examinations in young patients with abdominopelvic pain caused by gonadal pathologies was evaluated based on a systematic literature review using PubMed (Medline, National Library of Medicine, Bethesda, MD), Cochrane library, and the National Guideline Clearinghouse. All searches were performed in July 2008 without any time restrictions. The clinical examination search strategy used the following statements: (1) abdominal or abdominopelvic or pelvic and pain; (2) clinical examination; (3) epidemiology; (4) physical examination; (5) imaging (including MRI, ultrasound, scintigraphy, and acronyms of these terms); (6) diagnosis; as well as combinations of these search strings. Animal studies and non-English and non-German studies were excluded.

I. What Is the Diagnostic Performance of the Different Imaging Studies for the Diagnosis or Exclusion of Ovarian Torsion?

Summary of Evidence: Sonography is the first-line modality in children and adolescents with abdominal and/or pelvic pain suspected to be of gynecological origin (limited evidence).

The most common finding in ovarian torsion is an enlarged heterogeneous ovary (limited evidence).

Presence or absence of arterial or venous flow is neither sensitive nor specific for the diagnosis of ovarian/adnexal torsion (limited evidence). Therefore, close clinical correlation is mandatory and if suspected, laparoscopy confirmation and treatment are required.

Supporting Evidence: Chiou et al. reviewed surgically proven cases of adnexal torsion between 1990 and 2006 (71). A correct preoperative diagnosis was made in 15 (71%) of 21 with initial sonography versus 5 (38%) of 13 cases with initial CT. A correct imaging diagnosis was made more frequently in premenopausal than in menopausal patients ($p = 0.02$) (Table 39.1). Common imaging findings were an adnexal mass (65% on sonography, 87% on CT, and 75% on MRI), a displaced adnexal mass/enlarged ovary (53% on sonography, 87% on CT, and 75% on MRI), and ascites (53% on sonography, 73% on CT, and 50% on MRI) (71).

A retrospective study with surgically and pathologically proven ovarian torsions found in 100% of the patients an enlarged torsed ovary, with the median volume 12 times (range 4.4–27.3) that of the normal contralateral side (72). In 62%, venous or arterial flow was present in the torsed ovary (72). A twisted vascular pedicle (whirlpool sign) was found in up to 88% of twisted ovaries (44, 73).

The sensitivity of sonography was 100% and specificity was 93% in a small study of 28 girls, using an enlarged ovary as the criterion for abnormal (limited evidence). The volume of the enlarged ovaries ranged from 34 to 365 cm³ (mean 130 ± 99 cm³) (37).

The classical description of a torsed ovary on sonography is enlargement with peripheral small cysts (follicles) and a small amount of pelvic free fluid. However, this finding is not common.

II. What Is the Best Imaging Technique for the Diagnosis of PID?

Summary of Evidence: Transvaginal US is superior to transabdominal US in the diagnosis of PID (limited evidence). For the depiction and management planning of pelvic abscesses, cross-sectional imaging with US, CT, or MRI is often required. Comparisons between US, CT, and MRI are not available (limited evidence).

Supporting Evidence: Studies evaluating the value of imaging techniques in young patients with PID are very limited. Bulas et al. studied the diagnostic performance of transabdominal and transvaginal sonography in 84 patients aged 12–21 years with the clinical diagnosis of acute PID (74). Transvaginal sonography demonstrated superior resolution of 25 dilated fallopian tubes. Heterogeneous pelvic masses, described as tubo-ovarian abscesses on transabdominal sonograms, could be separated on transvaginal sonograms into various stages of PID including pyosalpinx, hydrosalpinx, tubo-ovarian complex, and tubo-ovarian abscess. Thirty-one transabdominal and transvaginal studies were normal despite patients fulfilling strict clinical criteria for PID. The level of severity of PID, as determined at transabdominal sonography, was altered in 28 cases, with medical therapy changed in 23 cases because of additional transvaginal sonographic findings. Transvaginal sonography provided superior anatomic details in the evaluation of patients with PID, demonstrating abnormalities that were not seen at transabdominal sonography in 71% of patients.

CT (and MRI) findings in early PID include obscuration of the normal pelvic floor fascial planes, thickening of the uterosacral ligaments, cervicitis, oophoritis, salpingitis, and accumulation of simple fluid in the endometrial canal, fallopian tubes, and pelvis. As the disease progresses, the simple fluid may become complex and the inflammatory changes may progress to frank tubo-ovarian or pelvic abscesses (75).

III. What Is the Best Imaging Technique for the Diagnosis of Endometriosis?

Summary of Evidence: Transvaginal sonography is the imaging test of choice for the evaluation of endometriosis. MRI is more expensive but performs similarly to transvaginal sonography for the diagnosis of intestinal endometriosis. For some less common imaging findings, MRI has higher sensitivity and diagnostic likelihood ratios for uterosacral ligament and vaginal endometriosis (limited evidence). Transrectal sonography is also a sensitive test but is less well tolerated by patients and less widely used for this diagnosis.

Supporting Evidence: Bazot et al. compared physical examination, transvaginal sonography, rectal endoscopic sonography, and magnetic resonance imaging for the diagnosis of endometriosis in 92 adult patients prior to surgery in a retrospective study (76). MRI performed similarly to US for the diagnosis of intestinal endometriosis but had higher sensitivity and likelihood ratios for uterosacral ligament and vaginal endometriosis. This study has limited value for the diagnosis of endometriosis in children, because transvaginal and rectal endoscopic sonography are not the imaging techniques of choice in this age group (Table 39.1). However, since MRI was the superior technique compared to US and physical examination, the results are also valuable for a younger age group.

IV. What Is the Best Technique for the Diagnosis of an Ectopic Pregnancy?

Summary of Evidence: Pregnancy and ectopic pregnancy are both best imaged by sonography. Initially, abdominal sonography is performed and when there are unclear findings that suggest pregnancy or ectopic pregnancy, transvaginal sonography improves diagnostic accuracy (moderate evidence).

Supporting Evidence: Beta-hCG levels assist in interpreting sonographic findings. Ectopic pregnancy is suspected if transabdominal sonography does not show an intrauterine gestational sac and the patient's β-hCG level is greater than 6,500 IU/L or if transvaginal sonography does not show an intrauterine gestational sac and the patient's β-hCG is 1,500 IU/L or greater. Combined transvaginal sonography and serial quantitative β-hCG measurements are approximately 96% sensitive and 97% specific for diagnosing ectopic pregnancy (77–79) (moderate evidence) (Table 39.1).

Take-Home Tables

Table 39.1 discusses the diagnostic performance of US in pediatric female pelvic conditions.

Table 39.1. Diagnostic performance of ultrasound in pediatric female pelvic conditions

	Ovarian torsion	Pelvic inflammatory disease	Endometriosis	Ectopic pregnancy
Sensitivity	1.00	0.72	0.75–0.95[a]	0.96[a]
Specificity	0.93	N/A	0.83–1.00[a]	0.97[a]
Accuracy	0.71	N/A	0.83[a]	N/A

Data from (37, 44, 72, 73, 76–79) (limited evidence).

Reprinted with kind permission of Springer Science+Business Media from Puig S. Imaging of Female Children and Adolescents with Abdominopelvic Pain Caused by Gynecological Pathologies. In Medina LS, Applegate KE, Blackmore CC (eds): *Evidence-Based Imaging in Pediatrics: Optimizing Imaging in Pediatric Patient Care.* New York: Springer Science+Business Media, 2010.

N/A Not available.

[a]Using endovaginal ultrasound (adolescents and adults).

Imaging Case Studies

Case 1

Figure 39.1 illustrates a very large ovarian cyst in a 10-year-old girl who presented with acute abdominal pain and urinary retention.

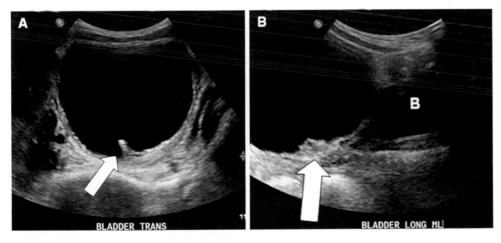

Figure 39.1. Very large ovarian cyst. A 10-year-old girl presented with acute abdominal pain and urinary retention. At sonography, she had a very large simple cyst measuring up to 11 cm [(**A**) in trans, (**B**) in long]. Note the wall of the cyst had a few focal thickened strands (*white arrows*). The bladder is visualized inferior to the cyst in B (*B* bladder). At surgery, the ovary had torsed and was removed. (Reprinted with kind permission of Springer Science+Business Media from Puig S. Imaging of Female Children and Adolescents with Abdominopelvic Pain Caused by Gynecological Pathologies. In Medina LS, Applegate KE, Blackmore CC (eds): *Evidence-Based Imaging in Pediatrics: Optimizing Imaging in Pediatric Patient Care.* New York: Springer Science+Business Media, 2010.)

Case 2

Figure 39.2 illustrates a hemorrhagic ovarian cyst in an 11-year-old girl who presented with severe left lower quadrant abdominal pain.

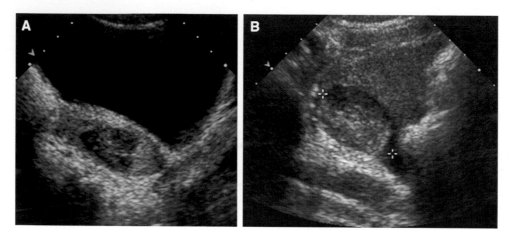

Figure 39.2. Hemorrhagic ovarian cyst. An 11-year-old girl presented with severe left lower quadrant abdominal pain. Her ultrasound revealed a debris-fluid level [(**A**), *arrow*] within her left ovary, which represents acute hemorrhage into an ovarian cyst. (**B**) shows the left ovary with the echogenic blood and faintly seen in the periphery are some normal follicles. Both her pain and the fluid resolved without the need for surgery. (Reprinted with kind permission of Springer Science+Business Media from Puig S. Imaging of Female Children and Adolescents with Abdominopelvic Pain Caused by Gynecological Pathologies. In Medina LS, Applegate KE, Blackmore CC (eds): *Evidence-Based Imaging in Pediatrics: Optimizing Imaging in Pediatric Patient Care*. New York: Springer Science+Business Media, 2010.)

Suggested Imaging Protocols

Plain Radiographs

Plain radiographs are not recommended.

Ultrasound

Ultrasound is the key screening tool and often the only examination indicated. US with a 7 MHz probe is ideal for children (5 MHz for older children). For obese children or adolescents, 3 MHz may be required. To evaluate the female reproductive tract, a full urinary bladder is essential. If the bladder is not adequately full, it might be useful to repeat the examination every 15 min. Further evaluation with CT or MRI may depend on the results of the sonograms, the clinical examination, and acuity of the problem.

Multi-Detector Computed Tomography

Intravenous contrast is essential to visualize infection or inflammation and abscess. Oral or rectal contrast may help to distinguish fluid-filled bowel loops in the pelvis.

Magnetic Resonance Imaging

Axial and coronal T1-spin echo, axial and sagittal T2 FSE with fat saturation, coronal STIR or HASTE, and axial and coronal T1 2D SPGR with fat saturation before and after intravenous gadolinium (in patients with acceptable renal function). Alternative to imaging with CT. Not as sensitive for calcification but can provide functional data.

Future Research

- What are the clinical predictors for ovarian pathology that leads to appropriate use of sonography?
- What is the appropriate use of MR imaging in girls with gynecologic disorders?

References

1. Carrico CW, Fenton LZ, Taylor GA, DiFiore JW, Soprano JV. AJR Am J Roentgenol 1999;172: 513–516.
2. Hollmann AS, Macdonald S. In Carty H (ed.): Emergency Pediatric Radiology. Berlin: Springer, 1999;217–232.
3. Klein MD, Rabbani AB, Rood KD et al. J Pediatr Surg 2001;36:1375–1380.
4. Puig S, Hörmann M, Rebhandl W, Felder-Puig R, Prokop M et al. Radiology 2003;226:101–104.
5. Strouse PJ. Singapore Med J 2003;44:312–322.
6. Bailez MM. Semin Pediatr Surg 2007;16:278–287.
7. Rock JA, Schlaff WD. Fertil Steril 1985;43:681–692.
8. Bhatt S, Kocakoc E, Dogra VS. Ultrasound Q 2006;22:273–280.
9. Woodward PJ, Sohaey R, Mezzetti TP, Jr. Radiographics 2001;21:193–216; questionnaire 288–294.
10. Chatman DL, Ward AB. J Reprod Med 1982;27: 156–160.
11. Guo SW, Wang Y. Gynecol Obstet Invest 2006;62:121–130.
12. Guo SW, Wang Y. Fertil Steril 2006;86:1584–1595.
13. Black AY, Jamieson MA. Curr Opin Obstet Gynecol 2002;14:467–474.
14. Vinatier D, Orazi G, Cosson M, Dufour P. Eur J Obstet Gynecol Reprod Biol 2001;96:21–34.
15. Laufer MR, Sanfilippo J, Rose G. J Pediatr Adolesc Gynecol 2003;16:S3–S11.
16. Ozkan S, Murk W, Arici A. Ann N Y Acad Sci 2008;1127:92–100.
17. Eskenazi B, Warner ML. Obstet Gynecol Clin North Am 1997;24:235–258.
18. Houston DE, Noller KL, Melton LJ III., Selwyn BJ, Hardy RJ. Am J Epidemiol 1987;125:959–969.
19. Matalliotakis IM, Cakmak H, Fragouli YG, Goumenou AG, Mahutte NG et al. Arch Gynecol Obstet 2008;277:389–393.
20. Kontoravdis A, Hassan E, Hassiakos D, Botsis D, Kontoravdis N et al. Clin Exp Obstet Gynecol 1999;26:76–77.
21. Laufer MR, Goitein L, Bush M, Cramer DW, Emans SJ. J Pediatr Adolesc Gynecol 1997;10: 199–202.
22. Reese KA, Reddy S, Rock JA. J Pediatr Adolesc Gynecol 1996;9:125–128.
23. Vercellini P, Fedele L, Arcaini L, Bianchi S, Rognoni MT et al. J Reprod Med 1989;34:827–830.
24. Osuga Y, Koga K, Tsutsumi O et al. Gynecol Obstet Invest 2002;53(suppl 1):33–39.
25. Paterson A. In Carty H (ed.): Imaging Children. Edinburgh, NY: Elsevier Churchill Livingstone, 2005;915–941.
26. Gray-Swain MR, Peipert JF. Curr Opin Obstet Gynecol 2006;18:503–510.
27. Ross J, Judlin P, Nilas L. Int J STD AIDS 2008; 12:84–87.
28. Low N, McCarthy A, Macleod J et al. Health Technol Assess 2007;11:iii–iv, ix–xii, 1–165.
29. Bevan CD, Johal BJ, Mumtaz G, Ridgway GL, Siddle NC. Br J Obstet Gynaecol 1995;102: 407–414.
30. CDC. MMWR Recomm Rep 2002;51:1–78.
31. Morcos R, Frost N, Hnat M, Petrunak A, Caldito G. J Reprod Med 1993;38:53–56.
32. Chang HC, Bhatt S, Dogra VS. Radiographics 2008;28:1355–1368.
33. Albayram F, Hamper UM. J Ultrasound Med 2001;20:1083–1089.
34. Breech LL, Hillard PJ. Curr Opin Obstet Gynecol 2005;17:483–489.
35. Quillin SP, Siegel MJ. Radiographics 1993;13: 1281–1293; discussion 1294.
36. Bouguizane S, Bibi H, Farhat Y et al. J Gynecol Obstet Biol Reprod (Paris) 2003;32:535–540.
37. Graif M, Itzchak Y. AJR Am J Roentgenol 1988;150:647–649.
38. Hata K, Hata T, Senoh D et al. Br J Obstet Gynaecol 1990;97:163–166.
39. Stark JE, Siegel MJ. AJR Am J Roentgenol 1994;163:1479–1482.
40. Burnett LS. Surg Clin North Am 1988;68:385–398.
41. Hibbard LT. Am J Obstet Gynecol 1985;152: 456–461.
42. Houry D, Abbott JT. Ann Emerg Med 2001;38: 156–159.
43. Mordehai J, Mares AJ, Barki Y, Finaly R, Meizner I. J Pediatr Surg 1991;26:1195–1199.
44. Lee EJ, Kwon HC, Joo HJ, Suh JH, Fleischer AC. J Ultrasound Med 1998;17:83–89.
45. Littman ED, Rydfors J, Milki AA. Hum Reprod 2003;18:1641–1642.
46. Beaunoyer M, Chapdelaine J, Bouchard S, Ouimet A. J Pediatr Surg 2004;39:746–749.
47. Warner MA, Fleischer AC, Edell SL et al. Radiology 1985;154:773–775.

48. Pomeranz AJ, Sabnis S. Pediatr Emerg Care 2004;20:172–174.
49. Cohen HL, Shapiro MA, Mandel FS, Shapiro ML. AJR Am J Roentgenol 1993;160:583–586.
50. Orbak Z, Kantarci M, Yildirim ZK, Karaca L, Doneray H. J Pediatr Endocrinol Metab 2007;20: 397–403.
51. Webb EM, Green GE, Scoutt LM. Radiol Clin North Am 2004;42:329–348.
52. Park SB, Kim JK, Kim KR, Cho KS. Radiographics 2008;28:969–983.
53. Comerci JT, Jr., Licciardi F, Bergh PA, Gregori C, Breen JL. Obstet Gynecol 1994;84:22–28.
54. Kido A, Togashi K, Konishi I et al. AJR Am J Roentgenol 1999;172:445–449.
55. Outwater EK, Siegelman ES, Hunt JL. Radiographics 2001;21:475–490.
56. Zane SB, Kieke BA, Jr., Kendrick JS, Bruce C. Matern Child Health J 2002;6:227–236.
57. RCOG. Why Mothers Die 1997–1999. The Fifth Report of the Confidential Enquiries into Maternal Deaths in the United Kingdom. London: RCOG Press, 2001.
58. Menon S, Sammel MD, Vichnin M, Barnhart KT. J Pediatr Adolesc Gynecol 2007;20:181–185.
59. Yeh JM, Hook EW, III, Goldie SJ. Sex Transm Dis 2003;30:369–378.
60. Gao X, Outley J, Botteman M, Spalding J, Simon JA et al. Fertil Steril 2006;86:1561–1572.
61. Zhao SZ, Wong JM, Davis MB, Gersh GE, Johnson KE. Am J Manag Care 1998;4:1127–1134.
62. Simoens S, Hummelshoj L, D'Hooghe T. Hum Reprod Update 2007;13:395–404.
63. Kunz K, Kuppermann M, Moynihan C, Williamson A, Mazonson PT. Am J Manag Care 1995;1:25–29.
64. Husby GK, Haugen RS, Moen MH. Acta Obstet Gynecol Scand 2003;82:649–653.
65. Pandian Z, Bhattacharya S, Vale L, Templeton A. Cochrane Database Syst Rev 2005:CD003357.
66. Pashayan N, Lyratzopoulos G, Mathur R. BMC Health Serv Res 2006;6:80.
67. Philips Z, Barraza-Llorens M, Posnett J. Hum Reprod 2000;15:95–106.
68. Stones RW, Selfe SA, Fransman S, Horn SA. Baillieres Best Pract Res Clin Obstet Gynaecol 2000;14:415–431.
69. Ballard K, Lowton K, Wright J. Fertil Steril 2006; 86:1296–1301.
70. Schenken RS. Fertil Steril 2006;86:1305–1306; discussion 1317.
71. Chiou SY, Lev-Toaff AS, Masuda E, Feld RI, Bergin D. J Ultrasound Med 2007;26: 1289–1301.
72. Servaes S, Zurakowski D, Laufer MR, Feins N, Chow JS. Pediatr Radiol 2007;37:446–451.
73. Vijayaraghavan SB. J Ultrasound Med 2004;23: 1643–1649; quiz 1650–1651.
74. Bulas DI, Ahlstrom PA, Sivit CJ, Blask AR, O'Donnell RM. Radiology 1992;183:435–439.
75. Sam JW, Jacobs JE, Birnbaum BA. Radiographics 2002;22:1327–1334.
76. Bazot M, Lafont C, Rouzier R, Roseau G, Thomassin-Naggara I et al. Fertil Steril 2009;92: 1825–1833.
77. Mol BW, van der Veen F, Bossuyt PM. Hum Reprod 1999;14:2855–2862.
78. Gracia CR, Barnhart KT. Obstet Gynecol 2002;97:464–470.
79. Buckley RG, King KJ, Disney JD, Ambroz PK, Gorman JD et al. Acad Emerg Med 1998;5: 951–960.

40

Imaging of Boys with an Acute Scrotum: Differentiation of Testicular Torsion from Other Causes

Stefan Puig

Issues

I. What are the clinical findings that raise the suspicion of testicular torsion in children with acute scrotal pain?
II. What is the diagnostic performance of the different imaging studies in children with acute scrotal pain?
III. In cases of testicular torsion, is manual reduction required?

Key Points

- Testicular torsion is a clinical emergency. Time is the major factor responsible for salvage of testes (moderate evidence).
- The first-line imaging of patients with suspected testicular torsion is Doppler sonography, which is highly sensitive and specific (moderate evidence).
- Scintigraphy using technetium 99m to assess blood flow to the testes is no longer a common imaging tool due to the more available, less expensive, and rapid test with Doppler sonography (limited to moderate evidence).
- If imaging cannot exclude testicular torsion, surgical exploration is recommended (moderate evidence).
- Successful manual detorsion of testicular torsion leads to reperfusion, which is immediately visible with Doppler sonography. In cases of successful manual detorsion, surgical exploration with orchiopexy is still necessary (limited evidence).
- Absolute dependence on clinical features can lead to a misdiagnosis of testicular torsion. Therefore, ultrasound (US) examination should be part of the presurgical evaluation, if promptly available (limited evidence).

S. Puig (✉)
Paracelsus Medical University, Strubergasse 21, Salzburg 5020, Austria
e-mail: stefan.puig@pmu.ac.at

L.S. Medina et al. (eds.), *Evidence-Based Imaging: Improving the Quality of Imaging in Patient Care, Revised Edition*,
DOI 10.1007/978-1-4419-7777-9_40, © Springer Science+Business Media, LLC 2011

Definition and Pathophysiology

A testicular torsion is a clinical emergency (1, 2). It occurs when the testicle is abnormally mobile and twists on its vascular pedicle and may result in testicular infarction (2). According to the mechanism, torsion of a testis can be divided into extravaginal (prenatal or neonatal) and the more common intravaginal torsion (3, 4). The exact cause for extravaginal or neonatal torsion is unknown and usually no anatomic defect can be identified to explain the torsion (5). It is a rare event and accounts for approximately 10% of all testicular torsions (6). In patients with an intravaginal torsion, the most common anatomical anomaly identified is a narrow attachment of the tunica vaginalis from the spermatic cord to the testes secondary to high insertion of the tunica on the spermatic cord. This results in the "Bell-Clapper" deformity characterized by increased testicular mobility (5). In an autopsy series of 51 males, the Bell-Clapper deformity was found in 12%. Since this is a much higher prevalence than the incidence of testicular torsion, factors other than this anatomical predisposition may be involved (7) (limited evidence).

Testicular torsion should be differentiated from other acute scrotal diseases, such as acute epididymo-orchitis, torsion of appendage of testis, or acute idiopathic scrotal edema (8, 9) (Table 40.1). The cause for the torsion might be several minor traumas, as they occur during sport activities (8). Of the etiologies for acute scrotal pain, testicular torsion is the only real emergency (10–12). Immediate detorsion within a very narrow time window is necessary to provide a high testicle salvage rate, since irreversible ischemia may start after 6 h (3) (moderate evidence). Dunne and O'Loughlin reported a series of 56 patients between 13 and 36 years of age, in which the average duration of pain in patients with viable testes was 9 h compared to 56 h of average duration of pain in those patients with nonviable testes (1). Previous reports found 80% infarcted testes 10 h after pain onset, and after 24 h all testes were lost (1, 13). Nearly 75% of patients need an orchiectomy if detorsion is delayed for more than 12 h (14) (limited evidence).

Sessions et al. reported a median duration of torsion of 5 h (0.5 h–6 days) in patients (116 testes) undergoing orchiopexy and 2.2 days (2.5 h–2 weeks) in those (70 testes) undergoing orchiectomy, which reveals the weakness of time as an accurate predictor for salvageable testes. The same group noted a median of 540° (range: 180°–1,080°) in patients with orchiectomy compared to a median of 360° (range: 180°–1,080°) in those with orchiopexy (15).

Epidemiology

The incidence of spermatic cord torsion in patients presenting with an acute scrotum varies between 18 and 45%, depending on the age of patients (15–17). The overall incidence is 1 in 4,000 in young males under the age of 25, with a peak age of 12–18 years. Cummings et al. reported that nearly 61% of patients were under 21 years of age (18). In children and adolescents under 17 years of age, the incidence of spermatic cord torsion in patients with an acute scrotum is about 26%. There is a peak in the first year of life with 39% and a second peak in young adolescents with 30% during puberty when the testes grow (19, 20).

The most common cause of acute scrotal pain in patients younger than age 18 is epididymitis (21). In prepubertal boys, acute scrotal pain occurs most frequently from torsion of the testicular appendages (21, 22).

Overall Cost to Society

No data were found on the overall cost to society from the diagnosis, treatment, and complications of testicular torsion. However, in cases of testicular torsion, imaging of the scrotum will increase the costs, since surgery is required in those patients anyway. But, this is counter-balanced by imaging eliminating unnecessary surgery in subjects found not to have torsion. Günther et al. calculated in 2006 (according to the German diagnosis-related group's catalog) a cost reduction of 1,000 (2,300 vs. 1,300) per patient if torsion can be ruled out and unnecessary surgical exploration is avoided (8, 9). Furthermore, orchiectomy will result in the implantation of testicular prostheses, which might reduce the psychological impact of a testicle loss, but has some complication rates and will lead to further costs (23) (limited evidence).

Goals

In cases of acute scrotal pain, the main goal is the differentiation of testicular torsion, which requires emergency surgery, from nonsurgical causes of acute scrotal pain, such as epididymitis (epididymo-orchitis) and torsion of the testicular appendix, because clinical presentation may overlap (24–27). In testicular torsion, manual detorsion may reduce time of ischemia before surgical evaluation is possible (3).

Methodology

The diagnostic performance of the clinical examination (history and physical exam) and surgical outcome was based on a systematic literature review using PubMed (National Library of Medicine, Bethesda, MD), Cochrane library, and the National Guideline Clearinghouse for data relevant to the diagnostic performance and accuracy of both clinical and radiographic examinations in patients with testicular torsion performed between January 1967 and July 2008. The clinical examination search strategy used the following statements: (1) testicular torsion or acute scrotum; (2) clinical examination; (3) epidemiology; (4) physical examination; (5) imaging [including *Magnetic resonance imaging (MRI), US, scintigraphy,* as well as acronyms of these terms]; (6) diagnosis; (7) detorsion; as well as combinations of these search strings. Animal studies and non-English and non-German studies were excluded.

I. What Are the Clinical Findings that Raise the Suspicion of Testicular Torsion in Children with Acute Scrotal Pain?

Summary of Evidence: Clinical presentation and physical examination are nonspecific and include previous trauma, pain attacks, nausea, vomiting, elevation and transverse position of the testis, anterior rotation of epididymitis, and absence of the cremaster reflex. These findings have the highest sensitivity, specificity, positive, and negative predictive values for testicular torsion, and the lowest for epididymitis

(moderate evidence). Karmazyn et al. scored the following three key historical elements as predictors for testicular torsion: onset of pain less than 6 h, absence of cremasteric reflex, and diffuse testicular tenderness (25). Out of 141 subjects, in the absence of any of these elements, none of the subjects had testicular torsion. When these three clinical findings were present, 87% were diagnosed with testicular torsion.

Supporting Evidence: Clinical presentation and physical examination do not differ significantly in children and adolescents with testicular torsion, torsion of testicular appendage, or epididymitis. However, children with testicular appendage torsion are typically younger with a peak age of 7–14 years. Previous history of trauma and pain attacks, presence of nausea and vomiting, and absence of urinary complaints are the main predictors of testicular torsion (11) (limited evidence). A so-called pathognomonic finding, the blue dot sign (tender nodule with blue discoloration on the upper pole of the testis), is only infrequently encountered (11, 21, 28). Physical findings consisting of elevation and transverse location of testis, anterior rotation of epididymis, and absence of cremaster reflex are highly suggestive for testicular torsion (3, 11, 24, 25, 29) (limited to moderate evidence). A Finnish study published in 2007 analyzed the clinical findings in 388 boys under 17 years of age with acute scrotum, in which the "blue dot sign" was only found in 10% (17/174) with torsion of the testicular appendage (20). Boys with acute scrotal pain of uncertain etiology based on clinical exam should undergo sonography to exclude the diagnosis of torsion as well as identify other reasons for the pain.

II. What Is the Diagnostic Performance of the Different Imaging Studies in Children with Acute Scrotal Pain?

Summary of Evidence: US with power Doppler has become the imaging modality of choice to diagnose or exclude torsion (moderate evidence). It is a useful addition to the clinical examination, specifically to avoid unnecessary surgery (moderate evidence). Other imaging tools, such as the near-obsolete nuclear medicine test, are not superior to US (27) (limited evidence). If Doppler sonography is equivocal, MRI or scintigraphy can add diagnostic information, but due to both higher costs and the relative delay to obtain these studies, particularly after hours, the clinical value is limited (limited evidence).

Supporting Evidence

Doppler Ultrasound

In clinical practice, US is preferred over other imaging tools (30–32). Several cohort studies reported a sensitivity of at least 90% and a specificity of more than 95% (33–42) (moderate evidence). In combination with certain clinical conditions such as blunt trauma, specificity may reach 100% (40). Ideally, both pulsed and color Doppler US should be used. The real-time whirlpool sign on gray scale sonography in combination with the absence of flow in the distal spermatic cord, testis, and epididymitis were found to be the most specific and sensitive signs of torsion. However, published data on these findings are limited to a few studies (43–45). In general, the first US sign in patients with testicular torsion is hypo- or avascularity of the testicle with preserved homogeneous echotexture in the acute phase (Figs. 40.1 and 40.2) (27). A false-negative finding might be due to flow in the capsule that is from a different arterial supply than the twisted spermatic cord (46).

Data on contrast-enhanced Doppler US are limited as well, and these contrast agents are not available for clinical use in the USA. In 1996, Coley et al. published their results of an animal study including 40 testes of 20 rabbits (47). They compared unenhanced and contrast-enhanced power Doppler sonography, color Doppler sonography, and radionuclide scintigraphy. The best results were achieved with color Doppler sonography (Figs. 40.1 and 40.2). Contrast-enhanced power Doppler sonography, using Levovist® (Schering, Germany), did not improve the diagnostic accuracy of power Doppler, which was below color Doppler and equal to scintigraphy. However, due to several technical developments, these data from 1996 have limited value today, and power Doppler

has the ability to show slower flow than color Doppler (47–49). Therefore, power Doppler can be especially useful in prepubertal boys who have lower blood flow (21, 50, 51) (limited to moderate evidence). Gray scale US of the scrotum without color or power Doppler is relatively insensitive and therefore not recommended in the evaluation of boys with acute scrotum (21).

Magnetic Resonance Imaging

Several experimental studies showed the value of MRI in detecting hypoperfused testes. After torsion of testes, the gadolinium enhancement and apparent diffusion coefficient values in diffusion-weighted images are decreased (52, 53). In case of inconclusive US and physical examination, MRI might be helpful (54). Watanabe et al. calculated a sensitivity of 93% and a specificity of 100% in 39 patients with inconclusive previous clinical examinations (55) (limited evidence). MRI can also visualize hemorrhagic necrosis in testicular torsion using contrast-enhanced and blood-sensitive sequences (56) (limited evidence).

However, due to the relatively expensive, less available, and time-consuming examination, including anesthesia in some children, MRI has no value in a potential emergency setting (8).

Radionuclide Imaging

Color Doppler sonography and technetium 99m scintigraphy show similar sensitivities in the diagnosis of testicular torsion in boys (57). Nussbaum Blask and colleagues prospectively compared color Doppler sonography and scintigraphy in 46 children, age 1 day to 18 years, reported in 2002 (57). Sonography correctly diagnosed 11 of 14 surgical conditions and 31 of 32 nonsurgical conditions. There was one indeterminate sonogram, no false-positive examinations, and three false-negative examinations (sensitivity = 79% [95% CI, 67–91%], specificity = 97% [95% CI, 94–99%], accuracy = 91%). Color flow was demonstrated in the asymptomatic testis in 34 of 44 boys. Scintigraphy correctly diagnosed 11 of 14 surgical conditions and 29 of 32 nonsurgical conditions. There were two indeterminate scintigrams, two false-positive and two false-negative examinations (sensitivity = 79% [95% CI, 67–91%], specificity = 91% [95% CI, 82–99%], accuracy = 87%) (57). However, the reported sensitivity in this study is lower than in other cohort studies. Technical advancements in Doppler make these results lower than current practice.

Scintigraphy has a high potential in differentiating ischemic from infectious disease (36). The specificity in the diagnosis of ischemia versus other photon-deficient lesions is slightly lower (21, 58) (limited to moderate evidence). Photon-deficient areas secondary to hydrocele, spermatocele, edematous appendix testis, and inguinal hernia can be mistaken for an avascular testis and therefore produce false positives (58). Also, the size of testes in infants and small children increases the risk of both false positives and false negatives (21). For these reasons, and because of the longer preparation and exam performance time, lower availability, and higher costs relative to Doppler sonography, scintigraphy is no longer favored. Radionuclide scintigraphy also uses ionizing radiation and requires intravenous access while Doppler does not (3, 57).

III. In Cases of Testicular Torsion, Is Manual Reduction Required?

Summary of Evidence: Manual detorsion of the testicle leads to immediate reperfusion of the affected testis and might be helpful to salvage the organ (limited evidence). If the US examination is performed by a physician with such experience, this procedure can be performed during the examination (Figs. 40.1 and 40.2). However, it is successful in only 30–70% of patients. This procedure must be followed by bilateral orchiopexy to prevent future repeat testicular torsion (strong evidence).

Supporting Evidence

Detorsion

Successful manual detorsion can lessen the surgical urgency of a twisted spermatic cord (3, 15, 59–61). Most testes are torsed in the medial direction. Therefore, experienced clinicians such as the urologist can detorse these testes from the medial to the lateral side (3). The subjective endpoint is the dramatic resolution of scrotal pain (3). One has to consider that the testis can be torsed up to 1,080° (15). A detorsed testis shows blood flow at US or scintigraphy immediately after the maneuver (Figs. 40.1 and 40.2) (15, 60, 61). Adequate sedation and/or spermatic cord anesthesia should be administered, since this procedure is painful (3). Surgical exploration and orchiopexy remain necessary despite symptomatic improvement with manual detorsion (3, 15, 60).

The number of reports in the literature is small, with reported success rates varying from 30 to nearly 100%. Garel et al. reported successful six out of seven patients in which manual detorsion led to immediate reperfusion of the organ at Doppler interrogation. The failed attempt in the seventh patient was due to a failure to manipulate beyond initial 1.5 rotations (540°) (60). Cattolica manually detorsed 34 out of 35 testes successfully in 104 patients during a 10-year period (59).

Take Home Figures and Tables

Figure 40.1 is an algorithm showing the workup for a patient suspected of acute scrotum.

Tables 40.1 and 40.2 discuss causes of acute scrotum in a child and a summary of the diagnostic performance of clinical examination versus imaging for the diagnosis of acute testicular torsion, respectively.

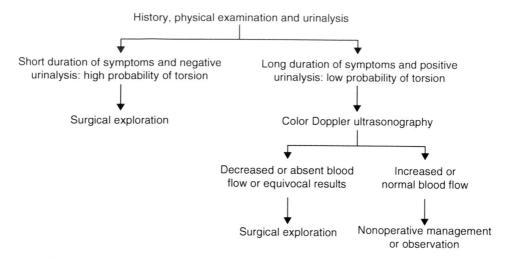

Figure 40.1. Flowchart for patient workup. Note that if the clinician (i.e., an urologist) is experienced in making the diagnosis of acute torsion, they may skip the ultrasound. However, in most situations, the ultrasound is recommended prior to surgery. The age of the patient is important. Testicular torsion is most common in neonates and postpubertal boys, although it can occur in males of any age. Schönlein–Henoch purpura and torsion of a testicular appendage typically occur in prepubertal boys, whereas epididymitis most often develops in postpubertal boys. (Adapted with permission from Galejs LE, Kass EJ. Diagnosis and Treatment of the Acute Scrotum. American Family Physician Feb 15, 1999; 817, 59; 4. Copyright © 1999 American Academy of Family Physicians. All Rights Reserved.)

Table 40.1. Causes for an acute scrotum in childhood

Torsion	Inflammation	Trauma	Generalized illness	Other causes
Torsion of the testicular appendages	Epididymitis	Hematoma Hematocele	Schönlein–Henoch purpura	Inguinal hernia Perforated appendicitis
Testicular torsion	Orchitis	Testicle rupture	Leukemia Lymphoma	Emphysema, edema of the scrotum, testicular tumor, and meconium orchitis

Adapted with kind permission of Springer Science+Business Media from Günther and Schenk (8).

Table 40.2. Summary of diagnostic performance of clinical examination versus imaging for the diagnosis of acute testicular torsion

Test for torsion	Sensitivity (%)	Specificity (%)	References
Clinical exam[a]	87	100	(24)
Technetium scintigraphy	79	>90	(24, 29, 62, 63)
Doppler sonography	>90	>95	(33–40, 42, 62, 63)

[a]Onset of pain less than 6 h, absence of cremasteric reflex, and diffuse testicular tenderness.
Reprinted with kind permission of Springer Science+Business Media from Puig S. Imaging of Boys with an Acute Scrotum: Differentiation of Testicular Torsion from Other Causes. In Medina LS Applegate KE Blackmore CC (eds): *Evidence-Based Imaging in Pediatrics: Optimizing Imaging in Pediatric Patient Care.* New York: Springer Science+Business Media 2010.

Imaging Case Studies

Case 1

Figure 40.2 presents color Doppler sonography of an 18-year-old patient with acute scrotum.

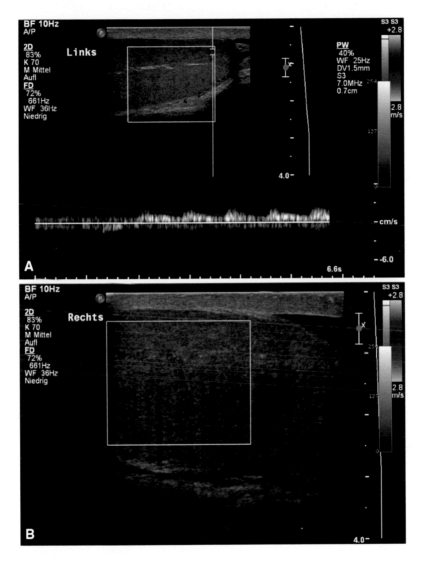

Figure 40.2. Color Doppler sonography of an 18-year-old patient with acute scrotum. (**A**) shows the unaffected left side with regular arterial and venous blood flow. In comparison, there is no blood flow on the right side (**B**). The parenchyma of the twisted testis is normal, and symmetric to the unaffected left testes, a small hydrocele can be seen. After manual detorsion, reperfusion (hyperperfusion) of the right testis is visible (**C**). After this maneuver, the patient underwent orchiopexy. (Reprinted with kind permission of Springer Science+Business Media from Puig S. Imaging of Boys with an Acute Scrotum: Differentiation of Testicular Torsion from Other Causes. In Medina LS, Applegate KE, Blackmore CC (eds): *Evidence-Based Imaging in Pediatrics: Optimizing Imaging in Pediatric Patient Care.* New York: Springer Science+Business Media, 2010.)

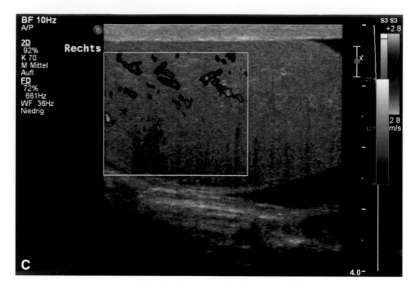

Figure 40.2. *Continued*

Suggested Imaging Protocols for Acute Scrotum

Timely diagnosis and intervention is critical to decrease the chances of testicular loss (3, 15).

Ultrasound

Linear transducer high-frequency transducer (7–12 MHz). Compare with opposite testis for blood flow and parenchymal homogeneity (Figs. 40.1 and 40.2). If possible, try to visualize the twisted spermatic cord "whirlpool sign." Spectral, color, and power Doppler should be used to evaluate the lack of blood flow within the testicular parenchyma. Doppler frequencies range from 3.5 to 10 MHz. Standoff pads can be used, if necessary, to improve imaging (64).

Manual Detorsion

Successful manual detorsion leads to immediate reperfusion of the testis. Since in most torsions the spermatic cord is twisted from lateral to medial, detorsion has to be performed from medial to lateral (the right testis counterclockwise, the left testis clockwise). Doppler is used both during this procedure and immediately afterward to assess testicular blood flow.

Future Research

- Accuracy of second-generation contrast media (e.g., SonoVue®, Bracco, Milan, Italy) that might improve diagnosis, specifically in combination with modern US scanners with harmonic imaging (65, 66).
- Prospective comparison of Doppler sonography with near-infrared spectroscopy, which is capable of noninvasively measuring a mixed venous and arterial hemoglobin tissue saturation of hemoglobin that might allow noninvasive, bedside emergency diagnosis of testicular torsion (67).

References

1. Dunne PJ, O'Loughlin BS. Aust N Z J Surg 2000;70:441–442.
2. Hollmann AS, Macdonald S. In Carty H (ed.): Emergency Pediatric Radiology. Berlin: Springer, 1999;217–232.
3. Kapoor S. Int J Clin Pract 2008;62:821–827.
4. Samnakay N, Tudehope D, Walker R. J Paediatr Child Health 2006;42:734–736.
5. Favorito LA, Cavalcante AG, Costa WS. Int Braz J Urol 2004;30:420–424.
6. Kaye JD, Levitt SB, Friedman SC, Franco I, Gitlin J et al. J Urol 2008;179:2377–2383.

7. Caesar RE, Kaplan GW. Urology 1994;44:114–116.
8. Günther P, Schenk JP. Radiologe 2006;46:590–595.
9. Günther P, Schenk JP, Wunsch R et al. Eur Radiol 2006;16:2527–2532.
10. Ben-Sira L, Laor T. Pediatr Radiol 2000;30:125–128.
11. Ciftci AO, Senocak ME, Tanyel FC, Buyukpamukcu N. Eur J Pediatr Surg 2004;14:333–338.
12. Somekh E, Gorenstein A, Serour F. J Urol 2004;171:391–394; discussion 394.
13. Munro I. Lancet 1981;2:76–77.
14. Anderson JB, Williamson RC. Br J Surg 1988;75:988–992.
15. Sessions AE, Rabinowitz R, Hulbert WC, Goldstein MM, Mevorach RA. J Urol 2003;169:663–665.
16. Caldamone AA, Valvo JR, Altebarmakian VK, Rabinowitz R. J Pediatr Surg 1984;19:581–584.
17. Clift VL, Hutson JM. Pediatr Surg Int 1989;4:185–188.
18. Cummings JM, Boullier JA, Sekhon D, Bose K. J Urol 2002;167:2109–2110.
19. Lewis AG, Bukowski TP, Jarvis PD, Wacksman J, Sheldon CA. J Pediatr Surg 1995;30:277–281; discussion 281–282.
20. Mäkelä E, Lahdes-Vasama T, Rajakorpi H, Wikström S. Scand J Surg 2007;96:62–66.
21. Remer EM, Francis IR, Baumgarten DA et al. Acute Onset of Scrotal Pain-Without Trauma, Without Antecedent Mass. Reston, VA: American College of Radiology (ACR), 2007:5.
22. Karmazyn B, Steinberg R, Livne P et al. J Pediatr Surg 2006;41:500–504.
23. Bodiwala D, Summerton DJ, Terry TR. Ann R Coll Surg Engl 2007;89:349–353.
24. Kadish HA, Bolte RG. Pediatrics 1998;102:73–76.
25. Karmazyn B, Steinberg R, Kornreich L et al. Pediatr Radiol 2005;35:302–310.
26. Kass EJ, Lundak B. Pediatr Clin North Am 1997;44:1251–1266.
27. Nussbaum Blask AR, Rushton HG. AJR Am J Roentgenol 2006;187:1627–1635.
28. Ringdahl E, Teague L. Am Fam Physician 2006;74:1739–1743.
29. Rabinowitz R. J Urol 1984;132:89–90.
30. Sparano A, Acampora C, Scaglione M, Romano L. Emerg Radiol 2008;15:289–294.
31. Kapasi Z, Halliday S. Emerg Med J 2005;22:559–560.
32. Varga J, Zivkovic D, Grebeldinger S, Somer D. Urol Int 2007;78:73–77.
33. Baker LA, Sigman D, Mathews RI, Benson J, Docimo SG. Pediatrics 2000;105:604–607.
34. Dewire DM, Begun FP, Lawson RK, Fitzgerald S, Foley WD. J Urol 1992;147:89–91.
35. Hendrikx AJ, Dang CL, Vroegindeweij D, Korte JH. Br J Urol 1997;79:58–65.
36. Kravchick S, Cytron S, Leibovici O et al. Eur Radiol 2001;11:1000–1005.
37. Schwaibold H, Fobbe F, Klan R, Dieckmann KP. Urol Int 1996;56:96–99.
38. Stehr M, Boehm R. Eur J Pediatr Surg 2003;13:386–392.
39. Yuan Z, Luo Q, Chen L, Zhu J, Zhu R. Ann Nucl Med 2001;15:225–229.
40. Pepe P, Panella P, Pennisi M, Aragona F. Eur J Radiol 2006;60:120–124.
41. Hod N, Maizlin Z, Strauss S, Horne T. Isr Med Assoc J 2004;6:13–15.
42. Patriquin HB, Yazbeck S, Trinh B et al. Radiology 1993;188:781–785.
43. Arce JD, Cortes M, Vargas JC. Pediatr Radiol 2002;32:485–491.
44. Baud C, Veyrac C, Couture A, Ferran JL. Pediatr Radiol 1998;28:950–954.
45. Vijayaraghavan SB. J Ultrasound Med 2006;25:563–574.
46. Atkinson GO, Jr., Patrick LE, Ball TI, Jr., Stephenson CA, Broecker BH et al. AJR Am J Roentgenol 1992;158:613–617.
47. Coley BD, Frush DP, Babcock DS et al. Radiology 1996;199:441–446.
48. Sidhu PS. Clin Radiol 1999;54:343–352.
49. Zinn HL, Cohen HL, Horowitz M. J Ultrasound Med 1998;17:385–388.
50. Bader TR, Kammerhuber F, Herneth AM. Radiology 1997;202:559–564.
51. Luker GD, Siegel MJ. Radiology 1996;198:381–385.
52. Cheng HC, Khan MA, Bogdanov A, Jr., Kwong K, Weissleder R. Invest Radiol 1997;32:763–769.
53. Kaipia A, Ryymin P, Makela E, Aaltonen M, Kahara V et al. Int J Androl 2005;28:355–359.
54. Fernandez-Perez GC, Tardaguila FM, Velasco M et al. AJR Am J Roentgenol 2005;184:1587–1593.
55. Watanabe Y, Dohke M, Ohkubo K et al. Radiology 2000;217:219–227.
56. Watanabe Y, Nagayama M, Okumura A et al. J Magn Reson Imaging 2007;26:100–108.
57. Nussbaum Blask AR, Bulas D, Shalaby-Rana E, Rushton G, Shao C et al. Pediatr Emerg Care 2002;18:67–71.
58. Lutzker LG, Zuckier LS. Semin Nucl Med 1990;20:159–188.
59. Cattolica EV. J Urol 1985;133:803–805.
60. Garel L, Dubois J, Azzie G, Filiatrault D, Grignon A et al. Pediatr Radiol 2000;30:41–44.
61. Sparks JP. Ann R Coll Surg Engl 1971;49:77–91.
62. Middleton WD, Siegel BA, Melson GL, Yates CK, Andriole GL. Radiology 1990;177:177–181.
63. Paltiel HJ, Connolly LP, Atala A, Paltiel AD, Zurakowski D et al. Radiology 1998;207:223–231.
64. ACR Guidelines and Standards Committee. ACR Practice Guideline for the Performance of Scrotal Ultrasound Examinations. Reston, VA: American College of Radiology, 2006.
65. Kollmann C. Eur J Radiol 2007;64:164–172.
66. Krestan C. Radiologe 2005;45:513–519.
67. Capraro GA, Mader TJ, Coughlin BF et al. Ann Emerg Med 2007;49:520–525.

Index

A

Abdomen, blunt trauma
bowel/mesentery imaging,
445–446
case studies (images), 159,
448–449
costs, 442–443
CT, 448–450, 463
Doppler ultrasound, 446
epidemiology, 442
future directions, 450
imaging protocol, 367
literature search, 443
pathophysiology, 442
retroperitonal injuries
imaging, 446–448
spleen/liver imaging, 445
types of injuries, 441–450
ultrasound, 450
Abdominal aortic aneurysms
(AAA)
endovascular vs. surgical,
418–419
treatment, 418–419
imaging cost-effectiveness, 417
mortality and screening,
417–418
pathophysiology, 416
stent-graft endoleaks,
420–421
Abdominal pain, acute
appendicitis, 468
colonic diverticulitis, 471–473
common causes, 468
costs, 469
epidemiology, 468–469
imaging goals, 469
literature search, 469
small bowel ischemia,
470–471, 474

small bowel obstruction,
469–471, 474
See also specific disorders
Acute abdomen. See Abdominal
pain, acute
Acute afebrile symptomatic
seizures
incidence, 247
See also Seizures neuroimaging
Acute aortic dissection
CT angiography, 420
imaging cost-effectiveness, 417
imaging goals, 416–417
pathophysiology, 416
Acute appendicitis. See
Appendicitis, acute
Acute calculous cholecystitis
case studies (images), 564–565
cholescintigraphy, 506–507
costs, 505
CT, 507
epidemiology, 505
imaging goals, 505
imaging strategy, 506–507
MR
cholangiopancreatography,
507
MRI, 507
pathophysiology, 504–505
ultrasound, 506
Acute hematogenous
osteomyelitis
clinical signs, 301
costs, 299
epidemiology, 298–299
long-term effects, 298, 299, 301
medical therapy versus
surgery, 301
pathogens, 300
pathophysiology, 298

Acute hematogenous
osteomyelitis imaging
case studies (images), 303–306
and diabetic foot, 302
diagnostic accuracy, 300–301
future directions, 306
goals of, 299
imaging protocols, 303
literature search, 299
MRI, 300
radionuclide bone
scintigraphy, 300
repeat imaging, 301–302
ultrasound, 301
Acute limb ischemia, 416
Adolescent idiopathic scoliosis,
371–372, 374–376
Adrenal gland
blunt trauma, imaging,
363–364
metastasis, and lung cancer,
95, 96
Alzheimer's disease
clinical criteria, accuracy of,
169–170
costs, 168
epidemiology, 168
genetic susceptibility, 172
Alzheimer's disease
neuroimaging
at-risk persons, identifying, 168
cost effectiveness, 173–174
CT, 190–191
for disease progression, 170
functional imaging, 171
goals of, 168
literature search, 169
MRI, 171–172
PET, 171, 175–176
PET FDG, 175

L.S. Medina et al. (eds.), *Evidence-Based Imaging: Improving the Quality of Imaging in Patient Care, Revised Edition*, **669**
DOI 10.1007/978-1-4419-7777-9, © Springer Science+Business Media, LLC 2011

Alzheimer's disease
        neuroimaging (*cont.*)
    proton MR spectroscopy
        (1HMRS), 190
    SPECT, 171
    structural neuroimaging,
        170–172
    for therapeutic efficacy,
        174–175
Analytical studies, 6
Aneurysms. *See* Abdominal aortic
        aneurysms; Intercranial
        aneurysms
Angiography
    pulmonary, 403
    See also Computed
        tomography angiography
        (CTA); Coronary
        angiography; Magnetic
        resonance angiography
        (MRA)
Angioplasty and stenting, carotid
        stenosis, 430, 433–434
Ankylosing spondylitis,
        MRI, 344
    radionuclide bone
        scintigraphy, 303
    SPECT, 344
    X-rays, 347
Anterior spinal meningocele, 370
Aorta
    abdominal aortic aneurysms
        (AAA), 417–418
    acute aortic dissection, 417
    aortic rupture, 416
    See also specific disorders
Aortic dissection. *See* Acute aortic
        dissection
Appendicitis, acute,
    case studies (images), 462–464
    costs, 458
    CT, 458–459
    defined, 458
    diagnostic accuracy, 459
    future directions, 465
    graded compression
        ultrasound, 458–460
    imaging protocol, 460
    literature search, 460
    pathophysiology, 458
    pediatric cases, 458
    ultrasound, 458–460
Arthritis, septic. *See* Septic
        arthritis

B
Back pain. *See* Low back pain
Barium, negative aspects of use,
        482, 485

Bayes' theorem, 12, 13, 15–16
Bias, 7, 11, 19–26, 66, 68, 92, 98,
        119, 219, 264, 313, 314,
        338–340, 342–344, 364, 374,
        405, 419, 422, 431, 432, 459,
        460, 470–472, 618
    lead-time, 23
    length-time, 23
    observer, 7, 22, 24
    reference standard, 22, 24,
        340, 459
    screening selection, 23
    selection, 11, 22–25, 66, 219,
        264, 342, 405, 419, 460
    slippery linkage, 23
    sticky diagnosis, 23
Bile duct obstruction, 503–524
    computed tomography (CT),
        507–517, 520, 523
    endoscopic ultrasonography,
        511, 512, 514–515, 517
    epidemiology, 505
    magnetic resonance
        cholangiopancreatography
        (MRCP), 507, 509–516,
        521–524
    magnetic resonance imaging
        (MRI), 507, 513–515, 523
    pathophysiology, 504–505
    ultrasound, 506
Bile duct stricture, 503–524
    computed tomography (CT),
        507–517, 520, 523
    endoscopic retrograde
        cholangiopancreatography
        (ERCP), 509–515, 521, 523
    endoscopic ultrasonography,
        511, 512, 514–515, 517
    imaging strategy, 506–523
    Klatskin tumor, 515–516, 522
    magnetic resonance
        cholangiopancreatography
        (MRCP), 507, 509–516,
        521–524
    percutaneous transhepatic
        cholangiography (PTC),
        514, 522
    ultrasonography, 506–517,
        519–521, 523
Biliary disorders
    acute calculous cholecystitis
        (ACC), 505–508, 517, 519
    bile duct obstruction, 505, 506,
        508, 510–511, 515, 516, 523
    bile duct stricture, 505,
        513–524
    choledocholithiasis, 505,
        511–513, 517, 521, 523
    chronic calculous cholecystitis,
        508–509, 521

    costs, 505, 515
    epidemiology, 505
    future directions, 524
    imaging goals, 505
    literature search, 507, 512
    pathophysiology, 504–505
    See also specific disorders
Bladder
    blunt trauma, imaging, 445
    disorders. *See* Urinary tract
        disorders
Blinding
    clinical studies, 6–7
    vs. not blinding, 22
Blunt trauma
    aortic rupture, 416
    thoracolumbar spine imaging,
        363–367
    See also Abdomen, blunt
        trauma; Chest, blunt
        trauma
Bone metastasis
    from lung cancer, 95–97
    from prostate cancer, 156–159
Bone scan. *See* Radionuclide bone
        scintigraphy
Bowel
    blunt trauma, imaging,
        445–446
    invagination. *See*
        Intussusception
    ischemia. *See* Small bowel
        ischemia
    obstruction. *See* Small bowel
        obstruction
Brain
    atropy, 170, 172–174, 178, 201,
        225, 234, 249, 251, 256
    imaging. *See* Neuroimaging
Brain cancer
    clinical signs, 128, 130–133,
        135–138, 140, 141, 145
    costs, 130, 137, 145
    epidemiology, 128–130, 132
    forms of, 128
    pediatric cases, 129–130, 132,
        133, 136, 145
    unique nature of, 128
Brain cancer neuroimaging
    case studies (images), 129, 131,
        134–135
    cost effectiveness, 130, 132,
        133, 136–138, 145
    CT, 130, 132–134, 137–142
    decision-making flowchart,
        140
    diffusion-weighted imaging
        (DWI), 135, 139, 142, 145
    goals of, 130
    indications for, 136

literature review, 131, 135
MRI, 130, 132–139, 144, 145
PET FDG, 133, 134, 136–138
proton MR spectroscopy,
    134–136, 139
SPECT, 133, 134, 136–138, 145
symptomatology criteria, 131
tumors *vs.* tumor-mimicking
    lesions, 135
Brain ischemia, imaging methods,
    187–189
Brain metastasis
    and headache, 265
    from lung cancer, 129, 137
Brain swelling, traumatic brain
    injury imaging, 223
Breast cancer
    at-risk persons, 32, 37, 63, 65,
        67–69, 85, 375
    costs, 64, 68
    epidemiology, 63
    grades, 63, 69
    scoliosis imaging as cause,
        32, 375
Breast cancer imaging
    and BIRADS category 3
        lesions, 71
    case studies (images), 63, 64,
        66–68, 71–73
    future directions, 85
    goals of, 64
    image-guided percutaneous
        biopsy, 64, 71, 80
    literature review, 64
    literature search, 64
    magnetic resonance imaging
        (MRI), 69, 70, 73
    mammographic screening, 47,
        63–66, 68, 85
    and nipple discharge, 70
    and radial scars, 71, 78, 80
    ultrasound, 64, 68–69, 76

C
Calcification scoring, coronary
    artery, 389–390
Calculous cholecystitis. *See* Acute
    calculous cholecystitis;
    Chronic calculous
    cholecystitis
Canadian C-spine rule, 359, 360,
    364, 365
Cancer risk, scoliosis
    imaging, 375
Cardiac imaging
    coronary angiography,
        390–392
    cost-effectiveness, 394
    CT, 394

CT calcium scoring, 389
future directions, 399
goals of, 388–389
literature search, 388
MRI, 394
PET, 391
SPECT, 393, 394
stress echocardiography, 388
stress electrocardiography, 392
Carotid imaging
    of asymptomatic patients,
        432–433
    catheter angiography (CA),
        432
    cost-effectiveness, 433, 436
    CT angiography, 428, 437
    Doppler ultrasound (DUS),
        432, 438
    goals of, 429
    literature review, 431
    MR angiography, 431
    multiple overlapping thinslab
        acquisition (MOTSA), 431
    transcranial Doppler
        (TCD), 434
Carotid stenosis
    and stroke risk, 435–436
    angioplasty and stenting,
        433–434
    carotid endarterectomy,
        effectiveness, 433
    cerebral blood flow
        assessment, 435
    cerebral blood volume
        assessment, 233
    complete occlusion, 431
    costs, 433, 436
    epidemiology, 429
    pathophysiology, 428
Case-control studies, 111
Catheter angiography (CA),
    carotid imaging, 432
Cauda equina syndrome, 338
Caudal regression syndrome,
    370, 372
CBTRUS database, 131
Cerebral blood flow assessment,
    carotid stenosis, 435
Cerebral blood volume
    assessment, carotid
    stenosis, 233
Cervical spine imaging
    Canadian C-spine rule,
        359, 364
    children, 360, 362
    cost-effectiveness, 360–362
    CT, 360–362, 366, 367
    goals of, 358
    Harborview high-risk cervical
        spine criteria, 362, 365

in high-risk patients, 360–362
indications for, 367
literature search, 359
NEXUS prediction rule, 359
and unconscious patient, 365
Cervical spine injury
    costs, 358
    epidemiology, 358
Chest, blunt trauma
    chest wall imaging, 102
    costs, 442–443
    CT, 443
    CT angiography, 443
    definition, 442
    diaphragm imaging, 444
    epidemiology, 442
    goals, 443
    literature search, 443
    MRI, 444
    pathophysiology, 442
    pleura/lung imaging, 443–444
    X-rays, 443
Children
    appendicitis, acute, 459–461
    brain cancer, 131–132
    cervical spine imaging, 360
    gastrointestinal tract
        obstruction. *See*
        Intussusception
    headache/headache
        neuroimaging, 268
    Ottawa knee rule, 328, 332
    seizures/seizures
        neuroimaging, 248–250
    sinusitis imaging, 279–281
    spinal disorders. *See* Occult
        spinal dysraphism;
        Scoliosis
    and stroke, 206–207
    thoracolumbar spine
        imaging, 363
    traumatic brain injury
        imaging, 225–229
Cholecystitis. *See* Acute calculous
    cholecystitis; Chronic
    calculous cholecystitis
Choledocholithiasis
    CT, 511–512
    endoscopic retrograde
        cholangiopancreatography
        (ERCP), 514
    endoscopic ultrasonography,
        514–515
    epidemiology, 495
    imaging strategy, 511–513, 516
    magnetic resonance
        cholangiopancreatography
        (MRCP), 512
    pathophysiology, 505
    ultrasound, 513

Cholescintigraphy
  acute calculous cholecystitis,
    506–507, 509–510
  chronic calculous cholecystitis,
    509–510
Chronic calculous cholecystitis
  cholescintigraphy, 509–510
  costs, 505
  endoscopic retrograde
    cholangiopancreatography,
    510
  epidemiology, 505
  imaging goals, 508
  imaging strategy, 509, 510
  magnetic resonance
    cholangiopancreatography
    (MRCP), 509
  pathophysiology, 505
  ultrasound, 509
Cirrhosis
  costs, 530
  epidemiology, 531
  pathophysiology, 530
  See also Hepatocellular
    carcinoma
Clinical prediction rules, 12, 220,
  324, 363, 367, 461
Clinical question, formulation for
  EBI, 5
Clinical studies
  analytical, 6
  bias, 21–22
  case-control, 6
  clinical trials, 5
  cohort, 6
  cross-sectional, 5
  descriptive, 6
  experimental, 5
  prospective, 6
  randomized, blinded, 7
  retrospective, 6
Cohort studies, 6
Colonic diverticulitis
  case studies (images), 472–473
  costs, 469
  CT, 472–473
  diagnostic accuracy, 471
  literature search, 469
  pathophysiology, 468
  ultrasound, 472
Colonoscopy, 111–124, 269,
  549–551, 554, 555
Colorectal cancer
  adenoma-carcinoma
    sequence, 110
  at-risk populations, 110, 113,
    114, 118
  costs, 110
  epidemiology, 110
  familial factors, 115

fecal occult blood testing
    (FOBT), 111, 112
  after first occurrence, 116
  hypothesis, 110
  and inflammatory bowel
    disease, 116
  and liver metastases, 539
  Lynch syndrome, 116
  sigmoidoscopy, 111–117
Colorectal cancer imaging
  asymptomatic patient imaging
    protocol, 120
  asymptomatic patients,
    screening protocol, 98
  colonoscopy, 122, 124
  comparison of methods,
    113–117
  computer-assisted detection
    (CAD) algorithms, 119
  cost-effectiveness, 118–119
  CT colonography (CTC),
    113–114
  double contrast barium enema
    (DCBE), 113
  false-negative (image), 121
  false-positive (image), 122
  future directions, 124
  goals of, 110
  literature review, 114
  prepless colonography, 119
  protocol, 120
  staging, 117–118
  true-positive (image), 120
Compression fractures
  bone scanning, 344
  computed tomography, 343
  magnetic resonance, 343–344
  osteoporotic type, 346
  plain radiographs, 343
  SPECT, 344
  vertebroplasty, 346
Computed tomography (CT)
  abdomen, blunt trauma,
    444–447
  acute calculous cholecystitis,
    507, 508
  Alzheimer's disease, 170, 175
  appendicitis, acute,
    459–461, 463
  bile duct obstruction, 511
  bile duct stricture, 513–514
  brain cancer, 132–134,
    137–138
  calcium scoring, 389–390
  cardiac, 393–394
  cervical spine, 5, 187, 360–362,
    365, 366
  chest, blunt trauma, 443–444
  choledocholithiasis,
    511–512, 523

colonic diverticulitis, 471,
    472, 475
  headache, 35, 137–138,
    227, 264–270
  hepatocellular carcinoma,
    540, 542
  herniated disk, 338, 339
  intracranial hemorrhage, 132,
    185–186, 248
  knee injury, 312
  liver metastases, 96, 532, 534,
    535, 537, 538
  lung cancer, 92–95, 97
  prostate cancer, 151–153, 159
  seizures, 220, 248–250
  sinusitis, 280–288
  small bowel ischemia,
    470, 471
  small bowel obstruction,
    469–470
  spinal stenosis, 344–345
  temporal lobe epilepsy, 250
  thoracolumbar spine, 364
  traumatic brain injury,
    220–224, 226–229, 239
  urolithiasis, 575, 576
Computed tomography
    angiography (CTA)
  acute aortic dissection, 417
  aneurysm, intercranial,
    267–268
  carotid imaging, 429
  chest, blunt trauma, 443
  headache, 267–268
  peripheral vascular disease,
    420, 424
  pulmonary embolism
    evaluation, 404, 413
  subarachnoid hemorrhage, 267
Computed tomography arterial
    portography (CTAP)
  hepatocellular carcinoma, 537
  liver metastases, 534
Computed tomography hepatic
    arteriography (CTHA)
  hepatocellular carcinoma,
    535–536
Computer-assisted detection
    (CAD) algorithms,
    colorectal cancer
    imaging, 119
Confidence intervals (CI)
  construction of, 20–21
Confounding factors, 7, 36, 566
Congenital scoliosis. See Scoliosis
CONSORT initiative, 19
Coronary angiography
  cost-effectiveness, 391
  decision tree, 391
  initial use, factors in, 392

Coronary artery calcification
    scoring, 389–390, 399
Coronary artery disease
    costs, 397
    epidemiology, 388
    pathophysiology, 388
    See also Cardiac imaging
Cortical rim sign, 447
Cost-benefit analysis (CBA), 9
Cost-effectiveness analysis (CEA),
    9, 12, 47, 48, 137, 145, 173,
    174, 203, 269, 274, 284, 312,
    314–315, 342, 360–362, 373,
    374, 417–419, 421–422, 433,
    436, 461, 485
Cost-minimization analysis, 9
Costs, types of, 10, 11
Cost-utility analysis
    quality-adjusted life
        year(QALY), 10
    quantification of health in, 10
Crescent sign,
    intussusception, 480
Cross-sectional studies, 6, 480
Cryoablation, 531

D
Data analysis
    meta-analysis, 11
    qualitative and quantitative,
        11
Deep venous thrombosis, clinical
    signs, 409
Descriptive studies, 6, 24, 481
Diabetic foot, osteomyelitis in, 302
Diagnostic tests
    evaluation of, 7, 22
    receiver operating
        characteristics (ROC)
        curve, 7–9, 281
    sensitivity of, 7–9, 373
    specificity of, 7–9, 373
Diaphragm, blunt trauma,
    imaging, 442
Diastematomyelia, 370, 376
Differential Outcome Scale
    (DOS), 218
Diffusion-tensor imaging,
    traumatic brain injury
    imaging, 219, 222
Diffusion-weighted imaging
    brain cancer, 139
    traumatic brain injury
        imaging, 222
Digital rectal exam (DRE),
    prostate cancer, 149
Digital subtraction angiography,
    peripheral vascular
    disease, 205

Direct costs, 10, 50, 64, 219, 253,
    279, 360, 549, 628
Disability Score (DS), 218
Diverticulitis. *See* Colonic
    diverticulitis
Doppler ultrasound (DUS)
    abdomen, blunt trauma, 446
    carotid imaging, 21, 432, 437
Dorsal dermal sinus, 370, 372,
    373, 377
Double contrast barium enema
    (DCBE), 113, 121
Dysraphism. *See* Occult spinal
    dysraphism

E
Echocardiography
    pulmonary embolism
        evaluation, 406
    stress, 388, 391–394, 397
Economic evaluations, 9–10
    cost-benefit analysis (CBA), 9
    cost-effectiveness analysis
        (CEA), 9, 12, 269
    cost-minimization analysis, 9
    costs, types of, 9–10
    cost-utility analysis, 9–10
Electron beam computed
    tomography (EBCT),
    pulmonary embolism
    evaluation, 405
Embolism. *See* Pulmonary
    embolism; Pulmonary
    embolism imaging
    evaluation
Endoleaks, abdominal aortic
    aneurysm (AAA) graft,
    418, 420–421
Endoscopic retrograde
    cholangiopancreatography
    (ERCP)
    bile duct stricture, 510,
        512, 514
    choledocholithiasis, 511–513
    chronic calculous cholecystitis,
        508–509
Endoscopic ultrasonography
    (EUS)
    bile duct obstruction, 511, 512,
        514–515
    bile duct stricture, 511, 512,
        514–515
    choledocholithiasis, 511,
        512, 517
    -guided fine-needle aspiration,
        513, 515
Endovascular repair, abdominal
    aortic aneurysms (AAA),
    418, 419, 422

Enema, intussusception. *See*
    Intussusception
Errors, 19, 25, 152
    and bias, 19–20
    random, 19–21, 24, 25
    systematic, 19, 20, 24, 25
    Type I, 20, 21, 24
    Type II, 20, 21, 24
Evidence-based imaging (EBI)
    clinical question in, 5
    defined, 3–5
    evidence, application of,
        11–14
    guiding principles, 8–16
    imaging effectiveness
        hierarchy, 11
    literature review. *See* Medical
        literature
Experimental studies, 6, 638

F
False-negatives, elimination of, 21
False-positives, elimination of, 21
Febrile seizures. *See* Seizures
    neuroimaging
Fecal occult blood testing (FOBT),
    111, 121
Fixed costs, 10
Fluid-attenuated inversion
    recovery (FLAIR)
    and intracranial
        hemorrhage, 186
    and temporal lobe
        epilepsy, 188
    traumatic brain injury, 219,
        229–233
Fluoroscopy, intussusceptions
    enema reduction, 483, 484
Flurodeoxyglucose PET. *See*
    Positron emission
    tomography with
    flurodeoxyglucose
    (PETFDG)
Functional endoscopic sinus
    surgery, before/after
    imaging, 286
Functional magnetic resonance
    imaging (fMRI)
    Alzheimer's disease, 171
    seizures, 247, 252, 253
    traumatic brain injury, 219, 235
Functional Status Examination
    (FSE), 219, 288, 347, 377,
    518, 580, 632

G
Gadobenate dimeglumine
    (Gd-BOPTA), 535

Gadolinium enhancement
  herniated disk, 338
  liver metastases, 531
  osteomyelitis, 306
Gallbladder disease. *See* Biliary
  disorders
Gastrointestinal tract obstruction.
  See Intussusception
Glasgow Coma Scale, 218, 448
Glasgow Outcome Scale, 218
Gleason score, 153, 154, 156–159
Graded compression ultrasound,
  appendicitis, acute, 459,
  460, 468, 471
Gradient echo sequences,
  traumatic brain injury, 207,
  208, 222

H
Harborview high-risk cervical
  spine criteria, 362, 365
Headache
  and children, 182
  epidemiology, 182
  primary/secondary etiologies,
  181, 183
Headache neuroimaging
  for brain metastases, 265
  case studies (images), 270
  cost effectiveness, 269
  CT, 266–267
  CT angiography, 267–268
  goals of, 203
  indications for, 208
  literature review, 265
  for migraine/chronic
  headache, 265
  MR angiography, 204
  MRI, 271
  for new-onset headache, 271
  pediatric imaging, 266, 269, 271
  sensitivity/specificity of
  methods, 266–268
  and subarachnoid
  hemorrhage, 267–268
  suspected intracranial
  aneurysm, 272
Head injury
  types of, 235
  See also Traumatic brain injury;
  Traumatic brain injury
  imaging
Health status, quantification of, 10
Helical CT, nephrolithiasis, 572
Hematogenous osteomyelitis.
  See Acute hematogenous
  osteomyelitis
Hepatic disorders
  cirrhosis, 530–531

hepatocellular carcinoma,
  530–531
  literature search, 531
  liver metastases, 530
  See also specific disorders
Hepatitis, and hepatocellular
  carcinoma, 529–543
Hepatocellular carcinoma
  case studies (images), 537
  cost-effectiveness, 538–542
  costs, 532, 549
  CT, 535–536
  CT arterial portography
  (CTAP), 534
  CT hepatic arteriography
  (CTHA), 536, 537, 539
  diagnostic accuracy, 553
  epidemiology, 531–532
  hematologic testing, 531
  imaging goals, 571
  MRI, 543
  prognosis, 530
  ultrasound, 555–556
  whole-body PET, 535
Herniated disk, 338–340
  bulge *vs.* herniation, 302–303
  CT, 302, 312
  gadolinium enhancement, 341
  MRI, 341–342
  MR myelography (MRM),
  338, 340
  protrusions and extrusions,
  339–340
  X-rays, 330, 333
Hierarchical framework, imaging
  effectiveness, 12–13

I
Image-guided biopsy. *See*
  Percutaneous image-
  guided breast biopsy
Indirect costs, 11
Inflammatory bowel disease, and
  colorectal cancer, 88–89
Intercranial aneurysms
  CT angiography, 185
  MR angiography, 204–205
Intracranial hemorrhage. *See*
  Intracranial hemorrhage
  imaging; Stroke
Intracranial hemorrhage imaging
  and bolus nonionic
  contrast, 186
  brain ischemia, identifying,
  187–189
  case studies (images), 157–159
  CT, 162–163, 165–167, 171–172
  CT angiography, 175
  diffusion-weighted MRI, 172

and fluid-attenuated inversion
  recovery (FLAIR), 186
  future directions, 196
  goals of, 168
  literature review, 162
  MR angiography, 175–176
  MRI, 173–174, 177
  MRI spectroscopy, 169
  noninvasive vascular
  imaging, 192
  and pediatric patients, 210
  perfusion-weighted MRI,
  188–189
  PET, 192–193
  SPECT, 193
  stroke mimics, exclusion of,
  174–175
  xenon gas in, 190
Intradural lipoma, 370, 377
Intraoperative ultrasound (IOUS),
  liver metastases, 534
Intussusception, 479–482
  alternative treatments, 483–484
  bowel necrosis, predictors of,
  479–480
  case study (images), 481
  clinical predictors of, 479–480
  cost-effectiveness, 485–486
  costs, 479–480
  crescent sign, 480
  delayed repeat enema, 478,
  483, 484, 489
  diagnostic accuracy, 508
  enema, air *vs.* liquid, 482–483,
  486–488
  enema reduction effectiveness,
  485–486
  enema reduction procedure,
  483, 484
  enema rule of threes, 483, 487
  enema therapy complications,
  484–485
  epidemiology, 492
  fluoroscopy and enema
  reduction, 488
  future directions, 489
  imaging goals, 479
  imaging protocol, 487–489
  linear transducer
  sonography, 481
  literature search, 479
  pathologic lead points,
  478, 482
  pathophysiology, 496
  radiation dose, 483–484
  recurrent, management of, 497
  rotavirus vaccine, relationship
  to, 479
  small bowel
  intussusception, 486

surgical complications, 484
treatment setting, 483
ultrasound, 480, 482
Klatskin tumor, 515–516

K
Kidney
    blunt trauma, imaging, 442–444
    cortical rim sign, 447
    renal artery stenosis, 422–425
    transplant donor, evaluation
        of, 403–407
    Klatskin tumor, 515–516
Knee injury
    costs, 314–315
    epidemiology, 278
    Ottowa knee rule, 311
Knee injury imaging
    children, 311–313
    cost effectiveness, 314–316, 318
    CT, 280–281
    decision rules, 320
    diagnostic accuracy, 282, 284
    future directions, 324
    goals of, 328
    imaging protocols, 330
    literature review, 299
    meniscal/ligamentous
        injuries, 330, 337
    MRI, 313–314
    osteoarthritic knee, 315
    of prosthesis, 315–316
    X-rays, 336, 338

L
Laser photocoagulation, 531
Lead-time bias, 23
Length-time bias, 23
Ligament tears. See Knee injury
        imaging
Likelihood ratios (LR)
    positive and negative, 460
Limb ischemia, acute, 416
Linear transducer sonography
        intussusception, 481
Lipomyelocele, 370
Lipomyelomeningocele, 370
Literature review. See Medical
        literature search
Liver
    blunt trauma, imaging, 445
    See also Hepatic disorders
Liver metastases
    and colorectal cancer, 529–543
    CT, 533–534
    CT arterial portography, 534, 539
    epidemiology, 531
    gadolinium enhancement,
        535, 537

image-guided therapies, 531
intraoperative ultrasound, 533
MRI, 534–535
multirow detector helical CT, 534
organ-specific contrast, 535
pathophysiology, 530
PET, 532–533
staging, 532
ultrasound, 536
whole-body PET, 535, 537–538
Low back pain
    costs, 338
    differential diagnosis, 337
    epidemiology, 337
Low back pain imaging
    ankylosing spondylitis, 344
    cauda equina syndrome, 337, 338
    compression fractures,
        343–344, 346–347
    diagnostic accuracy, 336,
        345, 346
    future directions, 353
    goals of, 338
    herniated disk, 338–341
    imaging protocols, 347
    infection, 342–343
    literature review, 338
    metastatic disease, 341–342
    osteoporotic vertebral, 346
    compression fractures,
        343–344
    and outcome, 340, 345, 346, 349
    patient expectations/
        satisfaction, 346
    spinal stenosis, 344–345
    vertebroplasty, 346
    See also individual conditions
Lung cancer
    categories of, 89–90
    costs, 90
    epidemiology, 90
    occupational causes, 90
    radiologic follow-up, 97–99
Lung cancer imaging
    for adrenal metastasis, 96
    for bone metastasis, , 96–97
    for brain metastasis, 97
    chest X-ray, 91–92
    cost effectiveness, 94–95
    CT, 92–94
    literature search, 90
    for liver metastasis, 96
    mediastinum evaluation,
        95–96
    MRI, 90, 95, 97
    PET, 90
    PET FDG, 96
    primary tumor evaluation, 95
    small cell lung cancer
        (SCLC), 97

staging, 99
video-assisted thoracotomy
    (VATS), 93
Lynch syndrome
    diagnostic criteria, 117
    colorectal cancer imaging,
        109–124
    See also Colorectal cancer

M
Magnetic resonance angiography
    (MRA)
    carotid imaging, 429–432,
        437, 439
    headache, 267, 270, 272
    peripheral vascular disease,
        416, 417, 419–423, 425
    pulmonary embolism
        evaluation, 405, 413
    knee injury imaging, 317–320,
        322, 324
Magnetic resonance
    cholangiopancreatography
    (MRCP)
    acute calculous cholecystitis
        (ACC), 507
    bile duct obstruction, 507,
        509–516, 521–524
    bile duct stricture, 507,
        509–516, 521–524
    choledocholithiasis, 511–513,
        521, 523
    chronic calculous cholecystitis
        (CCC), 521
Magnetic resonance imaging
    (MRI)
    acute calculous cholecystitis
        (ACC), 507
    acute hematogenous
        osteomyelitis (AHO)
        imaging, 298–304, 306
    Alzheimer's disease,
        169–177, 180
    ankylosing spondylitis, 344
    bile duct obstruction, 507,
        513–515, 523
    brain cancer, 130, 132–139,
        144, 145
    breast cancer, 69, 70, 73, 85
    cardiac, 388, 393–395, 399
    chest, blunt trauma, 444
    diffusion-weighted, 135, 139,
        142, 172, 184, 187, 196, 200,
        222, 638
    fluid-attenuated inversion
        recovery (FLAIR), 139,
        141–144, 175, 186, 193, 194,
        219, 222, 229, 233–235, 239,
        250, 251, 257, 270, 288

Magnetic resonance imaging (MRI) (*cont.*)
functional. *See* Functional magnetic resonance imaging
headache, 35, 132, 202, 224, 265–269, 271–273
hepatocellular carcinoma, 531–537, 539–541, 543
herniated disk, 338–341, 348
intracranial hemorrhage imaging, 132, 185–187
knee injury, 313–315, 321, 324
liver metastases, 96, 532, 533, 535, 537, 539
lung cancer, 90, 95, 97, 101
magnetization transfer MRI, 172
occult spinal dysraphism (OSD) imaging, 372–374, 377–379
osteomyelitis, 298–304, 306
perfusion-weighted, 188, 196
prostate cancer, 148, 151–155, 157–160
scoliosis, 372–379, 382
seizures, 132, 188, 224, 247–258, 265,
shoulder injury, 310–319, 321–324
sinusitis, 281, 284, 288
small bowel ischemia, 470, 471
single photon emission computed tomography (SPECT), 133, 134, 136–138, 145, 160, 169, 172–174, 180, 185, 189, 203–205, 209, 229–233, 235, 247, 252, 388, 389, 393, 394, 434
spinal metastasis, 341–342
spinal stenosis, 338, 340, 345
temporal lobe epilepsy, 250–253, 256–258
traumatic brain injury, 219, 221–225, 229–235, 239
Magnetic resonance myelography (MRM), herniated disk, 340
Magnetic resonance spectroscopy (MRS)
prostate cancer, 155, 160
seizures, 231, 247, 252, 253
single-voxel proton. *See* Single-voxel spectroscopy
traumatic brain injury, 230, 231, 234, 235
Mammographic screening, 47, 63–66, 68
age and benefits, 63, 65–68, 70, 84, 110, 118, 269

age factors, 65–68, 70, 84, 110, 118
in community setting, 65
cost effectiveness, 47–48, 68
effectiveness, 64–66
frequency of, 74, 75
Mangafodipir trisodium (MnDPDP), 535
Marfan syndrome, 371
Medical literature, 5, 9, 11, 19, 22, 130, 299, 402
clinical studies, types of, 6–7
cost-effectiveness analysis (CEA), 9, 130, 299
data-analysis, 11
diagnostic tests, evaluation of, 6–9, 12–14
National Guideline Clearinghouse, 220, 506, 532, 629, 637
See also Clinical studies
Medical literature search
Central Brain Tumor Registry of the United States (CBTRUS) data, 131
Medline/PubMed, 4, 5, 11, 31, 64, 90, 110, 130, 148, 169, 185, 203, 219, 247, 263, 280, 299, 311, 328, 338, 359, 372, 389, 402, 417, 429, 458, 469, 479, 493, 506, 532, 549, 550, 571, 588, 614, 629, 637
MESH headings, 359, 458, 469, 479
National Cancer Data Base (NCDB), 131
National Guideline Clearinghouse, 220, 506, 532, 629, 637
on-line sources, 5
Ovid search engine, 148, 185, 263, 372
Surveillance, epidemiology, and end results (SEER) program, 129, 131, 613
See also specific medical conditions
Medicine
economic evaluations, 9, 513
literature. *See* Medical literature
Medline/PubMed, 4, 5, 11, 31, 64, 90, 110, 130, 148, 169, 185, 203, 219, 247, 263, 280, 299, 311, 328, 338, 359, 372, 389, 402, 417, 429, 458, 469, 479, 493, 506, 532, 549, 550, 571, 588, 614, 629, 637
Meningitis, and occult spinal dysraphism, 373

Meningocele, 370
Meniscal injuries. *See* Knee injury imaging
Mesentery, blunt trauma, imaging, 445–446
MESH headings, 359, 458, 469, 479
Meta-analysis, 11, 14, 24, 65, 66, 95, 113, 115, 118, 252, 282, 311, 344, 345, 389, 432, 459, 460, 472, 506, 511, 512, 532, 535, 538, 558, 559, 592, 618
Metastatic disease
adrenal, 96, 102
bone, 96–97
brain, 97, 129, 133–135, 137, 138, 265
liver, 96, 513, 530–535, 537, 539
spinal, 341
Microwave ablation, 531
Midline shift, traumatic brain injury imaging, 221–223, 225
Migraine. *See* Headache neuroimaging
Multidetector computed tomography (MDCT)
peripheral vascular disease, 420, 422
pulmonary embolism evaluation, 404–405, 413
Multiplanar imaging (MPI), renal artery stenosis, 422
Multiple overlapping thinslab acquisition (MOTSA), carotid imaging, 431
Multirow detector helical CT, liver metastases, 534
Multivoxel resonance spectroscopy, traumatic brain injury, 231
Myelodysplasia, 370
Myelomeningocele, 370

N
National Cancer Data Base (NCDB), 131
National Guideline Clearinghouse, 220, 506, 532, 629, 637
Negative likelihood ratio (NLR), 12, 321, 322, 445, 459, 460, 619, 620
Negative predictive value (NPV), 15, 16, 72, 76, 135, 137, 138, 149, 188, 220, 226, 232, 267, 363, 402–406, 408, 409, 419, 420, 422, 445, 459, 460, 463,

470–472, 474, 475, 495, 550, 554, 555, 560, 575, 637
Nephrolithiasis
 case studies (images), 579
 costs, 571
 diagnostic accuracy, 574–576
 epidemiology, 570–571
 helical CT, 572
 imaging goals, 571
 and pregnancy, 573
 X-rays, 574
Neural tube defects. See Occult spinal dysraphism
Neurofibromatosis, 129, 371, 377
Neurogenic bladder
 pathophysiology, 586–587
 urologic workup, 587
Neuroimaging. See Alzheimer's disease neuroimaging; Headache neuroimaging; Seizure neuroimaging; Traumatic brain injury imaging
Newborn evaluation, occult spinal dysraphism imaging, 377
NEXUS prediction rule, 359
Nipple discharge, imaging, 70
Noninvasive vascular imaging, intracranial hemorrhage, 192–193

O
Observer bias, 7, 22, 24
Occult spinal dysraphism
 closed spina bifida entities, 370
 conus medullaris position issue, 371
 early intervention benefits, 373
 epidemiology, 371–372
 open spina bifida entities, 370
 pathophysiology, 370–371
 spectrum of manifestations, 372
 surgical intervention, 373
Occult spinal dysraphism imaging
 at-risk groups, 372
 cost-effectiveness, 373–374
 diagnostic accuracy, 372
 goals of, 372
 literature search, 389
 MRI, 375–376
 newborn evaluation, 372–373
 ultrasound, 377
On-line sources, medical literature. See Medical literature search

Osteoarthritis, knee imaging, 315
Osteomyelitis
 in diabetic foot, 302
 MRI, 300
 radionuclide bone scintigraphy, 300, 303
 SPECT, 303
 X-rays, 300
 See also Acute hematogenous osteomyelitis
Osteoporotic vertebral compression fractures, 346
Ottowa knee rule, 311, 320, 324
Overhead costs, 10
Ovid search engine, 148

P
Pancreas, blunt injury, imaging, 446–447
Pathologic lead points, intussusception, 478, 482
Patient outcome efficacy, 12
Percutaneous image-guided breast biopsy
 benefits of, 71–72
 cost-effectiveness, 68
 imaging guidance, type of, 72
Percutaneous transhepatic cholangiography (PTC), bile duct stricture, 514
Perfect test, 8
Perfusion studies, traumatic brain injury, 221–225
Peripheral vascular disease
 CT angiography, 420
 digital subtraction angiography, 422, 423
 future directions, 425
 imaging goals, 416–417
 literature search, 420, 421
 MR angiography, 419–420
 multidetector CT, 422
 pathophysiology, 416
Pleura, blunt trauma, imaging, 406
Positive likelihood ratio (PLR), 12–14, 321, 322, 459, 619, 620
Positive predictive value (PPV), 12, 15, 16, 35, 63, 71, 135, 149, 188, 223, 267, 363, 403, 404, 409, 420, 459, 460, 470, 472, 474, 475, 495, 506, 515, 534, 555, 556, 561, 627
Positron emission tomography (PET)
 Alzheimer's disease, 169, 171, 173, 174
 brain cancer, 133, 134

cardiac imaging, 389, 391–393
 hepatocellular carcinoma, 531–533, 535, 537, 538
 intracranial hemorrhage, 191
 liver metastases, 535
 lung cancer, 90, 95, 96, 98
 prostate cancer, 155–156
 seizures, 252, 253
 traumatic brain injury, 232–233
 whole-body, 101, 535, 537–538
Positron emission tomography with flurodeoxyglucose (PET FDG)
 Alzheimer's disease, 175
 brain cancer, 136–138
 lung cancer, 96, 97
 prostate cancer, 155, 156
 traumatic brain injury imaging, 232
Power analysis, and sample size, 21
Predictive values
 negative, 15, 16, 72, 76, 135, 137, 138, 149, 188, 210, 226, 232, 267, 363, 402–406, 408, 409, 419, 420, 422, 445, 459, 460, 463, 470–472, 474, 475, 495, 550, 554, 555, 561, 565, 637
 positive, 12, 15, 16, 35, 63, 71, 135, 149, 188, 223, 267, 363, 403, 404, 409, 420, 459, 460, 470, 472, 474, 475, 495, 506, 515, 534, 555, 556, 561, 627
Pregnancy
 and nephrolithiasis, 573
 and urinary tract infection, 587, 592, 593, 604
Prepless colonography, 119
Prospective studies, 6, 7, 185, 186, 192, 220, 241, 274, 346, 403, 460, 469, 484, 572, 592
Prostate cancer
 costs, 148
 digital rectal exam (DRE), 149, 150
 epidemiology, 148
 Gleason score, 153, 154, 156–159
 prostate-specific antigen (PSA) testing, 149–151, 153–159
 treatment flow chart, 158
Prostate cancer imaging
 for bone metastases, 156–157
 case studies (images), 157–159
 CT, 152–153, 159
 future directions, 160
 goals of, 148
 image-guided biopsy, 150–151

Prostate cancer imaging (*cont.*)
    imaging evaluation
        flowchart, 158
    literature review, 151, 152
    MRI, 153–154, 159
    MR spectroscopy (MRS),
        154–155
    PET-FDG, 155, 156, 160
    radionuclide bone scan,
        159–160
    staging, 151–156
    transrectal ultrasound
        (TRUS), 159
    ultrasound, 151–152
Prosthesis, knee, imaging of, 315
Proton magnetic resonance
    spectroscopy (1H MRS)
    brain cancer, 135–136
PubMed. *See* Medline/PubMed
Pulmonary embolism
    costs, 402
    epidemiology, 402
    pathophysiology, 402
Pulmonary embolism imaging
    evaluation
    case studies (images), 411–412
    CT pulmonary
        angiography, 404
    and diagnosis, 407
    diagnostic accuracy, 407
    echocardiography, 406
    electron beam CT, 405
    future directions, 413
    goals of, 402
    limitations of studies of, 402
    literature review, 413
    MR angiography, 405
    multidetector computed
        tomography (MDCT),
        404–405
    pulmonary angiography, 404
    recurrence rate, 402–407
    ultrasound, 406
    ventilation-perfusion imaging
        (VQ), 403–404
P value, 20, 21, 94, 337, 488
Pyleonephritis, future
    directions, 606

Q
Qualitative analysis, 11
Quality-adjusted life year
    (QALY), 10, 12, 362, 374,
    397, 418, 433, 531

R
Radial scars, breast cancer
    imaging, 71

Radio frequency ablation, 530
Radionuclide bone scintigraphy
    acute hematogenous
        osteomyelitis, 300–301
    osteomyelitis, 298–306
    septic arthritis, 298–306
Random error, 19–21, 24, 25
Randomized controlled trial
    bias related to, 21–22
    blinded clinical trial, 22
Rappaport Disability Rating Scale
    (DRS), 218
Receiver operating characteristics
    (ROC) curve, 281
Recurrence rate, pulmonary
    embolism, 402
Reference standards, and bias, 22
Renal artery stenosis, multiplanar
    imaging, 422
Retroperitonal injuries, blunt
    trauma, imaging, 445–447
Retrospective studies, 6, 24, 99,
    221, 265, 461, 462
Rotator cuff tears, 317, 322
Rotavirus vaccine, and
    intussusception, 479
Rule of threes, liquid enema,
    482–484

S
Sample size
    confidence intervals (CI), 20–21
    and power analysis, 21
Scoliosis
    classification of, 370
    epidemiology, 371–372
    pathophysiology, 370–371
Scoliosis imaging
    adverse reproductive outcome
        risk, 375
    cancer risk, 375
    CIs, degrees of, 374
    goals of, 372
    literature search, 370
    MRI, 377–381
    severe idopathic scoliosis,
        375–376
Screening selection bias, 23
SEER program, 129, 131
Seizures
    categories of, 246, 248
    children, 247
    costs, 247
    epidemiology, 246–247
    febrile, 247
    Wada test, 252–253
Seizures neuroimaging
    for acute symptomatic
        seizures, 246

    children, 247, 249, 250, 256,
        248–251
    decision-making
        algorithm, 253
    and febrile seizures, 247
    for first unprovoked seizures,
        248–250
    functional MRI, 247
    goals of, 247
    literature review, 247
    MRI, 247–252
    MR spectroscopy (MRS), 252
    PET, 252
    SPECT, 252
    for temporal lobe epilepsy,
        250–252
Selection bias, 22–24, 66, 219, 264,
    405, 419, 460
Sensitivity of tests, 7–9
Septic arthritis
    clinical signs, 301
    costs, 299
    epidemiology, 298–299
    future directions, 306
    long-term effects, 301
    medical therapy versus
        surgery, 301
    pathogens, 300
    pathophysiology, 298
    predictors of, 300
    ultrasound, 300–303, 306
Septic arthritis imaging
    and diabetic foot, 302
    diagnostic accuracy, 299
    future directions, 306
    imaging protocols, 303
    and IV drug users, 302
    MRI, 298–303
    radionuclide bone
        scintigraphy, 300,
        302–304, 306
    repeat imaging, 301–302
Shoulder injury
    costs, 310
    differential diagnosis, 317
    epidemiology, 310
Shoulder injury imaging
    dislocations, 316–317
    future directions, 324
    goals of, 311
    high-risk patients, 311
    imaging protocols, 319–320
    indications for, 284–285
    literature review, 311
    MR arthrography
        (MRA), 317
    MRI, 311–319
    rotator cuff tears, 317
    soft tissue diagnosis, 317–319
    ultrasound, 322

Sickle cell anemia, stroke
    prevention, 193
Sigmoidoscopy, 111–113, 117, 119
Single photon emission computed
    tomography (SPECT)
    Alzheimer's disease, 169, 173,
        174
    ankylosing spondylitis, 344
    brain cancer, 133–134
    cardiac imaging, 391
    intracranial hemorrhage, 191
    osteomyelitis, 303
    seizures, 252
    spinal metastasis, 341
    thallium, 392
    traumatic brain injury, 229–233
Single-voxel spectroscopy (SVS)
    seizures, 253
    traumatic brain injury, 233
Sinusitis
    antibiotic treatment, 280, 284
    at-risk persons, 278
    costs, 279
    defined, 278, 283
    epidemiology, 278–279
Sinusitis imaging
    case studies (images), 288
    children, 279
    chronic, diagnosis of, 279–280,
        282, 284–286
    cost-effectiveness, 284–285
    CT, 280–288
    diagnostic accuracy, 282, 285
    before/after functional
        endoscopic sinus
        surgery, 286
    goals of, 279–280
    imaging findings, 288–289, 302
    indications for, 286
    MRI, 281, 284, 288
    to predict clinical
        outcome, 280
Slippery linkage bias, 23
Small bowel ischemia, 470–471
    CT, 470
    MRI, 470
Small bowel obstruction, 468–475,
    478, 480, 485, 553–560, 563
    case studies (images), 472–473
    costs, 469
    CT, 468–470
    diagnostic accuracy, 471
    imaging protocol, 487
    literature search, 469
    pathophysiology, 468
    ultrasound, 468
Small cell lung cancer (SCLC)
    metastatic disease, 96
    staging, 97
    whole-body MRI, 97

Sonography, intussusception, 481
Specificity of tests, 7–9
Spina bifida. See Occult spinal
    dysraphism
Spinal metastasis, 341
    MRI, 341–342
    radionuclide bone
        scintigraphy, 342
    SPECT, 341
Spinal stenosis, 337, 338, 340,
    344–345
    CT, 338
    MRI, 338
    X-rays, 338
Spinal trauma. See Cervical spine
    imaging; Thoracolumbar
    spine imaging
Spine disorders, children. See
    Occult spinal dysraphism;
    Scoliosis
Spleen, blunt trauma,
    imaging, 445
STARD initiative, 19
Stenting and angioplasty, carotid
    stenosis, 433–434
Sticky diagnosis bias, 23
Stress echocardiography, 388,
    391–394
Stress electrocardiography, 392
Stroke
    and carotid stenosis, 190
    classification of, 218
    costs, 184
    defined, 184
    epidemiology, 184
    pediatric, 193
    treatment, 184
    See also Carotid imaging;
        Carotid stenosis;
        Intracranial hemorrhage
        imaging
Structural neuroimaging,
    Alzheimer's
    disease, 170
Subarachnoid hemorrhage, CT
    angiography, 267
Superparamagnetic iron oxide
    (SPIO), 535–537, 539
Supervision Rating Scale
    (SRS), 219
Susceptibility-weighted imaging
    (SWI), traumatic brain
    injury, 222, 229
Systematic error, 19–20, 24, 25.
    See also Bias

T
Temporal lobe epilepsy
    CT, 247, 254

and fluid-attenuated inversion
    recovery (FLAIR), 250, 251
magnetic resonance
    imaging(MRI), 257, 258
Therapeutic efficacy, 174–175
Thoracolumbar spine imaging
    blunt trauma patients, 363–364
    children, 363
    clinical prediction rules,
        359–360
    CT, 359
    diagnostic accuracy, 364–366
    future directions, 367
    imaging protocols, 367
    indications for, 76
Thoracolumbar spine injury
    costs, 358
    epidemiology, 358
    goals of, 358
    literature review, 359
Transcranial Doppler (TCD),
    carotid imaging, 432–436
Transient ischemic attacks (TIA).
    See Carotid imaging;
    Carotid stenosis
Transrectal ultrasound (TRUS)
    color Doppler imaging, 149
    prostate cancer, 148–150
Trauma Coma Databank
    (TCDB), 222
Traumatic brain injury
    causes of, 219
    costs, 219
    epidemiology, 219
    Glasgow Coma Scale, 218,
        236, 237
    Glasgow Outcome Scale, 218
    outcome scales, 218
Traumatic brain injury imaging
    in acute care setting, 220
    atrophy, quantification of, 225
    brain swelling, 223
    case studies (images), 233
    children, 225–229
    CT, 231–233
    diffuse axonal injury, 238, 239
    diffusion-tensor imaging,
        219, 222
    diffusion-weighted
        imaging, 222
    FLAIR, 219, 222
    functional MRI, 229–233
    future directions, 241
    goals of, 219
    gradient echo sequences,
        219, 222
    hemorrhage, 223
    image classification, 222–223
    and immediate, 221–222
    treatment/surgery, 220

Traumatic brain injury
imaging (*cont.*)
lesions, number/size/depth,
223–224
literature review, 219–220
methods, summary of,
234–235
midline shift, 221
MRI, 224, 229
MR spectroscopy, 230–231
multivoxel resonance
spectroscopy, 231
normal scans, 221
and outcome prediction, 222
perfusion studies, 229–230
PET, 232–233
PET FDG, 232
sensitivity/specificity of, 221
single-voxel spectroscopy
(SVS), 233, 240
SPECT, 231–232
susceptibility-weighted
imaging (SWI), 239
Type I error, 20
Type II error, 21

U
Ultrasound
abdomen, blunt trauma, 441,
443, 445
acute calculous
cholecystitis, 504,
506–507, 519
acute hematogenous
osteomyelitis imaging, 297,
299–303, 305, 306
bile duct obstruction, 504, 506
bile duct stricture, 504
choledocholithiasis, 504
chronic calculous
cholecystitis, 506
colonic diverticulitis, 471, 475
endoscopic. *See* Endoscopic
ultrasonography
hepatocellular carcinoma

intussusception, 467, 480,
482, 487
liver metastases, 535–536
occult spinal dysraphism
imaging, 369, 372–374,
377–379
prostate cancer, 147–152,
157, 159
pulmonary embolism
evaluation, 401, 402,
406–409
septic arthritis, 297, 299–303,
305, 306
shoulder injury, 319
small bowel obstruction,
469–471, 474, 480,
485, 555
See also Doppler ultrasound
Ultrasound, breast cancer, 68–69
interpretation issue, 534
local extent, detection of, 70,
77, 151, 515
as supplemental screening, 62
Unconscious patient, cervical
spine imaging, 362–363
Urinary tract disorders
literature search, 338
nephrolithiasis, 570–577,
579, 580
neurogenic bladder, 573,
574, 576
urinary tract infection, 10,
498, 573, 574, 577, 579, 580,
585–606
urolithiasis, 570, 571,
573–577
Urinary tract infection, 10, 498,
573, 574, 577, 579, 580,
584–606
case studies (images), 498,
579, 580
costs, 10, 574, 587
epidemiology, 587, 589
pathophysiology, 586
and pregnancy, 587, 593, 604
treatment, 587–589, 591, 593

Urolithiasis
CT, 570, 573–578, 581
pathophysiology, 570
types of stones, 571, 577
See also Nephrolithiasis

V
Variable costs, 10
Ventilation-perfusion imaging
(VQ), pulmonary embolism
evaluation, 401, 403–404,
408, 410, 411
Vertebroplasty, 336, 338, 346
Video-assisted thoracotomy
(VATS), lung cancer, 92

W
Wada test, 9, 252, 253
Whole-body MRI, small cell lung
cancer (SCLC), 97
Whole-body PET
hepatocellular
carcinoma, 535
liver metastases, 535
William's criteria, 280

X
X-rays
ankylosing spondylitis, 350
cancer risk and radiation, 32
chest, blunt trauma, 443
hematopoietic cancer risks,
33, 38
herniated disk, 336, 338,
348, 350
inherited human syndromes,
28, 37
lung cancer screening,
90–92
radiation terminology, 28
radiation mechanisms, 28
scoliosis, 32
spinal stenosis, 338